MAYO CLINIC INTERNAL MEDICINE BOARD REVIEW

ELEVENTH EDITION

MAYO CLINIC SCIENTIFIC PRESS

MAYO CLINIC INTERNAL MEDICINE BOARD REVIEW

ELEVENTH EDITION

EDITOR-IN-CHIEF

Christopher M. Wittich, MD, PharmD

Consultant, Division of General Internal Medicine
Mayo Clinic, Rochester, Minnesota
Associate Professor of Medicine
Mayo Clinic College of Medicine

SENIOR ASSOCIATE EDITOR

Thomas J. Beckman, MD

Consultant, Division of General Internal Medicine
Mayo Clinic, Rochester, Minnesota
Professor of Medicine and of Medical Education
Mayo Clinic College of Medicine

ASSOCIATE EDITORS

Nerissa M. Collins, MD   Nina M. Schwenk, MD
Jason H. Szostek, MD   Amy T. Wang, MD

MAYO CLINIC SCIENTIFIC PRESS   OXFORD UNIVERSITY PRESS

OXFORD
UNIVERSITY PRESS

Oxford University Press is a department of the University of Oxford. It furthers the University's objective of excellence in research, scholarship, and education by publishing worldwide. Oxford is a registered trade mark of Oxford University Press in the UK and certain other countries.

Published in the United States of America by Oxford University Press
198 Madison Avenue, New York, NY 10016, United States of America.

Library of Congress Cataloging-in-Publication Data
Names: Wittich, Christopher M., editor | Mayo Clinic. | Mayo Foundation for
   Medical Education and Research.
Title: Mayo Clinic internal medicine board review / editor-in-chief,
   Christopher M. Wittich ; senior associate editor, Thomas J. Beckman;
   associate editors, Nerissa M. Collins, Nina M. Schwenk, Jason H. Szostek,
   Amy T. Wang.
Other titles: Internal medicine board review | Mayo Clinic scientific press
   (Series)
Description: Eleventh edition. | Oxford ; New York, NY : Oxford University
   Press, [2016] | Series: Mayo Clinic scientific press | Includes
   bibliographical references and index.
Identifiers: LCCN 2016006611 | ISBN 9780190464868 (alk. paper)
Subjects: | MESH: Internal Medicine | Examination Questions | Outlines
Classification: LCC RC58 | NLM WB 18.2 | DDC 616.0076—dc23
LC record available at http://lccn.loc.gov/2016006611

9 8 7 6 5 4 3 2 1

Printed by Walsworth, USA

Cover images, clockwise from the upper left: Figure 47.2. chaining of β-hemolytic *Streptococcus* in a blood culture (Gram stain); Figure 26.9. pemphigus vulgaris; Figure 11.5. aortogram of contained rupture of proximal descending thoracic aorta; Figure 37.11. spur cells (acanthocytes).

Foreword

The Department of Medicine at Mayo Clinic has a long and rich history of educating physicians in training and practice. The Mayo Clinic School of Graduate Medical Education, which began in 1915, has celebrated its centennial of training resident physicians. Additionally, the Department of Medicine's continuing medical education courses are nearing their 90th consecutive year of educating physicians in practice. An ongoing key mission of the Department of Medicine is to provide lifelong learning programs to educate learners across the medical education continuum. The *Mayo Clinic Internal Medicine Board Review*, Eleventh Edition, is one such learning program resource designed to teach internists and update them on the ever-changing field of internal medicine.

For the Eleventh Edition, the chapters have been completely revised and reorganized to cover the breadth of internal medicine. In addition, the new edition has an updated design to simplify study and improve readability. All chapters were written by Mayo Clinic physicians whose primary mission is to care for patients. The editors added their depth of experience in general internal medicine and medical education to develop a text that is relevant to practice. This textbook will be of value to those preparing for the American Board of Internal Medicine Certification and Maintenance of Certification examinations and as a general reference for those striving to provide outstanding clinical care for patients.

Morie A. Gertz, MD, MACP

Chair, Department of Internal Medicine, Mayo Clinic, Rochester, Minnesota
Roland Seidler Jr Professor of the Art of Medicine
Mayo Clinic College of Medicine

Preface

The *Mayo Clinic Internal Medicine Board Review*, Eleventh Edition, is the result of the dedicated efforts of Mayo Clinic physicians in multiple specialties whose primary mission is to put the needs of the patient first. The field of internal medicine is constantly changing as science is advanced. The goal of this textbook is to provide the reader with the essential elements for the practice of internal medicine. Readers preparing for the American Board of Internal Medicine (ABIM) Certification and Maintenance of Certification examinations will find the textbook comprehensive and easy to study. Additionally, readers who want a reference or a general knowledge review in internal medicine will find this textbook an important addition to their medical library.

The Eleventh Edition uses a new design to improve readability with color-coded chapter tabs and key facts and key definitions highlighted separately from the main text. The oncology and neurology chapters have been completely reorganized according to disease site. New chapters have been added on complementary and integrative medicine and quality improvement. Several major topics have been divided into shorter chapters for ease of study, and all chapters have been completely revised with a focus on covering content in the ABIM Certification Examination Blueprint. The editors have worked diligently to remove extraneous material that would not be useful for the practice of general internal medicine, yet the book is comprehensive and easy to study.

I wish to thank all the authors for their careful attention to detail and hard work. The associate editors, all members of the Division of General Internal Medicine at Mayo Clinic, provided incredible insights into what information is truly needed to practice general internal medicine. I would like to especially thank Thomas J. Beckman, MD, senior associate editor, for his years of mentorship, during which he taught me to be a scholar and medical writer. I would like to thank Morie A. Gertz, MD, Chair of the Department of Internal Medicine at Mayo Clinic in Rochester, Minnesota, and Paul S. Mueller, MD, Chair of the Division of General Internal Medicine, who provided the encouragement and resources to make this textbook possible. I also thank Michael O'Brien for his administrative support. This book would not exist without the dedication of the Mayo Clinic Section of Scientific Publications staff, including Joseph G. Murphy, MD, Chair; Randall J. Fritz, DVM, and LeAnn M. Stee, with assistance from Patricia M. Flynn and Colleen M. Sauber, editors; Kenna L. Atherton, manager; Jane M. Craig, editorial assistant; and John P. Hedlund and Ann M. Ihrke, proofreaders. I gratefully acknowledge the support of Mayo Clinic Scientific Press and Oxford University Press. Finally, I thank Laura M. Sadosty, in the Department of Medicine, who organized over 70 physician authors—a remarkable feat indeed!

In the spirit of the previous editions, I trust that *Mayo Clinic Internal Medicine Board Review,* Eleventh Edition, will serve those in the pursuit of mastering the art and science of internal medicine.

Christopher M. Wittich, MD, PharmD

Contents

[a] Other Section editors reviewed a single chapter in this section.

Section IV: Gastroenterology and Hepatology
Section editor, Nina M. Schwenk, MD[a]

Section V: General Internal Medicine
Section editors, Thomas J. Beckman, MD; Jason H. Szostek, MD; Amy T. Wang, MD; and Christopher M. Wittich, MD, PharmD

Section VI: Hematology
Section editor, Amy T. Wang, MD

[a] Other Section editors reviewed a single chapter in this section.

[a] Other Section editors reviewed a single chapter in this section.

---

[a] Other Section editors reviewed a single chapter in this section.

Contributors[a]

Timothy R. Aksamit, MD
Consultant, Division of Pulmonary and Critical Care
  Medicine, Mayo Clinic; Associate Professor of Medicine

Nandan S. Anavekar, MB, BCh
Consultant, Division of Cardiovascular Diseases,
  Mayo Clinic; Associate Professor of Medicine

Brent A. Bauer, MD
Consultant, Division of General Internal Medicine,
  Mayo Clinic; Professor of Medicine

Thomas J. Beckman, MD
Consultant, Division of General Internal Medicine, Mayo
  Clinic; Professor of Medical Education and of Medicine

Eduardo E. Benarroch, MD
Consultant, Department of Neurology, Mayo Clinic;
  Professor of Neurology

Elie F. Berbari, MD
Consultant, Division of Infectious Diseases, Mayo Clinic;
  Professor of Medicine

Lori A. Blauwet, MD
Consultant, Division of Cardiovascular Diseases, Mayo
  Clinic; Associate Professor of Medicine

Robert D. Brown Jr, MD
Consultant, Department of Neurology, Mayo Clinic;
  Professor of Neurology

John B. Bundrick, MD
Consultant, Division of General Internal Medicine, Mayo
  Clinic; Assistant Professor of Medicine

Rodrigo Cartin-Ceba, MD, MSc
Consultant, Division of Pulmonary and Critical
  Care Medicine, Mayo Clinic, Scottsdale, Arizona;
  Assistant Professor of Medicine

Tony Y. Chon, MD
Consultant, Division of General Internal Medicine,
  Mayo Clinic; Assistant Professor of Medicine

C. Scott Collins, MD
Consultant, Division of General Internal Medicine,
  Mayo Clinic; Assistant Professor of Medicine

Nerissa M. Collins, MD
Consultant, Division of General Internal Medicine,
  Mayo Clinic; Instructor in Medicine

Brian A. Costello, MD, MS
Consultant, Department of Oncology, Mayo Clinic;
  Associate Professor of Urology and of Oncology

Brian A. Crum, MD
Consultant, Department of Neurology, Mayo Clinic;
  Assistant Professor of Neurology

Floranne C. Ernste, MD
Consultant, Division of Rheumatology, Mayo Clinic;
  Assistant Professor of Medicine

Fernando C. Fervenza, MD, PhD
Consultant, Division of Nephrology and Hypertension,
  Mayo Clinic; Professor of Medicine

---

[a] Unless otherwise noted, clinical appointments refer to Rochester, Minnesota, and academic appointments refer to Mayo Clinic College
of Medicine.

Naseema Gangat, MBBS
Consultant, Division of Hematology, Mayo Clinic;
  Instructor in Oncology and Assistant Professor
  of Medicine

Tufia C. Haddad, MD
Consultant, Department of Oncology, Mayo Clinic;
  Assistant Professor of Oncology

Anhar Hassan, MB, BCh
Consultant, Department of Neurology, Mayo Clinic;
  Assistant Professor of Neurology

C. Christopher Hook, MD
Consultant, Division of Hematology, Mayo Clinic;
  Associate Professor of Medicine

Joleen M. Hubbard, MD
Consultant, Department of Oncology, Mayo Clinic;
  Instructor in Medicine and Assistant Professor of
  Oncology

Ryan T. Hurt, MD, PhD
Consultant, Division of General Internal Medicine, Mayo
  Clinic; Associate Professor of Medicine

Vivek N. Iyer, MD
Consultant, Division of Pulmonary and Critical Care
  Medicine, Mayo Clinic; Assistant Professor of
  Medicine

Lyell K. Jones Jr, MD
Consultant, Department of Neurology, Mayo Clinic;
  Associate Professor of Neurology

Mithri R. Junna, MD
Senior Associate Consultant, Department of Neurology
  and Division of Pulmonary and Critical Care Medicine,
  Mayo Clinic; Assistant Professor of Neurology

Ekta Kapoor, MBBS
Consultant, Divisions of General Internal Medicine and
  Endocrinology, Diabetes, Metabolism, & Nutrition,
  Mayo Clinic; Assistant Professor of Medicine

Kianoush B. Kashani, MD
Consultant, Divisions of Nephrology and Hypertension
  and Pulmonary and Critical Care Medicine, Mayo
  Clinic; Assistant Professor of Medicine

Mary J. Kasten, MD
Consultant, Divisions of General Internal Medicine and
  Infectious Diseases, Mayo Clinic; Assistant Professor of
  Medicine

Jordan M. Kautz, MD
Senior Associate Consultant, Division of General Internal
  Medicine, Mayo Clinic; Instructor in Medicine

Cassie C. Kennedy, MD
Consultant, Division of Pulmonary and Critical Care
  Medicine, Mayo Clinic; Assistant Professor of Medicine

James P. Klaas, MD
Senior Associate Consultant, Department of Neurology,
  Mayo Clinic; Assistant Professor of Neurology

Kyle W. Klarich, MD
Consultant, Division of Cardiovascular Diseases,
  Mayo Clinic; Professor of Medicine

Matthew J. Koster, MD
Fellow in Rheumatology, Mayo School of Graduate
  Medical Education; Instructor in Medicine

Scott C. Litin, MD
Consultant, Division of General Internal Medicine,
  Mayo Clinic; Professor of Medicine

Conor G. Loftus, MD
Consultant, Division of Gastroenterology and Hepatology,
  Mayo Clinic; Assistant Professor of Medicine

Fabien Maldonado, MD
Consultant, Division of Pulmonary and Critical Care
  Medicine, Mayo Clinic; Assistant Professor of Medicine
Present address: Vanderbilt University School of
  Medicine

Rekha Mankad, MD
Consultant, Division of Cardiovascular Diseases,
  Mayo Clinic; Assistant Professor of Medicine

Karen F. Mauck, MD, MSc
Consultant, Division of General Internal Medicine,
  Mayo Clinic; Associate Professor of Medicine

Robert D. McBane, MD
Consultant, Division of Cardiovascular Diseases,
  Mayo Clinic; Professor of Medicine

Andrew McKeon, MB, BCh, MD
Consultant, Department of Neurology and Division of
  Clinical Biochemistry, Mayo Clinic; Associate Professor
  of Laboratory Medicine and Pathology and of Neurology

Clement J. Michet, MD
Consultant, Division of Rheumatology, Mayo Clinic;
  Associate Professor of Medicine

Arya B. Mohabbat, MD
Senior Associate Consultant, Division of General Internal Medicine, Mayo Clinic; Assistant Professor of Medicine

Timothy J. Moynihan, MD
Consultant, Department of Oncology, Mayo Clinic; Associate Professor of Oncology

Michelle A. Neben Wittich, MD
Consultant, Divisions of Radiation Oncology and General Internal Medicine, Mayo Clinic; Assistant Professor of Radiation Oncology

Suzanne M. Norby, MD
Consultant, Division of Nephrology and Hypertension, Mayo Clinic; Associate Professor of Medicine

Peter A. Noseworthy, MD
Senior Associate Consultant, Division of Cardiovascular Diseases, Mayo Clinic; Assistant Professor of Medicine

Amy S. Oxentenko, MD
Consultant, Division of Gastroenterology and Hepatology, Mayo Clinic; Associate Professor of Medicine

Brian A. Palmer, MD
Consultant, Department of Psychiatry & Psychology, Mayo Clinic; Assistant Professor of Psychiatry

Sabrina D. Phillips, MD
Consultant, Division of Cardiovascular Diseases, Mayo Clinic; Assistant Professor of Medicine
Present address: Oklahoma University Cardiovascular Institute

Alyx B. Porter, MD
Consultant, Department of Neurology, Mayo Clinic Hospital, Phoenix, Arizona; Assistant Professor of Neurology

John J. Poterucha, MD
Consultant, Division of Gastroenterology and Hepatology, Mayo Clinic; Professor of Medicine

Katharine A. Price, MD
Consultant, Division of Medical Oncology, Mayo Clinic; Assistant Professor of Oncology

Rajiv K. Pruthi, MBBS
Consultant, Division of Hematology, Mayo Clinic; Associate Professor of Medicine

Qi Qian, MD
Consultant, Division of Nephrology and Hypertension, Mayo Clinic; Professor of Medicine and of Physiology

William Sanchez, MD
Consultant, Division of Gastroenterology and Hepatology, Mayo Clinic; Assistant Professor of Medicine

Nicole P. Sandhu, MD, PhD
Consultant, Division of General Internal Medicine, Mayo Clinic; Assistant Professor of Medicine

Carrie A. Schinstock, MD
Consultant, Division of Nephrology and Hypertension, Mayo Clinic; Assistant Professor of Medicine

Nina M. Schwenk, MD
Consultant, Division of General Internal Medicine, Mayo Clinic; Assistant Professor of Medicine

Pankaj Shah, MD
Consultant, Division of Endocrinology, Diabetes, Metabolism, & Nutrition, Mayo Clinic; Assistant Professor of Medicine

Lynne T. Shuster, MD
Consultant, Division of General Internal Medicine, Mayo Clinic; Associate Professor of Medicine

M. Rizwan Sohail, MD
Consultant, Divisions of Infectious Diseases and Cardiovascular Diseases, Mayo Clinic; Associate Professor of Medicine

Marius N. Stan, MD
Consultant, Division of Endocrinology, Diabetes, Metabolism, & Nutrition, Mayo Clinic; Assistant Professor of Medicine

Jacob J. Strand, MD
Consultant, Division of General Internal Medicine, Mayo Clinic; Assistant Professor of Medicine

Karna K. Sundsted, MD
Senior Associate Consultant, Division of General Internal Medicine, Mayo Clinic; Assistant Professor of Medicine

Seth R. Sweetser, MD
Consultant, Division of Gastroenterology and Hepatology, Mayo Clinic; Associate Professor of Medicine

Keith M. Swetz, MD, MA
Consultant, Division of General Internal Medicine, Mayo Clinic; Assistant Professor of Medicine
Present address: Birmingham Veterans Affairs Medical Center, Birmingham, Alabama

Jason H. Szostek, MD
Consultant, Division of General Internal Medicine, Mayo Clinic; Assistant Professor of Medicine

Zelalem Temesgen, MD
Consultant, Division of Infectious Diseases, Mayo Clinic; Professor of Medicine

Carrie A. Thompson, MD
Consultant, Division of Hematology, Mayo Clinic; Assistant Professor of Medicine

Farris K. Timimi, MD
Consultant, Division of Cardiovascular Diseases, Mayo Clinic; Assistant Professor of Medicine

Pritish K. Tosh, MD
Consultant, Division of Infectious Diseases, Mayo Clinic; Associate Professor of Medicine

Ericka E. Tung, MD, MPH
Consultant, Division of Primary Care Internal Medicine, Mayo Clinic; Assistant Professor of Medicine

Bert B. Vargas, MD
Consultant, Department of Neurology, Mayo Clinic Hospital, Phoenix, Arizona; Assistant Professor of Neurology
Present address: University of Texas Southwestern Medical Center

Gerald W. Volcheck, MD
Chair, Division of Allergic Diseases, Mayo Clinic; Associate Professor of Medicine

Andrea E. Wahner Hendrickson, MD
Consultant, Department of Oncology, Mayo Clinic; Assistant Professor of Oncology and of Pharmacology

Amy T. Wang, MD
Consultant, Division of General Internal Medicine, Mayo Clinic; Assistant Professor of Medicine
Present address: Harbor-UCLA Medical Center

Kenneth J. Warrington, MD
Chair, Division of Rheumatology, Mayo Clinic; Professor of Medicine

Carilyn N. Wieland, MD
Consultant, Department of Dermatology, Mayo Clinic; Assistant Professor of Dermatology

Christopher M. Wittich, MD, PharmD
Consultant, Division of General Internal Medicine, Mayo Clinic; Associate Professor of Medicine

Lily C. Wong-Kisiel, MD
Consultant, Department of Neurology, Mayo Clinic; Assistant Professor of Neurology

Allergy

1 Allergic Diseases[a]

GERALD W. VOLCHECK, MD

Allergy Testing

Standard allergy testing relies on identifying the immunoglobulin (Ig) E antibody specific for the allergen in question. Two classic methods of doing this are the immediate wheal-and-flare skin prick tests (in which a small amount of antigen is introduced into the skin and the site is evaluated after 15 minutes for the presence of an immediate wheal-and-flare reaction) and in vitro (blood) testing.

Methods of allergy testing that do not have a clear scientific basis include cytotoxic testing, provocation-neutralization testing or treatment, and "yeast allergy" testing.

Patch Tests and Prick (Cutaneous) Tests

Patch testing of skin is not the same as immediate wheal-and-flare skin prick testing. Patch testing is used to investigate only contact dermatitis, a type IV hypersensitivity skin reaction. Patch tests require 72 to 96 hours for complete evaluation. Many substances cause contact dermatitis. Common contact sensitivities include those to nickel, formaldehyde, fragrances, and latex.

Skin prick testing, in comparison, identifies inhalant allergens that cause respiratory symptoms, such as allergic rhinitis and asthma. These allergens include dust mites, cats, dogs, cockroaches, molds, and tree, grass, and weed pollens. Food allergy is also assessed by skin prick testing.

Skin prick testing and intradermal testing involve introducing allergen into the skin layers below the external keratin layer. Intradermal testing, the deeper technique, is used to evaluate allergy to stinging insect venoms, penicillin, and other medications. Intradermal tests are preceded by skin prick tests.

Drugs with antihistamine properties, such as histamine$_1$ (H$_1$) receptor antagonists, and many anticholinergic and tricyclic antidepressant drugs can suppress the immediate response to allergy skin tests. Use of nonsedating antihistamines should be discontinued 5 days before skin testing. The histamine$_2$ (H$_2$) receptor antagonists have a small suppressive effect. High-dose corticosteroids can suppress the delayed-type hypersensitivity and the immediate response.

In Vitro Allergy Testing

In vitro (blood) allergy testing initially involves chemically coupling allergen protein molecules to a solid-phase substance and ultimately measuring the patient's specific IgE to the allergen via radiolabeling, colorimetry, or other markers.

This test identifies the presence of allergen-specific IgE antibody in the same way that the allergen skin test does. Generally, in vitro allergy testing is not as sensitive as skin testing and has some limitations because of the potential for chemical modification of the allergen protein while it is being coupled to the solid phase. Generally, it is more expensive than allergen skin tests and has no advantage in routine clinical practice. In vitro allergy testing may be useful clinically for patients who have been taking antihistamines and are unable to discontinue their use or for patients who have primary cutaneous diseases that make allergen skin testing impractical or inaccurate (eg, severe atopic eczema with most of the skin involved in a flare).

[a] Portions previously published in Volcheck GW. Clinical allergy: diagnosis and management. Totowa (NJ): Humana; c2009. Used with permission of Mayo Foundation for Medical Education and Research.

Chronic Rhinitis

Medical History

The differential diagnosis of chronic rhinitis is given in Box 1.1. **Nonallergic rhinitis** is defined as nasal symptoms occurring in response to nonspecific, nonallergic irritants. Vasomotor rhinitis is the most common form. Common triggers of vasomotor rhinitis are strong odors, respiratory irritants such as dust or smoke, changes in temperature, changes in body position, and ingestants such as spicy food or alcohol.

Key Definition

Nonallergic rhinitis: *nasal symptoms occurring in response to nonspecific, nonallergic irritants.*

Historical factors favoring a diagnosis of *allergic* rhinitis include a history of nasal symptoms that have a recurrent seasonal pattern (eg, every August and September) or symptoms provoked by being near specific sources of allergens, such as animals. Factors favoring *vasomotor* rhinitis include symptoms provoked by strong odors and changes in humidity and temperature.

Factors common to allergic rhinitis and nonallergic rhinitis (thus, without differential diagnostic value) include perennial symptoms, intolerance of cigarette smoke, and history of "dust" sensitivity. Factors that suggest fixed nasal obstruction (which should prompt physicians to consider other diagnoses) include unilateral nasal obstruction, unilateral facial pain, unilateral nasal purulence, nasal voice but no nasal symptoms, disturbances of olfaction without any nasal symptoms, and unilateral nasal bleeding. Nasal polyps, septal deviation, and tumor may present with unilateral symptoms. Further evaluation with computed tomographic (CT) scan of the sinuses or rhinolaryngoscopy is indicated.

Box 1.1 • Differential Diagnosis of Chronic Rhinitis

Bilateral presentation
  Allergic rhinitis
  Vasomotor rhinitis
  Rhinitis medicamentosa
  Sinusitis
Unilateral presentation
  Nasal polyposis
  Nasal septal deviation
  Foreign body
  Tumor

Allergy Skin Tests in Allergic Rhinitis

Interpretation of allergy skin test results must be tailored to the unique features of each patient: For patients with perennial symptoms and negative results on allergy skin tests, the diagnosis is nonallergic rhinitis. For patients with seasonal symptoms and appropriately positive results on allergy skin tests, the diagnosis is seasonal allergic rhinitis. For patients with perennial symptoms, positive results on allergy skin tests for house dust mite suggest house dust mite allergic rhinitis. In this case, dust mite allergen avoidance should be recommended.

Corticosteroid Therapy for Rhinitis

The need for systemic corticosteroid treatment of rhinitis is limited. Occasionally, patients with severe symptoms of allergic rhinitis may benefit greatly from a short course of prednisone (10 mg 4 times daily by mouth for 5 days). Improvement may be sufficient to allow topical corticosteroids to penetrate the nose and satisfactory levels of antihistamine to be established in the blood. Severe nasal polyposis, a separate condition, may warrant a longer course of oral corticosteroid therapy. Sometimes the recurrence of nasal polyps can be prevented by continued use of topical corticosteroids. Polypectomy may be required if nasal polyps do not respond to treatment with systemic and intranasal corticosteroids, but nasal polyps often recur after surgical intervention.

In contrast to systemic corticosteroids, topical corticosteroid agents for the nose are easy to use and have few adverse systemic effects.

KEY FACTS

✓ Patch testing—used to investigate only contact dermatitis

✓ Skin prick testing—identifies inhalant allergens that cause respiratory symptoms

✓ Nasal symptoms with a recurrent seasonal pattern favor a diagnosis of allergic rhinitis

✓ Intranasal corticosteroids—easy to use; few adverse systemic effects

---

Long-term treatment with decongestant nasal sprays may have "addictive" potential (a vicious cycle of rebound congestion called *rhinitis medicamentosa* caused by topical vasoconstrictors). In contrast, intranasal corticosteroid therapy does not induce this type of dependence.

A substantial number of patients with nonallergic rhinitis also have a good response to intranasal (topical aerosol) corticosteroid therapy, especially if they have the nasal eosinophilia form of nonallergic rhinitis.

A patient who has allergic rhinitis and does not receive adequate relief with topical corticosteroid plus antihistamine therapy may need systemic corticosteroid treatment and immunotherapy.

An unusual adverse effect of intranasal corticosteroids is nasal septal perforation. Spray canisters deliver a powerful jet of particulates, and a few patients have misdirected the jet to the nasal septum. Instruction on correct nasal inhaler technique can help in prevention.

Antihistamines and Other Treatments

Antihistamines antagonize the interaction of histamine with its receptors. Histamine may be more causative of nasal itch and sneezing than other mast cell mediators. These are the symptoms most often responsive to antihistamine therapy.

Pseudoephedrine is the most common decongestant agent in nonprescription drugs for treating cold symptoms and rhinitis and usually is the active decongestant agent in widely used prescription agents. Phenylpropanolamine has been removed from the market because of its association with hemorrhagic stroke in women. Several prescription and nonprescription combination agents combine an antihistamine and a decongestant. Saline nasal rinses may provide symptomatic improvement in patients with chronic rhinitis by helping to remove mucus from the nares.

In men who are middle-aged or older, urinary retention may be caused by antihistamines (principally the older drugs that have anticholinergic effects) and decongestants. Although there has been concern for years that decongestants may exacerbate hypertension because they are α-adrenergic agonists, a clinically significant hypertensive response is rare in patients with hypertension that is controlled medically.

Immunotherapy for Allergic Rhinitis

Until topical nasal glucocorticoid sprays were introduced, allergen immunotherapy was considered first-line therapy for allergic rhinitis when the relevant allergen was seasonal pollen of grass, trees, or weeds. Immunotherapy became second-line therapy after topical corticosteroids were introduced, because immunotherapy requires a larger time commitment during the buildup phase and carries a small risk of anaphylaxis due to the immunotherapy injection itself. However, immunotherapy for allergic rhinitis can be appropriate first-line therapy for selected patients and is highly effective.

Immunotherapy is often reserved for patients who do not receive satisfactory relief from intranasal corticosteroids or who cannot tolerate antihistamines. Controlled trials have shown a benefit for pollen, dust mite, and cat allergies and a variable benefit for mold allergy. Immunotherapy is not used for food allergy or nonallergic rhinitis. Immunotherapy has also been shown to decrease the incidence of the development of asthma in children with allergic rhinitis and to decrease the onset of new allergen sensitivities in those treated for a single allergen.

Environmental Modification

House Dust Mites

The home harbors the most substantial dust mite populations in bedding, fabric-upholstered furniture (heavily used), and carpeting over concrete (when concrete is in contact with the ground). To decrease mite exposure, bedding (and sometimes, when practical, furniture cushions) should be encased in mite-impermeable encasements. To some degree, encasements also prevent infusion of water vapor into the bedding matrix. These 2 factors, a mite barrier and decreased humidity, combine to markedly decrease the amount of airborne mite allergen. In contrast, recently marketed acaricides that kill mites or denature their protein allergens have not proved useful in the home. Measures for controlling dust mites are listed in Box 1.2.

Pollen

Air-conditioning, which enables the home to remain tightly closed, is the principal defense against pollinosis. Most masks purchased at local pharmacies cannot exclude pollen particles and are not worth the expense. Some masks can protect the wearer from allergen exposure. These are industrial-quality respirators designed specifically to pass rigorous testing by the Occupational Safety and Health Administration and the National Institute for Occupational Safety and Health and meet certification requirements for excluding a wide spectrum of particulates, including pollen and mold. These masks allow wearers to mow the lawn and do yard work, which would be intolerable otherwise because of sensitivity to pollen allergen. It is important to shower and change clothes when entering the home after spending significant time outdoors during allergy season.

Animal Dander

No measure for controlling animal dander can compare with complete removal of the animal from the home. If complete removal is not tenable, some partial measures must be considered. Recommendations include keeping the animal out of the bedroom entirely and attempting to keep the animal in 1 area of the home. A high-efficiency

---

Box 1.2 • Dust Mite Control

Encase bedding and pillows in mite-impermeable encasements
Wash sheets and pillowcases in hot water weekly
Remove carpeting from bedroom
Remove upholstered furniture from bedroom
Run dehumidifier

Box 1.4 • Causes of Persistent or Recurrent Sinusitis

Nasal polyposis

Mucormycosis

Allergic fungal sinusitis

Ciliary dyskinesia

Granulomatosis with polyangiitis (Wegener)

Hypogammaglobulinemia

Tumor

particulate air (HEPA) room air purifier should be placed in the bedroom. The person should avoid close contact with the animal and should consider using a mask if handling the animal or entering the room where the animal is kept. Bathing cats about once every other week may reduce the allergen load in the environment.

Sinusitis

Sinusitis is closely associated with edematous obstruction of the sinus ostia (ostiomeatal complex). Poor drainage of the sinus cavities predisposes to infection, particularly by microorganisms that thrive in low-oxygen environments (eg, anaerobes). In adults, *Streptococcus pneumoniae, Haemophilus influenzae,* anaerobes, and viruses are common pathogens. In addition, *Moraxella (Branhamella) catarrhalis* is an important pathogen in children.

Important clinical features of acute sinusitis are purulent nasal discharge, tooth pain, cough, and poor response to decongestants. Findings on paranasal sinus transillumination may be abnormal.

Physicians should be aware of the complications of sinusitis, which can be life threatening (Box 1.3). Mucormycosis can cause recurrent or persistent sinusitis refractory to antibiotics. Allergic fungal sinusitis is characterized by persistent sinusitis, eosinophilia, increased total IgE level, antifungal (usually *Aspergillus*) IgE antibodies, and fungal colonization of the sinuses. Granulomatosis with polyangiitis (Wegener), ciliary dyskinesia, and hypogammaglobulinemia are medical conditions that can cause refractory sinusitis (Box 1.4).

Box 1.3 • Complications of Sinusitis

Meningitis

Subdural abscess

Extradural abscess

Orbital infection

Cellulitis

Cavernous sinus thrombosis

Untreated sinusitis may lead to osteomyelitis, orbital and periorbital cellulitis, meningitis, and brain abscess. Cavernous sinus thrombosis, an especially serious complication, can lead to retrobulbar pain, extraocular muscle paralysis, and blindness.

Chronic noninfectious sinusitis is most often due to eosinophilic inflammation of the sinus tissue with or without polyp formation. Treatment consists primarily of topical and systemic corticosteroids and saline irrigations. Sinus surgery can be helpful but is not curative, given the recurrent inflammatory component of this disease.

Persistent, refractory, and complicated sinusitis should be evaluated by a specialist. Sinus CT is the preferred imaging study for these patients (Figure 1.1).

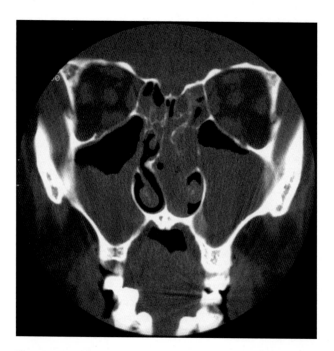

Figure 1.1 Sinusitis. Sinus computed tomogram shows opacification of the osteomeatal complex on the left, subtotal opacification of the right maxillary sinus, and an airfluid level in the left maxillary antrum.

Amoxicillin (500 mg 3 times daily) or trimethoprim-sulfamethoxazole (1 double-strength capsule twice daily) for 10 to 14 days is the treatment of choice for uncomplicated maxillary sinusitis.

Plain radiography of the sinuses is less sensitive than CT (using the coronal sectioning technique). CT scans show greater detail about sinus mucosal surfaces, but CT usually is not necessary in acute, uncomplicated sinusitis. CT is indicated, though, for patients in whom a sinus operation is being considered and for those in whom standard treatment of sinusitis fails. However, patients with extensive dental restorations that contain metal may generate too much artifact for CT to be useful. For these patients, magnetic resonance imaging techniques are indicated.

Urticaria and Angioedema

Duration of Urticaria

The distinction between *acute urticaria* and *chronic urticaria* is based on duration. If urticaria has been present for 6 weeks or longer, it is called chronic urticaria.

Secondary Urticaria

In most patients, urticaria is simply a skin disease (*chronic idiopathic urticaria*). Many of these patients have an antibody that interacts with their own IgE or IgE receptor and produces the urticaria. Occasionally urticaria is the presenting sign of more serious internal disease. It can be a sign of lupus erythematosus and other connective tissue diseases, particularly the "overlap" syndromes that are more difficult to categorize. Thyroid disease, malignancy (mainly of the gastrointestinal tract), lymphoproliferative diseases, and occult infection (particularly of the intestines, gallbladder, and dentition) may be associated with urticaria. Immune complex disease has been associated with urticaria, usually with urticarial vasculitis; hepatitis B virus has been identified as an antigen in cases of urticaria and immune complex disease.

A common cause of acute urticaria and angioedema (other than the idiopathic variety) is drug or food allergy. However, drug or food allergy usually does not cause chronic urticaria.

Relationship Between Urticaria and Angioedema

In common idiopathic urticaria, the hives last 2 to 18 hours, and the lesions itch intensely because histamine is the primary cause of wheal formation.

The pathophysiologic mechanism is similar for urticaria and angioedema. The critical factor is the type of tissue in which the capillary leak and mediator release occur. Urticaria occurs when the capillary events are in the tissue wall of the skin—the epidermis. Angioedema occurs when the capillary events affect vessels in the loose connective tissue of the deeper layers—the dermis. Virtually all patients with common idiopathic urticaria also have angioedema at some point.

Hereditary Angioedema

Hereditary angioedema (HAE), a rare genetic condition due to C1 esterase inhibitor dysfunction, is characterized by recurrent episodes of angioedema, typically without urticaria. The duration, size, and location of individual swellings vary. Many patients with HAE have also had symptoms resembling intestinal obstruction. These symptoms usually resolve in 3 to 5 days. HAE episodes may be related to local tissue trauma in a high percentage of cases, with dental work often regarded as the classic precipitating factor. The response to epinephrine is a useful differential point: HAE lesions do not respond well to epinephrine.

If HAE is strongly suspected, the diagnosis can be proved by appropriate measurement of complement factors (decreased levels of C1 esterase inhibitor [quantitative and functional] and C4 [also C2, during an episode of swelling]).

Treatment of C1 esterase inhibitor dysfunction includes plasma-derived C1 esterase inhibitor given intravenously and bradykinin antagonists: ecallantide, a kallikrein inhibitor, and icatibant, a bradykinin receptor antagonist.

Physical Urticaria

Heat, light, cold, vibration, and trauma or pressure can cause hives in susceptible persons. Obtaining the history is the only way of suspecting the diagnosis, which can be confirmed by applying each of the stimuli to the patient's skin. Heat can be applied by placing coins soaked in hot water for a few minutes on the patient's forearm. Cold can be applied with coins kept in a freezer or with ice cubes. For vibration, a laboratory vortex mixer or any common vibrator can be used. A pair of sandbags connected by a strap can be draped over the patient to create enough pressure to cause symptoms in those with delayed pressure urticaria. Unlike most cases of common idiopathic urticaria, in which the lesions affect essentially all skin surfaces, many cases of physical urticaria seem to involve only certain areas of skin. Thus, results of challenges will be positive only in the areas usually involved and negative in other areas.

Food Allergy in Chronic Urticaria

Food allergy almost never causes chronic urticaria. However, urticaria (or angioedema or anaphylaxis) can be an acute manifestation of true food allergy.

Histopathologic Features of Chronic Urticaria

Chronic urticaria is characterized by mononuclear cell perivascular cuffing around dermal capillaries, particularly involving the capillary loops that interdigitate with the rete pegs of the epidermis. Urticarial vasculitis shows the usual histologic features of leukocytoclastic vasculitis.

Management of Urticaria

The history is of utmost importance for discovering the 2% to 10% of cases of chronic urticaria due to secondary causes. A complete physical examination is needed, with particular attention paid to the skin (including testing for dermatographism) to evaluate for the vasculitic nature of the lesions and to the liver, lymph nodes, and mucous membranes. Laboratory testing need not be exhaustive but may include the following: chest radiography, a complete blood cell count with differential count (to discover eosinophilia), measurement of liver enzymes, tests for thyroid function and antibodies, erythrocyte sedimentation rate, serum protein electrophoresis (in patients older than 50 years), urinalysis, and stool examination for parasites. Allergy skin testing is indicated only if the patient has an element in the history suggesting an allergic cause. However, patients with idiopathic urticaria often have fixed ideas about an allergy causing their problem, and skin testing often helps to dissuade them of this idea.

Management of urticaria and angioedema consists of blocking histamine, beginning usually with nonsedating H_1 antagonists. The addition of leukotriene antagonists may be helpful. The role of H_2 antagonists is unclear; they may help a small percentage of patients. Doxepin, a tricyclic antidepressant, has potent antihistamine effects and is useful. Systemic corticosteroids can be administered for acute urticaria and angioedema.

Anaphylaxis

There is no universally accepted clinical definition of *anaphylaxis*. The manifestations of anaphylaxis vary,

---

Box 1.5 • Most Common Causes of Anaphylaxis

Foods (peanuts, tree nuts, fish, and shellfish)

Medications (antibiotics, neuromuscular blockers, and anticonvulsants)

Insect stings (bee, fire ant, and vespid)

Latex

Aspirin and other nonsteroidal anti-inflammatory agents

---

depending on the severity, and can include any combination of urticaria, angioedema, flushing, pruritus, upper airway obstruction, lower airway obstruction, diarrhea, nausea, vomiting, syncope, hypotension, tachycardia, and dizziness. Approximately 90% of anaphylactic episodes include urticaria or angioedema. A cellular and molecular definition of *anaphylaxis* is a generalized allergic reaction characterized by activated basophils and mast cells releasing many mediators (preformed and newly synthesized). The dominant mediators of acute anaphylaxis are histamine and prostaglandin D_2. The serum levels of tryptase peak at 1 hour after the onset of anaphylaxis and may stay elevated for 5 hours. Physiologically, the hypotension of anaphylaxis is caused by peripheral vasodilatation and not by impaired cardiac contractility. Anaphylaxis is characterized by a hyperdynamic state. For these reasons, anaphylaxis can be fatal in patients with preexisting fixed vascular obstructive disease in whom a decrease in perfusion pressure leads to a critical reduction in flow (stroke) or in patients in whom laryngeal edema develops and completely occludes the airway.

The most common causes of anaphylaxis are listed in Box 1.5. The vast majority of anaphylactic events occur within 1 hour, often within minutes, after exposure to the offending agent.

Food Allergy

Clinical History

The clinical syndrome of food allergy may include the following: Very sensitive persons experience tingling, itching, and a metallic taste in the mouth while the food is still in the mouth. Within 15 minutes after the food is swallowed, epigastric distress may occur. There may be nausea and rarely vomiting. Abdominal cramping is felt chiefly in the periumbilical area (small-bowel phase), and lower abdominal cramping and watery diarrhea may occur. Urticaria or angioedema may occur in any distribution, or there may be only itching of the palms and soles. With increasing clinical sensitivity to the offending allergen,

Box 1.6 • Common Causes of Food Allergy

Eggs

Milk

Nuts

Peanuts

Shellfish

Soybeans

Wheat

anaphylactic symptoms may emerge, including tachycardia, hypotension, generalized flushing, and alterations of consciousness.

In extremely sensitive persons, generalized flushing, hypotension, and tachycardia may occur before the other symptoms. Most patients with a food allergy can identify the offending foods. The diagnosis should be confirmed by skin testing or in vitro measurement of allergen-specific IgE antibody. Items considered to be the most common causes of food allergy are listed in Box 1.6.

Food-Related Anaphylaxis

Food-induced anaphylaxis is the same process as acute urticaria or angioedema induced by food allergens, except that the reaction is more severe in anaphylaxis. Relatively few foods are commonly involved in food-induced anaphylaxis; the main ones are peanuts, shellfish, and nuts, although any food has the potential to cause anaphylaxis. In patients with latex allergy, food allergy can develop to banana, avocado, kiwifruit, and other fruits.

KEY FACTS

✓ Hereditary angioedema—recurrent angioedema, typically without urticaria

✓ Heat, light, cold, vibration, and trauma or pressure can cause physical urticaria

✓ Urticaria and angioedema are managed by blocking histamine

✓ Food-induced anaphylaxis—same process but more severe reaction than acute food-induced urticaria or angioedema

Allergy Skin Testing in Food Allergy

Patients presenting with food-related symptoms may have food allergy, food intolerance, irritable bowel syndrome, nonspecific dyspepsia, or a nonallergic condition. A careful and detailed history on the nature of the "reaction," the reproducibility of the association of food and symptoms, and the timing of symptoms in relation to the ingestion of food can help the clinician form a clinical impression.

In many cases, allergy skin tests to foods can be helpful. If the results are negative (and the clinical suspicion for food allergy is low), the patient can be reassured that food allergy is not the cause of the symptoms. If the results are positive (and the clinical suspicion for food allergy is high), the patient should be counseled about management of the food allergy. The patient should strictly avoid the food and possible cross-reactive foods. These patients should also be given an epinephrine kit for self-administration in an emergency. Although some food allergies may be outgrown, peanut, tree nut, fish, and shellfish allergies are typically lifelong.

If the diagnosis of food allergy is uncertain or if the symptoms are mild and nonspecific, oral food challenges may be helpful. An open challenge is usually performed first. If the results are negative, the diagnosis of food allergy is excluded. If the results are positive but there is suspicion about them, a blinded placebo-controlled challenge test can be performed.

Stinging Insect Allergy

In patients clinically sensitive to Hymenoptera, reactions to a sting can be either large local reactions or systemic, anaphylactic reactions. With a large local sting reaction, swelling at the sting site may be dramatic, but there are no symptoms distant from that site. Stings of the head, neck, and dorsum of the hands are particularly prone to large local reactions.

Anaphylaxis caused by allergy to stinging insects is similar to all other forms of anaphylaxis. Thus, the onset of anaphylaxis may be very rapid, often within 1 or 2 minutes. Pruritus of the palms and soles is the most common initial manifestation. Frequently, 1 or more of the following occur next: generalized flushing, urticaria, angioedema, or hypotension. The reason for attaching importance to whether a stinging insect reaction is a large local or a generalized one is that allergy skin testing and allergen immunotherapy are recommended only for generalized reactions. Patients who have a large local reaction are not at significantly increased risk for future anaphylaxis.

Bee and Vespid Allergy

Yellow jackets, wasps, and hornets are vespids, and their venoms cross-react to a substantial degree. The venom of honeybees (family, Apidae) does not cross-react with that of vespids. Thus, it usually is appropriate to conduct skin testing for allergy to honeybee and to each of the vespids. In most cases, the patient will not be able to identify the causative stinging insect.

Box 1.7 • Indications for Insect Venom Immunotherapy

History of mild, moderate, or severe anaphylaxis to a sting

Positive results on skin tests to the venom that was implicated historically in the anaphylactic reaction

Urticaria distant from the site of the sting (adults only)

Allergy Testing

Patients who have had a generalized reaction need allergen skin testing. Patients who have had a large local reaction to a Hymenoptera sting do not need allergen skin testing because they are not at significantly increased risk for future anaphylaxis.

In many cases, skin testing should be delayed for at least 1 month after a sting-induced generalized reaction because tests conducted closer to the time of the sting have a substantial risk of false-negative results. Positive results that correlate with the clinical history are sufficient evidence for considering Hymenoptera venom immunotherapy.

Venom Immunotherapy

General indications for venom immunotherapy are listed in Box 1.7. Patients must understand that after immunotherapy is begun, the injection schedule must be maintained and that immunotherapy itself has a small risk of allergic reaction. Patients also need to understand that despite receiving allergy immunotherapy, they must carry epinephrine when outdoors because of the possibility (from 2% with vespid stings to 10% with apid stings) that immunotherapy will not provide suitable protection. Most, but not all, patients can safely discontinue venom immunotherapy after 5 years of treatment.

Avoidance

The warnings that every patient with stinging insect hypersensitivity should receive are listed in Box 1.8. A patient's specific circumstances may require additions to this list. Also, patients need to know how to use self-injectable epinephrine. Many patients wear an anaphylaxis identification bracelet.

Drug Allergy

Drug Allergy Not Involving IgE or Immediate-Type Reactions

Patients with drug allergy not involving IgE or immediate-type reactions have negative results on skin prick and intradermal testing.

Box 1.8 • *Do's* and *Don'ts* for Patients With Hypersensitivity to Insect Stings

Avoid looking or smelling like a flower

Avoid wearing flowered-print clothing

Avoid using cosmetics and fragrances, especially ones derived from flowering plants

Never drink from a soft-drink can outdoors during the warm months—a yellow jacket can land *on* or *in* the can while you are not watching, go inside the can, and sting the inside of your mouth (a dangerous place for a sensitive patient to be stung) when you take a drink

Never reach into a mailbox without first looking inside it

Never go barefoot

Always look at the underside of picnic table benches and park benches before sitting down

---

Stevens-Johnson Syndrome

Stevens-Johnson syndrome is a bullous skin and mucosal reaction; very large blisters appear over much of the skin surface, in the mouth, and along the gastrointestinal tract. Because of the propensity of the blisters to break down and become infected, the reaction often is life-threatening. Treatment consists of stopping use of the drug that causes the reaction, giving corticosteroids systemically, and providing supportive care. The patients are often treated in burn units. Penicillin, sulfonamides, barbiturates, diphenylhydantoin, warfarin, and phenothiazines are well-known causes. A drug-induced Stevens-Johnson reaction is an absolute contraindication to administering the causative drug to the patient in the future.

Toxic Epidermal Necrolysis

Clinically, toxic epidermal necrolysis is almost indistinguishable from Stevens-Johnson syndrome. Histologically, the cleavage plane for the blisters is deeper than in Stevens-Johnson syndrome. The cleavage plane is at the basement membrane of the epidermis, so even the basal cell layer is lost. This makes toxic epidermal necrolysis even more devastating than Stevens-Johnson syndrome, because healing occurs with much scarring. Often, healing cannot be accomplished without skin grafting, so the mortality rate is even higher than for Stevens-Johnson syndrome. Patients with toxic epidermal necrolysis should always be cared for in a burn unit because of full-thickness damage over 80% to 90% of the skin. The very high mortality rate is similar to that for burn patients with damage of this extent.

KEY FACTS

✓ Venoms of vespids (yellow jackets, wasps, hornets) cross-react; vespid venom and honeybee venom do not

✓ Patients with stinging insect allergy need to know how to use self-injectable epinephrine

✓ Stevens-Johnson syndrome—very large blisters on the skin, in the mouth, and along the gastrointestinal tract

✓ Toxic epidermal necrolysis and Stevens-Johnson syndrome are almost indistinguishable clinically

Morbilliform Skin Reaction

Morbilliform skin reaction is the most common dermatologic manifestation of a drug reaction. It is an immune-mediated drug rash without IgE involvement, manifested by a macular-papular exanthem. The rash can be accompanied by pruritus but has no other systemic symptoms. It typically occurs more than 5 days after use of a medication was begun. It is not associated with anaphylaxis or other serious sequelae.

Ampicillin-Mononucleosis Rash

Ampicillin-mononucleosis rash is a unique drug rash that occurs when ampicillin is given to an acutely ill, febrile patient who has mononucleosis. The rash is papular, nonpruritic, and rose colored. It occurs usually on the abdomen and feels granular when the fingers brush lightly over the surface of the involved skin. It is not known why the rash is specific for ampicillin and mononucleosis. This rash does not predispose to allergy to penicillin.

Key Definition

Ampicillin-mononucleosis rash: unique drug rash that occurs when ampicillin is given to an acutely ill, febrile patient who has mononucleosis.

Fixed Drug Eruptions

Fixed drug eruptions are red to red-brown macules that appear on a certain area of the patient's skin; any part of the body can be affected. The macules do not itch or have other signs of inflammation, although fever is associated with their appearance in a few patients. The unique aspect of this phenomenon is that if a patient is given the same drug in the future, the rash develops in exactly the same skin areas. Resolution of the macules often includes postinflammatory hyperpigmentation. Except for cosmetic problems due to skin discoloration, the phenomenon does not seem serious. Antibiotics and sulfonamides are the most frequently recognized causes.

Erythema Nodosum

Erythema nodosum is a characteristic rash of red nodules about the size of a quarter, usually nonpruritic and appearing only over the anterior aspects of the lower legs. Histopathologically, the nodules are plaques of infiltrating mononuclear cells. Erythema nodosum is associated with several connective tissue diseases, viral infections, and drug allergy.

Contact Dermatitis

Contact dermatitis can occur with various drugs. Commonly, it is a form of drug allergy that is an occupational disease in medical or health care workers. In some patients receiving topical drugs, allergy develops to the drug or to various elements in its pharmaceutical formulation (eg, fillers, stabilizers, antibacterials, emulsifiers). Contact dermatitis is a manifestation of type IV hypersensitivity. Clinically, it appears as an area of reddening on the skin that progresses to a granular, weeping eczematous eruption with some dermal thickening; the surrounding skin has a plaquelike quality. When patients are receiving treatment for dermatitis and contact hypersensitivity develops to corticosteroids or other drugs used in treatment, a particularly difficult diagnostic problem arises unless the physician is alert to this possibility. When contact hypersensitivity to a drug occurs, it does not increase the probability of acute type I hypersensitivity and is not associated with serious exfoliative syndromes. However, exquisite cutaneous sensitivity of this type can develop to a degree that almost no avoidance technique in the workplace completely eliminates dermatitis; even protective gloves are only partly helpful. Thus, it can be occupationally disabling.

Drug Allergy Involving IgE or Immediate-Type Reactions

Penicillin Allergy

Penicillin can cause anaphylaxis in sensitive persons. Penicillin allergy is an IgE-mediated process that can be evaluated with skin testing to the major and minor determinants of penicillin.

Penicillin skin tests can be helpful in determining whether it is safe to administer penicillin to a patient with suspected penicillin allergy. About 85% of patients who give a history of penicillin allergy have negative results of skin tests to the major and minor determinants of penicillin. These patients are not at increased risk for anaphylaxis and can receive penicillin safely. If penicillin skin test results are positive, there is a 40% to 60% chance that an allergic reaction will develop if the patient is challenged with penicillin. These patients should avoid penicillin and related drugs. However, if there is a strong indication for penicillin treatment, desensitization can be performed. The desensitization procedure involves administration of progressively increasing doses of penicillin. Desensitization can be accomplished by the oral or intravenous route and is usually performed in a hospital setting.

Ampicillin, amoxicillin, nafcillin, and other β-lactam antibiotics cross-react strongly with penicillin. Early studies suggested that up to 20% to 30% of patients with penicillin allergy were also allergic to cephalosporins. More recent studies have suggested that the cross-sensitivity of penicillin with cephalosporins is much less (about 5%). Most studies have suggested that aztreonam does not cross-react with penicillin.

Radiocontrast Media Reactions

Radiocontrast media can cause reactions that have the clinical appearance of anaphylaxis. Estimates of the frequency of these reactions are 2% to 6% of procedures involving intravenous contrast media. The incidence of intra-arterial contrast-induced reactions is lower. Anaphylactoid reactions do not involve IgE antibody (thus the term *anaphylactoid*). Radiocontrast media appear to induce mediator release on the basis of some other property intrinsic to the contrast agent. The tonicity or ionic strength of the medium seems particularly related to anaphylactoid reactions. Since nonionic and low-osmolar media became available, the incidence of reactions has decreased.

The frequency of radiocontrast media reactions can be reduced with the use of nonionic or low-osmolar media in patients with a history of asthma or atopy. Patients who have a history of reaction to radiocontrast media and who subsequently need procedures that use radiocontrast media can be pretreated with a protocol of prednisone, 50 mg orally every 6 hours for 3 doses, with the last dose given 1 hour before the procedure. At the last dose, addition of 50 mg of diphenhydramine or an equivalent H_1 antagonist is recommended. Some studies show that the addition of oral ephedrine can be beneficial. Most studies show that the addition of an H_2 antagonist is unnecessary.

Other Allergic or Immunologic Conditions

Mastocytosis

Systemic mastocytosis is a disorder of abnormal proliferation of mast cells. The skin, bone marrow, liver, spleen, lymph nodes, and gastrointestinal tract can be affected. The clinical manifestations vary but can include flushing, pruritus, urticaria, unexplained syncope, fatigue, and dyspepsia. Bone marrow biopsies with stains for mast cells (toluidine blue, Giemsa, or chloral acetate esterase) and immunochemical stains for tryptase are the most direct diagnostic studies. Serum levels of tryptase and urinary concentrations of histamine, histamine metabolites, and prostaglandins are typically increased.

Treatment initially consists of antihistamines. Cromolyn sodium given orally can be beneficial, especially in patients with gastrointestinal tract symptoms. Corticosteroids should be considered in severe cases, and interferon is a promising investigational treatment.

Eosinophilia

Eosinophilia is idiopathic, primary, or secondary (reactive). Hypereosinophilia syndrome is an idiopathic eosinophilic disorder characterized by an absolute eosinophil count of more than 1.5×10^9/L; a course of 6 months or longer; organ involvement as manifested by eosinophilia-mediated tissue injury (cardiomyopathy, dermatitis, pneumonitis, sinusitis, gastrointestinal tract inflammation, left or right ventricular apical thrombus, or stroke); and no other causes of eosinophilia. The syndrome typically affects persons in the third through sixth decades of life; women are affected more often than men. Symptoms include fatigue, cough, shortness of breath, or rash. Cardiac involvement in hypereosinophilia syndrome is especially significant: Endomyocardial fibrosis, mural thrombi, and mitral and tricuspid incompetence can occur. The clinical syndrome is manifested as restrictive cardiomyopathy with congestive heart failure. Echocardiography and endomyocardial biopsy are important diagnostic tests.

Secondary causes include the following: infectious (tissue-invasive parasitosis); drugs; toxins; inflammation; atopy and allergies (asthma); malignancy (lymphoma, Hodgkin lymphoma, cutaneous T-cell lymphoma, and metastatic cancer); collagen vascular disease (eosinophilic vasculitis); pulmonary (hypereosinophilic pneumonitis and Löffler syndrome); and eosinophilic myalgia syndrome.

The clinical diagnostic approach is to exclude secondary eosinophilic disorders; to evaluate bone marrow aspirates and biopsy specimens with genetic and molecular studies; and to perform tests to assess eosinophilia-mediated tissue injury (chest radiography, pulmonary function tests, echocardiography, complete blood cell count, and liver enzyme and serum tryptase levels). The differential diagnosis of eosinophilia is given in Box 1.9.

Hypereosinophilia syndrome is treated with prednisone, 1 mg/kg daily, alone or in combination with hydroxyurea. Second-line therapy includes recombinant interferon-alfa.

Common Variable Immunodeficiency

Common variable immunodeficiency (CVID) affects males and females of all ages. It is the most common primary immunodeficiency in adults. Patients have recurrent sinopulmonary infections, primarily with encapsulated organisms. The primary laboratory abnormality is hypogammaglobulinemia (low IgG levels). IgA and IgM levels may be normal or decreased. Recurrent pyogenic infections include chronic otitis media, chronic or recurrent sinusitis, pneumonia, and bronchiectasis.

Box 1.9 • Common Causes of Eosinophilia

Typically mild eosinophilia ($0.5–1.0\times10^9$/L)

    Atopic
    Allergic bronchopulmonary aspergillosis
    Asthma
    Atopic dermatitis
    Drug hypersensitivity (sometimes very high
      eosinophil levels)
    Vasculitis/connective tissue disease

Typically moderate to severe eosinophilia ($>1.0\times10^9$/L)

    Proliferative/neoplastic
    Idiopathic hypereosinophilic syndrome
    Churg-Strauss vasculitis
    Eosinophilic fasciitis
    Eosinophilic gastroenteritis
    Helminth infection
    Eosinophilia-myalgia syndrome

KEY FACTS

✓ Penicillin can cause anaphylaxis in sensitive persons; evaluate with skin testing

✓ About 85% of patients who give a history of penicillin allergy have negative skin test results

✓ Radiocontrast media reactions—estimated frequency, 2% to 6% of procedures

✓ Clinical manifestations of mastocytosis vary; bone marrow biopsy and staining are most direct diagnostic studies

✓ CVID affects both sexes and all ages; most common primary immunodeficiency in adults

---

Patients with CVID often have autoimmune or gastrointestinal tract disturbances. About one-half of patients have chronic diarrhea and malabsorption. They may have steatorrhea, protein-losing enteropathy, ulcerative colitis, or Crohn disease. Other gastrointestinal tract problems associated with the disease are atrophic gastritis, pernicious anemia, giardiasis, and chronic active hepatitis. Pathologic changes in the gastrointestinal tract mucosa include loss of villi, nodular lymphoid hyperplasia, and diffuse lymphoid infiltration.

Autoimmune anemia, thrombocytopenia, or neutropenia is present in 10% to 50% of the patients and can occur before CVID is diagnosed. Inflammatory arthritis and lymphoid interstitial pneumonia are other associated conditions. Also, patients have an increased risk of a malignancy, particularly a lymphoid malignancy such as non-Hodgkin lymphoma.

The diagnosis of CVID should be considered if patients have recurrent pyogenic infections and hypogammaglobulinemia. Associated gastrointestinal tract or autoimmune disease and the exclusion of hereditary primary immunodeficiencies support the diagnosis. Treatment is with intravenous or subcutaneous γ-globulin. The typical dosage is 400 to 600 mg/kg monthly.

Terminal Complement Component Deficiencies

Patients with deficiency of the terminal complement component C5, C6, C7, or C8 have an increased susceptibility to meningococcal infections.

Terminal complement component deficiency should be suspected if patients have recurrent meningococcal disease, a family history of meningococcal disease, systemic meningococcal infection, or infection with an unusual serotype of meningococcus. Diagnosis is confirmed with assay of total hemolytic complement and measurement of individual complement components.

2 Asthma[a]

GERALD W. VOLCHECK, MD

Pathophysiology

Bronchial hyperresponsiveness and airway inflammation are common to all forms of asthma. Hyperresponsiveness is measured by assessing pulmonary function before and after exposure to albuterol, methacholine, histamine, cold air, or exercise. A decrease in forced expiratory volume in 1 second (FEV_1) of 20% or more with challenge or an increase in FEV_1 of 12% or more with albuterol is considered a sign of airway hyperreactivity.

Persons who have allergic asthma generate mast cell and basophil mediators that have important roles in the development of endobronchial inflammation and smooth muscle changes that occur after acute exposure to allergen. Mast cells and basophils are prominent during the immediate-phase reaction. In the late-phase reaction to allergen exposure, the bronchi show histologic features of chronic inflammation and eosinophils become prominent in the reaction.

Patients who have chronic asthma and negative results on allergy skin tests usually have an inflammatory infiltrate in the bronchi and histologic findings dominated by eosinophils when asthma is active. Patients with sudden asphyxic asthma may have a neutrophilic rather than an eosinophilic infiltration of the airway. The pathologic features of asthma have been studied chiefly in fatal cases; some bronchoscopic data are available for mild and moderate asthma. The histologic hallmarks of asthma include mucous gland hypertrophy, mucus hypersecretion, epithelial desquamation, widening of the basement membrane, and infiltration by eosinophils (Box 2.1).

Important characteristics of cytokines are summarized in Table 2.1. Interleukin (IL)-1, IL-6, and tumor necrosis factor are produced by antigen-presenting cells and start the

---

Box 2.1 • Histologic Hallmarks of Asthma

Mucous gland hypertrophy

Mucus hypersecretion

Alteration of tinctorial and viscoelastic properties of mucus

Widening of basement membrane zone of bronchial epithelial membrane

Increased number of intraepithelial leukocytes and mast cells

Round cell infiltration of bronchial submucosa

Intense eosinophilic infiltration of submucosa

Widespread damage to bronchial epithelium

  Large areas of complete desquamation of epithelium into airway lumen

  Mucous plugs filled with eosinophils and their products

---

acute inflammatory reaction; IL-4 and IL-13 stimulate IgE synthesis; IL-5 stimulates eosinophils; IL-2 and interferon-γ stimulate a cell-mediated response; and IL-10 is the primary anti-inflammatory cytokine.

Presentation and Diagnosis

Medical History

A medical history for asthma includes careful inquiry about symptoms, provoking factors, alleviating factors, and severity. The hallmark symptoms for asthma are wheeze, cough, and shortness of breath. Patients with marked respiratory allergy have symptoms when exposed

---

[a] Portions previously published in Volcheck GW. Clinical allergy: diagnosis and management. Totowa (NJ): Humana Press; c2009. Used with permission of Mayo Foundation for Medical Education and Research.

Table 2.1 • Characteristics of Cytokines

Cytokine	Major Actions	Primary Sources
IL-1	Lymphocyte activation Fibroblast activation Fever	Macrophages Endothelial cells Lymphocytes
IL-2	T- and B-cell activation	T cells (TH1)
IL-3	Mast cell proliferation Neutrophil and macrophage maturation	T cells Mast cells
IL-4	IgE synthesis	T cells (TH2)
IL-5	Eosinophil proliferation and differentiation	T cells (TH2)
IL-6	IgG synthesis Lymphocyte activation	Fibroblasts T cells
IL-8	Neutrophil chemotaxis	Fibroblasts Endothelial cells Monocytes
IL-10	Inhibition of IFN-γ and IL-1 production	T cells Macrophages
IL-13	IgE synthesis	T cells
IFN-α	Antiviral activity	Leukocytes
IFN-γ	Macrophage activation Stimulation of MHC expression Inhibition of TH2 activity	T cells (TH1)
TNF-γ	Antitumor cell activity	Lymphocytes Macrophages
TNF-β	Antitumor cell activity	T cells
GM-CSF	Mast cell, granulocyte, and macrophage stimulation	Lymphocytes Mast cells Macrophages

Abbreviations: GM-CSF, granulocyte-macrophage colony-stimulating factor; IFN, interferon; IL, interleukin; MHC, major histocompatibility complex; TH, helper T cell; TNF, tumor necrosis factor.

to aeroallergens and often have seasonal variation of symptoms. If allergy skin test results are negative, one can be reasonably certain that the patient does not have allergic asthma, but rather intrinsic or nonallergic asthma. Respiratory infections (particularly viral); cold, dry air; exercise; and respiratory irritants can trigger allergic and nonallergic asthma.

Methacholine Bronchial Challenge

If a patient has a history suggestive of episodic asthma but has normal results on pulmonary function tests on the day of the examination, the patient is a reasonable candidate for a methacholine bronchial challenge. The methacholine bronchial challenge is also useful in evaluating patients for cough if baseline pulmonary function appears normal. Positive results indicate that bronchial hyperresponsiveness is present, although results can be positive in conditions besides asthma (Box 2.2). Some consider isocapnic hyperventilation with subfreezing dry air (by either

exercising or breathing a carbon dioxide–air mixture) or exercise testing as alternatives to a methacholine challenge.

A methacholine challenge should not be performed in patients who have severe airway obstruction or a clear diagnosis of asthma. Usually, a 20% decrease in FEV_1 is considered a positive result.

Box 2.2 • Medical Conditions Associated With Positive Findings on Methacholine Challenge

Current asthma
Past history of asthma
Chronic obstructive pulmonary disease
Smoking
Recent respiratory infection
Chronic cough
Allergic rhinitis

Exhaled Nitric Oxide

Exhaled nitric oxide has been studied as a noninvasive measure of airway inflammation. The fraction of nitric oxide in the exhaled air increases in proportion to inflammation of the bronchial wall, sputum eosinophilia, and airway hyperresponsiveness. Exhaled nitric oxide levels increase with deterioration in asthma control and decrease in a dose-dependent manner with anti-inflammatory treatment. The usefulness of measuring exhaled nitric oxide may be in monitoring asthma control, guiding therapy, and predicting response to corticosteroid therapy.

Differential Diagnosis

The differential diagnosis of wheezing is given in Box 2.3.

Assessment of Severity

Asthma is **intermittent** if 1) the daytime symptoms are intermittent (<2 times weekly), 2) continuous treatment is not needed, and 3) the flow-volume curve during formal pulmonary function testing is normal between episodes of symptoms. Even for patients who meet these criteria, inflammation (albeit patchy) is present in the airways and corticosteroid inhaled on a regular basis diminishes bronchial hyperresponsiveness.

Asthma is **mild persistent** or **moderate persistent** when 1) the symptoms occur with some regularity (>2

Box 2.3 • Differential Diagnosis of Wheezing

Pulmonary embolism
Cardiac failure
Foreign body
Central airway tumors
Aspiration
Carcinoid syndrome
Chondromalacia or polychondritis
Löffler syndrome
Bronchiectasis
Tropical eosinophilia
Hyperventilation syndrome
Laryngeal edema
Vascular ring affecting trachea
Factitious (including psychophysiologic vocal cord adduction)
α_1-Antitrypsin deficiency
Immotile cilia syndrome
Bronchopulmonary dysplasia
Bronchiolitis (including bronchiolitis obliterans), croup
Cystic fibrosis

---

times weekly) or daily, 2) there is nocturnal occurrence of symptoms, or 3) asthma exacerbations are troublesome. For many of these patients, the flow-volume curve is rarely normal and complete pulmonary function testing may show evidence of hyperinflation, as indicated by increased residual volume or an increase above expected levels for the diffusing capacity of the lung for carbon dioxide. Asthma is *severe persistent* when symptoms are present almost continuously and the usual medications must be given in doses at the upper end of the dose range to control the disease.

Key Definition

Intermittent asthma: *daytime symptoms are intermittent (<2 times weekly), continuous treatment is not needed, and flow-volume curve during pulmonary function testing is normal between episodes.*

Key Definition

Mild persistent or moderate persistent asthma: *symptoms occur with some regularity (>2 times weekly) or daily, symptoms occur at night, or exacerbations are troublesome.*

Patients with mild, moderate, or severe persistent asthma should receive treatment daily with anti-inflammatory medications, usually inhaled corticosteroids. Most patients with severe asthma require either large doses of inhaled corticosteroid or oral prednisone daily for adequate control. A majority have been hospitalized more than once for asthma. The severity of asthma can change over time, and an early sign that asthma is not well controlled is the emergence of nocturnal symptoms.

Conditions Contributing to Asthma

Assessment of Contributors to Asthma

The mnemonic *AIR-SMOG* provides a concise checklist of possible contributors to asthma (Box 2.4). In addition, patient adherence to therapy and ability to use the inhaler correctly should be reviewed for all patients with persistent asthma.

Gastroesophageal Reflux and Asthma

The precise role of gastroesophageal reflux in asthma is not known. There appears to be a subgroup of patients whose asthma is exacerbated by gastroesophageal reflux.

Asthma-Provoking Drugs

It is important to recognize the potentially severe adverse response that patients with asthma may show to β_1- and β_2-blockers, including β_1-selective blockers such as atenolol. Patients with asthma who have glaucoma treated with ophthalmic preparations of timolol or betaxolol may experience bronchospasm. β-Blockers are not absolutely contraindicated in asthma, but observation is warranted.

KEY FACTS

✓ A decrease in FEV_1 ≥20% with challenge—sign of airway hyperreactivity

✓ Hallmark symptoms for asthma—wheeze, cough, and shortness of breath

✓ If the history suggests episodic asthma but results of pulmonary function tests are normal on examination day, consider methacholine bronchial challenge

✓ Exhaled nitric oxide—useful in monitoring asthma control, guiding therapy, and predicting response to corticosteroids

✓ β-Blockers not absolutely contraindicated in asthma, but observation is warranted

A chronic, dry cough that mimics asthma may develop in persons taking angiotensin-converting enzyme inhibitor drugs. Wheeze and dyspnea, however, do not accompany the cough.

Aspirin ingestion can cause acute, severe, and fatal asthma in a small subset of patients with asthma. Most of the affected patients have nasal polyposis, hyperplastic pansinus mucosal disease, and moderate to severe persistent asthma. However, not all patients with this reaction to aspirin fit the profile. Many nonsteroidal anti-inflammatory drugs can trigger the reaction; the likelihood correlates with a drug's potency for inhibiting cyclooxygenase. Only nonacetylated salicylates such as choline salicylate (a weak cyclooxygenase inhibitor) seem not to provoke the reaction. Leukotriene-modifying drugs may be particularly helpful in aspirin-sensitive asthma.

Traditionally, patients with asthma have been warned not to take antihistamines because the anticholinergic activity of some antihistamines was thought to cause drying of lower respiratory tract secretions, further worsening the asthma. However, antihistamines do not worsen asthma, and some studies have shown a beneficial effect.

Cigarette Smoking and Asthma

The combination of asthma and cigarette smoking leads to accelerated chronic obstructive pulmonary disease. Because of the accelerated rate of irreversible obstruction, all patients with asthma who smoke should be counseled to stop smoking.

Environmental tobacco smoke is an important asthma trigger. In particular, children with asthma who are exposed to environmental smoke have more respiratory infections and asthma attacks.

Subtypes of Asthma

Occupational Asthma

The incidence of occupational asthma is estimated to be 6% to 15% of all cases of adult-onset asthma. A large fraction of occupational asthma escapes diagnosis because physicians often obtain an inadequate occupational history. A wide range of possible industrial circumstances may lead to exposure and resultant disease. The most widely recognized causes of occupational asthma are listed in Box 2.5. Breathing tests performed in the workplace and away from the workplace aid in the diagnosis.

Allergic Bronchopulmonary Aspergillosis

Allergic bronchopulmonary aspergillosis is an obstructive lung disease caused by an immunologic reaction to *Aspergillus* in the lower airway. The typical patient presents with severe steroid-dependent asthma. Most patients with this condition have coexisting asthma or cystic fibrosis. The diagnostic features of allergic bronchopulmonary aspergillosis are summarized in Box 2.6. Fungi other than *Aspergillus fumigatus* can cause an allergic bronchopulmonary mycosis similar to allergic bronchopulmonary aspergillosis.

Chest radiography can show transient or permanent infiltrates and central bronchiectasis, usually affecting the upper lobes (Figure 2.1). Advanced cases show extensive pulmonary fibrosis. Allergic bronchopulmonary aspergillosis is treated with systemic corticosteroids. Total serum IgE (elevated >1,000 kU/L when active) may be helpful in following the course of the disease. Antifungal therapy alone has not been effective.

Medications for Asthma

Medications for asthma are listed in Box 2.7. They can be divided into bronchodilator compounds and anti-inflammatory compounds.

Box 2.5 • Industrial Agents That Can Cause Asthma

Metals
 Salts of platinum, nickel, and chrome
Wood dusts
 Mahogany
 Oak
 Redwood
 Western red cedar (plicatic acid)
Vegetable dusts
 Castor bean
 Cotton
 Cottonseed
 Flour
 Grain (mite and weevil antigens)
 Green coffee
 Gums
Industrial chemicals and plastics
 Ethylenediamine
 Phthalic and trimellitic anhydrides
 Polyvinyl chloride
 Toluene diisocyanate
Pharmaceutical agents
 Phenylglycine acid chloride
 Penicillins
 Spiramycin
Food industry agents
 Egg protein
 Polyvinyl chloride
Biologic enzymes
Bacillus subtilis (laundry detergent workers)
Pancreatic enzymes
Animal emanations
 Canine or feline saliva
 Horse dander (racing workers)
 Rodent urine (laboratory animal workers)

Box 2.6 • Diagnostic Features of Allergic Bronchopulmonary Aspergillosis

Clinical asthma

Bronchiectasis (usually proximal)

Increased total serum IgE

IgE antibody to *Aspergillus* (by skin test or in vitro assay)[a]

Precipitins or IgG antibody to *Aspergillus*

Radiographic infiltrates (often in upper lobes)

Peripheral blood eosinophilia

[a] Required for diagnosis.

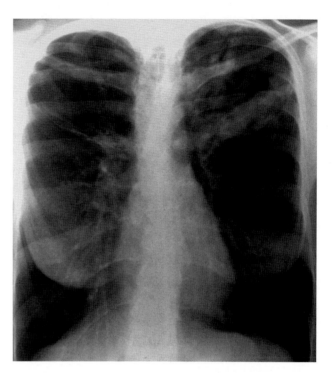

Figure 2.1 *Allergic Bronchopulmonary Aspergillosis. Chest radiograph shows cylindrical infiltrates involving the upper lobes.*

Bronchodilator Compounds

Currently, the only anticholinergic drug available in the United States for treating asthma is ipratropium bromide, although it is approved for treating only chronic obstructive pulmonary disease. A number of short-acting β-adrenergic compounds are available, but albuterol, levalbuterol, and pirbuterol are prescribed most often. More adverse effects occur when these medications are given orally than when they are given by inhalation. Nebulized β-agonists are rarely used long-term in adult asthma, although they may be used in acute attacks. For home use, the metered dose inhaler or dry powder inhaler is the preferred delivery system. Salmeterol and formoterol are 2 long-acting inhaled β-agonists. Both should be used only in combination with inhaled corticosteroids. Theophylline is effective for asthma, but it has a narrow therapeutic index, and interactions with other drugs (cimetidine, erythromycin, and quinolone antibiotics) can increase the serum level of theophylline.

Anti-inflammatory Compounds

Cromolyn and nedocromil are inhaled anti-inflammatory (mast cell–stabilizing) medications that are appropriate for treatment of mild or moderate asthma. The 5-lipoxygenase inhibitor zileuton and the leukotriene receptor antagonists zafirlukast and montelukast are approved for treatment

Box 2.7 • Medications for Asthma

Bronchodilator compounds

    Anticholinergic drugs (ipratropium bromide, tiotropium)

    β_2-Agonist drugs

        Short-acting (albuterol, pirbuterol, levalbuterol)

        Long-acting (salmeterol, formoterol, indacaterol, vilanterol)

    Methylxanthines (theophylline)

"Antiallergic" compounds

    Cromolyn

    Nedocromil

Glucocorticoids

    Systemic

        Prednisone

        Methylprednisolone

    Topical

        Beclomethasone

        Budesonide

        Ciclesonide

        Flunisolide

        Fluticasone

        Mometasone

        Triamcinolone acetonide

Antileukotrienes

    Leukotriene receptor antagonists (zafirlukast, montelukast)

    Lipoxygenase inhibitors (zileuton)

Glucocorticoids in combination with long-acting β_2-agonists

    Budesonide with formoterol

    Mometasone with formoterol

    Fluticasone with salmeterol

    Fluticasone with vilanterol

of mild persistent asthma. These agents work by decreasing the inflammatory effects of leukotrienes. Zileuton can cause increased liver function test results. Cases of Churg-Strauss vasculitis have also been linked to zafirlukast and montelukast, although a clear cause-and-effect relationship has not been established.

KEY FACTS

✓ Aspirin can cause acute, severe, and fatal asthma in a small subset of patients with asthma

✓ Asthma plus cigarette smoking—leads to accelerated chronic obstructive pulmonary disease

✓ Occupational asthma accounts for about 6% to 15% of all adult-onset asthma

✓ Allergic bronchopulmonary aspergillosis typically presents as severe steroid-dependent asthma

✓ Ipratropium bromide—the only anticholinergic drug available in the United States for treating asthma

Corticosteroids

Many experts recommend inhaled glucocorticoids for all severities of persistent asthma because of the potential long-term benefits of reduced bronchial hyperresponsiveness and reduced airway remodeling (fibrosis). Long-term use of β-agonist bronchodilators alone may adversely affect asthma; this also argues for earlier use of inhaled glucocorticoids. Asthma mortality has been linked to the heavy use of β-agonist inhalers, but this effect appears to be decreased when inhaled corticosteroids are concomitantly used.

The inflammatory infiltrate in the bronchial submucosa of patients with asthma probably depends on cytokine secretory patterns. Corticosteroids may interfere at several levels in the cytokine cascade, and they offer several benefits (Box 2.8).

The most common adverse effects of inhaled corticosteroids are dysphonia and thrush. These unwanted effects occur in about 10% of patients and can be reduced by using a spacer device and rinsing the mouth after administration. Usually, oral thrush can be treated successfully with oral antifungal agents. Dysphonia, when persistent, may be treated by decreasing or discontinuing the use of inhaled corticosteroids.

Detailed study of the systemic effects of inhaled corticosteroids shows that these agents are much safer than oral corticosteroids. Nevertheless, there is evidence that high-dose inhaled corticosteroids can affect the hypothalamic-pituitary-adrenal axis and bone metabolism. Also, high-dose inhaled corticosteroids may increase the risk of glaucoma, cataracts, and osteoporosis. Inhaled corticosteroids can decrease growth velocity in children and adolescents. The effect of inhaled corticosteroids on final adult height is not known but appears to be minimal.

Poor inhaler technique and poor adherence to therapy can result in poor control of asthma. Therefore, all patients using a metered dose inhaler or dry powder inhaler should be taught the proper technique for using these devices. Patients using metered dose inhaled corticosteroids should use a spacer device with the inhaler.

Box 2.8 • Benefits of Corticosteroids in Treatment of Asthma

Reduce airway inflammation by modulating cytokines interleukin (IL)-4 and IL-5

Can inhibit inflammatory properties of monocytes and platelets

Increase eosinophil apoptosis

Have vasoconstrictive properties

Decrease mucous gland secretion

Anti-IgE Treatment

Omalizumab is the first recombinant humanized anti-IgE monoclonal antibody approved for use in asthma. It blocks IgE binding to mast cells and is indicated for refractory moderate to severe persistent allergic asthma. It is approved for use in patients 12 years or older who have positive results of skin or in vitro allergy testing to relevant allergens. Dosing is based on the patient's IgE level and body weight. The dosage is typically 150 to 375 mg subcutaneously every 2 to 4 weeks.

Asthma Management

The goals of asthma management are listed in Box 2.9.

Management of Chronic Asthma

Baseline spirometry is recommended for all patients with asthma, and home peak flow monitoring is recommended for those with moderate or severe asthma (Figure 2.2). Environmental triggers and conditions contributing to asthma (AIR-SMOG; Box 2.4) should be discussed with all patients with asthma, and allergy testing should be offered to those with suspected allergic asthma or with asthma that is not well controlled. Although allergy immunotherapy is effective, it is recommended only for patients with allergic asthma who have had a complete evaluation by an allergist.

Management of Acute Asthma

Inhaled β-agonists, measurements of lung function at presentation and during therapy, and systemic corticosteroids (for most patients) are the cornerstones of managing acute asthma (Figure 2.3). Generally, nebulized albuterol, administered repeatedly if necessary, is the first line of treatment. Delivery of β-agonist by metered dose inhaler can be substituted in less severe asthma attacks. Inhaled β-agonist delivered by continuous nebulization may be appropriate for more severe disease.

It is important to measure lung function (usually peak expiratory flow rate but also FEV_1 whenever possible) at presentation and after administration of bronchodilators. These measurements provide invaluable information that allows the physician to assess the severity of the asthma attack and the response (if any) to treatment.

Patients who do not have a prompt and full response to inhaled β-agonists should receive a course of systemic corticosteroids. Patients with the most severe and poorly responsive disease (FEV_1 <50%, oxygen saturation <90%, and moderate to severe symptoms) should be treated on a hospital ward or in an intensive care unit.

Box 2.9 • Goals of Asthma Management

No asthma symptoms

No asthma attacks

Normal activity level

Normal lung function

Use of safest and least amount of medication necessary

Establishment of therapeutic relationship between patient and provider

---

KEY FACTS

✓ Cromolyn and nedocromil—inhaled anti-inflammatory drugs appropriate for treating mild or moderate asthma

✓ Inhaled glucocorticoids recommended for all severities of persistent asthma because of potential long-term benefits (reduced bronchial hyperresponsiveness, reduced airway remodeling)

✓ Omalizumab—first recombinant humanized anti-IgE monoclonal antibody approved for use in asthma

✓ Baseline spirometry recommended for all patients with asthma; home peak flow monitoring recommended for those with moderate or severe asthma

✓ Cornerstones of managing acute asthma—inhaled β-agonists, lung function measurements (at presentation, during therapy), and systemic corticosteroids (for most patients)

✓ If response to inhaled β-agonists not prompt and full, give course of systemic corticosteroids

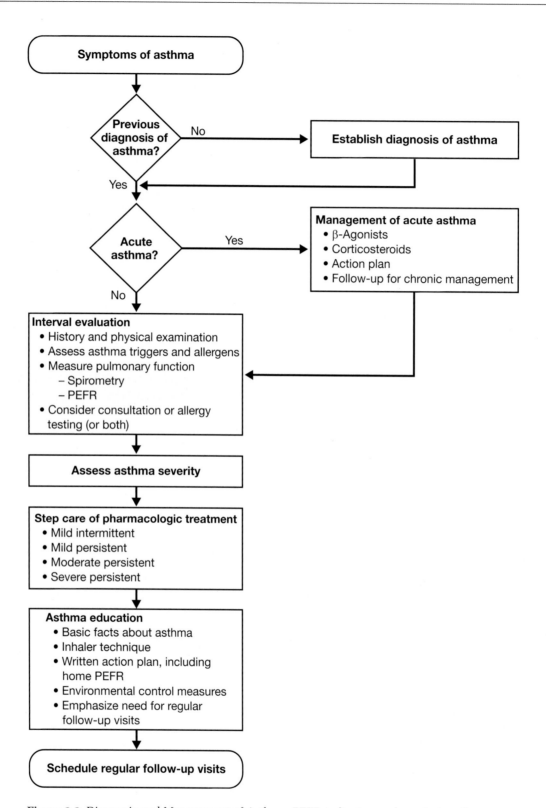

Figure 2.2 *Diagnosis and Management of Asthma. PEFR indicates peak expiratory flow rate.*

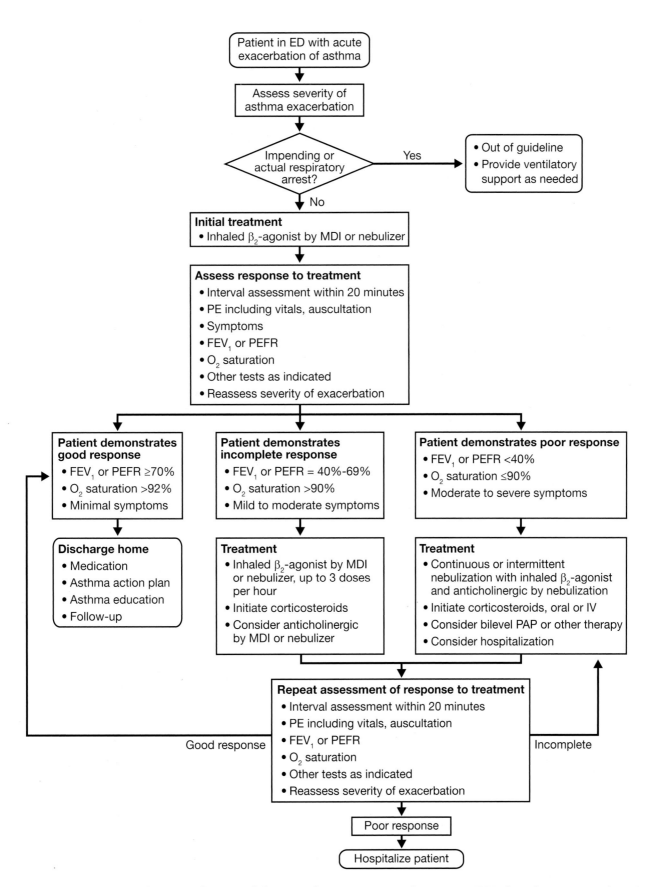

Figure 2.3 *Management of Acute Asthma in Adults. ED indicates emergency department; FEV₁, forced expiratory volume in 1 second; IV, intravenous; MDI, metered dose inhaler; O₂, oxygen; PAP, positive airway pressure; PE, physical examination; PEFR, peak expiratory flow rate.*

(Adapted from Sveum R, Bergstrom J, Brottman G, Hanson M, Heiman M, Johns K, et al. Diagnosis and management of asthma. 10th ed. Bloomington [MN]: Institute for Clinical Systems Improvement [updated 2012 Jul]. Available from: http://www.icsi.org/_asset/rsjvnd/ Asthma.pdf. July c2012. Used with permission.)

Questions and Answers

Questions

Multiple Choice (choose the best answer)

I.1. A 26-year-old woman is treated for *Neisseria gonorrhoeae* infection. She has had 2 episodes of infection with *Neisseria meningitidis*. She had 1 episode of pneumonia as a child. She has not had a history of skin infections or abscesses. What is the most likely underlying immunologic abnormality?
a. C2 deficiency
b. Terminal complement component deficiency
c. Low level of immunoglobulin G
d. Neutrophil chemotaxis
e. Lymphocyte count

I.2. A 32-year-old man is stung on the distal portion of the right forearm by what he describes as a bee. No stinger is visible. Within minutes, the area becomes red, painful, pruritic, and swollen. During the next several hours, the redness and swelling extend to the elbow. He has no other symptoms; specifically, he reports having no dyspnea, light-headedness, nausea, vomiting, or diarrhea. He does not have skin manifestations elsewhere. What is the most appropriate management?
a. Apply ice to the arm, provide symptomatic relief, and review strategies to avoid stinging insects.
b. Perform skin testing to apids (honeybee) only, and administer immunotherapy if results are positive.
c. Perform skin testing to apids (honeybee) and vespids (yellow jacket, wasp, and hornet), and administer immunotherapy if any of the results are positive.
d. Perform an in vitro test for immunoglobulin E that is specific for apid (honeybee) and vespid (yellow jacket, wasp, and hornet), and administer immunotherapy if results are positive.
e. Administer 0.3 mL of 1:1,000 epinephrine intramuscularly and observe.

I.3. A 31-year-old woman presents in her fifth month of pregnancy with increasing asthma symptoms. Her asthma had been controlled well throughout pregnancy but worsened over the past 4 days with the onset of an upper respiratory tract infection. She has daily symptoms and nighttime awakenings due to dyspnea. She uses her albuterol inhaler every 3 hours and has adhered to her usual inhaler regimen of budesonide 2 puffs daily. She reports having no fever or purulent mucus. On examination, scattered expiratory wheezes are heard throughout all lung fields, the respiratory rate is 18 breaths per minute, oxygen saturation is 97%, and forced expiratory volume in 1 second (FEV_1) is 64% of the predicted value, which improves to 72% of the predicted value after albuterol. How should you treat this exacerbation?
a. Add montelukast 10 mg daily.
b. Increase use of budesonide to 2 puffs twice daily.
c. Start amoxicillin 500 mg 3 times daily.
d. Discontinue use of budesonide inhaler.
e. Add prednisone 40 mg daily for 5 days.

I.4. A 62-year-old man presents with a 3-year history of recurrent sinopulmonary infections documented with chest radiography and computed tomography of his sinuses. He does not recall having recurrent infections, allergic rhinitis, or asthma before the past 3 years. Sputum cultures have shown growth of *Streptococcus pneumoniae* and *Haemophilus influenzae*. He reports having a chronic productive cough. Which laboratory test is most likely to be abnormal in this patient?
a. Total white blood cell count
b. Immunoglobulin (Ig)G level
c. Neutrophil chemotaxis assay
d. Total complement level
e. IgE level

Answers

I.1. Answer b.

The patient has had recurrent *Neisseria* infections, which are most commonly associated with deficiencies in the terminal complement components (C5-C9). Deficiencies in the other components of the immune system are associated with other types of infections. Hypogammaglobulinemia is associated primarily with upper and lower respiratory infections caused by encapsulated bacteria. Neutrophil deficiencies are associated with skin and pulmonary abscesses.

I.2. Answer a.

The patient has a large local reaction to a stinging insect. A large local reaction to a stinging insect is not considered a risk factor for a more serious reaction with a subsequent sting. Therefore, only symptomatic treatment is required. Skin testing to apids and vespids would be required only if immunotherapy were contemplated. Skin testing should be considered for all adults who have had a systemic reaction to a sting. A large local reaction, in the absence of other symptoms, does not require the use of epinephrine.

I.3. Answer e.

This pregnant woman is having a clinically significant flare of her asthma, and aggressive treatment is warranted by her decreased FEV_1, her increased use of albuterol, and her wheezing. In this situation, systemic corticosteroids are required. The main risk to the mother and child is hypoxia. Systemic corticosteroids, inhaled corticosteroids, long- and short-acting inhaled β-agonists, and leukotriene receptor blockers are acceptable for use in the management of asthma in a pregnant patient. For ongoing management, adding montelukast or increasing her use of budesonide may be helpful, but these options are not the most effective in treating an acute exacerbation.

I.4. Answer b.

Recurrent sinopulmonary infections with common respiratory microorganisms are the primary manifestations of common variable immunodeficiency (CVID). The major laboratory abnormality in CVID is a decreased level of IgG. The hypogammaglobulinemia predisposes to recurrent sinus and pulmonary infections. Other manifestations include autoimmune processes and infectious diarrhea. The neutrophil chemotaxis assay is decreased in chronic granulomatous disease, which is characterized by recurrent skin and pulmonary abscesses. Deficiencies of the terminal complement components C5 through C9 typically manifest as recurrent infections with meningococci and gonococci.

Section II

Cardiology

3 Arrhythmias and Syncope

PETER A. NOSEWORTHY, MD

Mechanism of Arrhythmias

Cardiac arrhythmias are due to disorders of impulse propagation (reentry) or impulse formation (abnormal automaticity or triggered activity). Reentry is the most common mechanism of arrhythmia and is further classified as macroreentrant or microreentrant. Macroreentrant arrhythmias have a discrete, definable circuit such as atrioventricular (AV) reentrant tachycardia (sustained over AV nodal, ventricular, accessory pathway, and ventricular tissue) or ventricular tachycardia (sustained around an area of myocardial scar or infarcted tissue). Microreentry occurs within a circuit that is too small to be mapped and thus appears to arise from a single point in the myocardium. Three conditions are needed for reentry to occur: 1) more than 2 anatomically or functionally distinct pathways (eg, AV nodal reentry via slow and fast AV nodal pathways), 2) transient, unidirectional block in 1 pathway, and 3) slowed conduction in the second pathway that allows the impulse to reenter the previously blocked limb of the circuit.

Automatic arrhythmias result from a single myocardial focus that has enhanced impulse formation activity and are more sensitive to sympathetic tone, hypoxia, acid-base and electrolyte disturbances, or atrial or ventricular stretch (eg, exacerbations of congestive heart failure). Triggered arrhythmias result from membrane potential oscillations following an action potential (so-called afterdepolarizations) that reach threshold and result in impulse formation. A common triggered arrhythmia is digoxin toxicity or ventricular fibrillation that occurs in the setting of a prolonged QT interval.

Evaluation of Suspected Rhythm Disorders

Electrocardiography

Electrocardiography (ECG) is the most simple and cost-effective tool for evaluating rhythm disorders. Most arrhythmias can be diagnosed on ECG and, even between episodes, it can provide important clues to the predisposing substrate (eg, ventricular preexcitation in Wolff-Parkinson-White syndrome or repolarization abnormalities in long QT syndrome).

Ambulatory ECG Monitoring

Ambulatory ECG (Holter) monitoring allows evaluation of rhythm disturbances and their relationship to daily activities. It is useful to have patients keep a diary and correlate symptoms with the recorded heart rhythm. Normal results on Holter monitoring, however, do not rule out infrequent arrhythmias. Ambulatory ECG monitoring is also useful for assessing the impact of medical or ablative therapies.

Event Recording

Transtelephonic event recording is similar to ambulatory ECG monitoring but is more useful for documenting rhythm when episodes are less frequent (<1 episode per 24–48 hours) but the events are symptomatic. The device is activated by the patient during symptoms. Continuous loop recorders record the ECG obtained 30 seconds to 4 minutes before the activation button is depressed.

Implantable loop recorders can be implanted when symptoms are very infrequent (as infrequently as 1 or 2 times per year) and are programmed to record at prespecified thresholds or with patient-triggered events.

Electrophysiologic Testing

Electrophysiologic (EP) testing is an invasive method that is useful for assessing the substrate for arrhythmia. Indications for EP testing include palpitations likely due to a cardiac rhythm disorder (supraventricular tachycardia or ventricular tachycardia) or syncope suggestive of a cardiogenic mechanism. It can be used in combination with tilt-table testing for the evaluation of patients with suspected cardioinhibitory or vasodepressor syncope or the evaluation of abnormal postural blood pressure and heart rate responses. EP testing is not required in most patients with symptomatic bradycardia for whom a permanent pacemaker is indicated.

KEY FACTS

✓ Reentry—most common mechanism of arrhythmia; classified as macroreentrant or microreentrant

✓ Three conditions needed for reentry to occur—1) more than 2 anatomically or functionally distinct pathways, 2) transient, unidirectional block in 1 pathway, and 3) slowed conduction in second pathway that allows impulse to reenter previously blocked limb of circuit

✓ EP testing—invasive method useful for assessing substrate for arrhythmia

✓ EP testing—not required in most patients with symptomatic bradycardia for whom permanent pacemaker is indicated

---

Therapy for Heart Rhythm Disorders

Several therapeutic options are available for heart rhythm disorders. These include drug therapy, radiofrequency ablation or cryoablation, and device therapy (pacing for brady-arrhythmias and implantable cardioverter-defibrillators [ICDs] for tachyarrhythmias).

Antiarrhythmic Drugs

Antiarrhythmic drugs are frequently used as first-line therapy for rhythm control in atrial fibrillation, for the treatment of ventricular arrhythmia (often as an adjunct to ICD therapy), and occasionally for suppression of supraventricular arrhythmias.

Amiodarone

Amiodarone is highly effective, but its use is limited by multiple noncardiac effects, including potential thyroid (hyperthyroidism and hypothyroidism), hepatic, ocular, and pulmonary toxicities. Nevertheless, amiodarone is generally considered reasonable in high-risk patients in whom the potential risks are justified. In patients with congestive heart failure (CHF), amiodarone has an essentially neutral effect on survival. It is not indicated for primary prevention of sudden death.

Amiodarone does not increase mortality in patients with symptomatic premature ventricular contractions or ventricular tachycardia and is most often used as an adjunct to an ICD for the control of symptoms and prevention of ICD shocks. Routine use of amiodarone after myocardial infarction or in unselected patients with CHF is not recommended.

Adenosine

Adenosine can terminate reentrant tachycardia that relies on conduction through the AV node by interrupting AV node conduction. It has a half-life of 10 seconds. Adenosine will not terminate arrhythmias such as atrial fibrillation or flutter in which the AV node is not a critical part of the reentrant circuit, but it may help in diagnosis of these arrhythmias (ie, by slowing AV conduction to allow visualization of flutter waves). Adenosine may terminate some ventricular arrhythmias (adenosine-sensitive ventricular tachycardia) that originate from the right ventricular outflow tract. Adenosine (and verapamil) is contraindicated in patients presenting with a wide QRS tachycardia and atrial fibrillation associated with Wolff-Parkinson-White syndrome because of the risk of rapid conduction across the accessory pathway (which is not sensitive to adenosine) and induction of ventricular fibrillation.

Adverse Effects of Antiarrhythmic Drugs

Most antiarrhythmic drugs can have proarrhythmic effects. The most worrisome proarrhythmic effect, increased ventricular arrhythmia, can sometimes limit antiarrhythmic drug use in patients with structural heart disease. A classic example of proarrhythmia is quinidine syncope, in which polymorphic ventricular tachycardia results in repeated syncopal events after initiation of quinidine therapy (Figure 3.1).

Transcatheter Radiofrequency Ablation

Transcatheter radiofrequency ablation has revolutionized the treatment of heart rhythm disorders. Narrow complex tachycardias, such as AV nodal reentrant tachycardia or tachycardia due to an accessory pathway (eg, Wolff-Parkinson-White syndrome), are curable with radiofrequency ablation in more than 95% of cases. Atrial tachycardias are curable in more than 90% of cases. Table 3.1 lists arrhythmias amenable to catheter ablation therapy. Atrial fibrillation (especially paroxysmal atrial fibrillation) and ventricular tachycardia (either reentrant or automatic) can also be successfully treated with radiofrequency ablation. Complications include vascular injury, cardiac perforation, and cardioembolic stroke and occur in 1% to 4% of patients. Occasionally, the target of ablation may be in proximity to the AV node (eg, parahisian accessory pathways) and ablation may be associated with a risk of complete heart block requiring pacemaker implantation.

Device Therapy

Device therapy is appropriate for symptomatic bradycardia (permanent pacemaker) and for the primary and secondary prevention of sudden cardiac death (ICD). Indications for a permanent pacemaker implantation in specific conduction system diseases are listed in Box 3.1.

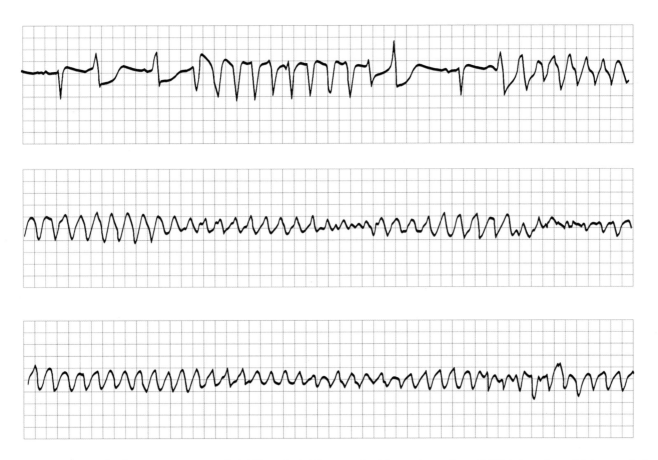

Figure 3.1 *Proarrhythmic Response to Quinidine. Quinidine resulted in prolongation of QT interval, and late-coupled premature ventricular complex initiated polymorphic ventricular tachycardia, termed* torsades de pointes.

Permanent Pacemaker Implantation

An internationally used 4-letter system is used to classify different types of permanent pacemakers (Table 3.2). The choice of device used depends on the clinical circumstances.

Table 3.1 • Heart Rhythms Amenable to Catheter Ablation

Rhythm	Curable	Treatable
SVT	AVNRT	AF
	AVRT (bypass tract)	
	EAT	
	AFL (without fibrillation)	
Ventricular	RV outflow tract tachycardia	VT due to coronary disease and scar after MI
	Idiopathic LV tachycardia	

Abbreviations: AF, atrial fibrillation; AFL, atrial flutter; AVNRT, atrioventricular node reentry tachycardia; AVRT, atrioventricular reentry tachycardia; EAT, ectopic atrial tachycardia; LV, left ventricular; MI, myocardial infarction; RV, right ventricular; SVT, supraventricular tachycardia; VT, ventricular tachycardia.

In general, all pacemakers pace the heart if the heart rate falls below a programmed lower rate limit. Dual-chamber pacemakers allow sequential atrial and ventricular pacing (as opposed to ventricular pacing, which can be asynchronous with the atrial impulse) or tracking of atrial rhythms to the ventricle in cases of heart block. Physiologic pacing attempts to maintain heart rate with normal AV synchrony and to increase heart rate in response to physical activity and can be used to treat chronotropic incompetence (inability to reach a heart rate required for physical activity). Patients fitted with this type of pacemaker may have improved exercise endurance during treadmill testing. A sensor that responds to body motion, respiratory rate, blood temperature, or some other variable can be used to drive the pacemaker so that the rate at which pacing occurs is appropriate to metabolic demands.

Early complications (within 30 days of implantation) are usually related to vascular injury, hematoma, pneumothorax, dislodgment of the lead, and extracardiac stimulation. *Late complications* include lead fracture or insulation defect, infection, pacemaker syndrome (simultaneous atrial and ventricular contraction resulting in symptomatic cannon A waves), and pacemaker-mediated tachycardia.

Box 3.1 • Indications for Pacemaker Implantation

Sinus node dysfunction

    Class I

        Documented symptomatic bradycardia

    Class II

        HR <40 bpm, symptoms present but not clearly
           correlated with bradycardia

    Class III

        Asymptomatic bradycardia (HR <40 bpm)

AV block

    Class I

        Symptomatic 2° or 3° AV block, permanent or
           intermittent

        Congenital 3° AV block with wide QRS

        Advanced AV block 14 days after cardiac surgery

    Class II

        Asymptomatic type II 2° or 3° AV block
           with ventricular rate >40 bpm

    Class III

        Asymptomatic 1° and type I 2° AV block

Myocardial infarction

    Class I

        Recurrent type II 2° AV block and 3° AV block
           with wide QRS

        Transient advanced AV block in presence of BBB

    Class II

        Persistent advanced AV block with narrow QRS

        Acquired BBB in absence of AV block

    Class III

        Transient AV block in absence of BBB

Abbreviations: AV, atrioventricular; BBB, bundle branch block; bpm, beats per minute; HR, heart rate.

Pacemaker-mediated tachycardia is a well-recognized complication of dual-chamber pacemakers (DDD pacing). It occurs during DDD pacing when there is intact retrograde conduction between the ventricle and atrium. A spontaneous premature ventricular contraction occurs that conducts retrogradely to the atrium and is then tracked to the ventricle. This sets up an endless loop tachycardia. The tachycardia rate is typically close to the upper rate limit of the device. Most pacemakers can recognize and attempt

Table 3.2 • Code of Permanent Pacing

Chamber(s) Paced	Chamber(s) Sensed	Mode(s) of Response	Programmable Capabilities
V = ventricle	V = ventricle	T = triggered	R = rate modulated
A = atrium	A = atrium	I = inhibited	
D = dual (atrium and ventricle)	D = dual (atrium and ventricle)	D = dual (triggered and inhibited)	
	O = none	O = none	

to abort pacemaker-mediated tachycardia, or it can be avoided by programming changes of the pacemaker generator that result in the device ignoring the retrograde atrial impulse.

Implantable Cardioverter-Defibrillator

An ICD continuously monitors heart rhythm and can detect and treat abnormal ventricular arrhythmia with overdrive pacing (antitachycardia pacing) or with up to 30- to 40-J shocks. ICDs have been shown to improve mortality outcomes among patients who survive sudden cardiac death and in those at high risk for sudden death (most typically those with an ejection fraction <35%). Some common indications for ICD implantation are listed in Box 3.2.

KEY FACTS

✓ Therapeutic options for heart rhythm disorders—drug, radiofrequency ablation or cryoablation, device

✓ Adenosine (and verapamil)—contraindicated for wide QRS tachycardia and atrial fibrillation with Wolff-Parkinson-White syndrome

✓ Transcatheter radiofrequency ablation—cures narrow complex tachycardias in >95% of cases and atrial tachycardias in >90% of cases

✓ Pacemaker implantation, early complications (≤30 days of implantation)—usually related to vascular injury, hematoma, pneumothorax, dislodgment of lead, extracardiac stimulation

✓ Pacemaker implantation, late complications—lead fracture or insulation defect, infection, pacemaker syndrome, pacemaker-mediated tachycardia

Box 3.2 • Indications for Placement of an Implantable Cardioverter-Defibrillator

Secondary prevention

    Cardiac arrest caused by ventricular fibrillation or
    ventricular tachycardia in the absence of acute
    ischemic or other reversible cause

Primary prevention

    Known conditions with a high risk of life-threatening
    ventricular tachycardia (eg, high-risk patients
    with long QT syndrome or hypertrophic
    cardiomyopathy)

    Ischemic and nonischemic cardiomyopathy (left
    ventricular ejection fraction [LVEF] <35%)
    plus congestive heart failure (New York Heart
    Association [NYHA] class II or III)

    Ischemic cardiomyopathy due to prior myocardial
    and LVEF <30%

Specific Arrhythmias

The Bradycardias

Bradycardia is defined as a heart rate less than 60 beats per minute at rest. Bradycardia can be a normal finding (associated with high vagal tone in asymptomatic and often fit and healthy persons), can be related to a diseased sinus node (sinus node dysfunction), or can be due to other insults (eg, drug therapy, conduction disease with heart block, myocardial infarction).

Key Definition

Bradycardia: *heart rate <60 beats per minute at rest.*

Sinus Node Dysfunction

Sinus node dysfunction includes sinus bradycardia, sinus pauses, tachycardia-bradycardia syndrome (Figure 3.2), sinus arrest, and chronotropic incompetence. In most cases, sinus node dysfunction is diagnosed on the basis of the history and results of ECG and Holter monitoring. Invasive EP testing is usually not necessary. Prolonged monitoring with an event recorder may be required to correlate symptoms with bradycardia. Treadmill testing can distinguish true sinus node dysfunction (chronotropic incompetence in this case), in which a blunted heart rate occurs in response to exercise, from high vagal tone, in which the heart rate increases appropriately during exercise to meet metabolic need. EP testing is reserved for a minority of patients in whom the arrhythmia mechanism cannot be determined by noninvasive means.

Asymptomatic patients with sinus node dysfunction do not require specific therapy, whereas symptomatic patients usually require a pacemaker. Patients with tachycardia-bradycardia often have atrial fibrillation that can present with rapid ventricular rates or with symptomatic bradycardia. Pacemakers are used to prevent bradycardia and allow titration of medications to slow conduction through the AV node and to prevent episodes of rapid ventricular rate during atrial fibrillation.

Conduction System Disorders

A conduction system disorder occurs when impulses from the sinus node reaching the ventricle are delayed. Delay can occur in the right bundle (right bundle branch block), left bundle (left bundle branch block), or one of the hemifascicles of the left bundle (left anterior or posterior hemiblock). Bifascicular block usually refers to right bundle branch block with left anterior fascicular block (marked left axis deviation) or to right bundle branch block with left posterior fascicular block (right axis deviation). Patients presenting with syncope and bifascicular block may have intermittent complete heart block due to conduction system disease or ventricular tachycardia caused by underlying myocardial disease and may require pacing. Patients who have aymtomatic bifascicular block can usually be observed because progression to complete heart block is slow and may never occur in the majority of patients.

Conduction system disorders can be divided into first-degree, second-degree, and third-degree (complete) heart block.

First-Degree AV Block

In first-degree AV block, the PR interval on the ECG is prolonged (>200 milliseconds). In most cases, the block occurs in the AV node.

Second-Degree AV Block

There are 2 subtypes of second-degree AV block: Mobitz I and Mobitz II. Mobitz I second-degree AV block (Wenckebach) manifests as gradual prolongation of the PR interval before a nonconducted P wave. The PR interval after the nonconducted P wave is shorter than the PR interval before the nonconducted P wave (Figures 3.3 and 3.4). The RR interval that encompasses the nonconducted P wave is shorter than 2 RR intervals between conducted beats (the long PR before the block "eats into" the RR interval). Wenckebach conduction occurs as a result of high vagal tone and often occurs after an inferior myocardial infarction or during vagal stimuli such as obstructive sleep apnea or vomiting. Wenckebach conduction almost never requires pacing.

Mobitz II second-degree AV block is caused by conduction block within the His-Purkinje system and may be

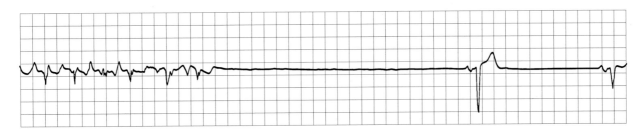

Figure 3.2 Tachycardia-Bradycardia Syndrome. In this case, episode of atrial fibrillation terminated spontaneously, followed by a 4.5-second pause until the sinus node recovered.

(Adapted from MKSAP IX: Part C, Book 1, c1992. American College of Physicians. Used with permission.)

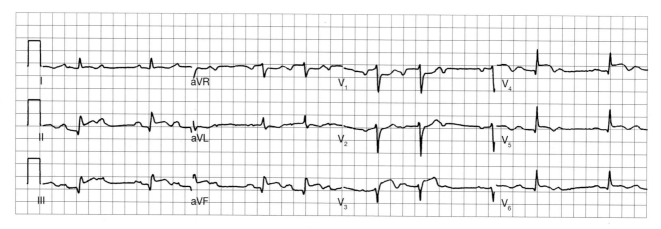

Figure 3.3 *3:2 Mobitz I (or Wenckebach) Second-Degree Atrioventricular Block. Patient had acute inferior myocardial infarction.*

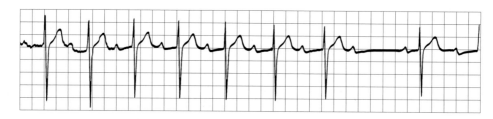

Figure 3.4 *Mobitz I Second-Degree Atrioventricular Block. Note gradual PR prolongation. The PR interval after a nonconducted P wave is shorter than the PR interval preceding the nonconducted P wave.*

associated with bundle branch block. The ECG shows a sudden failure of conduction of a P wave, with no change in the PR interval either before or after the nonconducted P wave (Figure 3.5). The ventricular escape rhythm is either a junctional escape focus, with a conduction pattern similar to that seen during normal rhythm, or a ventricular escape focus, with a wide QRS conduction pattern. Mobitz II block may herald complete heart block, and permanent pacing should be considered.

Third-Degree (Complete) Heart Block

Complete heart block is diagnosed when there is no relationship between atrial rhythm and ventricular rhythm, and atrial rhythm is faster than ventricular escape rhythm (Figure 3.6). The ventricular rhythm is usually regular. Treatment usually is permanent pacing.

Carotid Sinus Hypersensitivity Syndrome

Carotid sinus hypersensitivity is caused by significant bradycardia occurring during pressure of the carotid body (a 3-second pause or a decrease in systolic blood pressure of 50 mm Hg) (Figure 3.7). Carotid sinus hypersensitivity syndrome is common in the elderly and can rarely be caused by anatomical abnormalities in the region of the carotid body (lymph node enlargement, prior surgery). Most patients do not have spontaneous syncope, but those who do

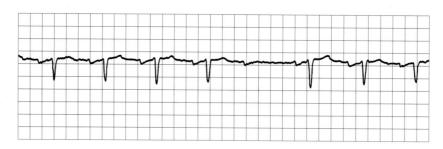

Figure 3.5 *Mobitz II Second-Degree Atrioventricular Block. There was no change in the PR interval before or after a nonconducted P wave.*

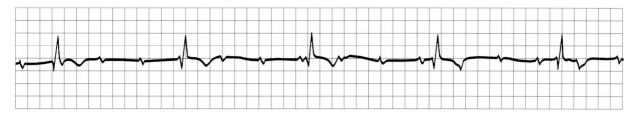

Figure 3.6 Complete Heart Block. Atrial rate was 70 beats per minute and ventricular escape rhythm was 30 beats per minute.

may require pacing. The abnormal response can be 1) pure cardioinhibitory manifested only by bradycardia, 2) pure vasodepressor manifested only with hypotension, or 3) combined cardioinhibitory-vasodepressor response. Permanent pacing treats only the cardioinhibitory response.

KEY FACTS

✓ First-degree AV block—PR interval on ECG is prolonged (>200 milliseconds)

✓ Second-degree AV block—2 subtypes are Mobitz I and Mobitz II

✓ Mobitz I block (Wenckebach)—gradual prolongation of PR interval before nonconducted P wave

✓ Mobitz II block—caused by conduction block within His-Purkinje system and may be associated with bundle branch block

✓ Third-degree (complete) heart block—no relationship between atrial rhythm and ventricular rhythm, and atrial rhythm is faster than ventricular escape rhythm

✓ Carotid sinus hypersensitivity—common in elderly and can rarely be caused by anatomical abnormalities in region of carotid body

---

The Tachycardias

Atrial Flutter

Atrial flutter is identified on the ECG by the characteristic sawtooth pattern of atrial activity at a rate of 240 to 320 beats per minute. Patients with normal conduction may have rapid ventricular rates. Higher degrees of AV block (3:1 or higher) in the absence of drugs that slow AV nodal conduction (digoxin, β-adrenergic blockers, calcium channel antagonists) suggest the presence of intrinsic AV conduction disease (Figure 3.8). In patients with 2:1 AV conduction and a heart rate of 150 beats per minute, 1 of the flutter waves is often buried in the QRS complex. Carotid sinus massage (or transient AV node blockade with adenosine) may help reveal the flutter waves to establish the diagnosis.

Pharmacologic therapy for atrial flutter is used to slow AV node conduction and control the ventricular rate or to control the flutter itself. The same medications used to treat atrial fibrillation are used to treat atrial flutter. Catheter ablation targets the most common arrhythmia circuit around the tricuspid annulus and has a success rate of more than 90%.

Atrial Fibrillation

Atrial fibrillation, characterized by continuous and chaotic atrial activity, is the most common arrhythmia. Its prevalence increases with age; 5% of patients 65 years or older are affected. Common associated conditions include hypertension, cardiomyopathy, valvular heart disease (particularly mitral stenosis), sleep-disordered breathing, sick sinus syndrome, Wolff-Parkinson-White syndrome (especially in young patients), alcohol use ("holiday heart"), and thyrotoxicosis.

The therapeutic approach to patients with atrial fibrillation is determined by the severity of symptoms and comorbid conditions. Therapeutic options include rate control (pharmacologic agents or ablation to slow AV node conduction), stroke prophylaxis in patients at risk of stroke, and rhythm control (treatments aimed at restoring and maintaining sinus rhythm). Stroke risk can be assessed using the CHADS2 scoring system (1 point each for *c*ongestive heart failure, *h*ypertension, *a*ge >75 years, and *d*iabetes, and 2 points for previous *s*troke or transient ischemic attack). Anticoagulation is usually indicated if the CHADS score is 2 or more (and can be considered if the CHADS2

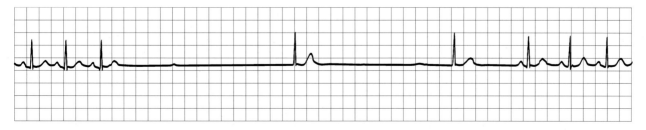

Figure 3.7 Sinus Pause With Junctional Escape Beats Before Sinus Rhythm Returns. Test was done during carotid sinus massage.

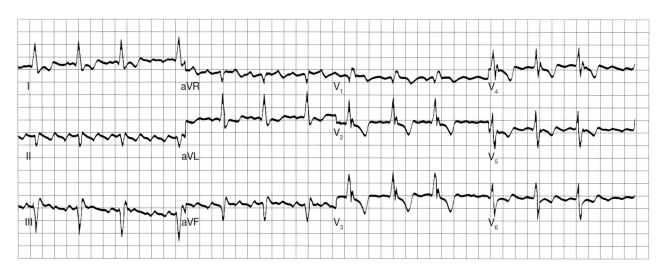

Figure 3.8 *Atrial Flutter With 3:1 Conduction. Patient had atrioventricular conduction disease.*

score is 1). Rhythm control is most appropriate in patients with symptoms due to atrial fibrillation despite adequate rate control but is generally not thought to reduce mortality. In all patients, initial management should be rate control using AV nodal blocking agents and an assessment of stroke risk and need for anticoagulation before deciding on a long-term strategy. Pharmacologic agents useful for rate control and rhythm control are shown in Table 3.3.

Table 3.3 • Pharmacologic Therapy For Atrial Fibrillation

Agents	Comments
Control of ventricular rate	
β-Blockers (eg, atenolol, metoprolol, propranolol, carvedilol)	Ideal postoperatively and in hyperthyroidism, acute MI, and chronic CHF (especially carvedilol)
Calcium channel blockers (eg, verapamil, diltiazem)	Nifedipine, amlodipine, and felodipine are not useful for slowing AV conduction
Digoxin	Less effective than β-blockers and calcium channel blockers, especially with exercise
	Useful in heart failure
Maintenance of sinus rhythm	
Class IA: quinidine, disopyramide, procainamide	Enhance AV conduction—rate must be controlled before use
	Monitor QTc
Class IC: propafenone, flecainide	Slow AV conduction
	Often first choice for patients with normal heart
	Monitor QRS duration
Class III: sotalol, amiodarone	Amiodarone is agent of choice for ventricular dysfunction and after MI

Abbreviations: AV, atrioventricular; CHF, congestive heart failure; MI, myocardial infarction.

Digoxin acts indirectly by increasing vagal tone and at therapeutic concentration has no direct effect in slowing AV node conduction. Because of its mechanism of action, digoxin is less effective than β-blockers or calcium channel blockers, particularly with exercise, when an increase in sympathetic tone results in more rapid AV node conduction. The optimal role for digoxin in atrial fibrillation is therapy for patients with left ventricular dysfunction (because of the drug's positive inotropy) or as adjunctive therapy for patients with chronic atrial fibrillation receiving β-blockers or calcium channel blockers. Digoxin alone is no better than placebo for terminating atrial fibrillation.

β-Blockers (eg, propranolol, metoprolol, atenolol) slow AV node conduction and may be particularly useful when atrial fibrillation complicates hyperthyroidism or myocardial infarction.

Calcium channel blockers are divided into 2 groups: dihydropyridines (eg, nifedipine, amlodipine, and felodipine) and non-dihydropyridines (eg, diltiazem and verapamil). Dihydropyridine agents have little or no effect on AV node conduction and no role in the management of atrial fibrillation. Verapamil and diltiazem are both available as intravenous and oral preparations and are well suited for acute and chronic rate control. Both agents have negative inotropic effects and must be used cautiously in CHF.

When pharmacologic rate control fails (due to persistent symptoms or intolerance of medications), catheter ablation of the AV junction may be considered as a "bail-out" rate control strategy. This approach is more than 95% effective for controlling symptoms and has minimal risk. The major disadvantage is creation of pacemaker dependence. In patients with paroxysmal atrial fibrillation, a dual-chamber pacemaker is implanted (to allow AV synchrony during time of sinus rhythm), whereas in patients with persistent atrial fibrillation a single-chamber ventricular pacemaker (programmed to VVIR mode) is implanted. Dual-chamber pacemakers have a mode-switching function that permits tracking of P waves during sinus rhythm and reverts to VVIR (or DDIR) mode pacing when atrial fibrillation recurs.

Rhythm control (maintenance of sinus rhythm) is useful to manage symptoms attributable to atrial fibrillation. Common pharmacologic agents include the class IC antiarrhythmic agents propafenone and flecainide (sodium channel blockers) and the class II agents sotalol, dofetilide, and amiodarone (potassium channel blocker). Class IC agents are often used as first-line therapy because they are generally well tolerated and can be initiated in the outpatient setting but should be avoided in patients with structural heart disease (risk of proarrhythmia). Sotalol and dofetilide are generally safe in patients with prior myocardial infarction and those with systolic dysfunction but necessitate hospitalization for initiation. Amiodarone is an effective medication, but it has the potential for significant long-term adverse effects (thyroid, liver, and pulmonary toxicities among them).

Cardioversion for atrial fibrillation is commonly used when patients remain symptomatic despite efforts to achieve rate control. Patients with atrial fibrillation of more than 2 days in duration should receive anticoagulation before cardioversion. Warfarin therapy for 3 weeks before cardioversion substantially decreases the incidence of cardioversion-associated thromboembolism, and anticoagulation should be continued for a minimum of 4 weeks after cardioversion. Current guidelines do not mandate anticoagulation in the setting of cardioversion for atrial fibrillation of recent onset (<48 hours). Anticoagulation guidelines for atrial flutter are identical to those for atrial fibrillation. An alternative approach for patients with atrial fibrillation of more than 2 days in duration is transesophageal echocardiography and cardioversion if no thrombus is found followed by anticoagulation for 3 to 4 weeks.

For prevention of stroke, warfarin therapy should be used in patients who have other risk factors for stroke. Risk of thromboembolism can be determined using the CHADS2 score (Table 3.4), and anticoagulation is considered with 1 risk factor and is indicated (unless there is a significant contraindication) if the CHADS2 score is 2 or more. For patients in whom warfarin therapy is indicated, the international normalized ratio should be maintained in the range of 2.0 to 3.0. Anticoagulation decreases the incidence of thromboembolism by close to 70% in this population.

Other Supraventricular Tachycardias

Tachycardia (rate >100 beats per minute) is characterized as a narrow complex or a wide complex tachycardia.

Paroxysmal Supraventricular Tachycardia

Paroxysmal supraventricular tachycardia (PSVT) is due to a reentrant mechanism with an abrupt onset and termination, a regular rate, and a narrow QRS complex (Figure 3.9), unless there is a rate-related or preexisting bundle branch block. Acutely, PSVT responds to vagal maneuvers; adenosine (or verapamil if PSVT is recurrent) terminates the arrhythmia in 90% of patients. PSVT generally is not a life-threatening arrhythmia; it often occurs in an otherwise normal heart. The preferred method for management of symptomatic PSVT is catheter ablation,

Table 3.4 • Risk Factors for Thromboembolism in Nonrheumatic Atrial Fibrillation

CHADS2 Criteria	Points	Stroke Risk Score	Recommended Therapy
Congestive heart failure	1	Low=0	Aspirin 100–300 mg daily
Hypertension	1	Moderate=1	Warfarin or aspirin
Age ≥75 years	1		
Diabetes mellitus	1		
Previous stroke or TIA	2	High=2–6	Warfarin (INR 2–3)

Abbreviations: INR, international normalized ratio; TIA, transient ischemic attack.

Data from Gage BF, Waterman AD, Shannon W, Boechler M, Rich MW, Radford MJ. Validation of clinical classification schemes for predicting stroke: results from the National Registry of Atrial Fibrillation. JAMA. 2001 Jun 13;285(22):2864–70.

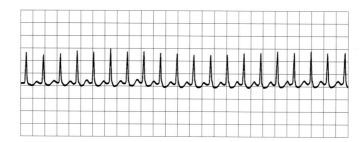

Figure 3.9 Paroxysmal Supraventricular Tachycardia.

which has success rates of more than 90%. For patients in whom catheter ablation is not feasible or preferred, β-blockers or calcium channel blockers may be useful.

Multifocal atrial tachycardia is an automatic atrial rhythm diagnosed when 3 or more distinct atrial foci (P waves of different morphologic forms) are present and the rate exceeds 100 beats per minute (Figure 3.10). This rhythm occurs primarily in patients with decompensated lung disease and associated hypoxia, increased catecholamines (exogenous and endogenous), atrial stretch, and local tissue acid-base and electrolyte disturbances. Digoxin worsens multifocal atrial tachycardia (shortens atrial refractoriness). Multifocal atrial tachycardia is best treated with calcium channel blockers and correction of the underlying medical illnesses, including increasing oxygenation.

Differentiating Supraventricular Tachycardia
With Aberrancy From Ventricular Tachycardia
Wide QRS tachycardia may be due to supraventricular tachycardia with aberrancy or to ventricular tachycardia (Figure 3.11). Findings useful for identifying ventricular tachycardia are listed in Box 3.3.

Wide QRS tachycardias are ventricular in origin in more than 85% of cases and are often well tolerated. The absence of hemodynamic compromise during tachycardia does not prove the tachycardia is supraventricular in origin.

A simple approach to a wide complex tachycardia is to review the morphologic features of the complex in lead V$_1$ and decide whether the pattern is that of right or left bundle branch block. If the morphologic pattern exactly matches a normal right or left bundle branch block, then it might be supraventricular with rate-related aberrant conduction. The safest approach to any wide complex tachycardia is to assume that it is due to ventricular tachycardia and treat it accordingly.

Wolff-Parkinson-White Syndrome
Wolff-Parkinson-White (WPW) syndrome is defined as symptomatic tachycardia occurring in a patient with evidence of anterograde accessory pathway conduction during sinus rhythm on the surface ECG (the WPW pattern). WPW pattern is characterized by a short PR interval (<0.12 second), a delta wave, and a prolonged QRS interval (>0.12 second) resulting from preexcitation of the ventricle by conduction across an accessory pathway. However, not all patients with preexcitation have a short PR interval. Normal PR conduction may occur if the accessory pathway is distant from the AV node (as can be the case with a left lateral pathway).

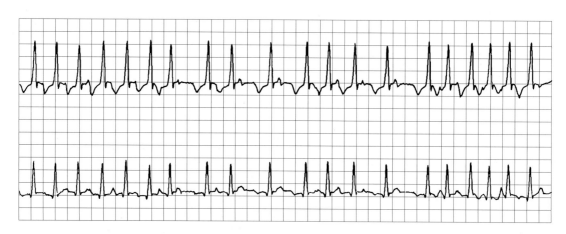

Figure 3.10 Multifocal Atrial Tachycardia. Simultaneous recordings show 3 or more P waves of different morphologic patterns.
(Lower tracing, adapted from MKSAP IX: Part C, Book 1, c1992. American College of Physicians. Used with permission.)

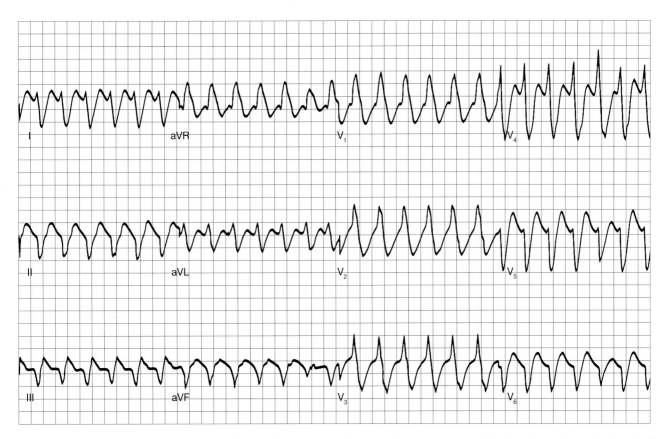

Figure 3.11 *Ventricular Tachycardia With a Wide QRS Complex, Northwest Axis, and Fusion Complexes. Patient had normal blood pressure.*

Key Definition

Wolff-Parkinson-White syndrome: *symptomatic tachycardia occurring in a patient with evidence of anterograde accessory pathway conduction during sinus rhythm on surface ECG.*

Box 3.3 • Findings That Differentiate Ventricular Tachycardia From Supraventricular Tachycardia With Aberrancy

Evidence of AV dissociation with P waves "marching through" the QRS complexes

A QRS width >0.14 s if the tachycardia has a right bundle branch block pattern and >0.16 s if the tachycardia has a left bundle branch block pattern

Northwest axis (axis between −90° and −180°)

A different QRS morphologic pattern in patients with a preexisting bundle branch block

A history of structural heart disease

Abbreviation: AV, atrioventricular.

Preexcitation occurs in about 2 of 1,000 patients; tachycardia subsequently develops in 70%. The most serious rhythm disturbance is atrial fibrillation with rapid ventricular conduction over the accessory pathway leading to ventricular fibrillation (Figure 3.12). Patients who are asymptomatic have a negligible chance of sudden death. For patients who are symptomatic, the incidence of sudden death is 0.0025 per patient-year.

The tachycardia in WPW syndrome can occur with a circuit that travels either down the AV node and then back to the atrium via the accessory pathway (orthodromic, most common circuit and results in a narrow complex tachycardia, Figure 3.13) or down the accessory pathway and then

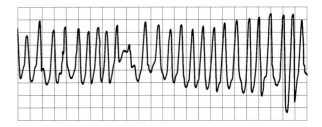

Figure 3.12 *Atrial Fibrillation in Wolff-Parkinson-White Syndrome. Recording shows a wide QRS complex and irregular RR intervals.*

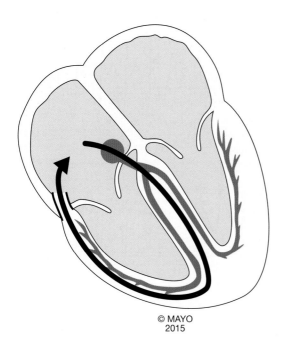

Figure 3.13 *Typical Mechanism of Supraventricular Tachycardia in Wolff-Parkinson-White Syndrome (Orthodromic Atrioventricular Reentry). Result is a narrow QRS complex because ventricular activation is over the normal conduction system.*

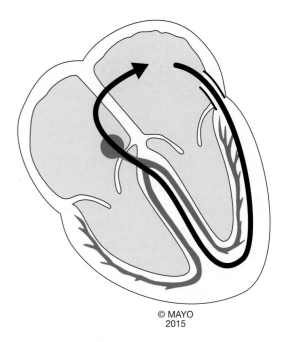

Figure 3.14 *Unusual Mechanism of Supraventricular Tachycardia in Wolff-Parkinson-White Syndrome. Result is a wide QRS complex because ventricular activation is over an accessory pathway. This arrhythmia is difficult to distinguish from ventricular tachycardia.*

back up the AV node (antidromic, results in a wide complex tachycardia, Figure 3.14).

EP testing and radiofrequency ablation of the accessory pathway are indicated in patients with symptomatic WPW syndrome.

WPW syndrome is associated with an increased frequency of atrial fibrillation related to the presence of the accessory pathway (Figure 3.12). After successful catheter ablation of the accessory pathway, atrial fibrillation resolves in most cases. During "preexcited" atrial fibrillation, wide, irregular, and rapid ventricular complexes are seen because activation down the accessory pathway does not use the normal His-Purkinje system (Figure 3.15). In preexcited atrial fibrillation, the drug of first choice is procainamide, which slows the accessory pathway and intra-atrial conduction. Acute administration of digoxin, adenosine, β-blockers, or calcium channel blockers in patients who present with atrial fibrillation and WPW syndrome is contraindicated because of the risk of ventricular fibrillation. If the heart rate is rapid and there is hemodynamic compromise, cardioversion should be performed.

Narrow complex tachycardias that involve the AV node in the circuit (atrioventricular node reentry tachycardia, orthodromic or antidromic atrioventricular reentry tachycardia) are often terminated with vagal maneuvers or intravenously administered adenosine or verapamil because

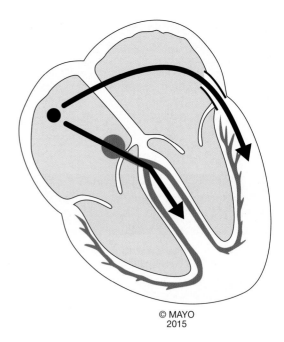

Figure 3.15 *Conduction of Sinus Impulses in Wolff-Parkinson-White Syndrome. The ventricles are activated over the normal atrioventricular node–His-Purkinje system and accessory pathway; the result is a fusion complex (QRS and delta wave).*

the circuit is interrupted at the AV node. Recurrence can be prevented with a β-blocker, a calcium antagonist, and class IA (eg, quinidine, procainamide, and disopyramide), class IC (eg, propafenone and flecainide), and class III (eg, amiodarone and sotalol) antiarrhythmic drugs. Radiofrequency ablation is used to cure tachycardia and should be strongly considered for symptomatic patients.

Ventricular Ectopy and Nonsustained Ventricular Tachycardia

Management of frequent ventricular ectopy and nonsustained ventricular tachycardia is based on the underlying cardiac lesion. In symptomatic patients, management includes β-blockers or calcium channel blockers for symptom control and, in rare cases of frequent monomorphic symptomatic ventricular ectopy, catheter ablation. Patients with a structurally normal heart and complex ectopy or nonsustained ventricular tachycardia have an excellent prognosis. Management includes reassurance or, if bothersome symptoms persist, calcium channel blockers, β-blockers, or ablation.

Ventricular Tachycardia and Fibrillation

Survivors of sudden cardiac death have a risk of death approaching 30% in the first year after hospital dismissal. Antiarrhythmic drug therapy has not been shown to have benefit. ICD therapy, however, improves survival outcomes.

Torsades de Pointes

Torsades de pointes is a form of ventricular tachycardia with a characteristic polymorphic morphologic pattern described as a "twisting of the points" (torsades de pointes) (Figure 3.16).

It occurs in the setting of QT interval prolongation. Common causes include medications that prolong the QT interval (eg, quinidine, procainamide, disopyramide, sotalol, and tricyclic antidepressants), electrolyte disturbance (hypokalemia), or bradycardia (especially after myocardial infarction). Acute treatment options include

isoproterenol infusion (to increase heart rate and shorten QT interval), temporary overdrive pacing (if due to bradycardia), and correction of electrolyte abnormalities. QT interval prolongation may be due to an inherited disorder of cardiac ion channels such as the long QT syndrome. Patients with this abnormality require evaluation and, in some cases, implantation of a cardioverter-defibrillator.

Tachycardia-Mediated Cardiomyopathy

Persistent tachycardia (usually due to poorly controlled atrial fibrillation) may lead to progressive ventricular dysfunction (termed *tachycardia-mediated cardiomyopathy*). It is reversible in most cases because control of the ventricular rate improves ventricular function.

Ventricular Arrhythmias During Acute Myocardial Infarction

Prevention of myocardial ischemia and the use of β-blockers are essential during and after acute myocardial infarction to decrease the frequency of life-threatening ventricular arrhythmias. Asymptomatic complex ventricular ectopy, including nonsustained ventricular tachycardia, should not be treated empirically with lidocaine or amiodarone in the acute phase because the risk of proarrhythmia outweighs the potential benefit of therapy for reducing the incidence of sudden cardiac death after hospital dismissal. Ventricular tachycardia and fibrillation occurring within 24 hours after myocardial infarction are independent risk factors for in-hospital mortality but not for subsequent total mortality or mortality due to an arrhythmic event after hospital dismissal and do not require antiarrhythmic therapy. Ventricular tachycardia and fibrillation occurring more than 24 hours after an acute myocardial infarction (without ongoing ischemia or reinfarction) are independent risk factors for increased total mortality and death due to an arrhythmic event after hospital dismissal. Patients may be assessed with EP testing; treatment is usually with an ICD. Use of a prophylactic ICD after myocardial infarction is not supported

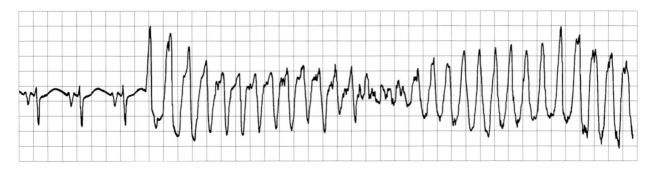

Figure 3.16 *Torsades de Pointes in a Patient With Long QT Syndrome.*

(Adapted from Hammill SC. Electrocardiographic diagnoses: criteria and definitions of abnormalities. In: Murphy JG, Lloyd MA, editors. Mayo Clinic cardiology: concise textbook. 4th ed. Rochester [MN]: Mayo Clinic Scientific Press and New York [NY]: Oxford University Press; c2013. p. 205–38. Used with permission of Mayo Foundation for Medical Education and Research.)

by available data. Refractory ventricular tachycardia and fibrillation during acute myocardial infarction should be treated with intravenously administered lidocaine or amiodarone.

Role of Pacing in Acute Myocardial Infarction

Among patients with an acute inferior myocardial infarction, 5% to 10% have Mobitz I second-degree or third-degree block in the absence of bundle branch block. This finding usually is transient, tends not to recur, and usually does not require pacing. Patients in whom transient complete heart block develops in association with a bundle branch block are at risk for recurrent complete heart block and should undergo permanent pacing. A new bundle branch block that never progresses to complete heart block is not an indication for permanent pacing, however. Second-degree (Mobitz II) block with bilateral bundle branch block and third-degree (complete) AV block warrant pacing.

Box 3.4 • Major Causes of Syncope

Cardiogenic	Noncardiogenic
Cardiogenic syncope	Neurologic
Structural heart	Metabolic
disease	Psychiatric
Coronary artery	
disease	
Rhythm disturbances	
Reflex syncope	
Vasovagal	
Carotid sinus	
hypersensitivity	
Situational	
Micturition	
Deglutition	
Defecation	
Glossopharyngeal	
neuralgia	
Postprandial	
Tussive	
Valsalva maneuver	
Oculovagal	
Sneeze	
Instrumentation	
Diving	
After exercise	
Orthostatic hypotension	

Adapted from Shen W-K, Gersh BJ. Fainting: approach to management. In: Low PA, editor. Clinical autonomic disorders: evaluation and management. 2nd ed. Philadelphia (PA): Lippincott-Raven; c1997. p. 649–79. Used with permission of Mayo Foundation for Medical Education and Research.

Syncope

Syncope is defined as a transient loss of consciousness with spontaneous recovery. It can be categorized as cardiogenic (about 30% of cases are due to bradycardia or tachycardia) or noncardiogenic (neurologic, metabolic, or psychiatric) (Box 3.4).

Key Definition

Syncope: *transient loss of consciousness with spontaneous recovery.*

KEY FACTS

- ✓ Multifocal tachycardia—best treated with calcium channel blockers and correction of underlying medical illnesses
- ✓ Wide QRS tachycardias—ventricular in origin in ≥85% of cases and are well tolerated
- ✓ Safest approach to wide complex tachycardia—assume it is due to ventricular tachycardia and treat accordingly
- ✓ Persistent tachycardia—may lead to progressive ventricular dysfunction; is reversible in most cases because control of ventricular rate improves ventricular function
- ✓ During and after myocardial infarction—prevention of myocardial ischemia and use of β-blockers are essential
- ✓ Syncope—can be categorized as cardiogenic (~30% of cases are due to bradycardia or tachycardia) or noncardiogenic (neurologic, metabolic, psychiatric)

Evaluation of Syncope

The history and physical examination are highly valuable for the evaluation of syncope. Risk factors for a cardiogenic cause of syncope are listed in Box 3.5. Recommendations for evaluation of patients with syncope are outlined in Figure 3.17. Consider EP testing in patients at increased risk for cardiogenic syncope. EP testing is usually not indicated if an arrhythmogenic cause (bradycardia or tachycardia) of syncope has been established unless other arrhythmias are suspected. A noninvasive approach should be considered in patients at low risk for cardiogenic syncope. Tilt-table testing can confirm the diagnosis in suspected vasovagal syncope. Tilt-table testing is not usually indicated after a single episode of syncope without injury or in cases with obvious vasovagal clinical features.

Box 3.5 • Risk Stratification in Patients With Unexplained Syncope[a]

High-Risk Factors

Coronary artery disease, previous myocardial infarction
Structural heart disease
Left ventricular dysfunction
Congestive heart failure
Older age
Abrupt onset
Serious injuries
Abnormal ECG (presence of Q wave, bundle branch
   block, or atrial fibrillation)

Low-Risk Factors

Isolated syncope without underlying cardiovascular
   disease
Younger age
Symptoms consistent with a vasovagal cause
Normal ECG

Abbreviation: ECG, electrocardiogram.

[a] In patients who present with a prodrome (eg, nausea, diaphoresis), a neurocardiogenic mechanism is likely. Patients who experience rapid
   recovery (less than 5–10 minutes) rarely have a neurologic cause for syncope and are most likely to have syncope due to seizure or "brain
   hypoperfusion" because recovery in such circumstances takes hours. Thus, for cases in which recovery from syncope is rapid and no
   residual neurologic signs or symptoms are present, detailed (and expensive) neurologic evaluation should be avoided.

Adapted from Shen W-K, Gersh BJ. Fainting: approach to management. In: Low PA, editor. Clinical autonomic disorders: evaluation and
   management. 2nd ed. Philadelphia (PA): Lippincott-Raven; c1997. p. 649–79. Used with permission of Mayo Foundation for Medical
   Education and Research.

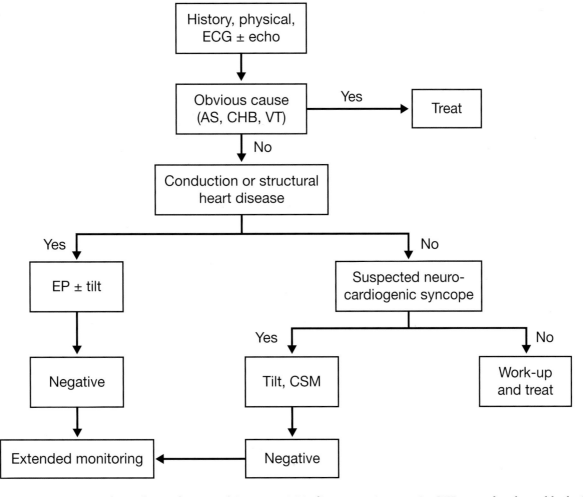

Figure 3.17 *Diagnostic Pathway for Evaluation of Syncope. AS indicates aortic stenosis; CHB, complete heart block; CSM, carotid sinus massage; ECG, electrocardiography; echo, echocardiography; EP, electrophysiologic study; tilt, tilt-table testing; VT, ventricular tachycardia.*

Management of Syncope

Pacemaker therapy is appropriate for sinus node dysfunction and AV conduction disease. Management of recurrent neurocardiogenic syncope (vasovagal syncope) includes education about the mechanism and triggering factors, instruction regarding appropriate action (eg, sitting or lying down to avert episodes), instruction regarding maintenance of increased intravascular volume, and instruction on maneuvers to prevent venous pooling. Midodrine, which promotes increased venous return, may be considered. Serotonin reuptake blockers may be effective in a subgroup of patients. β-Blockers have limited or no benefit. Pacemaker therapy has a limited role in preventing vasovagal syncope.

Cardiac Manifestations of Systemic Diseases and Pregnancy

LORI A. BLAUWET, MD; REKHA MANKAD, MD;
SABRINA D. PHILLIPS, MD; AND KYLE W. KLARICH, MD

The Heart and Systemic Disease

Hyperthyroidism

Effects

Cardiovascular manifestations of hyperthyroidism include increased heart rate, stroke volume, and cardiac output. Peripheral vascular resistance is decreased, and thus pulse pressure is widened. As a result, myocardial oxygen consumption increases, which may precipitate angina. Other symptoms include palpitations, presyncope or syncope, and exertional dyspnea. Arrhythmias may occur.

Clinical Features

Common symptoms include weight loss, weakness (especially in the elderly), and tachycardia or palpitations.

Common physical findings are tachycardia and a bounding pulse with a wide pulse pressure, a forceful apical impulse, and a systolic ejection murmur due to increased flow. Supraventricular tachycardia and atrial fibrillation are the most common arrhythmias. Angina may occur. Atrial fibrillation occurs in 10% to 20% of patients. Indeed, thyrotoxicosis should be excluded in patients with atrial fibrillation. Examination may also show tremor, and a goiter may be present.

Treatment

Treatment of hyperthyroidism usually leads to reversal of cardiac symptoms. If atrial fibrillation is present, the risk of embolization is high and anticoagulation should be instituted. Cardioversion should not be attempted until a euthyroid state is achieved.

Hypothyroidism

Effects

Mucoprotein infiltration of the myocardium due to hypothyroidism can lead to cardiac enlargement and decreased function. Hypothyroidism decreases metabolic rate and circulatory demand and can cause bradycardia, decreased contractility and stroke volume, and increased peripheral resistance. One-third of patients have pericardial effusion. The cardiomyopathy is reversible if detected early. Hypothyroidism is associated with increased cholesterol levels and atherosclerosis.

Symptoms

Patients may present with depression, lethargy, and slowed mentation. Hair loss on the scalp and lateral aspect of the eyebrows and a thick tongue may occur. Many patients report constipation and weight gain.

Physical Examination

Cardiac enlargement can be caused by myocardial disease or a pericardial effusion. The pulse volume is decreased as a result of reduced contractility. Sinus bradycardia usually is present. Other findings may include macroglossia, thinning or loss of the lateral third of the eyebrows, coarse hair and dry skin, and myxedema. Chest radiography shows increased cardiac size. Electrocardiography shows low voltage of QRS with prolonged intervals of QRS, PR, and QT.

Treatment

Reversal of cardiac involvement occurs with early treatment of hypothyroidism.

Diabetes Mellitus

Effects

Diabetes mellitus is associated with premature atherosclerosis, which is twice as prevalent in diabetic men and 3 times more prevalent in diabetic women than in a nondiabetic population. Patients with diabetes have a higher prevalence of hypertension and hyperlipidemia. Angina and myocardial infarction manifest with nonclassic symptoms, or patients may have silent ischemia. Congestive heart failure may be the first manifestation of coronary artery disease among diabetics. Cardiomyopathy not associated with epicardial coronary atherosclerosis may also exist; this may be caused by small-vessel disease. Fatal myocardial infarction is more common in patients with diabetes than in those who do not have diabetes.

Treatment

Aggressive management of traditional risk factors for coronary artery disease lowers mortality. Diabetic-specific risk factors for coronary artery disease may include poor glycemic control and urinary protein excretion. However, strict blood sugar control has come into question in recent years. The use of antihypertensive agents for aggressive lowering of blood pressure (systolic pressure ≤120 mm Hg, diastolic pressure ≤80 mm Hg) reduces mortality. Statins are effective for primary and secondary prevention of coronary artery disease in patients with both diabetes and age between 40 and 75 years (J Am Coll Cardiol. 2014 Jul 1;63[25 Pt B]:2889–934 and Circulation. 2014 Jun 24;129[25 Suppl 2]:S1–45). Angiotensin-converting enzyme inhibitors reduce cardiovascular events and mortality in patients with diabetes who are older than 55 years and have additional risk factors. To date, glycemic control has not been shown to lower the incidence of cardiovascular events.

Amyloidosis

Effects

Amyloidosis leads to extracellular deposition of insoluble proteins in organs and is classified by the precursor plasma proteins forming the extracellular fibril deposits. The primary systemic type, AL, is due to monoclonal immunoglobulin free light chains. The hereditary (familial) type is due to mutant transthyretin deposition, and its inheritance is autosomal dominant. The wild-type transthyretin type (wild-type TTR, previously referred to as senile type) is due to abnormal deposition of wild-type transthyretin. The secondary type (AA type) is related to amyloid A protein, often the result of multiple myeloma. The heart is frequently involved, especially by the AL type. Nearly 90% of patients with primary amyloidosis have clinical manifestations of cardiac dysfunction.

Cardiomyopathy results from protein infiltration, which causes thickened ventricular myocardium. Amyloid deposition in the atrioventricular cardiac valves may occur. Amyloid can also deposit in small vessels and lead to ischemia.

Cardiac involvement may occur in secondary amyloidosis, but it is usually not a prominent feature. Secondary amyloidosis occurs in association with chronic diseases such as rheumatoid arthritis, tuberculosis, chronic infection, neoplasm (especially multiple myeloma), and chronic renal failure. In wild-type TTR amyloidosis, the heart is the most commonly involved organ, and prevalence increases after age 60 years.

Clinical Features

Cardiac amyloidosis may cause congestive heart failure, arrhythmias, sudden death, angina, chest pain, pericardial effusion (usually not hemodynamically significant), and regurgitant murmurs. The natural history is usually intractable because of ventricular failure. Diastolic abnormalities are common and the earliest manifestation in the disease process. Although cardiac amyloidosis has been classified as a restrictive cardiomyopathy, any abnormality of diastolic dysfunction can signal early amyloid infiltration. Restrictive physiology (grade 3–4 diastolic dysfunction) indicates a poor prognosis. Newer imaging techniques, including strain echocardiography and cardiac magnetic resonance imaging, have been useful in helping to identify the disease.

Amyloidosis should be considered when a patient (usually >40–70 years old) presents with dyspnea and progressive edema of the lower extremities. Associated conditions such as vocal hoarseness, carpal tunnel syndrome, or peripheral neuropathy may be present and point to the systemic nature of the disease. A key finding is a low-voltage (or even normal voltage in up to 25%) QRS complex with or without other conduction abnormalities (such as increased PR interval or bundle branch block) coupled with echocardiographic findings of thick walls and usually preserved ventricular ejection fraction.

Diagnosis

Cardiac involvement is suggested by the classic electrocardiographic finding of a low-voltage QRS complex. However, this is a nonspecific finding, and 20% to 25% of patients with cardiac amyloid may have normal electrocardiographic findings. Echocardiography is particularly useful, showing increased left ventricular wall thickness, in contradistinction to the small (or normal) voltage on electrocardiography (Figure 4.1). The atria generally are dilated. The cardiac valves may show some thickening and regurgitation. A small pericardial effusion may be present. Diastolic function generally is abnormal; in the early stages of the disease, findings consistent with prolonged relaxation are found, whereas restrictive filling (consistent with high left ventricular filling pressures) is found in later stages.

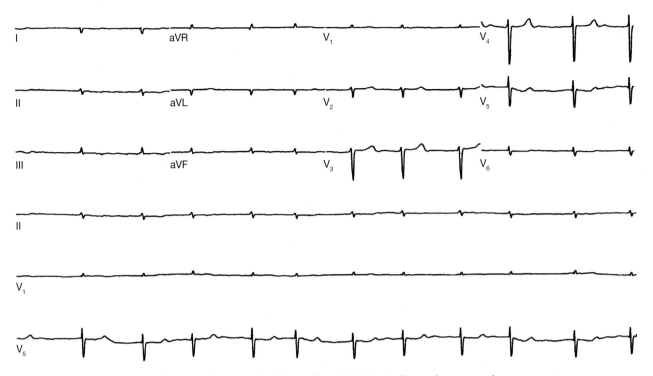

Figure 4.1 *Electrocardiography in Cardiac Amyloidosis. Classic finding is low-voltage complexes.*

Treatment

Although cardiac amyloidosis has a generally poor prognosis, it is important to have patients referred to centers experienced in typing the amyloid because, depending on the type, there are successful established and emerging therapies. Referral to a tertiary center with expertise in amyloidosis is warranted because prior experimental protocols have evolved into treatment options, such as stem cell transplant or chemotherapy in primary amyloidosis, liver transplant in familial amyloidosis, and emerging therapies in wild-type (or senile) amyloidosis.

Hemochromatosis

Effects

Hemochromatosis, an iron-storage disease, may be primary or secondary (related to exogenous iron, usually from repeated transfusions). Iron may deposit within the cardiac cells. Cardiac hemochromatosis is usually accompanied by other organ involvement, primarily pancreas, liver, and skin, leading to the classic tetrad of diabetes, liver disease, brown skin pigmentation, and congestive heart failure. Affected patients may present with cardiomegaly, congestive heart failure (with features of systolic and diastolic dysfunction), and arrhythmias.

Clinical Features

Many patients are asymptomatic or minimally symptomatic. Often the earliest manifestation is fatigue, hair loss, arthralgia, palpitations and syncope, impotence or loss of libido, and amenorrhea. Clinically, patients may present with new-onset diabetes or glucose intolerance. Symptoms and signs of heart failure may be present. Patients will not infrequently present with arrhythmias (both supraventricular and ventricular), even sudden cardiac death or out-of-hospital arrest. A clinical clue is the discovery of a dilated heart with reduced function in a patient who presents with cardiac arrest.

Diagnosis

The 2 key tests are serum transferrin saturation and serum ferritin. Transferrin saturation values more than 45% are considered too high. Increased serum ferritin values establish the diagnosis of hemochromatosis. Liver function tests can help identify liver damage that may be coexistent in hemochromatosis. Recently, cardiac magnetic resonance imaging has been established as a fast and noninvasive way to measure the degree of iron overload in the heart and other organs. Genetic testing for this autosomal recessive genetic disorder is indicated if it is suspected from the results of clinical testing. A liver biopsy may be indicated in patients with evidence of cirrhosis.

Treatment

Once clinical cardiac symptoms appear, the prognosis is very poor unless treatment is initiated with a combination of phlebotomy and iron chelation.

KEY FACTS

✓ Cardiac manifestations of hyperthyroidism—increased heart rate, stroke volume, and cardiac output

✓ Diabetes mellitus—associated with premature atherosclerosis

✓ Diabetes mellitus—prevalence of hypertension and hyperlipidemia is increased; angina and myocardial infarction manifest with nonclassic symptoms (or silent ischemia is present)

✓ Amyloidosis-associated cardiomyopathy—results from protein infiltration, which causes thickened ventricular myocardium; classic finding of cardiac involvement is low-voltage QRS complex on electrocardiography

✓ Hemochromatosis—may be primary or secondary; iron may deposit within cardiac cells

Carcinoid Heart Disease

Effects

Liver or lung metastases from carcinoid tumors can produce a classic syndrome (in only about 4% of patients) due to production of serotonin-like substances. These substances cause cutaneous flushing, wheezing, and diarrhea (the carcinoid syndrome) and are toxic to cardiac valves. Cardiac involvement occurs in approximately 50% of patients with hepatic or pulmonary metastasis; toxic effects generally affect right-sided cardiac valves. Left-sided valves can be affected if a cardiac shunt is present; such a shunt allows right-to-left movement of serotonin-like substances via the bloodstream. Also, left-sided valves may be affected in the presence of bronchial carcinoid. Carcinoid lesions are fibrous plaques that form on valvular endocardium. The valve leaflets become thickened, relatively immobile, and retracted. Regurgitation results, with some stenosis of the tricuspid and the pulmonary valves.

Clinical Features

Patients may complain of weight loss, fatigue, watery diarrhea (>10 stools daily), dyspnea on exertion, and intermittent hot flashes.

Typical findings on examination are an increased jugular venous pressure profile, a prominent *v* wave, a cardiac murmur, a pulsatile liver that may be enlarged, ascites, and usually peripheral edema. Audible wheezes may be present, and patients may have a ruddy complexion.

Diagnosis

Electrocardiography typically shows right ventricular hypertrophy and right bundle branch block. Diagnosis is made by identification of a thickened tricuspid valve and pulmonary valve (and left-sided valves if a shunt is present).

Lung and liver metastasis may be found if computed tomography is performed. The diagnosis is confirmed by a 24-hour urine measurement of 5-hydroxyindoleacetic acid. Acquired tricuspid and pulmonary stenosis with or without regurgitation is rare and should always raise the possibility of carcinoid heart disease.

Treatment

Treatment of the underlying tumor is important for symptom relief. In the setting of right heart failure (eg, intractable edema, ascites, and dyspnea), surgery may be warranted. Treatment of carcinoid syndrome may include octreotide and lanreotide, which may reduce the signs and symptoms of carcinoid syndrome, including skin flushing and diarrhea. Octreotide may also slow the growth of carcinoid tumors. Surgical therapies can include tricuspid valve replacement and pulmonary valve resection. Other treatments such as hepatic embolization and chemotherapy should be instituted in collaboration with oncology, radiology, and cardiology teams experienced in treatment of this rare syndrome.

Hypereosinophilic Syndrome

Effects

This syndrome affects young, usually male, patients. Causes include idiopathic hypereosinophilia known as Löffler endocarditis, reactive or allergic eosinophilia, leukemic or neoplastic eosinophilia, and Churg-Strauss syndrome. All of these may have cardiac manifestations.

Clinical Features

Patients typically present with weight loss, fatigue, dyspnea, syncope, and systemic embolization. Pulmonary involvement should prompt consideration of Churg-Strauss syndrome. Cardiac manifestations include arrhythmias, myocarditis, conduction abnormalities, and thrombosis. Cardiac eosinophilic deposition may occur, and clot formation occurs in the ventricular apices and the inflow surfaces of the mitral and tricuspid valves. Matting down of the atrioventricular valves occurs, causing considerable regurgitation. Scarring occurs where the clot formed, leading to endomyocardial fibrosis and a restrictive cardiomyopathy.

Diagnosis

The finding of persistent eosinophil concentrations of more than 1.5×10^9/L is typically associated with hypereosinophilia and end-organ damage.

Treatment

The treatment strategy should be aimed at the underlying cause of the increased eosinophil count. This may be due to primary disease of the bone marrow or systemic illness such as Churg-Strauss syndrome.

Systemic Lupus Erythematosus

Systemic lupus erythematosus may involve any of the cardiac structures. Cardiac involvement may include pericarditis, characterized by a positive antinuclear antibody in the pericardial fluid, myocarditis (more common in patients with anti-Ro antibody), valvulopathy, and coronary arteritis. Libman-Sacks endocarditis (nonbacterial thrombotic endocarditis), which results in noninfective vegetations, occurs in a high percentage of patients with systemic lupus erythematosus. These vegetations are more common if there is concomitant antiphospholipid antibody syndrome. The vegetations may embolize and, less frequently, interfere with valvular function. Congenital heart block may occur in newborns of mothers with lupus who have anti-La and anti-Ro antibodies due to myocarditis and to inflammation and fibrosis of the conduction system (neonatal lupus).

Scleroderma

Cardiac involvement is manifested by intramural coronary involvement and immune-mediated endothelial injury, which is often associated with the Raynaud phenomenon clinically (due to peripheral small-vessel involvement). Other systemic features include sclerotic skin changes and esophageal abnormalities. Cardiac involvement is the third most common cause of mortality in patients with scleroderma, usually due to pulmonary hypertension and cor pulmonale. Conduction defects occur in up to 20% of patients. A pericardial effusion, which is usually clinically silent, is found in one-third of patients.

Rheumatoid Arthritis

Nearly all cardiac components, including pericardium, myocardium, valves, coronary arteries, and aorta, may be affected in patients with rheumatoid arthritis. Granulomatous inflammation and nongranulomatous inflammation of valve leaflets occur but rarely lead to severe valvular incompetence. Associated pericarditis is typically associated with a low glucose level and complement depletion in the pericardial fluid. Cardiac tamponade is rare, however. Rheumatoid nodules in the conduction system can lead to heart block. Aortitis and pulmonary hypertension due to pulmonary vasculitis are very rare complications. Patients with rheumatoid arthritis have a higher risk of coronary artery disease and heart failure (specifically heart failure with preserved ejection fraction) than patients without rheumatoid arthritis.

Ankylosing Spondylitis

Approximately 10% of patients with ankylosing spondylitis have aortic dilatation and aortic regurgitation. Aortic valve cusp distortion and retraction also may cause considerable aortic regurgitation. Fibrosis and inflammation of the conduction system may occur.

Marfan Syndrome

Degeneration of elastic tissues occurs in this autosomal dominant condition. Features include arachnodactyly, tall stature, pectus excavatum, kyphoscoliosis, and lenticular dislocation. Cardiac involvement is common, including mitral valve prolapse, aortic regurgitation due to aortic dilatation, and an increased risk of aortic dissection. Long-term β-adrenergic blockade decreases the rate of aortic dilatation and the risk of aortic dissection. Angiotensin receptor blockade is emerging as a treatment to prevent aortic dilatation and dissection. Dissection can occur at any aortic dimension, but risk increases with increasing aortic dimension. Currently, operative intervention for aortic replacement is indicated for aortic dimension more than 50 mm or for rapid aortic dilatation (>5 mm increase in dimension in 1 year).

Cardiac Trauma

Cardiac contusion may lead to arrhythmia, increased cardiac enzyme values, transient regional wall motion abnormalities, and pericardial effusion or tamponade. It may also cause disruption of the aorta or valves (tricuspid valve most often) or right ventricular rupture. Commotio cordis is sudden cardiac death due to trauma, characteristically mild trauma to the chest wall. This is generally due to a nonpenetrating blow (eg, by a baseball or softball) leading to instantaneous cardiac arrest. Cardiac disease is often absent. The trauma must be delivered during the vulnerable phase of the cardiac cycle, described as the 15 to 30 milliseconds before and after the T wave.

KEY FACTS

✓ Carcinoid heart disease—liver or lung metastases from carcinoid tumors produce classic syndrome due to production of serotonin-like substances (toxic to cardiac valves)

✓ Carcinoid syndrome—cutaneous flushing, wheezing, diarrhea

✓ Systemic lupus erythematosus—may involve any cardiac structure; features of involvement include Libman-Sacks endocarditis (which is more common in patients with antiphospholipid antibody syndrome)

✓ Scleroderma—cardiac involvement manifested by intramural coronary involvement and immune-mediated endothelial injury

✓ Rheumatoid arthritis—nearly all cardiac components may be affected; rheumatoid nodules in conduction system can lead to heart block

✓ Marfan syndrome—cardiac involvement is common (mitral valve prolapse, aortic regurgitation due to aortic dilatation, increased risk of aortic dissection)

The Heart and Pregnancy

Physiologic Changes of Pregnancy

Hormonal changes that begin at conception and continue throughout gestation result in an increase in plasma volume and red cell mass. However, the increase in plasma volume is larger than the increase in red cell mass; therefore, a relative anemia occurs. In addition to an increase in total intravascular volume, systemic vascular resistance decreases and heart rate slightly increases. This increase in preload and decrease in afterload allow for an increase in cardiac output by 30% to 50% to supply the increased metabolic needs required to sustain the pregnancy. Overall blood pressure does not change substantially related to these physiologic changes. Related to these physiologic changes, the physical examination during a normal pregnancy may have some features to suggest cardiac compromise, including lower extremity edema, mildly increased jugular venous pressure, a soft short systolic murmur in the pulmonary area, an S_3, and a brisk and full carotid pulse.

Pregnancy and Cardiac Disease

Physical examination features that should be considered abnormal in pregnancy include a diastolic murmur, a loud (3/6 or greater) systolic murmur, and an S_4. The physiologic changes that occur during pregnancy may unmask previously unrecognized maternal cardiac disease or may result in decompensation of previously known cardiac anomalies. In general, cardiac lesions that do not allow for increased cardiac output (ie, valvular stenosis and ventricular dysfunction) are not well tolerated. Several situations provide such a high risk to the mother that pregnancy should be discouraged. These include pulmonary hypertension (pulmonary artery pressure >75% systemic systolic blood pressure), maternal aortopathy such as Marfan syndrome with an aortic dimension more than 40 mm, New York Heart Association class IV heart failure, and symptomatic severe aortic valve stenosis. The risk of a cardiac complication (pulmonary edema, sustained arrhythmia requiring treatment, stroke, cardiac arrest, or cardiac death) during pregnancy in mothers without the above contraindications can be estimated using the CARPREG risk model (Circulation. 2001 Jul 31;104[5]:515–21) with refinements validated in a population of women with congenital heart disease (Circulation. 2006 Jan 31;113[4]:517–24). The risk factors to consider in this modified model include 1) New York Heart Association class III or IV or cyanosis, 2) previous cardiac event (arrhythmia, stroke, or heart failure), 3) left heart obstruction (mitral valve area <2 cm², aortic valve area <1.5 cm², left ventricular outflow tract obstruction gradient >30 mm Hg), 4) systemic ventricular dysfunction (ejection fraction <40%), and 5) subpulmonary ventricular dysfunction or severe pulmonary valve regurgitation. Each risk factor present is given equal weight. The estimated risk of a cardiac event during pregnancy is 5% with 0 risk factors, 27% with 1 risk factor, and 75% with more than 1 risk factor; the most likely cardiac complication is pulmonary edema or arrhythmia.

Mothers who experience cardiac complications during pregnancy need specialized care that may include initiation or titration of medication, bed rest, cardioversion, catheter-based intervention, cardiac surgery, and early delivery. Cardioversion can be performed with low risk to the fetus. If catheter-based intervention such as balloon valvuloplasty is performed, the fetus should be shielded from the ionizing radiation. Cardiac surgical procedures can be performed with good maternal and fetal outcomes, but fetal outcomes are best if the surgical intervention is performed during the second trimester.

Medical Therapy During Pregnancy

Many cardiac drugs cross the placenta but can be used safely when necessary. These include digoxin, quinidine, procainamide, β-adrenergic blockers, and verapamil. β-Adrenergic blockers are associated with fetal growth retardation, neonatal bradycardia, and hypoglycemia and should be used cautiously. Patients with hypertrophic cardiomyopathy may require high doses of β-adrenergic blockers, and thus fetal growth must be monitored in these patients.

Angiotensin-converting enzyme inhibitors (which may cause fetal renal dysgenesis), phenytoin (which may cause hydantoin syndrome and teratogenicity), and statins should be avoided in pregnancy. Warfarin is associated with fetal malformations and fetal loss and should be avoided during the first trimester, but it can be used in the second and third trimesters if there is a compelling need. If warfarin is used during pregnancy, alternative anticoagulation should be used during the last 4 weeks of gestation to prevent the fetus from being anticoagulated at the time of delivery. If warfarin is being used at the time of labor, a Cesarean-section delivery is indicated with general (not regional) anesthesia.

Delivery in the Setting of Cardiac Disease

Rapid hemodynamic swings occur during delivery. About 500 mL of blood is released into the circulation with each uterine contraction. Cardiac output increases with advancing labor, and oxygen consumption increases threefold. High-risk patients need careful monitoring, maternal and fetal electrocardiographic monitoring, careful analgesia and anesthesia to avoid hypotension, and limited Valsalva maneuver ("pushing"). Facilitated delivery may be needed.

Vaginal delivery is safer for most women with cardiac disease; the average blood loss is 500 mL with vaginal delivery and 800 mL with cesarean section. Cesarean section is typically performed only for obstetric indications, urgent delivery for a mother in symptomatic heart failure, delivery in a pregnancy complicated by progressive aortic enlargement, and mothers who are anticoagulated with warfarin at the time of delivery. American Heart Association guidelines state that there is no need for antibiotic prophylaxis in an uncomplicated vaginal delivery.

Hypertension and Pregnancy

Four major hypertensive disorders occur in pregnant women (Box 4.1). Treatment of chronic or gestational hypertension during pregnancy with lebatolol, nifedipine, or methyldopa is recommended. β-Adrenergic blockers are safe and efficacious but may cause growth retardation and fetal bradycardia. The use of angiotensin-converting enzyme inhibitors, angiotensin receptor blockers, renin inhibitors, and mineralocorticoid receptor antagonists is not recommended unless there is a compelling reason, such as the presence of proteinuric renal disease. Diuretics are effective because the hypertension of pregnancy is "salt-sensitive." The Working Group on Hypertension in Pregnancy allows continuation of the use of diuretics if they had been prescribed before gestation.

Peripartum Cardiomyopathy

Peripartum cardiomyopathy (also known as pregnancy-associated cardiomyopathy) is a relatively rare form of systolic heart failure that occurs during the latter months of pregnancy or the first 6 months after delivery. Multiple causes have been proposed, but none are validated. Patients generally present with dyspnea, edema, and reduced exercise tolerance. Because these symptoms mimic those of normal pregnancy and the early postpartum period, a high degree of suspicion is needed to make the diagnosis. Echocardiography generally shows left ventricular dilatation and reduced left ventricular ejection fraction. The clinical course ranges from rapid, complete recovery to end-stage heart failure requiring heart transplant to even death. Standard treatment of heart failure, with adjustments for women who are pregnant or lactating, is used. Disease-specific therapeutic strategies, including prolactin blockade, are currently under investigation. Subsequent pregnancy may result in heart failure relapse, particularly in patients with persistent systolic dysfunction.

Box 4.1 • Hypertensive Disorders That Occur During Pregnancy

Preeclampsia-eclampsia
  Blood pressure increase after 20 weeks of gestation with proteinuria or any severe features of preeclampsia, including the following:
    Thrombocytopenia
    Impaired liver function
    New-onset renal insufficiency
    Pulmonary edema
    New-onset cerebral or visual disturbances
Chronic hypertension (of any cause that predates pregnancy)
Chronic hypertension with superimposed preeclampsia
Gestational hypertension
  Blood pressure increase after 20 weeks of gestation in the absence of proteinuria or any of the severe features of preeclampsia

---

Key Definition

Peripartum cardiomyopathy: *rare form of systolic heart failure that occurs during latter months of pregnancy or the first 6 months after delivery (also known as pregnancy-associated cardiomyopathy).*

KEY FACTS

✓ In pregnancy, abnormal physical examination findings include diastolic murmur, loud systolic murmur, S_4
✓ High blood pressure during pregnancy—treat with lebatolol, nifedipine, or methyldopa
✓ In pregnancy, avoid angiotensin-converting enzyme inhibitors, angiotensin receptor blockers, renin inhibitors, mineralocorticoid receptor antagonists
✓ Peripartum cardiomyopathy—relatively rare form of systolic heart failure; occurs during latter months of pregnancy or first 6 months after delivery

5 Cardiovascular Physical Examination

KYLE W. KLARICH, MD; LORI A. BLAUWET, MD;
AND SABRINA D. PHILLIPS, MD

Jugular Venous Pressure

Jugular venous pressure reflects right atrial pressure and the relationship between right atrial filling and emptying into the right ventricle (Figure 5.1). Changes in wave amplitude may indicate structural disease and rhythm changes. Normal jugular venous pressure is 6 to 8 cm H_2O. It is best evaluated with the patient supine at an angle of at least 45°. The right atrium lies 5 cm below the sternal angle, and thus the estimated jugular venous pressure equals the height of the jugular venous pressure above the sternal angle + 5 cm (Figure 5.1). The normal venous profile contains 3 positive waves and 2 negative waves. *Positive* waves are *a*, atrial contraction; *c*, closure of tricuspid valve; and *v*, atrial filling. *Negative* waves are the *x* descent (the downward motion of the right ventricle) and the *y* descent (the early right ventricular filling phase). The *a* wave comes just before the first heart sound, and the *v* wave comes during the ejection phase of the left ventricle.

The examiner must distinguish jugular venous pressure from carotid pulsations: jugular venous pressure varies with respiration, is nonpalpable, and can be eliminated by applying gentle pressure at descent (diastole). When the pressure is increased, consider biventricular failure, constrictive pericarditis, pericardial tamponade, cor pulmonale (especially pulmonary embolus), and superior vena cava syndrome.

Abnormalities of the venous waves suggest various cardiac conditions. Increased jugular venous pressure indicates possible fluid overload (common in congestive heart failure). The likelihood of congestive heart failure is increased 4 times if jugular venous pressure is increased. Increased jugular venous pressure can be associated with pulmonary embolus, superior vena cava syndrome, tamponade, and constrictive pericarditis. The inspection of individual wave profile may lend to the differential diagnosis. Large *a* waves may indicate tricuspid stenosis, right ventricular hypertrophy, or pulmonary hypertension (ie, increased right ventricular end-diastolic pressure).

Pronounced or "cannon" *a* waves are due to atria contracting intermittently against a closed atrioventricular valve, a finding consistent with atrioventricular dissociation. Observation of a rapid *x* + *y* descent indicates constrictive pericarditis. Kussmaul sign, the paradoxic increase in jugular venous pressure with inspiration, occurs in pericardial tamponade, constriction, and right ventricular failure. Large, fused *cv* waves are due to tricuspid regurgitation.

Arterial Pulses

Palpation of the radial pulse is useful for heart rate. The brachial or carotid pulse is checked for contour and timing. It is important to assess the upstroke and volume. **Tardus** is the timing and rate of rise of upstroke, and **parvus** is the pulse volume. Assess for radial- or brachial-femoral delay in patients with hypertension by checking radial, or brachial, and femoral pulses simultaneously. A delay is consistent with aortic coarctation.

Abnormalities of the arterial pulse and their associated conditions are listed in Table 5.1.

Key Definitions

Tardus: *timing and rate of rise of upstroke of arterial pulses.*

Parvus: *pulse volume of arterial pulses.*

Apical Impulse

This is normally a discrete area of localized contraction, usually maximal at the fifth intercostal space in the midclavicular line and the size of a quarter (25-cent piece). Abnormalities of the apical impulse and their associated conditions are listed in Table 5.2.

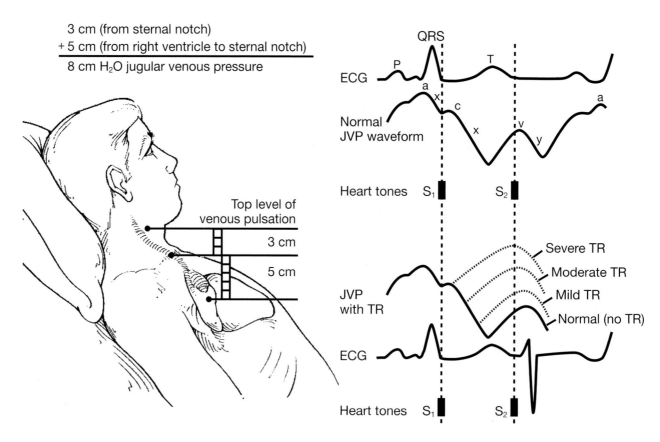

3 cm (from sternal notch)
+ 5 cm (from right ventricle to sternal notch)

8 cm H_2O jugular venous pressure

Figure 5.1 *Evaluation of Jugular Venous Pressure (JVP). ECG indicates electrocardiogram; S_1, first heart sound; S_2, second heart sound; TR, tricuspid regurgitation.*

Table 5.1 • Abnormalities of the Arterial Pulse and Their Associated Conditions

Abnormality	Associated Condition
Parvus (low volume) and tardus (delayed and slowed upstroke)	Aortic stenosis
Parvus only	Low output cardiomyopathy
Bounding upstroke	Aortic regurgitation or arterioventricular fistulas and shunts
Bifid (2 systolic peaks)	Hypertrophic obstructive cardiomyopathy (from midsystolic obstruction)
Bisferiens (2 systolic peaks and a distinct systolic dip, occurs when a large volume is ejected rapidly into aorta)	Aortic regurgitation
Dicrotic (a systolic peak followed by diastolic pulse wave)	Left ventricular failure with hypotension, low output, and increased peripheral resistance
Pulsus paradoxus (exaggerated inspiratory decrease [>10 mm Hg] in pulse pressure)	Tamponade
Pulsus alternans (alternating strong and weak pulse)	Severely reduced left ventricular function

Additional Cardiac Palpation

A palpable aortic valve component (A_2) at the right upper sternum suggests a dilated aorta (eg, aneurysm, dissection, severe aortic regurgitation, poststenotic dilatation in aortic stenosis, hypertension). Severe tricuspid regurgitation may cause a pulsatile liver palpable in the right

Table 5.2 • Abnormalities of the Apical Impulse and Their Associated Conditions

Abnormality	Associated Condition
Displaced (laterally, downward, or both) with a weak, diffuse impulse	Cardiomyopathy
Sustained (may not be displaced)	Left ventricular hypertrophy Aortic stenosis (often with large *a* wave)
Trifid (or multifid)	Hypertrophic cardiomyopathy
Hyperdynamic, descended, and enlarged with rapid filling wave	Mitral regurgitation Aortic regurgitation
Tapping quality, localized, nondisplaced	Normal but may indicate mitral stenosis

epigastrium. Hepatojugular reflux (distention of the external jugular vein 3 or 4 beats after compression of the liver) may also occur in congestion of the liver with substantial fluid overload or tricuspid regurgitation. The apical impulse rotates medially and may be appreciated in the epigastrium (which can be confused with a pulsatile liver) in patients with severe emphysema. Right ventricular hypertrophy results in sustained lift, best appreciated in the fourth intercostal space along the left parasternal border. Diastolic overload (eg, atrial septal defect, anomalous pulmonary venous return) results in a vigorous outward and upward motion but may not be sustained. The pulmonary valve component (P_2) may be palpable in the second right intercostal space in marked pulmonary hypertension. This may be physiologic in slender people with a small anteroposterior diameter.

Thrills

Thrills indicate marked turbulent flow (eg, aortic stenosis, severe mitral regurgitation, and ventricular septal defect) and distinction of a grade 4 murmur.

Heart Sounds

Knowledge of how the heart sounds are related to the cardiac cycle allows an understanding of cardiac auscultation (Figure 5.2). The cardiac cycle starts with atrial contraction; this increases ventricular pressure just before closure of the atrioventricular valves, which generates the first heart sound (S_1). There is a period of time while the

left ventricle generates pressure, known as the isovolumic contraction time, when the atrioventricular and semilunar valves are closed. Normally silent semilunar valve openings then occur, followed by blood ejection from the left ventricle to the aorta, which creates the pulse. As the ventricle relaxes, aortic pressure decreases; this decrease closes the semilunar valves, creating the second heart sound (S_2). Another period follows when both sets of valves are closed. Pressure decreases to less than the left atrial pressure, leading to the usually silent opening of the atrioventricular valves. Early rapid filling followed by slow filling of the ventricles is followed by atrial contraction. The mnemonic for valve sequence—S_1-S_2 (right ventricular-left ventricular sequence)—is "**Many Things Are Possible**" (MTAP): S_1 = *m*itral opens before *t*ricuspid, and S_2 = *a*ortic closes before *p*ulmonary, under normal conditions.

First Heart Sound

S_1 consists of audible mitral valve closure followed by tricuspid valve closure. A loud S_1 occurs with mitral stenosis and short PR intervals (the mitral valve is open when the left ventricle begins to contract and then slaps shut). S_1 also is augmented in hypercontractile states (eg, fever, exercise, thyrotoxicosis, pheochromocytomas, anxiety, and anemia). Conversely, S_1 is decreased if the mitral valve is heavily calcified and immobile (severe mitral stenosis) and with a long PR interval, poor left ventricular function, and rapid diastolic filling (due to premature mitral valve closure) as in aortic regurgitation.

Second Heart Sound

S_2 consists of aortic valve closure (A_2) followed by pulmonary valve closure (P_2). Intensity is increased by hypertension (ie, loud or tympanic A_2 with systemic hypertension; loud P_2 with pulmonary hypertension, with P_2 audible at apex). Intensity is decreased with heavily calcified valves (severe aortic stenosis). Normally, the split between A_2 and P_2 widens on inspiration and narrows on expiration

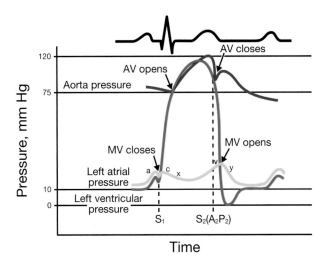

Figure 5.2 *The Normal Cardiac Cycle. A_2 indicates the aortic valve component of S_2; AV, aortic valve; MV, mitral valve; P_2, pulmonary valve component of S_2; S_1, first heart sound; S_2, second heart sound.*

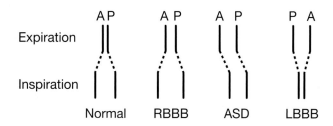

Figure 5.3 Effects of Respiration and Conduction on the Second Heart Sound. The A indicates aortic closure; ASD, atrial septal defect; LBBB, left bundle branch block; P, pulmonary closure; RBBB, right bundle branch block.

due to relatively increased blood return to the right heart during inspiration and greater capacitance of the lungs (Figure 5.3). This is reversed during expiration and is normal physiologic splitting of S_2. This is best heard in the left second intercostal space with the patient seated.

The interplay of multiple factors can affect the timing of the closure of semilunar valves: electrical activation, duration of ventricular ejection, gradient across semilunar valves, and elastic recoil properties of the great vessels. Common types of splitting of the S_2 and their indicated conditions are listed in Table 5.3.

Third Heart Sound

The third heart sound (S_3) occurs in early diastole, coinciding with maximal early diastolic left ventricular filling. It is low-pitched and best heard with the stethoscope bell. S_3 is

Table 5.3 • Common Types of Splitting of the Second Heart Sound and Their Indicated Conditions

Type	Indicated Condition
Physiologic	Normal splitting due to respiratory variation of blood flow On inspiration, P_2 moves farther from A_2, widening the split
Fixed	Atrial septal defect Widest split occurs with a combination of atrial septal defect and pulmonary stenosis
Paradoxic (delayed atrial closure, pulmonary valve closes first)	Left bundle branch block
Persistent	Right bundle branch block A_2 and P_2 are separated because of delayed electromechanical activation of right ventricle Inspiration accentuates the effect

Abbreviations: A_2, aortic valve closure; P_2, pulmonary valve closure; S_1, first heart sound.

associated with left ventricular volume overload (eg, aortic regurgitation, mitral regurgitation, and cardiomyopathy). It is a normal variant in very fit young adults.

Fourth Heart Sound

The fourth heart sound (S_4) is low-pitched, best heard with the stethoscope bell and loudest at the apex. This sound occurs with the atrial "kick" as blood is forced into the left ventricle by atrial contraction against a stiff and noncompliant left ventricle. An S_4 may be heard in aortic stenosis, systemic hypertension, hypertrophic cardiomyopathy, and ischemia. It cannot occur in atrial fibrillation because of the loss of atrial contraction.

KEY FACTS

✓ First heart sound—a loud S_1 occurs with mitral stenosis and short PR intervals (mitral valve is open when left ventricle begins to contract and then slaps shut)

✓ Second heart sound—intensity is increased by hypertension (loud or tympanic A_2 with systemic hypertension; loud P_2 with pulmonary hypertension, with P_2 audible at apex)

✓ Second heart sound—intensity is decreased with heavily calcified valves (severe aortic stenosis)

✓ Third heart sound—associated with left ventricular volume overload (eg, aortic regurgitation, mitral regurgitation, and cardiomyopathy)

✓ Fourth heart sound—may be heard in aortic stenosis, systemic hypertension, hypertrophic cardiomyopathy, and ischemia

✓ Fourth heart sound—cannot occur in atrial fibrillation because of loss of atrial contraction

---

Opening Snap

Opening snap is an early diastolic sound caused by opening of the pathologic rheumatic mitral valve. It is virtually always caused by mitral stenosis. With severe mitral stenosis, the left atrial pressure is very high and thus the valve opens earlier, and the interval is less than 60 milliseconds.

Murmurs

The specific murmurs are discussed with the individual valvular lesions described in Chapter 10, "Valvular and Congenital Heart Diseases," but some broad guidelines are presented here.

A systolic ejection murmur begins after S_1 and ends before S_2. It may have a diamond-shaped quality with crescendo and decrescendo components. In general, a more severe obstruction (a narrower valve orifice) causes a louder, later-peaking murmur. An *ejection click* may precede a bicuspid (aortic or pulmonary) valve murmur if the valve pliability is preserved. A holosystolic murmur engulfs S$_1$ and S$_2$ and occurs when blood moves from a very high-pressure to a low-pressure system, such as in mitral regurgitation

and ventricular septal defect. Diastolic murmurs are always abnormal. Echocardiography should be considered in this setting if a systolic murmur of grade 3 or higher is heard or if there are other signs or symptoms of cardiac disease (Figure 5.4).

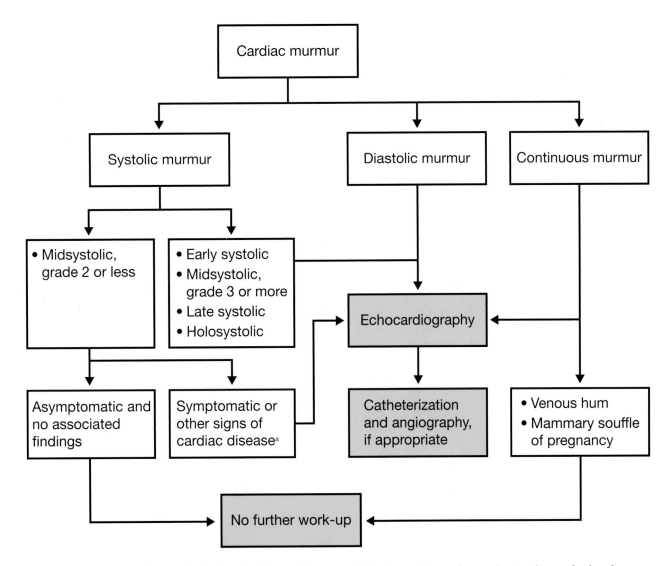

Figure 5.4 *Recommendations for Evaluating Heart Murmurs.* [a]*If electrocardiography or chest radiography has been performed and the results are abnormal, echocardiography is recommended.*

(Adapted from Bonow RO, Carabello BA, Chatterjee K, de Leon AC Jr, Faxon DP, Freed MD, et al; American College of Cardiology/American Heart Association Task Force on Practice Guidelines. 2008 Focused update incorporated into the ACC/ AHA 2006 guidelines for the management of patients with valvular heart disease: a report of the American College of Cardiology/American Heart Association Task Force on Practice Guidelines [Writing Committee to revise the 1998 guidelines for the management of patients with valvular heart disease]. Endorsed by the Society of Cardiovascular Anesthesiologists, Society for Cardiovascular Angiography and Interventions, and Society of Thoracic Surgeons. J Am Coll Cardiol. 2008 Sep 23;52[13]:e1–142 and Bonow RO, Carabello BA, Chatterjee K, de Leon AC Jr, Faxon DP, Freed MD, et al; 2006 Writing Committee Members; American College of Cardiology/American Heart Association Task Force. 2008 Focused update incorporated into the ACC/AHA 2006 guidelines for the management of patients with valvular heart disease: a report of the American College of Cardiology/American Heart Association Task Force on Practice Guidelines [Writing Committee to Revise the 1998 Guidelines for the Management of Patients With Valvular Heart Disease]: endorsed by the Society of Cardiovascular Anesthesiologists, Society for Cardiovascular Angiography and Interventions, and Society of Thoracic Surgeons. Circulation. 2008 Oct 7;118[15]:e523–661. Epub 2008 Sep 26. Used with permission.)

Table 5.4 • Effects of Physical Maneuvers and Other Factors on Valvular Diseases

Maneuver or Factor	Result	Mitral Regurgitation	MVP	Aortic Stenosis	HOCM
Amyl nitrite	↓ afterload	↓	↑/0	↑	↑
Valsalva	↓ preload	↓	↑	↓	↑
Handgrip	↑ afterload	↑	↓/0	↓	↓
Post-PVC	↑ contractility ↓ afterload	=	↓	↑	↑[a]

Abbreviations: HOCM, hypertrophic obstructive cardiomyopathy; MVP, mitral valve prolapse; PVC, premature ventricular complex.

[a]Although the murmur increases, the peripheral pulse decreases because of the increase in outflow obstruction.

Certain maneuvers alter cardiac murmurs. *Inspiration* increases venous return, increasing right-sided sounds (S_3 and S_4) and murmurs (tricuspid and pulmonary stenosis, and tricuspid and pulmonary regurgitation). The *Valsalva maneuver* increases intrathoracic pressure, inhibiting venous return and thus decreasing preload. Most cardiac murmurs and sounds diminish in intensity during the Valsalva maneuver because of decreased ventricular filling and cardiac output. The exception is hypertrophic obstructive cardiomyopathy, in which the murmur increases because of dynamic left ventricular outflow obstruction accentuated by decreased preload. The Valsalva maneuver is the classic way to distinguish between the murmurs of aortic stenosis and hypertrophic cardiomyopathy. *Handgrip* increases cardiac output and systemic arterial pressure, decreasing the gradient across a stenotic aortic valve. A *change in posture* from supine to upright causes decreased venous return, reducing stroke volume and thus a reflex increase in heart rate and peripheral resistance. *Squatting* and the Valsalva maneuver have opposite hemodynamic effects. Squatting increases peripheral resistance and venous return. *Amyl nitrite* pharmacologically decreases afterload. The amyl nitrite is inhaled and transiently lowers blood pressure, increasing the murmurs of hypertrophic cardiomyopathy and aortic stenosis. Its main use is to determine the gradient in patients with dynamic left ventricular outflow obstruction due to hypertrophic cardiomyopathy. The effects of maneuvers are shown in Table 5.4.

6 | Heart Failure and Cardiomyopathies

FARRIS K. TIMIMI, MD

Heart Failure

Heart failure is a clinical syndrome characterized by inability of the heart to maintain adequate cardiac output to meet the metabolic demands of the body while still maintaining normal or near-normal ventricular filling pressures. Heart failure may be present at rest, but often it is symptomatic only during exertion due to the dynamic nature of cardiac demands. For the optimal treatment of heart failure, the mechanism, underlying cause, and any reversible precipitating factors must be identified. Typical manifestations of heart failure are dyspnea and fatigue limiting activity tolerance and fluid retention leading to pulmonary or peripheral edema. These abnormalities do not always occur simultaneously. Dyspnea may be due to impaired cardiac output, increased filling pressures, or both.

> ### Key Definition
>
> Heart failure: *a clinical syndrome characterized by inability of the heart to maintain adequate cardiac output to meet the metabolic demands of the body while still maintaining normal or near-normal ventricular filling pressures.*

Heart failure, the symptomatic expression of cardiac disease, usually arises sometime after cardiac disease is established. The American College of Cardiology and the American Heart Association stages of heart failure (Figure 6.1) emphasize that symptoms follow an asymptomatic phase of cardiac dysfunction, highlighting the opportunity to preclude the development of heart failure by early intervention. In symptomatic patients, it can often be challenging to determine whether symptoms are cardiac due to structural disease or whether they are coincidental noncardiac symptoms coexisting with asymptomatic structural disease.

Heart failure may result from abnormalities of the pericardium, myocardium, endocardium, cardiac valves, or vascular or renal systems (eg, hyperreninemic pulmonary edema). Most commonly it is due to impaired left ventricular myocardial function. In approximately 50% of cases, the left ventricle is enlarged and there is abnormal contractile function with reduced ejection fraction (less than 50%). This type is referred to as dilated cardiomyopathy. The ejection fraction is normal in the remaining 50%. This type is referred to as heart failure with preserved ejection fraction. Isolated right ventricular failure can occur; however, the majority of cases of heart failure involve either the left ventricle alone or the left ventricle with associated right ventricular dysfunction. High ventricular filling pressures can cause dyspnea and edema.

Presentation

Patients may present with asymptomatic ventricular dysfunction (usually dilated ventricles with reduced ejection fraction). These patients do not have heart failure, and they can usually be managed as outpatients; their treatment is discussed later in this chapter. Patients with heart failure (ie, symptoms and signs) may present either as outpatients or to acute care facilities, often depending on the severity of their symptoms. This heterogeneous group is said to have acute decompensated heart failure and includes both patients presenting for the first time with heart failure and patients presenting with a decompensation of known heart failure.

Hospitalization is advisable when hypotension, worsening renal function, altered mentation, dyspnea at rest, significant arrhythmias (eg, new atrial fibrillation), or other complications such as disturbed electrolytes are present or outpatient care options are lacking (Box 6.1). Patients without these factors who have exclusively exertional symptoms, are not severely congested on examination, and have adequate vascular perfusion (warm extremities, adequate blood pressure) may receive treatment as outpatients. The stages of heart failure development and management are outlined in Figure 6.1.

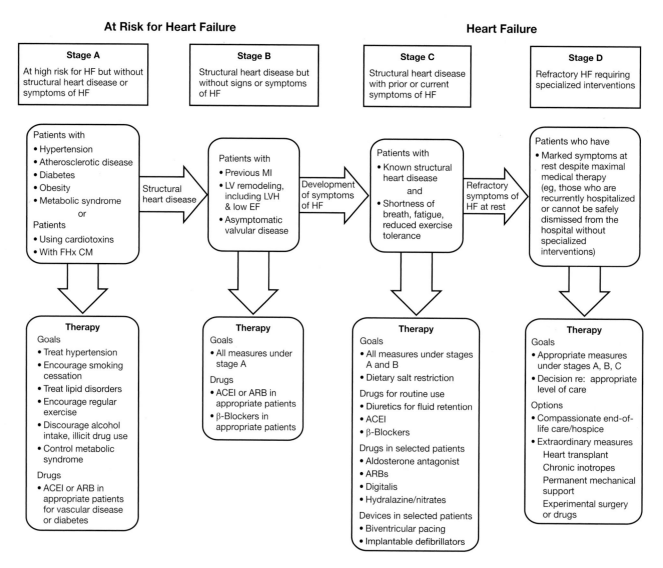

Figure 6.1 *Stages in the Development of Heart Failure and Recommended Therapy by Stage. ACEI indicates angiotensin-converting enzyme inhibitor; ARB, angiotensin receptor blocker; EF, ejection fraction; FHx CM, family history of cardiomyopathy; HF, heart failure; LV, left ventricular; LVH, left ventricular hypertrophy; MI, myocardial infarction.*
(Adapted from Hunt SA, Abraham WT, Chin MH, Feldman AM, Francis GS, Ganiats TG, et al; American College of Cardiology Foundation; American Heart Association. 2009 Focused update incorporated into the ACC/AHA 2005 guidelines for the diagnosis and management of heart failure in adults: a report of the American College of Cardiology Foundation/American Heart Association Task Force on Practice Guidelines Developed in Collaboration With the International Society for Heart and Lung Transplantation. J Am Coll Cardiol 2009 Apr 14;53[15]:e1–90. Erratum in: J Am Coll Cardiol. 2009 Dec 15;54[25]:2464 and Hunt SA, Abraham WT, Chin MH, Feldman AM, Francis GS, Ganiats TG, et al. 2009 Focused update incorporated into the ACC/AHA 2005 Guidelines for the Diagnosis and Management of Heart Failure in Adults: a report of the American College of Cardiology Foundation/American Heart Association Task Force on Practice Guidelines: developed in collaboration with the International Society for Heart and Lung Transplantation. Circulation. 2009 Apr 14;119[14]:e391–479. Epub 2009 Mar 26. Erratum in: Circulation. 2010 Mar 30;121[12]:e258. Used with permission.)

Diagnosis

Heart failure is a clinical diagnosis based on symptoms, physical findings, and chest radiography. The symptoms typically include some combination of dyspnea, fatigue, and fluid retention. The dyspnea may be with exertion or with recumbency. Physical findings include evidence of low output, volume overload, or both. Such evidence includes narrow pulse pressure, poor peripheral perfusion, jugular venous distention, hepatojugular reflux, peripheral edema, ascites, and dull lung bases suggestive of pleural effusions. Lung crackles usually represent atelectatic compression rather than fluid in the alveoli,

---

Box 6.1 • Conditions That Prompt Hospitalization in Heart Failure

Hypotension

Worsening renal function

Altered mentation

Dyspnea at rest

Significant arrhythmias

Disturbed electrolytes

Lack of outpatient care

---

the latter being more common in *acute* heart failure. In contrast, exacerbation of chronic heart failure may be associated with less notable pulmonary findings as a product of chronic pulmonic lymphatic recruitment. Edema usually affects the lower extremities but can also affect the abdomen. Cardiac findings include abnormalities of the cardiac apex (enlarged, displaced, sustained point of maximal impulse) and gallop rhythms. The liver may be enlarged, pulsatile, and tender if there is right heart failure. Clinical signs indicating high- and low-output heart failure could aid in patient management (Table 6.1). Both the symptoms and the signs of heart failure described above are nonspecific and can occur in other conditions. Heart failure is a probabilistic clinical diagnosis best made by use of the modified Framingham criteria (Box 6.2).

Table 6.1 • Management of High-Output and Low-Output Heart Failure

Perfusion at Rest	Congestion at Rest	
	No	**Yes**
Normal	Warm and dry PCWP normal CI normal (compensated)	Warm and wet PCWP increased CI normal ↓ Hospitalize ± Nesiritide or vasodilators[a] Diuretics
Low	Cold and dry PCWP low or normal CI decreased ↓ Hospitalize Cautious hydration Inotropic drugs[b]	Cold and wet PCWP increased CI decreased ↓ Hospitalize Nesiritide or vasodilators[a] Diuretics

Abbreviations: CI, cardiac index; PCWP, pulmonary capillary wedge pressure; ±, patient may or may not require hospitalization, depending on clinical assessment.

[a]Vasodilators: nitroglycerin or nitroprusside.

[b]Inotropic drugs: milrinone or dobutamine.

Box 6.2 • Framingham Criteria for Clinical Diagnosis of Congestive Heart Failure[a]

Major Criteria	*Minor Criteria*
PND	Peripheral edema
Orthopnea	Night cough
Increased JVP	DOE
Rales	Hepatomegaly
Third heart sound	Pleural effusion
Chest radiography	Heart rate >120 beats per minute
Cardiomegaly Pulmonary edema	Weight loss ≥4.5 kg in 5 days with diuretic

Abbreviations: DOE, dyspnea on exertion; JVP, jugular venous pressure; PND, paroxysmal nocturnal dyspnea.

[a]Validated congestive heart failure if 2 major or 1 major and 2 minor criteria are present concurrently.

Adapted from Ho KK, Anderson KM, Kannel WB, Grossman W, Levy D. Survival after the onset of congestive heart failure in the Framingham Heart Study subjects. Circulation. 1993 Jul;88(1):107–15. Used with permission.

According to the modified Framingham criteria, the simultaneous presence of 2 major or of 1 major and 2 minor criteria satisfies the clinical diagnosis of congestive heart failure. Exertional dyspnea does not have the same weight as paroxysmal nocturnal dyspnea or orthopnea, and edema does not have the same weight as increased venous pressure. Patients with low-output heart failure may not have findings of volume overload (congestion) and thus may not satisfy Framingham criteria.

Increased intracardiac pressure or chamber dilatation leads to increased production of natriuretic peptides, substances produced by the heart. Accordingly, measurement of B-type natriuretic peptide or N-terminal prohormone of brain natriuretic peptide complements the clinical diagnosis of heart failure. In general, the degree of increase reflects the degree of myocardial dysfunction. However, increased levels of these peptides do not distinguish systolic from diastolic, left from right, or acute from chronic cardiac dysfunction. Interpreting these levels has caveats (Box 6.3). In addition, there is substantial variability of levels in stable patients, up to 50%.

The utility of the natriuretic peptide values for diagnosing heart failure has been best shown in patients without prior known cardiac disease. Interpretation of intermediately increased levels can be difficult in patients with a prior history of ventricular dysfunction or heart failure who are receiving medical treatment. The negative predictive value of normal natriuretic peptide levels (in the absence of constriction, morbid obesity, or mitral stenosis) is more powerful than their positive predictive value. Natriuretic

Box 6.3 • Pitfalls in the Interpretation of Natriuretic Peptide Value

NP Higher Than Expected	*NP Lower Than Expected*
Women	Obesity
Elderly	Acute heart failure
Renal failure	Heart failure due to mitral stenosis
	Constriction

Abbreviation: NP, natriuretic peptide.

peptide values are most useful in patients without a prior diagnosis of heart failure and in patients not receiving treatment for heart failure.

Management of Acute Heart Failure

At the time of initial diagnosis, the common alternative diagnoses of pulmonary embolism or exacerbation of chronic obstructive pulmonary disease must be excluded. Clinical stratification guides initial treatment (usually parenteral) (Figure 6.2).

Once clinical improvement begins, treatment is adjusted to optimize hemodynamics, minimize symptoms, and allow transition to oral medications. The mechanism of heart failure and precipitating factors are defined, patient and family education are provided, and dismissal (including timely follow-up) is planned.

Mechanisms

Selection of proper therapy depends on correctly identifying the mechanism of heart failure. A simple categorical framework is given in Table 6.2. Left ventricular myocardial dysfunction is the most common cause of heart failure. Accurate diagnosis is essential because treatment and prognosis are based on the cause of heart failure. Diagnosis is initially based on physical examination and noninvasive testing, such as echocardiography or radionuclide angiography.

Precipitating Factors

New-onset or worsening symptoms of heart failure may represent only natural disease progression. However, 1 or more precipitating factors may be responsible for symptomatic deterioration (Box 6.4). If these factors are not identified and corrected, symptoms of heart failure often return after initial therapy. The most common precipitants

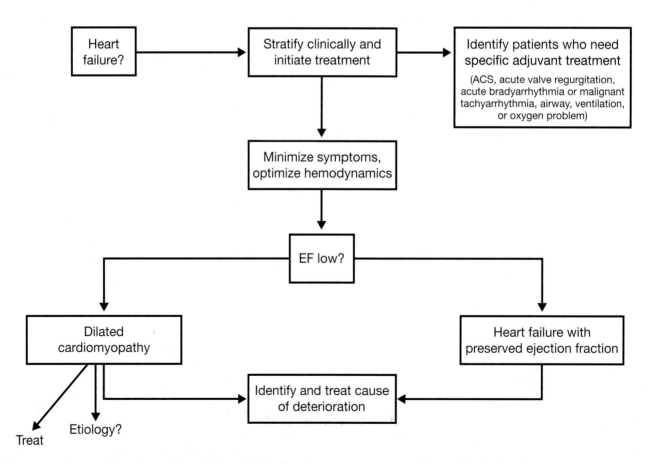

Figure 6.2 *Approach to Acute Heart Failure. ACS indicates acute coronary syndrome; EF, ejection fraction.*

Table 6.2 • Causes of Heart Failure and Treatment

Cause	Treatment
Myocardial	
Dilated cardiomyopathy (including ischemic)	Angiotensin-converting enzyme inhibitors, angiotensin receptor blockers, β-adrenergic blockers (eg, carvedilol, metoprolol succinate, bisoprolol), diuretics, aldosterone antagonists, nitrates, digoxin, nitrates and hydralazine in combination, transplant, coronary revascularization, left ventricular aneurysmectomy (surgical ventricular remodeling), cardiac resynchronization therapy, cardiac defibrillator
Hypertrophic cardiomyopathy	β-Adrenergic blockers, verapamil, disopyramide, surgical myectomy, septal alcohol ablation, dual-chamber pacing
Restrictive cardiomyopathy	Diuretics, heart transplant, treatment of underlying systemic disease
Pericardial	
Tamponade	Pericardiocentesis
Constrictive pericarditis	Pericardiectomy
Valvular	Valve repair or replacement
Hypertension	Antihypertensive treatment
Pulmonary hypertension	Prostacyclin infusion, calcium channel blockers, heart-lung transplant, endothelin antagonists, phosphodiesterase type 5 inhibitor
High output	
Hyperthyroidism, Paget disease, arteriovenous fistula	Correction of underlying cause

are dietary indiscretion (eg, sodium, excess fluid, and alcohol), medication nonadherence (due to cost, regimen complexity, lack of patient understanding), and suboptimally controlled hypertension.

Evaluation should consist of 1) a medical history, which includes sodium and fluid intake, medication use and compliance, and sleep history from bedroom partners; 2) chest radiography to look for pneumonitis or pleural effusions; 3) electrocardiography and measurement of cardiac biomarkers to document heart rhythm and identify myocardial ischemia or injury; and 4) cultures of blood, urine, and sputum as suggested by history. Other tests should include determination of complete blood count and thyroid-stimulating hormone and creatinine levels.

Box 6.4 • Precipitating Factors in Heart Failure

Diet (excessive sodium or fluid intake, alcohol)
Noncompliance with medication or inadequate dosing
Sodium-retaining medications (NSAIDs)
Infection (bacterial or viral)
Myocardial ischemia or infarction
Arrhythmia (atrial fibrillation, bradycardia)
Breathing disorders of sleep
Worsening renal function
Anemia
Metabolic (hyperthyroidism, hypothyroidism)
Pulmonary embolus

Abbreviation: NSAIDs, nonsteroidal anti-inflammatory drugs.

KEY FACTS

✓ In symptomatic heart failure—can often be challenging to determine whether symptoms are cardiac due to structural disease or whether they are coincidental noncardiac symptoms coexisting with asymptomatic structural disease

✓ In heart failure—hospitalization is advised when hypotension, worsening renal function, altered mentation, dyspnea at rest, significant arrhythmias, or other complications are present or patient care options are lacking

✓ Heart failure—a clinical diagnosis based on symptoms, physical findings, and chest radiography

✓ Symptoms of heart failure—some combination of dyspnea, fatigue, and fluid retention

✓ Modified Framingham criteria—used to make a probabilistic clinical diagnosis of heart failure

✓ B-type natriuretic peptide or N-terminal pro-brain natriuretic peptide—measurement of these complements the clinical diagnosis of heart failure; their degree of increase reflects the degree of myocardial dysfunction

✓ Increased levels of B-type natriuretic peptide or N-terminal pro-brain natriuretic peptide—do not distinguish systolic from diastolic, left from right, or acute from chronic cardiac dysfunction

✓ Negative predictive value of normal natriuretic peptide levels—more powerful than their positive predictive value

Cardiomyopathies

Cardiomyopathies are divided into primary and secondary cardiomyopathies, and the primary disorders are further subdivided as genetic, acquired, or mixed. This classification scheme accounts for progressive understanding of this heterogeneous group of disorders. However, the previous phenotypic classification scheme of dilated, hypertrophic, and restrictive diseases can be more useful for guiding clinical understanding and management. The different anatomical and pathophysiologic processes for each cardiomyopathy are listed in Table 6.3.

Dilated Cardiomyopathy

Pathology and Etiology

The major abnormality in dilated cardiomyopathy is a remodeled left ventricle characterized by dilatation and reduced ejection fraction. Left ventricular end-diastolic pressure is typically increased. The increased filling pressures and low cardiac output cause dyspnea and fatigue. *Idiopathic* dilated cardiomyopathy indicates left ventricular dysfunction without any known cause. The right ventricle may be normal, hypertrophied, or dilated.

In many patients with dilated cardiomyopathy, the cause is genetic, and up to 30% have at least 1 identifiable affected family member. Other causes of left ventricular dysfunction include severe coronary artery disease—the most common cause in the United States—(hibernating myocardium), previous infarction, uncontrolled hypertension, ethanol abuse, myocarditis, hyperthyroidism or hypothyroidism, postpartum cardiomyopathy, toxins and drugs (including doxorubicin and trastuzumab), tachycardia-induced cardiomyopathy, infiltrative cardiomyopathy (ie, hemochromatosis, sarcoidosis), AIDS, and pheochromocytoma.

Clinical Presentation

The presentation is highly variable. The patient may be asymptomatic and the diagnosis prompted by examination, chest radiography, electrocardiography (ECG), or imaging findings. Patients may have symptoms of mild to severe heart failure (New York Heart Association [NYHA] functional class II-IV). Atrial and ventricular arrhythmias are common in dilated cardiomyopathy. Physical examination may indicate increased jugular venous pressure, a right ventricular lift (if there is right heart involvement), low-volume upstroke of the carotid artery, displaced and sustained left ventricular impulse (possibly with a rapid filling wave), audible third or fourth heart sounds, and an apical systolic murmur of mitral regurgitation. Pulsus alternans may occur in patients with advanced heart failure. Pulmonary examination may have normal results or indicate crackles or evidence of pleural effusion.

The ECG is almost always abnormal and frequently indicates left ventricular hypertrophy, intraventricular conduction delay, or bundle branch block. Rhythm abnormalities may include premature atrial contractions, atrial fibrillation, premature ventricular contractions, or short bursts of ventricular tachycardia. The chest radiograph often shows left ventricular enlargement and pulmonary venous congestion. The diagnosis is based on clinical signs and symptoms coupled with the findings of left ventricular enlargement and reduced ejection fraction, which can be measured with echocardiography, radionuclide angiography, left ventriculography, cine computed tomography, or magnetic resonance imaging.

Evaluation

After diagnosis, treatable secondary causes of left ventricular dysfunction should be sought. Tests of thyroid function should be done to exclude hyperthyroidism or hypothyroidism. Transferrin levels should be measured to screen for hemochromatosis. Measurement of the serum angiotensin-converting enzyme level should be considered if sarcoidosis is a possibility. Metanephrine levels should be measured if there is a history of severe labile hypertension or unusual spells. Ethanol or drug abuse history should be obtained.

In severe coronary artery disease, reversible left ventricular dysfunction can be caused by hibernating myocardium. With revascularization, left ventricular function may improve gradually. Identifying patients with significant hibernating myocardium is difficult. Currently, the reference standard is positron emission tomography to evaluate metabolic activity. Viability protocols used in

---

Table 6.3 • Anatomical and Pathophysiologic Processes for Each Cardiomyopathy

Type	Left Ventricular Cavity Size	Left Ventricular Wall Thickness	Ejection Fraction	Diastolic Function	Other
Dilated cardiomyopathy	↑	N/↑	↓	↓	
Hypertrophic cardiomyopathy	↓/N	↑	↑	↓	Left ventricular outflow obstruction
Restrictive cardiomyopathy	N/↑	N	N	↓	

Abbreviation and symbols: ↓, decreased; N, normal; ↑, increased.

stress echocardiography and radionuclide perfusion imaging are more widely available than positron emission tomography and are useful for identifying hibernating myocardium.

Tachycardia-induced cardiomyopathy can occur in patients with prolonged periods of tachycardia (usually atrial fibrillation or flutter or prolonged atrial tachycardia). Because systolic dysfunction can be completely reversed with treatment of tachycardia, identifying these causes is important.

Acute myocarditis may cause left ventricular dysfunction; the natural history is unknown. Many patients have development of persistent left ventricular dysfunction, whereas others have improvement with time. Thus, it is necessary to remeasure left ventricular function 3 to 6 months after diagnosis and treatment. Endomyocardial biopsy may help diagnose myocarditis. Immunosuppressive therapy does not improve outcome and should be reserved for patients with giant cell myocarditis, concomitant skeletal myositis, or clinical deterioration despite standard pharmacologic therapy.

Pathophysiology

The hemodynamic, pathophysiologic, and biologic aspects of heart failure must be appreciated to understand treatment of dilated cardiomyopathy. **Preload** is the ventricular volume at the end of diastole (end-diastolic volume). Typically, when it is increased, stroke volume increases. The relationship of stroke volume to preload is illustrated by the preload Starling curve (Figure 6.3). **Afterload** is the tension, force, or stress on the ventricular wall muscle fibers after fiber shortening begins. Left ventricular afterload is increased by aortic stenosis and systemic hypertension but is decreased by mitral regurgitation. Ventricular enlargement increases afterload.

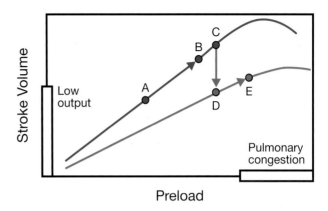

Figure 6.3 *Starling Curve. Blue line is patient with normal contractility, and red line is one with depressed systolic function. Normally, stroke volume depends on preload of the heart. Increasing preload increases stroke volume (A to B). Myocardial dysfunction causes a shift of the curve downward and to the right (C to D), causing a severe decrease in stroke volume, which leads to symptoms of fatigue and lethargy. The compensatory response to decrease in stroke volume is an increase in preload (D to E). Because the diastolic pressure-volume relationship is curvilinear, increased left ventricular volume produces increased left ventricular end-diastolic pressure, causing symptoms of pulmonary congestion. Note flat portion of the curve at its upper end; here, there is little increase in stroke volume for increase in preload.*

> ### Key Definition
>
> Preload: *the ventricular volume at the end of diastole (end-diastolic volume).*
>
> Afterload: *the tension, force, or stress on the ventricular wall muscle fibers after fiber shortening begins.*

Figure 6.4 illustrates the neurohormonal response to decreased myocardial contractility. Decreased cardiac output activates baroreceptors and the sympathetic nervous system. Sympathetic nervous system stimulation causes increased heart rate and contractility. α-Stimulation of the arterioles causes increases in afterload. The renin-angiotensin system is activated by sympathetic stimulation, decreased renal blood flow, and decreased renal sodium, in turn activating aldosterone, causing increased renal retention of sodium, which leads to pulmonary congestion. Low renal blood flow causes renal sodium retention. Increased angiotensin II causes vasoconstriction and increased afterload. In congestive heart failure, the compensatory mechanisms that increase preload eventually cause a malcompensatory increase in afterload, in turn causing further decrease in stroke volume.

In the subacute and chronic stages of heart failure, neurohormonal (adrenergic, angiotensin II) and other signaling pathways lead to myocyte dysfunction and cell death. Increased collagen production results in progressive cardiac fibrosis. Progressive myocardial dysfunction and remodeling are the natural history of untreated myocardial disease.

Treatment

Nonpharmacologic Treatment

For adequate treatment of dilated cardiomyopathy, precipitating factors must be identified and addressed. Nonpharmacologic treatment is crucial and includes sodium and fluid restriction, alcohol avoidance, daily weight monitoring with action plan, and regular aerobic exercise. Ongoing patient and family education and regular outpatient follow-up reduce heart failure exacerbations, emergency department visits, and hospitalizations.

KEY FACTS

✓ Dilated cardiomyopathy—in many patients the cause is genetic, and up to 30% have at least 1 identifiable affected family member

✓ Atrial and ventricular arrhythmias—common in dilated cardiomyopathy

✓ After diagnosis of dilated cardiomyopathy—treatable secondary causes of left ventricular dysfunction should be sought

✓ In severe coronary artery disease—reversible left ventricular dysfunction can be caused by hibernating myocardium. With revascularization, left ventricular dysfunction may improve gradually

✓ Significant hibernating myocardium—identification of affected patients is difficult; reference standard is positron emission tomography to evaluate metabolic activity

Pharmacologic Treatment

Angiotensin-converting enzyme (ACE) inhibitors, β-adrenergic blockers, and diuretics are the mainstays of pharmacologic therapy. ACE inhibitors decrease afterload, decrease sodium retention by inhibiting aldosterone formation, and directly affect myocyte growth and myocardial remodeling (Figure 6.5).

ACE inhibitors provide symptomatic improvement in patients with NYHA functional class II-IV failure and improve mortality in patients with moderate and severe heart failure. In asymptomatic patients, ACE inhibitors prevent onset of heart failure and reduce the need for hospitalization. The dose of the ACE inhibitor used should be titrated up as tolerated on the basis of symptoms and blood pressure. Upward dose adjustment as tolerated is beneficial even in clinically compensated patients receiving low to intermediate doses. Common adverse effects include hypotension, hyperkalemia, azotemia, cough, angioedema (mild or severe), and dysgeusia. The benefits and potential adverse effects of ACE inhibitors are thought to be a class effect.

Angiotensin II receptor blockers provide hemodynamic benefits similar to those of ACE inhibitors in patients with dilated cardiomyopathy. They can be used in patients who have cough and angioedema with use of ACE inhibitors because they do not inhibit the breakdown of bradykinin (the cause of cough and angioedema). They are less beneficial than ACE inhibitors in the reverse remodeling of the myocardium, and thus they remain second-line treatment.

β-Adrenergic blockers (β-blockers) improve symptoms and ejection fraction and decrease hospitalizations and mortality in patients with systolic heart failure. They may

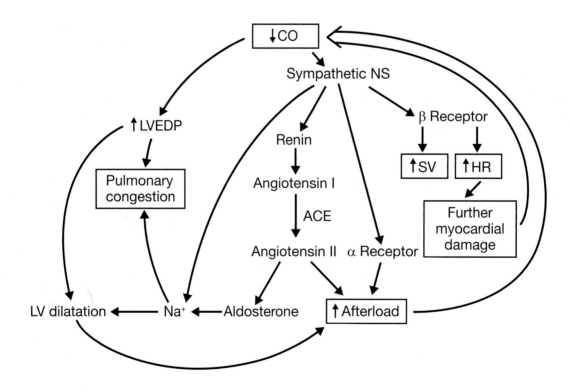

Figure 6.4 *Neurohormonal Response to Decreased Myocardial Contractility. ACE indicates angiotensin-converting enzyme; CO, cardiac output; HR, heart rate; LV, left ventricular; LVEDP, left ventricular end-diastolic pressure; NS, nervous system; SV, stroke volume.*

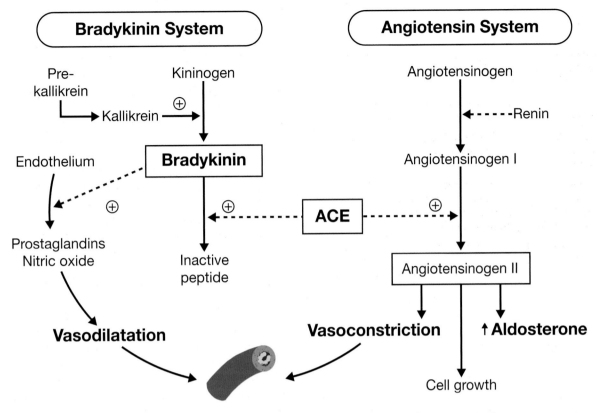

Figure 6.5 *Action of Angiotensin-Converting Enzyme (ACE) on the Bradykinin and Angiotensin Systems.*

have unwanted hemodynamic effects in the acute setting (negative inotropic effects, attenuation of heart rate response that may be maintaining cardiac output in the setting of reduced stroke volume), but they provide long-term benefit by modifying the unfavorable biologic effects of enhanced adrenergic tone. This benefit may take up to 6 months to observe. These drugs are most useful for patients with asymptomatic left ventricular dysfunction after myocardial infarction and NYHA class II or III symptoms. They can be given cautiously to patients with class IV symptoms but should *not* be given to patients with substantial volume overload and cardiogenic shock. Initial dosing should be low, with close clinical follow-up. Upward titration of the β-blocker dose should be slow and cautious. Critically, the likelihood of patients continuing treatment with β-blockers is much higher when treatment is initiated during a hospitalization for heart failure. Well-studied β-blockers with established benefit for patients with heart failure include metoprolol succinate, carvedilol, and bisoprolol.

Diuretics are part of the routine management in patients with symptoms and signs of systemic and pulmonary congestion. Diuretic doses should be minimized when possible because of associated neurohormonal activation and electrolyte imbalance. Fluid overload can be treated initially with thiazide or loop diuretics. Occasionally, a combination of thiazides and loop diuretics is needed for severe fluid retention. The addition of spironolactone can help in patients

with hypokalemia and may provide additional benefit by blocking aldosterone-mediated effects.

Drugs directly affecting myocardial contractility include digoxin, phosphodiesterase inhibitors (milrinone), and β-agonists (dopamine and dobutamine). Digoxin provides symptomatic relief when the ejection fraction is less than 40%, but it does not improve survival. It is useful for ventricular rate control and atrial fibrillation and in patients who are symptomatic despite treatment with ACE inhibitors and β-blockers. Because digoxin is excreted by the kidneys, dosage must be decreased in older patients and patients with renal dysfunction. Because of drug-drug interactions, digoxin dosage should be decreased with concomitant administration of amiodarone, verapamil, and quinidine. Short-term use of parenteral inotropic agents (milrinone and dobutamine) may improve symptoms, but long-term use *increases* mortality, and therefore these drugs should be used transiently in the hospital for low-output states and occasionally for palliative purposes in refractory end-stage heart failure.

Aldosterone antagonists may provide additional benefit by inhibiting fibrosis and combating mechanical and electrical remodeling. Significant survival benefit has been shown in patients with NYHA class III-IV heart failure. Eplerenone, a selective aldosterone inhibitor, provides survival benefit at 30 days and 1 year in patients who have had infarction and who have left ventricular dysfunction and either heart failure or diabetes. However, aldosterone antagonists have considerable risk of hyperkalemia and thus must be given carefully with cautious follow-up, avoidance of nonsteroidal anti-inflammatory drugs, and prompt attention to illnesses predisposing to dehydration.

High-dose nitrates and hydralazine in combination provide symptomatic improvement and improved mortality in patients with heart failure, but this approach is inferior to ACE inhibitors when used alone. It is used in patients who are unable to tolerate ACE inhibitors or angiotensin receptor blockers because of renal insufficiency or hyperkalemia. The combination has been shown to increase survival in African-American patients when given as adjunctive therapy to ACE inhibitors and β-blockers.

Amlodipine and felodipine are safe in patients with dilated cardiomyopathy. They can be used to treat hypertension that persists despite optimal dosages of ACE inhibitors and β-blockers, but they do not provide a survival benefit. First-generation calcium channel blockers (verapamil, diltiazem, nifedipine) are *contraindicated* because of their negative inotropic effects.

Anticoagulation with warfarin is recommended for patients in atrial fibrillation and those with intracardiac thrombus or a history of systemic or pulmonary thromboembolism, but it is not recommended as prophylaxis in the setting of ventricular dysfunction. Retrospective studies have suggested that aspirin may diminish the benefits of ACE inhibitors by blocking prostaglandin-induced vasodilatation. An increased incidence of hospitalizations for heart failure in patients with dilated cardiomyopathy receiving aspirin was also observed. The most common recommendation is to use low-dose aspirin in patients with heart failure and coronary artery disease.

Device Therapy

Implanted defibrillators improve survival when used at least 40 days after a myocardial infarction in patients with ischemic and nonischemic dilated cardiomyopathies who have ejection fractions less than 35% despite optimal medical therapy. They should be offered to patients who have a reasonable functional status with at least 1 year of survival. Patients in sinus rhythm with ventricular dyssynchrony may benefit from biventricular pacing (cardiac resynchronization therapy). Current implantation criteria are sinus rhythm, QRS duration more than 120 milliseconds, NYHA class III-IV, ejection fraction less than 35%, and optimal medical management. Cardiac resynchronization therapy results in improvement in symptoms, exercise capacity, and left ventricular ejection fraction and survival in well-selected patients.

Cardiac Replacement Therapy

Heart transplant is the procedure of choice for patients with dilated cardiomyopathy and severe, refractory symptoms. With a successful transplant, the 1-year survival rate can exceed 90%. Early referral to a heart transplant center is recommended for patients with refractory heart failure. Long-term complications include rejection, infection, hypertension, hyperlipidemia, malignancy, and accelerated coronary vasculopathy. Donor availability is the major limiting factor. In selected patients, left ventricular assist devices have now been approved by the US Food and Drug Administration and are used either as a bridge to transplant or as final (destination) therapy.

KEY FACTS

✓ Treatment of dilated cardiomyopathy—pharmacologic mainstays are ACE inhibitors, β-blockers, and diuretics

✓ Short-term use of parenteral inotropic agents in dilated cardiomyopathy—may improve symptoms, but long-term use *increases* mortality; thus, these agents should be used transiently in the hospital for low-output states and occasionally palliatively in refractory end-stage heart failure

✓ Amlodipine and felodipine—safe to use for dilated cardiomyopathy; can be used to treat hypertension that persists despite use of ACE inhibitors and β-blockers, but they do not provide a survival benefit

✓ First-generation calcium channel blockers—contraindicated for dilated cardiomyopathy because of their negative inotropic effects

✓ Aspirin use in dilated cardiomyopathy—may diminish effects of ACE inhibitors by blocking prostaglandin-induced vasodilatation; increased incidence of hospitalizations for heart failure has been found in patients receiving aspirin

✓ Current recommendation for aspirin use in dilated cardiomyopathy—use in patients with heart failure and coronary artery disease

✓ Heart transplant—procedure of choice for dilated cardiomyopathy with severe, refractory symptoms

---

Heart Failure With Preserved Ejection Fraction

Approximately half of hospitalized patients with newly diagnosed heart failure have a normal ejection fraction. Many of these patients have contractile abnormalities that could be identified by more sophisticated evaluation techniques, but ejection fraction is the most widely available measure of systolic function and remains the standard. Heart failure with preserved ejection fraction is a heterogeneous group of disorders and includes hypertrophic and restrictive cardiomyopathies, infiltrative cardiac disorders, and constrictive pericarditis.

Many patients have a history of hypertension. Some have fairly normal diastolic filling properties at rest, but exertional hypertension, ischemia, or both cause deterioration of diastolic filling properties, resulting in increased filling pressure. Others have abnormal baseline diastolic compliance with superimposed volume overload, which increases diastolic filling pressures. Other patients have exuberant heart rate responses to exercise with inadequate diastolic filling periods, and others rely on the atrial contribution to ventricular filling and suffer when atrial fibrillation develops. Some patients have low output due to severe regurgitant valve disease (including severe tricuspid regurgitation) or bradycardia. Severe occult renal insufficiency is also a common finding in this condition.

It is important to try to understand the mechanism of diastolic dysfunction in any given patient to tailor the most effective treatment, which might include some combination of antihypertensive or coronary revascularization strategies, diuretic treatment, ventricular rate slowing or support (pacemaker), restoration of sinus rhythm, valvular intervention, or renal replacement therapy. Morbidity and mortality in this group of patients are high, approaching the rates in patients with reduced ejection fraction.

Hypertrophic Cardiomyopathy

Hypertrophic cardiomyopathy is a rare (approximately 0.2% prevalence in the general population), heterogeneous group of disorders characterized by increased thickness of the ventricle and preserved ejection fraction. The hypertrophy may be regional (involving the septum, mid left ventricle, or apex) or concentric. Obstruction may occur in the left ventricular outflow tract or mid-ventricular cavity. Diagnosis is based on increased myocardial wall thickness on echocardiogram in the absence of an underlying cause such as hypertension, aortic stenosis, chronic renal failure, or infiltrative disease. Because of its hereditary nature, first-degree relatives of patients should be screened, and genetic counseling is advised for patients considering childbearing.

> ### Key Definition
>
> Hypertrophic cardiomyopathy: *a rare, heterogeneous group of disorders characterized by increased thickness of the ventricle and preserved ejection fraction.*

Symptoms

Hypertrophic cardiomyopathy appears to have a bimodal distribution of age at presentation. Affected young males (typically teens or early 20s) often present with syncope and sudden death. Recently, an X-linked variant known as *LAMP2* cardiomyopathy (Danon disease) was described in young patients. Affected older patients (sixth and seventh decades of life) typically present with shortness of breath and angina and may have a better prognosis than young patients. The classic presentation in the younger group is a young athlete undergoing a physical examination found

to have a heart murmur or left ventricular hypertrophy on ECG. The classic presentation in the older group is an older woman who has development of pulmonary edema after noncardiac surgery and worsening with diuresis, afterload reduction, and inotropic support (due to worsening dynamic left ventricular outflow tract obstruction). The classic symptom triad is syncope, angina, and dyspnea. The symptoms are similar to those of valvular aortic stenosis. The per-year frequency of evolution from hypertrophic to dilated cardiomyopathy is 1.5%. This may reflect either the natural history or a superimposed secondary process such as ischemia. The treatment of a "burnt-out hypertrophic" is then the same as that of other dilated cardiomyopathies.

Pathophysiology

Signs and symptoms of hypertrophic cardiomyopathy are caused by 4 major abnormalities: diastolic dysfunction, left ventricular outflow tract obstruction, mitral regurgitation, and ventricular arrhythmias.

Diastolic dysfunction is caused by many mechanisms, including marked abnormalities in calcium metabolism (abnormal ventricular relaxation), high afterload due to left ventricular tract obstruction (also delays ventricular relaxation), and severe hypertrophy and increased muscle mass (decreased compliance). Diastolic dysfunction leads to increased left ventricular diastolic pressure, angina, and dyspnea. Coronary microvascular dysfunction also contributes to angina and dyspnea. In many patients, dynamic left ventricular tract obstruction is caused by the hypertrophied septum encroaching into the left ventricular outflow tract. Subsequently, the anterior leaflet of the mitral valve is "sucked in" (systolic anterior motion), and left ventricular outflow tract obstruction is created. Because of this pathophysiologic process, dynamic outflow tract obstruction increases dramatically with decreased preload, decreased afterload, or increased contractility.

Systolic anterior motion of the mitral valve distorts the mitral valve apparatus during systole and may cause considerable mitral regurgitation. Thus, the degree of mitral regurgitation is also dynamically influenced by the degree of left ventricular outflow tract obstruction. Patients with severe mitral regurgitation usually have severe symptoms of dyspnea. Cellular disorganization leads to abnormalities in the conduction system; thus, patients are prone to ventricular arrhythmias. Frequent ventricular arrhythmias may cause sudden death or syncope.

Left ventricular outflow tract obstruction and mitral regurgitation are caused by distortion of the mitral valve apparatus (systolic anterior motion), and they are dynamically influenced by preload, afterload, and contractility.

Examination

The carotid artery upstroke and left ventricular impulse are abnormal in patients with hypertrophic cardiomyopathy. The carotid artery upstroke is more rapid than that in aortic stenosis. If left ventricular outflow tract obstruction is extensive, the carotid artery upstroke has a bifid quality. In the setting of considerable left ventricular hypertrophy, the left ventricular impulse is sustained and there is often a palpable *a* wave. The first heart sound is normal, but the second heart sound is paradoxically split. Patients with excessive left ventricular outflow tract obstruction may have a triple apical impulse and a loud systolic ejection murmur. The murmur changes in intensity with changes in loading conditions (Box 6.5). A holosystolic murmur of mitral regurgitation may be present; it increases in intensity with increases in the dynamic left ventricular outflow tract obstruction.

Maneuvers affect the mitral regurgitant murmur of hypertrophic obstructive cardiomyopathy differently than other mitral regurgitant murmurs. When mitral regurgitation is *not* due to hypertrophic obstructive cardiomyopathy, the murmur increases with increasing afterload and varies little with changes in contractility and preload. When mitral regurgitation *is* due to hypertrophic cardiomyopathy, increased afterload decreases the dynamic left ventricular outflow obstruction and thus the degree of mitral regurgitation. In patients with hypertrophic cardiomyopathy with obstruction, the intensity of the ejection murmur increases, whereas the arterial pulse volume *decreases* on

the beat following a premature ventricular contraction (the Brockenbrough sign) as a result of postectopic increased contractility and decreased afterload, resulting in more dynamic obstruction. These changes differ from those in patients with fixed left ventricular outflow tract obstruction (eg, aortic stenosis) in whom *both* the murmur intensity and the pulse volume increase with the beat following a premature ventricular contraction.

Diagnostic Testing

A marked left ventricular hypertrophy pattern on ECG (Figure 6.6) is usually seen in patients with hypertrophic cardiomyopathy, whereas patients with apical hypertrophy have deep, symmetric T-wave inversions across the precordium (Figure 6.7). ECG abnormalities may precede echocardiographic abnormalities; thus, surveillance echocardiography is appropriate in patients with suspicious ECG results.

Echocardiography shows severe hypertrophy of the myocardium (left ventricular wall thickness >16 mm in diastole) without any other identified cause. Hypertrophy may be in any part of the myocardium. Doppler echocardiography can be used to diagnose left ventricular outflow tract obstruction, measure its severity, and detect mitral regurgitation. Cardiac catheterization is no longer necessary to diagnose dynamic left ventricular outflow tract obstruction.

Patients with hypertrophic cardiomyopathy may have sudden death. Because of the strong association between ventricular arrhythmias and sudden death, 48- to 72-hour Holter monitoring is recommended for all patients with hypertrophic cardiomyopathy. Predictors of sudden death include a personal or family history of sudden death, severe left ventricular hypertrophy, ventricular tachycardia on Holter monitoring or electrophysiologic study, and history of syncope. Genetic markers may identify patients with a strong propensity for sudden death. In some patients, carefully supervised stress testing may be indicated to search for induced ventricular tachycardia, to determine exercise tolerance, and to evaluate the variables contributing to symptoms.

Treatment

Symptomatic Patients

For symptomatic patients, initial treatment is with drugs that decrease contractility in an attempt to decrease left ventricular outflow tract obstruction (Figure 6.8). The most effective medication is a high dose of β-blockers (equivalent of >240 mg propranolol/day). Although verapamil may be used if β-adrenergic blockade fails, it may cause sudden hemodynamic deterioration in patients with high resting left ventricular outflow tract gradients because of its vasodilating properties. Disopyramide may improve symptoms by decreasing left ventricular outflow tract obstruction, but anticholinergic

---

Box 6.5 · Dynamic Left Ventricular Outflow Tract Obstruction

Increased obstruction

    Decreased afterload

        Amyl nitrite

        Vasodilators

    Increased contractility

        Postpremature ventricular contraction beat

        Digoxin

        Dopamine

    Decreased preload

        Squat-to-stand

        Nitrates

        Diuretics

        Valsalva maneuver (strain phase)

Decreased obstruction

    Increased afterload

        Handgrip

        Stand-to-squat

    Decreased contractility

        β-Adrenergic blockers

        Verapamil

        Disopyramide

    Increased preload

        Fluids

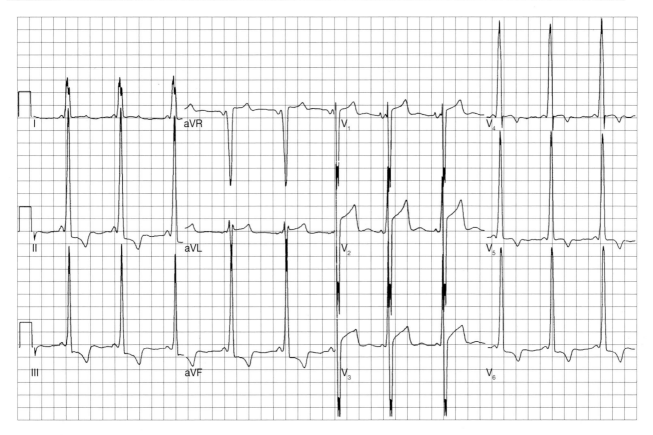

Figure 6.6 *Electrocardiogram in Hypertrophic Cardiomyopathy. Marked left ventricular hypertrophy is noted.*

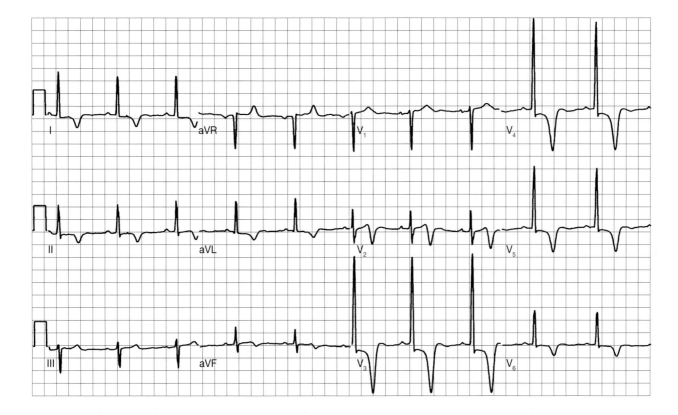

Figure 6.7 *Electrocardiogram in Apical Hypertrophic Cardiomyopathy. Deep, symmetric T-wave inversions are shown in precordial leads.*

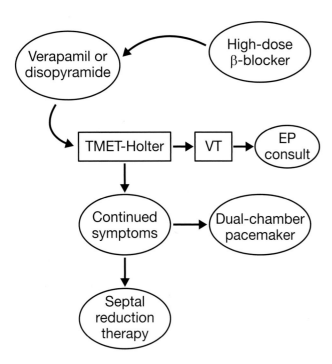

Figure 6.8 Treatment of Symptomatic Hypertrophic Cardiomyopathy. EP indicates electrophysiologic; TMET, treadmill exercise test; VT, ventricular tachycardia.

adverse effects limit its use. All drugs that reduce afterload or preload and those that increase contractility *must* be avoided in patients with hypertrophic cardiomyopathy. Diuretics may be cautiously used for volume-overloaded states.

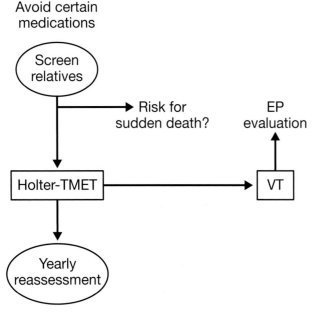

Figure 6.9 Treatment of Asymptomatic Hypertrophic Cardiomyopathy. EP indicates electrophysiologic; TMET, treadmill exercise test; VT, ventricular tachycardia.

Asymptomatic Patients

Asymptomatic patients should be assessed for risk of sudden cardiac death. Treatment of asymptomatic nonsustained ventricular tachycardia is controversial (Figure 6.9). No antiarrhythmic agent is uniformly effective, and any agent may make the arrhythmia worse. In select patients with multiple risk factors for sudden death, empiric implantation of a cardiac defibrillator may be chosen. In patients who have had an out-of-hospital arrest, the treatment of choice is an implantable cardiac defibrillator.

KEY FACTS

✓ Heart failure with preserved ejection fraction—about half of hospitalized patients with newly diagnosed heart failure have a normal ejection fraction

✓ Hypertrophic cardiomyopathy—affected young males often present with syncope and sudden death

✓ ECG findings in hypertrophic cardiomyopathy— marked left ventricular hypertrophy pattern is usually seen (deep, asymmetric T-wave inversions across the precordium are seen in apical hypertrophy)

✓ ECG abnormalities in hypertrophic cardiomyopathy— may precede echocardiographic abnormalities and thus surveillance echocardiography is appropriate in patients with suspicious ECG results

✓ Recommendation for all patients with hypertrophic cardiomyopathy—affected patients may have sudden death; because of the strong association between ventricular arrhythmias and sudden death, 48- to 72-hour Holter monitoring is recommended

Restrictive Cardiomyopathy

Diastolic dysfunction is the primary abnormality in restrictive cardiomyopathy and is usually due to abnormal relaxation, abnormal ventricular filling, and ineffectual atrial contribution to filling, which in turn affect the pulmonary and systemic circulations, causing shortness of breath and edema. In addition, because the ventricle cannot fill adequately to meet its preload requirements, low cardiac output (Starling mechanism), fatigue, and lethargy result. Normal or near-normal left ventricular ejection fraction and volumes are present in most patients with restrictive cardiomyopathy.

The cause of primary restrictive cardiomyopathy is unknown. The 2 major categories are idiopathic restrictive cardiomyopathy and endomyocardial fibrosis. Progressive fibrosis of the myocardium occurs in idiopathic restrictive cardiomyopathy. Familial cases, often with associated peripheral myopathy, have been reported. Endomyocardial fibrosis is probably an end stage of eosinophilic syndromes in which there is intracavitary thrombus filling of the left ventricle. This restricts filling and causes increased diastolic pressures. Fibrosis also may involve the mitral valve, causing severe mitral regurgitation. There may be 2 different forms of endomyocardial fibrosis: active inflammatory eosinophilic myocarditis (temperate zones) and chronic endomyocardial fibrosis (tropical zones).

Infiltration diseases involving the myocardium (eg, amyloidosis) have a presentation and pathophysiology similar to those of primary restrictive cardiomyopathy. Signs and symptoms similar to those of restrictive cardiomyopathy also may develop after radiation therapy and anthracycline chemotherapy. Although other infiltrative diseases (eg, sarcoidosis, hemochromatosis) initially may mimic restrictive cardiomyopathy, they usually progress to a dilated cardiomyopathy by the time they cause cardiac symptoms.

Signs and Symptoms

Patients with restrictive cardiomyopathy usually present with symptoms of right heart failure such as edema, dyspnea, and ascites. Atrial arrhythmias due to passive atrial enlargement are frequently present, and the patient may present with atrial fibrillation. Jugular venous pressure is almost always increased, with rapid *x* and *y* descents. The precordium is quiet, and heart sounds are soft. There may be an apical systolic murmur of mitral regurgitation and a left sternal border murmur of tricuspid regurgitation. A third heart sound may be present. Dullness at the bases of the lungs is consistent with bilateral pleural effusions. ECG is usually low or normal voltage with atrial arrhythmias. Chest radiography may show pleural effusions with a normal cardiac silhouette or atrial enlargement.

Diagnosis

Restrictive cardiomyopathy is diagnosed with echocardiography. Typical findings are normal left ventricular cavity size, preserved ejection fraction, and marked biatrial enlargement. In the setting of right heart failure, the inferior vena cava is enlarged. In amyloid heart disease, echocardiography demonstrates thickened myocardium with a scintillating appearance, a pericardial effusion, and thickened regurgitant valves. In endomyocardial fibrosis, there is an apical thrombus (without underlying apical akinesis) or thickening of the endocardium under the mitral

valve, which often tethers the valve, causing mitral regurgitation. Other causes of restrictive cardiomyopathy have nonspecific echocardiographic features. Cardiac catheterization shows increase and end-equalization of all end-diastolic pressures. A typical "square-root sign" or "dip-and-plateau" pattern consistent with early rapid filling is present. Endomyocardial biopsy usually is not helpful, except to confirm the diagnosis of amyloidosis.

Treatment

Treatment of idiopathic restrictive cardiomyopathy is usually symptom-based. Diuretics decrease filling pressures and give symptomatic relief, but these effects may be at the expense of further decreasing cardiac output. Heart transplant is the only proven therapy for patients with severe restrictive cardiomyopathy. Corticosteroids are appropriate during the early stages of eosinophilic endocarditis. Endomyocardial fibrosis can be surgically resected and the mitral valve can be replaced, although mortality is significant.

It is important to differentiate restrictive cardiomyopathy from constrictive pericarditis. Both have similar presentations and findings on clinical examination and diagnostic studies. However, in constrictive pericarditis, pericardiectomy produces symptomatic improvement and, frequently, survival. Therefore, exploratory thoracotomy may be indicated in patients with normal left ventricular systolic function, large atria, and severe increase of diastolic filling pressures if doubt remains after anatomical (computed tomography or magnetic resonance imaging) and other tests (echocardiography, cardiac catheterization).

KEY FACTS

✓ Severe restrictive cardiomyopathy—heart transplant is the only proven therapy

✓ Restrictive cardiomyopathy and constrictive pericarditis—differentiation of these 2 conditions is important; they have similar presentations and findings on clinical examination and diagnostic studies, but, in constrictive pericarditis, pericardiectomy produces symptomatic improvement and, frequently, survival

Hypertension

C. SCOTT COLLINS, MD AND CHRISTOPHER M. WITTICH, MD, PharmD

Definition

Hypertension is the most common condition seen in primary care. Hypertension can lead to myocardial infarction, stroke, renal failure, and death if not adequately treated. A normal blood pressure is defined as less than 120/80 mm Hg. Prehypertension is defined as a blood pressure of 120–139/80–89 mm Hg. Stage 1 hypertension is a blood pressure of 140–159/90–99 mm Hg, and stage 2 hypertension is a blood pressure of 160 or more/100 or more mm Hg (Table 7.1).

Initial Evaluation

Initial evaluation of hypertension should focus on 1) determining contributing lifestyle and genetic risk factors,

2) ordering basic laboratory tests, 3) identifying and treating secondary causes of hypertension, and 4) identifying target organ damage.

Lifestyle and Individual Risk Factors

Lifestyle risk factors include family history of hypertension, African American race, obesity, physical inactivity, excess sodium and alcohol intake, dyslipidemia, and type A personality traits.

Basic Laboratory Testing

Laboratory testing in the initial evaluation of hypertension is aimed at looking for end-organ damage. This should include complete blood count, urinalysis, glucose, creatinine, electrolytes, lipid profile, and electrocardiography.

Secondary Causes of Hypertension

Causes of secondary hypertension and key features of each condition are listed in Table 7.2. Physical examination and history should be tailored to ruling out these diseases.

Target Organ Damage

Target organ damage that can occur as a result of hypertension is summarized in Table 7.3. Organs typically involved include the heart, brain, kidney, arteries, and eye. Physical examination should focus on these organs, looking for signs of heart failure, vascular disease, and retinopathy.

Treatment

Goals of Treatment

The goal of therapy for hypertension is to eliminate the morbidity and mortality of disease attributable to long-standing hypertension. Blood pressure treatment targets

Table 7.1 • Classification of Blood Pressure for Adults 18 Years or Older[a]

Category	Blood Pressure, mm Hg		
	Systolic		Diastolic
Normal	<120	and	<80
Prehypertension	120–139	or	80–89
Hypertension			
Stage 1	140–159	or	90–99
Stage 2	≥160	or	≥100

[a] Not taking antihypertensive drugs and not acutely ill. When a patient's systolic and diastolic blood pressures are in different categories, the higher category should be selected to classify the blood pressure status.

Adapted from Chobanian AV, Bakris GL, Black HR, Cushman WC, Green LA, Izzo JL Jr, et al; Joint National Committee on Prevention, Detection, Evaluation, and Treatment of High Blood Pressure. National Heart, Lung, and Blood Institute; National High Blood Pressure Education Program Coordinating Committee. Seventh report of the Joint National Committee on Prevention, Detection, Evaluation, and Treatment of High Blood Pressure. Hypertension. 2003 Dec;42(6):1206–52. Epub 2003 Dec 1. Used with permission.

Table 7.2 • Secondary Causes of Hypertension

Cause	Key Features
Endocrine	
Pheochromocytoma	Presents with headaches, diaphoresis, and palpitations If appropriate, screen with plasma metanephrine value
Primary aldosteronism	Presents with hypokalemia and HTN If appropriate, screen with aldosterone-renin ratio
Cushing disease	Presents with hyperglycemia, hypokalemia, and HTN If appropriate, screen with 24-hour urinary cortisol value
Hyperparathyroidism	Screen with serum calcium value
Hypothyroidism	Presents with diastolic HTN
Cardiac	
Coarctation of the aorta	Examine for weak, delayed, or absent femoral pulse Rib notching on chest radiography
Obstructive sleep apnea	Presents in overweight persons with loud snoring, large neck circumference, morning headaches, and daytime sleepiness Confirm diagnosis with polysomnography
Renal	
Renal artery stenosis	Presents in smokers, persons with CAD, or new-onset HTN after age 50 years Examine for high-pitched systolic-diastolic abdominal bruit
Fibromuscular dysplasia	Presents in females, usually younger than age 30 years without family history of HTN
Renal parenchymal disease	Check creatinine value and results of urinalysis

Abbreviations: CAD, coronary artery disease; HTN, hypertension.

Adapted from Chobanian AV, Bakris GL, Black HR, Cushman WC, Green LA, Izzo JL Jr, et al; Joint National Committee on Prevention, Detection, Evaluation, and Treatment of High Blood Pressure. National Heart, Lung, and Blood Institute; National High Blood Pressure Education Program Coordinating Committee. Seventh report of the Joint National Committee on Prevention, Detection, Evaluation, and Treatment of High Blood Pressure. Hypertension. 2003 Dec;42(6):1206–52. Epub 2003 Dec 1. Used with permission.

for adults aged 18 years or older have been defined in the eighth report of the Joint National Committee (JNC 8). It is noteworthy that the JNC 8 committee did not redefine hypertension, and our definitions in this chapter are based on the JNC 7 report. In the hypertension management algorithm of the JNC 8 (Figure 7.1), adults are divided into 2 groups: 1) the general population and 2) those with diabetes or chronic kidney disease (CKD) present. Once divided, adults in the general population who are younger than 60 years have a blood pressure goal of less than 140/90 mm Hg. Those 60 or older have a blood pressure goal of less than 150/90 mm Hg. Adults of all ages with diabetes and CKD have a blood pressure goal of less than 140/90 mm Hg.

Lifestyle Modification

Lifestyle modifications (Table 7.4) are the initial step for any patient found to have prehypertension, stage 1 hypertension, or stage 2 hypertension. The modifications may be sufficient as initial therapy for some persons. They are adjunctive therapy for those with continued hypertension and should be continued throughout hypertension management.

Pharmacologic Treatment

The JNC 8 report recommends initiation of medication therapy in patients in whom lifestyle modifications are inadequate to reach their desired blood pressure goal. Initial medication recommendations are based on age, race, compelling indications, and diabetes or CKD status (Figure 7.1).

In the general population, nonblack patients and diabetic patients without CKD should be started on a thiazide diuretic, angiotensin-converting enzyme inhibitor, angiotensin receptor blocker, or calcium channel blocker, alone or in combination, as initial therapy. Black patients with or without diabetes and without CKD should be given a thiazide diuretic or calcium channel blocker alone or in combination as initial therapy. All patients regardless of race who have CKD should have an angiotensin-converting enzyme inhibitor or angiotensin receptor blocker used as initial therapy alone or with another drug class.

KEY FACTS

✓ Hypertension—most common condition seen in primary care; can lead to myocardial infarction, stroke, renal failure, and death if not adequately treated

✓ Target organ damage in hypertension—typically involves heart, brain, kidneys, arteries, and eye

✓ Treatment of hypertension—blood pressure goal for adults in the general population <60 years old is <140/90 mm Hg, and blood pressure goal for adults ≥60 years old is <150/90 mm Hg. Adults of all ages with diabetes and CKD have blood pressure goal of <140/90 mm Hg

✓ Treatment of hypertension—nonblack patients and diabetic patients without CKD should be started on a thiazide diuretic, angiotension-converting enzyme inhibitor, angiotensin receptor blocker, or calcium channel blocker, alone or in combination, as initial therapy

✓ Treatment of hypertension—black patients with or without diabetes and without CKD should be given a thiazide diuretic or calcium channel blocker alone or in combination as initial therapy

Table 7.3 • Hypertensive Target Organ Injury

Target Organ	Injury	Clinical Marker/Diagnosis
Heart	Left ventricular hypertrophy	S_4 gallop, forceful and prolonged apical thrust Displacement of point of maximal intensity Chest radiography, ECG, echocardiography
	Angina Prior myocardial infarction Prior revascularization	History, ECG
	Heart failure (systolic or diastolic)	History Lung rales S_3 gallop Edema Chest radiography, echocardiography
Brain	Stroke Leukoaraiosis Transient ischemic attack Dementia	History CT or MRI History History Cognitive testing
Kidney	Chronic kidney disease	Creatinine, serum urea nitrogen, urinalysis, eGFR
Arteries	Peripheral artery disease	History of claudication Bruits Diminished pulses
Eye	Retinopathy	Funduscopic examination: Generalized and focal arteriolar narrowing "Copper wiring" of arterioles Arteriovenous nicking Cotton-wool spots Microaneurysms and macroaneurysms Flame and blot-shaped retinal hemorrhages Retinal vein occlusion Optic disc swelling

Abbreviations: CT, computed tomography; ECG, electrocardiography; eGFR, estimated glomerular filtration rate; MRI, magnetic resonance imaging; S_3, third heart sound; S_4, fourth heart sound.

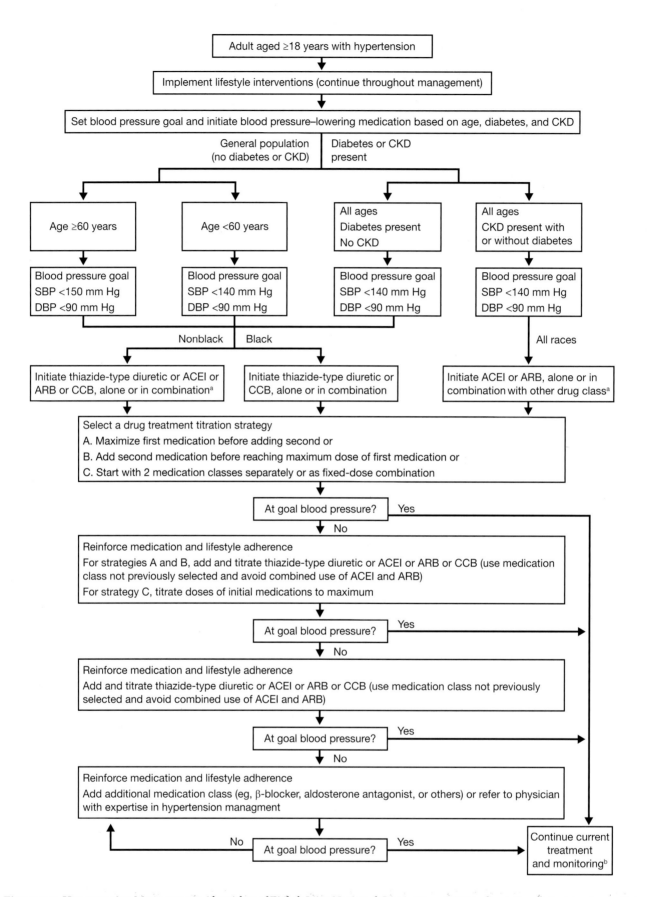

Figure 7.1 *Hypertension Management Algorithm of Eighth Joint National Committee. ACEI indicates angiotensin-converting enzyme inhibitor; ARB, angiotensin receptor blocker; CCB, calcium channel blocker; CKD, chronic kidney disease; DBP, diastolic blood pressure; SBP, systolic blood pressure. [a] ACEIs and ARBs should not be used in combination. [b] If blood pressure fails to be maintained at goal, reenter the algorithm where appropriate based on the current individual therapeutic plan.* (Adapted from James PA, Oparil S, Carter BL, Cushman WC, Dennison-Himmelfarb C, Handler J, et al. 2014 evidence-based guideline for the management of high blood pressure in adults: report from the panel members appointed to the Eighth Joint National Committee [JNC 8]. JAMA. 2014 Feb 5;311[5]:507–20. Erratum in: JAMA. 2014 May 7;311[17]:1809. Used with permission.)

Table 7.4 • Effect of Lifestyle Modifications on Systolic Blood Pressure

Modification	Recommendation	Expected Decrease in Systolic Blood Pressure, mm Hg[a]
Adopt DASH eating plan	Consume a diet rich in fruits, vegetables, and low-fat dairy products with a reduced content of saturated and total fat	8–14
Reduce weight	Normal body weight (BMI, 18.5–24.9)	5–20 (per 10 kg)
Restrict dietary sodium	Restrict daily sodium intake to ≤2.4 g (6 g sodium chloride)	2–8
Increase physical activity	Regular aerobic exercise (eg, brisk walking for 30 min) most days of the week	4–9
Limit alcohol intake	For most men: ≤2 drinks daily (30 mL alcohol) For women: ≤1 drink daily	2–4

Abbreviations: BMI, body mass index; DASH, Dietary Approaches to Stop Hypertension.

[a] Effects on blood pressure may be greater in some individuals.

Adapted from Chobanian AV, Bakris GL, Black HR, Cushman WC, Green LA, Izzo JL Jr, et al; Joint National Committee on Prevention, Detection, Evaluation, and Treatment of High Blood Pressure. National Heart, Lung, and Blood Institute; National High Blood Pressure Education Program Coordinating Committee. Seventh report of the Joint National Committee on Prevention, Detection, Evaluation, and Treatment of High Blood Pressure. Hypertension. 2003 Dec;42(6):1206–52. Epub 2003 Dec 1. Used with permission.

Secondary Hypertension

Secondary causes of hypertension should be considered when there is an unusual age at onset, when there is a sudden change in blood pressure, and when hypertension is refractory to treatment.

Renovascular Hypertension

Renovascular hypertension is a potentially curable form of secondary hypertension. Generally, renovascular hypertension can be grouped into 1) renal artery stenosis and 2) fibromuscular dysplasia.

Clues that suggest renovascular hypertension include lack of a family history of hypertension, onset of hypertension before age 30 years (consider fibromuscular dysplasia, especially in white women), onset of hypertension after age 50 years (consider atherosclerotic renovascular disease, especially in a smoker or a person with coronary or peripheral arterial disease), or presentation with accelerated hypertension.

The most important physical finding is an abdominal bruit, especially a high-pitched systolic-diastolic bruit in the upper abdomen or flank. However, 50% of persons with renovascular hypertension do not have this finding.

Options for the management of renovascular hypertension include interventional therapies when feasible and medical therapy for persons who are not candidates for interventions. Percutaneous transluminal angioplasty is the treatment of choice for amenable lesions caused by fibromuscular dysplasia and is an option in some cases of atherosclerotic renovascular disease. The medical treatment of renovascular hypertension is similar to that of essential hypertension.

Renal Parenchymal Disease

Renal parenchymal disease is a common secondary cause of hypertension. The major mechanisms of hypertension in renal disease include volume expansion from impaired renal elimination of salt and water, oversecretion of renin, and decreased production of renal vasodilators. Angiotensin-converting enzyme inhibitors and angiotensin receptor blockers reduce proteinuria and high glomerular transcapillary pressures, slowing further loss of renal function. However, they can cause hyperkalemia and an acute decline in renal function. Modest acute decreases in renal function (<30%) should be tolerated because they are often followed by stabilization and preservation of renal function. Calcium channel blockers are effective blood pressure–lowering agents in persons with CKD. It is important to note that nondihydropyridine calcium channel blockers reduce proteinuria, but dihydropyridine calcium channel blockers do not.

Primary Aldosteronism

The syndrome of primary aldosteronism is characterized by overproduction of aldosterone by the adrenal glands leading to hypertension, hypokalemia, alkalosis, hyperglycemia, and increased aldosterone levels. Prevalence estimates range from 2% to 15% of the hypertensive population.

Primary aldosteronism should be suspected in hypertensive patients who have spontaneous hypokalemia or marked hypokalemia precipitated by usual doses of diuretics. However, in many patients with primary aldosteronism, the potassium level is normal. Additionally, it should be suspected in those with an adrenal mass, a history of early-onset hypertension, or a first-degree relative with primary aldosteronism.

Screening for primary aldosteronism is done using the aldosterone-renin ratio. This should be measured when the patient is not taking any aldosterone-blocking medications. In essential hypertension, the average value of the ratio is 5.5.

A ratio more than 15 to 20 suggests the diagnosis of primary aldosteronism.

Treatment of primary aldosteronism can involve spironolactone, eplerenone, other antihypertensive medications, or surgery.

Pheochromocytoma

Pheochromocytoma is a tumor that causes hypertension due to excess catecholamines. Pheochromocytoma is rare; its incidence is 2 to 8 cases per million persons per year. The prevalence is 0.5% among persons with hypertension.

A "rule of 10" describes the typical locations of pheochromocytomas: 10% are extra-adrenal; 10% of extra-adrenal gland tumors are extra-abdominal; 10% occur in children; 10% are multiple or bilateral; 10% recur after the initial resection; 10% are malignant; 10% are found in persons without hypertension; and 10% are familial.

Patients can present with paroxysms of hypertension, but most have sustained hypertension. Paroxysms can be associated with headache, diaphoresis, and palpitations. The presentation of pheochromocytoma corresponds to 5 Ps: *pressure, pain, palpitations, perspiration,* and *pallor*. Patients can also present with symptoms mimicking an anxiety attack. Additionally, pheochromocytomas can be discovered as an incidental adrenal mass on an imaging study.

Pheochromocytoma is associated with multiple endocrine neoplasia 2A (medullary thyroid carcinoma, pheochromocytoma, and parathyroid tumors), multiple endocrine neoplasia 2B (medullary thyroid cancer, pheochromocytoma, and neuroma), neurofibromatosis, von Hippel-Lindau disease (pheochromocytoma, retinal hemangiomatosis, cerebellar hemangioblastomas, epididymal cystadenoma, renal and pancreatic cysts, and renal cell carcinoma), and familial paraganglioma syndrome.

Diagnosis of pheochromocytoma consists of biochemical confirmation with 24-hour urine collection to measure fractionated metanephrines and fractionated catecholamines and blood testing to measure plasma levels of fractionated metanephrines.

Computed tomography or magnetic resonance imaging of the abdomen and pelvis is the initial test used to locate a tumor after biochemical testing has confirmed the presence of the disorder. Treatment is surgical. Preoperatively, administration of a phenoxybenzamine is needed to control blood pressure and cardiac rhythm. Because pheochromocytomas can recur in 10% of cases, long-term biochemical follow-up is required.

Coarctation of the Aorta

Coarctation of the aorta is a constriction of the vessel usually just beyond the takeoff of the left subclavian artery. It is usually detected in childhood when blood pressure in the upper extremities is increased and blood pressure in the lower extremities is low. Weak or delayed lower extremity pulses can also be present. Patients can experience signs of lower extremity claudication. Dilated collateral vessels can cause bruits and characteristic rib notching on chest radiography. Treatment is surgical repair.

Obstructive Sleep Apnea

Obstructive sleep apnea is associated with hypertension that may be severe and resistant to control. Upper body obesity is a risk factor for obstructive sleep apnea and is common in hypertensive persons. Consider the diagnosis of obstructive sleep apnea in persons who are overweight, snore loudly, have a large neck circumference, and complain of morning headaches and daytime sleepiness.

Other Causes of Hypertension

Cushing syndrome should be considered in the hypertensive person who has impaired fasting glucose and unexplained hypokalemia.

Hypothyroidism is associated with diastolic hypertension due to decreased cardiac output and contractility. Tissue perfusion is maintained by an increase in peripheral vascular resistance mediated by increased activity of the sympathetic nervous system.

Hyperparathyroidism may increase blood pressure directly via hypercalcemia, which increases peripheral vascular resistance, and indirectly by increasing vascular sensitivity to catecholamines.

KEY FACTS

✓ Clues that suggest renovascular hypertension—lack of family history of hypertension, onset of hypertension before age 30 years (consider fibromuscular dysplasia, especially in white women), onset of hypertension after age 50 years (consider atherosclerotic renovascular disease, especially in a smoker or a person with coronary or peripheral arterial disease), or presentation with accelerated hypertension

✓ Primary aldosteronism—should be suspected in hypertensive patients who have spontaneous hypokalemia or marked hypokalemia precipitated by usual doses of diuretics

✓ Pheochromocytoma—presentation corresponds to 5 Ps: *pressure, pain, palpitations, perspiration,* and *pallor*

Special Cases of Hypertension

Pregnancy

Blood pressure typically decreases early in pregnancy (first 16–18 weeks) and then gradually increases. Hypertension during pregnancy is defined as a systolic blood pressure of 140 mm Hg or greater or diastolic blood pressure of 90 mm Hg or greater on 2 separate occasions. Hypertension during pregnancy is associated with increased neonatal morbidity and mortality.

Preeclampsia is defined as a blood pressure greater than 140/90 mm Hg and proteinuria (24-hour urine protein excretion >0.3 g) that develops after the 20th week of gestation. Eclampsia is defined by seizures that occur in the presence of preeclampsia and cannot be attributed to other causes. Patients with preeclampsia can also have headache, blurry vision, epigastric pain, nephrotic-range proteinuria (>3.5 g in 24 hours), oliguria, creatinine level greater than 1.2 mg/dL, low platelet count, evidence of microangiopathic hemolytic anemia (abnormal blood smear or increased lactate dehydrogenase value), increased liver transaminase values, and pulmonary edema.

Key Definition

Preeclampsia: *blood pressure >140/90 mm Hg and proteinuria (24-hour urine protein excretion >0.3 g) that develops after the 20th week of gestation.*

The HELLP syndrome (*h*emolysis, *e*levated *l*iver enzymes, and *l*ow *p*latelet count) occurs when intravascular coagulation and liver ischemia develop in preeclampsia. The HELLP syndrome can rapidly develop into a life-threatening disorder of liver failure and worsening thrombocytopenia in the presence of only mild or moderate hypertension. The most serious complication of the HELLP syndrome is liver rupture, which is associated with high maternal and fetal mortality.

Hypertensive Crisis

Hypertensive crisis can be subdivided into hypertensive urgency and emergency.

Hypertensive urgency is severe hypertension without evidence of acute target organ injury. It should be treated to decrease blood pressure to safer levels over 24 to 48 hours. This decrease can usually be achieved in the outpatient setting with oral agents.

Hypertensive emergency is severe hypertension with evidence of acute injury to target organs. It implies the need for hospitalization to immediately lower blood pressure with parenteral therapy. Parenteral medications such as sodium nitroprusside, nitroglycerin, clevidipine, nicardipine, fenoldopam, labetalol, esmolol, hydralazine, enalaprilat, and phentolamine are the drugs of choice that are available for hypertensive emergencies.

Key Definition

Hypertensive urgency: *severe hypertension without evidence of acute target organ injury.*

Hypertensive emergency: *severe hypertension with evidence of acute injury to target organs.*

---

8 Ischemic Heart Disease[a]

NANDAN S. ANAVEKAR, MB, BCH

Ischemic heart disease is cardiac disease that results in diminished myocardial blood supply and its attendant clinicopathologic manifestations. It may be clinically silent or present with syndromes categorized as stable angina, unstable angina, non–ST-elevation acute coronary syndrome, ST-elevation myocardial infarction (MI), or sudden death. Ischemic heart disease causes nearly 800,000 deaths annually. Notably, about a third of deaths annually in the United States are due to MI. Primary prevention and new treatments have led to a substantial decrease in death from acute MI since 1970 (Figure 8.1).

> ## Key Definition
>
> Ischemic heart disease: *cardiac disease that results in diminished myocardial blood supply and its attendant clinicopathologic manifestations.*

Prevention

The Framingham risk score is the most commonly used model to calculate the 10-year risk for development of ischemic heart disease (http://cvdrisk.nhlbi.nih.gov/calculator.asp). The score is derived from pre-specified risk factors: age, sex, low-density lipoprotein (LDL) cholesterol level, high-density lipoprotein (HDL) cholesterol level,

systemic blood pressure, diabetes mellitus, and smoking history (Circulation. 1998 May 12;97[18]:1837–47).

The risk factors for which interventions have been proved to reduce cardiac events include tobacco use, serum LDL cholesterol level, serum HDL cholesterol level, and hypertension (Box 8.1). Factors that clearly increase the risk

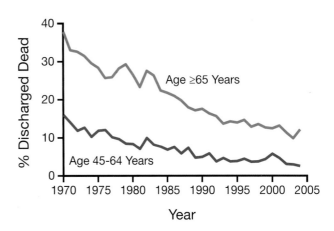

Figure 8.1 *Case-Fatality Rate for Acute Myocardial Infarction in the United States, 1970–2004.*

(Adapted from National Heart, Lung, and Blood Institute. Morbidity and mortality: 2007 chart book on cardiovascular, lung, and blood diseases. Bethesda [MD]: National Institutes of Health; c2007.)

---

[a] Portions previously published in Stone NJ, Robinson JG, Lichtenstein AH, Bairey Merz CN, Blum CB, Eckel RH, et al; American College of Cardiology/American Heart Association Task Force on Practice Guidelines. 2013 ACC/AHA guideline on the treatment of blood cholesterol to reduce atherosclerotic cardiovascular risk in adults: a report of the American College of Cardiology/American Heart Association Task Force on Practice Guidelines. Circulation. 2014 Jun 24;129(25 Suppl 2):S1–45. Epub 2013 Nov 12. Erratum in: Circulation. 2014 Jun 24;129(25 Suppl 2):S46–8 and Stone NJ, Robinson JG, Lichtenstein AH, Bairey Merz CN, Blum CB, Eckel RH, et al; American College of Cardiology/American Heart Association Task Force on Practice Guidelines. 2013 ACC/AHA guideline on the treatment of blood cholesterol to reduce atherosclerotic cardiovascular risk in adults: a report of the American College of Cardiology/American Heart Association Task Force on Practice Guidelines. J Am Coll Cardiol. 2014 Jul 1;63(25 Pt B):2889–934. Epub 2013 Nov 12. Erratum in: J Am Coll Cardiol. 2014 Jul 1;63(25 Pt B):3024–25. Used with permission.

Box 8.1 • Risk Factors for Ischemic Heart Disease

Modifiable Factor	Nonmodifiable Factor	Novel Factor
Increased LDL cholesterol level	Age	Inflammatory markers (eg, C-reactive protein)
Low HDL cholesterol level	Male sex	Small, dense LDL
Cigarette smoking	Family history of premature CAD[a]	Lipoprotein(a)
Hypertension		Homocysteine
Diabetes mellitus		Fibrinogen
Sedentary lifestyle		
Obesity		
Metabolic syndrome		
Stress and depression		
Socioeconomic factors		

Abbreviations: CAD, coronary artery disease; HDL, high-density lipoprotein; LDL, low-density lipoprotein.

[a] Age at onset <55 years in men and <65 years for primary relatives.

of ischemic heart disease and for which therapeutic interventions are likely to be effective include diabetes mellitus, physical inactivity, obesity, metabolic syndrome, and serum triglyceride levels. Factors for which intervention may improve subsequent risk include psychosocial factors (eg, anxiety and depression).

Smoking more than doubles the risk of ischemic heart disease and increases mortality by 50%. The relative risk in smokers who quit smoking decreases rapidly, approaching the level in nonsmokers within 2 to 3 years. Plasma levels of total and LDL cholesterol are important risk factors for ischemic heart disease. A 1% decrease in total serum cholesterol reduces risk by 2% to 3%. Lowering the LDL cholesterol level slows progression and may result in regression of coronary atherosclerosis. Lowering the LDL cholesterol level also prevents coronary events, possibly due to atherosclerotic plaque stabilization.

Hypertension is an important modifiable risk factor for coronary artery disease. Traditionally the goal of antihypertensive therapy is the prevention of atherosclerotic cardiovascular and renal complications. In a review of several thousand patients with hypertension treated before 1990, mainly with diuretics or β-adrenergic blockers (β-blockers) for a mean duration of 5 years, a reduction in systolic blood pressure of 10 to 12 mm Hg or in diastolic blood pressure of 5 to 6 mm Hg resulted in a decrease in incidences of stroke of 35% to 40%, coronary artery disease of 20% to 25%, congestive heart failure of 45% to 55%, and cardiovascular death of 20% to 25% (Lancet. 1999 Feb 20;353[9153]:611–6).

The risk for MI is decreased 35% to 55% with maintenance of an active vs a sedentary lifestyle. Adjusted mortality rates for ischemic heart disease are 2 to 3 times higher in men and 3 to 7 times higher in women with diabetes mellitus compared with the rates in men and women without diabetes. Heavy alcohol use increases the risk of ischemic heart disease, but moderate consumption decreases risk. Metabolic syndrome is present in 20% of

the US population, and it is associated with a twofold to threefold increase in mortality from cardiovascular disease. Aspirin is recommended for persons at intermediate risk for ischemic heart disease and at low risk for bleeding. This recommendation includes patients with an absolute risk of more than 15% over 10 years by Framingham score or patients with diabetes with a risk of more than 10% over 10 years. The role of aspirin in the primary prevention of stroke or overall cardiovascular *mortality* is uncertain. Estrogen replacement therapy is *not* indicated in women with cardiovascular disease, and it may be harmful.

Secondary prevention aims to prevent recurrent ischemic events in patients with known ischemic heart disease. Smoking cessation and optimum treatment of hyperlipidemia, hypertension, and diabetes mellitus are essential. Statins reduce ischemic events after MI more than would be expected from their effect on atherosclerosis progression alone, possibly due to stabilization of lipid-rich, rupture-prone plaques. Statins decrease overall mortality by 30% and coronary event-related mortality by 42% in patients with a prior MI and a high cholesterol level (>220 mg/dL). Statins reduce the risk for fatal heart disease or recurrent MI by 24% in patients with a prior MI and average levels of cholesterol (total cholesterol, <240 mg/dL; LDL, >125 mg/dL).

The clinical indications for cholesterol-lowering therapies were radically revised in the most recent American College of Cardiology/American Heart Association clinical guidelines (2013); the most striking changes were related to the dismissal of LDL cholesterol and non–HDL cholesterol target levels. Instead, a focus on the groups of patients that would benefit from pharmacologic therapies and categorizing therapies as high-, moderate-, or low-intensity, depending on the proportion of decrease in LDL cholesterol with therapy, has been the evidence-based recommendation. The pharmacologic therapy emphasizes statins as the mainstay of lipid-lowering therapies. With regard to the intensity of therapy, rather than focusing on cutoff targets for cholesterol levels, the current recommendations high-light high-intensity therapy as that which decreases LDL cholesterol by more than 50%, moderate-intensity therapy as that which decreases LDL cholesterol by 30% to 50%, and low-intensity therapy as that which decreases LDL cholesterol by less than 30%. These recommendations formulate 4 groups of patients who are deemed to benefit from lipid-lowering, specifically statin, therapy:

1. Patients with clinical atherosclerotic disease as defined by a prior history of MI, stable or unstable angina, history of coronary or other arterial revascularization, stroke or transient ischemic attack, or atherosclerotic peripheral vascular disease
2. Patients 21 years or older with primary elevations in LDL cholesterol 190 mg/dL or more
3. Patients between 40 and 75 years old with diabetes mellitus but without clinical atherosclerotic disease and an LDL cholesterol level of 70 to 189 mg/dL
4. Patients between 40 and 75 years old without atherosclerotic disease or diabetes mellitus but with an LDL cholesterol level of 70 to 189 mg/dL and an estimated 10-year risk of atherosclerotic heart disease of 7.5% or more

There are currently no evidence-based recommendations for or against specific LDL or non–HDL cholesterol targets for the primary or secondary prevention of atherosclerotic cardiovascular disease. For secondary prevention, high-intensity statin therapy should be initiated or continued as first-line therapy in women and men 75 years or younger who have clinical atherosclerotic heart disease, unless contraindicated. A moderate-intensity regimen may be reasonable in persons older than 75 years or who cannot tolerate the high-intensity regimen. For primary prevention in persons 21 years or older with an LDL cholesterol level of 190 mg/dL or more, statin therapy is indicated, and a high-intensity regimen or maximal tolerated dose is recommended, unless otherwise contraindicated. After maximum statin therapy has been achieved, addition of a nonstatin drug may be considered to further lower the level of LDL cholesterol, after evaluation of the potential for atherosclerotic cardiovascular disease risk-reduction benefits, adverse effects, and drug-drug interactions and after consideration of patient preferences. In persons with diabetes mellitus and an LDL cholesterol level of 70 to 189 mg/dL, moderate-intensity statin therapy should be initiated or continued for adults (40–75 years old). A high-intensity regimen is reasonable in patients with a 7.5% or more estimated 10-year risk of atherosclerotic heart disease. In adults with diabetes who are younger than 40 years or older than 75 years, it is reasonable to evaluate the potential for atherosclerotic cardiovascular disease benefits, adverse effects, and drug-drug interactions and to consider patient preferences.

Lifestyle changes, including a low-fat, low-cholesterol diet, weight management, and physical activity are essential for cholesterol lowering and remain in the background of management on which is superimposed the pharmacologic strategies mentioned above. Soluble fiber (10–25 g/day) and plant stanols or sterols (2 g/day) should be considered as therapeutic options.

Novel risk factors proposed for ischemic heart disease, especially in patients who do not have the conventional risk factors, include increased blood levels of lipoprotein(a), homocysteine, small, dense LDL particle (phenotype B), and fibrinogen. Additionally, acute and chronic inflammation and possibly lifetime exposure to pathogens (eg, *Chlamydia*, cytomegalovirus, and *Helicobacter*) have been proposed as potential factors in the pathophysiology of atherosclerosis.

KEY FACTS

✓ Ischemic heart disease—causes nearly 800,000 deaths annually

✓ MI—accounts for about a third of deaths annually in the United States

✓ Smoking—more than doubles the risk of ischemic heart disease and increases mortality by 50%

✓ Relative risk of ischemic heart disease in smokers who quit smoking—decreases rapidly and approaches the level in nonsmokers within 2 to 3 years

✓ Statins—

- reduce ischemic events after MI more than would be expected from their effect on atherosclerosis progression alone, possibly due to stabilization of lipid-rich, rupture-prone plaques

- decrease overall mortality by 30% and coronary event-related mortality by 42% in patients with a prior MI and a high cholesterol level (>220 mg/dL)

- reduce the risk for fatal heart disease or recurrent MI by 24% in patients with a prior MI and average levels of cholesterol (total cholesterol, <240 mg/dL; LDL, >125 mg/dL)

Mechanism of Atherosclerosis

The response-to-injury hypothesis is the most prevalent explanation of atherosclerosis. The stages of the process are as follows:

Stage I: Chronic injury to the arterial endothelium due to risk factors such as hypercholesterolemia, hypertension, diabetes mellitus, tobacco abuse, inflammation, and possibly infections

Stage II: Release of toxic products by macrophages, leading to platelet adhesion and smooth muscle cell migration and proliferation resulting in formation of fibrointimal lesions or lipid plaques

Stage III: Disruption of the lipid-rich plaque leads to thrombus formation. Acute coronary syndrome (unstable angina or MI) results from thrombus organization and atherosclerosis or vessel occlusion (Figure 8.2).

The most frequent site of atherosclerotic plaque disruption is lipid-laden coronary artery lesions with mild to moderate angiographic stenosis—not severely stenotic lesions.

The culprit lesion is at a site with less than 50% stenosis in up to two-thirds of cases of unstable angina or MI.

Chronic Stable Angina

Pathophysiology

A mismatch between myocardial oxygen demand and supply causes myocardial ischemia. Demand is determined

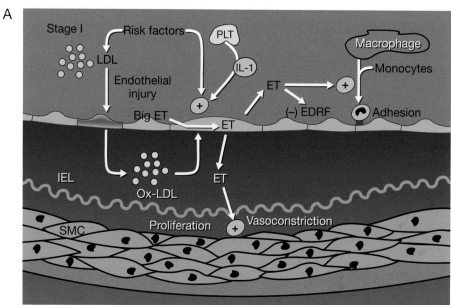

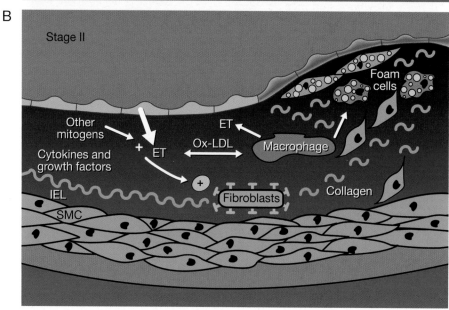

Figure 8.2 *Stages of Vascular Injury. A, Stage I. B, Stage II. Interaction of endothelin (ET) and the atherosclerotic plaque. EDRF indicates endothelium-derived relaxing factor; IEL, internal elastic lamina; IL-1, interleukin 1; LDL, low-density lipoprotein particles; Ox-LDL, oxidized LDL particles; PLT, platelet; SMC, smooth muscle cell. "+" indicates stimulation.*
(Adapted from Lerman A. The endothelium. In: Murphy JG, editor. Mayo Clinic cardiology review. 2nd ed. Philadelphia [PA]: Lippincott Williams & Wilkins; c2000. p. 99–112. Used with permission of Mayo Foundation for Medical Education and Research.)

by heart rate, contractility, and wall stress (determined by afterload and preload).

Normally, coronary blood flow can increase up to 5 times to meet effort-related increases in myocardial oxygen demands. The double product [(heart rate) × (systolic blood pressure)] is a useful index for quantifying myocardial oxygen demand. Ischemia occurs when flow reserve is inadequate, usually the result of fixed coronary artery disease.

Restriction of resting blood flow sufficient to cause resting ischemia does not occur unless vessel stenosis is more than 95%. However, decreased overall flow reserve begins to occur at about 60% vessel stenosis, and symptoms of exercise-induced ischemia may begin. The temporal sequence of events during ischemia are diastolic dysfunction→regional wall motion abnormalities→electrocar-diographic (ECG) changes→pain.

Clinical Presentation

Symptomatic Chronic Stable Coronary Artery Disease

Typical angina is characterized by retrosternal pain occurring with cardiovascular stress and relieved by rest or nitroglycerin. Atypical angina is defined by the presence of 2 of these 3 features. Noncardiac chest pain is defined by the presence of 1 or none of these features.

Angina may be precipitated by any activity that increases myocardial oxygen consumption. The pain or discomfort has various descriptions such as pressure, burning, stabbing, ache, hurt, or heaviness, or it may be described only as shortness of breath. It can be substernal or epigastric, and it may radiate to the neck, jaw, shoulder, back, elbow, or wrist. In stable angina, the pain lasts 2 to 30 minutes and is usually relieved by rest. Uncommon findings that may occur with ischemia include a fourth heart sound and mitral regurgitant murmur due to papillary muscle dysfunction. ST-segment depression may be found on the ECG, indicating subendocardial ischemia.

Silent Ischemia

Silent ischemia is common in patients with chronic stable coronary artery disease, with unstable angina, or after MI. Patients with diabetes may have silent ischemia, possibly due to neuropathy. It is also more common in the elderly. **Silent ischemia** is defined as the presence of dynamic ST-segment depression in the absence of symptoms. Medical therapy is similar to that for symptomatic ischemia. Whether percutaneous coronary intervention or coronary artery bypass grafting should be performed for silent ischemia in the absence of other markers of high risk is unknown. The prognosis for this condition is the same as that for symptomatic ischemia.

> ### Key Definition
>
> Silent ischemia: *the presence of dynamic ST-segment depression in the absence of symptoms.*

Testing in Ischemic Heart Disease

Ancillary testing for ischemic heart disease is strongly imaging-based and focuses on cardiac performance at rest and with stress, whether physical or chemically induced. The standard assessment for coronary artery disease remains invasive coronary angiography. The imaging studies that are commonly used in the evaluation of patients with ischemic heart disease include the following:

1. ECG: This study is inexpensive and is performed at the bedside. It assesses underlying rhythm. Voltage changes may indicate the presence of ventricular hypertrophy, and dynamic ST-segment changes may point to the presence of underlying ischemic heart disease. The ECG may be coupled with an exercise stress test to assess for dynamic ST-segment changes that may indicate stress-induced ischemia. The stress ECG is positive for ischemia if there is a flat or downsloping ST-segment depression of 1 mm or more with exertion, whereas it is uninterpretable when there is more than 1 mm of *resting* ST-segment depression, left bundle branch block, left ventricular hypertrophy, paced rhythm, or preexcitation (Wolff-Parkinson-White syndrome). Digoxin therapy results in an uninterpretable stress ECG.
2. Chest radiography: This study is useful to gauge cardiac size and pulmonary vascular markings, which may be prominent in the setting of congestive heart disease.
3. Echocardiography: Typically, transthoracic echocardiography is the mainstay of cardiac function in the evaluation of ischemic heart disease. A resting study provides information regarding cardiac structure and function, including valve function. In the appropriate clinical setting, echocardiography may also be coupled with either a physical or a chemical stress to assess for stress-induced ischemia.
4. Nuclear cardiac stress testing is a nuclear-based cardiac imaging test that uses either physical or chemical stress to assess for changes in myocardial perfusion, comparing resting vs stress perfusion images. This test can reliably evaluate for prior MI, active ischemia, and the presence of viable myocardium in the setting of coronary artery disease associated with profound ventricular dysfunction.
5. Cardiac magnetic resonance imaging: This is an emerging noninvasive cardiac imaging test with superior spatial resolution that allows assessment of both cardiac structure and function. Its unique ability to characterize tissue inflammation allows for quantification of myocardial scar and viability. The ability to perform stress cardiac magnetic resonance imaging is also an emerging tool in cardiac imaging.

6. Cardiac computed tomography: This is an emerging noninvasive cardiac imaging test that has greatest power in coronary artery imaging. It is especially powerful in its negative predictive value. The coronary calcium score allows for further risk stratification of patients who are at intermediate risk of coronary events. It is also extremely useful for identifying coronary artery anomalies that may pose risk of development of ischemia, such as anomalies of origin or myocardial bridging. Computed tomography requires the use of iodinated intravenous contrast media. It is of limited value in patients with greater than mild to moderate coronary calcification or an irregular rhythm. These current limitations likely represent transient phenomena as computed tomography technology advances.

7. Left heart catheterization: This is an invasive test that directly assesses coronary artery anatomy. It involves access to the arterial side of the circulation with special catheters designed to engage the coronary ostia. This technique uses intra-arterial injection of iodinated contrast agent to delineate vascular structures. Additionally, ventricular function can be assessed with direct left ventricular angiography. Although coronary angiography has limitations, it is the standard for defining the severity and extent of coronary artery disease. Subjective visual estimation of the percentage of stenosis may underestimate the severity of disease, especially if it is diffuse, because angiography outlines the vessel lumen. The risk of serious complications of coronary angiography is approximately 0.1%, including MI, stroke, and death. Patients with advanced age, severe left ventricular dysfunction, left main coronary artery disease, or other comorbidities have a somewhat higher risk of complications. Other complications include vascular complications (0.5%) and contrast nephropathy.

Risk Stratification by Stress Testing

Treadmill exercise testing can identify high-risk patients. Results that indicate high risk are listed in Box 8.2.

Patients who achieve a good workload with appropriate blood pressure and heart rate responses without marked ST-segment depression have an excellent prognosis; therefore, medical management may be preferred in these patients.

Imaging-based stress testing slightly increases the sensitivity and specificity of ECG exercise testing. In nuclear perfusion imaging, the tracer is injected at peak exercise and labels areas of hypoperfusion as a defect or "cold spot." Scanning is repeated a few hours later at rest, and persistent cold spots indicate infarction, whereas reperfused areas indicate areas of inducible ischemia. In patients with left bundle branch block or severe left ventricular hypertrophy,

---

Box 8.2 • Treadmill Exercise Results Indicating High Risk of Ischemic Heart Disease

A positive electrocardiogram in stage I of the Bruce protocol or at a heart rate less than 120 beats per minute

ST-segment depression more than 2 mm

ST-segment depression more than 6 minutes in duration after stopping exercise

Decrease in blood pressure

Multiple perfusion or wall motion defects (>25% of segments with exercise) and an increase in left ventricular end-systolic volume with exercise

---

thallium and sestamibi scanning can give false-positive results during exercise stress.

In exercise echocardiography, 2-dimensional echocardiography is performed at rest and at peak exercise. The test is positive for ischemia if new regional wall motion abnormalities develop, global systolic function decreases, or left ventricular end-systolic volume increases.

Stress testing should *not* be performed for patients with high-risk unstable angina, patients who have had acute MI in the prior 2 days, or patients with symptomatic severe aortic stenosis, uncontrolled heart failure, or uncontrolled arrhythmia. Consider invasive angiography to define coronary artery anatomy, and evaluate the need for revascularization in patients with poor prognostic factors.

Imaging stress tests are considerably more expensive than the ECG exercise test and should not be routinely used instead of ECG exercise testing for diagnostic purposes, except when the result of resting ECG is uninterpretable, the ECG result is possibly false-positive, or specific regions of ischemia need to be localized (for planning revascularization procedures).

Pharmacologic stress tests are used for patients who cannot exercise. These tests include the use of vasodilators such as adenosine and dipyridamole (redistribute flow away from ischemic myocardium). The tests are generally performed with perfusion agents such as thallium or sestamibi. Alternatively, dobutamine is used as a chronotropic and inotropic agent to increase myocardial oxygen demand, and imaging is performed with echocardiography.

Stress tests should not be used for the diagnosis of ischemic heart disease in patients at high or low risk. Stress testing is appropriate for patients at intermediate risk to rule in or rule out ischemia. The pretest probability of ischemic heart disease is estimated using the following criteria: age (men >40 years and women >60 years), male sex, and symptom status (in decreasing order of risk: typical angina, atypical angina, noncardiac chest pain, asymptomatic) (Table 8.1 and Figure 8.3).

KEY FACTS

✓ Coronary blood flow—normally can increase up to 5 times to meet effort-related increases in myocardial oxygen demands

✓ Double product [(heart rate) × (systolic blood pressure)]—useful index for quantifying myocardial oxygen demand

✓ Restriction of resting blood flow sufficient to cause resting ischemia does not occur unless vessel stenosis is >95%. But, decreased overall flow reserve begins to occur at about 60% vessel stenosis, and symptoms of exercise-induced ischemia may begin

✓ Temporal sequence of events during ischemia— diastolic dysfunction→regional wall motion abnormalities→ECG changes→pain

✓ Stress testing—should *not* be performed for patients with high-risk unstable angina, patients who have had acute MI in the prior 2 days, or patients with symptomatic severe aortic stenosis, uncontrolled heart failure, or uncontrolled arrhythmia

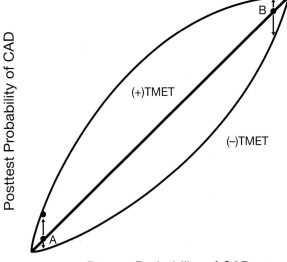

Pretest Probability of CAD

Figure 8.3 *The Effect of Bayes Theorem on the Ability of Treadmill Exertion Testing (TMET) to Diagnose Coronary Artery Disease (CAD). Patient A, a young patient with atypical chest pain and no risk factors. Pretest probability (5%) of coronary artery disease is low. If the test results are negative, the probability decreases to 3%. However, if the results are positive, the probability is less than 15%. Patient B, an older man with typical chest pain and multiple risk factors. Pretest probability of coronary artery disease is high (90%), and even with negative test results the probability is higher than 70%. Thus, stress tests should not be used for the diagnosis of coronary artery disease in patients at high or low risk.*

Medical Therapy of Angina

Medical therapy for chronic stable angina includes risk factor modification, antiplatelet therapy, and medication-based therapy of myocardial ischemia. Antiplatelet agents are essential. Aspirin reduces the likelihood of acute MI and mortality, but it does not prevent progression of atherosclerosis. Aspirin therapy provides greater benefit for secondary than for primary prevention. Treatable underlying

---

Table 8.1 • Pretest Probability of Coronary Artery Disease by Age, Sex, and Symptoms[a]

Age, y	Sex	Typical/Definite Angina Pectoris	Atypical/Probable Angina Pectoris	Non-anginal Chest Pain	Asymptomatic
30–39	Males	Intermediate	Intermediate	Low (<10%)	Very low (<5%)
	Females	Intermediate	Very low (<5%)	Very low	Very low
40–49	Males	High (>90%)	Intermediate	Intermediate	Low
	Females	Intermediate	Low	Very low	Very low
50–59	Males	High (>90%)	Intermediate	Intermediate	Low
	Females	Intermediate	Intermediate	Low	Very low
60–69	Males	High	Intermediate	Intermediate	Low
	Females	High	Intermediate	Intermediate	Low

[a] High indicates more than 90%; intermediate, 10% to 90%; low, less than 10%; very low, less than 5%.

Data from Gibbons RJ, Balady GJ, Bricker JT, Chaitman BR, Fletcher GF, Froelicher VF, et al; American College of Cardiology/American Heart Association Task Force on Practice Guidelines (Committee to Update the 1997 Exercise Testing Guidelines). ACC/AHA 2002 guideline update for exercise testing: summary article: a report of the American College of Cardiology/American Heart Association Task Force on Practice Guidelines (Committee to Update the 1997 Exercise Testing Guidelines). Circulation. 2002 Oct 1;106(14):1883–92 and Gibbons RJ, Balady GJ, Bricker JT, Chaitman BR, Fletcher GF, Froelicher VF, et al; American College of Cardiology/American Heart Association Task Force on Practice Guidelines. Committee to Update the 1997 Exercise Testing Guidelines. ACC/AHA 2002 guideline update for exercise testing: summary article. A report of the American College of Cardiology/American Heart Association Task Force on Practice Guidelines (Committee to Update the 1997 Exercise Testing Guidelines). J Am Coll Cardiol. 2002 Oct 16;40(8):1531–40. Erratum in: J Am Coll Cardiol. 2006 Oct 17;48(8):1731.

factors that contribute to ischemia (eg, anemia, thyroid abnormalities, and hypoxia) should always be sought.

A stepwise approach should be used when introducing a pharmacologic strategy to treat myocardial ischemia. Medications should be titrated according to symptoms. The dose of a first-line drug should be optimized before adding additional agents.

β-Blockers are the most effective and are first-line drugs for ischemic heart disease. They relieve angina by decreasing heart rate, reducing contractility, and decreasing afterload (blood pressure). They are the most effective drugs for reducing the double product (heart rate × blood pressure) with exercise. β-Blockers improve survival, especially in patients with prior MI or depressed left ventricular systolic function. β-Blockers should not be used in the setting of *marked* bronchospastic disease, decompensated heart failure, or bradycardia. However, they should be given to patients with left ventricular systolic dysfunction in the absence of overt heart failure. The target resting heart rate is 70 beats per minute or less, and dose should be titrated to effect.

Nitrates should be added if symptoms continue despite optimal β-blocker therapy. Nitrates cause venodilatation and decreasing wall tension, thus relieving angina. Nitrate tolerance can develop with continuous exposure. Thus, a nitrate-free interval is important, particularly when using short-acting preparations. Sublingual nitroglycerin should be given to all symptomatic patients for use as needed.

Calcium channel blockers decrease afterload, heart rate, and contractility. Diltiazem and verapamil have more heart rate–lowering effects than the dihydropyridine group of calcium channel blockers and may be used when β-blockers are contraindicated. Short-acting calcium channel blockers, specifically the dihydropyridines (eg, amlodipine, nifedipine), may cause reflex tachycardia and increased mortality; therefore, they are relatively contraindicated in patients with ischemic heart disease. This detrimental effect probably does not occur with the longer-acting calcium channel blockers or in patients with normal systolic function, but they should be avoided in patients with left ventricular systolic dysfunction. If a calcium channel blocker is required for patients with left ventricular systolic dysfunction, amlodipine is preferred.

Ranolazine is a second-line drug used as an adjunct to one of the aforementioned drugs. Experience with its use is limited. The exact mechanism of action remains to be clearly elucidated, although purported mechanisms suggest an effect on membrane ion channels.

For patients with left ventricular dysfunction or nocturnal angina, diuretics and angiotensin-converting enzyme inhibitors decrease wall tension. They may be beneficial for secondary prevention in ischemic heart disease regardless of the degree of systolic function.

Percutaneous Coronary Intervention

Percutaneous coronary intervention (PCI) for chronic stable angina relieves symptoms but does not reduce the risk of MI or death. It is indicated for treatment in symptomatic patients, particularly those who remain symptomatic despite optimized medical therapy. An initial medical strategy is reasonable for most patients at low to moderate risk of an event (based on symptoms and the findings on stress testing or angiography). There is no clear role for PCI in management of asymptomatic disease.

PCI is performed at the time of coronary angiography. During percutaneous transluminal coronary angioplasty, the device is placed across a coronary stenosis and a balloon is inflated to increase the area of the lumen. This procedure "splits" the atheroma and stretches the vessel. The major problem is restenosis, occurring in 30% to 40% of patients within 6 months. Antiplatelet agents may decrease the rate of acute closure, but they do not prevent restenosis.

Other catheter-based therapies such as atherectomy and laser have high restenosis rates and are infrequently used.

Intracoronary stent placement at the time of PCI decreases restenosis. Stents are used in approximately 90% of PCIs. The restenosis rate after successful bare-metal stent implantation is 20% to 30%. Stents also are used to treat acute complications of percutaneous transluminal coronary angioplasty such as acute dissection and have decreased the need for emergency coronary artery bypass grafting (CABG). However, for patients who have restenosis within a stent, the rate of recurrent restenosis is high (>60%) if another procedure is performed.

Drug-eluting stents are coated with and release drugs that considerably decrease restenosis (5%–10%). They are the most commonly used stents. They are associated with a higher risk for very late (>1 year) stent thrombosis than bare-metal stents.

Dual antiplatelet therapy is initiated at the time of stent deployment to prevent early restenosis. Duration varies according to the type of stent (Table 8.2). Recommendations regarding discontinuation of dual antiplatelet therapy for noncardiac surgery are outlined in Box 8.3.

The success rate for PCI is greater than 95%. Potential complications include MI (<5%), vascular complications (1%), emergency CABG (0.2%), and mortality (<0.5%). The risks of the procedure are higher during emergency procedures, in the elderly, and in patients with severely reduced ejection fraction, acute coronary syndromes, or severe diffuse coronary artery disease.

PCI is the preferred revascularization strategy for single-vessel disease, young patients (age <50 years), elderly patients with significant comorbid conditions, and patients who are not surgical candidates.

Table 8.2 • Antiplatelet Therapy Used With Coronary Stents

Therapy	Duration
Aspirin	Indefinitely
Clopidogrel or prasugrel Bare-metal stent	At least 1 month for patient with stable disease At least 12 months for an acute coronary syndrome (unstable angina and myocardial infarction). If the risk of substantial bleeding outweighs the anticipated benefit, earlier discontinuation should be considered
Drug-eluting stent	12 months (a subset of patients may require long-term therapy). If the risk of morbidity because of bleeding outweighs the anticipated benefits afforded by thienopyridine therapy, earlier discontinuation should be considered

Surgical Treatment

CABG uses the saphenous vein (occlusion rate of 20% at 1 year and 50% at 5 years) and internal mammary artery (occlusion rate <10% at 10 years). CABG provides excellent symptom relief (partial relief in >90%, complete relief in >70%).

The indications for CABG (over medical therapy or PCI) are symptom relief in patients whose limiting symptoms are unresponsive to other management strategies and prolonging the life of patients with severe disease.

CABG reduces mortality in patients with severe disease, including left main coronary artery disease, 3-vessel disease with moderately depressed left ventricular function, 3-vessel disease with severe ischemic symptoms at a low workload, and multivessel disease with proximal left anterior descending artery involvement. Recommendations for surgery are derived from randomized trials of CABG vs medical therapy. In meta-analyses, a survival benefit in favor of CABG compared with medical therapy has been observed for all patients with 3-vessel disease.

In-hospital mortality after CABG varies widely (about 1% in most elective cases to 30% in high-risk cases). Mortality increases with age, female sex, reduced left ventricular function, diffuse multivessel disease, recent acute coronary syndrome, diabetes mellitus, repeat CABG, and emergency surgery. Complications of CABG include sternal wound infection (especially in patients with diabetes mellitus), severe left ventricular dysfunction (from perioperative MI or inadequate cardioprotection during cardiopulmonary bypass), and late constrictive pericarditis.

Postcardiotomy Syndrome

Postcardiotomy syndrome occurs 2 weeks to 2 months postoperatively and consists of fever, pericarditis, and increased erythrocyte sedimentation rate. Rarely, it presents as pericardial tamponade. It is likely an autoimmune process. Treatment is with aspirin and other nonsteroidal anti-inflammatory drugs. Rarely, constrictive pericarditis may be a late complication. The diagnosis should be suspected in patients presenting months to years after cardiac surgery with congestive heart failure with predominantly right-sided signs of fluid overload, including increased jugular venous pressure but normal left ventricular ejection fraction.

Medical vs Catheter-Based vs Surgical Therapy

The decision about which therapy to use for a patient with chronic stable angina must be individualized. Factors to consider include disease severity, ischemia, symptoms, and the patient's age, lifestyle, and personal preference. The incidence of MI and emergency CABG with PCI is similar to that with medical management. PCI neither decreases risk for MI nor improves resting left ventricular function or survival. Procedure-related mortality is lower with PCI than with CABG.

There are more procedure-related infarctions and strokes with CABG than with PCI, and the duration of hospitalization is longer after CABG. The overall rates of death or MI at 5-year follow-up are similar for PCI and CABG (85%–90% free of death and 80% free of MI), except for patients with severe disease. This subgroup includes patients with left

Box 8.3 • Management of Patients With Drug-Eluting Stents Who Need Noncardiac Surgery or an Invasive Procedure Within 1 Year of Percutaneous Coronary Intervention

Defer elective procedures for 1 year after stent placement and consider less invasive alternatives that may be performed in patients receiving dual antiplatelet therapy

Aspirin therapy must be continued during the perioperative period, unless absolutely contraindicated

For urgent procedures, consider performing them without discontinuing dual antiplatelet therapy or with aspirin alone. The relative risks of perioperative bleeding vs stent thrombosis must be discussed with the surgical team. The risk of postoperative stent thrombosis is low, but it increases if use of one or both of the antiplatelet agents is discontinued. If stent thrombosis occurs, the associated morbidity and mortality are high

If clopidogrel therapy must be withheld for an urgent operation, withhold therapy for 5 days preoperatively. Ideally, clopidogrel therapy should be resumed with a 300-mg loading dose on the day of operation

main coronary artery disease, 3-vessel disease with moderately depressed left ventricular function, 3-vessel disease with severe ischemic symptoms at a low workload, and multivessel disease with proximal left anterior descending artery involvement. CABG offers a survival benefit in these patients. Patients with multivessel or anatomically complex disease who have CABG have less angina, require less antianginal medication, and are less likely to need a repeat revascularization procedure. For patients with diabetes mellitus and diffuse multivessel disease, survival is higher with CABG than with PCI. Increased survival is related to having a patent internal mammary artery graft to the left anterior descending artery.

KEY FACTS

✓ β-Blockers—most effective agents and are first-line drugs for ischemic heart disease

✓ β-Blockers—relieve angina by decreasing heart rate, reducing contractility, and decreasing afterload (blood pressure)

✓ Percutaneous coronary intervention for chronic stable angina—relieves symptoms but does not reduce the risk of MI or death

✓ CABG—reduces mortality in patients with severe disease, including left main coronary artery disease, 3-vessel disease with moderately depressed left ventricular function, 3-vessel disease with severe ischemic symptoms at a low workload, and multivessel disease with proximal left anterior descending artery involvement

---

Coronary Artery Spasm

The vasomotor tone of coronary arteries is important in the pathogenesis of coronary artery disease. Arterial injury leads to coronary artery vasoconstriction. The vascular endothelium regulates vasomotor tone by releasing relaxing factors (eg, prostacyclin and nitric oxide), preventing vasoconstriction and platelet deposition. Endothelial dysfunction leads to depletion of these factors, and the coronary arteries become prone to spasm. Most clinical episodes of coronary artery spasm are superimposed on atherosclerotic plaques. However, coronary artery spasm may also develop in patients with angiographically normal coronary arteries.

Coronary artery spasm classically consists of recurrent episodes of rest pain with associated ST-segment elevation, which reverses with administration of nitrates (Prinzmetal angina). However, many patients present with atypical chest pain without ECG changes. Coronary angiography with acetylcholine provocation is used to diagnose coronary artery spasm, but the sensitivity and specificity are not known. Coronary artery spasm is treated with long-acting nitrates or calcium channel blockers.

Acute Coronary Syndromes

Acute coronary syndromes include unstable angina and acute MI (both ST-segment elevation and non–ST-segment elevation MI). At the time of initial presentation, the differentiation of these patients from those with noncardiac chest pain is based on clinical assessment.

The resting ECG is essential for the evaluation and triage of a patient presenting with an acute coronary syndrome. Those without ST-segment elevation have unstable angina or non–ST-segment elevation MI, usually the result of subtotal coronary artery occlusion. Patients with ST-segment elevation generally have complete coronary artery occlusion leading to transmural injury.

Patients presenting with a suspected acute coronary syndrome require prompt evaluation. Patients with ST-segment elevation must be treated on an emergency basis. Patients without ST-segment elevation can be evaluated in the chest pain unit of an emergency department; this approach allows discharge of low-risk patients, observation of intermediate-risk patients, and admission of high-risk patients (Box 8.4 and Figures 8.4 and 8.5).

Unstable Angina and Non–ST-Segment Elevation MI

Pathophysiology

These conditions are due to mismatched myocardial oxygen demand and supply, most often precipitated by conditions of decreased myocardial oxygen supply—usually due to coronary stenosis from non-occlusive thrombus at the site of a disrupted atherosclerotic plaque. Episodes may also be caused by increased myocardial oxygen demand in the presence of a fixed myocardial oxygen supply. Coronary spasm may also precipitate episodes. Nocturnal ischemic symptoms are generally due to unstable angina and may be

---

Box 8.4 • Baseline Characteristics Analyzed for TIMI Risk Score for Unstable Angina and Non–ST-Segment Elevation Myocardial Infarction

Age ≥65 y

≥3 CAD risk factors

Known CAD (stenosis ≥50%)

Aspirin use in past 7 days

Recent (≤24 h) severe angina

↑ Cardiac markers

ST deviation ≥0.5 mm

Abbreviations: CAD, coronary artery disease; TIMI, Thrombolysis in Myocardial Infarction trial.

Adapted from Antman EM, Cohen M, Bernink PJLM, McCabe CH, Horacek T, Papuchis G, et al. The TIMI risk score for unstable angina/non–ST elevation MI: a method for prognostication and therapeutic decision making. JAMA. 2000 Aug 16;284(7):835–42. Used with permission.

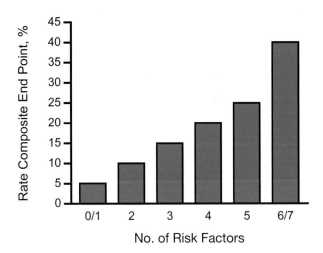

Figure 8.4 *The 14-Day Risk of Death, Myocardial Infarction, and Severe Ischemia Requiring Urgent Revascularization. Rates are based on number of risk factors present (Thrombolysis in Myocardial Infarction [TIMI] trial cohort).* (Adapted from Antman EM, Cohen M, Bernink PJLM, McCabe CH, Horacek T, Papuchis G, et al. The TIMI risk score for unstable angina/non–ST elevation MI: a method for prognostication and therapeutic decision making. JAMA. 2000 Aug 16;284[7]:835–42. Used with permission.)

due to altered coronary tone or increased wall tension in patients with left ventricular dysfunction.

Biomarkers

Cardiac biomarkers are used to differentiate unstable angina from non–ST-segment elevation MI. Cardiac-specific troponin T and I are the preferred biomarkers. MI is defined by increased troponin T and I levels in the presence of symptoms of ischemia, and biomarker increases identify patients at high risk for future events.

Management

All patients with a possible acute coronary syndrome should have continuous ECG monitoring and treatment to improve the myocardial oxygen demand-supply mismatch. Sedation may decrease anxiety and catecholaminergic stimulation of the heart. β-Blockade is the treatment of choice to decrease myocardial oxygen demand.

Antiplatelet agents, such as aspirin, are given immediately and decrease the incidence of progression to ST-segment elevation MI. Clopidogrel is an adenosine diphosphate-receptor antagonist that can be administered as an alternative in patients with aspirin allergy or intolerance. Other such antagonist agents include prasugrel and ticagrelor. Typically, dual antiplatelet support is provided during acute coronary syndrome and is a guideline-based recommendation. At the time of coronary angiography, however, findings such as triple-vessel disease or critical

left main artery disease may suggest the benefit of CABG in such settings. The administration of dual antiplatelet therapy before CABG predicts increased bleeding in the perioperative period; given this risk, if the patient is otherwise hemodynamically and electrically stable, surgery may be delayed up to 5 days to alleviate this increased perioperative bleeding risk. However, in clopidogrel-treated patients, urgent CABG may have an acceptable bleeding risk when performed by experienced surgeons.

Anticoagulation decreases the incidence of progression to MI and should be given to all patients without contraindications. Continuous intravenous administration of unfractionated heparin or subcutaneous injections of low-molecular-weight heparin may be used. Bivalirudin (direct thrombin inhibitor) and fondaparinux (activated factor X inhibitor) are alternative anticoagulants. One important caveat is that the agent fondaparinux is contraindicated at the time of percutaneous intervention because it has an increased risk of catheter-related thrombosis.

Conservative vs Invasive Strategy

There are 2 accepted therapeutic pathways for patients presenting with unstable angina or non–ST-segment elevation MI, depending on risk stratification. Patients at high risk should undergo an early invasive strategy (within 4–48 hours of admission) with revascularization (PCI or CABG) performed when appropriate. High-risk patients include those with a Thrombolysis in Myocardial Infarction trial (TIMI) risk score of more than 3, ongoing chest pain, ST-segment depression on the resting ECG, and an increase in troponin levels. Use of clopidogrel or a glycoprotein IIb/IIIa inhibitor should be initiated before coronary angiography (Figure 8.6A and 8.6B).

A conservative (or selective invasive) strategy is indicated for non–high-risk patients. Initially, medical management is used for treatment. Coronary angiography is indicated if 1) recurrent ischemia occurs despite optimal medical therapy, 2) results of the pre-discharge stress test are positive, 3) there is left ventricular dysfunction (ejection fraction ≤40%) or heart failure, or 4) serious arrhythmias occur.

ST-Segment Elevation MI

Pathophysiology

An **ST-segment elevation MI** is the result of events occurring after rupture of an intracoronary plaque. Plaque rupture causes platelet adhesion and aggregation, thrombus formation, and sudden, complete occlusion of the artery. Without collateral circulation, 90% of the myocardium supplied by the occluded coronary artery is infarcted within 3 hours. Transmural MI develops if the condition is untreated. Patients with ST-segment elevation MI require urgent diagnosis and therapy to preserve the myocardium because prompt reperfusion therapy improves survival.

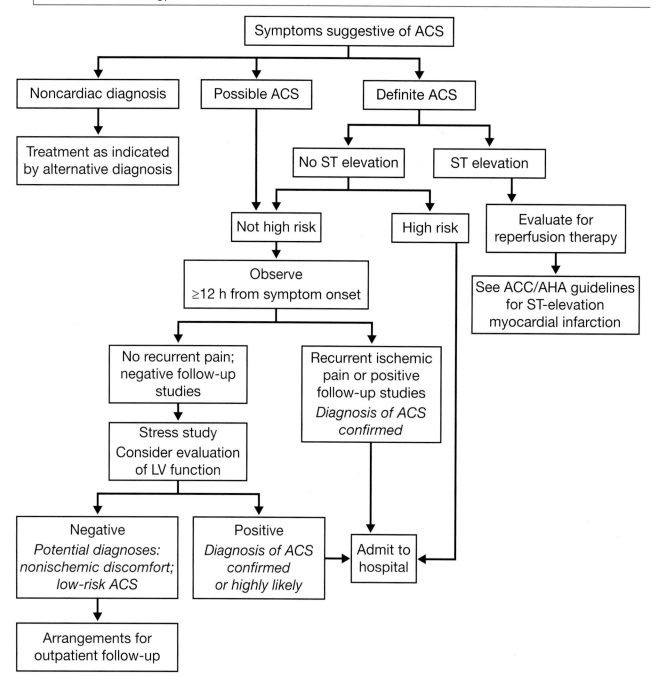

Figure 8.5 *Algorithm for Evaluation and Management of Patients Suspected of Having Acute Coronary Syndrome (ACS). ACC indicates American College of Cardiology; AHA, American Heart Association; LV, left ventricular.*

(Adapted from Anderson JL, Adams CD, Antman EM, Bridges CR, Califf RM, Casey DE Jr, et al. ACC/AHA 2007 guidelines for the management of patients with unstable angina/non–ST-elevation myocardial infarction: a report of the American College of Cardiology/American Heart Association Task Force on Practice Guidelines [Writing Committee to Revise the 2002 Guidelines for the Management of Patients With Unstable Angina/Non–ST-Elevation Myocardial Infarction]. J Am Coll Cardiol. 2007 Aug 14;50[7]:e1–157 and Anderson JL, Adams CD, Antman EM, Bridges CR, Califf RM, Casey DE Jr, et al; American College of Cardiology; American Heart Association Task Force on Practice Guidelines [Writing Committee to Revise the 2002 Guidelines for the Management of Patients With Unstable Angina/Non ST-Elevation Myocardial Infarction]; American College of Emergency Physicians; Society for Cardiovascular Angiography and Interventions; Society of Thoracic Surgeons; American Association of Cardiovascular and Pulmonary Rehabilitation; Society for Academic Emergency Medicine. ACC/AHA 2007 guidelines for the management of patients with unstable angina/non ST-elevation myocardial infarction: a report of the American College of Cardiology/American Heart Association Task Force on Practice Guidelines [Writing Committee to Revise the 2002 Guidelines for the Management of Patients With Unstable Angina/Non ST-Elevation Myocardial Infarction]: developed in collaboration with the American College of Emergency Physicians, the Society for Cardiovascular Angiography and Interventions, and the Society of Thoracic Surgeons: endorsed by the American Association of Cardiovascular and Pulmonary Rehabilitation and the Society for Academic Emergency Medicine. Circulation. 2007 Aug 14;116[7]:e148–304. Epub 2007 Aug 6. Erratum in: Circulation. 2008 Mar 4;117[9]:e180. Used with permission.)

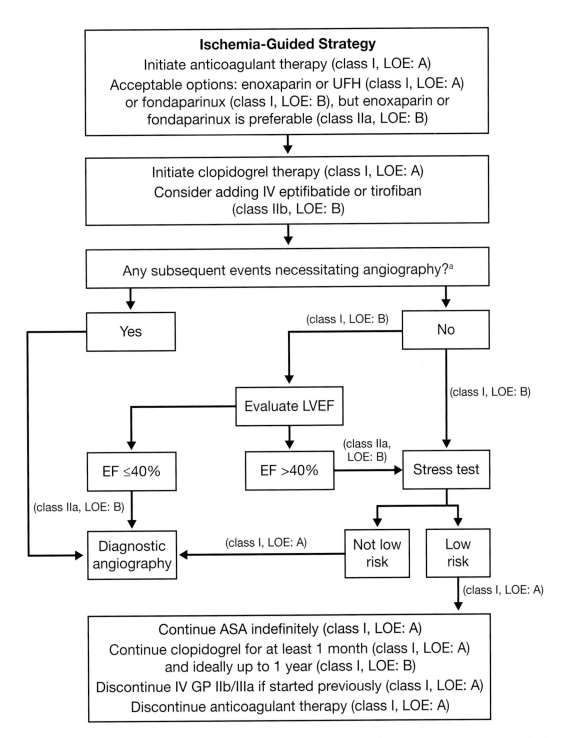

Figure 8.6A. *Therapeutic Pathways for Acute Ischemia: Ischemia-Guided Strategy.* [a] *Recurrent symptoms/ischemia, heart failure, or serious arrhythmia. Abbreviations are defined in the legend for Figure 8.6B.*

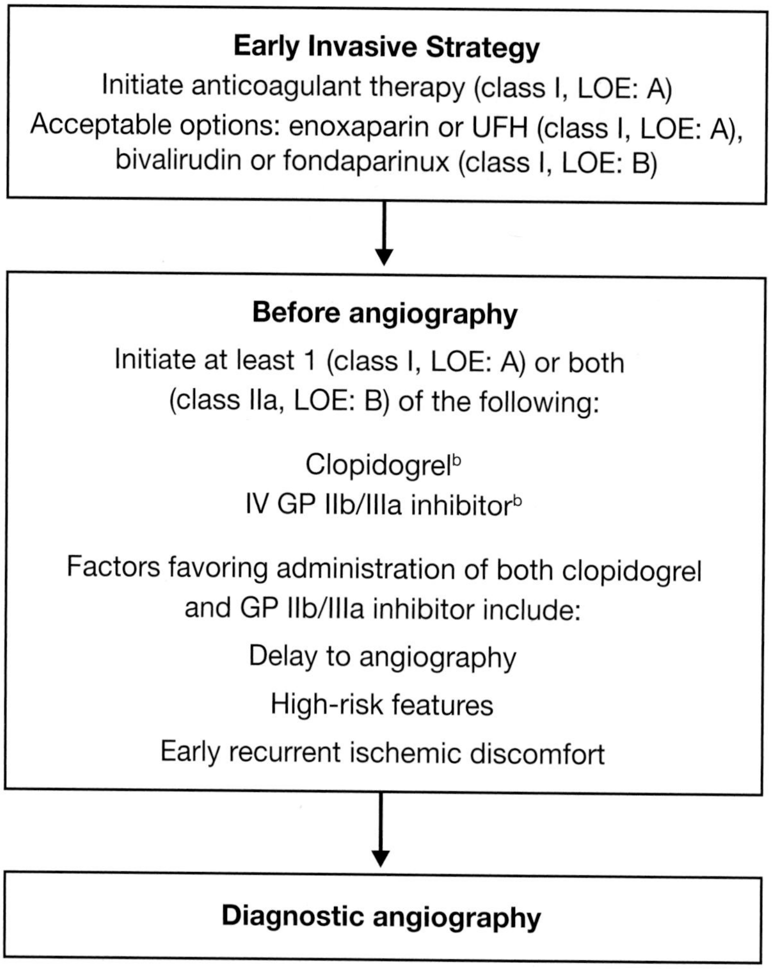

Figure 8.6B. *Therapeutic Pathways for Acute Ischemia: Early Invasive Strategy.* [b] *Evidence exists that glycoprotein (GP) IIb/IIIa inhibitors may not be necessary if a patient received a preloading dose of at least 300 mg of clopidogrel at least 6 hours earlier (class I level of evidence, [LOE] B for clopidogrel administration) and bivalirudin is selected as the anticoagulant (class IIa, LOE B). ASA indicates acetylsalicylic acid; EF, ejection fraction; IV, intravenous; LVEF, left ventricular ejection fraction; UFH, unfractionated heparin.*
(Both A and B adapted from Anderson JL, Adams CD, Antman EM, Bridges CR, Califf RM, Casey DE Jr, et al. ACC/AHA 2007 guidelines for the management of patients with unstable angina/non–ST-elevation myocardial infarction: a report of the American College of Cardiology/American Heart Association Task Force on Practice Guidelines [Writing Committee to Revise the 2002 Guidelines for the Management of Patients With Unstable Angina/Non–ST-Elevation Myocardial Infarction]. J Am Coll Cardiol. 2007 Aug 14;50[7]:e1–157 and Anderson JL, Adams CD, Antman EM, Bridges CR, Califf RM, Casey DE Jr, et al. ACC/AHA 2007 guidelines for the management of patients with unstable angina/non–ST-elevation myocardial infarction: a report of the American College of Cardiology/American Heart Association Task Force on Practice Guidelines [Writing Committee to Revise the 2002 Guidelines for the Management of Patients With Unstable Angina/Non–ST-Elevation Myocardial Infarction]. Circulation. 2007 Aug 14;116[7]:e148-e304. Epub 2007 Aug 6. Erratum in: Circulation. 2008 Mar 4;117[9]:e180. Used with permission.)

Key Definition

ST-segment elevation MI: *the result of events occurring after rupture of an intracoronary plaque.*

MI is a major public health problem in the United States—about 1 million patients annually are admitted for an acute coronary syndrome, including MI. ST-segment elevation accounts for 20% of these cases. More than 30% of patients with MI die before reaching a hospital. With improved cardiac care, mortality from MI has declined, primarily due to treatment of ventricular arrhythmias. β-Blockade has also decreased in-hospital and post-hospital mortality by 30% to 40%. Reperfusion therapy has contributed to improved survival. Currently, the overall in-hospital mortality for patients with an ST-segment elevation MI is 5% to 10%.

Stunned myocardium occurs when reversible systolic dysfunction of the myocardium follows transient, nonlethal ischemia. With early reperfusion, contraction of the affected myocardium may be decreased and the myocardium remains viable. Systolic contraction returns hours to days later.

Infarct remodeling occurs mainly after a large anteroapical MI. An area of infarction may undergo thinning, dilatation, and dyskinesis. Myocardial remodeling may lead to congestive heart failure and increased mortality. Adverse infarct remodeling may be reduced with early initiation of therapy with angiotensin-converting enzyme inhibitors or angiotensin receptor blockers (if angiotensin-converting enzyme inhibitors are contraindicated). β-Blockers can also help reduce long-term adverse infarct remodeling, but they must be administered cautiously in the patient presenting with acute heart failure, in which further decompensation may be precipitated by the institution of β-blockade in the acute phase.

Presentation and Diagnosis

Patients with ST-segment elevation MI commonly present with angina-like pain lasting longer than 20 minutes associated with typical ECG changes and increased levels of cardiac biomarkers (Figure 8.7). However, more than 25% to 30% of MIs are silent, and silent MIs often occur in patients with diabetes mellitus and in the elderly. In addition, women having an MI often present without typical angina-like pain. Symptoms such as nausea, jaw pain, upper back pain, and shortness of breath should be considered possible indicators of ischemia, in addition to chest pain or pressure.

An acute MI is usually diagnosed on the basis of ECG changes (ST elevation or depression or pathologic Q-wave development that meets criteria for diagnosis) in the setting of ischemic symptoms, biochemical markers of myocardial damage, or other evidence of myocardial damage not due to another potential cause.

KEY FACTS

✓ Acute coronary syndromes—include unstable angina and acute MI (both ST-segment elevation and non–ST-segment elevation MI)

✓ Cardiac biomarkers—used to differentiate unstable angina from non–ST-segment elevation MI

✓ More than 25% of MIs are silent, and silent MIs often occur in patients with diabetes mellitus and in the elderly

✓ Women having an MI often present without typical angina-like pain

---

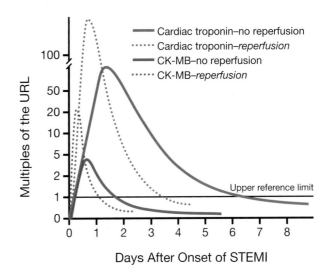

Figure 8.7 *Cardiac Biomarkers in ST-Segment Elevation Myocardial Infarction (STEMI). Typical cardiac biomarkers that are used to evaluate patients with STEMI include the MB isoenzyme of creatine kinase (CK-MB) and cardiac-specific troponins. The horizontal line depicts the upper reference limit (URL) for the cardiac biomarker in the clinical chemistry laboratory. The URL is that value representing the 99th percentile of a reference control group without STEMI. The kinetics of release of CK-MB and cardiac troponin in patients who do not undergo reperfusion are shown in the solid blue and red curves as multiples of the URL. Note that when patients with STEMI undergo reperfusion, as depicted in the dotted blue and dotted red curves, the cardiac biomarkers are detected sooner, increase to a higher peak value, but decline more rapidly, resulting in a smaller area under the curve and limitation of infarct size.* (Adapted from Antman EM, Anbe DT, Armstrong PW, Bates ER, Green LA, Hand M, et al. ACC/AHA guidelines for the management of patients with ST-elevation myocardial infarction: a report of the American College of Cardiology/American Heart Association Task Force on Practice Guidelines [Committee to Revise the 1999 Guidelines for the management of patients with acute myocardial infarction]. J Am Coll Cardiol. 2004 Aug 4;44[3]:E1-E211 and Antman EM, Anbe DT, Armstrong PW, Bates ER, Green LA, Hand M, et al; American College of Cardiology; American Heart Association Task Force on Practice Guidelines; Canadian Cardiovascular Society. ACC/AHA guidelines for the management of patients with ST-elevation myocardial infarction: a report of the American College of Cardiology/American Heart Association Task Force on Practice Guidelines [Committee to Revise the 1999 Guidelines for the Management of Patients with Acute Myocardial Infarction]. Circulation. 2004 Aug 31;110[9]:e82–292. Errata in: Circulation. 2005 Apr 19;111[15]:2013–4. Circulation. 2007 Apr 17;115[15]:e411. Circulation. 2010 Jun 15;121[23]:e441. Used with permission.)

Management

Bed rest, pain management, and sedation are essential and beneficial in the acute stage of MI to decrease myocardial oxygen demand. Oxygen has little benefit after 2 or 3 hours unless hypoxia (oxygen saturation <90%) is present. Modest hypoxemia is common as a result of ventilation-perfusion lung mismatch, even with uncomplicated MI. Continuous ECG monitoring is required to detect tachyarrhythmias and bradyarrhythmias.

Reperfusion therapy is the mainstay of management of ST-segment elevation MI. This is achieved chemically with fibrinolytic therapy or directly via percutaneous therapy. Both approaches require pharmacologic support with antiplatelet and anticoagulant medicines.

With regard to the antiplatelet therapy, a dual approach is invoked, including aspirin in addition to an adenosine diphosphate-receptor antagonist (clopidogrel, prasugrel, or ticagrelor). If fibrinolytic therapy is the reperfusion strategy that is used, then clopidogrel is the adenosine diphosphate-receptor antagonist of choice, simply because the other agents have not been adequately studied in this setting. Aspirin (325 mg) reduces recurrent MI and mortality when given in addition to thrombolytic therapy and should be administered on admission. Clopidogrel (75 mg daily) is an alternative in patients with aspirin allergy or intolerance. After lytic therapy, clopidogrel therapy should be started on day 1 and continued during the hospitalization and for at least 1 month; ideally, it is continued for up to a year.

Anticoagulation prevents recurrent infarction (especially after thrombolytic therapy, when it should be administered for at least 48 hours), deep vein thrombosis, and intracardiac thrombus formation. Long-duration anticoagulation is indicated for higher-risk patients (large anterior MI for which reperfusion therapy was not given or was unsuccessful, atrial fibrillation, previous thromboembolic complication, presence of mechanical prosthetic valves). Thromboembolism is uncommon in patients in whom reperfusion therapy is successful. Unfractionated heparin or low-molecular-weight heparin can be used.

Nitroglycerin is useful for certain patients with MI: those with pulmonary edema, severely increased blood pressure, or persistent myocardial ischemia. Intravenous nitroglycerin should be given instead of long-acting oral nitrates. Nitrate intolerance develops with infusions of more than 24 hours in duration. Intravenous nitroglycerin should not be given in the setting of low blood pressure (systolic <90 mm Hg) or right ventricular infarction or in patients who have used a phosphodiesterase inhibitor (eg, sildenafil) within the previous 24 hours (48 hours for tadalafil).

β-Blockade during and after MI lowers mortality in the hospital and after discharge. Oral β-blockers should be administered at presentation to patients who do not have contraindications. Intravenous administration may be considered in hypertensive patients. Contraindications to β-blockers are bradycardia (heart rate <60 beats per minute), second- or third-degree atrioventricular block, hypotension (systolic blood pressure <100 mm Hg), acute heart failure, cardiogenic shock, and cocaine-induced MI. The need for continued treatment should be reassessed periodically. Beneficial effects include decreased pain, decreased myocardial oxygen demand, reduced ventricular fibrillation, decreased platelet aggregability, and decreased sympathetic effects on the myocardium. β-Blockers are most beneficial for patients with a large infarction who are at higher risk for complications.

Calcium channel blockers are generally not used in patients with an acute MI. However, diltiazem may be used to control ventricular rate in atrial fibrillation, especially if β-blockers are contraindicated. Amlodipine may be used to treat hypertension after the acute phase.

Angiotensin-converting enzyme inhibitors prevent ventricular remodeling, especially after a large anterior MI. Oral therapy may be initiated within the first 24 hours if blood pressure and renal function are stable. Angiotensin-converting enzyme inhibitors are indicated in patients with anterior infarction, congestive heart failure, diabetes mellitus, or left ventricular ejection fraction less than 40%. It is reasonable to treat all patients after ST-segment elevation MI in the absence of hypotension or contraindications. Angiotensin-receptor blockers are recommended as an alternative in patients who are intolerant of or allergic to angiotensin-converting enzyme inhibitors.

Long-term aldosterone blockade (spironolactone or eplerenone) is indicated for patients without renal dysfunction (creatinine, <2.0 mg/dL for women and <2.5 mg/dL for men) or hyperkalemia (potassium, <5.0 mEq/L) who are receiving therapeutic doses of angiotensin-converting enzyme inhibitors and β-blockers and have a left ventricular ejection fraction of less than 40% with either symptomatic heart failure or diabetes mellitus.

Glycoprotein IIb/IIIa inhibitors are given only if primary PCI is performed, and their use is generally initiated in the cardiac catheterization laboratory. They are not indicated in patients treated with thrombolytics because of the associated increase in bleeding risk. With the advent and widespread use of potent adenosine diphosphate-receptor antagonists, the role of glycoprotien IIb/IIIa antagonists is currently limited in contemporary practice and typically involves situations in which a large thrombus burden is found at the time of angiography or when inadequate loading with an adenosine diphosphate-receptor antagonist has occurred.

Magnesium does not seem to have a therapeutic role after MI and should be given only for the treatment of torsades de pointes or if a patient has documented hypomagnesemia of potential clinical significance.

Reperfusion Therapy

Early reperfusion therapy decreases mortality by approximately 25%. The extent of myocardial salvage and degree of beneficial effect on mortality are measurably improved the earlier reperfusion occurs. Mortality is as low as 1% when fibrinolysis is given less than 90 minutes after the onset of pain. The majority of delays to reperfusion lie in time to patient presentation, transport, and in-hospital institution of therapy. Reperfusion at 2 to 6 hours results in a lesser effect on myocardial salvage but still has an important effect on survival.

Reperfusion therapy with fibrinolytics (thrombolytics) or primary PCI is indicated for patients presenting within 12 hours of onset of symptoms with the following findings: more than 1 mm of ST-segment elevation in 2 adjacent leads, a new (or presumably new) left bundle branch block, or a true posterior MI.

PCI is more effective than fibrinolysis for restoring normal coronary blood flow (TIMI grade 3) (90% vs 65%–70%). However, intravenous fibrinolysis allows faster administration and is more widely available. The preferred strategy depends on time since the onset of symptoms, transportation time to a skilled PCI laboratory, risk profile of the patient, and contraindications to fibrinolytics. Primary PCI is indicated for patients with immediate access to a high-volume catheterization laboratory, a contraindication to intravenous fibrinolysis, high-risk ST-segment elevation MI (eg, cardiogenic shock or pulmonary edema), or continued ischemia after thrombolytic therapy (rescue PCI).

Routine immediate PCI after successful fibrinolytic therapy is not indicated in the absence of ongoing symptoms or ischemia. Reperfusion therapy is not indicated for patients with ST-segment depression or those who present late (>12 hours after symptom onset) and are asymptomatic without hemodynamic compromise or serious arrhythmia. Fibrinolytic therapy is less beneficial for patients 75 years or older.

Major complications of intravenous fibrinolysis include major bleeding (5%–6%), intracranial bleeding (0.5%), major allergic reaction (0.1%–1.7%), and hypotension (2%–10%). The incidence of myocardial rupture may be higher in patients who are given thrombolytic therapy late (>12 hours after pain onset). Several agents are available for intravenous fibrinolysis, including streptokinase (a nonselective thrombolytic agent) and tissue plasminogen activator (selectively binds to and lyses preformed fibrin). Tissue plasminogen activator has the fastest onset of action. The dosage is 100 mg over 90 minutes. Thrombolytic agents such as reteplase and tenecteplase offer better selectivity for active thrombus, but their efficacy is equivalent to that of tissue plasminogen activator in clinical trials. Their greatest advantage is the ability to administer them as a bolus, which reduces drug errors and speeds delivery. Streptokinase is rarely used in the United States, and tenecteplase and reteplase are now the most commonly used fibrinolytics.

After administration of an intravenous fibrinolytic, a high-grade residual lesion is usually present. Re-occlusion or ischemia occurs in 15% to 20% of patients and re-infarction occurs in 2% to 3%. Heparin should be given in conjunction with intravenous fibrinolysis with tissue-specific plasminogen activators used to prevent re-infarction. The indications for coronary angiography or PCI after intravenous fibrinolysis are spontaneous or inducible ischemia, cardiogenic shock, pulmonary edema, ejection fraction less than 40%, and serious arrhythmias. Routine angiography after fibrinolysis is indicated, typically within 24 hours but after 2 to 4 hours of lytic administration in a strategy referred to as the pharmacoinvasive approach.

Acute Mechanical Complications of ST-Segment Elevation MI

Mechanical complications are relatively uncommon in patients who receive prompt reperfusion therapy. Mechanical complications include cardiogenic shock, myocardial free wall rupture, papillary muscle rupture, and ventricular septal defects. Right ventricular infarct may also occur after an inferior MI.

Most cases of cardiogenic shock are due to extensive left ventricular dysfunction. Echocardiography is helpful to determine the mechanism of cardiogenic shock. The mortality from cardiogenic shock is 50% (Table 8.3).

Right ventricular infarction occurs in up to 40% of patients with inferior MI and typically involves occlusion of the proximal right coronary artery. It can present hours to days after the infarction and is diagnosed from increased jugular venous pressure in the presence of clear lung fields. ST-segment elevation in lead V_4R is diagnostic of a large right ventricular infarction and portends increased mortality. In extreme circumstances, right ventricular infarction can cause cardiogenic shock due to compromised filling of the left ventricle. Treatment includes intravenous fluid resuscitation; if this is inadequate, consideration of the addition of an inotropic agent may be reasonable. In the setting of a right ventricular infarction, dobutamine is the inotropic agent of choice. When right ventricular infarction is recognized early, reperfusion therapy is indicated. Once the acute complication is treated and the patient is supported through the illness, recovery is usually the rule.

Myocardial free wall rupture causes abrupt decompensation. Free wall rupture occurs in 85% of all ruptures. It usually occurs 2 to 14 days after transmural MI, most commonly in elderly hypertensive women, and usually presents as electromechanical dissociation or death. Tamponade may occur if the rupture is contained in the pericardium. If the diagnosis can be made with emergency echocardiography, surgery should be performed. If the rupture is sealed

Table 8.3 • Diagnosis of Cause of Cardiogenic Shock

	Test Results				
	Pulmonary Artery Catheterization				
Cause	RA	PAWP	CO	Catheterization	Two-Dimensional Echocardiography
Left ventricular dysfunction	↑	↑↑	↓↓	NA	Poor left ventricle
Right ventricular infarction	↑↑	↓	↓↓	NA	Dilated right ventricle
Tamponade	↑↑	↑↑	↓↓	End-equalization	Pericardial tamponade
Papillary muscle rupture	↑	↑↑	↓↓	Large V	Severe mitral regurgitation
Ventricular septal defect	↑	↑↑	↑	Step-up	Defect seen
Pulmonary emboli	↑↑	=	↓	PADP >PAWP	Dilated right ventricle

Abbreviations: CO, cardiac output; NA, not applicable; PADP, pulmonary artery diastolic pressure; PAWP, pulmonary artery wedge pressure; RA, right atrial pressure.

off, a pseudoaneurysm may occur. Surgical treatment is required because of the high incidence of further rupture. Unfortunately, mortality in this setting is extremely high.

Papillary muscle rupture usually occurs 2 to 10 days after MI. It is associated with inferior MI because of the single blood supply to the posteromedial papillary muscle. Rupture of papillary muscle is heralded by the sudden onset of dyspnea and hypotension. Although a murmur may be present, it may not be audible because of equalization of left atrial and left ventricular pressures. An intra-aortic balloon pump can be used to temporarily stabilize the patient, and emergency surgery is done for definitive therapy.

Ventricular septal defects usually occur 1 to 20 days after MI and are equally frequent in inferior and anterior MIs. Ventricular septal defects associated with inferior MIs have a poorer prognosis because of the serpiginous nature of the rupture and associated ventricular infarction. They are indicated by the abrupt onset of dyspnea and hypotension. A loud murmur and systolic thrill are almost always present. The diagnosis is made with echocardiography. Treatment is similar to the circumstance of papillary muscle rupture, wherein the hemodynamic status is temporarily stabilized with use of an intra-aortic balloon pump while awaiting definitive emergency surgical management.

Pre–Hospital-Discharge Evaluation

Risk stratification for long-term outcomes is required before hospital discharge and typically includes left ventricular function determination, assessment of risk for arrhythmias, and identification of inducible ischemia. A submaximal treadmill test can be performed before discharge, 4 to 6 days after MI. Alternatively, a symptom-limited treadmill test can be performed safely 10 to 21 days after MI. If a submaximal treadmill test is performed before discharge, a late symptom-limited treadmill test should be performed at follow-up evaluation 3 to 6 weeks after MI. High-risk patients identified by treadmill exertion testing have an ST-segment depression more than 1 mm, a decrease in blood pressure, or an inability to achieve 4 metabolic equivalents on the exercise test. Imaging exercise tests may identify additional high-risk patients by demonstrating multiple areas of ischemia. Pharmacologic stress tests (dobutamine echocardiography, dipyridamole thallium scanning, or adenosine thallium scanning) may be useful for patients unable to exercise.

Increasingly, rather than a stress test, a delayed invasive (pharmacoinvasive) strategy is being practiced in which coronary angiography is performed at least 4 hours after fibrinolysis and before hospital discharge in the setting of ST-segment elevation MI. PCI is performed in the majority of patients, and few undergo CABG or medical therapy alone. The choice between PCI and CABG is based on factors similar to those used to make the decision in patients with stable coronary artery disease. This strategy is associated with lower recurrent ischemia and infarction compared with the ischemia-guided approach described above.

Optimal risk factor modification is essential, including an exercise program, weight loss, and dietary modifications. The goal of treatment is to decrease the low-density lipoprotein cholesterol level to 100 mg/dL or less (optimal <70). If the level is more than 100 mg/dL, statin treatment should be initiated before discharge. All tobacco users should be counseled and nicotine cessation must be stressed.

Aspirin and statins decrease recurrent MI and mortality and should be given to all patients unless contraindicated. β-Blockers improve survival after MI and are most effective in high-risk patients (ie, decreased left ventricular function and ventricular arrhythmias). Chronic therapy may not be required for low-risk patients. Antiarrhythmic agents are associated with increased mortality and should not be used to suppress ventricular ectopy. Angiotensin-converting enzyme inhibitors decrease mortality after anterior MI and depressed left ventricular function, presumably by inhibiting infarct remodeling. A rehabilitation program is essential for the patient's well-being and cardiovascular fitness. An automatic implantable cardioverter-defibrillator should be considered if the ejection fraction is less than 35% 40 days after MI in patients with an expected survival of at least 1 year.

KEY FACTS

✓ Early reperfusion therapy for ST-segment elevation MI—decreases mortality by approximately 25%

✓ Routine angiography after fibrinolysis for ST-segment elevation MI—indicated, typically within 24 hours but after 2–4 hours of lytic administration in a strategy referred to as the pharmacoinvasive approach

✓ Risk stratification for long-term outcomes after ST-segment elevation MI—required before hospital discharge and typically includes left ventricular function determination, assessment of risk for arrhythmias, and identification of inducible ischemia

✓ Automatic implantable cardioverter-defibrillator—should be considered if the ejection fraction is <35% 40 days after MI in patients with an expected survival of ≥1 year

9 Pericardial Disease and Cardiac Tumors

KYLE W. KLARICH, MD

Pericardial Disease

The space between the visceral and parietal pericardium normally contains 15 to 25 mL of clear fluid. The pericardium functions to prevent cardiac distention, limit cardiac displacement (by its attachment to neighboring structures), and protect the heart from inflammation.

Acute or Subacute Inflammatory Pericarditis

Symptoms

The chest pain of pericarditis is aggravated by movement of the trunk, inspiration, and coughing. The pain can be relieved by sitting up. Low-grade fever and malaise may occur.

Diagnosis

Pericardial friction rub may be variable. Chest radiography is usually normal, but globular enlargement may be found if the effusion is marked (>250 mL). A pulmonary infiltrate or small pleural effusion may be present. Left pleural effusion predominates for unknown reasons. Electrocardiography shows acute, concave ST elevation in all ventricular leads. The PR segment is depressed in the early stages. Echocardiography is diagnostic and helps determination of hemodynamic significance.

Causes

Causes include viral or idiopathic pericarditis, autoimmune and collagen vascular diseases, and postmyocardial infarction. Postcardiotomy syndrome may occur weeks to months after open heart procedures. It presents with pyrexia, increased sedimentation rate, and pleural or pericardial chest pain. Incidence decreases with age. Management is with anti-inflammatory agents. Pericarditis is also associated with radiation and neoplasm (especially Hodgkin disease, leukemia, and lymphoma). Melanoma and breast, thyroid, and lung tumors can metastasize to the pericardium and cause pericarditis or pericardial effusion. Uremia and tuberculosis also can cause pericarditis. Idiopathic viral pericarditis is the most likely diagnosis in the absence of a definable cause, and treatment with high-dose aspirin or other nonsteroidal anti-inflammatory agents usually resolves the condition.

Pericardial Effusion

The pericardium exudes fluid, fibrin, and blood cells in response to inflammation, causing a pericardial effusion. It cannot be seen on chest radiography until the effusion is 250 mL. With slow fluid accumulation, the pericardial sac distends slowly with no cardiac compression. With rapid accumulation (eg, bleeding), tamponade can occur with relatively small amounts of fluid. Tamponade restricts ventricular filling, decreasing ventricular volume. Increased intrapericardial pressure increases ventricular end-diastolic pressure, and increased mean atrial pressure increases the venous pressure. Decreased ventricular volume and filling diminish cardiac output. Any cause of pericarditis can cause tamponade, but acute causes of hemopericardium should be considered (eg, ruptured myocardium after infarction, aortic dissection, ruptured aortic aneurysm, and sequelae of cardiac operation).

Clinical Features

Tamponade produces a continuum of features, depending on severity. Typical findings are low blood pressure, a small and quiet heart, tachycardia, increased jugular venous pressure, and pulsus paradoxus (enhanced systemic blood pressure drop during inspiration due to decreased left ventricular filling). Kussmaul sign (increased distention of the neck veins during inspiration) may occur, as with constrictive pericarditis.

Treatment

Emergency pericardiocentesis guided by echocardiography is necessary in hemodynamically compromised patients.

Constrictive Pericarditis

Constrictive pericarditis is characterized by dissociation of respiratory-induced changes in intrathoracic and intracardiac pressures. Ventricular filling is limited by the constraining pericardium, an effect leading to lower ventricular volume, higher end-diastolic pressures, and decreased cardiac output. The most common causes are recurrent viral pericarditis, irradiation, previous open heart operation, tuberculosis, and neoplastic disease.

Symptoms

Symptoms of constrictive pericarditis are predominantly right-sided failure, peripheral edema, ascites, and often dyspnea and fatigue.

Physical Examination

In constrictive pericarditis, the jugular venous pressure is increased (best observed when the patient is sitting or standing) and neck veins are distended on inspiration (Kussmaul sign). The jugular venous pressure may show rapid descents; a pericardial knock is present in fewer than half of the cases. Ascites and peripheral edema are usually present. Chest radiography may show pericardial calcification and cardiac enlargement. No specific changes are found on electrocardiography.

Diagnosis

A high degree of clinical suspicion is necessary because the diagnosis of constrictive pericarditis can be challenging. Echocardiography, particularly with Doppler, shows the hemodynamic effects of respiratory changes in mitral and tricuspid inflow velocities and other classic changes. Pericardial thickness may be delineated by computed tomography and magnetic resonance imaging, but up to 20% of constraining pericardium may not be thickened according to computed tomographic criteria. Magnetic resonance scanning can show pericardial inflammation. Restrictive cardiomyopathy is the main differential diagnosis, and differentiation can be difficult. Myocardial disease is likely if pulmonary artery systolic pressure is more than 50 mm Hg or if end-diastolic pulmonary artery pressure is more than 30% of systolic pressure, but both are nonspecific findings. In very difficult cases, cardiac catheterization for hemodynamic measurements may be necessary to show the intraventricular dependence and dissociation of intracardiac and intrathoracic pressures. Constrictive pericarditis is a reversible cause of heart failure and should be considered in all patients presenting with symptoms of predominantly right heart failure.

Treatment

The treatment of choice for constrictive pericarditis is pericardiectomy.

KEY FACTS

✓ Acute or subacute inflammatory pericarditis—pericardial friction rub may be variable, chest radiography is usually normal, but globular enlargement may be found if effusion is marked (>250 mL)

✓ Acute or subacute inflammatory pericarditis—idiopathic viral pericarditis is the most likely diagnosis in the absence of a definable cause, and treatment with high-dose aspirin or other nonsteroidal anti-inflammatory agents and colchicine usually resolves the condition

✓ Pericardial effusion—any cause of pericarditis can cause tamponade, but acute causes of hemopericardium should be considered (eg, ruptured myocardium after infarction, aortic dissection, ruptured aortic aneurysm, and sequelae of cardiac operation)

✓ Constrictive pericarditis

- jugular venous pressure is increased (best observed when patient is sitting or standing) and neck veins are distended on inspiration (Kussmaul sign)

- a high degree of clinical suspicion is necessary because the diagnosis can be challenging

- is a reversible cause of heart failure and should be considered in all patients presenting with symptoms of predominantly right heart failure

---

Cardiac Tumors

Metastatic tumors are far more common than primary cardiac tumors (>40-fold). The most frequent metastases to the heart are melanoma, lymphoma, and breast, lung, and esophageal tumors. More than half of patients with malignant melanoma have metastases to the heart. This occurrence carries a poor prognosis.

The most common primary benign tumors of the adult heart are cardiac myxoma, papillary fibroelastoma, lipoma, and fibroma. Primary tumors are extremely rare. Cardiac tumors may cause circulatory problems, valve dysfunction, myocardial infiltration–related complications, invasion into local structures, or embolization.

The most common primary cardiac tumor is myxoma, a benign tumor. Most cardiac myxomas are sporadic, but a subset of these tumors are familial. The majority (75%–85%) are located in the left atrium, 18% are in the right atrium, and the rest are ventricular. Most atrial tumors arise from the atrial septum, usually adjacent to the fossa ovalis. About 95% are solitary. Most have a short stalk, are gelatinous and friable, and tend to embolize.

They occasionally calcify and may be visible on chest radiography.

A familial syndrome, **Carney complex**, involves multiple, often recurrent, cardiac and extracardiac myxomas, lentiginosis (spotty pigmentation) and other blue nevi, endocrine tumors, and schwannomas. Myxomas present at a young age compared with sporadic myxomas.

> ### Key Definition
>
> Carney complex: *a familial myxoma syndrome that involves multiple endocrine neoplasias and multiple myxomas.*

Blood flow obstruction, embolization, and systemic effects are the most common complications. Systemic emboli may occur in 30% to 60% of patients with left-sided myxoma, frequently to the brain and lower extremities. Coronary embolization is rare, but it should be considered in a young patient with no known previous cardiac disease. Systemic effects are fatigue, fever, weight loss, and arthralgia. Systemic effects may be associated with an increased sedimentation rate, leukocytosis, hypergammaglobulinemia, and anemia. Increased immunoglobulins are usually of immunoglobulin G class.

Left atrial tumors prolapse into the mitral valve orifice, producing symptoms of mitral stenosis (dyspnea, orthopnea, cough, pulmonary edema, and hemoptysis) and can even lead to syncope or sudden cardiac death. Classically, symptoms occur with a change in body position. Physical findings suggest mitral stenosis. Pulmonary hypertension may occur. An early diastolic sound, the tumor "plop," may be heard, with the timing of a third heart sound. The later timing and lower frequency differentiate it from an opening snap.

Echocardiography allows accurate diagnosis. Once diagnosed, myxomas should be surgically excised.

KEY FACTS

- ✓ Cardiac tumors—metastatic tumors are far more common than primary cardiac tumors (>40-fold)
- ✓ Most common primary benign tumors of adult heart—cardiac myxoma, papillary fibroelastoma, lipoma, and fibroma
- ✓ Left atrial tumors prolapse into the mitral valve orifice, producing symptoms of mitral stenosis (dyspnea, orthopnea, cough, pulmonary edema, and hemoptysis) and can even lead to syncope or sudden cardiac death

10 Valvular and Congenital Heart Diseases[a]

KYLE W. KLARICH, MD; LORI A. BLAUWET, MD;
AND SABRINA D. PHILLIPS, MD

Valvular Heart Disease

Aortic Stenosis

The **pathophysiologic effect** of aortic stenosis on the heart is pressure overload, leading to left ventricular hypertrophy. The vast majority of cases of aortic stenosis are due to valvular stenosis.

Types

The *congenital bicuspid* type of aortic stenosis occurs in 2% of the population; the male to female ratio is 3:1. It is inherited in an autosomal dominant pattern. First-degree relatives should be screened. Bicuspid aortic valve is the most common cause of aortic stenosis in adults younger than 55 years. Frequently, when a patient is young and the valve is still pliable, the auscultation is different from that of degenerative aortic valve disease. An ejection click classically precedes the systolic murmur and may be heard even in the absence of murmur or before the murmur is present. This is a high-pitched sound that comes early in systole, right after the first heart sound. The ejection click represents opening of the less pliable bicuspid valve and is heard best in the aortic listening post, the second intercostal space. It is a high-pitched sound that is best heard with the diaphragm of the stethoscope. As aortic stenosis worsens, aortic valve closure is delayed; when aortic stenosis is severe, there may even be paradoxic splitting of the second heart sound.

Bicuspid aortic valve may be associated with coarctation of the aorta in about 10% of patients. Conversely, if coarctation is noted, there is a 30% to 50% chance of bicuspid aortic valve. Even with a normally functioning aortic valve, the ascending aorta may not be normal. The aortopathy associated with bicuspid aortic valve can cause dilatation of the sinus of Valsalva and the ascending aorta. Both of these phenomena should be specifically screened for with imaging of the aorta. If bicuspid aortic valve is suspected, the diagnosis usually can be made with 2-dimensional and Doppler echocardiography without the need for cardiac catheterization in young people. If the diagnosis is confirmed, the aorta should be imaged with ultrasonography, magnetic resonance imaging, or computed tomography to rule out coarctation and aortic dilatation or aneurysm. *Degenerative aortic valve disease* due to calcification is the most common cause of aortic stenosis in adults older than 55 years. The valve is tricuspid. When calcification is extensive, the aortic valve component becomes inaudible.

The *rheumatic* type of aortic valve disease is less common. It is associated with thickening and fusion of the aortic cusps at the commissures. It always occurs with a rheumatic mitral valve, although considerable mitral stenosis or regurgitation may not always be evident. It usually occurs in adulthood (age 40–60 years), usually 15 ± 5 years after acute rheumatic fever.

Symptoms

The classic symptoms of the valvular type of aortic stenosis (regardless of type) include exertional dyspnea, syncope, angina, and sudden cardiac death. The onset of symptoms is an ominous sign and portends a very poor prognosis. Patients with symptomatic aortic stenosis need rapid

[a] Portions previously published in Bonow RO, Carabello BA, Chatterjee K, de Leon AC Jr, Faxon DP, Freed MD, et al; 2006 Writing Committee Members; American College of Cardiology/American Heart Association Task Force. 2008 Focused update incorporated into the ACC/AHA 2006 guidelines for the management of patients with valvular heart disease: a report of the American College of Cardiology/American Heart Association Task Force on Practice Guidelines (Writing Committee to Revise the 1998 Guidelines for the Management of Patients With Valvular Heart Disease): endorsed by the Society of Cardiovascular Anesthesiologists, Society for Cardiovascular Angiography and Interventions, and Society of Thoracic Surgeons. Circulation. 2008 Oct 7;118(15):e523–661. Epub 2008 Sep 26. Used with permission.

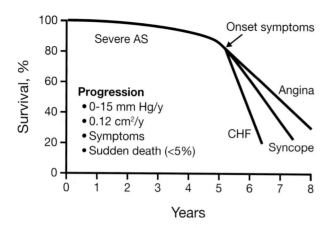

Figure 10.1 *Natural History of Aortic Stenosis (AS). CHF indicates congestive heart failure.*
(Adapted from Ross J Jr, Braunwald E. Aortic stenosis. Circulation. 1968 Jul 1;38 Suppl 1:61–7. Used with permission.)

surgical intervention (Figure 10.1); there is no medical treatment. The presence of angina does not necessarily indicate coexisting coronary disease; rather, it is related to increased left ventricular filling pressure causing subendocardial ischemia. The chest pain syndrome, in the absence of coronary artery disease, is due to supply-demand mismatch.

Physical Examination

The arterial pulse is parvus (small and difficult to feel) and tardus (delayed) in hemodynamically significant aortic stenosis. The left ventricular impulse is localized, lateralized, and sustained. Arterial thrills may be palpable at the carotid artery, suprasternal notch, second intercostal space, or left and right sternal borders. An audible and palpable fourth heart sound may be present. The aortic valve component is diminished and delayed and may even become absent with decreasing pliability of the aortic cusps. The ejection systolic murmur becomes louder and peaks later with increasing severity, radiating to the carotid arteries and the apex.

Diagnosis

Electrocardiography in aortic stenosis may show left ventricular hypertrophy; echocardiography is more sensitive and specific. Left bundle branch block is common; in later stages of the condition, conduction abnormalities may develop (eg, complete heart block) if calcium impinges on the conducting system. On chest radiography, the heart size is usually normal even when the stenosis is severe and the left ventricle fails; enlargement of the heart may not be evident until late stages and left ventricular remodeling occurs. The aortic root may show "poststenotic" dilatation, now recognized as an aortopathy when the valvular abnormality is bicuspid. In degenerative aortic valve disease, calcium may be seen in the valve leaflets and in the intervalvular fibrosa, especially on a lateral view.

The differential diagnosis of aortic stenosis includes 1) hypertrophic cardiomyopathy (note different carotid upstroke and change in murmur with Valsalva maneuver) and 2) mitral regurgitation (murmur may radiate anteriorly and upward along the aorta, particularly if there is rupture of chordae of the posterior mitral valve leaflet; no radiation to the carotid arteries).

Aortic stenosis can be diagnosed with bedside physical examination. The most important physical finding is the parvus and tardus pulse contour. The degree of aortic stenosis can be difficult to determine, particularly in older patients. Noninvasive Doppler echocardiography is useful for assessing aortic valve area and gradients and correlates well with invasive catheter-based assessment of the same. Severe aortic stenosis is present when the mean Doppler gradient is more than 40 mm Hg, the valve area is less than 1.0 cm^2, and the valve index is 0.6 cm^2/m^2 or less. Progression of aortic stenosis is highly variable; on average, it is about 0.12 cm^2 per year with wide individual variation. Progression to symptoms can be insidious; the onset of clinical symptoms is an ominous prognostic sign. Survival after symptom onset is 1 to 3 years (Figure 10.1).

Treatment

All patients should be educated about worrisome symptoms that may develop. Dyspnea, chest pain, angina, syncope, or newly diagnosed congestive heart failure are important clinical evidence for surgical intervention and should be promptly evaluated (Table 10.1). Aortic valve replacement is the only effective treatment for patients with severe obstruction (Figure 10.2).

Aortic Regurgitation

The pathophysiology of aortic regurgitation is that of volume and pressure overload on the left ventricle, leading to hypertrophy and dilatation. It can be related to either the aortic valve or the aortic root, and the condition can be acute or chronic (Table 10.2). Acute aortic regurgitation may be associated with an aortic dissection.

Valvular Aortic Regurgitation

Causes of valvular aortic regurgitation include 1) congenital bicuspid valve, 2) rheumatic fever, 3) endocarditis, 4) degenerative aortic valve disease, 5) seronegative arthritis, 6) ankylosing spondylitis, and 7) rheumatoid arthritis.

Aortic Root Dilatation

Various conditions have been associated with aortic root dilatation. Advancing age is one factor; hypertension accelerates this process. Aortic regurgitation associated with age or hypertension is common and usually mild. Marfan syndrome may cause progressive dilatation of the aortic root and sinuses (cystic medial necrosis). Prophylactic β-adrenergic blocker therapy slows the rate of aortic

Table 10.1 • Quantitation of the Severity of Aortic Stenosis and Treatment Guidelines

Severity	AVA, cm²	AVA Index, cm²/m²	Gradient, mm Hg	Follow-up or Treatment
Normal	3.0–4.0		<10	
Mild	>1.5	>0.8	<30	Echo every 5 y or if symptoms
Moderate	1.0–1.5	0.5–0.8	30–40	Monitor for symptoms Echo every 1–2 y
Severe	<1.0	<0.5	>40	Symptoms: operate No symptoms: echo every 6–12 mo

Abbreviations: AVA, aortic valve area; echo, echocardiography.

Data from Bonow RO, Carabello BA, Chatterjee K, de Leon AC Jr, Faxon DP, Freed MD, et al; American College of Cardiology/American Heart Association Task Force on Practice Guidelines. 2008 focused update incorporated into the ACC/AHA 2006 guidelines for the management of patients with valvular heart disease: a report of the American College of Cardiology/American Heart Association Task Force on Practice Guidelines (Writing Committee to revise the 1998 guidelines for the management of patients with valvular heart disease). Endorsed by the Society of Cardiovascular Anesthesiologists, Society for Cardiovascular Angiography and Interventions, and Society of Thoracic Surgeons. J Am Coll Cardiol. 2008 Sep 23;52(13):e1–142 and Bonow RO, Carabello BA, Chatterjee K, de Leon AC Jr, Faxon DP, Freed MD, et al; 2006 Writing Committee Members; American College of Cardiology/American Heart Association Task Force. 2008 Focused update incorporated into the ACC/AHA 2006 guidelines for the management of patients with valvular heart disease: a report of the American College of Cardiology/American Heart Association Task Force on Practice Guidelines (Writing Committee to Revise the 1998 Guidelines for the Management of Patients With Valvular Heart Disease): endorsed by the Society of Cardiovascular Anesthesiologists, Society for Cardiovascular Angiography and Interventions, and Society of Thoracic Surgeons. Circulation. 2008 Oct 7;118(15):e523–661. Epub 2008 Sep 26.

dilatation and reduces the development of aortic complications in some patients with Marfan syndrome. When the aortic root reaches 5 to 5.5 cm or more in diameter, it should be replaced. Syphilis is an uncommon cause of aortic regurgitation and usually causes aortic root dilatation above the sinuses, sparing the sinuses. Syphilis is associated with aortic root calcium on chest radiography.

Symptoms

The symptoms of *acute* aortic regurgitation are extreme: pulmonary edema, shock, and, often, chest pain (in the setting of aortic dissection). The symptoms of *chronic* aortic regurgitation can develop insidiously because of compensatory mechanisms of the heart. The most common symptoms of *severe* aortic regurgitation include fatigue, dyspnea, palpitations, and exertional angina.

Physical Examination

Severe aortic regurgitation is associated with physical findings that include a bounding, rapidly collapsing Corrigan pulse resulting from wide pulse pressure; bisferiens pulse (may be present); de Musset head nodding; Duroziez sign (systolic and diastolic ["to-and-fro"] murmur on gentle compression with stethoscope) over the femoral artery; and Quincke sign (pulsatile capillary nail bed). Müller sign (systolic pulsations of the uvula) is often noted. The left ventricular impulse is diffuse and hyperdynamic. The apical impulse is often displaced downward. A diastolic decrescendo murmur is heard at either the left or the right sternal border, and the second heart sound may be paradoxically split because of increased left ventricular volume.

Murmur duration is related to the rate of pressure equilibration between the aorta and the left ventricle. Aortic regurgitation with physiologic diastolic pressures results in a holodiastolic murmur. The shorter the aortic regurgitation murmur, the faster the pressure equilibration, and thus the more severe the aortic regurgitation (higher left ventricular end-diastolic pressure). The loudness of the murmur does not correlate with the severity of aortic regurgitation, particularly in acute aortic regurgitation (such as with dissection). A systolic flow murmur is common, because of the increased ejection volume. It does not necessarily indicate aortic stenosis.

Diagnosis

Acute aortic regurgitation may not be identified on bedside examination if a patient presents with little or no murmur. Electrocardiography often shows left ventricular hypertrophy. Echocardiography is best suited to gather the important functional and hemodynamic data needed to make management decisions in patients with aortic regurgitation.

Because chronic aortic regurgitation has a long, silent, well-compensated natural history, left ventricular size, aortic root size and morphology, valve morphology, and left ventricular function (ejection fraction) should be followed with echocardiography.

Chest radiography shows an enlarged cardiac shadow and prominence of the left ventricle in a leftward and inferior pattern. The aorta also may be enlarged, especially in Marfan syndrome. Table 10.3 outlines the natural history of severe aortic regurgitation.

Treatment

Acute severe aortic regurgitation is a surgical emergency. If untreated, severe pulmonary congestion, arrhythmias, and circulatory collapse will develop. As a bridge to operation, nitroprusside to reduce peripheral resistance and encourage forward flow or inotropic agents to augment cardiac

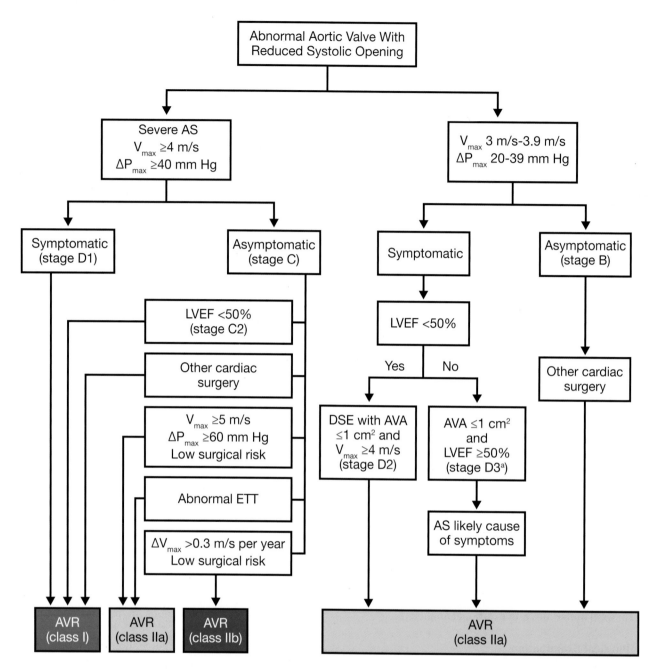

Figure 10.2 *Indications for Aortic Valve Replacement (AVR), Surgically or Transcatheter Approach, in Patients With Aortic Stenosis (AS). Arrows show the decision pathways that result in a recommendation for AVR. Periodic monitoring is indicated for all patients in whom AVR is not yet indicated, including those with asymptomatic AS (stage D or C) and those with low-gradient AS (stage D2 or D3) who do not meet the criteria for intervention. AVA indicates aortic valve area; DSE, dobutamine stress echocardiography; ETT, exercise treadmill test; LVEF, left ventricular ejection fraction; ΔP_{max}, maximum pressure gradient; V_{max}, maximum velocity. [a]AVR should be considered with stage D3 AS only if valve obstruction is the most likely cause of symptoms, stroke volume index is less than 35 mL/m², indexed AVA is less than or equal to 0.6 cm²/m², and data are recorded when the patient is normotensive (systolic blood pressure <140 mm Hg).*

(Adapted from Nishimura RA, Otto CM, Bonow RO, Carabello BA, Erwin JP 3rd, Guyton RA, et al; ACC/AHA Task Force Members. 2014 AHA/ACC Guideline for the Management of Patients With Valvular Heart Disease: a report of the American College of Cardiology/ American Heart Association Task Force on Practice Guidelines. Circulation. 2014 Jun 10;129[23]:e521–643. Epub 2014 Mar 3. Errata in: Circulation. 2014 Jun 10;129[23]:e651. Circulation. 2014 Sep 23;130[13]:e120. Dosage error in article text and Nishimura RA, Otto CM, Bonow RO, Carabello BA, Erwin JP 3rd, Guyton RA, et al; American College of Cardiology/American Heart Association Task Force on Practice Guidelines. 2014 AHA/ACC guideline for the management of patients with valvular heart disease: a report of the American College of Cardiology/American Heart Association Task Force on Practice Guidelines. J Am Coll Cardiol. 2014 Jun 10;63[22]:e57–185. Epub 2014 Mar 3. Erratum in: J Am Coll Cardiol. 2014 Jun 10;63[22]:2489. Dosage error in article text. Used with permission.)

Table 10.2 • Aortic Regurgitation: Symptoms and Findings on Examination

	Acute	Chronic
Symptoms	Pulmonary edema Shock Arrhythmia Chest pain Dissection, RCA infarct	Dyspnea Fatigue Exercise intolerance Night sweats Palpitations
Examination	Faint, short murmur	Peripheral pulses Quincke and Duroziez signs, pistol-shot pulse Enlarged, diffuse, hyperdynamic LV Murmur LSB—valve etiology RSB—root etiology
Chest radiography	Wide mediastinum Pulmonary edema	Enlarged heart Enlarged aorta
Electrocardiography	Low voltage (if pericardial effusion) ST elevation II, III, F (if aortic dissection into RCA)	LVH

Abbreviations: LSB, left sternal border; LV, left ventricle; LVH, left ventricular hypertrophy; RCA, right coronary artery; RSB, right sternal border.

Table 10.3 • Natural History of Severe Aortic Regurgitation

Status of Patient	% of Patients/y
Asymptomatic with normal LV systolic function	
Progression to symptoms or LV dysfunction	<6
Progression to asymptomatic LV dysfunction	<3.5
Sudden death	<0.2
Asymptomatic with LV dysfunction	
Progression to cardiac symptoms	>25
Symptomatic	
Mortality rate	>10

Abbreviation: LV, left ventricular.
Adapted from Bonow RO, Carabello BA, Chatterjee K, de Leon AC Jr, Faxon DP, Freed MD, et al; American College of Cardiology/American Heart Association Task Force on Practice Guidelines. 2008 focused update incorporated into the ACC/AHA 2006 guidelines for the management of patients with valvular heart disease: a report of the American College of Cardiology/American Heart Association Task Force on Practice Guidelines (Writing Committee to revise the 1998 guidelines for the management of patients with valvular heart disease). Endorsed by the Society of Cardiovascular Anesthesiologists, Society for Cardiovascular Angiography and Interventions, and Society of Thoracic Surgeons. J Am Coll Cardiol. 2008 Sep 23;52(13):e1–142 and Bonow RO, Carabello BA, Chatterjee K, de Leon AC Jr, Faxon DP, Freed MD, et al; 2006 Writing Committee Members; American College of Cardiology/American Heart Association Task Force. 2008 Focused update incorporated into the ACC/AHA 2006 guidelines for the management of patients with valvular heart disease: a report of the American College of Cardiology/American Heart Association Task Force on Practice Guidelines (Writing Committee to Revise the 1998 Guidelines for the Management of Patients With Valvular Heart Disease): endorsed by the Society of Cardiovascular Anesthesiologists, Society for Cardiovascular Angiography and Interventions, and Society of Thoracic Surgeons. Circulation. 2008 Oct 7;118(15):e523–661. Epub 2008 Sep 26. Used with permission.

output may be considered. An intra-aortic balloon pump is contraindicated because it will worsen regurgitation.

Key Definition

Chronic aortic regurgitation: *combined volume and pressure overload on left ventricle.*

Chronic aortic regurgitation is a combined volume and pressure overload on the left ventricle. The left ventricle compensates by dilating and increasing compliance. Patients with aortic regurgitation may remain asymptomatic for decades. The development of symptoms usually reflects left ventricular dysfunction, and survival is limited (10% annual mortality) unless surgical intervention is prompt. Medical management (eg, angiotensin-converting enzyme inhibitor or nifedipine) slows ventricular dilatation in patients with severe aortic regurgitation and may help delay operation. Compensation is not maintained indefinitely, and eventually left ventricular filling pressure increases, coronary flow reserve diminishes, and left ventricular dysfunction develops insidiously. Angina, even in the absence of epicardial coronary stenosis, may be present as a result of supply-and-demand mismatch.

Asymptomatic left ventricular dysfunction may develop in a subset of patients. Several factors have been suggested to prompt surgical intervention before left ventricular dysfunction develops: an end-systolic dimension more than 50 mm, an end-diastolic dimension more than 65 mm, or an ejection fraction of 50% or less (Figure 10.3).

KEY FACTS

✓ Bicuspid aortic valve—may be associated with coarctation of the aorta in ~10% of patients; conversely, if coarctation is noted, the chance of bicuspid aortic valve is 30%–50%

✓ In hemodynamically significant aortic stenosis—the arterial pulse is parvus (small and difficult to feel) and tardus (delayed)

✓ Causes of valvular aortic regurgitation—1) congenital bicuspid valve, 2) rheumatic fever, 3) endocarditis, 4) degenerative aortic valve disease, 5) seronegative arthritis, 6) ankylosing spondylitis, and 7) rheumatoid arthritis

✓ Acute severe aortic regurgitation—

  • a surgical emergency that, if untreated, will lead to severe pulmonary congestion, arrhythmias, and circulatory collapse

  • as a bridge to operation, nitroprusside to reduce peripheral resistance and encourage forward flow or inotropic agents to augment cardiac output may be considered

---

Asymptomatic patients with a dilated left ventricle must be followed carefully. Evidence of left ventricular systolic dysfunction at rest, progressive diastolic dysfunction, or rapidly progressive left ventricular dilatation should prompt surgical treatment. The ability to repair (rather than replace) the valve may favor earlier operation (before left ventricular dilatation has occurred).

Mitral Stenosis

Etiology and Pathophysiology
Rheumatic fever is the cause of rheumatic heart disease, which leads to leaflet thickening with fusion of the commissures and later calcification. These effects result in mitral stenosis, and prophylaxis against rheumatic fever is therefore strongly recommended. Mitral stenosis results in obstruction of blood flow from the left atrium to the left ventricle, preventing proper diastolic filling and leading to pulmonary congestion.

Symptoms
Symptoms of mitral stenosis usually develop decades after rheumatic fever. The murmur of mitral stenosis is apparent on physical examination about 10 years after rheumatic fever. After another decade, symptoms develop, usually dyspnea and later orthopnea with paroxysmal nocturnal dyspnea, which can be insidious. Atrial fibrillation leads to deterioration of clinical status. Hemoptysis and pulmonary hypertension with signs of right-sided failure (ie, ascites and peripheral edema) are late manifestations. There is an increased risk of systemic emboli, especially with the development of atrial fibrillation. Not uncommonly, patients with previously undiagnosed mitral stenosis initially present with an embolic event or atrial fibrillation.

Physical Examination
The first heart sound in mitral stenosis is loud as long as the leaflets remain pliable. The shorter the interval from the aortic valve component to the opening snap, the more severe the mitral stenosis. An opening snap occurs only with a pliable valve, and it disappears if the valve calcifies. The stenosis is mild if this interval is more than 90 milliseconds, moderate if it is 80 milliseconds, and severe if it is less than 60 milliseconds. The diastolic murmur is a low-pitched, holodiastolic rumble, heard best at the apex with the bell of the stethoscope and with the patient in the left lateral decubitus position. The murmur may have presystolic accentuation if sinus rhythm is present. Right ventricular lift and increased pulmonic valve component are associated with pulmonary hypertension.

Diagnosis
Electrocardiography can show left atrial enlargement, P mitrale (notched P wave in leads I and II with a duration ≥0.12 millisecond due to characteristic left atrial

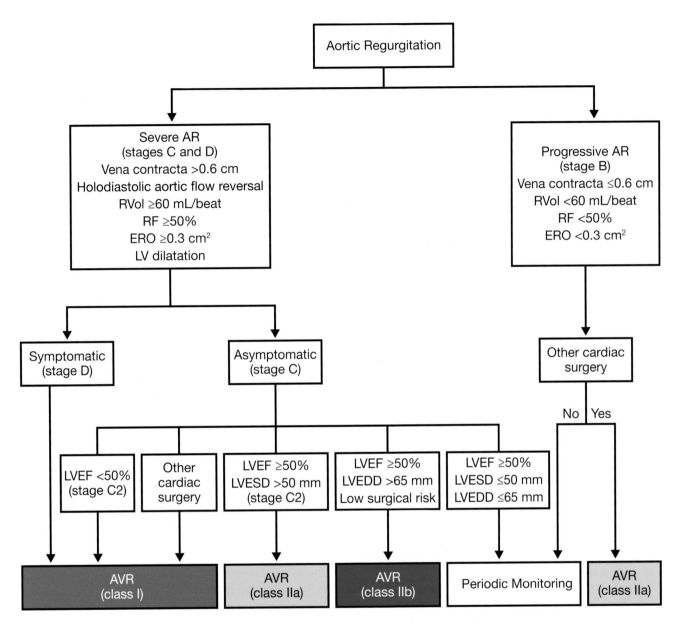

Figure 10.3 *Indications for Aortic Valve Replacement in Chronic Aortic Regurgitation. AR indicates aortic regurgitation; AVR, aortic valve replacement (valve repair may be appropriate in selected patients); ERO, effective regurgitant orifice; LV, left ventricular; LVEDD, left ventricular end-diastolic dimension; LVEF, left ventricular ejection fraction; LVESD, left ventricular end-systolic dimension; RF, regurgitant fraction; RVol, regurgitant volume.*

(Adapted from Nishimura RA, Otto CM, Bonow RO, Carabello BA, Erwin JP 3rd, Guyton RA, et al; ACC/AHA Task Force Members. 2014 AHA/ACC Guideline for the Management of Patients With Valvular Heart Disease: a report of the American College of Cardiology/ American Heart Association Task Force on Practice Guidelines. Circulation. 2014 Jun 10;129[23]:e521–643. Epub 2014 Mar 3. Errata in: Circulation. 2014 Jun 10;129[23]:e651. Circulation. 2014 Sep 23;130[13]:e120. Dosage error in article text and Nishimura RA, Otto CM, Bonow RO, Carabello BA, Erwin JP 3rd, Guyton RA, et al; American College of Cardiology/American Heart Association Task Force on Practice Guidelines. 2014 AHA/ACC guideline for the management of patients with valvular heart disease: a report of the American College of Cardiology/American Heart Association Task Force on Practice Guidelines. J Am Coll Cardiol. 2014 Jun 10;63[22]:e57–185. Epub 2014 Mar 3. Erratum in: J Am Coll Cardiol. 2014 Jun 10;63[22]:2489. Dosage error in article text. Used with permission.)

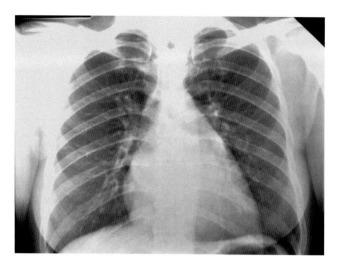

Figure 10.4 Chest Radiograph From a Patient With Severe Mitral Stenosis. The straight left heart border, prominent pulmonary artery, large left atrium, right ventricular contour, and pulmonary venous hypertension are typical findings.

enlargement), and right ventricular hypertrophy. Chest radiography (Figure 10.4) shows straightening of the left heart border with a large left atrial shadow and dilated upper lobe pulmonary veins. With pulmonary hypertension, the central pulmonary arteries become prominent. In severe stenosis, pulmonary congestion characterized by Kerley B lines may be present, indicating a pulmonary wedge pressure of more than 20 mm Hg.

Two-dimensional and Doppler echocardiography is the test of choice to diagnose mitral stenosis and determine its severity. Information is gained about valve gradient and valve area (Table 10.4), and pulmonary artery pressures can be noninvasively assessed. Cardiac catheterization is usually unnecessary unless the coronary arteries need to be studied or the echocardiographic findings do not concur with the clinical situation. Severe stenosis usually correlates with a mean gradient of 12 mm Hg or more.

Treatment
Because mitral stenosis represents obstruction to diastolic filling, anything that shortens diastolic filling time will worsen the severity and symptoms of the disease (eg, tachycardia,

atrial fibrillation, and exercise). Therefore, β-adrenergic blockers and calcium channel blockers can be used to slow heart rate and improve left ventricular filling. Salt restriction and diuretic therapy are useful for early symptoms.

The left ventricle is unaffected in mitral stenosis. It is small, vigorous, and possibly underfilled (reduced preload) in late mitral stenosis. Intervention on the mitral valve is not recommended until there are symptoms of exertional dyspnea, pulmonary edema, or moderate pulmonary hypertension. Marked volume overload of the left atrium leads to increased stroke risk as a result of stagnation of blood flow and thrombus formation. Atrial fibrillation is frequent and intermittent in the early stages. Intermittent screening may be warranted, and anticoagulation should be considered early.

Once symptoms are present (Figure 10.5), treatment is with either surgical valve replacement or percutaneous balloon valvuloplasty. Percutaneous mitral valve balloon valvuloplasty is first-line therapy when mitral valve leaflets are pliable and noncalcified regurgitation is minimal, and no left atrial clot is present. Valve replacement is done when symptoms are more severe because of its associated morbidity and mortality. Intervention for mitral stenosis is indicated by 1) the severity of the valvular disease; 2) symptoms of exertional dyspnea, 3) development of atrial fibrillation, and 4) pulmonary capillary wedge pressure more than 25 mm Hg with exercise.

Mitral Regurgitation

Etiology and Pathophysiology
The mitral valve is a complex structure, and regurgitation can result from abnormalities of 3 anatomical locations: leaflet, tensor apparatus (chordal and papillary muscles), and myocardium. Common causes of mitral regurgitation include mitral valve prolapse syndrome and myxomatous degeneration, infective endocarditis, left ventricular dilatation in congestive heart failure, collagen vascular disease, ischemia, rheumatic heart disease, and left ventricular dilatation due to cardiomyopathy (Table 10.5). In the case of ischemic mitral regurgitation, the posterior medial papillary muscle with its single blood supply (compared with anterolateral, which has a dual blood supply) is more susceptible.

Symptoms
Chronic mitral regurgitation causes left ventricular volume overload with reduced afterload. Given time, the left ventricle compensates by increasing stroke volume. A long asymptomatic phase is thus possible. The most common symptoms include fatigue, dyspnea (due to increased left atrial pressure), and pulmonary edema. Symptoms often worsen with atrial fibrillation.

Physical Examination
Findings of mitral regurgitation include a diffuse and hyperdynamic left ventricular impulse, which may be visible, and a palpable rapid filling wave. The second heart sound

Severity	Valve Area, cm²	Mean Gradient, mm Hg	Systolic PAP, mm Hg
Mild	>1.5	<6	Normal
Moderate	≤1.5	6–11	≤50
Severe	<1	≥12	>50

Table 10.4 • Severity of Mitral Stenosis, by Valve Area, Gradient, and Pulmonary Pressure

Abbreviation: PAP, pulmonary artery pressure.

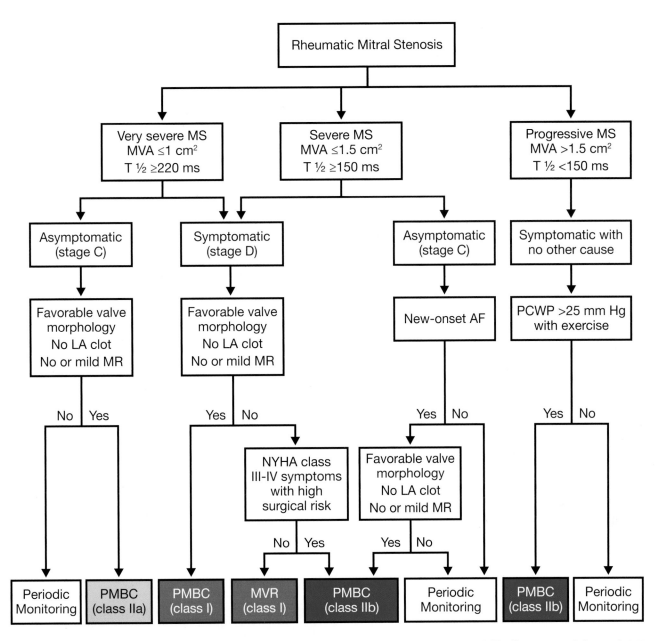

Figure 10.5 *Indications for Intervention for Rheumatic Mitral Stenosis. AF indicates atrial fibrillation; LA, left atrial; MR, mitral regurgitation; MS, mitral stenosis; MVA, mitral valve area; MVR, mitral valve surgery (repair or replacement); NYHA, New York Heart Association; PCWP, pulmonary capillary wedge pressure; PMBC; percutaneous mitral balloon commissurotomy; T ½, pressure half-time.*

(Adapted from Nishimura RA, Otto CM, Bonow RO, Carabello BA, Erwin JP 3rd, Guyton RA, et al; ACC/AHA Task Force Members. 2014 AHA/ACC Guideline for the Management of Patients With Valvular Heart Disease: a report of the American College of Cardiology/ American Heart Association Task Force on Practice Guidelines. Circulation. 2014 Jun 10;129[23]:e521–643. Epub 2014 Mar 3. Errata in: Circulation. 2014 Jun 10;129[23]:e651. Circulation. 2014 Sep 23;130[13]:e120. Dosage error in article text and Nishimura RA, Otto CM, Bonow RO, Carabello BA, Erwin JP 3rd, Guyton RA, et al; American College of Cardiology/American Heart Association Task Force on Practice Guidelines. 2014 AHA/ACC guideline for the management of patients with valvular heart disease: a report of the American College of Cardiology/American Heart Association Task Force on Practice Guidelines. J Am Coll Cardiol. 2014 Jun 10;63[22]:e57–185. Epub 2014 Mar 3. Erratum in: J Am Coll Cardiol. 2014 Jun 10;63[22]:2489. Dosage error in article text. Used with permission.)

Table 10.5 • Types of Mitral Regurgitation

Anatomical Type	Clinical Presentation	
	Chronic	Acute or Subacute
Leaflets	Rheumatic Prolapse Annular calcification Connective tissue disease Congenital cleft Drug-related	Infective endocarditis
Tensor apparatus (chordal and papillary muscles)	Prolapse	Rupture of chordae Myocardial infarction Papillary muscle rupture
Myocardium	Regional ischemia or infarctions Dilated cardiomyopathy Hypertrophic cardiomyopathy	

Adapted from McGoon MD, Schaff HV, Enriquez-Sarano M, Fuster V, Callahan MJ. Mitral regurgitation. In: Guiliani ER, Gersh BJ, McGoon MD, Hayes DL, Schaff HV, editors. Mayo Clinic practice of cardiology. 3rd ed. St. Louis (MO): Mosby; c1996. p. 1450–69. Used with permission of Mayo Foundation for Medical Education and Research.

may be obliterated, and there is a holosystolic murmur. There may be a third heart sound (or a third heart sound and a flow rumble) and a fourth heart sound. A third heart sound with a low-pitched early diastolic rumble indicates severe regurgitation; it represents a volume murmur, but coexisting mitral stenosis needs to be ruled out.

In acute mitral regurgitation, the murmur may be short because of increased left atrial pressure. In severe mitral regurgitation, the carotid upstroke may appear parvus, because of the low forward stroke volume, but not tardus. The left atrium may be palpable with systole, and the left ventricle, with diastole. The cause of mitral regurgitation may be suspected by the radiation of the auscultated murmur. A murmur that is due to a rupture of the anterior leaflet chordae leads to a posteriorly directed jet of mitral regurgitation and a murmur that radiates to the axilla and back. When posterior leaflet chordae rupture, the murmur radiates to the sternum and possibly the carotid arteries.

Diagnosis

Chest radiography may first show a dilated left atrium and then, as mitral regurgitation increases, dilatation of the left ventricle. A low or low-normal ejection fraction suggests substantial ventricular dysfunction. It is important to follow patients closely to determine the optimal timing of surgical intervention.

Treatment

There is no universally accepted medical treatment for mitral regurgitation. The onset of clinical symptoms warrants intervention (mitral valve repair or replacement). Asymptomatic patients with a normal or hyperdynamic ejection fraction can continue to have regular observation. Operation should be considered for symptomatic patients (preoperative left ventricular function considerably influences the postoperative outcome), and, because afterload is increased when the mitral valve is replaced, left ventricular function may actually deteriorate after mitral valve repair or replacement. In most patients, ejection fraction decreases approximately 10% after mitral valve repair or replacement.

In mildly symptomatic patients, operation may be considered, particularly if serial examinations show progressive cardiac enlargement. Earlier operation may be indicated in patients who are suitable for mitral valve repair rather than replacement, especially when the ejection fraction is less than 60% or the left ventricular end-systolic dimension is more than 40 mm (Figure 10.6).

KEY FACTS

✓ Mitral stenosis—2-dimensional and Doppler echocardiography is test of choice to diagnose the condition and determine its severity

✓ Intervention on mitral valve—is not recommended until there are symptoms of exertional dyspnea, pulmonary edema, or moderate pulmonary hypertension

✓ Mitral regurgitation—there is no universally accepted medical treatment

✓ In patients with mitral regurgitation who are suitable for mitral valve repair rather than replacement—earlier operation may be indicated, especially if ejection fraction is <60% or left ventricular end-diastolic dimension is >40 mm

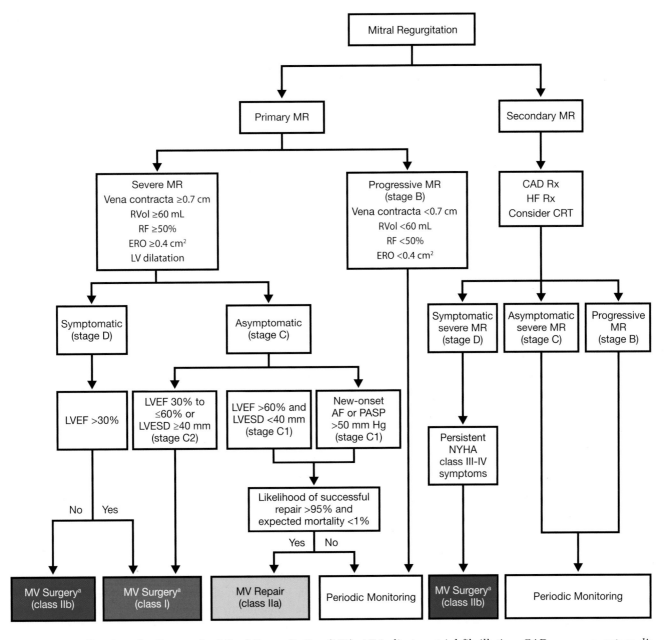

Figure 10.6 *Indications for Surgery for Mitral Regurgitation (MR). AF indicates atrial fibrillation; CAD, coronary artery disease; CRT, cardiac resynchronization therapy; ERO, effective regurgitant orifice; HF, heart failure; LV, left ventricular; LVEF, left ventricular ejection fraction; LVESD, left ventricular end-systolic dimension; MR, mitral regurgitation; MV, mitral valve; NYHA, New York Heart Association; PASP, pulmonary artery systolic pressure; RF, regurgitant fraction; RVol, regurgitant volume; Rx, therapy. ªMitral valve repair is preferred over replacement when possible.*

(Adapted from Nishimura RA, Otto CM, Bonow RO, Carabello BA, Erwin JP 3rd, Guyton RA, et al; ACC/AHA Task Force Members. 2014 AHA/ACC Guideline for the Management of Patients With Valvular Heart Disease: a report of the American College of Cardiology/American Heart Association Task Force on Practice Guidelines. Circulation. 2014 Jun 10;129[23]:e521–643. Epub 2014 Mar 3. Errata in: Circulation. 2014 Jun 10;129[23]:e651. Circulation. 2014 Sep 23;130[13]:e120. Dosage error in article text and Nishimura RA, Otto CM, Bonow RO, Carabello BA, Erwin JP 3rd, Guyton RA, et al; American College of Cardiology/American Heart Association Task Force on Practice Guidelines. 2014 AHA/ACC guideline for the management of patients with valvular heart disease: a report of the American College of Cardiology/American Heart Association Task Force on Practice Guidelines. J Am Coll Cardiol. 2014 Jun 10;63[22]:e57–185. Epub 2014 Mar 3. Erratum in: J Am Coll Cardiol. 2014 Jun 10;63[22]:2489. Dosage error in article text. Used with permission.)

Mitral Valve Prolapse

Pathophysiology and Natural History

Mitral valve prolapse is the most common cause of both valvular heart disease and mitral regurgitation in the United States. **Mitral valve prolapse** refers to a systolic billowing of one or both mitral leaflets into the left atrium with or without mitral regurgitation. In patients with mitral valve prolapse, as with other causes of mitral regurgitation, the degree of left atrial and left ventricular dilatation depends on the severity of mitral regurgitation. Mitral valve prolapse is associated with secundum atrial septal defect and supraventricular arrhythmias.

Key Definition

Mitral valve prolapse: *systolic billowing of one or both mitral leaflets into the left atrium with or without mitral regurgitation.*

In Marfan syndrome, the supporting apparatus is often involved with dilatation of the mitral annulus in addition to elongated chordae and redundant leaflets, abnormalities leading to mitral valve prolapse. Other valves also may be involved with the same myxomatous degeneration, which leads to tricuspid valve prolapse (occurring in approximately 40% of patients with mitral valve prolapse), pulmonic valve prolapse (about 10%), and aortic valve prolapse (2%). Other connective tissue disorders may be associated with mitral valve prolapse.

Mitral valve prolapse syndrome has a benign course in most patients. Patients with diagnostic findings of click-murmur on auscultation, thickened mitral leaflets on echocardiography, and left ventricular and atrial enlargement are at high risk for future complications, including atrial fibrillation, systemic embolism, and pulmonary hypertension. There is also a lifelong risk for ruptured mitral valve chordae, which may lead to acute decompensation. Infective endocarditis is a serious complication of mitral valve prolapse, although the overall incidence is low. There is a low risk for sudden cardiac death (Figure 10.7).

Physical Examination

Mitral valve prolapse is usually diagnosed with cardiac auscultation in asymptomatic patients or incidentally on echocardiography. The classic auscultatory finding is the midsystolic click, a high-pitched sound of short duration. There may be multiple clicks. Clicks result from sudden tensing of the mitral valve apparatus as the leaflets prolapse into the left atrium during systole. The midsystolic click(s) is frequently followed by a mid-late systolic

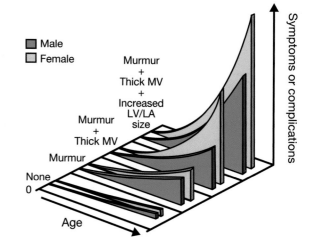

Figure 10.7 *Risk Factors for Complications in Mitral Valve Prolapse. LA indicates left atrial; LV, left ventricular; MV, mitral valve.*

(Adapted from Boudoulas H, Kolibash AJ Jr, Wooley CF. Mitral valve prolapse: a heterogeneous disorder. Primary Cardiol. 1991;17[2]: 29–43. Used with permission.)

murmur that is high-pitched, musical, or honking and often loudest at the cardiac apex. The character and intensity of the clicks and the murmur vary with left ventricle loading conditions. Dynamic auscultation helps establish the diagnosis. Changes in left ventricular end-diastolic volume result in changes in the timing of the click(s) and murmur. When end-diastolic volume is decreased (eg, with standing), the critical volume is achieved earlier in systole and the click-murmur complex occurs earlier after the first heart sound. By contrast, any maneuver that augments the volume of blood in the ventricle (eg, squatting), reduces myocardial contractility, or increases left ventricular afterload lengthens the time from onset of systole to initiation of mitral valve prolapse, and the systolic click or murmur moves toward the second heart sound (Figure 10.8).

Diagnosis

Results of electrocardiography most often are normal, although 24-hour ambulatory electrocardiographic recordings or event monitors may be useful for documenting arrhythmias. Echocardiography is the most useful noninvasive test for defining mitral valve prolapse. The definition includes more than 2 mm of posterior displacement of 1 or both leaflets into the left atrium. All patients with mitral valve prolapse should have initial echocardiography to establish the diagnosis, stratify risk, and define possible associated lesions (eg, atrial septal defect). Serial echocardiograms are not necessary in asymptomatic patients with mitral valve prolapse. Echocardiographic follow-up should be done if there are clinical indications of progression.

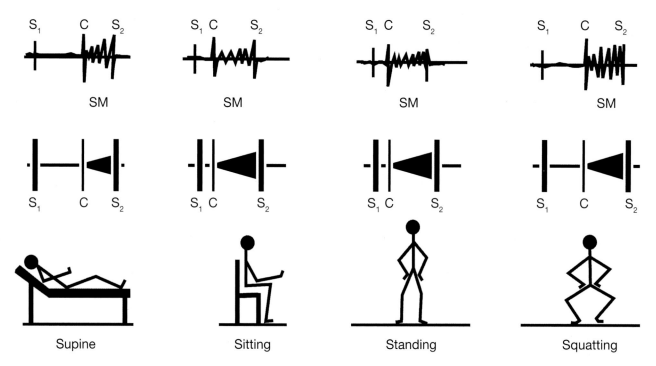

Figure 10.8 *Auscultation Findings in Mitral Valve Prolapse. C indicates click; S_1, S_2, heart sound (first, second); SM, systolic murmur; ◄, murmur.*

Treatment

Reassurance is a major part of the management of patients with mitral valve prolapse because most are asymptomatic and lack a high-risk profile. A normal lifestyle and regular exercise are encouraged. Patients should be educated about when to seek medical advice (worsening symptoms). Subacute bacterial endocarditis prophylaxis is no longer indicated for mitral valve prolapse without a history of endocarditis.

Common symptoms include palpitations, chest pain that rarely resembles classic angina pectoris, dyspnea, and fatigue. Patients should be advised to discontinue caffeine, alcohol, and tobacco use. Patients with recurrent palpitations often respond to β-adrenergic blockers or calcium channel blockers. Orthostatic symptoms due to postural hypotension and tachycardia are treated with volume expansion, preferably by liberalizing fluid and salt intake. Transient cerebral ischemic episodes occur with increased incidence in patients with mitral valve prolapse, and some patients need long-term anticoagulation.

Asymptomatic patients with mitral valve prolapse and no serious mitral regurgitation can be evaluated clinically every 3 to 5 years. Serial echocardiography is necessary only in patients who have high-risk features on the initial echocardiogram.

Surgery may be required in a small subset of patients. The thickened, redundant mitral valve often can be repaired rather than replaced; repair has a low operative mortality rate and excellent short- and long-term results. Repair is

KEY FACTS

✓ Mitral valve prolapse—most common cause of both valvular heart disease and mitral regurgitation in the United States

✓ Mitral valve prolapse—all patients should have initial echocardiography to establish diagnosis, stratify risk, and define possible associated lesions (eg, atrial septal defect)

✓ In asymptomatic patients with mitral valve prolapse—serial echocardiography is not necessary

✓ In patients with mitral valve prolapse and clinical indications of progression—echocardiographic follow-up should be done

often sufficient in patients who have a flail mitral leaflet due to rupture or marked elongation of the chordae tendineae. Recommendations for surgery in patients with mitral valve prolapse and mitral regurgitation are the same as those for patients with other forms of severe mitral regurgitation.

Tricuspid Stenosis

The cause of tricuspid stenosis is almost always rheumatic, and it is never an isolated lesion. Carcinoid syndrome may cause tricuspid valve retraction and a relative stenosis (usually causes worse tricuspid regurgitation), and in rare cases atrial tumors may be the cause.

Tricuspid Valve Prolapse

This may occur in isolation or be associated with other connective tissue abnormalities. The tricuspid valve may prolapse or become flail as a result of trauma or endocarditis (commonly fungal or staphylococcal in drug addicts).

Tricuspid Regurgitation

Mild tricuspid regurgitation is relatively common, occurring in up to 85% to 90% of patients. Significant tricuspid regurgitation is usually caused by right ventricle dilatation. Tricuspid regurgitation often accompanies mitral valve disease, but it may be related to 1) right ventricular infarction, 2) primary pulmonary hypertension (common), 3) congenital heart disease (eg, Ebstein anomaly), or 4) carcinoid syndrome—more commonly associated with tricuspid regurgitation than tricuspid stenosis.

Physical Examination

Findings on physical examination include jugular venous distention with a prominent *v* wave, a prominent right ventricular impulse, a pansystolic murmur at the left sternal edge, possibly a right-sided third heart sound, peripheral edema, ascites, and hepatomegaly.

Surgical Therapy

Tricuspid annuloplasty may be helpful if regurgitation is caused by right ventricular dilatation. However, if there is considerable pulmonary hypertension, tricuspid valve replacement is usually required with either a biologic or a mechanical valve. Biologic prostheses in the tricuspid position do not degenerate as quickly as left-heart prostheses. In patients with endocarditis, the tricuspid valve can be removed completely, and patients may tolerate this well for several years (Figure 10.9).

Prosthetic Valves

Bioprosthetic Valves

Tissue valves, or bioprostheses, include autografts (usually the patient's own pulmonary valve), homografts (aortic or pulmonary valves from human cadavers), and heterografts (either porcine valves or bovine pericardial tissue attached to a metal frame). Bioprosthesis implantation traditionally required open heart surgery, but, in recent years, patients deemed at too high a risk for surgical aortic valve replacement are increasingly undergoing transcatheter aortic valve replacement with implantation via a transfemoral or transapical catheter. Transcatheter pulmonary valve replacement in patients with congenital heart disease is also becoming increasingly common. Currently, no approved transcatheter mitral or tricuspid valve replacement options are available.

Because bioprostheses are not as thrombogenic as mechanical valves, most patients in sinus rhythm do not require anticoagulation after the first 3 to 6 months after implantation unless they have additional risk factors, such as atrial fibrillation. Tissue valves degenerate and calcify, particularly in patients who 1) are young, 2) have disordered calcium metabolism (eg, patients with end-stage renal disease, or 3) are pregnant, regardless of age. Approximately 50% of patients with a bioprosthesis require re-do valve replacement at 10 to 15 years due to structural deterioration. Prostheses in the tricuspid and pulmonary positions tend to last longer than those in left heart positions. Aortic bioprostheses are generally more durable than mitral bioprostheses. Prosthesis failure can be detected by clinical evaluation and 2-dimensional and Doppler echocardiography.

Mechanical Valves

Older-generation mechanical prostheses including the caged ball (eg, Starr-Edwards) and tilting disk (eg, Medtronic-Hall) were durable but quite thrombogenic. These prosthesis types are no longer being manufactured, but, because they are durable, many patients still have these prostheses in place. The newer-generation bileaflet mechanical valves (eg, St. Jude Medical) are less thrombogenic than prior models, but they still pose a risk for thromboembolism and necessitate long-term anticoagulation. Vitamin K antagonists (eg, warfarin) are the only systemic anticoagulants approved for mechanical heart valves. Anticoagulant therapy with oral direct thrombin inhibitors or anti-Xa agents should not be used in patients with mechanical valve prostheses because of their increased risk for valve thrombosis. The 2014 AHA/ACC Guideline for the Management of Patients With Valvular Heart Disease (Circulation. 2014 Jun 10;129[23]:e521–643 and J Am Coll Cardiol. 2014 Jun 10;63[22]:e57–185) recommend a single target international normalized ratio for therapeutic anticoagulation. All patients with mechanical heart valves should be given low-dose aspirin in addition to anticoagulation (Figure 10.10). Dual antiplatelet therapy with aspirin and a thienopyridine (eg, clopidogrel) is not an acceptable substitute for antiplatelet plus anticoagulant therapy in these patients.

Bridging Therapy

In patients with mechanical prostheses in any position who undergo minor procedures (such as dental extractions or cataract removal) in which bleeding can easily be controlled, continuation of anticoagulation with a therapeutic international normalized ratio is recommended. In patients with bileaflet mechanical aortic valve prostheses with no additional risk factors for thrombosis (ie, atrial fibrillation or flutter, history of stroke, left ventricular ejection fraction <30%, history of thromboembolism or hypercoagulable state), temporary interruption of anticoagulation without bridging therapy for surgical or other invasive procedures is recommended. Bridging anticoagulation with either intravenous unfractionated heparin or subcutaneous low-molecular-weight heparin is recommended in patients undergoing invasive or surgical procedures who have any

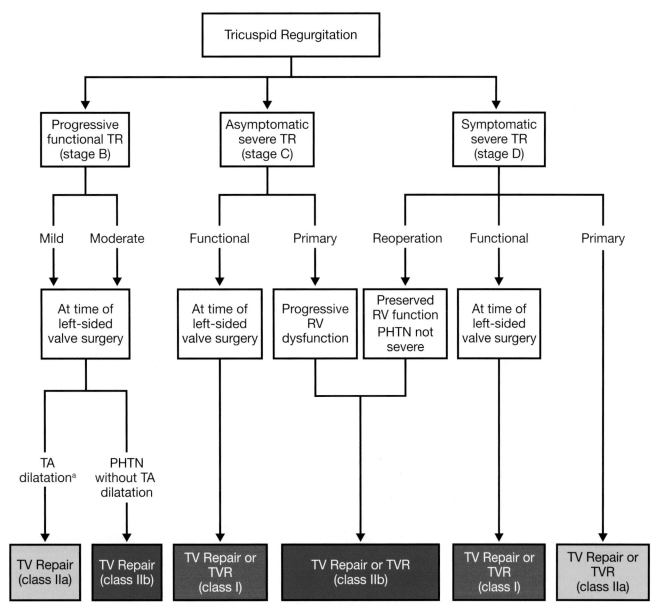

Figure 10.9 Indications for Surgery for Tricuspid Regurgitation (TR). PHTN indicates pulmonary hypertension; RV, right ventricular; TA, tricuspid annular; TV, tricuspid valve; TVR, tricuspid valve replacement. ªDilatation is defined as more than 40 mm on transthoracic echocardiography (>21 mm/m²) or more than 70 mm on direct intraoperative measurement.

(Adapted from Nishimura RA, Otto CM, Bonow RO, Carabello BA, Erwin JP 3rd, Guyton RA, et al; ACC/AHA Task Force Members. 2014 AHA/ACC Guideline for the Management of Patients With Valvular Heart Disease: a report of the American College of Cardiology/ American Heart Association Task Force on Practice Guidelines. Circulation. 2014 Jun 10;129[23]:e521–643. Epub 2014 Mar 3. Errata in: Circulation. 2014 Jun 10;129[23]:e651. Circulation. 2014 Sep 23;130[13]:e120. Dosage error in article text and Nishimura RA, Otto CM, Bonow RO, Carabello BA, Erwin JP 3rd, Guyton RA, et al; American College of Cardiology/American Heart Association Task Force on Practice Guidelines. 2014 AHA/ACC guideline for the management of patients with valvular heart disease: a report of the American College of Cardiology/American Heart Association Task Force on Practice Guidelines. J Am Coll Cardiol. 2014 Jun 10;63[22]:e57–185. Epub 2014 Mar 3. Erratum in: J Am Coll Cardiol. 2014 Jun 10;63[22]:2489. Dosage error in article text. Used with permission.)

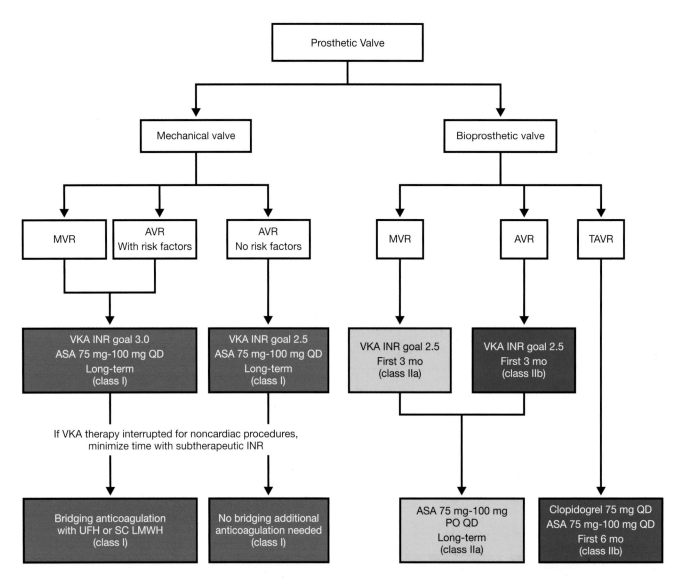

Figure 10.10 *Anticoagulation for Prosthetic Valves. Risk factors include atrial fibrillation, previous thromboembolism, left ventricular dysfunction, hypercoagulable condition, and older-generation mechanical aortic valve replacement (AVR). ASA indicates aspirin; INR, international normalized ratio; LMWH, low-molecular-weight heparin; MVR, mitral valve replacement; PO, by mouth; QD, every day; SC, subcutaneous; TAVR, transcatheter aortic valve replacement; UFH, unfractionated heparin; VKA, vitamin K antagonist.*

(Adapted from Nishimura RA, Otto CM, Bonow RO, Carabello BA, Erwin JP 3rd, Guyton RA, et al; ACC/AHA Task Force Members. 2014 AHA/ACC Guideline for the Management of Patients With Valvular Heart Disease: a report of the American College of Cardiology/ American Heart Association Task Force on Practice Guidelines. Circulation. 2014 Jun 10;129[23]:e521–643. Epub 2014 Mar 3. Errata in: Circulation. 2014 Jun 10;129[23]:e651. Circulation. 2014 Sep 23;130[13]:e120. Dosage error in article text and Nishimura RA, Otto CM, Bonow RO, Carabello BA, Erwin JP 3rd, Guyton RA, et al; American College of Cardiology/American Heart Association Task Force on Practice Guidelines. 2014 AHA/ACC guideline for the management of patients with valvular heart disease: a report of the American College of Cardiology/American Heart Association Task Force on Practice Guidelines. J Am Coll Cardiol. 2014 Jun 10;63[22]:e57–185. Epub 2014 Mar 3. Erratum in: J Am Coll Cardiol. 2014 Jun 10;63[22]:2489. Dosage error in article text. Used with permission.)

of the following: 1) mechanical aortic prosthesis and any thromboembolic risk factor, 2) older-generation mechanical aortic prosthesis, or 3) any type of mechanical mitral valve prosthesis. Aspirin therapy for all patients with prosthetic heart valves should be continued without interruption unless bleeding risk is considered prohibitive.

Infective Endocarditis Prophylaxis

Patients with any type of prosthetic heart valve have a high risk for infective endocarditis. Antibiotic therapy before all dental procedures that involve manipulation of gingival tissue or perforation of the oral mucosa is recommended. In the absence of suspected infection, prophylaxis before gastrointestinal or genitourinary procedures is not recommended. Morbidity and mortality rates for patients with prosthetic valve endocarditis are higher than rates associated with native valve endocarditis.

Prosthetic Valve Complications and Dysfunction

The risk for serious complications is approximately 3% per year. Potential complications include bleeding, valve obstruction due to thrombosis or pannus formation, systemic embolization, structural deterioration (primarily with bioprosthesis), hemolytic anemia, perivalvular regurgitation, and infective endocarditis.

Significant bleeding may occur in patients with mechanical prostheses, particularly in patients with a supratherapeutic international normalized ratio. The rate of minor hemorrhage is 2% to 4% per year, and that of major hemorrhage is 1% to 2% per year. When life-threatening bleeding occurs, fresh frozen plasma or prothrombin concentrate may be administered.

Thrombosis may occur on both bioprosthetic and mechanical valves, particularly with inadequate anticoagulation. Thrombosis occurs most commonly with tricuspid valve prostheses. Thrombolytic therapy or surgery may be indicated when significant obstruction of left-sided prostheses occurs. The risk for systemic embolization in patients with mechanical prostheses treated appropriately with anticoagulation is approximately 1.0% per year. Patients with mechanical mitral valves have twice the risk of embolization as patients with mechanical aortic valves.

Hemolytic anemia may occur in patients with prosthetic heart valves, particularly in the setting of a perivalvular leak. Diagnosis is based on a high degree of suspicion and laboratory evidence of intravascular hemolysis. Surgical or catheter closure of the perivalvular leak is indicated in patients who require repeated transfusions.

Infective endocarditis may occur at any time, but the risk is highest in the first few weeks and months after valve implantation. For a detailed discussion of infective endocarditis, please refer to Chapter 44.

Serial Follow-up of Patients With Prosthetic Valves

A baseline transthoracic echocardiogram should be obtained in all patients with prosthetic heart valves shortly after implantation. All patients with prosthetic heart valves should have an annual clinical evaluation, including symptom assessment and physical examination. According to the 2014 AHA/ACC Guideline for the Management of Patients With Valvular Heart Disease (Circulation. 2014 Jun 10;129[23]:e521–643 and J Am Coll Cardiol. 2014 Jun 10;63[22]:e57–185), patients with mechanical valves require no further echocardiographic testing if they remain stable with no clinical suspicion for valve dysfunction. Because of the risk of degeneration, patients with a surgically implanted bioprosthesis should undergo annual echocardiographic examinations starting 10 years after implantation, even in the absence of symptoms. Recommendations for echocardiographic follow-up of transcatheter valve replacements are evolving, but current guidelines suggest annual echocardiographic examinations.

KEY FACTS

✓ Tricuspid stenosis—cause is almost always rheumatic, and it is never an isolated lesion

✓ Carcinoid syndrome—may cause tricuspid valve retraction and a relative stenosis (usually causes worse tricuspid regurgitation), and in rare cases atrial tumors may be the cause

✓ Bioprosthesis—not as thrombogenic as mechanical valves and thus most patients in sinus rhythm do not require anticoagulation after first 3–6 months after implantation unless they have additional risk factors (eg, atrial fibrillation)

✓ Patients who have a prosthetic heart valve of any type—
- are at high risk for infective endocarditis
- antibiotic therapy is recommended before all dental procedures that involve manipulation of gingival tissue or perforation of oral mucosa
- prophylaxis is not recommended before gastrointestinal or genitourinary procedures in the absence of suspected infection

---

Congenital Heart Disease

Atrial Septal Defect

There are multiple types of atrial septal defects (Table 10.6).

Table 10.6 • Types of Atrial Septal Defects

Type	%	Location	Associated Findings	ECG Findings
Ostium secundum	75	Fossa ovalis	None	Incomp RBBB, R axis
Sinus venosus	10	Vena cava	Anomalous PV	Incomp RBBB, ectopic P wave, R axis
Ostium primum	10–15	Lower septum	Cleft MV, Down syndrome	Incomp RBBB, L axis (LAHB)

Abbreviations: ECG, electrocardiography; Incomp, incomplete; L axis, left axis deviation; LAHB, left anterior hemiblock; MV, mitral valve; P wave, atrial depolarization wave on ECG; PV, pulmonary veins; R axis, right axis deviation; RBBB, right bundle branch block.

Secundum Atrial Septal Defect

Secundum atrial septal defect is the most common type of atrial septal defect. Because physical examination findings are subtle and symptoms are nonspecific, patients with secundum atrial septal defect often survive to adulthood and the condition may be diagnosed for the first time later in life. The physical examination may demonstrate a fixed split second heart sound and a soft systolic murmur representing excess flow across the pulmonary valve.

Electrocardiography characteristically shows right bundle branch block and right axis deviation. Chest radiography shows pulmonary plethora, a prominent pulmonary artery, and right ventricular enlargement (Figure 10.11). Echocardiography is warranted for definitive diagnosis.

Primum Atrial Septal Defect (Partial Atrioventricular Canal)

Primum atrial septal defect is a defect at the crux of the heart with the tricuspid and mitral valves forming part of the border of the defect. It is also called a partial atrioventricular canal defect. The mitral valve is often congenitally cleft and produces various degrees of mitral regurgitation.

Key Definition

Primum atrial septal defect: *defect at crux of the heart; tricuspid and mitral valves form part of border of the defect.*

On electrocardiography, findings are different from those of secundum type; left axis deviation and right bundle branch block are evident. More than 75% of patients have first-degree atrioventricular block. The chest radiographic findings are the same as those for secundum atrial septal defect, but there may be left atrial enlargement due to mitral regurgitation.

Sinus Venosus Atrial Septal Defect

A sinus venosus defect occurs in atrial septal tissue at the junction of the vena cava to the right atrium, most commonly the superior vena cava. It is often associated with anomalous pulmonary venous return. If echocardiography shows right ventricular volume overload and no secundum defect (surface echocardiography can miss the sinus venosus area), consider sinus venosus atrial septal defect or anomalous pulmonary veins.

Treatment

Antibiotic prophylaxis is not recommended unless there is associated complex congenital heart disease. Patients with

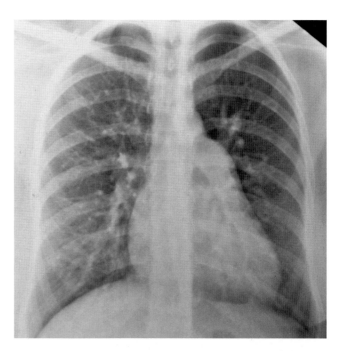

Figure 10.11 *Chest Radiograph From a Patient With a Large Left-to-Right Shunt Due to a Secundum Atrial Septal Defect. Note cardiac enlargement with right ventricular contour, prominent pulmonary artery, and pulmonary plethora.*

atrial septal defect have variable symptoms depending on the size of the shunt. Intervention should be considered in the setting of hemodynamic compromise (left-to-right shunting of more than 30% or evidence of right-sided chamber enlargement). Surgical closure is possible for all types of atrial septal defects, but only the secundum atrial septal defect can be treated with a transcatheter device closure.

Ventricular Septal Defect

Ventricular septal defect occurs in different parts of the ventricular septum, most commonly classified as either in the membranous septum or in the muscular septum. A small ventricular septal defect generally presents with a loud holosystolic murmur in an asymptomatic patient, and often a thrill at the left sternal edge, usually around the fourth interspace, is heard. Large defects may produce a mitral diastolic flow rumble (due to increased volume) at the apex, especially when the shunt is more than 2.5:1, and may cause considerable symptoms early in life. Ventricular septal defects are usually detected in early childhood, and in developed countries they are usually closed early if they are thought to be significant. If undiscovered until late childhood or adulthood, a large ventricular septal defect often results in pulmonary vascular disease with pulmonary hypertension (Eisenmenger syndrome) and cannot be closed (see Eisenmenger Syndrome below).

Diagnosis

Chest radiography shows a narrow pedicle with an enlarged globular silhouette and right atrial enlargement. The lung fields are normal or oligemic. Electrocardiographic findings include tall P waves (so-called Himalayan P waves) and right bundle branch block. Two-dimensional and Doppler echocardiography precisely delineate the anatomy. Cardiac magnetic resonance imaging can be useful to evaluate right ventricular size and function. Cardiac catheterization is unnecessary to make the diagnosis of Ebstein anomaly. Electrophysiologic study may be necessary to delineate a bypass tract.

Treatment

Surgical repair or replacement of the tricuspid valve is indicated to prevent right ventricular failure. Closure of an atrial septal defect, if present, should be performed at the time of valve surgery. Patients with accessory conduction pathways may benefit from catheter ablation techniques.

KEY FACTS

✓ Eisenmenger syndrome—
- develops in first few years of life when a large shunt (usually a ventricular septal defect or patent ductus arteriosus, less often atrial septal defect) produces pulmonary hypertension as a result of irreversible pulmonary vascular disease
- cyanosis results in appropriate secondary erythrocytosis to increase oxygen delivery to the tissues
- routine phlebotomy is never indicated and should not be performed on the basis of a hemoglobin value

✓ Coarctation of aorta has 5 major complications—1) cardiac failure, 2) aortic valve disease, 3) aortic rupture or dissection, 4) endarteritis, and 5) rupture of an aneurysm of the circle of Willis

11

Vascular Disease

ROBERT D. McBANE, MD

Disease of the Aorta

Aneurysmal Disease

Thoracic Aortic Aneurysm

Aneurysms of the ascending aorta are typically due to medial degeneration, whereas aneurysms of the descending thoracic aorta are primarily due to atherosclerosis. Men and women are equally affected, and the prevalence of thoracic aortic aneurysm (TAA) increases with advancing age. Overall, the incidence is approximately 1 per 10,000 individuals, and 20% of patients with TAA have at least 1 affected first-degree relative. Typical risk factors include tobacco exposure, hypertension, infection, and trauma.

Temporal arteritis (age >50 years), Takayasu arteritis (age <50 years), Behçet disease, ankylosing spondylitis, and syphilis are uncommon inflammatory causes to consider. Marfan, Loeys-Dietz, and Ehlers-Danlos syndromes should be considered in young patients (<40 years) with ascending aortic involvement (especially the root) and in patients with a family history of aortic dissection or sudden death. Specific clinical clues may include ectopia lentis (Marfan syndrome); bifid uvula; strong family history of aneurysms with rupture (Loeys-Dietz syndrome); visceral perforation such as gastrointestinal, uterine, or pneumothorax (Ehlers-Danlos syndrome); and webbed neck and short stature (Turner syndrome). A mid systolic click noted on cardiac auscultation should prompt echocardiographic evaluation for bicuspid aortic valve disease, which can have an associated aortopathy.

Early-onset hypertension, intermittent claudication in young patients, or delay from the radial or brachial pulse to the femoral pulse should bring to mind coarctation. Up to 50% of patients with coarctation will also have bicuspid aortic valve. The converse is not true, however; only 6% of patients with bicuspid aortic valve disease will have coarctation. Intracranial aneurysms are common, occurring in 10% of patients with coarctation. Coarctation is prominent in Turner syndrome.

Most TAAs are asymptomatic and incidentally discovered on chest radiography (Figure 11.1). If they are symptomatic, patients may report chest or back pain, vocal hoarseness, cough, dyspnea, stridor, or dysphagia. Hemoptysis or hematemesis may occur in the setting of erosion into adjacent structures. Findings on physical examination may include hypertension or fixed distention of a neck vein(s). Findings on cardiac examination may include mid systolic clicks (bicuspid aortic valve) and systolic or diastolic murmurs (aortic regurgitation). Other examination findings may include a fixed vocal cord, signs of cerebral or systemic embolism, or other aneurysmal disease (ie, abdominal aortic aneurysm [AAA]). It is important to search for synchronous aneurysms (AAA, femoral and popliteal aneurysms), which can be present in 25% of patients. The diagnosis is confirmed with magnetic resonance imaging (MRI) (Figure 11.2A), computed tomography (CT) (Figure 11.2B), or transesophageal echocardiography (TEE).

Complications of TAA include rupture, dissection, or, rarely, thromboembolism. There is a direct correlation between aneurysm size and risk of rupture (diameter <4.0 cm, 0%; 4.0–5.9 cm, 16%; ≥6.0 cm, 31%). Hypertension, large aneurysm size, traumatic aneurysm, and associated coronary and carotid artery disease worsen the prognosis.

Hypertension treatment should include β-blockers or angiotensin receptor blockers. β-Blockers in patients with Marfan syndrome have been shown to slow aortic enlargement and may improve survival. Angiotensin receptor blockers are preferred for patients with Loeys-Dietz syndrome. These drugs are also reasonable for patients with TAA and no defined connective tissue disease. Statin therapy to achieve a target low-density lipoprotein cholesterol value of 70 mg/dL or less is warranted (class IIa). Smoking cessation is always warranted.

Elective surgical repair is indicated for ascending TAA exceeding 5.5 cm, descending TAA exceeding 6.0 cm, or

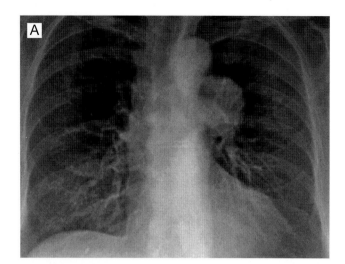

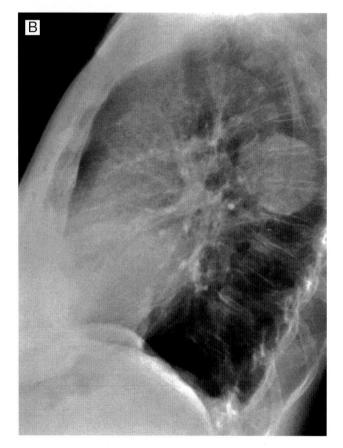

Figure 11.1 *Chest Radiographs for a Patient With Thoracic Aortic Aneurysm. Show a Large Mass in Left Posterior Aspect of Chest. A, Anteroposterior. B, Lateral.*

growth rate exceeding 0.5 cm per year. For patients with connective tissue diseases (Marfan syndrome, Loeys-Dietz syndrome, or Ehlers-Danlos syndrome), the size limit is 4.5 cm. For patients with bicuspid aortic valves, surgery is indicated if the aortic root or ascending aorta exceeds 5.0 cm or if growth rate exceeds 0.5 cm per year.

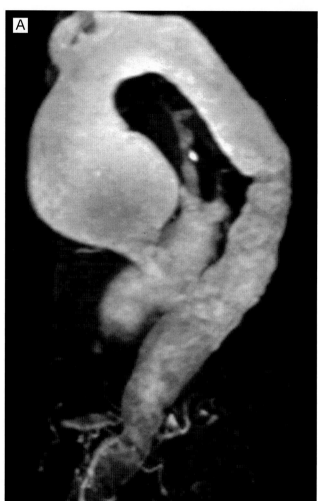

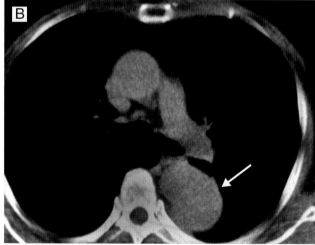

Figure 11.2 *Imaging of Thoracic Aortic Aneurysm. A, Magnetic resonance angiogram (longitudinal view) shows a large ascending aortic aneurysm and moderate aortic regurgitation. B, Computed tomogram shows a saccular aneurysm in the mid descending thoracic aorta (arrow).*

Abdominal Aortic Aneurysm

The abdominal aorta is the most common site of aneurysm. Men are affected 5 times more often than women, and the incidence increases with age. The prevalence of AAA is 3% among persons 50 years or older. Most aneurysms are due to atherosclerosis. Tobacco use is a major risk factor. However, other diseases must be considered, including connective tissue diseases (Marfan syndrome, Ehlers-Danlos syndrome, pseudoxanthoma elasticum), infection, trauma, or vasculitis (Takayasu arteritis and temporal arteritis). Twenty-five percent of patients with AAA have an affected relative; thus, a familial predisposition is suspected. Most AAAs are infrarenal. Juxtarenal and suprarenal AAAs (2%–5%) are less common but important to identify when considering management.

Most patients with AAA are asymptomatic. Livedo reticularis, painful blue toes with palpable pulses, hypertension, renal insufficiency, increased erythrocyte sedimentation rate, and transient eosinophilia imply AAA-associated atheroembolism (Figure 11.3). A history of new or worsening abdominal or low back pain suggests aneurysm instability. The triad of severe abdominal pain, hypotension, and a tender abdominal mass characterize AAA rupture. The annual risk of rupture is directly related to aneurysm size: 4.0 cm, <2%; 5.0 cm, 5%; 6.0 cm, 10%; and 7.0 cm or more, 20%.

The most common physical finding is a pulsatile abdominal mass; however this lacks sensitivity, particularly for smaller aneurysms. A one-time screening ultrasonography for men aged 65 to 75 years old who have ever smoked is recommended, and AAA screening is indicated for men 60 years or older who have a first-degree family history of AAA. Screening women is not guideline-endorsed. Ultrasonography (Figure 11.4A), CT and CT angiography (Figure 11.4B), or MRI and MR angiography are reliable for diagnosis.

Medical management includes modification of atherosclerotic risk factors, including blood pressure control (preferably with a β-blocker), tobacco cessation, and statin therapy. If the aneurysm size is 4.0 cm or more, serial

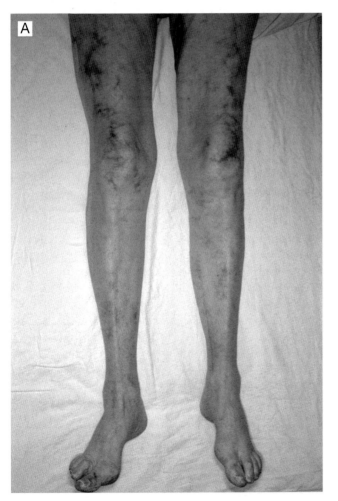 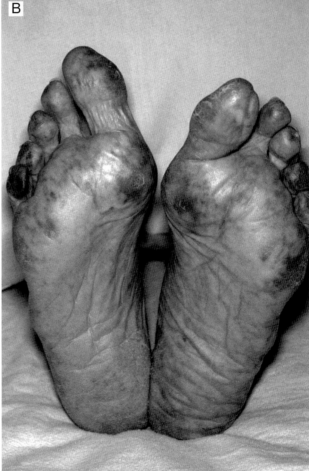

Figure 11.3 *Findings in a Patient With Atheroembolism. A and B, Livedo reticularis (upper aspect of thighs, plantar surface of feet) and multiple blue toes.*

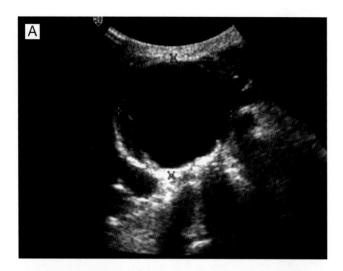

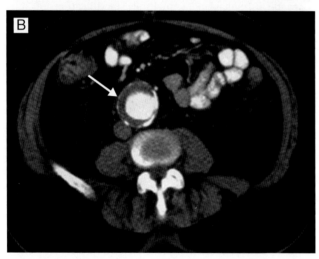

Figure 11.4 *Imaging of Abdominal Aortic Aneurysm. A, Ultrasonogram (transverse view) shows a 4.7-cm aneurysm. B, Computed tomogram (contrast-enhanced) shows aneurysm (arrow).*

ultrasonography should be done every 6 to 12 months. For aneurysms less than 4.0 cm, imaging intervals can be extended to every 2 to 3 years. Repair is recommended for aneurysms of 5.5 cm or more, growth rate of 0.5 cm or more per year, atheroembolism, or any suggestion of instability.

Endovascular repair of AAA with stent grafts is an alternative to open surgical repair. Endovascular and surgical repair are associated with similar risks of overall and aneurysm-related mortality. Graft-related complications are higher for endovascular AAA repair. An endoleak (ie, persistent flow into the aneurysm sac, most often due to patent branch vessels feeding the aneurysm sac) is the most common graft-related complication. It is usually repaired by catheter-based techniques. Because of the risk of endovascular leak, serial CT angiography surveillance is required indefinitely. For this reason, endovascular repair is often

reserved for older patients with increased surgical risk, whereas open repair is recommended for younger patients at low to average surgical risk.

Thoracic Aortic Dissection

Acute thoracic aortic syndromes include aortic dissection (80%), intramural hematoma (10%) and penetrating aortic ulcer (10%). Aortic dissection begins with a tear through the arterial intima that allows pulsating blood to penetrate along the media longitudinally, separating the arterial wall. The dissection extends before either reentering the lumen through a second intimal tear or exiting the artery through an adventitial tear. Dissection can be catastrophic, including organ infarction or frank rupture. Causes include atherosclerosis, hypertension, cystic medial necrosis (ascending aorta, including connective tissue disease processes such as Marfan syndrome), bicuspid aortic valve disease, or trauma (blunt or penetrating). Dissection may also be iatrogenic (cardiac surgery or invasive angiography). Aortic dissection may complicate pregnancy in at-risk women; when this occurs, it is usually in the third trimester.

An intramural hematoma occurs when bleeding develops within the media without a demonstrable intimal tear or flowing blood within a false lumen. A penetrating aortic ulcer results from ulceration that penetrates through the internal elastic lamina with bleeding into the media, often in a segment of atheromatous plaque. These syndromes are treated in the same manner as dissections and depend on where the injury occurs (ascending vs descending thoracic aorta). Incomplete rupture of the thoracic aorta (in the region of the aortic isthmus) results from a sudden deceleration injury, frequently a motor vehicle crash (Figure 11.5).

Symptoms of aortic dissection include sudden-onset, severe, often migratory pain in the anterior aspect of the chest, back, or abdomen; these occur in 70% to 80% of patients (sensitivity 90%, specificity 84%). The pain is often described as "ripping," "tearing," or "stabbing." Hypertension is present in 70% of patients. For patients who have an ascending thoracic aortic dissection, additional findings may include a diastolic murmur due to aortic regurgitation (from disruption of the aortic annulus; 20%), pulse deficits (30%), neurologic changes (20%), and syncope (13%). A pulse deficit portends a worse outcome; in-hospital mortality rates are 45% (compared with 15% when pulses are present). Focal neurologic deficits imply carotid transection. Hypotension, tachycardia, jugular venous distention, systemic vascular congestion, and pulsus paradoxus suggest pericardial tamponade due to rupture into the pericardium. Congestive heart failure is usually due to acute, severe aortic regurgitation. Acute myocardial infarction, pericarditis, and complete heart block may also occur.

Chest radiography may show widening of the superior mediastinum (Figure 11.6), deviation of the trachea

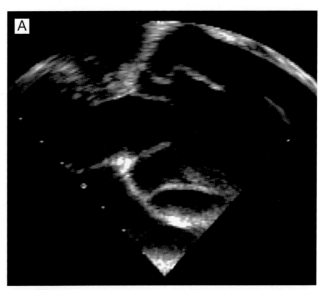

Figure 11.5 *Aortogram of Contained Rupture of Proximal Descending Thoracic Aorta Just Distal to Origin of Left Subclavian Artery. Patient was involved in a severe motor vehicle crash.*

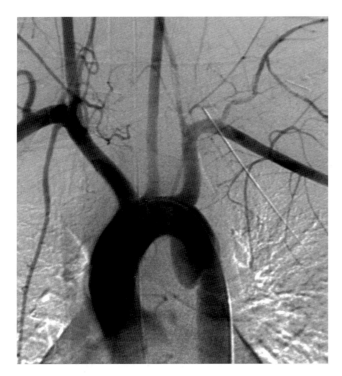

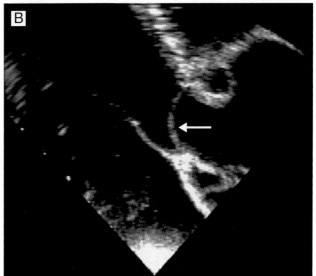

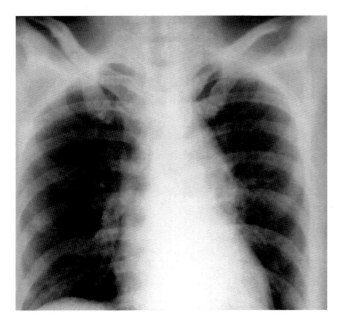

Figure 11.6 *Chest Radiograph of Aortic Dissection. Superior mediastinum is widened.*

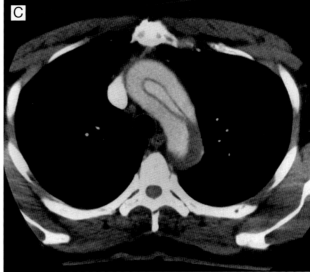

Figure 11.7 *Imaging of Aortic Dissection. A and B, Multiplane transesophageal echocardiograms. Longitudinal view (A) shows an intimal flap in the ascending aorta. In diastole (B), the intimal flap prolapses through the aortic valve (arrow). C, Computed tomogram (contrast-enhanced) shows a spiraling intimal flap in the transverse aortic arch.*

from the midline, a discrepancy in diameter between the ascending aorta and the descending aorta, and pleural effusion. Electrocardiography most commonly shows left ventricular hypertrophy, but ST-segment depression, ST-segment elevation, T-wave changes, and the changes of acute pericarditis and complete heart block occur in up to 55% of patients. Diagnosis is readily and accurately confirmed with TEE, CT angiography, and MR angiography (Figure 11.7). Test choice is determined by availability and local expertise.

Aortic dissections are classified by location relative to the ascending aorta and aortic arch (Figure 11.8). There are 2 commonly used classification systems: DeBakey and Stanford. Aortic dissection involving the ascending aorta is designated as DeBakey type I or II (proximal, Stanford type A). Descending aortic dissection begins distal to the left subclavian artery orifice and is designated as DeBakey type III (distal, Stanford type B). Clinical clues to DeBakey type I and type II (ascending) aortic dissection include substernal pain, aortic valve incompetence, decreased pulse or blood pressure in the right arm, decreased right carotid pulse, pericardial friction rub, syncope, and ischemic electrocardiographic changes. Clinical clues to descending thoracic aortic dissection include interscapular pain, hypertension, and left pleural effusion.

Acute dissections of the ascending thoracic aorta are surgical emergencies because of mortality rates exceeding 1% per hour within the first 48 hours in untreated patients. In contrast, acute dissections of the descending thoracic aorta are typically managed medically with aggressive blood pressure and heart rate control. Intravenous β-blockers (goal heart rate <70 beats per minute) are indicated in the acute setting. Pharmacologic therapy should be instituted as soon as the diagnosis of any aortic dissection is suspected (Box 11.1). If systolic blood pressure remains more than 120 mm Hg, angiotensin-converting enzyme inhibitors or other vasodilators should be administered. Indications for surgical repair for a descending thoracic aortic dissection include organ malperfusion, progression of the dissection despite aggressive heart rate and blood pressure control, aneurysm enlargement, and inability to control blood pressure or symptoms of the dissection. There is now a growing trend to consider aortic stent grafts for descending thoracic aortic dissections in order to limit aortic injury, promote occlusion of the false lumen, and prevent late aortic ruptures.

Factors predicting a poor prognosis for descending thoracic aortic dissections and the need for surgical repair include aortic diameter more than 4.0 cm or a persistently patent false lumen. Preoperative coronary angiography in acute ascending aortic dissection is *not* indicated because of an association with an increased mortality rate. Treatment of an intramural hematoma or penetrating aortic ulcer is similar to treatment of dissection of the corresponding thoracic aortic segment (surgical if ascending, medical if descending). Once the patient is stabilized, serial imaging is necessary to monitor progression and development of aneurysmal disease. The management of acute aortic dissection is summarized in Figure 11.9.

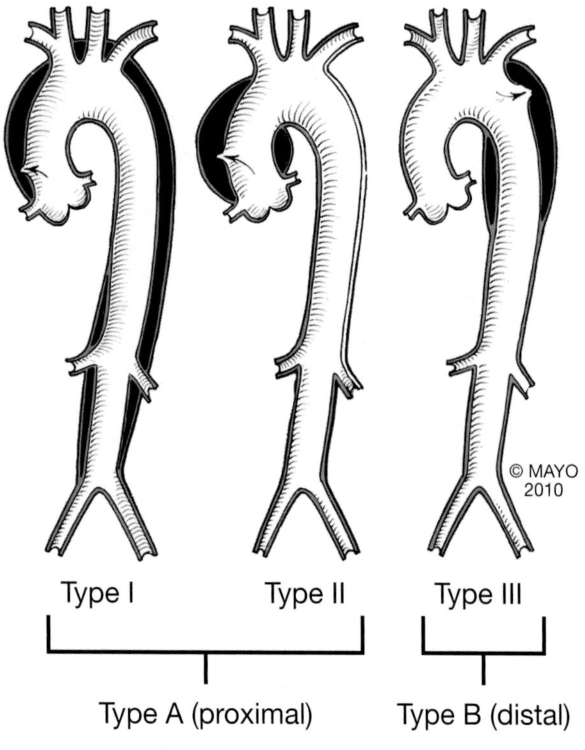

© MAYO 2010

Type I   Type II   Type III

Type A (proximal)   Type B (distal)

Figure 11.8 Classification System for Aortic Dissection.

Box 11.1 • Initial Pharmacologic Therapy for Acute Aortic Dissection

Hypertensive patients

    Sodium nitroprusside intravenously (2.5–5.0 mcg/kg per min)

    with

    Propranolol intravenously (1 mg every 4–6 h)

    Goal: Systolic blood pressure in the range of 110 mm Hg (or the lowest level maintaining a urine output of 25–30 mL/h) until oral medication is started

    or

    Esmolol, metoprolol, or atenolol intravenously (in place of propranolol)

    or

    Labetolol intravenously (in place of sodium nitroprusside and a β-blocker)

Normotensive patients

    Propranolol intravenously (1 mg every 4–6 h) or orally (20–40 mg every 6 h) (metoprolol, atenolol, esmolol, or labetalol may be used in place of propranolol)

KEY FACTS

✓ Aneurysms of ascending aorta—typically due to medial degeneration

✓ Aneurysms of descending thoracic aorta—primarily due to atherosclerosis

✓ Indications for elective surgical repair of TAA—ascending TAA ≥5.5 cm, descending TAA ≥6.0 cm, or growth rate ≥0.5 cm per year

✓ AAA—
  • men are affected 5 times more often than women, and incidence increases with age
  • ≥4.0 cm: ultrasonography every 6–12 months
  • <4.0 cm: ultrasonography every 2–3 years
  • repair recommended for size ≥5.5 cm, growth rate ≥0.5 cm per year, atheroembolism, any suggestion of instability

✓ All ascending thoracic aortic dissections (Stanford type A or DeBakey type I or II)—surgical emergencies (mortality rate is 1% per hour within the first 48 hours if left untreated)

✓ Descending thoracic aortic dissection (Stanford type B or DeBakey type III)—treated medically unless there is organ ischemia, dissection progression, enlarging aneurysm, or inability to control pain or hypertension

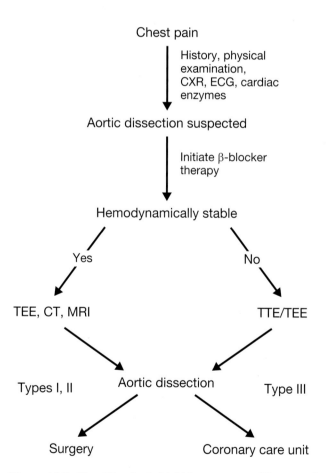

Figure 11.9 Algorithm for Initial Management of Suspected Acute Aortic Dissection. CT indicates computed tomography; CXR, chest radiography; ECG, electrocardiography; MRI, magnetic resonance imaging; TEE, transesophageal echocardiography; TTE, transthoracic echocardiography.

Peripheral Arterial Conditions

Aneurysms

Iliac artery aneurysms are usually associated with AAA, but they may occur as an isolated finding. Symptoms at presentation may include urinary obstruction, iliac vein obstruction, and unexplained groin or perineal pain. Repair is indicated when the aneurysm size exceeds 3.5 cm. Femoral artery aneurysm repair is indicated at a size of 3.0 cm or more. Popliteal artery aneurysm may lead to thromboembolization, neuropathy, or thrombophlebitis. Repair is indicated when the aneurysm is more than 2 cm or when thrombus is present. The greatest concern for popliteal aneurysm is thromboembolism to distal arteries. Popliteal artery aneurysm is bilateral in 50% of patients, and 40% may have synchronous aneurysms elsewhere, most commonly the abdominal aorta.

Arterial Occlusive Disease

Peripheral artery disease of the legs may be symptomatic at presentation (50%) or may be found incidentally (50%). Of symptomatic patients, 40% have intermittent claudication and 10% have critical limb ischemia at diagnosis. **Intermittent claudication** is the most common symptom and is defined as "exertional pain involving the calf that impedes walking, resolves within 10 minutes of rest, and neither begins at rest nor resolves on walking" (Monogr Ser World Health Organ. 1968;56:1–188). Pseudoclaudication (due to lumbar spinal stenosis) is the condition most commonly confused with intermittent claudication. Clinical clues suggesting pseudoclaudication include day-to-day variability of distance to symptom onset, symptom onset with prolonged standing (spinal extension), and need to sit for symptom relief (spinal flexion) (Table 11.1). Other

Table 11.1 • Differential Diagnosis of Intermittent Claudication and Pseudoclaudication

Factor	Claudication	Pseudoclaudication
Onset	Walking	Standing and walking
Character	Cramp, ache	Paresthetic
Bilateral	Sometimes	Often
Walking distance	Fairly constant	More variable
Cause	Atherosclerosis	Spinal stenosis
Relief	Standing still	Sitting down, leaning forward

Table 11.2 • Grading System for Lower-Extremity Arterial Occlusive Disease

Grade	ABI	
	Supine Resting	Postexercise[a]
Normal	1.0–1.4	≥1.0
Minimal disease	0.9–1.0	0.8–1.0
Mild disease	0.8–0.9	0.5–0.8
Moderate disease	0.5–0.8	0.15–0.5
Severe disease	<0.5	<0.15

Abbreviation: ABI, ankle-to-brachial systolic pressure index.
[a] After treadmill exercise (1–2 mph, 10% grade for 5 minutes or until limited by symptoms) or active pedal plantar flexion (50 repetitions or until limited by symptoms).

clues may include a history of back pain or prior spinal operations. Lumbar spinal stenosis can be confirmed with a normal or minimally abnormal ankle-to-brachial systolic pressure index (ABI) before and after exercise in combination with characteristic findings on electromyography and CT or MRI of the lumbar spine.

Symptoms of walking impairment for patients with peripheral artery disease remain stable in 75% of affected patients, and less than 2% per year require amputation. However, mortality is high (5 years 30%, 10 years 50%, 15 years 70%), reflecting coexisting atherosclerosis: severe coronary artery disease (40%–60%), carotid artery disease (25%–50%), and renal artery disease (25%–40%).

Key Definition

Intermittent claudication: *exertional pain involving the calf that impedes walking, resolves within 10 minutes of rest, and neither begins at rest nor resolves on walking.*

ABI screening should be performed in patients with exertional leg symptoms, patients 50 to 60 years old with atherosclerosis risk factors (especially diabetes mellitus or smoking), patients older than 70 years, or patients with a Framingham risk score of more than 10%. Disease severity assessed by ABI criteria correlate directly with overall survival such that the PAD severity of peripheral artery disease is an independent predictor of all-cause mortality. Patients with diabetes mellitus should be screened every 5 years. Supine ABIs before and after exercise testing (treadmill walking or active pedal plantar flexion) confirm the diagnosis (Table 11.2). An ABI index between 1.0 and 1.4 is considered normal. Values of 0.5 or less are considered severely reduced. If ABIs are normal at rest but symptoms are suggestive of intermittent claudication, ABIs should be determined before and after treadmill exercise. Heavily calcified peripheral arteries may result in a falsely increased Doppler-derived

systolic pressure and invalidate the ABI (≥1.4). In these cases, an accurate pressure may be obtained by measuring the toe pressure and calculating the toe-brachial index (a pressure gradient of 20–30 mm Hg is normally present between the ankle and the toe). An abnormally high ABI (≥1.4) implies arterial calcification and is associated with diabetes and with an increased cardiovascular risk.

Smoking cessation and lipid-lowering, diabetes mellitus, and hypertension treatment according to national treatment guidelines are recommended for all patients with peripheral artery disease. In patients who continue to use tobacco, the risk for major amputation is increased 10-fold and the mortality rate is increased more than 2-fold. Diabetes mellitus accounts for most amputations (12-fold increased risk of below-knee amputation).

All patients with peripheral artery disease should receive aspirin (81–325 mg daily) or clopidogrel if they are aspirin-allergic. Clopidogrel (75 mg daily) has been shown to be more effective than aspirin for preventing major atherosclerotic vascular events in patients with peripheral artery disease. Cilostazol can be used for relief of claudication symptoms and improves walking distance to claudication compared with pentoxifylline or placebo, but it is *contraindicated* in patients with heart failure. Although there is no evidence that treatment of hypertension alters the progression of claudication, blood pressure should be controlled to reduce morbidity and death due to cardiovascular and cerebrovascular disease. The angiotensin-converting enzyme inhibitor ramipril reduces the risk of ischemic cardiovascular events in patients with peripheral artery disease and may increase walking distance in select patients, in addition to its renal protective effects in diabetes. Statins reduce cardiovascular events in patients with peripheral artery disease, reduce new or worsening claudication, and improve walking distance and pain-free walking time. All patients with peripheral artery disease should receive treatment to reduce the low-density lipoprotein cholesterol value to less than 100 mg/dL (<70 mg/dL in patients with atherosclerosis in other circulatory beds).

Systemic antibiotic therapy should be initiated promptly in patients with critical limb ischemia, skin ulcerations, and evidence of limb infection. Patients at risk of critical limb ischemia (ABI <0.4 in a nondiabetic patient or any diabetic with known lower-extremity peripheral artery disease) should undergo regular foot inspection to detect objective signs of critical limb ischemia. Foot care and protection are of paramount importance in patients with diabetes mellitus who have peripheral artery disease. The combination of peripheral neuropathy, small-vessel disease, and peripheral artery disease in patients with diabetes mellitus makes foot trauma more likely to be associated with a nonhealing wound or ulcer.

Supervised walking should be part of the initial treatment for all patients with peripheral artery disease (Circulation. 2012 Jan 3;125[1]:130–9). Maximal walking distance has been shown to improve 200% to 300% when treadmill or track walking is used to the point of symptom reproduction with rest intervals in 30- to 60-minute sessions, 3 times weekly for 3 months.

Absolute indications for revascularization (surgical bypass or angioplasty and stenting) include ischemic rest pain and nonhealing ulceration. Ischemic ulcers are typically found at pressure points on the foot (eg, between-toes "kissing ulcers") and point of contact with a shoe (eg, medial aspect of great toe, lateral aspect of fifth toe, and heels). A relative indication for revascularization includes lifestyle-limiting intermittent claudication. MR angiography and CT angiography define anatomic localization of disease and provide a roadmap necessary for endovascular or surgical therapeutic planning.

Indications for amputation are severe rest pain with no revascularization option, limb gangrene, or life-threatening infection. Below-knee amputation is associated with a mortality rate of 10% perioperatively and 25% at 1 year. The primary healing rate with below-knee amputation is 60%, and 15% of patients will eventually need above-knee amputation.

Acute Arterial Occlusion

Acute arterial occlusion is suggested by the sudden onset of extreme pain and paresthesia of the involved limb. These and other suggestive conditions are listed in Box 11.2. It is

---

Box 11.2 • The 6 *P*s Suggestive of Acute Arterial Occlusion

Pain

Pallor

Paresthesia

Paralysis

Poikilothermy (coldness)

Pulselessness

---

important to distinguish thrombus due to local plaque rupture from an embolic source because the natural histories of these 2 mechanisms differ. Features suggestive of local thrombus include known arterial occlusive disease of the involved limb, which can be identified by examining the pulse integrity of the opposite limb. Diminished or absent pulses in the "good" limb suggest underlying atherosclerosis and plaque rupture with associated thrombosis as the most likely mechanism. An embolic cause is suggested by the presence of cardiac disease (valvular or ischemic), atrial fibrillation, proximal aneurysm, or proximal atherosclerotic disease.

Therapeutic results from thrombectomy are much better if the acute arterial occlusion is due to embolism as opposed to plaque rupture with local thrombus. Amputation rates are considerably higher for patients with local thrombus. Infrequent causes of arterial occlusion include dissection, traumatic transection, vasculitis, sepsis or disseminated intravascular coagulation, compartment syndrome, vasospasm, foreign body embolization, or tumor. Tissue tolerance to ischemia varies by tissue type. Nerve injury occurs within 4 hours, whereas muscle (6 hours) and skin (10 hours) are relatively more resistant to ischemia. Angiography is performed after initiation of intravenous heparin therapy and foot protection. After confirmation of the diagnosis, initial therapeutic options include intra-arterial thrombolysis and surgery (thromboembolectomy). If thrombolysis is the initial treatment, percutaneous treatment or surgical therapy is usually indicated for the underlying stenosis (if present) for improvement of long-term patency rates.

Fluid resuscitation is needed to prevent reperfusion syndrome, including myoglobinuric renal failure, metabolic (lactic) acidosis, and hyperkalemia. Four-compartment fasciotomy is often required to prevent muscle and nerve injury associated with the compartment syndrome.

Carotid Artery Disease

Carotid artery disease is present in 5% to 9% of the US population older than 65 years and contributes substantially to transient ischemic attacks and strokes. Large-vessel disease, most commonly of the carotid artery, accounts for 30% of ischemic strokes. Cardiac embolism (especially atrial fibrillation) and small-vessel disease each account for an additional 30%. Carotid disease may initially be detected as a bruit. The prevalence of an asymptomatic bruit may be as high as 13% depending on the population examined. The prevalence increases with age.

The natural history of carotid artery disease varies by the clinical presentation (whether symptomatic or asymptomatic) and the severity of the underlying stenosis. When the clinical presentation is consistent with either transient ischemic attack or stroke, it is important to distinguish anterior from posterior circulation and right from left hemispheric injury to determine whether the carotid lesion is responsible for the symptoms. Symptomatic carotid artery lesions typically result in cortical neurologic deficits, whereas small-vessel mechanisms involve the deep parenchyma. A significant stenosis is typically defined as more than 70%. For asymptomatic carotid artery stenosis of more than 70%, the annual risk of stroke is between 3% and 4%. If the stenosis is less than 60%, the annual risk of stroke is less than 1%. For symptomatic patients with stenoses greater than 70%, the annual risk of stroke is 15%.

Medical management of all patients with carotid artery disease should include aggressive treatment of hypertension, hyperlipidemia, and diabetes mellitus, and cessation of the use of all tobacco products is strongly recommended. Antiplatelet therapy should be initiated.

Carotid endarterectomy reduces the annual risk of stroke in both asymptomatic and symptomatic patients. For asymptomatic patients, this annual risk can be reduced from 4% to 1.5%. For symptomatic patients, the annual stroke rate can be reduced from 15% to 5% and perhaps as low as 1.6% according to recent trial data. Risks associated with carotid surgery include stroke and cranial nerve injury. Compared with stenting, surgery is associated with slightly higher risk of myocardial infarction but perhaps a slightly lower risk of stroke.

The risk of adverse outcomes (stroke, myocardial infarction, or death) with carotid artery stenting is similar to that of carotid artery surgery in asymptomatic patients with significant carotid artery stenosis. For asymptomatic patients in the Carotid Revascularization Endarterectomy vs Stenting Trial (CREST), the risk of stroke or death was 4.5% with carotid stenting and 2.7% with surgery. For symptomatic patients in this trial, this combined outcome was 8.0% for stenting and 6.4% for surgery. According to the guidelines, both stenting and surgery are acceptable for symptomatic patients. In general, for symptomatic patients

at good risk for a surgical procedure, carotid endarterectomy should be pursued. For high-risk symptomatic patients who would not be good candidates for surgery, carotid stenting with an embolic protection device should be considered. For asymptomatic patients, revascularization should be determined on the basis of comorbidities, life expectancy, and other factors, including a thorough discussion of risks and potential benefits (untreated annual stroke risk, 4% per year).

Uncommon Types of Arterial Occlusive Disease

Thromboangiitis Obliterans (Buerger Disease)

Thromboangiitis obliterans (Buerger disease) (Table 11.3) should be considered in young smokers with foot claudication or ulceration of the feet or hands (Figure 11.10). These patients have early symptom onset, typically in the second or fourth decade of life. Foot claudication is nearly universal, and hand or finger involvement occurs in 33% to 63% of patients. All 4 limbs are involved in 40% of patients. Rest pain and ischemic ulceration are typically present in the lower extremity. Thromboangiitis obliterans affects distal arteries initially and primarily. Venous involvement (superficial phlebitis) is common. The disease was previously considered a male-dominated disease, but the incidence in women has increased in recent decades. A hallmark of the disease is addiction to tobacco. Smoking cessation ameliorates the course of the disease and reduces the risk of ulcer formation and amputation.

Evaluation must be thorough and distinguish between thromboangiitis obliterans and premature atherosclerosis. Distinguishing features of thromboangiitis obliterans include upper-extremity involvement, foot claudication, and

---

KEY FACTS

✓ Peripheral arterial disease: severity correlates strongly with mortality due to coexisting systemic cardiovascular disease

✓ Iliac artery aneurysm—repair is indicated when aneurysm size is >3.5 cm

✓ Femoral artery aneurysm—repair is indicated when aneurysm size is ≥3.0 cm

✓ ABI criteria—normal 1.0–1.4, severe <0.5

✓ Cilostazol—improves walking distance in patients with arterial occlusive disease but is contraindicated in patients with clinical heart failure

✓ Symptomatic carotid artery disease (>70% stenosis)—in good-risk patients, treatment is surgical endarterectomy; in high-risk patients, stenting is used for treatment

✓ Asymptomatic carotid artery disease (<70% stenosis)—treatment can be surgical, stenting, or medical (4% risk of stroke per year)

Table 11.3 • Clinical Criteria for Thromboangiitis Obliterans

Age	<40 y (often <30 y)
Sex	Males most often
Habits	Tobacco, cannabis use
History	Superficial phlebitis Claudication of arch or calf Raynaud phenomenon Absence of atherosclerotic risk factors other than smoking
Examination	Small arteries involved Upper extremity involved (positive Allen test) Infrapopliteal artery disease
Laboratory findings	Normal values of glucose, blood cell counts, sedimentation rate, lipids, and screening tests for connective tissue disease and hypercoagulable disorders
Radiography	No arterial calcification

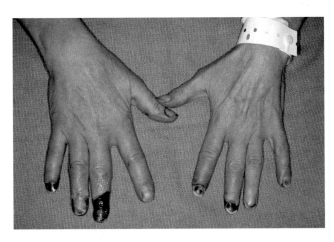

Figure 11.10 Gangrene of the Tips of Multiple Upper Extremity Digits in a Patient With Thromboangiitis Obliterans.

a history of superficial thrombophlebitis. Patients may present in their early 20s and 30s, whereas even profound premature atherosclerosis does not usually present until in the fifth decade of life.

Angiographic features include normal proximal vessels, distal artery occlusions, and skip lesions. "Tree root," "spider," and "corkscrew" are adjectives frequently applied to the angiographic appearance of collateral vessels and vasa vasorum; however, these findings are nonspecific and may be present in occlusive disease of other causes. Involved vessels may be thrombosed. Thrombi are infiltrated with inflammatory cells, but inflammatory marker values (ie, erythrocyte sedimentation rate) are nearly always normal.

Treatment is limited to tobacco cessation, wound care, limb protection, and amputation when needed. Arterial bypass grafting and angioplasty with stenting are rarely possible or effective.

Thoracic Outlet Compression Syndrome

The thoracic outlet syndromes are a group of often disabling disorders caused by mechanical compression or irritation of the neurovascular bundle as it leaves the chest cavity through the thoracic outlet. There are 3 unique clinical presentations of the syndromes: 1) neurogenic, 2) venous, and 3) arterial. The thoracic outlet boundaries consist of the superior surface of the first rib and the anterior and middle scalene muscles. The neurogenic type is the most common (80% of patients) and presents with numbness, pain, and tingling primarily involving the ulnar nerve. Patients complain of arm symptoms with arm elevation (abduction), such as when working with their arms above their heads. The differential diagnosis of neurogenic thoracic outlet syndrome is broad and includes multiple neurologic, orthopedic, and vascular diagnoses. Electromyographic results are normal. Cervical spine radiographs may be helpful to show the presence of cervical rib arising from the C7 pedicle (as opposed to T1). Arm lowering (adduction) relieves symptoms. Approximately 15% of patients present with venous

symptoms, including subclavian vein thrombosis (Paget-Schroetter syndrome or effort thrombosis). Approximately 5% of patients have an aneurysm of the subclavian artery as a result of trauma at the point where the artery crosses the outlet. Subclavian artery aneurysms tend to thrombose and embolize. Patients present with painful embolic digital artery occlusion and finger gangrene.

The diagnosis of neurogenic thoracic outlet syndrome (most common presentation) is complex and is primarily based on clinical presentation and physical findings. Thoracic outlet maneuvers (costoclavicular active, costoclavicular passive, hyperabduction, Adson, and elevated arm stress tests) are performed to aid in the diagnosis. These maneuvers induce dynamic compression of the axillary-subclavian artery, which is identified as dynamic obliteration of the radial pulse. Results of these maneuvers may be positive in up to 30% of the general population; thus, their specificity and positive predictive value are limited. Vascular imaging (ultrasonography, CT angiography, and MR angiography) for neurogenic thoracic outlet syndrome shows dynamic vascular compression with maneuvers in up to 30% of the general population; thus, the usefulness of imaging in diagnostic evaluation is limited. Electromyography is normal in the majority of patients, such that an abnormal result should prompt a search for alternative diagnoses.

Treatment for neurogenic thoracic outlet syndrome is primarily and initially conservative with physical therapy. Severe cases in which conservative therapy fails may benefit from thoracic outlet decompression and first rib resection. Patients with upper-extremity venous thrombosis related to thoracic outlet syndrome (Paget-Schroetter syndrome or effort thrombosis) receive aggressive thrombolytic therapy, anticoagulation, and first rib resection. Patients with upper-extremity arterial thrombosis related to thoracic outlet syndrome often present with digital ischemia related to thromboembolism from an axillary-subclavian artery aneurysm. These patients undergo aggressive treatment with surgical repair of the aneurysm, anticoagulation, and thoracic outlet decompression.

Vasospastic Disorders

Vasospastic disorders are characterized by episodic color changes of the skin resulting from intermittent spasm of the small arteries and arterioles of the skin and digits. These vascular disorders are important because they may be a clue to another underlying disorder, such as arterial occlusive disease, connective tissue disorders, arterial injury, neurologic disorders, or endocrine disease. Vasospastic disorders may also be caused by certain medications, particularly β-blockers. Ergot preparations, estrogen therapy, chemotherapeutic agents, interferon, cyclosporine, clonidine, narcotics, nicotine, and cocaine use are other possible causes.

Raynaud Syndrome

For this syndrome, it is important to differentiate vasospasm due to primary Raynaud "disease" from secondary Raynaud "phenomenon" (due to a fixed obstruction) (Table 11.4). The natural histories of these 2 disorders vary considerably.

Primary Raynaud Disease

Raynaud disease typically involves the digits of the upper extremity and, to a lesser extent, the lower extremity. Females are more often affected than males, and the typical patient is young at onset of the disease (<40 years). Vasospasm is induced by cold weather or emotional stress. Involvement is typically bilateral with multiple, if not all, digits involved. The symptoms are usually stable over time. Triphasic color changes (blanching, cyanosis, and hyperemic response to warming) may be present but are not universal. Other features of connective tissue disease such as systemic lupus erythematosus, rheumatoid arthritis, or scleroderma are absent. Arterial occlusion and digital ulcerations are rare. It is considered a benign condition, and treatment emphasizes avoiding cold exposure and vasoconstrictive triggers. Vasodilator therapy includes calcium channel blockers (dihydropyridine) and α-blockers (doxazosin).

Secondary Raynaud Phenomenon

In contrast to patients with Raynaud disease, those with secondary Raynaud phenomenon are more commonly male and older than 40 years. There is evidence of fixed digital artery obstruction, which may be due to various causes, including atherosclerosis, vasculitis, connective tissue diseases, hypothenar hammer syndrome, embolism, or drugs (especially β-blockers and ergotamine). Distribution of symptoms is asymmetric with involvement of few digits. Associated pulse deficits, ischemic changes (including digital ulcerations), and systemic signs and symptoms are often present. Identification of the underlying cause is essential for appropriate treatment.

Evaluation should focus on differentiating primary Raynaud "disease" from secondary Raynaud "phenomenon," including exclusion of connective tissue diseases and vasculitis. Vascular laboratory testing is important to differentiate vasospasm from arterial occlusion. Baseline laboratory tests include complete blood count, erythrocyte sedimentation rate, C-reactive protein, serum protein electrophoresis, antinuclear antibody, antiphospholipid antibody, and cryoglobulins. Conventional angiography (arch angiogram with upper-extremity runoff) is rarely needed for the evaluation of primary Raynaud disease but can often be helpful for the evaluation of secondary Raynaud phenomenon, particularly if the underlying disease is not apparent.

Livedo Reticularis

Livedo reticularis is due to spasm or occlusion of dermal arterioles leading to a bluish mottling of the skin in a lacy, reticular pattern (Figure 11.3). Primary livedo reticularis is idiopathic and not associated with an identifiable underlying disorder. Secondary livedo reticularis may result from atheroembolism from a proximal aneurysm or from proximal atheromatous plaques. Other causes of secondary livedo reticularis include connective tissue disease, antiphospholipid antibody syndrome, vasculitis, myeloproliferative disorders, dysproteinemias, reflex sympathetic dystrophy, cold injury, and an adverse effect of amantadine hydrochloride therapy.

Chronic Pernio

Chronic pernio is a vasospastic disorder characterized by sensitivity to cold and predominantly occurs in female patients with a past history of often intense cold exposure and injury. It may result in a blistering process with ulceration, particularly of the toes (Figure 11.11). It typically presents with symmetric blue discoloration and blistering and ulceration of the toes in cooler weather with resolution during warmer weather. Treatment with an α-blocker can be quite effective.

Table 11.4 • Characteristic Clinical Features of Primary and Secondary Raynaud Syndrome

Clinical Feature	Primary	Secondary
Symmetry	Bilateral	Unilateral or bilateral
Pulses	Normal	Abnormal
Skin ulcers	Absent	May be present
Gangrene, tissue loss	Absent	May be present
Vascular laboratory finding	Vasospasm	Fixed obstruction
Other underlying connective tissue disease	Absent	Present
Response to vasodilator or warming	Present	Minimal

KEY FACTS

✓ Thromboangiitis obliterans (Buerger disease)—should be considered in young smokers with foot claudication or digital ulceration of feet or hands

✓ Thoracic outlet compression syndromes—the 3 unique clinical presentations are 1) neurogenic, 2) venous, and 3) arterial

✓ Primary Raynaud disease—typically involves the digits of the upper extremity and, to a lesser extent, the lower extremity; females are affected more often than males; typical patient is young at disease onset (<40 years)

✓ Secondary Raynaud phenomenon—in contrast to patients with Raynaud disease, these patients are more commonly male and older than 40 years

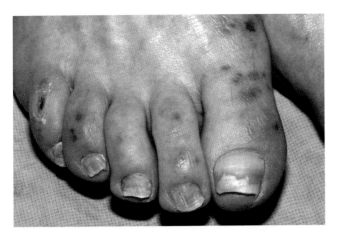

Figure 11.11 Characteristic Lesions of Chronic Pernio.

Erythromelalgia

Erythromelalgia is the occurrence of red, hot, painful, burning digits with exposure to warm temperatures or after exercise. It is not a true vasospastic disorder, but it is associated with color change of the skin. It may be primary (idiopathic) or due to an underlying disorder, most commonly myeloproliferative disorders (eg, polycythemia rubra vera), diabetes mellitus, or small-fiber neuropathy.

Treatment of the primary form includes warm temperature avoidance and aspirin therapy. Therapy with a nonselective β-blocker is helpful in some patients. Symptoms of secondary erythromelalgia are typically relieved with treatment of the underlying disorder.

Key Definition

Erythromelalgia: *occurrence of red, hot, painful, burning digits with exposure to warm temperatures or after exercise.*

Edema

Lower-extremity edema is commonly encountered in clinical practice and has several potential underlying causes. Noncardiac causes of regional edema usually can be identified from characteristic clinical features.

Lymphedema

Lymphedema can be primary (idiopathic) or due to an underlying disorder. Primary lymphedema (lymphedema praecox) is more common in women (9-fold greater frequency than in men) and typically begins before age 40 years and often before age 20 years. In women, symptoms often first appear at menarche or with the first pregnancy. Edema is bilateral in about half the cases (Table 11.5).

Table 11.5 • Differential Diagnosis of Regional Types of Edema

Feature	Venous	Lymphedema	Lipedema
Bilateral	Occasional	±	Always
Foot involved	+	+	−
Toes involved	−	+	−
Thickened skin	−	+	−
Stasis changes	+	−	−

Secondary lymphedema is broadly classified into obstructive (postsurgical, postradiation, or neoplastic) and inflammatory (infectious) types.

Obstructive lymphedema due to neoplasm typically begins after age 40 years and often is due to a pelvic neoplasm, lymphoma, or breast cancer. Initial evaluation should include a complete history and physical examination. CT of the abdomen and pelvis should be done to evaluate for a neoplastic cause of lymphatic obstruction. Women should undergo a pelvic examination and Papanicolaou smear. Men should be evaluated for prostate cancer. Inflammatory lymphedema occurs as a result of chronic or recurring lymphangitis or cellulitis. Dermatophytosis (tinea pedis) is the most common portal of entry for infection, which is often overlooked. The diagnosis of lymphedema can be evaluated noninvasively with lymphoscintigraphy.

Medical management of lymphedema includes edema reduction therapy using bandage wrapping, followed by daily use of custom-fitted, graduated-compression (usually 40–50 mm Hg) elastic support. Manual lymphatic drainage is a type of massage used in combination with skin care, support and compression therapy, and exercise to manage lymphedema. A combined multimodality approach may substantially reduce excess limb volume and improve quality of life. Dermatophytosis, if present, should be treated with antifungal agents. Weight reduction in obese patients is beneficial. Surgical treatment of lymphedema (eg, lymphaticovenous anastomosis, lymphedema reduction) may be helpful in carefully selected patients.

Leg Ulcer

The appropriate evaluation and care of skin ulcers involving the lower extremity must begin with identifying and treating the underlying cause when at all possible. Lower-extremity ulcers can be divided into 4 main categories: large-vessel arterial disease, small-vessel arterial disease, venous disease, and neuropathic disease. The cause of lower-extremity ulceration usually can be determined by a careful clinical examination. Clinical features of the 4 most common types of leg ulcer are summarized in Table 11.6 (Figure 11.12).

Table 11.6 • Clinical Features of the 4 Most Common Types of Leg Ulcer

Feature	Venous	Arterial	Arteriolar	Neurotrophic
		Type of Ulcer		
Onset	Trauma ±	Trauma	Spontaneous	Trauma
Course	Chronic	Progressive	Progressive	Progressive
Pain	No (unless infected)	Yes	Yes	No
Location	Medial aspect of leg	Toe, heel, foot	Lateral, posterior aspect of leg	Plantar
Surrounding skin	Stasis changes	Atrophic	Normal	Callous
Ulcer edges	Shaggy	Discrete	Serpiginous	Discrete
Ulcer base	Healthy	Eschar, pale	Eschar, pale	Healthy or pale

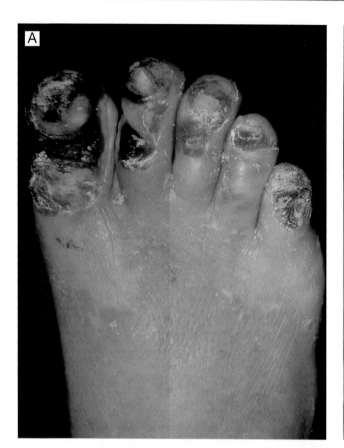

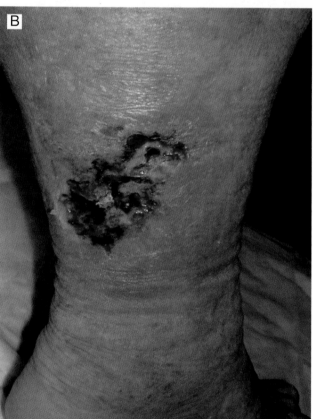

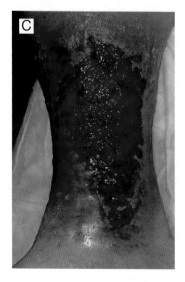

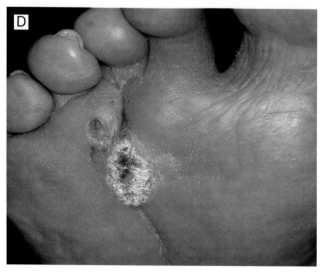

Figure 11.12 *Clinical Features of the 4 Most Common Types of Leg Ulcer. A, Critical limb ischemia due to peripheral artery disease. B, Small vessel "arteriolar" disease. C, Venous disease. D, Neurotrophic disease.*

Questions and Answers

Questions

Multiple Choice (choose the best answer)

II.1. A 30-year-old woman comes to your office to establish you as her primary care provider. She appears healthy and is not limited by physical activity. She admits to occasional chest pains that occur at rest, often with change in position. Her blood pressure is 110/70 mm Hg with a heart rate of 76 beats per minute and regular. Auscultatory findings are a midsystolic click followed by a 2/6 apical systolic murmur that radiates to her axilla. Which the following dynamic physical examination findings confirms your suspicion of mitral valve prolapse?

a. No change is heard in click with squat or stand.

b. A passive leg raise makes the click murmur earlier.

c. A squat maneuver makes the click murmur later.

d. The mitral regurgitant murmur does not change with positional maneuvers.

II.2. A 55-year-old patient in the emergency department has syncope that occurred during a pickup basketball game. Blood pressure is 132/76 mm Hg, heart rate is 77 beats per minute, carotid pulsations are brisk, and jugular venous pressure is normal. The apex is not displaced but is sustained. On auscultation, a grade 3/6 systolic murmur is best heard in the second interspace, right sternal border. It radiates to the neck. A fourth heart sound can be heard. The murmur becomes softer on handgrip, louder with Valsalva maneuver, and softer with the squat maneuver. The patient most likely has which of the following?

a. Hypertrophic cardiomyopathy with dynamic outflow obstruction

b. Bicuspid aortic valve stenosis with moderate stenosis

c. Mitral valve regurgitation due to mitral valve prolapse

d. Pulmonary valve stenosis with marked stenosis

e. Severe mitral valve stenosis

II.3. A 14-year-old girl comes for evaluation of a sudden syncopal spell that occurred while she was waiting in the dentist's office. Although the spell was sudden, she remembers feeling hot and clammy and having a sensation of tunnel vision and of "wanting to get out of there" shortly before losing consciousness. Afterward, she came around quickly and was fully oriented, although she felt somewhat fatigued. On examination in the office, she has no abnormal physical findings. No orthostatic symptoms or signs are apparent. Peripheral pulse and neurologic evaluation are normal. What is your advice?

a. Order a tilt-table test.

b. Give a β-adrenergic blocker to prevent further episodes of syncope.

c. Perform awake and sleep electroencephalography to rule out epilepsy.

d. Reassure the patient.

e. Advise an increased dietary salt intake.

II.4. A 55-year-old man presents for a routine physical examination. On examination, you find that his pulse is irregular but the rate is well controlled. He has no symptoms whatsoever and has good exercise tolerance. You diagnose atrial fibrillation on the basis of 12-lead electrocardiography. Which of the following historical factors elicited from the history increases his risk of stroke?

a. Persistent atrial fibrillation

b. Tobacco use

c. Family history of stroke

d. Left atrial enlargement

e. Hypertension

II.5. A 62-year-old man presents with atrial fibrillation and rapid ventricular response. He tells you this episode is his third in the past month. Which of the following drugs may be effective for preventing recurrence of symptoms?

a. Verapamil

b. Propafenone

c. Adenosine

d. Atenolol

e. Digoxin

II.6. A 57-year-old man with a history of diabetes mellitus and hypertension presents to the hospital with new orthopnea and edema. His blood presure is 95/60 mm Hg, and heart rate is 96 beats per minute. His lungs are clear. He has a displaced cardiac apex with a third heart sound but no cardiac murmurs and no lower extremity edema. Laboratory tests show his levels of hemoglobin at 14 g/dL, sodium at 137 mmol/L, potassium at 4.4 mmol/L, and serum creatinine at 1.7 mg/dL. Chest radiography shows pulmonary congestion with cardiomegaly. Electrocardiography shows sinus rhythm, nonspecific ST-T changes, and frequent premature ventricular complexes. He undergoes echocardiography that shows a left ventricular ejection fraction of 20% and a dilated left ventricle. The next step in evaluating this patient is to perform which of the following?

a. Endomyocardial biopsy

b. Stress testing

c. Coronary angiography

d. Holter monitoring

e. Sleep study

II.7. A 72-year-old woman presents to the emergency department with dyspnea and retrosternal chest pain of 3-hour duration that developed soon after she was in an intense argument with her daughter. Her past medical history is remarkable for hypertension and diabetes mellitus. The chest discomfort is not relieved by sublingual nitroglycerin. Her heart rate is 100 beats per minute, and blood pressure is 156/92 mm Hg. Jugular venous pressure, carotid pulse, and peripheral pulses are normal. Cardiac auscultation is normal; lungs are clear to auscultation. Cardiac troponin T level is 0.12 (reference range, ≥0.01). The 12-lead electrocardiography shows 0.5- to 1-mm ST-segment elevation in precordial leads V2 through V4. She is taken for an emergency coronary angiography, which demonstrates mild coronary atherosclerosis. A left ventriculography is performed, which shows severe hypokinesis of the apical and midsegments of the heart, with normal function at the base. Which of the following is the *most likely* diagnosis?

a. Myocarditis
b. Apical ballooning syndrome (takotsubo cardiomyopathy)
c. Acute coronary syndrome
d. Dilated cardiomyopathy
e. Pericarditis

II.8. A 46-year-old man with diabetes mellitus, ongoing tobacco use, hypertension, and hyperlipidemia reports claudication in both legs after walking 2 blocks. His ankle brachial index is 0.55 bilaterally. Angiography performed at his home hospital shows severe disease of the infrapopliteal arteries, with patent proximal vessels. His symptoms improve with standing and are consistent from 1 day to the next. He has no rest pain or ulceration. His symptoms have been stable for the past 2 years. His blood pressure is 150/70 mm Hg and his heart rate is 80 beats per minute with regularity. Chest is clear to auscultation. His carotid upstrokes are normal without bruit. Cardiac examination reveals normal jugular venous pressure and apical impulse. Auscultation is normal. His vascular examination shows normal pulses in the femoral and popliteal arteries bilaterally without bruit. The pedal pulses are not palpable. Extremity examination reveals no ulcers, ischemic fissures, dependent rubor, or elevation pallor. Ankle brachial indices are 0.55 on the right and 0.52 on the left. Angiography performed at his local medical facility 1 year ago showed severe infrapopliteal arterial occlusive disease with diseased, though patent, proximal arteries bilaterally. Which of the following is the *most appropriate* treatment regimen for this patient with intermittent claudication?

a. Computed tomographic angiography of the legs
b. Magnetic resonance angiography of the legs
c. Risk factor modification and participation in the Canadian Walking Program
d. Angioplasty and stenting
e. Bypass surgery

II.9. A 72-year-old woman is 2 days post total hip arthroplasty. She has long-term hypertension. Blood pressure is noted to be 220/110 mm Hg and is confirmed on a repeat measure. She reports substernal chest pressure and mild dyspnea. Electrocardiography shows ST-segment depression in the inferior leads. Which of the following is the *most appropriate* parenteral antihypertensive drug to consider in this clinical setting?

a. Sodium nitroprusside
b. Hydralazine
c. Labetalol
d. Nitroglycerin
e. Nicardipine

Answers

II.1. Answer c.

This 30-year-old patient presents with atypical chest pain, which may be associated with mitral valve prolapse. This prolapse is essentially a mismatch of the left ventricular cavity size and the mitral valve leaflets, which are redundant. The classic bedside maneuver is squat to standing; however, any maneuver that increases the left ventricular cavity size will delay the midsystolic clicks and the mitral regurgitant murmur. The Valsalva maneuver decreases venous return, which would thus result in a smaller left ventricle and an earlier mitral valve prolapse. A postextrasystolic beat (due to the compensatory pause), the passive leg raise, and the squat (all of which improve left ventricular filling) should actually delay midsystolic clicks and murmur (Figure II.A1).

II.2. Answer a.

Hypertrophic cardiomyopathy is characterized by a dynamic outflow obstruction that can be exacerbated by a small left ventricle; reduced filling is due to dehydration, exercise, position, or decreased venous return. Thus, the Valsalva maneuver is an excellent bedside test to distinguish the murmur of aortic stenosis from hypertrophic cardiomyopathy. The murmurs of aortic valve stenosis, pulmonary valve stenosis, and mitral valve regurgitation all get softer with the Valsalva maneuver. In addition, the other disease processes (eg, mitral valve prolapse, pulmonary valve stenosis) generally have different murmur locations on the chest wall and other associated physical findings. Mitral valve prolapse usually is associated with a systolic click. Pulmonary valve stenosis generally is associated with an opening click that gets softer on inspiration. In fact, the opening click of pulmonary stenosis is the only right-sided sound that decreases with inspiration (because of the premature opening of the pulmonary valve with an inspiratory increase in flow to the right ventricle).

II.3. Answer d.

Tilt-table testing is not needed unless the diagnosis is in doubt. Electroencephalography adds information, and increased salt intake and volume replacement are unnecessary unless symptoms are recurrent. Use of β-blocker therapy in most patients with neurocardiogenic syncope is not associated with a decrease in symptoms and is not routinely recommended, even for patients with recurrent episodes.

II.4. Answer e.

Hypertension is the only risk factor that has been associated with an increased risk of stroke in patients with atrial fibrillation.

II.5. Answer b.

Calcium channel blockers and β-blockers do not prevent atrial fibrillation; they merely control rate during episodes of atrial fibrillation. Digoxin does not prevent recurrences and has limited efficacy to control rate during exercise. Adenosine has no effect on the occurrence of atrial fibrillation.

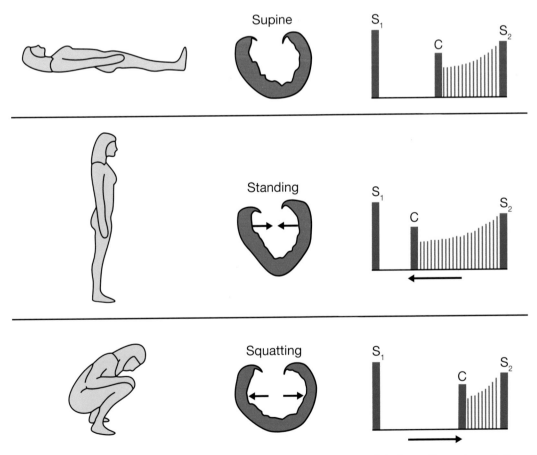

Figure II.A1 (Adapted from Shaver JA, Leonard JJ, Leon DF. Examination of the heart. Part 4: Auscultation of the heart. Dallas [TX]: American Heart Association; c1990. p. 13. Used with permission.)

II.6. Answer c.

The patient has dilated cardiomyopathy. The most common cause of this cardiomyopathy is coronary artery disease, especially in a person with atherosclerotic risk factors. The next most appropriate therapeutic step for this patient is coronary angiography—a gold standard diagnostic test in this circumstance. Stress testing may have false-positive or false-negative results in patients with dilated cardiomyopathy. Endomyocardial biopsy should not be routinely performed in the evaluation of patients with heart failure. Holter monitoring is useful in detecting the burden of premature ventricular contraction over 24 hours and, when its number is especially high, this burden could be implicated as a rare cause of heart failure. However, Holter monitoring would not be the next step in evaluation and should not be performed without initiating medical therapy because indicated medical treatment, such as β-blockers, can attenuate premature ventricular contractions. Sleep apnea could be a frequent accompaniment of decompensated heart failure, and its diagnostic evaluation should be performed only after patients are optimally treated.

II.7. Answer b.

The patient presents with symptoms consistent with an acute coronary syndrome with ST-segment elevation seen on electrocardiography. Therefore, emergency angiography was reasonable to perform, and it demonstrated normal coronary arteries. The differential diagnosis in such patients includes coronary spasm, coronary embolism, pericarditis, and myocarditis. However, this patient had a characteristic regional wall motion abnormality on left ventriculography, which involved the mid and apical segments of the left ventricle, with sparing of the basal segments. This entity has recently been recognized as the apical ballooning syndrome (takotsubo cardiomyopathy). Apical ballooning syndrome occurs predominantly in postmenopausal women and frequently is preceded by mental or physical stress. Acute coronary syndrome was ruled out by coronary angiography. Myocarditis is in the differential diagnosis, although it typically produces global left ventricular dysfunction. Pericarditis is not associated with systolic dysfunction.

II.8. Answer c.

This patient has classic presentation of infrapopliteal arterial occlusive disease in the clinical setting of long-term diabetes. Both the physical examination and the previous conventional angiography support this impression. It will not be helpful to repeat either magnetic resonance angiography or a computed tomographic angiography. Angioplasty and stenting of these distal arteries will have poor durability. At this point, no indication for surgical bypass is present because the patient has neither rest pain nor ulceration. The best option for this patient is risk factor modification (ie, smoking cessation, statin therapy, hypertension control, and diabetes therapy).

II.9. Answer d.

This clinical situation should be considered a hypertensive emergency because of evidence of organ injury (coronary ischemia and infarction). Therefore, an immediate reduction in blood pressure with a parenteral agent is indicated. Of the available drugs, nitroglycerin is preferred in the myocardial ischemia setting. Nitroglycerin is a balance arteriolar and venous dilator and lessens myocardial oxygen demand by reducing both preload and afterload. Hydralazine is a direct arteriolar vasodilator and may worsen myocardial ischemia. The other medications listed would be acceptable second-line agents in this case; of them, sodium nitroprusside is the best studied.

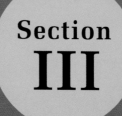

Section
III

Endocrinology

12 Calcium and Bone Metabolism Disorders

MARIUS N. STAN, MD

Hypercalcemia

The causes of hypercalcemia are categorized as either parathyroid hormone (PTH) dependent or PTH independent.

PTH-Dependent Hypercalcemia

Primary Hyperparathyroidism

Etiology

Primary hyperparathyroidism is the most common cause of hypercalcemia in ambulatory patients. A single parathyroid adenoma is the cause in 85% of patients, and multiglandular disease is the cause in the remainder. Parathyroid carcinoma is a rare cause of hypercalcemia. Primary hyperparathyroidism may be sporadic or familial. Familial hyperparathyroidism is usually multiglandular and most commonly a manifestation of multiple endocrine neoplasia (MEN) type 1 (MEN-1) or type 2 (MEN-2) syndromes.

Clinical Features

Most patients with hyperparathyroidism are asymptomatic and are identified with routine laboratory testing. Symptoms of hypercalcemia include polyuria, polydipsia, constipation, fatigue, and abdominal pain. Hypercalciuria can cause nephrolithiasis and nephrocalcinosis. Skeletal manifestations include osteopenia or osteoporosis and, in severe disease, bone pain, fractures, and osteitis fibrosa cystica (bone pain and characteristic areas of periosteal bone resorption).

Diagnosis

Elevated serum calcium and PTH levels are hallmarks of primary hyperparathyroidism. The serum PTH level is usually increased but may be inappropriately normal for the degree of hypercalcemia. Serum phosphate concentrations are normal or low. Urinary calcium excretion is high-normal or elevated; this test is also useful to assess risk for nephrolithiasis and exclude disorders characterized by low urinary calcium excretion (eg, familial hypocalciuric hypercalcemia and thiazide use). Characteristic skeletal radiographic changes include subperiosteal bone resorption, a salt-and-pepper appearance of the skull, and osteitis fibrosa cystica. Renal stones or nephrocalcinosis may be visible on abdominal radiographs.

Therapy

Surgical parathyroidectomy is the treatment of choice. Conservative therapy may be indicated for mild uncomplicated disease, especially in the elderly. Indications for surgical intervention are listed in Box 12.1. Imaging studies are helpful for guiding the surgeon, but they do not help in diagnosis. Preoperative imaging (parathyroid sestamibi scanning or ultrasonography) often identifies a solitary parathyroid adenoma, allowing minimally invasive surgery. Transient, mild hypocalcemia is common in the early postoperative period. However, in patients with severe preexisting parathyroid-induced bone disease, correction of hyperparathyroidism may lead to marked and prolonged hypocalcemia due to hungry bone syndrome.

Familial Hypocalciuric Hypercalcemia

Familial hypocalciuric hypercalcemia is an autosomal dominant disorder resulting from an altered set point of

---

Box 12.1 • Indications for Surgical Intervention for Primary Hyperparathyroidism

Age <50 y

Serum calcium level >1 mg/dL above the upper limit of the reference range

Nephrolithiasis

Osteoporosis

Renal insufficiency (creatinine clearance <60 mL/min)

---

the calcium-sensing receptor in the parathyroid glands and renal tubules. It manifests as mild, asymptomatic hypercalcemia in a patient with a normal or slightly increased level of PTH, low urinary calcium, and often a family history positive for hypercalcemia. The diagnosis is strongly supported by a ratio of urinary calcium to creatinine clearance that is less than 0.01, distinguishing it from primary hyperparathyroidism. Genetic testing is clinically available. Parathyroid surgery is not indicated because complications associated with hyperparathyroidism do not develop.

KEY FACTS

✓ Primary hyperparathyroidism—most common cause of hypercalcemia in ambulatory patients

✓ Hyperparathyroidism—usually asymptomatic; identified with laboratory testing

✓ Hallmarks of primary hyperparathyroidism—elevated levels of serum calcium and (usually) PTH

✓ Beware of severe preexisting parathyroid-induced bone disease—correction of hyperparathyroidism may cause marked, prolonged hypocalcemia (from hungry bone syndrome)

✓ Familial hypocalciuric hypercalcemia—ratio of urinary calcium to creatinine clearance <0.01 (unlike in primary hyperparathyroidism)

Thiazide-Induced Hypercalcemia

Mild hypercalcemia may occur in patients taking thiazide diuretics. The hypercalcemia is multifactorial (dehydration, decreased renal calcium clearance, and possibly increased PTH secretion). PTH levels are inappropriately normal or mildly increased. Unless it is coexistent with primary hyperparathyroidism, the hypercalcemia usually resolves within a few weeks after discontinuation of the drug.

Lithium

Lithium raises the threshold for serum calcium to inhibit PTH secretion. PTH levels are inappropriately normal or mildly increased. The hypercalcemia is likely to resolve after discontinuation of lithium therapy, yet 4-gland parathyroid hyperplasia can occur with long-term lithium administration, and hypercalcemia may then persist despite discontinuation of lithium therapy.

PTH-Independent Hypercalcemia

Hypercalcemia of Malignancy

Hypercalcemia of malignancy often develops acutely and may be severe and life-threatening. It is the most common cause of hypercalcemia in hospitalized patients. It results from 1 of 3 mechanisms: 1) the destructive effects of skeletal metastases through local cytokines, 2) the effect of increased production of 1,25-dihydroxyvitamin D by some tumors (eg, lymphomas), or 3) the paraneoplastic effect of a malignancy through increased production of PTH-related peptide. Serum PTH is suppressed in all cases of hypercalcemia due to malignancy.

Vitamin D Intoxication

Hypercalcemia, hypercalciuria, renal insufficiency, and soft tissue calcification can result from prolonged intake of high levels of vitamin D. Because vitamin D is stored in fat, this condition may persist for months after vitamin D supplementation has been discontinued.

Sarcoidosis, Granulomatous Disorders, and Lymphoma

Hypercalcemia and hypercalciuria in sarcoidosis, granulomatous disorders, and lymphoma are due to increased 1α-hydroxylase activity within the cells of the granuloma or lymphoma, which can autonomously generate 1,25-dihydroxyvitamin D (the active form of vitamin D). The serum 25-hydroxyvitamin D level is normal, whereas the 1,25-dihydroxyvitamin D level is increased. The PTH level is low, and the serum phosphorus level may be normal or elevated. The hypercalcemia is responsive to treatment of the underlying disease and glucocorticoid therapy (which inhibits 1α-hydroxylase activity).

Miscellaneous Causes

Hyperthyroidism enhances bone turnover and may lead to net bone loss. Hypercalcemia and, more often, hypercalciuria may be present. The hypercalcemia resolves with the treatment of thyrotoxicosis.

Addison disease can cause symptomatic hypercalcemia related to dehydration and increased albumin concentration. The hypercalcemia is reversible with glucocorticoid therapy.

Management of Hypercalcemia

When feasible, treatment of the primary cause of hypercalcemia is the best intervention. Glucocorticoids are the drugs of choice for the hypercalcemia of granulomatous disorders. Humoral hypercalcemia of malignancy may respond to complete resection of the tumor. In severe hypercalcemia or hypercalcemia in which the primary cause is not immediately treatable, calcium concentrations should be decreased. Aggressive rehydration with volume expansion is necessary because most patients are dehydrated and because it also promotes calciuresis. Loop diuretics (used *after* volume expansion) promote renal calcium excretion. A single-dose, intravenous infusion of pamidronate or zoledronic acid inhibits bone resorption and mobilization of calcium from bone and has a marked, prolonged effect on calcium concentrations. For patients with persistent disease not amenable to surgery, calcimimetic agents (eg, cinacalcet) are an acceptable medical option. Dialysis with a low-calcium dialysate bath is reserved for patients with renal failure or when a rapid decrease in calcium is needed that cannot be achieved by the above methods.

Hypocalcemia

Etiology

The causes of hypocalcemia include hypoparathyroidism, decreased vitamin D production, vitamin D resistance, and disorders associated with decreased mobilization of calcium from bone or increased calcium deposition in tissues.

Hypoparathyroidism may be due to decreased PTH production (the most common cause) or to resistance of the target tissue to the actions of PTH. The parathyroid glands may be damaged during thyroidectomy, or they may be excised completely for the treatment of primary hyperparathyroidism due to parathyroid hyperplasia. Postoperative hypoparathyroidism may be transient or permanent. It appears within hours after the operation and, if transient, can take days to weeks for full recovery. Other causes of decreased PTH secretion are an autoimmune or infiltrative process involving the parathyroid glands (hemochromatosis or Wilson disease), congenital defect (DiGeorge syndrome), or hypomagnesemia (due to diuretic use, malabsorption, or malnutrition), which impairs the secretion and action of PTH.

Pseudohypoparathyroidism is characterized by end-organ (kidney and bone) resistance to the actions of PTH as a result of a receptor or postreceptor defect. In one type, patients have a characteristic appearance: short stature, round face, obesity, short fourth metacarpal bones, and mild mental retardation (Albright hereditary osteodystrophy). A defect in the Gs subunit of the receptor is commonly identified. Patients have hypocalcemia, hyperphosphatemia, and elevated PTH.

Pseudopseudohypoparathyroidism is a variant in which patients have the same characteristic phenotype as patients with Albright hereditary osteodystrophy but do not have the biochemical abnormalities.

Vitamin D deficiency may be caused by malnutrition, malabsorption, and liver or kidney disease. In acute or chronic renal failure, the pathogenesis of hypocalcemia is thought to be multifactorial, resulting from hyperphosphatemia and decreased 1,25-dihydroxyvitamin D production. In vitamin D deficiency, hypocalcemia triggers secondary hyperparathyroidism with renal phosphate wasting.

Increased tissue deposition occurs in *osteoblastic metastases* (eg, prostate cancer) and in the *hungry bone syndrome* occurring after parathyroidectomy for hyperparathyroidism with severe bone disease. Hypocalcemia and soft tissue calcification may also occur in *acute pancreatitis*. Increased calcium elimination is associated with the use of *loop diuretics*. An inability to maintain a normal serum calcium level can also occur after the administration of potent antiresorptive drugs, particularly in patients with preexisting vitamin D deficiency.

Laboratory and Clinical Features

Hypoparathyroidism leads to decreased mobilization of calcium from bone, decreased renal calcium reabsorption, decreased renal phosphate excretion, and decreased renal production of 1,25-dihydroxyvitamin D with subsequent hypocalcemia and hyperphosphatemia. In hypoparathyroidism, the PTH level is low or inappropriately normal in the presence of hypocalcemia. In contrast, the PTH level is increased in pseudohypoparathyroidism.

Hypocalcemia is often manifested by tingling in the fingers, perioral numbness, muscle cramping, or a positive Chvostek sign (facial nerve hyperirritability) or Trousseau sign (characteristic hand posture after blood pressure cuff inflation due to nerve hyperirritability and muscle spasm). Symptoms of hypocalcemia reflect its severity and rate of development. Laryngeal stridor and convulsions can occur when hypocalcemia is severe. Basal ganglia calcification, cataract formation, and benign intracranial hypertension can result from chronic hypoparathyroidism. QT-interval prolongation may be present. Mucocutaneous candidiasis may develop as a manifestation of polyglandular autoimmune syndrome type I (hypoparathyroidism, adrenal insufficiency, and mucocutaneous candidiasis).

Diagnostic Approach

Correct assessment of calcium requires a mathematical correction of the total calcium value based on serum albumin level or the measurement of ionized calcium. This assessment should be followed by measurement of the serum PTH level. In a hypocalcemic patient, a low PTH level is diagnostic of hypoparathyroidism. A high PTH level suggests vitamin D deficiency or pseudohypoparathyroidism. Serum concentrations of creatinine and magnesium help identify renal failure and magnesium deficiency states.

Therapy

For acute, severe hypocalcemia, urgent treatment with intravenous calcium is indicated to prevent tetany, laryngeal stridor, or convulsions. Extravasation of calcium can cause severe tissue necrosis, so administration through central intravenous access (*not* peripheral) is urged. Intravenous calcium should be infused slowly over 5 to 10 minutes. Continuous electrocardiographic monitoring is essential. For long-term treatment of hypocalcemia, oral calcium supplements (2.0–3.0 g daily) and vitamin D are given. In hypoparathyroidism and renal insufficiency, the PTH-mediated conversion of 25-hydroxyvitamin D to 1,25-dihydroxyvitamin D does not occur. Therefore, the preferred form of vitamin D therapy is calcitriol (the active form of vitamin D). Thiazide diuretics are used to decrease the risk of marked hypercalciuria, and oral phosphate binders may be given to control hyperphosphatemia. It is critical to monitor therapy closely since patients are at risk for hypercalciuria, nephrolithiasis, and nephrocalcinosis. Therapeutic doses are adjusted to keep the serum level of calcium *just below* the lower limit of the reference range and the urinary level of calcium at less than 300 mg in 24 hours.

KEY FACTS

✓ Thiazide diuretics—a cause of mild hypercalcemia with inappropriately normal or mildly increased PTH levels; usually resolves within weeks after stopping the drug

✓ Hypercalcemia of malignancy—most common cause of hypercalcemia in hospitalized patients; often acute and may be severe and life-threatening; serum PTH is suppressed

✓ Treatment of severe, symptomatic hypocalcemia requires intravenous calcium through a central line

---

Osteoporosis

Osteoporosis is the most common skeletal disorder encountered in clinical practice. It is characterized by decreased bone mass, leading to bone fragility and increased risk of fracture. Bone density can be quantified with dual energy x-ray absorptiometry (DEXA). **Osteopenia** is defined as bone mass that is between 1.0 and 2.5 SDs below the mean peak bone mass of a sex-matched control population and is designated by a T score between –1.0 and –2.5. **Osteoporosis** is defined as bone mass of at least 2.5 SDs below the mean peak bone mass of a sex-matched control population and is designated by a T score of –2.5 or less (eg, –3.0 or –4.0).

Key Definitions

Osteopenia: *bone mass between 1.0 and 2.5 SDs below mean peak bone mass of a sex-matched control population; T score between –1.0 and –2.5.*

Osteoporosis: *bone mass ≥2.5 SDs below mean peak bone mass of a sex-matched control population; T score ≤ –2.5.*

Etiology

Osteoporosis may be primary or secondary. Primary osteoporosis (postmenopausal osteoporosis and senile osteoporosis, which occurs in older men and women) is more common. Secondary osteoporosis may result from endocrine, nutritional, intestinal, neoplastic, or genetic disorders or from certain drugs and immobilization (Box 12.2).

Box 12.2 • Causes of Secondary Osteoporosis

Endocrine: hypogonadism, hyperparathyroidism, hyperthyroidism, hypercortisolism

Nutritional and intestinal: calcium deficiency, protein malnutrition, alcoholism, malabsorption, current smoking, primary biliary cirrhosis

Neoplastic disorders: multiple myeloma, leukemia, lymphoma, systemic mastocytosis

Genetic disorders: osteogenesis imperfecta

Culprit drugs: corticosteroids, heparin, anticonvulsants, gonadotropin-releasing hormone analogues (suppress sex steroid production), aromatase inhibitors

---

Clinical Features

Fractures can occur with minor trauma. Osteoporotic fractures heal normally. Vertebral fractures lead to loss of height and spinal deformity. Serum levels of calcium, phosphate, and alkaline phosphatase are normal (with the exception of acute fracture changes).

Diagnosis

The diagnosis of osteoporosis is based on the finding of low bone mass by DEXA (T score ≤ –2.5) or the presence of insufficiency fractures. Other causes of low bone mass, such as osteomalacia, multiple myeloma, and metastatic disease, must be excluded. Osteomalacia may coexist with osteoporosis. Myeloma and metastatic disease should be excluded as causes of pathologic fracture.

Secondary causes of osteoporosis should be excluded. Evaluation should include serum levels of calcium, 25-hydroxyvitamin D, testosterone (free, bioavailable, and total) for males, and thyrotropin. The medication list should be thoroughly reviewed for possible culprit drugs (eg, glucocorticoids), and there should be a low threshold for ruling out endogenous Cushing syndrome and multiple myeloma. DEXA should be used as a screening study for patients at risk for osteoporosis (eg, women 65 years or older, younger women or men with risk factors for osteoporosis or osteoporotic fracture, and men with a fragility fracture). Routine screening in other populations (eg, men older than 70 years) is currently debated.

Prevention and Treatment

Bone loss can be prevented through adequate lifestyle activities, including regular weight-bearing exercise, tobacco avoidance, and avoidance of excessive alcohol use. All adults should consume an adequate amount of vitamin D (400–800 international units) and calcium (1,000–1,200 mg) daily. Estrogen replacement in women at or after menopause is effective, but it is not indicated for this purpose (there are more effective options for therapy) and, if used, must be balanced against its known risks.

Pharmacotherapy should be recommended to patients with a history of fragility fracture or with osteoporosis based on a T score of −2.5 or less. For the decision on whether to initiate pharmacotherapy for patients with osteopenia, one should consider the use of FRAX, a tool developed by the World Health Organization to quantify the fracture risk for individual patients. It is derived from studies of population-based cohorts in different parts of the world, thus allowing a more individualized assessment. It includes the known risk factors in a weighted formula and generates a number that represents the probability (a percentage) of a fragility fracture occurring in the next 10 years. Pharmacotherapy is recommended for patients with osteopenia who have a probability of 20% or more for any major osteoporotic fracture or a probability of 3% or more for a hip fracture.

Therapy requires adequate calcium and vitamin D supplementation, similar to preventive approaches. Bisphosphonates are considered first-line therapy for osteoporosis. Alendronate, risedronate, and ibandronate are oral bisphosphonates with potent antiresorptive effects that prevent bone loss. They reduce fracture risk and are effective in preventing steroid-induced bone loss. Side effects include dyspeptic symptoms and esophagitis, particularly if the medication is taken incorrectly. Ibandronate and zoledronic acid are intravenous bisphosphonates approved for treatment of osteoporosis when oral forms are not tolerated or cannot be administered. Osteonecrosis of the jaw is a rare complication of bisphosphonate therapy; the risk is significantly higher among patients given frequent intravenous bisphosphonates while being treated for a malignancy. Bisphosphonates should not be given to patients who have creatinine clearances of less than 30 to 35 mL/min because of the risk of renal osteodystrophy.

Estrogen replacement is effective for treating osteoporosis in postmenopausal women, yet this approach is not indicated as primary therapy because other therapies are more effective and because estrogen therapy has known risks (breast cancer, venous thrombosis, and cardiovascular disease). Raloxifene is a selective estrogen receptor modulator (SERM) effective in the prevention of both osteoporosis and breast cancer. It is less effective than bisphosphonates and estrogens with regard to bone benefits, and it increases the risk of thrombotic events. Denosumab is a monoclonal antibody and another potent antiresorptive agent that blocks the action of RANK ligand (RANKL), thus reducing osteoclastogenesis. It is administered intravenously every 6 months, and it can be used in patients with renal insufficiency. Recombinant PTH (teriparatide) is a potent enhancer of bone formation by increasing bone turnover. Patients who have increased bone turnover (eg, Paget disease) or an increased risk of osteosarcoma (eg, prior radiotherapy to bone) are not candidates for this therapy. It is administered as a daily subcutaneous injection for a maximum of 2 years. Nasal calcitonin is a weak antiresorptive agent with some analgesic properties. The best assessment

of therapeutic efficacy is clinical, yet further decrease in bone mineral density should prompt a reevaluation of the treatment plan.

Osteomalacia

Definition and Etiology

Osteomalacia is characterized by inadequate mineralization of newly formed bone. Normal bone mineralization requires adequate calcium and phosphate concentrations, functional osteoblasts, and optimal conditions for the mineralization of mature osteoid. Osteomalacia ensues when these conditions are not met. Vitamin D deficiency is the most common cause of osteomalacia. It results from inadequate oral intake, malabsorption (celiac disease), limited sun exposure, or decreased liver production of 25-hydroxyvitamin D (due to liver disease or drug side effect). Renal disease and inherited disorders affecting activation or action of vitamin D can also cause osteomalacia. Phosphate deficiency may result from malnutrition or increased renal losses. This is seen in inherited conditions such as hypophosphatemic rickets. An acquired tubular phosphate leak can occur with some mesenchymal tumors (oncogenic osteomalacia) or with multiple myeloma (generalized tubular defect in renal Fanconi syndrome).

> **Key Definition**
>
> Osteomalacia: *inadequate mineralization of newly formed bone.*

Clinical Features

Typical symptoms of osteomalacia include diffuse bone pain and tenderness along with muscle weakness. Calcium levels (serum and urinary) and serum phosphorus levels are low or low-normal, and the serum bone alkaline phosphatase level is usually increased. With vitamin D deficiency, secondary hyperparathyroidism also occurs. Radiographs can display fractures or pseudofractures in later stages of osteomalacia (Figure 12.1). Pseudofractures appear as narrow lines of radiolucency perpendicular to the cortical bone surface; they are typically bilateral and symmetrical. They are found most commonly in the pubic rami and the medial aspect of the femur near the femoral head.

Therapy

Effective therapy requires treating the underlying disorder and providing adequate calcium and phosphate to the areas of inadequate mineralization. This usually is achieved with calcium, vitamin D, and, when indicated, phosphate supplementation. Vitamin D dosing regimens

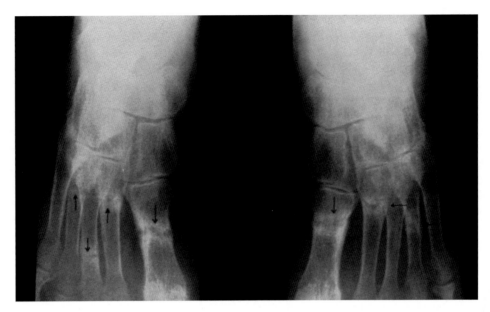

Figure 12.1 *Osteomalacia. Plain radiograph of metatarsal pseudofractures in a patient with osteomalacia shows bilateral, symmetrical, radiolucent lines (arrows) perpendicular to the bone cortex. In general, they are thought to represent either stress fractures repaired with inadequately mineralized osteoid or bone erosions generated by nearby arterial pulsations.*
(Courtesy of Bart L. Clarke, MD, Mayo Clinic, Rochester, Minnesota. Used with permission.)

vary, but a common approach is 50,000 international units weekly for 8 weeks followed by 800 international units daily for maintenance. Osteomalacia is considered adequately treated when urinary calcium excretion and bone density start to increase. The goal of therapy is to achieve bone healing while normalizing the serum concentrations of calcium, phosphate, vitamin D, and alkaline phosphatase. The alkaline phosphatase level can remain elevated for several months after correction of vitamin D deficiency. During therapy, serum and urinary calcium levels should be monitored closely to avoid hypercalcemia, hypercalciuria, and nephrocalcinosis.

Paget Disease

Paget disease affects 3% of the population older than 45 years and is characterized by increased bone resorption with disorganized bone remodeling. Its pathogenesis is not fully understood.

Clinical Features

Most patients are asymptomatic and present with increased serum levels of alkaline phosphatase or a radiographic abnormality. Serum alkaline phosphatase is the most useful marker of disease activity and response to therapy. The main clinical features are bone pain and deformity. Disorganized bone remodeling results in decreased tensile strength, skeletal pain, and bone deformities. Pain may also be related to fracture, degenerative changes in adjoining joints, or, rarely, the development of osteosarcoma. Commonly affected sites include the sacrum, spine, femur, tibia, skull, and pelvis. Other complications include nerve entrapment, hydrocephalus due to the development of platybasia, osteosarcoma, and high-output cardiac failure due to increased vascularity of affected bones.

Diagnosis

Paget disease should be suspected if the serum alkaline phosphatase level is increased and the serum calcium, phosphate, and 25-hydroxyvitamin D levels are normal. A bone scan is the most sensitive test for identifying bone lesions of Paget disease. Plain radiographs (Figure 12.2) are best for further definition of the affected bones (expansion, sclerosis, and deformity) and surrounding joints.

Therapy

Many patients require only monitoring of alkaline phosphatase levels. The decision to initiate therapy relates to the presence of symptoms, the location of the bone lesions, and the disease activity. Indications for therapy are

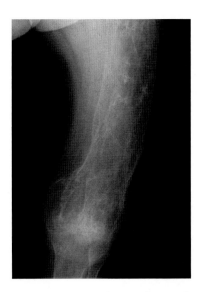

Figure 12.2 Paget Disease. *Plain radiograph of bone involved by Paget disease shows a mixture of sclerotic and lytic lesions with distortion and overgrowth of the involved bone.*
(Courtesy of Bart L. Clarke, MD, Mayo Clinic, Rochester, Minnesota. Used with permission.)

bone pain, disease involving bones where complications could occur (skull, spine, weight-bearing bone, or bones near joints), or a significant increase in the serum alkaline phosphatase level. Medical therapy consists of bisphosphonates, most commonly intravenous zoledronic acid. Alkaline phosphatase levels are used to monitor therapy. Orthopedic surgery is rarely needed to treat deformity, fracture, or degenerative joint disease. Neurosurgical intervention may be required for nerve entrapment syndromes.

KEY FACTS

✓ Pharmacotherapy for osteopenia is recommended according to patient's fracture probability: ≥20% probability for any major osteoporotic fracture or ≥3% probability for a hip fracture

✓ First-line therapy for osteoporosis—bisphosphonates

✓ Most common cause of osteomalacia—nutritional vitamin D deficiency

✓ Paget disease—elevated serum bone alkaline phosphatase with normal serum calcium and vitamin D levels

13 Diabetes Mellitus

EKTA KAPOOR, MBBS

Etiology and Classification

Diabetes mellitus, characterized by increased levels of plasma glucose (fasting or postprandial or both), is the most common metabolic disorder, affecting approximately 10% of the US population. Type 1 diabetes mellitus (T1D), previously known as insulin-dependent diabetes mellitus, is caused by autoimmune destruction of insulin-producing beta cells of the pancreatic islets, resulting in an absolute insulin deficiency. About 10% of diabetic patients have T1D. It usually occurs in children or lean young adults, but T1D can develop at any age. The onset is usually abrupt and dramatic, with symptoms of marked hyperglycemia (polyuria, polydipsia, fatigue, weight loss, and dehydration) or diabetic ketoacidosis (in patients with more severe insulin deficiency).

A complex interaction between genes and the environment leads to the development of T1D. Autoantibodies to islet cells or their products (anti–glutamic acid decarboxylase 65 and anti-insulin antibodies) are frequently present, and they may help to differentiate T1D from the more common type 2 diabetes mellitus (T2D). A "honeymoon" period, marked by restoration of euglycemia, may occur soon after disease onset. However, the duration of this phase is highly variable, and all patients eventually require insulin. Oral agents are not useful in the management of T1D.

T2D, previously known as non–insulin-dependent diabetes mellitus, is characterized by beta cell dysfunction (resulting in impaired insulin secretion) and insulin resistance in target tissues (liver, muscle, and adipose). Genetic factors are thought to be more important in the development of T2D compared to T1D. Patients with T2D are typically older and are nearly always overweight or obese. The cases of childhood T2D, however, are increasing with the obesity epidemic in children. Excess body fat, particularly when concentrated intra-abdominally, leads to insulin resistance, which is the hallmark of T2D. Patients with T2D have high insulin levels in the initial stages of their disease as the pancreas tries to compensate for the insulin resistance. Eventually, however, the beta cells start failing, leading to relative insulin deficiency and hyperglycemia. Even with that, patients with T2D do not have the absolute insulin deficiency that occurs in patients with T1D; therefore, diabetic ketoacidosis is rare in patients with T2D.

Secondary causes of diabetes include pancreatic disease (pancreatitis, cystic fibrosis, and hemochromatosis); endocrinopathies (Cushing syndrome, pheochromocytoma, and acromegaly); drugs (corticosteroids) or chemicals; and infections. Certain genetic syndromes are sometimes associated with diabetes (Down syndrome, Klinefelter syndrome, Turner syndrome, and Prader-Willi syndrome).

Gestational diabetes mellitus is diabetes that develops in pregnancy. The hormonal changes during pregnancy induce a state of insulin resistance, which can lead to hyperglycemia in susceptible women (ie, overweight or obese women with a family history of T2D). Therapy may involve dietary modification, oral medications, or insulin. Gestational diabetes mellitus may or may not persist after pregnancy, but it portends an increased risk of subsequent development of T2D.

Clinical Features

The onset of T1D is usually rapid, with weight loss, polyuria, and polydipsia due to an abrupt, severe insulin deficiency. The manifestation is often precipitated by an infection or another severe physical stress. Dehydration and ketoacidosis may occur.

T2D usually has a more insidious onset than T1D and is often diagnosed during routine laboratory testing that identifies glucosuria or hyperglycemia. Patients may report blurry vision, nearsightedness, recurrent skin infections, or candidal vaginitis (females) or balanitis (males). Patients sometimes present with chronic diabetic complications (eg, neuropathy, nephropathy, retinopathy, or vascular disease)

157

without symptoms of hyperglycemia. Polyuria, polydipsia, and polyphagia may develop only at times of increased insulin resistance (eg, pregnancy, infection, or corticosteroid use). Patients occasionally present with hyperosmolar nonketotic coma.

KEY FACTS

✓ Cause of T1D—
- autoimmune destruction of insulin-producing beta cells of the pancreatic islets, resulting in an absolute deficiency of insulin
- autoantibodies to islet cells or their products are frequently present

✓ Development of T2D—
- genetic factors are more important than in T1D
- patients are usually older than patients with T1D
- patients are nearly always overweight or obese

✓ Onset of T1D—usually rapid, with weight loss, polyuria, and polydipsia due to an abrupt, severe insulin deficiency

✓ Onset of T2D—
- more insidious than onset of T1D
- often diagnosed during routine laboratory testing that identifies glucosuria or hyperglycemia

---

Diagnosis

The normal fasting plasma glucose concentration is less than 100 mg/dL. Impaired fasting glucose, or **prediabetes**, is defined by fasting glucose values from 100 to 125 mg/dL. A glucose tolerance test is not required for the diagnosis. Diabetes mellitus is diagnosed with elevated levels of plasma glucose or hemoglobin A_{1c} (Box 13.1).

Key Definition

Prediabetes: *fasting glucose values of 100–125 mg/dL.*

The diagnosis of gestational diabetes mellitus requires an oral glucose tolerance test (see the Diabetes and Pregnancy section).

Therapy for T1D

Insulin replacement is necessary for treatment of T1D; oral agents are not useful in its management. Therapy is aimed at preventing acute and chronic complications of diabetes while allowing the patient to maintain a healthy and active lifestyle with optimal glycemic control and minimal

---

Box 13.1 • Diagnosis of Diabetes Mellitus

Diabetes mellitus is diagnosed if 1 of the following is met:

Fasting plasma glucose ≥126 mg/dL documented on ≥2 occasions

Casual plasma glucose ≥200 mg/dL in the presence of classic symptoms of hyperglycemia

Plasma glucose ≥200 mg/dL 2 h after a 75-g oral glucose load

Hemoglobin A_{1c} ≥6.5% documented on 2 occasions (values of 5.7%–6.4% are consistent with impaired glycemia)

---

hypoglycemia. Intensive insulin therapy requires considerable commitment from the patient to self-monitor plasma glucose concentrations and adjust the insulin dosage accordingly. Intensive therapy with tight glycemic control prevents or markedly decreases the risks of chronic microvascular complications of diabetes and reduces mortality.

An amylin analogue (pramlintide) can be used to manage both T1D and insulin-requiring T2D. Amylin is a peptide that is cosecreted with insulin by beta cells. Like insulin, it is deficient in patients with T1D and relatively so in patients with T2D. Amylin has several mechanisms for lowering glucose levels, including delayed gastric emptying, suppression of postprandial glucagon secretion, and decreased appetite. Its effect in lowering blood glucose is complementary to that of insulin. Pramlintide is injected before meals of at least 250 kcal, and it is always used as an adjunct to insulin therapy. It shows modest efficacy at improving glycemic control (decreasing hemoglobin A_{1c} <1%), with nausea being the most common side effect. Mealtime insulin doses should be decreased by 50% when pramlintide therapy is initiated. Pramlintide therapy does not cause weight gain, and it may even lead to some weight loss.

Nutrition

Intake should allow for maintenance of a healthy weight, with 10% to 20% of the total calories from protein, less than 30% of the calories from fat (saturated fat <10%), and the remainder from complex carbohydrates. Insulin doses for meals depend on the carbohydrate content of the meal. Patients are advised to maintain a consistent intake of carbohydrates or adjust the insulin dose according to carbohydrate intake at each meal (ie, "carbohydrate counting").

Exercise

The glycemic response to exercise depends on the glucose level before exercise, the duration and type of exercise, the patient's physical fitness, the relation of exercise to meals and insulin injections. Glucose levels should be monitored before and after exercise. If strenuous exercise is initiated while the patient is hyperglycemic, the serum glucose concentration may increase further. Patients should always carry appropriate identification and have access to glucose or sugar.

Insulin Therapy

Intensive insulin therapy mimics insulin secretion by the healthy pancreas. Short-acting insulin (regular, lispro, aspart, or glulisine insulin) is injected at mealtimes, and a once- or twice-daily long-acting insulin (glargine or detemir insulin) provides basal insulin.

An insulin pump provides programmable continuous subcutaneous insulin infusion and meal-stimulated insulin secretion. It allows the patient to adjust the infusion rate of basal insulin (during exercise or at night).

The insulin dosage required for a typical patient with T1D (within 20% of ideal body weight and without intercurrent illness) is approximately 0.5 to 1.0 U/kg daily. Insulin requirements may increase markedly during illness.

Glycemic goals are individualized according to the presence of other disease (ischemic heart disease or cerebrovascular disease), diabetic complications, and the ability to perceive hypoglycemia. For women with T1D who are considering pregnancy, tight glucose control starting weeks to months before pregnancy is critical to decrease the risk of birth defects. Tight glycemic control during pregnancy prevents macrosomia.

Glycemic Goals of Optimal Therapy

The target preprandial plasma glucose level is 90 to 130 mg/dL. Hemoglobin A_{1c} should be less than 7.0%. Higher target levels are recommended for children, adolescents, older patients with comorbidities and limited life expectancy, and patients at risk of hypoglycemia who have a limited ability to recognize it.

Monitoring

Glucose concentration should be self-monitored 4 times daily—before meals and at bedtime. If the patient has unexplained morning hypoglycemia or hyperglycemia, blood glucose should be measured between 2 am and 4 am. Hemoglobin A_{1c} should be measured every 3 months.

Therapy for T2D

Most patients with T2D are obese, have a sedentary lifestyle, and often have multiple cardiovascular risk factors, such as hypertension and dyslipidemia. Therapy should include modification of risk factors (including exercise, weight loss, and improved nutrition) and achievement of appropriate glycemic control with a near-normal hemoglobin A_{1c} in the absence of hypoglycemia.

A goal of losing 5% to 10% of initial body weight is recommended for patients with body mass index (BMI) values greater than 25 (calculated as weight in kilograms divided by height in meters squared). Exercise improves insulin action, facilitates weight loss, increases a sense of well-being, and reduces cardiovascular risks (increases high-density lipoprotein cholesterol [HDL-C] and decreases very low-density lipoprotein [VLDL] and triglycerides). Exercise recommendations should be modified appropriately for patients with preexisting coronary or peripheral vascular disease.

Drug Therapy for T2D

Metformin

Metformin is the first-line agent for managing T2D. Unless a contraindication for its use exists, all patients receiving pharmacotherapy for T2D should receive metformin. Its most important action is suppression of hepatic glucose production. It also enhances the sensitivity of peripheral tissues (muscle and adipose) to insulin. Metformin is effective as monotherapy and in combination therapy with other glucose-lowering drugs. It lowers hemoglobin A_{1c} by 1% to 2%. The main side effect is diarrhea, but that can be minimized by taking it with meals. Patients taking metformin do not usually gain weight and may even lose some weight. Metformin may improve lipid levels, lowering adverse vascular outcomes and reducing mortality. The drug may lead to vitamin B_{12} deficiency due to decreased absorption. It should generally be held when patients are hospitalized. The risk of lactic acidosis is a concern, but the condition is extremely rare. Nevertheless, given the high fatality rate of patients with lactic acidosis, metformin is contraindicated in several situations, including renal impairment, decompensated heart failure, severe infection, and liver disease (Box 13.2).

Box 13.2 • Contraindications for Metformin

The following situations may increase the risk of lactic acidosis:

Renal impairment (creatinine ≥1.5 mg/dL for men and ≥1.4 mg/dL for women)

Cardiac disease (decompensated heart failure) or respiratory disease likely to cause central hypoxia or reduced peripheral perfusion

History of lactic acidosis

Severe infection that could lead to reduced tissue perfusion

Liver disease

Alcohol abuse with binge drinking

Use of intravenous radiographic contrast agents

Sulfonylureas

Sulfonylureas (eg, glyburide, glipizide, and glimepiride) are insulin secretagogues. Their efficacy depends on the presence of adequate beta cell function and endogenous insulin secretion. Secondary failure occurs with progression of disease and loss of beta cell function, when sulfonylureas become ineffective. They lower hemoglobin A_{1c} by 1% to 2%. Despite the advantage of low cost, sulfonylureas have fallen out of favor because of the risk of hypoglycemia, weight gain, and perhaps increased cardiovascular risk. They should be used with caution in patients who have advanced hepatic or renal disease. The risk of hypoglycemia from sulfonylureas increases with longer-acting sulfonylureas (eg, glyburide) and in patients with renal failure.

Meglitinides

Meglitinides (eg, repaglinide and nateglinide) also stimulate insulin release like sulfonylureas. They have extremely short half-lives and are taken before each meal to target postprandial glycemic excursions. Concerns with their use include hypoglycemia, their relatively higher cost, and weight gain.

Thiazolidinediones

Thiazolidinediones (TZDs) (eg, rosiglitazone and pioglitazone) enhance peripheral insulin sensitivity by activating peroxisome proliferator-activated receptor (PPAR)-γ. They do not cause hypoglycemia, and they lower hemoglobin A_{1c} by 1% to 2%. Pioglitazone causes marked fluid retention, increasing the risk of heart failure, and should not be prescribed for patients who have congestive heart failure. Pioglitazone has not been associated with other cardiovascular risks. Significant weight gain and osteoporosis have been reported with TZD use.

α-Glucosidase Inhibitors

α-Glucosidase inhibitors (eg, acarbose and miglitol) inhibit upper intestinal glucosidases, limiting the conversion of complex carbohydrates to monosaccharides. Modest efficacy (lowering hemoglobin A_{1c} by <1%) and significant gastrointestinal tract adverse effects (flatulence in 70% of users) limit their clinical use. Glucose is necessary to treat hypoglycemia in patients taking an α-glucosidase inhibitor.

Glucagon-Like Peptide-1 Analogues

Glucagon-like peptide-1 (GLP1) analogues (eg, exenatide and liraglutide) augment insulin secretion and glucagon suppression in response to glucose. They also slow gastric emptying, reduce appetite, and lead to moderate weight loss. They are approved for use with metformin and sulfonylureas. Nausea and vomiting occur in a substantial proportion of users early in therapy but often subside. Used in combination with sulfonylurea, these agents can lead to hypoglycemia. Although all the newer agents seem to be effective in improving the level of hemoglobin A_{1c}, the effect on clinical outcomes (vascular disease and microvascular complications) is unknown.

Dipeptidyl-peptidase-4 Inhibitors

Dipeptidyl-peptidase-4 (DPP4) inhibitors (eg, sitagliptin and saxagliptin) potentiate the effect of GLP1 by inhibiting its degradation by DPP4. Glucose lowering occurs by enhancing GLP1-mediated insulin secretion. DPP4 inhibitors do not have a strong effect on gastric emptying or food intake and do not affect the patient's weight. They are associated with a lower risk of hypoglycemia and are approved for use as monotherapy and combination therapy with sulfonylureas, metformin, and TZDs.

Insulin

Insulin is often reserved for 1) patients with T2D when diet and oral agents (monotherapy and combination therapy) provide inadequate glycemic control, 2) sick patients or patients with advanced hepatic or renal disease when oral agents may be contraindicated, 3) patients who require rapid glycemic control, and 4) patients who are pregnant, under perioperative care, or severely ill. Patients with T2D often have some degree of meal-stimulated endogenous

---

KEY FACTS

✓ Therapy for T1D—
- amylin analogue (pramlintide) can be used to manage both T1D and insulin-requiring T2D
- insulin dosage for a typical patient (within 20% of ideal body weight and without intercurrent illness): 0.5–1.0 U/kg daily
- target preprandial plasma glucose level: 90–130 mg/dL
- target hemoglobin A_{1c}: <7.0%

✓ Therapy for T2D—
- metformin: first-line agent for all patients who are receiving pharmacotherapy and who have no contraindications; may lead to vitamin B_{12} deficiency (from decreased absorption)
- sulfonylureas: risk of hypoglycemia, weight gain, and perhaps increased cardiovascular risk
- TZDs: pioglitazone should not be prescribed for patients who have congestive heart failure (causes marked fluid retention)
- α-Glucosidase inhibitors: limited clinical use because of modest efficacy (lowers hemoglobin A_{1c} by <1%) and gastrointestinal tract adverse effects (flatulence)
- GLP1: nausea and vomiting may occur early in therapy but often subside
- insulin: regimens are simpler than for patients with T1D (often patients with T2D have meal-stimulated endogenous insulin secretion)

insulin secretion, which allows treatment with simpler insulin regimens than for T1D. Once-daily injections of intermediate-acting insulin in combination with an oral agent or twice-daily injections of intermediate-acting insulin are commonly used to manage T2D. Insulin therapy is associated with some degree of weight gain in most patients. Insulin can also be given in combination with metformin. Patients who have a more severe insulin deficiency may use an intensive insulin program, as in T1D. Intensive insulin therapy with basal and bolus doses gives more flexibility with meal schedules; the split-mix regimen requires scheduled meals.

An amylin analogue (pramlintide) is also approved for T2D patients receiving insulin therapy (see the Therapy for T1D section).

Hypoglycemia in Diabetes

Hypoglycemia may result from unplanned exercise, inappropriate dosing of insulin, or inadequate carbohydrate intake. Patients with long-standing T1D are prone to hypoglycemia unawareness due to repeated neuroglycopenia. Prevention of hypoglycemia has been shown to reverse or ameliorate hypoglycemia unawareness in some patients. Hypoglycemia can occur at night (*nocturnal hypoglycemia*) and may not be apparent if glucose is checked at bedtime and at breakfast. Patients may report symptoms such as nightmares, morning headache, or night sweats. Periodic monitoring of blood glucose between 1 am and 3 am is essential, especially if the patient is taking intermediate insulin in the evenings. Preventive strategies include increasing the bedtime snack or modifying the insulin regimen.

In patients with long-standing T1D, inability to secrete glucagon leads to defective counterregulation, and patients become dependent on the autonomic nervous system to respond to hypoglycemia. The use of β-blockers in these situations can abolish the warning palpitations that are caused by hypoglycemia.

Lower doses of insulin may be needed in patients with renal impairment. Alcohol may interfere with gluconeogenesis and the perception of hypoglycemic symptoms. Hypoglycemia may also be a manifestation of cortisol deficiency (eg, Addison disease or autoimmune hypophysitis).

Acute Complications of Diabetes Mellitus

Diabetic Ketoacidosis

Diabetic ketoacidosis (DKA) may be the initial presentation for patients with T1D. Rarely, DKA occurs in patients who have T2D and a major intercurrent illness, including infection, myocardial infarction, or other major stresses.

DKA results from a profound insulin deficiency and an excess of counterregulatory hormones such as glucagon. Thus, it may be caused by a failure to take insulin or to increase the insulin dose when the need is increased in times of physiologic stress. The major manifestations of DKA are the direct result of severe insulin deficiency: hyperglycemia, ketosis (due to unrestrained lipolysis and conversion of fatty acids to ketone bodies), and severe dehydration (due to osmotic diuresis). The ketoacids cause an anion gap metabolic acidosis. Patients with DKA may be severely volume contracted.

Patients usually present with polyuria, polydipsia, poor appetite, nausea and vomiting, abdominal pain, tachypnea, mental obtundation, and coma. Physical findings include evidence of dehydration, decreased mentation, deep and rapid Kussmaul respiration, and a characteristic breath odor (fruity odor of acetone).

The diagnosis is based on the presence of moderate to severe hyperglycemia (plasma glucose >250 mg/dL), ketonemia, and anion gap metabolic acidosis. Associated biochemical abnormalities include hyponatremia, azotemia, and hyperamylasemia. Large body losses of electrolytes occur, but serum levels of potassium, phosphate, and magnesium are often within the reference range or even elevated. Their concentrations often decrease precipitously as the acidosis is corrected.

Treatment

Treatment of DKA requires administration of fluids and insulin to correct the metabolic acidosis and dehydration. Electrolyte levels should be carefully monitored and corrected, and precipitating factors ameliorated. The average fluid deficit in adults is 5 to 8 L. The risk of cerebral edema is decreased through careful rehydration and correction of ketoacidosis, thereby avoiding a rapid decrease in serum osmolality.

Insulin infusion doses should be modified according to the degree of glycemia, and they should be continued until the ketonemia and acidosis resolve. The preferred initial fluid is 0.9% saline because it can expand intravascular volume. However, when plasma volume is restored, the fluids can be changed to 0.45% saline with 5% dextrose, which also provides dextrose and prevents hypoglycemia that may result from continued use of an insulin infusion to manage the ketonemia and acidosis.

The potassium deficit is typically 300 to 500 mmol, reflecting low total body stores. Serum potassium levels decrease with correction of the acidosis. Potassium should be added to the intravenous fluids as soon as renal perfusion and urine flow are ensured. Phosphate repletion is indicated at phosphate levels less than 1 mg/dL. The serum level of phosphate must be monitored carefully owing to the risk of hypocalcemia, seizures, and death with hypophosphatemia.

DKA is a life-threatening condition. Most deaths result from cerebral edema, which carries a mortality rate of over

20%. Other complications of DKA include myocardial infarction, acute respiratory distress syndrome, stroke, deep vein thrombosis and pulmonary embolism, and arrhythmias. After successful therapy, the goal is to avoid recurrence by educating the patient.

Hyperglycemic Hyperosmolar Nonketotic Coma

Hyperglycemic hyperosmolar nonketotic coma is characterized by hyperglycemia (more profound than the hyperglycemia in DKA) and hyperosmolar dehydration *without* ketoacidosis. This typically occurs in poorly treated T2D when insulin levels are sufficient to inhibit excess lipolysis and ketogenesis but not to suppress hyperglycemia. High concentrations of urinary glucose provoke an osmotic diuresis, resulting in marked dehydration and decreased renal function. It is commonly precipitated by an acute illness, such as myocardial infarction, pancreatitis, infection, or surgery.

Diagnosis

Hyperglycemic hyperosmolar nonketotic coma should be suspected in any patient with diabetes who presents with an altered level of consciousness and severe dehydration. Laboratory abnormalities include hyperglycemia (blood glucose often >600 mg/dL), absence of ketones, and plasma hyperosmolality (>320 mOsm/kg).

Therapy

The objectives of treatment are to restore volume and osmolarity, and to control the hyperglycemia. Total fluid loss is often larger in hyperglycemic hyperosmolar nonketotic coma than in DKA. Fluid resuscitation and insulin infusion are necessary but must be done with caution. Renal failure can complicate electrolyte replacement. Repeated neurologic evaluation is essential because focal deficits or seizures may become apparent during therapy. Always correct the underlying disorder.

Complications include vascular events such as myocardial infarction or stroke, cerebral edema, and hypokalemia. The mortality rate can be up to 50%.

Chronic Complications of Diabetes Mellitus

Microvascular Disease in Diabetes

The microcirculation is damaged by chronic hyperglycemia and other metabolic abnormalities associated with diabetes. Clinical manifestations include retinopathy, nephropathy, and neuropathy. Diabetic retinopathy occurs in most patients with T1D within 10 years after diagnosis. Diabetic retinopathy is present in 15% to 20% of patients when T2D is diagnosed and in 50% of patients by 15 years after the diagnosis. Background diabetic retinopathy is characterized by microaneurysms, hard exudates,

hemorrhages, and macular edema. Retinal ischemia leads to proliferative retinopathy, stimulating the growth of new vessels that are fragile and prone to hemorrhage; loss of vision may result. Proliferative retinopathy is treated with panretinal laser photocoagulation. Patients should undergo a dilated ophthalmic examination annually. Treatment of hypertension, hyperglycemia, glaucoma, and dyslipidemia is also important.

Infections and Diabetes

Skin infections can be a presenting feature of poorly controlled T2D. They include carbuncles (*Staphylococcus aureus*), malignant external otitis (*Pseudomonas*), and, in DKA, mucormycosis (*Mucor* species). Candidiasis and furunculosis also occur more frequently with poorly controlled diabetes.

Atherosclerotic Vascular Disease in Diabetes

Ischemic cardiovascular disease appears earlier and is more extensive in diabetic patients than in the general population. Coronary heart disease accounts for the majority of deaths among persons with diabetes, and patients may present with sudden cardiac death. Persons with T2D are thought to have the same risk of myocardial infarction as patients who have had a myocardial infarction. Treatment of dyslipidemia is therefore considered secondary prevention in this population. Patients with ischemic heart disease may present with atypical symptoms; angina may manifest as epigastric distress, heartburn, and neck or jaw pain. Myocardial infarction may be silent, and patients may present with sudden onset of left ventricular failure. Patients with diabetes have a higher risk of cerebrovascular and peripheral arterial diseases, but the role of screening for vascular disease in asymptomatic patients with diabetes is uncertain.

Hyperlipidemia in Diabetes

In poorly controlled T2D, the concentrations of triglyceride-rich lipoproteins are increased owing to overproduction of VLDL and decreased lipoprotein lipase activity. HDL-C levels are low, and control of glucose and triglyceride levels leads to levels that are improved but usually not normalized. Compositional changes in low-density lipoprotein (LDL) (small, dense LDL) that increase the atherogenicity of these particles are more likely to occur in patients with T2D. Aggressive management of hyperlipidemia is warranted for diabetic patients because they have a high risk of cardiovascular disease.

Diabetes and Pregnancy

Pregnancy is a diabetogenic state due to the insulin resistance conferred by various placental hormones, including growth hormone, human placental lactogen, progesterone, and corticotropin-releasing hormone. Women with preexisting diabetes may have worsening control during pregnancy. Inadequate glycemic control early in pregnancy increases the risk of congenital malformations; poor control in late pregnancy increases the risk of macrosomia, neonatal hypoglycemia, hypocalcemia, polycythemia, hyperbilirubinemia, and respiratory distress. Pregnancy may exacerbate diabetic retinopathy, and nephropathy may lead to pregnancy-induced hypertension and toxemia.

Gestational diabetes mellitus (GDM) complicates 6% to 7% of all pregnancies, but the rate varies significantly between different ethnic groups. Women at high risk for GDM include obese women, women who belong to a high-risk ethnic group, and women with glycosuria, a personal history of GDM, a previous adverse obstetric outcome, or a family history of T2D. These women should undergo screening for diabetes at the first prenatal visit. Other women should undergo screening at 24 to 28 weeks of gestation. Women of normal weight who are younger than 25 years are excluded from this recommendation because their risk of GDM is low. The screening test is a 50-g oral glucose challenge test. A plasma glucose level of 140 mg/dL or more 1 hour after ingestion of the glucose load is considered a positive result and should prompt formal testing with a 100-g oral glucose tolerance test (OGTT). GDM is diagnosed if 2 or more of the plasma glucose values are abnormal during the OGTT (fasting glucose >105 mg/dL; 1-hour glucose >190 mg/dL; 2-hour glucose >165 mg/dL; or 3-hour glucose >145 mg/dL).

Treatment

Home monitoring for blood glucose and urine ketones is important for women with GDM. Postprandial glucose concentrations are closely associated with macrosomia and neonatal complications, so they are often used to guide therapy. The fasting blood glucose concentration should be 95 mg/dL or less; the 1-hour postprandial level should be 140 mg/dL or less; and the 2-hour postprandial goal is 120 mg/dL or less.

Women with GDM who become euglycemic in the postpartum state remain at high risk for T2D. They should be encouraged to institute lifestyle changes to prevent onset of T2D, and they should be evaluated periodically.

Hypoglycemia in Nondiabetic Patients

Etiology

Hypoglycemic disorders may be classified as *insulin mediated* and *noninsulin mediated*. Causes of insulin-mediated hypoglycemia include insulinoma, sulfonylurea or exogenous insulin use, and autoimmune hypoglycemia mediated by insulin antibodies. These antibodies bind insulin and unpredictably release it from the insulin-antibody complexes, or they bind the insulin receptor and cause hypoglycemia. Noninsulin-mediated hypoglycemia may be related to drugs, alcohol use, or cortisol insufficiency. Renal failure, liver failure, and sepsis are common causes of noninsulin-mediated hypoglycemia in hospitalized patients. Insulinlike growth factor 2 (IGF-2)-producing tumors, such as mesenchymal or epithelial tumors, may also cause hypoglycemia.

Clinical Features

Hypoglycemia may cause hyperadrenergic symptoms (palpitations, sweating, tremor, and nervousness) and neuroglycopenic symptoms (confusion, inappropriate affect, blurred vision, diplopia, seizures, and loss of consciousness). Symptoms are relieved promptly after oral carbohydrate intake.

Diagnosis

The symptoms due to hypoglycemia are rather nonspecific, so their presence alone does not establish hypoglycemia as the cause. The Whipple triad must be present for a diagnosis of hypoglycemia: symptoms of hypoglycemia, presence of low plasma glucose during symptoms (*not* measured with fingerstick glucose testing), and reversal of symptoms with glucose administration.

Insulinoma

Insulinoma is an insulin-secreting islet cell tumor that usually causes fasting hypoglycemia. Diagnostic criteria for insulinoma are plasma insulin level of 3 mcIU/mL or more and C-peptide level of 0.6 ng/mL or more when plasma glucose is less than 50 mg/dL and plasma sulfonylurea is undetectable. A 72-hour fasting protocol is often required to induce hypoglycemia for diagnostic biochemical testing. Ultrasonography (transabdominal and endoscopic), spiral computed tomography, and magnetic resonance imaging of the pancreas are used to identify most insulinomas. When imaging is not conclusive, selective arterial catheterization with calcium stimulation of insulin release can help to differentiate a focal area of insulin overproduction from a diffuse process. The key to successful removal is surgical exploration of the pancreas by an experienced surgeon in combination with intraoperative ultrasonography. Almost all insulinomas can be identified and excised in this manner. Patients with insulinoma who decline surgical excision or who have persistent or recurrent malignant insulinoma may be treated with diazoxide, which inhibits insulin secretion, but side effects (edema and malaise) limit its tolerability.

Key Definition
Insulinoma: *an insulin-secreting islet cell tumor that usually causes fasting hypoglycemia.*

KEY FACTS

✓ DKA—
- rare in patients with T2D
- major manifestations (from severe insulin deficiency): hyperglycemia, ketosis, and severe dehydration
- ketoacids cause an anion gap metabolic acidosis

✓ Treatment of DKA—fluids and insulin to correct metabolic acidosis and dehydration

✓ Hyperglycemic hyperosmolar nonketotic coma—
- hyperglycemia (more profound than in DKA)
- hyperosmolar dehydration *without* ketoacidosis

✓ GDM—
- risk factors for women: obesity, glycosuria, member of a high-risk ethnic group, personal history of GDM or a previous adverse obstetric outcome, or a family history of T2D
- screening for women at high risk: at first prenatal visit
- screening for other women: at 24–28 weeks of gestation

✓ Whipple triad for diagnosis of hypoglycemia—
- symptoms of hypoglycemia
- low plasma glucose during symptoms
- reversal of symptoms with glucose administration

✓ Insulinoma diagnostic criteria—
- plasma insulin level ≥3 mcIU/mL
- C-peptide level ≥0.6 ng/mL when plasma glucose <50 mg/dL and plasma sulfonylurea is undetectable

Postprandial Hypoglycemia

Postprandial symptoms are not always caused by postprandial hypoglycemia. **Postprandial hypoglycemia** is defined as symptomatic hypoglycemia occurring within 4 hours after a meal. Patients with noninsulinoma pancreatogenous hypoglycemia syndrome can have postprandial hypoglycemia.

Key Definition

Postprandial hypoglycemia: *symptomatic hypoglycemia occurring within 4 hours after a meal.*

Therapy

Treatment of hypoglycemia is directed at correcting both the hypoglycemia and the underlying cause. For patients with serious hypoglycemia who cannot eat or drink, 1 mg of glucagon can be administered to stimulate endogenous glucose production. Alternatively, intravenous dextrose can be given, although this may be associated with superficial phlebitis and pain.

14 | Gonadal and Adrenal Disorders

PANKAJ SHAH, MD

Disorders of the Adrenal Glands

Adrenocortical Failure

Etiology

Adrenocortical failure most commonly is due to a decrease in production of 1 or more adrenal hormones. Clinically relevant deficiencies may involve cortisol or aldosterone or a combination of both. Decreased production of adrenocortical hormones may be a consequence of adrenocortical disease (primary failure) or tropic hormone loss (secondary failure).

Primary Adrenocortical Failure (Addison Disease)
Primary adrenocortical failure is usually associated with deficiencies of all adrenal cortical hormones, with clinical manifestations resulting from lack of both aldosterone and cortisol. It may be due to organ-specific autoimmune adrenalitis; granulomatous adrenalitis such as tuberculosis or histoplasmosis; bilateral adrenal hemorrhage with anticoagulant use, trauma, or sepsis (particularly meningococcemia); congenital adrenal enzyme deficiency (starting in childhood); AIDS (rarely); metastatic malignancies; or use of steroidogenesis-blocking drugs such as ketoconazole. In the United States, the most common causes are autoimmune adrenalitis and bilateral adrenal hemorrhage. Adrenal failure associated with infections may be due to the combined effects of adrenalitis and the use of drugs that inhibit steroidogenesis (eg, ketoconazole) or, especially in patients receiving replacement glucocorticoids, the use of drugs that accelerate cortisol clearance (eg, rifampin and phenytoin).

Secondary Adrenocortical Failure
Secondary cortisol deficiency is due to a lack of corticotropin (ACTH). Therefore, it does not affect aldosterone secretion.

Functional central ACTH deficiency, the most common cause of ACTH deficiency, is a consequence of suppression of the axis by the prolonged use of glucocorticoids in pharmacologic doses for nonendocrine purposes. The deficiency becomes clinically manifest after withdrawal of the glucocorticoid therapy.

Structural problems in the hypothalamic-pituitary region may cause ACTH deficiency as an isolated deficiency or, more commonly, in association with other features of hypopituitarism. The deficiency may occur in association with pituitary tumors, hypothalamic or extrasellar disease, surgery or radiotherapy to the hypothalamic-pituitary region, autoimmune hypophysitis, or head injury.

Hypoaldosteronism can occur independently of cortisol deficiency. It may result from a primary disorder of the zona glomerulosa, or it may be secondary to angiotensin II deficiency, which may be a consequence of decreased renal renin release.

Clinical Features

The clinical features of adrenocortical failure depend on the magnitude of the hormone deficiency, whether the failure is partial or complete, whether 1 or all hormones are involved, the rapidity of development of the deficiency, and, when present, changes in the levels of circulating ACTH. The usual manifestation of adrenocortical failure is that of a chronic, slowly evolving disorder (Box 14.1).

Acute Adrenocortical Failure or Adrenal Crisis
Adrenal crisis is suspected in the presence of dehydration, hypotension, or shock out of proportion to the severity of the current illness; nausea and vomiting, with a history of severe anorexia and weight loss; abdominal pain (may mimic acute abdomen); unexplained fever; and hyponatremia, hyperkalemia, azotemia, hypercalcemia, eosinophilia, and hypoglycemia. It often is precipitated by an illness in

---

Box 14.1 • Manifestations of Adrenocortical Failure

Cortisol deficiency: severe malaise, decreased vitality, energy, and stamina; muscle weakness; anorexia, weight loss, nausea, vomiting, or diarrhea (may mimic abdominal malignancy); mood changes; hyponatremia, fasting hypoglycemia, transient hypercalcemia, anemia, lymphocytosis, and eosinophilia

Aldosterone deficiency: hypovolemia, orthostatic hypotension, hyperkalemia, hyperchloremic acidosis, and azotemia

Androgen deficiency: not significant in males; associated with decreased libido and thinning of sexual hair in females

ACTH-related symptoms: ACTH excess in Addison disease is associated with hyperpigmentation and easy tanning; ACTH deficiency in secondary adrenocortical failure is associated with pallor and the inability to tan

Abbreviation: ACTH, corticotropin.

---

a patient who has unrecognized adrenocortical failure and who recently had glucocorticoid therapy withdrawn or has sustained bilateral hemorrhage of the adrenals.

Diagnosis

Endocrine Diagnosis

The symptoms and signs of adrenocortical failure are variable and nonspecific, and diagnosis requires a high degree of clinical awareness. Blood samples for determining plasma cortisol and ACTH levels should be drawn (preferably before 10 am) before presumptive therapy for glucocorticoid insufficiency is begun.

The reference range for morning serum cortisol is 7 to 27 mcg/dL. In the appropriate clinical setting, a value less than 3 mcg/dL strongly indicates adrenocortical failure. In a nonstressed ambulatory patient, a serum cortisol concentration greater than 10 mcg/dL indicates that cortisol deficiency is unlikely, and a value greater than 18 mcg/dL excludes the diagnosis.

In a patient receiving potent synthetic glucocorticoids who does not have clinical features suggestive of cortisol insufficiency, a very low cortisol level (eg, <3 mcg/dL) does not imply cortisol deficiency. However, a very low cortisol level in a patient with symptoms of glucocorticoid insufficiency and signs of cortisol excess (see below) suggests secondary adrenocortical deficiency after withdrawal of supraphysiologic doses of glucocorticoids.

The diagnosis of cortisol deficiency is confirmed most reliably and effectively with the cosyntropin test, which assesses the cortisol response to intravenous infusion of synthetic, rapidly acting ACTH (cosyntropin, 250 mcg). The normal response to cosyntropin is an absolute value of plasma cortisol greater than 18 mcg/dL. An impaired response to cosyntropin establishes the diagnosis of adrenocortical failure but does not specify the type. Defining whether the failure is primary or secondary rests on the measurement of serum ACTH: A high ACTH concentration indicates primary adrenal disease (Addison disease), and a low or "inappropriately normal" level indicates secondary failure from hypothalamo-pituitary insufficiency.

A normal response to cosyntropin rules out Addison disease but does not exclude recent-onset or partial ACTH deficiency. If the diagnosis is still suspected, a metyrapone test or an insulin-hypoglycemia test is rarely performed: A normal response to the provocative test excludes adrenocortical failure; an impaired response in a patient who has a normal response to cosyntropin indicates secondary failure. A low-dose cosyntropin test (1 mcg) has been advocated as a reliable alternative for the diagnosis of recent or partial ACTH deficiency, but its value for this purpose is debatable.

Etiologic Diagnosis

In Addison disease, an etiologic diagnosis depends on the clinical assessment and a search for other autoimmune disorders, infections, and neoplasms. Autoimmune adrenalitis is diagnosed by measuring antibodies against the steroidogenic enzyme 21-hydroxylase (*CYP21A2*). Computed tomographic (CT) imaging of the adrenal glands is helpful in the diagnosis of infectious disorders, adrenal hemorrhage, or malignancy. In secondary failure, other pituitary function is assessed and magnetic resonance imaging (MRI) or CT imaging of the head is performed to look for a space-occupying lesion in the hypothalamic-pituitary region.

Therapy

Primary adrenocortical failure requires replacement of glucocorticoid and mineralocorticoid hormones, whereas secondary failure requires only glucocorticoid replacement. Patient education is critical and must cover several topics: the need for disciplined daily lifelong therapy, the manner of dosage adjustments during acute illness, the use of injectable glucocorticoids when oral replacement therapy is not possible, and the use of a medical alert identification bracelet or necklace.

Primary Adrenocortical Failure

Glucocorticoid therapy consists of hydrocortisone (10–20 mg in the morning and 5–10 mg in the afternoon) or prednisone (4–5 mg in the morning and 0–2.5 mg in the afternoon). Unlike with other hormone replacement therapies, monitoring hormone concentrations (ACTH or cortisol) is not reliable for monitoring the adequacy of therapy. The adequacy of therapy is instead assessed by the patient's sense of well-being and the absence of manifestations of excessive glucocorticoid replacement.

Mineralocorticoid therapy consists of fludrocortisone (0.05–0.2 mg orally) and liberal salt intake. The adequacy of replacement is indicated by normal supine blood pressure without a postural decrease on standing up and by the absence of hypertension, edema, and an abnormal potassium concentration. Rarely, plasma renin activity is measured to titrate mineralocorticoid therapy. Adequate mineralocorticoid therapy reduces the dose needed for glucocorticoid replacement and therefore reduces the risks of adverse effects from glucocorticoids.

Acute Illness

In mild to moderate acute illness, the glucocorticoid dose is doubled or tripled and given at that increased dosage for the duration of the illness. If the patient cannot retain oral glucocorticoids because of vomiting, an intramuscular injection of glucocorticoids (eg, dexamethasone 4 mg, hydrocortisone 100 mg, or methylprednisolone 20 mg) is adminstered. In the presence of severe illness, patients should seek medical attention promptly and be treated with a parenteral glucocorticoid.

For minor procedures performed under local anesthesia and for most radiologic procedures, no special preparation is required beyond a doubling of the patient's oral glucocorticoid dose for that day. For moderately stressful procedures, such as endoscopy, hydrocortisone (100 mg intravenously) or another glucocorticoid in an equivalent dose should be given 1 hour before the procedure. For major surgery, 100 mg of hydrocortisone is given intravenously before the induction of anesthesia and repeated every 6 to 8 hours for the first 24 hours, after which the dose is tapered at a rate that depends on the patient's recovery (usually a decrease in dosage by 50% daily to maintenance levels). Because this stress-dosage of hydrocortisone has adequate mineralocorticoid effect, the use of a specific mineralocorticoid during the acute illness is not necessary.

Adrenal Crisis

When an adrenal crisis is suspected, intravenous access should be promptly established and blood samples collected for measuring electrolyte, glucose, plasma cortisol, and serum ACTH levels. An adrenal crisis requires prompt management before the availability of the test results. Infuse saline and dextrose (to restore intravascular and extracellular fluid volumes) and hydrocortisone (100 mg every 6 hours). With this dosage of hydrocortisone, specific mineralocorticoid therapy is not necessary. After the patient's condition has stabilized, continue infusions, but at a lower rate. Search for and treat possible infections and other precipitating causes.

If the patient is known to have glucocorticoid insufficiency, after the acute illness is over, the glucocorticoid dose is promptly increased to the stress dose until the acute illness is present (usually 3–5 days), and then the dose is promptly decreased to the maintenance dose. Mineralocorticoid replacement is initiated as soon as the daily dose of hydrocortisone is less than 100 mg.

If the patient is not known to have glucocorticoid insufficiency, after the acute illness is over, switch the glucocorticoid therapy to dexamethasone (it will not interfere with plasma cortisol measurements) and perform the cosyntropin stimulation test to evaluate for adrenocortical insufficiency. Taper the dosage of glucocorticoids to a maintenance dosage and begin mineralocorticoid replacement after the saline infusion is stopped.

KEY FACTS

- ✓ Adrenal crisis—dehydration, hypotension, or shock out of proportion to the severity of the current illness
- ✓ Therapy for primary adrenocortical failure—both glucocorticoid and mineralocorticoid replacement
- ✓ Therapy for secondary adrenocortical failure—only glucocorticoid replacement
- ✓ After an adrenal crisis has passed in a patient without glucocorticoid insufficiency, change the glucocorticoid therapy from hydrocortisone to dexamethasone and perform the cosyntropin stimulation test

---

Cushing Syndrome

Etiology

Cushing syndrome may have an exogenous or endogenous origin. *Exogenous Cushing syndrome* is more common and is usually caused by long-term use of supraphysiologic doses of cortisol or, more commonly, its analogues (eg, prednisone) in the management of inflammatory, allergic, or neoplastic disorders. It rarely is caused by the surreptitious use of these agents.

Endogenous Cushing syndrome is caused by cortisol overproduction by the adrenal cortex. Cortisol overproduction may result from 1) primary adrenal, autonomous, and ACTH-independent disorders, such as an adrenal adenoma (a small differentiated tumor usually <4 cm in diameter) that often produces a "pure glucocorticoid excess" syndrome; 2) an undifferentiated adrenal carcinoma (usually >6 cm in diameter) that is inefficient in steroidogenesis and produces (in addition to cortisol) large quantities of adrenal androgens (eg, dehydroepiandrosterone-sulfate [DHEA-S]); or, rarely, 3) macronodular or micronodular adrenal hyperplasia.

ACTH-dependent Cushing syndrome may be caused by excessive secretion of ACTH derived from the pituitary or from an ectopic neuroendocrine tumor. Pituitary ACTH overproduction is caused by a pituitary corticotroph cell adenoma (ie, *Cushing disease*). The adenoma usually is small; more than 50% of these tumors are not detected on MRI.

The most common causes of endogenous Cushing syndrome are Cushing disease (75%), ectopic-ACTH tumors (15%), and adrenal tumors (10%). Ectopic ACTH production from certain tumors (eg, carcinoid tumors) may be clinically indistinguishable from Cushing syndrome caused by ACTH overproduction from the pituitary. However, ectopic ACTH production from aggressive malignancies (eg, small cell lung cancer) may be associated with a rapid increase in cortisol concentrations to very high levels, leading to severe metabolic abnormalities (hypokalemia, metabolic alkalosis, hypertension and hyperglycemia) but not many classical physical features of Cushing syndrome (see below).

Clinical Features

Features of cortisol excess are the dominant features of the syndrome and are those of chronic indolent cortisol excess: weight gain and central obesity, thin skin with easy bruisability and wide violaceous striae, plethora, muscle weakness, osteoporosis, cessation of linear growth in growing children or adolescents, lanugo hair, hypertension, insulin resistance and secondary diabetes, hypercalciuria and renal stones, and propensity to fungal infections.

Features of adrenal androgen excess may be modest and lead to acne, hirsutism, and menstrual irregularities, as in the usual cases of Cushing disease and ACTH-producing bronchial carcinoids, or they may be more severe and lead to virilization, as in adrenal carcinoma. Features of androgen excess may be absent in patients with glucocorticoid-producing adrenal adenoma or exogenous Cushing syndrome.

ACTH produced in significant quantities, as in the usual malignant causes of ectopic-ACTH tumors, may lead to hyperpigmentation.

Anatomical effects of the underlying tumor include extrasellar effects with pituitary macroadenomas, bronchopulmonary effects of lung cancer, and abdominal pain caused by adrenocortical carcinoma or the metastatic effects of malignant causal tumors.

Diagnosis

The diagnostic approach to a patient with suspected Cushing syndrome has 2 central components: confirming the diagnosis of pathologically elevated cortisol production and concentration and identifying its cause. Several issues make establishing the diagnosis complex.

Many non-Cushing disorders can increase cortisol production and impair hypothalamic-pituitary-adrenal homeostatic mechanisms. These include acute illness of any type, stress, nutritional disorders, alcoholism, and depression.

Many drugs can alter diagnostic tests. For example, the use of oral contraceptives can be associated with an increase in cortisol-binding globulin (and therefore a falsely elevated plasma cortisol). Barbiturates, rifampin, and phenytoin can increase dexamethasone metabolism and therefore cause a falsely positive dexamethasone suppression test.

No single test is completely reliable to confirm or exclude the diagnosis of Cushing syndrome. Clinicians often rely on repeated measurements of several tests, which are sometimes repeated over an extended period.

Some patients with Cushing syndrome have only cyclic expression of the disease, with periods of activity extending over several weeks to months, interspersed with periods of disease inactivity. Laboratory test results during periods of disease inactivity may be normal, so that only repeated testing over several months may point to the underlying disease.

Identification of Cushing Syndrome

The best screening tests for Cushing syndrome are the overnight 1-mg dexamethasone suppression test, a 24-hour urine collection for free cortisol, and late-night salivary cortisol testing.

For the overnight dexamethasone suppression test, a tablet of 1-mg dexamethasone is taken orally at 11 pm and blood is drawn between 7:30 and 8 the next morning. A plasma cortisol level less than 1.8 mcg/dL rules out endogenous pathologic hypercortisolemia with a high degree of confidence. A plasma cortisol level less than 5 mcg/dL provides a false-positive result in 13% of patients with simple obesity and in 25% of patients with a chronic illness. Most patients with Cushing syndrome have a post-dexamethasone cortisol level of 10 mcg/dL or more.

Urinary free cortisol is increased in more than 97% of patients with Cushing syndrome. High urinary free cortisol is also present in the absence of Cushing syndrome in people with high urine output. It can be modestly increased in simple obesity, but a higher value strengthens support for Cushing syndrome.

A late-night (11 pm) elevated cortisol level suggests the loss of diurnal variation in cortisol concentrations, which occurs in people with Cushing syndrome.

Often 2 or 3 of these screening tests are performed if Cushing syndrome is suspected. Concordant results greatly increase confidence in the diagnosis.

Etiologic Diagnosis

The serum ACTH level is the test that differentiates between ACTH-dependent and ACTH-independent causes. Plasma ACTH levels are 1) suppressed (<5 pg/mL) in patients with adrenal tumors; 2) within the reference range (20–80 pg/mL) or modestly increased (<200 pg/mL) in patients with Cushing disease or ectopic ACTH caused by bronchial carcinoids; and 3) very high (>200 pg/mL) in most patients with the usual ectopic ACTH production from malignancies.

MRI of the hypothalamopituitary region is performed to evaluate the morphology of the pituitary if ACTH is not suppressed. If the clinical features and MRI findings are not definitive, inferior petrosal sinus sampling is performed to determine whether the source of the ACTH is the pituitary region or elsewhere.

Therapy

For Cushing disease, the treatment of choice is transsphenoidal surgical adenomectomy or subtotal hypophysectomy.

If the disease persists postoperatively, the therapeutic options include pituitary radiotherapy and the interim use of steroidogenesis blockers, such as ketoconazole, or bilateral adrenalectomy and postoperative targeted pituitary radiotherapy (eg, Gamma Knife [Elekta AB] stereotactic radiosurgery) if and when the location of the pituitary adenoma is identified on MRI. The treatment of adrenal adenoma is unilateral adrenalectomy. For adrenal carcinoma, the treatment is unilateral adrenalectomy. Blockers of steroidogenesis and mitotane are indicated for persistent or recurrent hypercortisolemia caused by adrenocortical carcinoma. Tumor excision is indicated for an ectopic ACTH-secreting tumor. If the tumor is unresectable or if it cannot be found, hypercortisolism can be managed short-term with blockers of steroidogenesis. For a rapid cure of hypercortisolism, bilateral adrenalectomy is recommended.

In all cases of Cushing syndrome, surgical excision of the causative tumor is followed by cortisol deficiency caused by the suppressed hypothalamic-pituitary adrenal axis. It may take up to 1 or 2 years for the axis to recover; during this period, the patient needs glucocorticoid replacement therapy.

Primary Aldosteronism

Etiology
Primary aldosteronism results from an autonomous renin-angiotensin–independent disorder of the zona glomerulosa. It may be caused by idiopathic bilateral hyperplasia (65%), an aldosterone-producing adenoma (30%), unilateral adrenal hyperplasia (<5%), adrenocortical carcinoma (<1%), and, very rarely, the familial disorder glucocorticoid-remediable aldosteronism (<0.1%).

> ### Key Definition
>
> Primary aldosteronism: *excessive secretion of aldosterone that results from an autonomous renin-angiotensin–independent disorder of the zona glomerulosa.*

Clinical Features
The prevalence of primary aldosteronism in the hypertensive population is about 10% (5%–13%). Most patients present with hypertension that is mild to severe (malignant hypertension is extremely rare). Unprovoked hypokalemia is a typical feature of primary aldosteronism, or it may be provoked with diuretic therapy. More than 70% of patients with primary aldosteronism may not have hypokalemia. Most patients are asymptomatic, but a few report the effects of hypokalemic alkalosis (fatigue and muscle weakness, paresthesias, nephrogenic diabetes insipidus, and glucose intolerance). Edema typically is absent.

Diagnosis
The diagnosis of primary aldosteronism rests on documenting autonomous aldosterone hypersecretion and on defining the underlying cause.

Endocrine Diagnosis
Hypokalemia is a classic finding in patients with primary aldosteronism; however, it may be absent (>70% of patients) and is nonspecific. In a patient with hypokalemia, a urinary potassium level greater than 30 mmol/24 h suggests renal potassium wasting and increases the likelihood that the patient has aldosteronism.

Primary aldosteronism autonomous of regulation by the renin-angiotensin system is associated with suppressed plasma renin activity. The best screening test is based on measurements of the plasma aldosterone concentration (PAC) (in nanograms per deciliter) and renin activity (PRA) (in nanograms per milliliter per hour), which are used to calculate the PAC:PRA ratio. It is important to remember that hypokalemia should be corrected before aldosterone levels are measured, because hypokalemia may reduce the aldosterone production in primary aldosteronism. The test can be done with the patient receiving antihypertensive drugs except spironolactone and eplerenone, which are aldosterone-receptor blockers. A PAC:PRA ratio greater than 20 in the presence of an elevated plasma aldosterone concentration (>15 ng/dL) is a positive test for primary aldosteronism. An increased PAC and an increased PRA with a PAC:PRA ratio less than 10 indicate secondary aldosteronism. A low PAC and a low PRA suggest that another corticosteroid being produced in excess (eg, 11-deoxycorticosterone or cortisol) is acting at the mineralocorticoid receptor and is the cause of hypertension and hypokalemia.

The diagnosis of primary aldosteronism is confirmed by demonstrating the nonsuppressible autonomous secretion of aldosterone despite salt loading (oral salt loading, saline infusion, or fludrocortisone suppression test), often with measurement of urinary sodium and aldosterone.

Etiologic Diagnosis
The major challenge is to differentiate between a unilateral adrenal disorder (an aldosterone-producing adenoma or unilateral adrenal hyperplasia) and bilateral adrenal hyperplasia. This differentiation has important therapeutic implications. Unilateral adrenal disease may be treated surgically by unilateral adrenalectomy. However, bilateral hyperplasia is treated medically by the use of a mineralocorticoid receptor antagonist (see below). This differentiation relies on CT of the adrenals and selective venous sampling.

A unilateral 1- to 2-cm adrenal mass on a CT scan usually indicates an aldosterone-producing adenoma and is diagnostic in a young person (age <35 years). In older patients, or if the mass is not clearly visible or not unilateral, selective adrenal venous sampling is the most helpful in localizing the source of aldosterone. After confirming reliable adrenal venous catheterization, a unilateral gradient suggests unilateral disease, and the absence of a gradient suggests bilateral hyperplasia. This technically difficult procedure should be performed in centers with radiologic expertise.

Differential Diagnosis

The main considerations in the differential diagnosis of primary aldosteronism are hypertensive variants of secondary aldosteronism and other causes of mineralocorticoid-induced hypertension.

Secondary aldosteronism associated with hypertension results from increased renin production as a consequence of renal artery stenosis, malignant hypertension, or a renin-producing tumor. Plasma renin activity, the angiotensin II level, and aldosterone production are increased, and patients present with renin-dependent hyperaldosteronism with hypertension and hypokalemia.

Therapy

Therapy has 3 objectives: control or reverse hypertension, correct hypokalemia, and prevent the toxic effects of excess aldosterone on the cardiovascular system.

Unilateral adrenalectomy is the treatment of choice for aldosteronoma or unilateral hyperplasia unless the patient is at high surgical risk. Surgery corrects the hypokalemia in all patients and normalizes the blood pressure or significantly improves the hypertension in most (98%). Patients with persistent postoperative hypertension should be treated with standard antihypertensive drug therapy.

Medical treatment is indicated for bilateral adrenal hyperplasia and for aldosteronoma if the patient is at high surgical risk. (Surgical treatment of bilateral hyperplasia would require bilateral adrenalectomy to normalize the serum potassium level, but it rarely restores blood pressure to normal levels.) Spironolactone, a mineralocorticoid receptor antagonist, is given at a dosage of 25 to 100 mg once or twice daily. The dose is adjusted for a target serum potassium level near the upper limit of the reference range without the aid of potassium supplements. Spironolactone restores normokalemia and normalizes blood pressure in most patients. Adverse effects include gastrointestinal tract upset, menstrual irregularity in women, and gynecomastia, impaired

libido, and impaired potency in men. Women of childbearing age who take spironolactone should use oral contraceptives because the drug may cause feminization of the male fetus through its androgen-blocking effects. Eplerenone, a highly selective mineralocorticoid receptor antagonist with fewer side effects, is a good alternative to spironolactone, although eplerenone is more expensive and shorter acting (so twice daily dosing is mandatory).

Pheochromocytoma and Paraganglioma

Clinical Features

Pheochromocytomas can be asymptomatic (10%–50%), especially with adrenal incidentalomas or when diagnosed during screening of relatives of a person with a genetic syndrome. More commonly, they are suspected because of the presence of hypertension (particularly if it is labile, paroxysmal, or refractory to treatment) or paroxysmal symptoms of headaches, forceful palpitations, sweating, and pallor. Flushing is not a feature of excess catecholamines. In most patients, the paroxysmal symptoms are stereotypical and vary only in severity or frequency, often getting more severe and more frequent with the duration of the disease. It is important to recognize that most patients with paroxysmal symptoms (spells) do not have pheochromocytoma.

Diagnosis

Endocrine Diagnosis

The biochemical diagnosis of pheochromocytoma requires measurement of fractionated catecholamines and metanephrines in urine over 24 hours and plasma fractionated metanephrines. Creatinine is measured in urine to ensure adequacy of 24-hour collection. In pheochromocytoma, these values are typically elevated to more than twice the upper limit of the reference range. A 24-hour urine collection for metanephrines and catecholamines has 90% sensitivity and 98% specificity. Plasma metanephrine levels have 97% to 99% sensitivity but only 85% to 89% specificity; they provide the best test for patients who have a high pretest probability of the disease, such as those with genetic syndromes. Therefore, whereas plasma fractionated metanephrine values in the reference range exclude the diagnosis of pheochromocytoma with a good degree of certainty, increased values often need further confirmation with more specific urinary catecholamines and metanephrines.

Radiologic Localization

Radiologic evaluation helps localize the source after the diagnosis has been established by the biochemical confirmation of catecholamine excess. CT and MRI of the abdomen (and, if findings are negative, CT and MRI of the pelvis, thorax, and neck) are the mainstays of radiologic localization. They have a sensitivity and specificity greater than 90%. On MRI, pheochromocytomas show high-signal

---

KEY FACTS

✓ Cushing syndrome screening tests—overnight 1-mg dexamethasone suppression test, free cortisol level in 24-hour urine collection, and late-night salivary cortisol testing

✓ Primary aldosteronism classic finding—hypokalemia (but it is a nonspecific finding and is absent in >70% of patients)

intensity on T2-weighted images. CT provides better spatial resolution. CT with nonionic contrast medium is considered the first radiologic procedure of choice. This imaging does not require adrenergic receptor blockade.

Therapy

Surgical excision of the tumor is curative. Blood pressure is controlled to diminish perioperative morbidity and mortality. α-Adrenergic blockade with phenoxybenzamine is instituted as soon as the diagnosis is made and is followed with calcium channel blockers (nifedipine or amlodipine) if needed to improve the control of blood pressure. The target for seated blood pressure is the low-normal range for the patient's age. β-Adrenergic blockers (propranolol or metoprolol) may be necessary to control tachycardia (target, 80 beats per minute), but β-blockade should be used only after adequate α-blockade has been established. β-Adrenergic blockade without α-adrenergic blockade could exacerbate or even precipitate malignant hypertension. For hypertensive emergencies, intravenous phentolamine (an α-blocker) is the drug of choice and can be given in 5- to 10-mg doses every 5 to 15 minutes as needed. Alternatively, nitroprusside can be used.

Adrenal Incidentaloma

Etiology

Small (1–6 cm) adrenal masses are found in up to 9% of unselected autopsies and in more than 2% of all abdominal imaging studies. Most are nonfunctioning adenomas; a few are functioning adenomas or carcinomas of the adrenal cortex or medulla. Metastatic disease to the adrenal glands is common. Identification of the nature of the mass is important: Nonfunctioning adenomas are harmless, a functioning adenoma or a carcinoma requires surgery, and metastasis requires oncologic care.

Diagnosis

The diagnosis of a functioning adrenal tumor rests on clinical evaluation, the use of screening tests, and, when appropriate, confirmatory tests. For all patients, hormonal evaluation should screen for pheochromocytoma (24-hour urinary fractionated catecholamines and metanephrines) and Cushing syndrome (overnight 1-mg dexamethasone suppression test). DHEA-S should also be measured. Plasma renin activity and plasma aldosterone concentration should be measured in hypertensive patients. If the results of these screening tests imply a particular hormonal abnormality, appropriate confirmatory tests are required.

Often CT scans without and with radiocontrast medium, with an adrenal protocol, are performed to further characterize the incidentally diagnosed adrenal mass. Radiodensity less than 10 Hounsfield units on CT, a homogeneous appearance, lack of vascularity, and a well-defined border are strong indicators that the tumor is benign. Other

than showing the fat density of an adrenal myelolipoma, imaging studies may not differentiate between benign and malignant neoplasms. A mass that is 4 cm or larger has a higher chance of being malignant. On dynamic contrast data of the CT scan, a contrast wash out of 50% or more within 10 minutes implies that the tumor is benign. On MRI, bright T2 images suggest pheochromocytoma or adrenal cancer.

If an incidental adrenal mass is identified in a patient who has an active malignancy with a chance that the mass is metastatic, further investigation is indicated only if the diagnosis of the mass will change the management strategy for the malignancy. Needle aspiration of the mass may then be performed but only after excluding pheochromocytoma. Otherwise, needle biopsy of the mass is never indicated.

Therapy

All functional adrenal masses and most masses 4 cm or larger should be excised after appropriate preparation as needed. A nonfunctional adrenal mass smaller than 4 cm with a benign imaging phenotype should be monitored with another CT scan in 3 to 6 months and again at 12 months to assess for growth of the mass. Every mass lesion that demonstrably increases in size (>1 cm) during the observation period should be surgically excised after appropriate tests and preparation. For patients with a nonfunctional adrenal mass, follow-up hormonal screening for 1 to 2 years may be performed as clinically indicated. Long-term routine testing for hormonal abnormality is not indicated.

KEY FACTS

✓ Pheochromocytoma biochemical diagnosis—24-hour urinary fractionated catecholamines and metanephrines and plasma fractionated metanephrines

✓ Pheochromocytoma therapy—if control of tachycardia requires β-blockers, first ensure the adequacy of α-blockade (to avoid exacerbation or precipitation of malignant hypertension)

✓ Small adrenal masses (1–6 cm) found incidentally in autopsies (≤9%) or abdominal imaging studies (>2%) are usually nonfunctioning adenomas

✓ Hormonal evaluation for diagnosis of functioning adrenal tumor—screen for pheochromocytoma and Cushing syndrome, and measure DHEA-S; for hypertensive patient, also measure plasma renin activity and plasma aldosterone concentration

✓ After pheochromocytoma has been excluded, needle biopsy of an incidental adrenal mass is indicated only if the mass may be metastatic in a patient who has active malignancy and the mass diagnosis would change the management of the malignancy

Disorders of the Testis

Male Hypogonadism in the Adult

Male hypogonadism refers to the clinical presentations resulting from testosterone deficiency (Box 14.2). Such deficiency usually is associated with defects in spermatogenesis and infertility. Spermatogenic failure may exist independently of any testosterone deficiency.

Etiology

Testosterone deficiency may result from decreased testosterone production by the testes or from target tissue resistance to testosterone action (Table 14.1).

Box 14.2 • Clinical Manifestations of Male Hypogonadism

More specific symptoms and signs

Incomplete or delayed sexual development, eunuchoidism (long limbs)

Reduced sexual desire (libido) and activity

Decreased spontaneous erections

Breast tenderness, gynecomastia

Loss of body hair (axillary and pubic), reduced shaving frequency

Very small (especially <5 mL) or shrinking testes

Infertility, sperm count low or zero, decreased ejaculate volume

Height loss, low-trauma fracture, low bone mineral density (osteoporosis)

Hot flushes, sweats (especially if rapid onset)

Less specific symptoms and signs

Decreased energy, motivation, initiative, and self-confidence

Feeling sad or blue, depressed mood, dysthymia

Poor concentration and memory

Sleep disturbance, increased sleepiness

Mild anemia (normochromic, normocytic; in the female range)

Reduced muscle bulk and strength

Increased body fat, feminine fat distribution, increased BMI

Diminished physical or work performance

Classic hypogonadal facies (with pallor and fine wrinkling around the mouth and eyes)

Abbreviation: BMI, body mass index.

Adapted from Bhasin S, Cunningham GR, Hayes FJ, Matsumoto AM, Snyder PJ, Swerdloff RS, et al; Task Force, Endocrine Society. Testosterone therapy in men with androgen deficiency syndromes: an Endocrine Society clinical practice guideline. J Clin Endocrinol Metab. 2010 Jun;95(6):2536–59. Used with permission.

Diagnosis

The diagnosis of hypogonadism can be established by documenting very low serum total testosterone concentrations in a patient with classic clinical features for severe hypogonadism and a high clinical suspicion. If the suspicion is moderate, low morning serum total testosterone concentration should be reconfirmed before making a diagnosis of hypogonadism. Evening testosterone is often "low" in healthy men, so measurement in the evening is not recommended. The total testosterone level may not always reflect testosterone status because of an abnormal concentration of sex hormone–binding globulin (SHBG) (eg, decreased with obesity and increased with aging). If the total testosterone concentration is borderline-low in a person suspected of having hypogonadism, free testosterone (or bioavailable testosterone) may be measured.

When convenient and possible, a semen analysis is performed. A normal semen analysis nearly always indicates a normal hypothalamic-pituitary-gonadal axis.

Total serum testosterone concentrations in men decrease with age, especially after 50 years. This apparent decrease is less than the decrease in the free testosterone concentration because the level of SHBG increases with age. A substantial proportion of older men have testosterone concentrations that are less than the reference range for young men. This decrease in testosterone is often associated with decreased libido, erectile dysfunction, and decreased muscle mass and energy level. This late-onset hypogonadism is often associated with weight gain, obesity, and lack of physical activity. Among men older than 60 years, 3% to 5% have low testosterone concentrations. It is not clear whether treatment is safer than no treatment for late-onset hypogonadism.

Therapy

Prostate and breast cancers are contraindications for testosterone therapy. Testosterone replacement therapy should not be considered an option for a person with an elevated hematocrit (>50%), uncontrolled obstructive sleep apnea (this can itself cause reversible hypogonadism), severe lower urinary tract symptoms, a prostate-specific antigen level of more than 4 ng/mL (or >3 ng/mL with a family history of prostate cancer), or poorly controlled heart failure. Relative contraindications include mental retardation and psychopathy.

In adults, androgen therapy is aimed at restoring and maintaining androgenic functions by replacing and normalizing the serum total testosterone concentration. In hypogonadal pubertal males, androgen therapy is designed to initiate and induce full pubertal development; therapy is started at a smaller dose and titrated upward over time to prevent behavioral changes associated with full replacement.

Androgen replacement may be given in the form of parenteral long-acting 17-hydroxyl esters of testosterone (enanthate or cypionate esters). They are effective and safe. The usual dosage for an adult male is 200 mg intramuscularly every 15 days. Intramuscular testosterone often leads to a

Table 14.1 • Causes of Testosterone Deficiency

| | | Testosterone Deficiency | |
| | | Primary Testicular Dysfunction (Hypergonadotropic Hypogonadism) | Hypothalamic-Pituitary Dysfunction (Central or Hypogonadotropic Hypogonadism) |
Feature	Testosterone Resistance		
Testosterone level	High-normal	Low	Low
LH and FSH level	High-normal	Very high	Normal or low
Causes			
Genetic	Androgen receptor defect	Klinefelter syndrome	. . .
Drugs	Spironolactone, flutamide, finasteride	Ketoconazole	Neuroleptic agents, antidepressants
Trauma	. . .	Bilateral testicular injury, bilateral orchidectomy, radiotherapy, chemotherapy (busulfan, vincristine)	. . .
Inflammatory	. . .	Mumps, autoimmune testicular failure	. . .
Structural	. . .	. . .	Hypothalamopituitary mass, inflammatory disease, hemorrhage
Functional	. . .	. . .	Constitutional delay in puberty
Degenerative	. . .	Myotonia dystrophica	. . .
Nutritional	. . .	. . .	Stress of major systemic illness
Endocrinopathy	. . .	. . .	Hyperprolactinemia, other hyperestrogenic states, hypothyroidism, hyperthyroidism, adrenocortical dysfunction

Abbreviations: FSH, follicle-stimulating hormone; LH, luteinizing hormone.

substantially high testosterone level soon after the injection and a decrease before the next dose. Alternatively, testosterone may be administered transdermally with a patch (2.5–7.5 mg) or a gel (2.5–7.5 mg) applied daily. These transdermal therapies are associated with stable physiologic serum testosterone concentrations. Buccal testosterone given twice daily is also available, but experience with it is limited. Testosterone pellets (3–6 pellets) can be implanted subcutaneously at a medical facility every 3 to 6 months, depending on the formulation.

Oral preparations of testosterone are not used for replacement in the United States. They are less effective and more costly, and they can be associated with the potentially serious adverse effects of hepatotoxicity, induction of peliosis hepatis, and hepatic tumors.

Adverse effects of testosterone replacement therapy include acne, mild weight gain, edema, increased erythropoiesis, and induction or worsening of obstructive sleep apnea. Monitoring of therapy is important (Tables 14.2 and 14.3).

Adequacy of therapy is best assessed clinically and by measurement of the serum testosterone concentration 2 to 3 months after the institution of therapy. The testosterone dose is titrated to achieve a total testosterone concentration in the middle of the reference range. If the patient has primary hypogonadism, normalization of the serum luteinizing hormone (LH) concentration is sometimes used as an indicator of the adequacy of therapy.

Table 14.2 • Monitoring Adverse Effects of Testosterone Replacement Therapy

Feature of Concern	Method of Monitoring
Polycythemia	Hematocrit: baseline, 3–6 mo, and yearly
Prostate	Digital rectal examination and PSA: baseline, 6 mo, and yearly PSA at 6 mo after initiation of treatment is considered the reference for monitoring Significant changes after 6 mo: PSA increase >1.4 ng/mL over 1-y period *or* PSA rate of increase >0.4 ng/mL yearly Lower urinary tract symptom assessment for significant change: AUA/IPSS >19
Obstructive sleep apnea	History (Epworth Sleepiness Scale); overnight oximetry, as indicated
Dyslipidemia	Fasting triglycerides
Gynecomastia	History, examination; mammography if indicated on examination
Local problems	History, examination of the site of testosterone delivery

Abbreviations: AUA, American Urological Association; IPSS, International Prostate Symptom Score; PSA, prostate-specific antigen.

Table 14.3 • Monitoring Testosterone Concentration During Testosterone Replacement Therapy

Treatment Modality	Schedule for Measuring Testosterone Level
Injectable testosterone (testosterone enanthate or testosterone cypionate)	Midway between injections
Transdermal patches	Within 3–12 h after application of the patch
Buccal testosterone	Immediately before or after application of a fresh system
Transdermal gels	Anytime after ≥1 wk of treatment
Testosterone pellets	At the end of the dosing interval

Box 14.3 • Causes of Gynecomastia

Primary hypogonadism (testicular failure)

Puberty

Aging

Refeeding in severe, long-standing malnutrition

Renal failure and dialysis

Hepatic cirrhosis

Hyperthyroidism

Hormonal abnormalities (excess estrogens, exogenous testosterone, elevated levels of hCG or prolactin)

Drugs (ketoconazole, spironolactone, metronidazole)

Other drugs (alcohol, marijuana)

Abbreviation: hCG, human chorionic gonadotropin.

Testosterone therapy reduces fertility. Treatment of fertility in a person with hypogonadotropic hypogonadism necessitates the use of LH, follicle-stimulating hormone (FSH), or their agonists.

Gynecomastia

Etiology

Gynecomastia refers to a benign enlargement of the male breast caused by an increase in glandular and stromal tissues. It is the most common breast disorder in males, accounting for more than 85% of breast masses in males. The basic pathophysiologic mechanism is an increase in the estrogen to androgen ratio, which may result from androgen deficiency, exposure to exogenous estrogen, exposure to exogenous testosterone (which is converted to estrogen in the body), or an endogenous increase in estrogen production. It is always important to attempt to identify a specific cause because it may have been a serious systemic illness (Box 14.3). In young pubertal males, the most likely cause is physiologic gynecomastia. In adults, the most common causes are drugs and alcohol-related liver disease. In about 10% of cases, the cause of gynecomastia is indeterminate or idiopathic.

Key Definition

Gynecomastia: *benign enlargement of the male breast caused by an increase in glandular and stromal tissues.*

Diagnosis

If gynecomastia is bilateral, exclude pseudogynecomastia (fatty enlargement). If it is unilateral, exclude cancer of the breast. Signs that should arouse suspicion of malignancy include an eccentric location in relation to the areola, unusual firmness, a distinct mass, fixation, ulceration, bloody discharge from the nipple, and the presence of axillary lymphadenopathy. Mammography and excisional biopsy may be necessary for definitive diagnosis.

A complete medical history, physical examination, and appropriate laboratory studies should be performed to determine the cause and therefore the path of management. Endocrine tests may include measurement of the serum levels of testosterone, estradiol, LH and FSH, β-human chorionic gonadotropin, sensitive thyrotropin, DHEA-S, and prolactin.

Treatment

Minimal gynecomastia of puberty is often only observed. Indications for surgery include cosmetic correction and malignancy (or suspicion of malignancy).

KEY FACTS

✓ Testosterone levels in many older men are less than those in young men, but the apparent decrease in total serum testosterone in men older than 50 is less than the decrease in free testosterone levels because SHBG increases with age

✓ Contraindications for testosterone therapy—prostate cancer or breast cancer

✓ Oral testosterone (not used in the United States)—less effective and more expensive than other forms (intramuscular injection, transdermal patch or gel) and associated with hepatotoxicity, peliosis hepatis, and hepatic tumors

✓ Gynecomastia—most common breast disorder in males (>85% of breast masses in males)

Disorders of the Ovary

Amenorrhea

Primary amenorrhea is present when menarche has not occurred by age 16 in a young female patient with normal secondary sex characteristics or by age 14 in the absence of secondary sex characteristics. *Secondary amenorrhea* is present when a woman with previously established menstrual function experiences the absence of menstruation for more than 3 of her previous cycle intervals or for 6 months.

Etiology

Normal regular menstrual function has several requirements (Box 14.4). Amenorrhea can be physiologic or pathologic. The most common causes of amenorrhea are physiologic (pregnancy, lactation, and prepubertal and perimenopausal states). Pathologic amenorrhea may result from several disorders (Box 14.5).

Primary Amenorrhea
Ovarian disorders, including developmental (eg, Turner syndrome, müllerian duct agenesis) and acquired disorders (eg, pelvic inflammatory disorders), account for most of the causes of primary amenorrhea. Outflow tract abnormalities are uncommon causes of primary amenorrhea. Developmental anomalies include imperforate hymen, isolated absence of the uterus, and vaginal aplasia or atresia. Hypothalamic-pituitary disease can cause gonadotropin deficiency and amenorrhea by 1) destruction of pituitary gonadotrophs or the hypothalamic gonadotropin-releasing hormone (GnRH) cell population by organic diseases or by 2) functional suppression of these cells. Functional suppression commonly occurs from a nutritional or psychiatric disorder, prolonged heavy exercise, systemic illness, malnutrition, and other endocrinopathies such as uncontrolled diabetes mellitus, hyperprolactinemia, and severe thyroid and adrenal disorders.

Box 14.4 • Requirements for Normal Regular Menstrual Function

Normal cyclic secretion of hypothalamic gonadotropin-releasing hormone (GnRH) and the pituitary gonadotropins, luteinizing hormone (LH) and follicle-stimulating hormone (FSH)

Normal ovarian follicular apparatus that responds to cyclic gonadotropin stimulation by ovulation and production of estrogen and progesterone in a cyclic fashion

Normal endometrium capable of responding to estradiol (follicular proliferative endometrium) and progesterone (luteal secretory endometrium) and then to their decreasing concentrations by the initiation of menstrual shedding

---

Box 14.5 • Causes of Pathologic Amenorrhea

A functional or organic hypothalamic disorder leading to loss of production of cyclic gonadotropin-releasing hormone (GnRH)

An organic pituitary disorder resulting in loss of the gonadotrope population

An organic ovarian disorder resulting in loss of the follicular apparatus or in anovulation, and in loss of the normal sequential secretion of estradiol and progesterone

Organic uterine disorders and loss of the endometrium or genital tract disorders, preventing egress of the shed endometrium

---

Secondary Amenorrhea
Ovarian disorders are common causes of secondary amenorrhea. The most common disorder is polycystic ovary syndrome (PCOS). Ovarian destructive processes are an uncommon cause of secondary amenorrhea and premature menopause. These processes include autoimmune oophoritis, abdominal radiotherapy, chemotherapy with agents such as cyclophosphamide and vincristine, and ovarian tumors that cause secondary amenorrhea by hormonal abnormalities (hypersecretion of estrogen, androgen, or human chorionic gonadotropin) or, if bilateral, by destruction of the ovarian tissue.

Hypothalamic-pituitary disorders are the most common pathologic causes of secondary amenorrhea and may be either functional or organic. *Functional hypothalamic dysfunction* is caused by a defect in the cyclic center, inhibition of the mid-cycle surge of GnRH and LH, and the failure of ovulation. Mild disorders of GnRH release may be triggered by situational stresses or mild weight loss. Moderate or severe disorders of GnRH release may occur with severe weight loss, severe emotional stresses, competitive athletics, systemic disease, thyroid disorders, uncontrolled diabetes mellitus, or a hyperandrogenic state caused by an adrenal or ovarian disorder.

Organic hypothalamic-pituitary disorder may be isolated or occur in association with other pituitary hormonal abnormalities, such as pituitary disorders, hypothalamic disorders, and disorders of extrasellar structures impinging on the hypothalamic-pituitary unit. Hyperprolactinemia is a common cause of secondary amenorrhea, accounting for 25% to 40% of all cases. The incidence of postpartum pituitary necrosis (Sheehan syndrome), previously a common cause, has decreased with improvements in obstetric care.

Clinical Features

In addition to amenorrhea, estrogen deficiency may cause decreased vaginal secretions and dyspareunia, hot flushes, osteopenia, and lack of development or loss of secondary sex characteristics. Other clinical features are related to the cause, such as hyperandrogenic features (eg, polycystic ovarian syndrome), expressible or spontaneous galactorrhea (high prolactin concentrations), and short stature or other features related to Turner syndrome, hypothyroidism, goiter, and other manifestations of hypopituitarism.

Diagnosis

The diagnostic approach to secondary amenorrhea is summarized in Box 14.6.

Therapy

Management of amenorrhea is directed at the underlying disorder and restoration of a eugonadal state. The cause should be identified and treated. If the cause cannot be treated successfully, hypogonadism (resulting in low estrogen concentration) should be corrected with estrogen replacement (with or without progesterone); if feasible, ovulation and fertility potential should be restored.

Estrogen Replacement

The goals of estrogen therapy include control of vasomotor instability, prevention of genitourinary atrophy, preservation of secondary sex characteristics, prevention of osteoporosis, and restoration of a sense of well-being.

Absolute contraindications to estrogen therapy include known or suspected estrogen-dependent neoplasm (breast or endometrial), cholestatic hepatic dysfunction, active thromboembolic disorder, history of thromboembolic disorder associated with previous use of estrogen, neuro-ophthalmologic vascular disease, and undiagnosed vaginal bleeding.

Estrogen therapy must be individualized and administered only after a thorough discussion with the patient about the benefits and risks of therapy. Therapy is initiated as soon as possible after the diagnosis of estrogen deficiency and is continued indefinitely or until the cause has been reversed.

Estrogen preparations include oral estradiol (0.5–2 mg daily), conjugated estrogens (0.625–1.25 mg daily), and transdermal estradiol patch (0.025–0.1 mg estradiol daily). Oral progestational agents are used for a woman with an intact uterus (medroxyprogesterone acetate, 10 mg daily, or progesterone, 200 mg daily) for days 1 to 12 of each month. Oral and transdermal hormonal combinations are also available.

Complications of estrogen replacement include an increased risk (4- to 8-fold) of endometrial cancer (usually stage I, with no excess mortality), which is dependent on dose and duration. This risk is prevented by progestin supplementation. Other possible adverse effects include a slightly increased risk of breast cancer (breast examination and mammography before treatment and annually thereafter are essential) and increased risk of surgical gallbladder disease.

Ovulation Induction

Women with infertility from anovulation can be given clomiphene citrate, exogenous gonadotropin, or GnRH therapy. The drug of choice for infertility with hyperprolactinemia is the dopamine-agonist bromocriptine.

Polycystic Ovary Syndrome

PCOS is the most common cause of nonvirilizing hyperandrogenicity. It is characterized by the presence of specific criteria (Box 14.7). The pathogenesis is poorly understood. Gonadotropin dynamics are abnormal, with loss of the LH surge and increased LH levels. Hyperandrogenicity is mild to moderate and LH dependent.

Box 14.6 • Diagnostic Approach to Secondary Amenorrhea

1. Rule out physiologic amenorrhea (pregnancy test), genital tract outflow disorders (clinical evaluation, hysteroscopy), and hyperandrogenic state (clinical evaluation, serum levels of testosterone and DHEA-S).

2. Measure serum levels of estradiol, LH, and FSH to distinguish ovarian disease from hypothalamic-pituitary disease.

3. Low serum levels of estradiol and increased levels of FSH and LH suggest primary ovarian failure. Obtain a karyotype if the patient is younger than 30 years.

4. Low serum levels of estradiol and inappropriately low levels of FSH and LH suggest a hypothalamic-pituitary disorder. Rule out a functional disorder and organic hypothalamic-pituitary disease.

5. If organic disease is not identified, consider amenorrhea to be of indeterminate cause and pursue long-term follow-up.

Abbreviations: DHEA-S, dehydroepiandrosterone-sulfate; FSH, follicle-stimulating hormone; LH, luteinizing hormone.

Box 14.7 • Polycystic Ovary Syndrome (PCOS)

PCOS is characterized by the presence of 2 of the following 3 criteria:

1. Ovulatory dysfunction (anovulation: infrequent bleeding with cycles >35 d, <8 cycles yearly, or, rarely, frequent bleeding with cycles <21 d); for adolescents, anovulatory cycles are normal and are not used as a criterion

2. Clinical or biochemical evidence of hyperandrogenism (hirsutism, male pattern baldness, or elevated serum testosterone level)

3. Polycystic changes in the ovaries (≥1 ovary with 12 follicles of 2–9 mm or a volume >10 mL in the absence of a dominant follicle >10 mm)

Many patients have an associated obesity and insulin resistance with consequent hyperinsulinism, which further contribute to the androgen excess. Insulin resistance may be present without obesity. The degree of insulin resistance varies. Many women have a mild form; severe insulin resistance is usually appreciated clinically by the presence of acanthosis nigricans.

The onset of the disorder is at puberty, and its progression is slow and of mild degree. Hirsutism (70% of patients), menstrual abnormality (88%), infertility and anovulation (75%), and obesity (50%) are usually present. The serum level of testosterone is within the reference range or modestly increased (70% of patients) and is nearly always less than 200 ng/dL. DHEA-S levels are within the reference range or mildly increased in 25% of patients. Changes on pelvic ultrasonography are characteristic (70%), and hyperprolactinemia may be present in 25% to 30% of patients. It is important to note that anovulation exposes the endometrium to unopposed estrogen, which increases the risk of endometrial hyperplasia and cancer.

The diagnosis of PCOS is one of exclusion of other causes of hyperandrogenism, such as hypothyroidism, hyperprolactinemia, late-onset congenital adrenal hyperplasia, pregnancy, Cushing syndrome, androgen-secreting tumors of the ovaries or adrenals, and primary ovarian failure.

Disorders of Prolactin: Hyperprolactinemia

Amenorrhea, galactorrhea, infertility, pituitary mass, or hirsutism often leads to measurement of prolactin. Hypogonadism caused by elevated prolactin levels can cause osteoporosis. Prolactin concentrations are normally higher in women than men; therefore, sex-specific reference ranges should be used to interpret the results.

If asymptomatic patients have high prolactin concentrations, macroprolactin should be measured. Macroprolactin is a biologically inactive immunoglobulin G–bound prolactin with no clinical significance.

After the history (including a drug history) and physical examination, common causes of hyperprolactinemia should be excluded with testing for thyrotropin level (to rule out primary hypothyroidism), pregnancy, and creatinine level (Box 14.8).

If no other cause of hyperprolactinemia is found, MRI of the head is performed to evaluate the pituitary-hypothalamic region.

Secondary causes of hyperprolactinemia should be appropriately treated. The treatment plan for hyperprolactinemia depends on the purpose of therapy (Box 14.9).

Box 14.8 • Causes of Hyperprolactinemia

Physiologic
- Lactation
- Pregnancy
- Sleep
- Stress
- Coitus
- Exercise

Pharmacologic
- Anesthetics
- Anticonvulsants
- Antidepressants and other psychotropic medicines
- Antihistamines (H_2 receptor antagonists)
- Antihypertensives
- Cholinergic agonists
- Estrogens: oral contraceptives, oral contraceptive withdrawal
- Opiates and opiate antagonists

Pathologic
- Hypothalamic–pituitary stalk damage: hypothalamic or suprasellar damage, pituitary mass or injury
- Pituitary disorders: acromegaly, plurihormonal adenoma, prolactinoma
- Systemic disorders: primary hypothyroidism, chest nerve irritation, chest wall trauma, herpes zoster, chronic renal failure, cirrhosis, epileptic seizures

Adapted from Melmed S, Kleinberg D. Anterior pituitary. In: Kronenberg HM, Melmed S, Polonsky KS, Larsen PR, editors. Williams textbook of endocrinology. 11th Ed. Philadelphia (PA): Saunders Elsevier; c2008. p. 155–261. Used with permission.

Box 14.9 • Treatment of Hyperprolactinemia

Prolactin-producing pituitary adenoma—treat with dopamine agonist (cabergoline or bromocriptine) at a dose that normalizes prolactin concentrations for ≥1 y; treatment is withdrawn if the tumor disappears and prolactin level remains within the reference range after discontinuation of the dopamine agonist

Galactorrhea—if socially embarrassing, treat with dopamine agonist

Amenorrhea caused by hyperprolactinemia—treat with cyclic estrogen-progesterone tablets to avert the harmful effects of hypogonadism

Asymptomatic, physiologic, drug-induced, or stress-induced hyperprolactinemia—no therapy (mild hyperprolactinemia, even with expressive galactorrhea, may normally occur in premenopausal women who have had babies)

Potentially vision-threatening pituitary macroadenoma in patients intolerant to dopamine agonists— pituitary surgery

KEY FACTS

✓ Estrogen therapy—absolute contraindications: estrogen-dependent neoplasm, cholestatic hepatic dysfunction, active thromboembolic disorder, previous thromboembolic disorder with use of estrogen, neuro-ophthalmologic vascular disease, and undiagnosed vaginal bleeding

✓ Diagnosis of PCOS—exclude other causes of hyperandrogenism (eg, hypothyroidism, hyperprolactinemia, late-onset congenital adrenal hyperplasia, pregnancy, Cushing syndrome, androgen-secreting tumors of the ovaries or adrenals, primary ovarian failure)

✓ High prolactin levels in asymptomatic patients may reflect macroprolactinemia

15 Lipid Disorders

EKTA KAPOOR, MBBS

Etiology

Lipid disorders result from genetic abnormalities in lipoprotein metabolism, other medical conditions (eg, type 2 diabetes mellitus, nephrotic syndrome, hypothyroidism, and excessive alcohol use), and the use of certain drugs (corticosteroids and immunosuppressants) (Box 15.1). The features of genetic dyslipidemias are outlined in Tables 15.1 and 15.2. The most common disorders in this group are the disorders of low-density lipoprotein (LDL) cholesterol (LDL-C), which often lead to premature atherosclerosis in patients and their family members.

Clinical Features

Hyperlipidemia is typically asymptomatic and diagnosed on screening. Patients usually do not have physical findings directly attributable to hyperlipidemia; however, some patients have eyelid xanthelasmata and arcus corneae.

Extreme increases in LDL-C, as noted in familial hypercholesterolemia, may cause **tendon xanthomas** (papules and nodules in the tendons of the hands and feet and the Achilles tendon). **Palmar xanthomas** (yellowish plaques involving the palms and flexural surfaces of the fingers) occur in hyperlipoproteinemia type II and type III. Hyperchylomicronemia can cause **eruptive xanthomas** (small, yellowish orange to reddish brown papules).

Increased LDL-C and lipoprotein (a), also known as Lp(a), and decreased high-density lipoprotein cholesterol (HDL-C) confer increased risk of atherosclerotic cardiovascular disease (ASCVD). Increased HDL-C is associated with decreased atherogenic risk. Hypertriglyceridemia

---

Key Definitions

Tendon xanthomas: *papules and nodules in the tendons of the hands and feet and the Achilles tendon.*

Palmar xanthomas: *yellowish plaques on the palms and flexural surfaces of the fingers.*

Eruptive xanthomas: *small, yellowish orange to reddish brown papules.*

Box 15.1 • Causes of Secondary Hyperlipidemia

Increased LDL-C

  Hypothyroidism
  Nephrotic syndrome
  Cholestatic liver disease
  Progestins
  Anabolic steroids, glucocorticoid therapy
  Anorexia nervosa
  Acute intermittent porphyria

Increased triglycerides

  Obesity
  Diabetes mellitus
  Hypothyroidism
  Sedentary lifestyle
  Alcohol
  Renal insufficiency
  Estrogens
  β-Blockers
  Thiazides, steroids
  Dysglobulinemia
  Systemic lupus erythematosus

Decreased HDL-C

  Hypertriglyceridemia
  Obesity
  Diabetes mellitus
  Cigarette smoking
  Sedentary lifestyle
  β-Blockers
  Progestins
  Anabolic steroids

Abbreviations: HDL-C, high-density lipoprotein cholesterol; LDL-C, low-density lipoprotein cholesterol.

Table 15.1 • Features of Primary Hyperlipidemias: Familial Hypercholesterolemia, Combined Hyperlipidemia, and Dysbetalipoproteinemia

Feature	Familial Hypercholesterolemia	Familial Combined Hyperlipidemia	Familial Dysbetalipoproteinemia
Pathophysiology	Defective LDL receptor or defective apo B-100; impaired catabolism of LDL	Complex; in some cases, overproduction of apo B-100	Defective or absent apo E; excess of CM remnants and VLDL in fasting state
Mode of inheritance	Autosomal codominant	Autosomal dominant	Autosomal recessive
Estimated population frequency	Heterozygotes: 1:500 Homozygotes: 1 per 1 million	1:50 to 1:100	1:5,000
Risk of CHD	+++	++	+
Physical findings	Arcus corneae Tendinous xanthomas	Arcus corneae	Arcus corneae Tuberoeruptive and palmar xanthomas
Associated findings	. . .	Obesity Glucose intolerance Hyperuricemia HDL-C deficiency Elevated apo B	Obesity Glucose intolerance Hyperuricemia
Treatment	Diet Statins Ezetimibe Bile acid–binding resins LDL apheresis	Diet Drugs singly or in combination with niacin, statin, gemfibrozil, resin	Diet Niacin Gemfibrozil Statin

Abbreviations: apo, apolipoprotein; CHD, coronary heart disease; CM, chylomicron; HDL-C, high-density lipoprotein cholesterol; LDL, low-density lipoprotein; VLDL, very low-density lipoprotein; +++, very high risk; ++, high risk; +, moderate risk.

Table 15.2 • Features of Primary Hyperlipidemias: Hypertriglyceridemia

Feature	Familial Hypertriglyceridemia	Severe Hypertriglyceridemia	
		Early-Onset	Adult-Onset
Pathophysiology	Overproduction of hepatic VLDL-Tg but not of apo B-100	Lipoprotein lipase deficiency Apo C-II deficiency; defect in CM and VLDL catabolism	Overproduction of hepatic VLDL-Tg Delayed catabolism of CMs and VLDL
Mode of inheritance	Autosomal dominant	Autosomal recessive	Autosomal recessive
Estimated population frequency	1:50	<1:10,000	Rare
Risk of CHD	+ In families in which HDL-C is deficient	−	+
Physical findings	None	Lipemia retinalis Eruptive xanthomas	Milky plasma Lipemia retinalis Eruptive xanthomas Pancreatitis
Associated findings	Obesity Glucose intolerance Hyperuricemia HDL-C deficiency	HDL-C deficiency Recurrent abdominal pain Pancreatitis Hepatosplenomegaly	Obesity Glucose intolerance Hyperuricemia HDL-C deficiency Pancreatitis
Treatment	Diet Niacin Gemfibrozil Abstinence from alcohol, estrogen	Diet Fish oil	Diet Control diabetes when present Avoidance of alcohol, estrogen Gemfibrozil Fish oil

Abbreviations: apo, apolipoprotein; CHD, coronary heart disease; CM, chylomicron; HDL-C, high-density lipoprotein cholesterol; Tg, triglyceride; VLDL, very low-density lipoprotein; +, moderate risk; −, no increased risk.

may be atherogenic by inducing alterations in other lipoproteins. Triglycerides likely also have an unidentified direct atherogenic action. Pancreatitis may develop with very high triglyceride concentrations (generally >1,000 mg/dL).

Diagnosis and Screening

Disorders of lipoprotein metabolism predispose to premature coronary heart disease (CHD) and vascular disease, and CHD is the leading cause of death in developed nations. Although dyslipidemia is a modifiable risk factor for cardiovascular disease (CVD), it is usually asymptomatic. Experts therefore recommend screening for it in appropriate patients. This strategy aids risk stratification of patients to identify those who would benefit from interventions, including lipid-lowering therapy. LDL-C has conventionally been the target of lipid-lowering therapy, but that alone is a poor predictor of CHD risk. Most risk-prediction models use total cholesterol and HDL-C levels in their calculations.

The updated American College of Cardiology (ACC)/American Heart Association (AHA) guidelines, released in 2013, replaced the Adult Treatment Panel (ATP III) guidelines. The ACC/AHA guidelines recommend assessment of risk factors, including smoking, hypertension, diabetes mellitus, total cholesterol, and HDL-C, every 4 to 6 years for patients aged 20 to 79 years who are free of CVD; this assessment is used to calculate the 10-year CVD risk (with the Pooled Cohort Equations Cardiovascular Risk Calculator). Further, for adults aged 20 to 59 years with a 10-year risk of CVD less than 7.5%, a 30-year or lifetime CVD risk "may be considered."

The US Preventive Services Task Force recommends screening every 5 years: for men, starting at age 35 years, and for women, starting at age 45 years.

Therapy

Lipid-Lowering Therapy for ASCVD Reduction

Statins are the cornerstone of lipid-lowering therapy for ASCVD reduction. This group is the only class of lipid-lowering drugs that have consistently decreased CVD risk. Statins are used for both primary and secondary prevention of CVD. They mainly decrease levels of LDL-C. Depending on the type of statin and the dose used, they can decrease triglyceride levels by 20% to 40%. Fibrates and niacin have not resulted in any convincing improvement in clinical outcomes, and niacin may actually increase adverse cardiovascular outcomes.

Candidates for Therapy

According to the latest ACC/AHA guidelines, 4 high-risk groups should be considered for statin therapy to reduce the ASCVD risk (Box 15.2).

High-intensity statin therapy (aimed at an LDL-C reduction of ≥50%) is recommended for patients with known ASCVD, for patients with an LDL-C level of 190 mg/dL or more, and for diabetes mellitus patients with a 10-year ASCVD risk of at least 7.5%. Moderate-intensity statin treatment (aimed at an LDL-C reduction of 30%–49%) is recommended for the other groups: diabetes mellitus patients with a 10-year risk of an event of less than 7.5% (based on the risk calculator) and patients without diabetes mellitus who have a 10-year risk of at least 7.5%. The relevant statin doses are provided in Table 15.3.

Treatment Goals

Unlike the ATP III guidelines, the ACC/AHA guidelines do not recommend treating to reach particular goal levels of LDL-C or non-HDL-C. Instead, they recommend that patients be followed to assess for an appropriate response to treatment as predicted according to the dose of statin used.

Box 15.2 • High-Risk Groups to Be Considered for Statin Therapy

Patients with known atherosclerotic cardiovascular disease

Patients with LDL-C level ≥190 mg/dL

Patients with diabetes mellitus who are 40–75 y old and have LDL-C levels of 70–189 mg/dL

Patients with a 10-year risk of cardiac event or stroke ≥7.5% (by the Pooled Cohort Equations Cardiovascular Risk Calculator)

Abbreviation: LDL-C, low-density lipoprotein cholesterol.

Adapted from Stone NJ, Robinson JG, Lichtenstein AH, Bairey Merz CN, Blum CB, Eckel RH, et al; American College of Cardiology/American Heart Association Task Force on Practice Guidelines. 2013 ACC/AHA guideline on the treatment of blood cholesterol to reduce atherosclerotic cardiovascular risk in adults: a report of the American College of Cardiology/American Heart Association Task Force on Practice Guidelines. Circulation. 2014 Jun 24;129(25 Suppl 2):S1–45. Epub 2013 Nov 12. Erratum in: Circulation. 2014 Jun 24;129(25 Suppl 2):S46–8 and Stone NJ, Robinson JG, Lichtenstein AH, Bairey Merz CN, Blum CB, Eckel RH, et al; American College of Cardiology/American Heart Association Task Force on Practice Guidelines. 2013 ACC/AHA guideline on the treatment of blood cholesterol to reduce atherosclerotic cardiovascular risk in adults: a report of the American College of Cardiology/American Heart Association Task Force on Practice Guidelines. J Am Coll Cardiol. 2014 Jul 1;63(25 Pt B):2889–934. Epub 2013 Nov 12. Erratum in: J Am Coll Cardiol. 2014 Jul 1;63(25 Pt B):3024–5. Used with permission.

Table 15.3 • Statin Therapy for Reducing the Risk of Atherosclerotic Cardiovascular Disease

Statin Therapy	Daily Dose, mg
High-dose	
Atorvastatin	40–80
Rosuvastatin	20–40
Moderate-dose	
Atorvastatin	10–20
Rosuvastatin	5–10
Simvastatin	20–40
Pravastatin	40–80
Lovastatin	40
Fluvastatin	80
Pitavastatin	2–4

If the response is less than expected, the guidelines recommend increasing the intensity of treatment. This approach reflects a paradigm shift in the strategy for lowering lipids to reduce CVD risk: Now the focus of treatment is on the baseline cardiovascular risk, as opposed to the traditional emphasis on a target LDL-C level.

KEY FACTS

✓ Causes of lipid disorders—genetic abnormalities, various medical conditions, and certain drugs

✓ Dyslipidemia—usually asymptomatic, but a modifiable risk factor for CVD

✓ ACC/AHA criteria for consideration of statin therapy in 4 high-risk groups—1) known ASCVD; 2) LDL-C ≥190 mg/dL; 3) diabetes mellitus, age 40–75 years, and LDL-C 70–189 mg/dL; and 4) ≥7.5% 10-year risk of cardiac event or stroke

✓ ACC/AHA recommendation—do not treat with statins to reach specific LDL-C or non-HDL-C goals

Nonstatin Medications

If a patient is intolerant of statins or does not achieve the desirable LDL-C reduction with statin monotherapy, medications such as ezetimibe, niacin, and bile-acid sequestrants can be considered. Also, fibric acid therapy is appropriate for patients who have diabetes mellitus and triglyceride levels above 400 mg/dL despite adequate lifestyle interventions and diabetes management. Bile acid sequestrants, however, may have significant gastrointestinal tract adverse effects (nausea, bloating, cramping) and can cause elevations in triglyceride levels.

Therapeutic Lifestyle Change

Healthy dietary habits, regular exercise, weight management, and smoking cessation should be recommended to all patients with elevated CVD risk regardless of whether they are candidates for statin therapy. The AHA step 1 diet recommends limiting dietary fat intake (to ≤30% of total calories, with <10% of calories from saturated fat and avoidance of *trans*-fatty acids). Alcohol restriction can decrease triglyceride concentrations. The AHA recommends moderate-intensity aerobic activity for at least 150 minutes weekly.

Monitoring Patients

Patients should be evaluated 4 to 12 weeks after statin initiation to assess for treatment response and adverse effects. A fasting lipid panel should be rechecked. There is no role for routine measurement of hepatic enzymes or markers of muscle injury (eg, creatine kinase level) unless the patient has concerning symptoms.

Management of Hypertriglyceridemia

Normal fasting triglyceride levels are less than 150 mg/dL. Triglyceride elevations are defined as *borderline high* (150–199 mg/dL), *high* (200–499 mg/dL), or *very high* (≥500 mg/dL).

Elevated triglycerides are associated with an increased risk of CVD, but it is unclear whether this association is causal. High triglycerides are also associated with other potential atherogenic abnormalities, including a low level of HDL-C, small dense LDL particles, and insulin resistance.

Pancreatitis is a rare complication of *severe* hypertriglyceridemia (usually >1,000 mg/dL). Therefore, treatment of mild to moderate hypertriglyceridemia (≤500 mg/dL), and perhaps even treatment of severe hypertriglyceridemia with levels less than 1,000 mg/dL, is mainly for CVD risk reduction and *not* for pancreatitis prevention or triglyceride lowering per se.

Lifestyle change is the cornerstone of management of elevated triglycerides. Triglyceride levels are exquisitely sensitive to diet and physical activity level. Consequently, limiting simple carbohydrate and alcohol intake, performing physical activity on a regular basis, and losing weight can significantly reduce triglyceride levels. Lowering total fat intake is necessary, however, for patients with severe hypertriglyceridemia to avoid chylomicronemia and the risk of pancreatitis. Strict glycemic control in patients with diabetes mellitus and avoidance of any medications causing hypertriglyceridemia (whenever possible) should be considered.

If a patient has persistently elevated triglycerides despite lifestyle interventions, and the goal of treatment is cardiovascular risk reduction, a statin is the treatment of choice, even though it is not primarily a triglyceride-lowering medication. Statins are the only class of lipid-lowering medications that have shown consistent benefit in lowering cardiovascular morbidity and mortality. However, if the goal of treatment is triglyceride reduction, as for patients with severe hypertriglyceridemia with its attendant risk of pancreatitis, patients are treated with a fibric acid derivative, nicotinic acid, or fish oil alone or in combination.

Fibric acid derivatives include gemfibrozil and fenofibrate. Gemfibrozil should be avoided in combination with a statin because of the increased chance of statin-induced myopathy. Fenofibrate is neutral from that standpoint.

Nicotinic acid may worsen glycemic control in patients with diabetes mellitus and may cause flushing, limiting its tolerability. Administering aspirin 30 to 60 minutes before the patient takes nicotinic acid can minimize flushing.

The use of ω-3 fatty acids (docosahexaenoic acid [DHA] and eicosapentaenoic acid [EPA]) effectively reduces triglycerides at doses greater than 3 g daily. Prescription formulations are nearly 100% ω-3 fatty acids, allowing for more effective dosing compared with over-the-counter formulations. The main side effects of ω-3 fatty acids are gastrointestinal (nausea and fishy taste). Their use should be limited to patients with refractory hypertriglyceridemia.

Management of Low HDL-C

The latest ACC/AHA guidelines on cholesterol reduction for ASCVD risk reduction do not recommend specific medical therapy for patients with low HDL-C per se. Statin therapy is indicated for such patients if they meet any of the criteria for treatment, as previously discussed in this chapter. Studies have not shown any cardiovascular benefit with the use of specific therapies for increasing HDL-C levels, including nicotinic acid and fibric acid derivatives.

Lifestyle changes, including exercise, weight loss (in overweight patients), substitution of monounsaturated fatty acids for saturated fatty acids, and smoking cessation can raise HDL-C levels. Drugs causing low HDL-C should be discontinued whenever possible.

KEY FACTS

✓ Recommend therapeutic lifestyle changes (healthy diet, exercise, weight management, and smoking cessation) to *all* patients with elevated CVD risk

✓ Key to managing elevated triglycerides—lifestyle change

✓ Severe hypertriglyceridemia—need to decrease total fat intake

16 Obesity and Nutritional Disorders

RYAN T. HURT, MD, PHD

Obesity

Etiology

The prevalence of overweight and obesity has been increasing in the United States and the westernized world. The cause of the recent obesity epidemic involves a complex interplay between genetic and environmental factors. Specific, rare genetic disruptions of the hypothalamic regulation of energy homeostasis pathways can cause obesity (eg, Prader-Willi syndrome). Most cases of obesity result from a group of gene variants exposed to environmental factors. The 2 major environmental factors that contribute to overweight and obesity are excess caloric intake and low physical activity. Additional risk factors include smoking cessation, sleep deprivation, contributory social networks, lower socioeconomic status, medications, and, less commonly, health conditions.

Health Risk Assessment

Body mass index (BMI) (calculated as weight in kilograms divided by height in meters squared) is used to assess the health risk of body weight. Waist circumference (WC), another variable used to predict health risk, is a surrogate for visceral fat. WC is most useful for persons who have a BMI between 25 and 35. Persons who have an increased BMI in combination with an increased WC, which indicates excess visceral fat, have a greater health risk than if the BMI alone is increased. BMI values greater than 35 are associated with high health risk anyway, so in that BMI range, WC is less meaningful (Table 16.1).

Overweight (BMI 25.0–29.9) and **obesity** (BMI ≥30) are associated with increased morbidity and mortality (Box 16.1). Some of the increased mortality risk may be negated by cardiovascular fitness. Screening for weight-related medical complications is indicated (measurement of blood pressure, fasting blood glucose or hemoglobin A_{1c}, lipid profile, and thyrotropin and evaluation for obstructive sleep apnea).

> ### Key Definitions
>
> Overweight: *BMI 25.0–29.9.*
> Obesity: *BMI ≥30.*

Obesity Management

Implementation of healthy lifestyle changes is the key factor to managing overweight and obesity. Dietary changes with caloric restriction (by 250–500 kcal daily) are required for weight loss. Macronutrient composition has minimal impact on weight loss at 12 months. Regular physical activity promotes weight loss by creating an additional caloric deficit but is insufficient alone. However, regular physical activity is a key determinant to maintaining weight loss.

Achieving an initial weight loss goal of 5% to 10% of initial body weight is associated with multiple benefits, including prevention of type 2 diabetes mellitus. Predictors of weight loss success include having a higher initial body weight, engaging in more minutes of physical activity weekly, recording caloric intake, and participating in group behavioral therapy. Considerable weight loss occurs with aggressive dietary restriction (very low-calorie diets of <800 kcal daily) and bariatric surgery, but with very low-calorie diets, the prevalence of weight regain is high.

Medications for Weight Loss

Use of medication improves the likelihood of losing 5% to 10% of initial body weight. The 4 medications that are approved by the US Food and Drug Administration for obesity are phentermine (for short-term use; <12 weeks), orlistat, lorcaserin, and phentermine-topiramate extended-release capsules (Table 16.2). Medications are generally reserved for patients who are obese or overweight and have at least 1 obesity-associated comorbidity.

Table 16.1 • Body Mass Index, Waist Circumference, and Health Risk

BMI	BMI Classification	WC	Health Risk BMI Alone	Health Risk BMI With WC
<18.5	Underweight			
18.5–24.9	Normal			
25.0–29.9	Overweight		Increased	
		Women: >88		High
		Men: >102		High
30.0–34.9	Class I obesity		High	
		Women: >88		Very high
		Men: >102		Very high
35.0–39.9	Class II obesity		Very high	
≥40.0	Class III obesity		Extremely high	

Abbreviations: BMI, body mass index (calculated as weight in kilograms divided by height in meters squared); WC, waist circumference in centimeters.

Adapted from National Institutes of Health, National Heart, Lung, and Blood Institute, North American Association for the Study of Obesity. The practical guide: identification, evaluation, and treatment of overweight and obesity in adults. Bethesda (MD): National Institutes of Health; c2000. NIH Publication No. 00-4084.

Phentermine is a sympathomimetic agent that suppresses appetite, but few long-term studies (>12 weeks) have been performed, and there are insufficient data detailing efficacy and safety. Phentermine has not been implicated in the development of cardiac valve abnormalities and pulmonary hypertension. Patients previously treated with fenfluramine or dexfenfluramine should be evaluated for cardiac valve abnormalities. Sibutramine was removed from the market after it was reported to increase the risk of nonfatal heart attacks and stroke in a high-risk population.

Orlistat is a lipase inhibitor that limits dietary fat absorption. Administered with a low-fat diet (fat <30% of calories),

it is associated with greater weight loss than placebo. The main side effects involve the gastrointestinal tract; diarrhea and flatulence often limit adherence to therapy. A daily multivitamin is recommended to prevent vitamin deficiencies. Concurrent use with medications influenced by fat absorption (eg, cyclosporine, amiodarone, warfarin) can limit the efficacy of those drugs.

Lorcaserin is a selective serotonin receptor agonist that can lead to satiety, hypophagia, and subsequent weight loss. In combination with a hypocaloric diet, lorcaserin was associated with greater weight loss than placebo in several large studies. Participants receiving lorcaserin did not have the valvular abnormalities that were identified in patients receiving other nonselective serotonin agonists (fenfluramine and dexfenfluramine). The use of lorcaserin can lead to serotonin syndrome, especially when combined with medications that increase serotonin levels.

Phentermine-topiramate extended-release capsules combine 2 medications known to lead to weight loss. The weight loss mechanism for topiramate is not known, but, like lorcaserin, topiramate in combination with a hypocaloric diet was associated with greater weight loss than placebo in several large studies. Phentermine-topiramate extended-release capsules are contraindicated in pregnancy because of the risk of cleft lip and cleft palate.

Bariatric Surgery

The indications for bariatric surgery include the following: 1) BMI greater than 40 *or* 2) BMI greater than 35 *and* weight-related medical comorbidities, documented efforts at medically supervised weight management, absence of

---

Box 16.1 • Health Risks Associated With Obesity

Type 2 diabetes mellitus
Hypertriglyceridemia
Hypertension
Obstructive sleep apnea
Coronary artery disease
Congestive heart failure
Atrial fibrillation
Thromboembolic disease
Degenerative joint disease
Gastroesophageal reflux disease
Nonalcoholic steatohepatitis
Cancer
Death

Table 16.2 • Approved Pharmacologic Agents for the Treatment of Obesity

Drug	Mechanism	Contraindications	Common Adverse Effects
Phentermine	Sympathomimetic	Pregnancy, breastfeeding, glaucoma, hyperthyroidism, use of MAOI within 14 d, history of cardiovascular disease	Insomnia, tremor, headache, risk of dependency, palpitations, elevated blood pressure
Orlistat	Pancreatic lipase inhibitor	Pregnancy, cholestasis, chronic malabsorption syndromes	Abdominal pain, bloating, diarrhea, acute pancreatitis, renal failure
Lorcaserin	Selective serotonin 2C receptor agonist	Pregnancy	Headache, back pain, nasopharyngitis, nausea, dizziness
Phentermine-topiramate ER	Sympathomimetic and anticonvulsant	Pregnancy, breastfeeding, glaucoma, hyperthyroidism, use of MAOI within 14 d, history of cardiovascular disease	Dizziness, dry mouth, constipation, depression, insomnia, tremor, headache, risk of dependency, palpitations, elevated blood pressure

Abbreviations: ER, extended-release; MAOI, monoamine oxidase inhibitor.

psychologic contraindications, and life expectancy of more than 5 years.

Mechanisms for weight loss after bariatric surgery vary (Box 16.2). The most commonly performed operation is the Roux-en-Y gastric bypass (RYGB), and data have demonstrated its beneficial effects, including prevention and resolution of type 2 diabetes mellitus. Resolution rates have been reported for other medical problems, including obstructive sleep apnea, gastroesophageal reflux disease, hypertriglyceridemia, and hypertension. Restrictive operations are generally associated with less weight loss and lower resolution rates for most obesity-related complications, and biliopancreatic diversion with a duodenal switch (BPD-DS) is associated with the greatest reported weight loss and the greatest effect on the complications of excess weight.

Early Complications of Bariatric Surgery

Reported perioperative mortality with bariatric surgery is less than 1%. The most common cause of death is pulmonary embolism. Anastomotic leak with subsequent peritonitis is the second most common cause of death with RYGB and BPD-DS. A high level of awareness is critical when assessing an ill patient presenting with dyspnea or abdominal pain within weeks after a bariatric operation.

Box 16.2 • Mechanisms for Weight Loss After Bariatric Surgery

Dietary restriction—vertical banded gastroplasty, laparoscopic adjustable gastric banding, and sleeve gastrectomy

Malabsorptive—biliopancreatic diversion with a duodenal switch

Combination of restriction and malabsorptive—Roux-en-Y gastric bypass

---

Sinus tachycardia is the most common physical finding in patients with an anastomotic leak. Risk factors associated with higher perioperative morbidity and mortality are male sex, age older than 60 years, BMI greater than 60, smoking, untreated obstructive sleep apnea, inactivity, and surgeon inexperience.

Anastomotic complications are also common after RYGB. Anastomotic ulcerations and stricture of the gastrojejunal anastomosis are the most common. Risk factors include use of nonsteroidal anti-inflammatory drugs, prior *Helicobacter pylori* infection, and smoking. Presenting symptoms include epigastric pain with or without nausea and vomiting. Esophagogastroduodenoscopy is the diagnostic study of choice; balloon dilation of a stricture can be performed. Anastomotic ulcers are effectively treated with proton pump inhibitors with or without sucralfate.

Nutrition After Bariatric Surgery

Nutritional deficiencies are recognized complications of bariatric surgery; therefore, empirical vitamin supplementation is recommended for all patients after surgery and should include vitamin B_{12}, a multivitamin, and calcium with vitamin D.

After any bariatric procedure, acute thiamine deficiency can occur in a patient who is vomiting and cannot maintain adequate oral intake over several days. In addition to gastrointestinal tract symptoms, neurologic complaints are common. Wernicke-Korsakoff syndrome may occur, so thiamine must be supplemented before intravenous infusion of dextrose-containing fluids.

Anemia is the most common manifestation of deficiencies of iron, vitamin B_{12}, or folate; it resolves with appropriate supplementation. Iron deficiency anemia is the most common vitamin deficiency reported, especially among menstruating women. Folate and vitamin B_{12} deficiencies are less common as a result of empirical supplementation, but a high level of awareness is needed because of the variable adherence to vitamin supplementation regimens. Neurologic complications due to vitamin B_{12} deficiency may not resolve. Care must be taken to assess folate status before supplementation. Measuring the ferritin level is a reliable screening test for iron deficiency. Low vitamin B_{12} levels should be confirmed with a methylmalonic acid level.

Inadequate diet, inadequate supplementation, and, often, persistent gastrointestinal tract symptoms such as diarrhea can lead to chronic nutritional deficiencies. Vitamin D deficiency is common among obese patients seeking bariatric surgery and may worsen during rapid weight loss after surgery. Hypocalcemia is a late finding and is often absent with mild or moderate deficiencies. The most common early findings may be increased parameters of bone turnover (elevated bone alkaline phosphatase level) and secondary hyperparathyroidism (elevated parathyroid hormone level). Secondary hyperparathyroidism is also influenced by decreased dietary calcium. The only way to detect calcium deficiency early is by identifying hypocalciuria in a 24-hour urine collection. Long-term vitamin D deficiency can lead to metabolic bone disease with low bone mineral density or mineralization defects (or both), resulting in osteomalacia. Deficiencies of other fat-soluble vitamins besides vitamin D (vitamins A, E, and K) are less common but may occur. Protein malnutrition is a worrisome complication of BPD-DS, which must be reversed in 1% to 2% of patients.

KEY FACTS

- ✓ Medications may be used in combination with lifestyle changes to treat obesity
- ✓ Obese patients can gain cardiovascular benefits from losing as little as 5% of their initial weight
- ✓ Vitamin deficiencies—a risk for patients after bariatric surgery
- ✓ Confirmation of low vitamin B_{12} level—high methylmalonic acid level

---

Late Complications of Bariatric Surgery

After bariatric surgery, cholelithiasis develops in one-third of patients; 40% become symptomatic. Prophylactic cholecystectomy was commonly performed at bariatric surgery when it was an open abdominal operation (before the laparoscopic approach became common). Administration of ursodeoxycholic acid for 6 months after surgery decreases the prevalence of gallstone development and is gaining popularity. Therefore, prophylactic cholecystectomy is no longer indicated.

Bacterial overgrowth is common after RYGB and BPD-DS. Abdominal pain and bloating associated with diarrhea are common symptoms. Esophagogastroduodenoscopy with small-bowel aspirates for culture or breath tests are usually diagnostic. When bacterial overgrowth is suspected or confirmed, antibiotic therapy should be instituted; various regimens are available. Resolution of symptoms occurs within 1 week. Bacterial overgrowth can recur, worsening the malabsorption of nutrients and increasing the risk of vitamin deficiencies.

Other complications include renal stone disease (primarily calcium oxalate stones). Fat malabsorption and dietary calcium allow increased absorption of intestinal oxalate, increasing the risk of calcium oxalate stone formation. Insulin-mediated hypoglycemia may occur in patients who have postprandial symptoms that suggest hypoglycemia. Symptoms may be difficult to differentiate from those of classic dumping syndrome. Further evaluation requires documentation of hypoglycemia (blood glucose <55 mg/dL), endogenous hyperinsulinemia (insulin >3 mcIU/mL; C peptide >0.2 ng/mL), and a negative sulfonylurea screen while the patient is symptomatic.

Nutrition

Ideal weight is reflected by BMI values from 18.5 to 24.9. Persons with BMI values less than 18.5 are considered underweight, and the risk of morbidity and mortality increases with BMI values less than 15.

An optimal diet should provide the caloric requirements to maintain the weight within an ideal BMI range and minimize the risk of illness. A high intake of fruits and vegetables has been consistently shown to provide multiple health benefits, particularly in lowering the risk of cardiovascular disease (Box 16.3).

Micronutrient Supplementation

Multivitamin supplementation has not been shown to provide health benefits to the population at large, and it is recommended only for persons not meeting their nutritional needs orally owing to illness or self-imposed dietary

---

Box 16.3 • Dietary Guidelines to Decrease the Risk of Cardiovascular Disease

Restrict dietary protein to <20% of total calories

Prefer lean meats

Restrict dietary fat to <35% of total calories

Avoid *trans* fats

Restrict saturated fats to <10% of total calories

Restrict dietary cholesterol to <300 mg daily

Prefer polyunsaturated fats

Restrict dietary carbohydrates to <55% of total calories

Prefer fruits, vegetables, and whole grains

Restrict the intake of refined carbohydrates, processed grains, and starches

restriction. The benefits of empirical vitamin supplementation have been reported for folic acid in women of childbearing age (to prevent neural tube defects) and for vitamin D (to prevent metabolic bone disease).

Empirical supplementation of antioxidant vitamins (β-carotene and vitamin E) to prevent cardiovascular disease is no longer advised owing to a lack of benefit and the potential risk of lung cancer in smokers and patients who have a history of asbestos exposure. Folic acid supplementation to decrease homocysteine levels is no longer advised owing to a lack of benefit in preventing cardiovascular disease.

Supplementation with ω-3 fatty acids (docosahexaenoic acid [DHA] and eicosapentaenoic acid [EPA]) lowers cardiovascular mortality. Eating at least 1 serving of a fatty fish (rich in ω-3 fatty acids) weekly or supplementing with DHA and EPA is beneficial, with studies suggesting that antiarrhythmic properties contribute to a lower risk of cardiovascular death. Higher doses lower triglyceride levels.

Micronutrient Deficiencies

In the general population, nutritional deficiencies of calcium, vitamin D, vitamin B_{12}, and iron are common. Current dietary intake of dairy products and other food sources of calcium is low. Recommended calcium intake varies by age, and calcium supplementation is effective. Various calcium preparations are available. Calcium carbonate requires gastric acid for optimal absorption, so dosing is advised with meals; efficacy may be lower with medications that decrease gastric acid secretion. Calcium citrate is generally better absorbed, and it is preferred if a patient has a gastrointestinal tract illness.

Vitamin D deficiency is associated with decreased sun exposure, inflammatory bowel disease, and renal disease. Vitamin D status is reflected by 25-hydroxyvitamin D levels (reference range, 20–50 ng/mL). Mild to moderate deficiencies (10–20 ng/mL) are common, are often asymptomatic, and can be associated with secondary hyperparathyroidism. Severe deficiency (<10 ng/mL) increases the risk of bone mineralization defects and osteomalacia. Patients often report deep bone pain and proximal muscle weakness.

Deficiences of vitamin D and other fat-soluble vitamins (vitamins A, E, and K) occur in patients with inflammatory bowel disease, short bowel syndrome, bariatric surgery, or other malabsorption disease states. Deficiency of vitamin A (retinol) can lead to night blindness or xerophthalmia. Vitamin E deficiency is rare, but it can lead to neuromuscular disease with clinical manifestations, including ataxia, decreased proprioceptive and vibratory sensations, and hyporeflexia. Clinical signs of vitamin K deficiency include easy bruising, mucosal bleeding, and any other symptoms of abnormal coagulation.

The cause of vitamin B_{12} deficiency can be 1) autoimmune (eg, pernicious anemia, which is characterized by the presence of anti–parietal cell antibodies); 2) gastrointestinal tract disease impairing vitamin B_{12} absorption (eg, inflammatory bowel disease or any gastrointestinal tract surgery or illness affecting the gastric antrum or ileum); or 3) medications (eg, metformin). A low vitamin B_{12} level (<100 ng/L) is consistent with a deficiency. Low-normal values should be evaluated with a methylmalonic acid measurement; a deficiency is indicated by an elevated level of methylmalonic acid. Macrocytic anemia is the most common presenting abnormality. Neurologic symptoms can occur and may not fully resolve if identification and supplementation are delayed. Patients with vitamin B_{12} deficiency should receive parenteral supplementation, particularly if they have neurologic symptoms or if the underlying cause is abnormal gastrointestinal tract absorption. Vitamin B_{12} levels should be monitored until they are in the reference range. To maintain adequate levels, vitamin B_{12} can be administered orally or parenterally. Folate levels should be checked before supplementing vitamin B_{12}.

Iron deficiency is another common micronutrient deficiency, and it is the most common abnormality in patients with celiac sprue. Other persons at risk include those with self-imposed dietary restrictions (including vegetarians and vegans), patients who have gastrointestinal tract illness or have had surgery affecting the duodenum (where most iron is absorbed), and women with heavy menses. Oral supplementation is sufficient unless more aggressive treatment with packed cell transfusion is needed or the patient is intolerant of oral iron.

Zinc and copper deficiencies can occur in patients with long-term parenteral nutrition, bariatric surgery, or malabsorptive diseases. Signs and symptoms of zinc deficiency include dysgeusia, alopecia, impaired wound healing, and dermatitis. Signs of copper deficiency include ataxia, neuropathy, anemia, and neutropenia. Patients with niacin deficiency can present with glossitis, dermatitis, dementia, and diarrhea.

Nutritional Support

During illness, patients often do not meet their nutritional needs orally. A weight loss of more than 5% of initial body weight suggests inadequate nutrition, and the need for nutritional support should be assessed.

If adequate oral intake can be resumed within 7 to 14 days, previously healthy patients generally do not benefit from nutritional support. Intravenous fluid hydration is adequate for most patients in an uncomplicated hospital setting. The potential need for nutritional support should be considered for critically ill patients and for patients with a BMI less than 18.5, a loss of 5% of initial body weight in 1 month, a loss of 10% of initial body weight in 6 months, more than 14 days of not meeting nutritional needs, or multiple organ failure.

Enteral feedings (delivered into the stomach with a nasogastric tube or as postpyloric feedings) are preferred unless contraindicated. Patients who benefit include perioperative patients with chronic liver disease, critically ill patients, and malnourished geriatric patients. Enteral feedings also reduce the risk of sepsis.

Gastric feedings should be avoided in clinical settings that may promote intolerance or potential complications, including any conditions that impair gastric emptying or increase the risk of aspiration. Most medications can be provided by this route.

Patients with contraindications or intolerance to gastric feedings or concerns with potential complications from gastric feeding should receive postpyloric feedings. Fewer medications can be safely administered by this route.

Parenteral nutrition is advised for patients who do not meet their nutritional needs for 7 to 14 days and have contraindications or intolerance to enteral feedings. Parenteral nutrition is associated with risks, and patients must be monitored appropriately.

Hyperglycemia is the most common complication, and glucose monitoring is advised. Hypertriglyceridemia is a recognized complication; limiting calories provided as fat is advised for patients with triglyceride levels greater than 300 mg/dL. An increased risk of bloodstream infection (bacterial and fungal organisms) is associated with parenteral nutrition. For patients receiving parenteral nutrition, the risk of fungal infection is up to 5-fold greater. Common risk factors include poor hygiene in managing venous access and formula, severity of illness, and duration of catheter insertion.

Ideally, nutritional needs are calculated with an accurate body weight, which is often difficult to measure if the patient is critically ill. Protein needs are higher in critically ill patients, but caution must be taken if patients have comorbidities contraindicating a high-protein load (eg, renal insufficiency, liver disease).

Refeeding syndrome is a recognized complication of aggressive nutritional support. It is most frequently observed in significantly underweight patients (BMI <15) who are receiving parenteral nutrition. Abnormalities due to hyperinsulinemia occur in response to feedings and include hypokalemia, hypophosphatemia, hypomagnesemia, volume overload, and edema, with hypophosphatemia being very common. Severe hypophosphatemia is associated with heart failure, arrhythmias, impaired diaphragmatic contractility, liver function test abnormalities, delirium, and seizures. Patients at risk of refeeding syndrome must be recognized so that the necessary precautions can be taken. Prevention includes gradual caloric progression, monitoring of clinical status, and correction of electrolyte abnormalities identified before the initiation of nutritional support.

KEY FACTS

✓ Iron deficiency anemia—common in patients with celiac sprue

✓ Copper deficiency—mimics neurologic signs of vitamin B_{12} deficiency

✓ Major complications of parental nutrition—hyperglycemia, central line infections, liver disease, and vitamin deficiencies

✓ Hypophosphatemia—a common sign of refeeding syndrome

17 Pituitary Disorders

PANKAJ SHAH, MD

Hypopituitarism

Etiology

Hypopituitarism usually results from a deficiency of anterior pituitary hormones or, rarely, from tissue resistance to these hormones. Deficiency may be from primary pituitary disease, pituitary stalk disorders, hypothalamic disease, or an extrasellar disorder impinging on, or infiltrating, the hypothalamic-pituitary unit.

Primary pituitary disease results from the loss of anterior pituitary cells and may be congenital or acquired. Common causes are pituitary tumors and their surgical or radiotherapeutic ablation. Infrequent causes include pituitary infarction (eg, postpartum pituitary necrosis, also known as Sheehan syndrome), pituitary apoplexy, lymphocytic hypophysitis, infiltrative diseases (eg, hemochromatosis), and metastatic disease (eg, from breast or lung).

Hypothalamic hypopituitarism results from hypothalamic or pituitary stalk disease associated with the loss of hypophysiotropic regulatory hormones of the anterior pituitary cells. Primary hypothalamic diseases are relatively rare and include disorders that are genetic (Kallmann syndrome); traumatic (accidental, surgical, or radiotherapeutic); inflammatory or infiltrative (eg, tuberculosis, sarcoidosis, and histiocytosis X); vascular (eg, bleeding disorders and vasculitis); or neoplastic, including primary neoplasms (eg, glioma, ependymoma, hamartoma, and gangliocytoma) and metastatic neoplasms.

Functional hypothalamic disorders are common (Box 17.1). A structural hypothalamic disorder is not evident in a functional hypothalamic disorder, and normal endocrine function is ultimately restored after the cause is managed or removed.

Extrasellar disorders impinge on and impair the function of the hypothalamic-pituitary unit. Examples include craniopharyngioma (most common), optic glioma, meningioma, nasopharyngeal carcinoma, sphenoid sinus mucocele, and carotid artery aneurysms.

Box 17.1 • Functional Hypothalamic Disorders and Related Causes

Functional suppression of gonadotropin-releasing hormone (GnRH)—weight disorders, exercise, psychiatric disorders, systemic disease, or endocrinopathy (eg, hyperprolactinemia, thyroid or adrenal disorders, and severely uncontrolled diabetes mellitus)

Functional lack of growth hormone (GH)—emotional deprivation syndrome

Functional lack of corticotropin (ACTH)—withdrawal of prolonged supraphysiologic glucocorticoid therapy

Functional lack of thyrotropin (TSH)—correction of a hyperthyroid state (first few weeks)

Clinical Features

Patients with hypopituitarism can present with features of deficiency of 1 or more of the anterior pituitary hormones. The clinical picture depends on the age at onset, hormones affected, extent and duration of deficiency, and acuteness of the process. The most common presentation is that of a chronic process of insidious onset.

Chronic Illness

Gonadotropin Deficiency

The features of gonadotropin deficiency are from deficiency of sex hormones and diminished fertility. Women may have infertility, oligomenorrhea or amenorrhea, loss of libido, vaginal dryness and dyspareunia, involution of the uterus and genitalia, and atrophy or loss of secondary sex characteristics. Male patients may have loss of libido, potency impairment, infertility, atrophy or loss of secondary sex characteristics, atrophy of the testes and prostate, and, occasionally, gynecomastia. In both sexes, fine wrinkling of the skin may be seen radially around the mouth or eyes, and osteoporosis may occur.

Corticotropin Deficiency

The features of corticotropin (ACTH) deficiency result primarily from a lack of cortisol. These features include malaise, anorexia, weight loss, gastrointestinal tract disturbances, rheumatologic aches and pains, hypoglycemia, hyponatremia, susceptibility to adrenocortical crises, pallor, an inability to tan or maintain a tan, and a loss of skin pigmentation. The features of mineralocorticoid deficiency are absent because aldosterone secretion depends on the renin-angiotensin system, not on ACTH; therefore, hyperkalemia and hypovolemia with orthostatism are typically absent. Partial ACTH deficiency may cause symptoms only during periods of acute medical or surgical illness, when elevated cortisol levels are needed.

Thyrotropin Deficiency

Thyrotropin (TSH) deficiency results in a lack of thyroid hormones (triiodothyronine [T_3] and thyroxine [T_4]) and the characteristic features of slowing of emotional, mental, and physical functions. The thyroid gland is atrophic.

Prolactin Deficiency

Postpartum women who have prolactin deficiency cannot lactate. Prolactin deficiency does not cause other symptoms in women or men.

Growth Hormone Deficiency

The features of growth hormone (GH) deficiency in adults are nonspecific and include ill health and asthenia, fatigue, muscle weakness, osteopenia, obesity, psychosocial difficulties, and increased cardiovascular risk.

Acute Illness

Adrenocortical crises may be precipitated by various events (Box 17.2). Manifestations of acute pituitary deficiency include fasting hypoglycemia (decreased hepatic glucose release due to lack of cortisol and GH); hyponatremic syndrome (decreased free water clearance with cortisol and thyroxine deficiency, renal water conservation

---

Box 17.2 • Causes of Adrenocortical Crises

Withdrawal of prolonged glucocorticoid therapy without proper glucocorticoid coverage during recovery of the hypothalamic-pituitary-adrenal axis

Pituitary surgery without optimal glucocorticoid stress coverage

Acute medical or surgical illness in a patient who has a lack of cortisol that is unrecognized or poorly managed

Pituitary apoplexy

Thyroid hormone replacement therapy in a patient who has an associated and unrecognized deficiency of corticotropin

---

due to decreased glomerular filtration rate and unchecked secretion of antidiuretic hormone [ADH]—ie, syndrome of inappropriate secretion of ADH [SIADH]); and increased sensitivity to central nervous system depressants (decreased metabolism and clearance due to lack of cortisol and thyroid hormones).

Diagnosis

Diagnosis of hypopituitarism requires documenting the presence of hypopituitarism *and* identifying the cause. In the appropriate clinical setting, provocative tests are used to accurately diagnose deficiencies of nontropic hormones, which act directly on target cells (eg, prolactin, oxytocin, and GH). For deficiencies of tropic hormones (eg, TSH, ACTH, luteinizing hormone [LH], follicle-stimulating hormone [FSH], and GH), which act on other endocrine glands, target gland function is evaluated: For TSH deficiency, measure free thyroxine; for ACTH deficiency, morning cortisol; for LH or FSH, testosterone or estrogen; and for GH, insulinlike growth factor 1 (Table 17.1). GH has both tropic and nontropic functions. In patients with target gland failure, tropic hormone levels must be determined to distinguish between primary target gland failure and failure due to hypothalamic-pituitary disease. Increased pituitary tropic hormone levels indicate target gland failure; normal or low tropic hormone levels indicate hypopituitarism.

Gonadotropin Axis

Male patients with hypopituitarism have a low serum testosterone level, inappropriately low serum LH and FSH levels, and a low sperm count. Testosterone is best measured in the morning because the testosterone concentration is lower in the afternoon and evenings.

Female patients have a low serum estradiol level and inappropriately low serum LH and FSH levels. Provocative tests for LH and FSH with gonadotropin-releasing hormone (GnRH) or clomiphene are rarely needed in clinical practice.

ACTH Axis

In the appropriate clinical setting, a cortisol value less than 3 mcg/dL strongly indicates adrenocortical failure. In an unstressed ambulatory patient, a serum cortisol concentration greater than 10 mcg/dL cortisol deficiency is unlikely, and a value greater than 18 mcg/dL excludes the diagnosis. If values are 3 to 10 mcg/dL, a provocative test should be used to assess adrenal function. Provocative tests may also be performed if clinical suspicion of glucocorticoid insufficiency is strong and the morning cortisol level is between 10 and 18 mcg/dL. Cortisol concentration is physiologically low and has no role in the diagnosis of cortisol deficiency.

In chronic ACTH deficiency, the adrenal cortices are atrophic and do not secrete cortisol in response to the

Table 17.1 • **Clinical Manifestations and Tests for Pituitary Hormone Deficiencies**

Hormone	Manifestation	Test
TSH	Cold intolerance, decreased appetite, dry skin, constipation, bradycardia, hyponatremia, depression	Free thyroxine level
ACTH	Malaise, lack of appetite, weight loss, nausea or vomiting, hyponatremia, hypoglycemia Women: decreased pubic and axillary hair	Morning cortisol level ACTH stimulation test
LH and FSH	Hypogonadism and infertility Men: decreased libido, erectile dysfunction, lack of energy, loss of pubic and axillary hair Women: amenorrhea, vaginal dryness, dyspareunia Men and women: fine wrinkles lateral to eyes and mouth	Men: sperm count—if normal, hypogonadism is ruled out; if abnormal, measure morning testosterone (total testosterone with or without bioavailable or free testosterone) Women: menstruation—if regular, hypogonadism is ruled out; if irregular, measure estradiol
GH	Nonspecific symptoms: lack of energy, muscle weakness, asthenia, fatigue, osteopenia, obesity, psychosocial difficulties, hypoglycemia	GH and IGF-1 Dynamic tests (arginine infusion or insulin hypoglycemia) are infrequently performed to confirm diagnosis and meet insurance needs
Prolactin	Failure to lactate	Testing for prolactin is rarely required
ADH	Polyuria, hypernatremia	24-h urine volume Serum and urine osmolality

Abbreviations: ACTH, corticotropin; ADH, antidiuretic hormone; FSH, follicle-stimulating hormone; GH, growth hormone; IGF-1, insulinlike growth factor 1; LH, luteinizing hormone; TSH, thyrotropin.

short-acting exogenous ACTH stimulation test (ie, the co-syntropin test). Adrenocortical failure is confirmed by the absence of an increased serum ACTH level and the absence of a cortisol response to exogenous ACTH stimulation.

In a patient with a recent-onset cortisol deficiency caused by a lack of ACTH from pituitary destruction (eg, from a postoperative cause, postpartum hemorrhage, or apoplexy), exogenous ACTH may stimulate cortisol production and produce a falsely reassuring test result despite glucocorticoid insufficiency.

TSH Axis

Low serum free T_4 and an inappropriately "normal" or low serum level of TSH support the diagnosis of central hypothyroidism. In contrast, in patients with primary hypothyroidism, TSH concentrations are high.

Growth Hormone

GH deficiency is likely present in a patient with demonstrable structural disease of the pituitary gland. A low age-specific serum level of insulinlike growth factor 1 (IGF-1) is a good screening test. In the absence of other pituitary hormone deficiencies, a provocative test is indicated if treatment with growth hormones is contemplated. The preferred test uses arginine in combination with GH-releasing hormone (GHRH). The insulin hypoglycemia test is performed with appropriate precautions; it is contraindicated in patients who have seizures or cerebrovascular or cardiovascular disease.

Prolactin

Tests for prolactin deficiency are rarely, if ever, needed in clinical practice.

Radiologic Evaluation

Radiologic evaluation includes imaging of the hypothalamic-pituitary region by magnetic resonance imaging (MRI) or computed tomography (CT) and, in the presence of suprasellar disease, neuro-ophthalmologic evaluation to assess visual fields, visual acuity, and optic discs. MRI is preferred.

In determining the cause of hypopituitarism, suspected functional causes must be removed or corrected. Normalization of pituitary function after correction of a functional cause lends support to "functional" hypopituitarism. If the functional causes are excluded, or if hypopituitarism persists despite removal or correction of a functional cause, evaluation for structural hypothalamic-pituitary disease is mandatory. This evaluation is based on the clinical setting and appropriate endocrine and anatomical studies.

Therapy

Therapy for hypopituitarism includes correction of the cause and, when applicable, administration of the hormones of the target glands or, in selected cases, pituitary hormones.

ACTH Deficiency

For ACTH deficiency, glucocorticoid replacement is critical. Instruct patients in dose modification during acute illness. In patients with a deficiency of both ACTH and TSH, initiate glucocorticoid therapy *before* thyroid hormone therapy to avoid a thyroid hormone–induced increased need for cortisol and precipitation of an acute adrenocortical crisis. Adequacy of therapy is judged by clinical criteria, resolution of symptoms, and the absence of signs and symptoms of supraphysiologic replacement. Serum ACTH levels cannot be used to assess adequacy of therapy.

The usual replacement dose of glucocorticoids is prednisone 4 to 7.5 mg in 1 or 2 doses or hydrocortisone 20 to 40 mg in 2 doses. The morning dose is taken soon after awakening and the evening dose in the afternoon. Mineralocorticoid replacement is not needed in glucocorticoid deficiency due to ACTH deficiency.

TSH Deficiency

For TSH deficiency, the drug of choice is levothyroxine. Assess the adequacy of therapy by the patient's feeling of well-being and the serum level of free T_4 in the mid-normal range. The serum TSH level should not be used to monitor the adequacy of the levothyroxine dose adjustment in hypothyroidism caused by TSH deficiency.

Gonadotropin Deficiency

Gonadotropin deficiency is treated with sex steroids. In female patients, estrogen therapy is used. Progestogens must be used for patients with an intact uterus. Birth control pills often provide adequate hormone replacement.

In male patients, testosterone can be given in the form of periodic injections, a transdermal gel or patch, or an inserted testosterone pellet. Assess the status of the prostate in middle-aged and elderly men before beginning therapy and recheck the status annually. If the testosterone concentration is in the goal range and the patient reports no symptomatic benefits, testosterone treatment is often withdrawn.

For restoration of fertility, FSH and LH (or GnRH therapy in patients with hypothalamic disorders and an intact pituitary) may be indicated. Evaluate the patient's psychosexual needs and lifestyle to assess the effect of therapy.

GH Deficiency

For GH deficiency, short-term GH therapy enhances a sense of well-being, improves body composition, increases muscle strength and exercise capacity, increases bone mineral density, and improves cardiac function. GH therapy is considered for patients with symptoms of GH deficiency especially if there is organic hypothalamic-pituitary disease. The goal of therapy is to restore the serum IGF-1 level to the reference range and to avoid side effects. If the IGF-1 concentration is in the goal range and the patient finds no symptomatic benefits, GH treatment is often withdrawn. The long-term effects of such therapy are unknown; thus, a benefit-risk profile cannot be determined.

KEY FACTS

✓ Hypopituitarism—usually from a deficiency of anterior pituitary hormones

✓ Diagnosis of hypopituitarism—document the cause in addition to documenting the presence of hypopituitarism

✓ Glucocorticoid (cortisol) deficiency should be corrected before correcting other hormone deficiencies

---

Pituitary Tumors

Pituitary tumors can be described by size, as microadenomas (≤10 mm) or macroadenomas (>10 mm); by extent, as sellar or as sellar and extrasellar; and by type, as functioning or nonfunctioning. These are almost always benign tumors. **Functioning pituitary tumors** include prolactinomas (40%–50%), GH-producing tumors (10%–15%), ACTH-producing tumors (10%–15%), and TSH-producing tumors (<5%). **Nonfunctioning pituitary tumors** (30%–40%) include the gonadotropin-producing tumors, tumors that make subunits (but not full hormones), and null-cell adenomas. Pituitary tumors are usually sporadic; rarely, they may be part of disorders such as multiple endocrine neoplasia type 1 (MEN-1), McCune-Albright syndrome, or Carney complex.

Key Definitions

Functioning pituitary tumors: *prolactinomas, GH-producing tumors, ACTH-producing tumors, and TSH-producing tumors.*

Nonfunctioning pituitary tumors: *gonadotropin-producing tumors, tumors that make hormone subunits, and null-cell adenomas.*

Clinical Features

The usual manifestation of a pituitary tumor is that of a chronic, slowly evolving disorder. The clinical features of pituitary tumors result from 3 components: 1) mass effect on surrounding structures; 2) hormone deficiency or excess caused by the mass effect; and 3) hormone excess from the tumor cells. These components may occur singly or in various combinations (Box 17.3). Rarely, pituitary tumors manifest acutely with pituitary apoplexy (acute hemorrhage into the pituitary gland), which may be the first clinical expression of the underlying tumor.

Diagnosis

The presence of a pituitary tumor is suggested by the clinical features and confirmed by pituitary imaging. MRI is the preferred imaging technique. Neuro-ophthalmologic

Box 17.3 • Clinical Features of Pituitary Tumors

Mass effects (headaches and evidence of tumor extension beyond the confines of the sella)

Superior tumor extension

Chiasma syndrome—impaired visual acuity and visual field defects

Hypothalamic syndrome—vegetative disturbance in thirst, appetite, satiety, sleep, and temperature regulation with diabetes insipidus or SIADH

Obstructive hydrocephalus

Frontal lobe dysfunction

Lateral tumor extension

Impairment of cranial nerves III, IV, V, and VI may result in diplopia, facial pain, and temporal lobe dysfunction

Inferior tumor extension

Nasopharyngeal mass

Cerebrospinal fluid rhinorrhea

Endocrine effects

Hypersecretory states

Gigantism or acromegaly (uncontrolled production of growth hormone)

Hyperprolactinemia (prolactin excess from interruption of the stalk or from prolactin produced by the tumor cells)

Cushing disease and Nelson-Salassa syndrome (corticotropin excess before and after adrenalectomy)

Thyrotoxicosis (thyrotropin excess), less often

Luteinizing hormone or follicle-stimulating hormone excess is usually clinically silent

Hypopituitarism

Caused by tumor growth that destroys the pituitary gland

Endocrine associations

MEN-1 (ie, parathyroid tumor or hyperplasia [primary hyperparathyroidism])

Endocrine pancreas tumor or hyperplasia (Zollinger-Ellison syndrome, hypoglycemia, or watery diarrhea)

Rarely, other endocrine gland tumors (thyroid or adrenal) and lipomas

Abbreviations: MEN-1, multiple endocrine neoplasia type 1; SIADH, syndrome of inappropriate secretion of antidiuretic hormone.

evaluation is important, particularly if suprasellar extension is present. Endocrine evaluation includes evaluation for hormonal excess or deficiency and for the presence of MEN-1. A pituitary tumor is diagnosed if a sellar mass is associated with an excess of anterior pituitary hormone (except for mild hyperprolactinemia, which can occur with nonpituitary masses and the "stalk effect"). Otherwise, the diagnosis is confirmed at surgical exploration.

Treatment

The first step in evaluation is to decide which type of treatment is appropriate for the patient. Pituitary tumors generally are treated with surgical excision or radiotherapy. Prolactinoma, a notable exception to this rule, is usually treated primarily with drug therapy. The conservative management approach of observation is an option for small tumors that have no effect on the quality or quantity of the patient's life, especially if the patient's expected lifespan is not long.

Dopamine agonists are often used as sole management for prolactinomas. Pituitary surgery is required for prolactinoma if the prolactin is not responding to dopamine agonists or if the patient cannot tolerate these agents. All other pituitary tumors are primarily treated with surgery.

Transsphenoidal surgery is the operation of choice for most tumors; the transcranial approach is used if there is a large suprasellar tumor extension. Surgical morbidity and mortality and the available neurosurgical expertise should be considered. Morbidity (eg, bleeding, infection, transient diabetes insipidus, and cerebrospinal fluid rhinorrhea) is less than 1% with microadenomas and less than 4% with macroadenomas; mortality is less than 1% with an experienced surgeon. Persistence or recurrence of the tumor is less than 20% to 30% for microadenomas and 50% to 70% for macroadenomas.

Options with radiotherapy include external beam radiotherapy and Leksell Gamma Knife (Elekta AB) stereotactic radiosurgery. However, radiotherapy results in a long latent period (a few months to years) before benefits are realized and in postradiotherapy hypopituitarism (in 10 years in >50% of patients, or in a smaller percentage with Gamma Knife therapy). Central nervous system damage and development of central nervous system tumors are rare.

Somatostatin analogues are used as adjuncts for the management of GH- or TSH-producing tumors. Pegvisomant, a GH-receptor blocker, is used to block the harmful metabolic effects of excess GH in the management of GH-producing tumors refractory to other management options.

Follow-up is essential to monitor for persistence or recurrence of the tumor, development of hypopituitarism in patients treated with surgery or radiotherapy, and the possible occurrence of MEN-1 in familial cases.

Prolactinoma and the Hyperprolactinemic Syndrome

Pituitary tumors associated with hyperprolactinemia may be prolactinomas, mixed tumors (eg, GH- and prolactin-producing tumors), or nonfunctioning tumors with suprasellar extension and the stalk effect. In stalk-effect hyperprolactinemia, impingement of the mass on the pituitary stalk interferes with the access of hypothalamic dopamine to the anterior pituitary and results in disinhibition of prolactin secretion by normal lactotrophs.

Clinical Features

Mass effects include hypopituitarism and expressions of extrasellar extension of the pituitary tumor. Persons with hyperprolactinemia, especially men, may be asymptomatic; women of childbearing age often present early. Hyperprolactinemia suppresses GnRH secretion and causes a lactogenic effect on the breasts.

In women, hyperprolactinemia is usually expressed as galactorrhea, ovulatory and menstrual dysfunction (short luteal phase or anovulation leading to infertility), oligomenorrhea or amenorrhea, hypogonadism, and decreased libido. In some women, hyperprolactinemia may be associated with hirsutism and acne.

In men, hyperprolactinemia results in hypogonadism, infertility due to oligospermia, and, rarely, galactorrhea or gynecomastia. Hyperprolactinemia is frequently unrecognized in men because decreased libido and impaired potency may be dismissed as aging or attributed to psychological factors. In men with a pituitary tumor, marked hyperprolactinemia and a macroadenoma are common at presentation.

Diagnosis

Prolactinoma must be distinguished from other causes of hyperprolactinemia and from other pituitary area masses. Hyperprolactinemia can be physiologic or pathologic in origin.

Physiologic hyperprolactinemia may occur in pregnancy and the postpartum state and in conditions of stress, such as surgery or acute illness. All women of reproductive age should have a pregnancy test performed.

Pathologic hyperprolactinemia may occur with primary hypothyroidism. TSH should be checked in all patients being evaluated for hyperprolactinemia. Pathologic hyperprolactinemia may also occur in patients with primary pituitary disease or hypothalamic or stalk disease and result in the loss of dopaminergic disinhibition of prolactin secretion by normal lactotrophs. Causes of primary pituitary disease include prolactinoma, "mixed tumors," nonfunctioning pituitary tumors with suprasellar extension and stalk effect hyperprolactinemia, hypophysitis, and primary empty sella.

Hypothalamic or stalk disorders can be functional or organic. *Functional hypothalamic disorders* lead to hyperprolactinemia because of interference with the synthesis, secretion, or action of dopamine or other hypothalamic regulators of prolactin secretion. These disorders may be caused by drugs (eg, neuroleptics, antidepressants, narcotics, and estrogens); primary hypothyroidism (15%–30%); chest wall irritative lesions (eg, herpes zoster, dermatitis, and thoracotomy) and nipple stimulation (eg, during sexual activity); renal failure; and cirrhosis or hepatic encephalopathy.

Organic hypothalamic disorders include traumatic disorders (eg, from surgery or radiotherapy), inflammatory disorders (eg, from sarcoidosis or histiocytosis X), or neoplastic disorders (eg, from craniopharyngioma, optic glioma, meningioma, or metastases such as those from the breast or lungs). Ectopic hyperprolactinemia (very rare) has been reported with hypernephroma, gonadoblastoma, and ovarian teratomas.

The diagnosis of prolactinoma is established with serum levels of prolactin that are greater than 10 times the upper limit of the reference range. However, prolactinomas, particularly microprolactinomas, may be associated with prolactin levels that exceed the upper limit of the reference range but by less than 10 times.

If the prolactin level is less than 10 times the upper limit of the reference range, functional causes should be ruled out. If a functional cause is suspected, reevaluation after addressing it is appropriate. If hyperprolactinemia does not resolve in about 3 months, the patient should be evaluated for hypothalamic-pituitary disease. If a functional cause is not suspected, organic hypothalamic-pituitary disease should be ascertained by imaging the hypothalamic-pituitary region, preferably by MRI. Other pituitary functions and the visual fields are evaluated, if appropriate, for the presence of tumor and closeness of the tumor to the optic nerve, optic chiasm, and optic tracts. MRI should be performed only after ruling out or addressing a functional cause of hyperprolactinemia, especially if the prolactin level is less than 10 times the upper limit of the reference range.

If a cause is not found, the hyperprolactinemia is considered to be of indeterminate origin. Follow-up evaluation may show evidence of a mass. The serum level of prolactin should be checked every 6 to 12 months, and imaging should be repeated in 1 to 2 years or sooner if new symptoms develop.

Differential Diagnosis

Macroprolactin may be measured as prolactin in prolactin assays. Macroprolactin is glycosylated prolactin circulating in aggregates that are not cleared well by the kidneys and therefore account for most of the circulating prolactin measured. Macroprolactinemia appears to be a benign condition requiring no specific therapy. However, it is sometimes misdiagnosed as hyperprolactinemia and treated inappropriately.

Macroprolactin is suspected as a cause of excess prolactin when prolactin levels are high in patients with no symptoms, functional cause, or pituitary-hypothalamic disorder that could indicate hyperprolactinemia. The blood is then tested for macroprolactin levels.

Treatment

Not every person who has a high prolactin level needs to be treated to normalize prolactin concentrations. If the person has a microadenoma causing hyperprolactinemia or idiopathic hyperprolactinemia, treatment is indicated if hyperprolactinemia is thought to be causing infertility, hypogonadism, or socially significant galactorrhea (ie, spontaneous galactorrhea staining clothes). Dopamine agonist therapy is first-line therapy. Transsphenoidal pituitary surgery is rarely needed for a microprolactinoma, but it is needed if dopamine agonists are not effective or not tolerated and if therapy for hyperprolactinemia is considered necessary. If hypogonadism is the indication for therapy and the patient's fertility does not need to be preserved, estrogen therapy may be used instead to prevent the adverse effects of hypogonadism in women (eg, bone loss, vaginal dryness). If none of the indications for therapy are present, patients may be observed without therapy with a check of serum prolactin annually and follow-up imaging every 2 to 3 years.

Macroprolactinoma

Therapy is indicated for all patients who have a large pituitary tumor (≥1 cm) that is making prolactin. These large tumors pose a dual threat: a mass lesion and the effects of hyperprolactinemia. Drug therapy with a dopamine agonist is the preferred treatment. Surgical excision or radiotherapy is reserved for patients with drug intolerance or drug resistance (10%–20% of patients receiving bromocriptine; 3%–7%, cabergoline).

Dopamine Agonists

Dopamine agonists are the mainstay of prolactinoma therapy. They suppress prolactin secretion and proliferation of prolactin-producing cells, restore gonadal function (in 70%–80% of patients), and decrease tumor size (in >50% of patients). Patients with Parkinson disease receiving cabergoline are monitored for cardiac valve disease. However, similar cardiac valve abnormalities have not been found in patients receiving smaller doses of dopamine agonists for hyperprolactinemia. Therapy with dopamine agonists is temporizing in most patients with macroadenoma, and discontinuation usually leads to recurrence of tumor growth and endocrine dysfunction. However, in some patients who have the outcomes of normoprolactinemia and significantly smaller tumor, use of the drug can be withdrawn after 1 to 2 years. In these patients, the tumor may have a long remission but need long-term monitoring.

Dopamine agonist therapy should be stopped if pregnancy is confirmed. In pregnancy, the risk of microprolactinoma growth is less than 5%, and the risk of macroprolactinoma growth, 20% to 40%. Patients are observed closely; if tumor growth is suspected, imaging (without gadolinium during pregnancy) should be performed. If significant tumor growth complicates pregnancy, surgical excision or reinstitution of dopamine agonist therapy is considered.

Surgical Treatment of Prolactinomas

For microadenomas, the surgical cure rates are 60% to 80%; for macroadenomas, 0% to 30%.

KEY FACTS

✓ Pituitary tumors—microadenomas (≤10 mm) or macroadenomas (>10 mm); sellar or both sellar and extrasellar; functioning or nonfunctioning

✓ Pituitary tumor mass effect—on surrounding structures (eg, optic chiasm) or on the normal pituitary, pituitary stalk, and hypothalamus (eg, ACTH deficiency and prolactin excess)

✓ Pituitary tumors may produce excess hormone (eg, prolactinoma and GH-producing tumor)

GH Tumors: Acromegaly and Gigantism

Etiology

Acromegaly is nearly always caused by a GH-producing pituitary tumor. These tumors usually secrete only GH; infrequently, they may simultaneously secrete prolactin, α-subunit of glycoprotein hormones (LH, FSH, and TSH), or ACTH. Rarely, acromegaly may be caused by ectopic GHRH-producing tumors (hypothalamic or ectopic). Very infrequently, it can be caused by ectopic GH-producing tumors.

GH-producing pituitary tumors are usually sporadic; rarely, they are familial and may occur in association with MEN-1, McCune-Albright syndrome, or Carney complex.

Clinical Features

The clinical features of GH tumors are related to excess levels of GH and IGF-1 and to the mass effect of the pituitary tumor on the pituitary and surrounding structures. Excess levels of GH and IGF-1 lead to tall stature (gigantism) in childhood and to characteristic acromegalic features in adults (Box 17.4). Pituitary mass–related manifestations include hypopituitarism, stalk-effect hyperprolactinemia, and anatomical effects related to the extrasellar extension of a macroadenoma.

Compared with survival among age-matched controls, survival among patients with untreated or poorly treated acromegaly is reduced by an average of 10 years (excess mortality primarily results from cardiovascular, cerebrovascular, and respiratory deaths). Patients with acromegaly have a 2- to 3-fold increased risk of cancer and a 3- to 8-fold increased risk of colon cancer and premalignant colon polyps.

Endocrine Diagnosis

Serum IGF-1 provides the best screening test for the diagnosis of acromegaly. Age- and sex-matched serum IGF-1 levels are almost universally increased. (IGF-1 levels are normally increased in pregnancy and in adolescence.) The diagnosis is confirmed by the demonstration of abnormal GH suppressibility within 1 to 2 hours after a 75-g glucose load (failure of GH suppression to <1 ng/mL

Box 17.4 • Clinical Features of Growth Hormone Tumors

Bone and soft-tissue overgrowth, with coarsening of facial features; frontal bossing; prognathism; widened spaces between teeth; macroglossia; increased hat, glove, ring, or shoe size; acroparesthesias; and nerve entrapment syndromes

Hyperhidrosis, heat intolerance, skin tags, and increased skin oiliness

Carbohydrate intolerance (20%); rarely, frank diabetes mellitus, hypercalciuria, and hyperphosphatemia; and urolithiasis

Fibromas or acanthosis nigricans

Sleep apnea (obstructive and central)

Cardiovascular effects, including hypertension, left ventricular hypertrophy, diastolic dysfunction, cardiomyopathy, arrhythmias, and coronary artery disease

Propensity to early and severe degenerative joint disease

---

or a paradoxical increase in GH secretion). A random serum level of GH is not helpful because of the pulsatile nature of GH secretion.

Radiologic Diagnosis

When the diagnosis is documented biochemically, imaging of the sella is indicated. MRI is the imaging study of choice. If a pituitary tumor is not delineated (a rare event) or if a symmetric pituitary enlargement is suggestive of hyperplasia, serum GHRH levels are measured to exclude a GHRH-producing tumor. If the GHRH level is high, a search is made for evidence of an ectopic GHRH-producing tumor. Evidence of an ectopic GH-producing tumor is sought if both the pituitary imaging findings and the GHRH level are normal.

Therapy

Because of the increased morbidity and mortality associated with untreated acromegaly, active management is indicated for all patients. Optimal therapy is directed at normalization of GH and IGF-1 levels, preservation or normalization of pituitary functions, and control of comorbidities with an aim to reduce excess mortality from increased GH. No single line of treatment can accomplish all these goals in all patients. Often several forms of therapy are needed for patients with acromegaly.

Ectopic GH or GHRH Tumors

Surgical resection is the therapy of choice for ectopic GH or GHRH tumors. For persistent or incurable disease, pharmacotherapy is considered.

ACTH-Producing Tumors

ACTH-producing tumors are discussed in Chapter 14 ("Gonadal and Adrenal Disorders").

Gonadotropin-Producing Tumors

Gonadotropin-producing tumors constitute the largest fraction of nonfunctioning pituitary tumors. Although more than 80% of them can synthesize the gonadotropins or their subunits, increased serum levels of FSH, LH, or their subunits are found in less than 35% of affected patients. Clinically, the tumors are macroadenomas at presentation; patients may present at any age, but they are usually middle-aged or elderly male patients. Extrasellar effects dominate the clinical picture, and some degree of hypopituitarism is usually present. The tumor mass may be associated with stalk-effect hyperprolactinemia. Imaging (MRI or CT) usually shows the sellar mass with extrasellar extension. Currently, no effective medical therapy is available. Treatment is usually surgical, with or without postoperative radiotherapy. Endocrine replacement therapy is given for the management of hypopituitarism.

TSH-Producing Tumors

The characteristic clinical presentations of patients who have primary TSH tumors are diffuse goiter and hyperthyroidism. Other presentations include extrasellar mass effects and deficiency of other pituitary hormones. Laboratory testing indicates the presence of a TSH-producing tumor in a thyrotoxic patient if the TSH value is normal or high with elevated thyroid hormone levels. Unlike Graves disease, TSH-producing tumors occur with equal frequency in both sexes without causing ophthalmopathy and dermopathy; in patients with TSH-producing tumors, the TSH concentration is normal or high in the presence of hyperthyroidism. Sometimes it is difficult to distinguish TSH-induced hyperthyroidism from T_4-resistance syndromes. TSH-producing tumors may have elevated α-glycoprotein subunit levels, and the TSH response to thyrotropin-releasing hormone is absent. MRI or CT shows a sellar mass with or without extrasellar extension.

Treatment options for TSH-producing tumor include ablation (surgically or with irradiation), pharmacologic therapy with the somatostatin analogue octreotide, and ancillary measures for the management of thyrotoxicosis.

Pituitary Incidentalomas

Pituitary incidentalomas are relatively common. Autopsy studies suggest that 10% to 20% of persons harbor small pituitary tumors. CT or MRI of the head performed for non-endocrine reasons shows mass lesions in the sella larger than 3 mm in 4% to 20% of persons. Potential threats to health from these incidentalomas include functioning pituitary tumors and incidentalomas with actual or potential mass effects. Masses larger than 10 mm are more likely to be associated with mass effects (hypopituitarism, hyperprolactinemia from a stalk effect, or chiasma syndrome) and are more likely to enlarge during observation.

The diagnostic approach includes assessing pituitary function and mass effects. Assessing for functioning pituitary tumors may include the overnight 1-mg dexamethasone suppression test or 24-hour urinary free cortisol test and measurement of prolactin, IGF-1, free T_4 and TSH, and FSH, LH, and their subunits. In the asymptomatic patient, only a serum prolactin level is measured. The other pituitary hormones are assessed only when suspicion is supported by clinical findings.

Active intervention is dictated by finding a functioning pituitary tumor that can cause morbidity or mortality (ie, all functioning pituitary tumors except a small microprolactinoma in a postmenopausal female patient) or identifying an incidentaloma larger than 1 cm in diameter with extrasellar extension. Otherwise the patient is observed and imaging studies are repeated in 6 to 12 months and then later at less frequent intervals. An increase in the size of the nonfunctioning incidentaloma under observation requires surgical intervention.

Miscellaneous Pituitary Disorders

Craniopharyngioma

Craniopharyngioma is a slow-growing, encapsulated squamous cell tumor originating from remnants of the Rathke pouch. It is the most common tumor in the pituitary region in childhood but can occur at any age. Two-thirds of the tumors are suprasellar, and one-third of the tumors originate in or extend into the sella. Most are cystic, and some are solid or mixed. These tumors have a propensity to calcify. The clinical presentation includes obstructive hydrocephalus, hypothalamic syndrome (diabetes insipidus and hyperprolactinemia), chiasmal defects, hypopituitarism, or calcification in or around the sella, as seen incidentally on radiography. Radiography shows calcification in intrasellar or suprasellar regions (75% of children; 25% of adults). CT or MRI shows a solid or cystic mass, calcification (on CT), and low attenuation values (cholesterol content).

Surgical excision is possible for only small craniopharyngiomas. Larger craniopharyngiomas are surgically decompressed. A ventriculoperitoneal shunt is used for obstructive hydrocephalus. Other treatments include postoperative radiotherapy and management of endocrine dysfunction.

Key Definition

Craniopharyngioma: *a slow-growing, encapsulated squamous cell tumor originating from Rathke pouch remnants.*

Pituitary Apoplexy

Pituitary apoplexy refers to hemorrhagic infarction of the pituitary gland, with or without underlying disease. The usual clinical setting is that of a pituitary tumor, irradiated pituitary tumor, pregnancy, postpartum state, anticoagulation therapy, increased intracranial pressure, vascular disease (eg, diabetes mellitus), or vasculitis (eg, temporal arteritis). Persons are asymptomatic if the bleeding is small or gradual. In the acute condition, hemorrhage is often sudden or large, with severe headache, ophthalmoplegia, visual defects, meningismus, depressed sensorium, and acute adrenocortical crisis leading to death if unrecognized and untreated. The diagnosis is made on the basis of the characteristic clinical, radiologic, and surgical findings. Therapy includes neurosurgical decompression and hormonal support. Late sequelae may include hypopituitarism, secondary empty sella syndrome, or regression of hypersecretory syndrome in an infarcted functioning pituitary tumor.

Key Definition

Pituitary apoplexy: *hemorrhagic infarction of the pituitary gland, with or without underlying disease.*

Sheehan Syndrome

Pituitary infarction in a patient with massive postpartum hemorrhage leads to panhypopituitarism, including failure of lactation and deficiencies of glucocorticoids, thyroid hormone, and sex hormones. This condition is called **Sheehan syndrome**. Early recognition and hormone replacement therapy are the keys to preventing the disabling adverse effects of hypopituitarism.

Key Definition

Sheehan syndrome: *panhypopituitarism from pituitary infarction with massive postpartum hemorrhage.*

Lymphocytic Hypophysitis

Lymphocytic hypophysitis is presumed to be of autoimmune origin. It usually occurs in association with other autoimmune endocrinopathies and affects adults, predominantly women, especially during pregnancy and the postpartum period. The clinical presentation may include hypopituitarism or the presence of a sellar mass associated with hyperprolactinemia. The main differential diagnoses are prolactinoma and Sheehan syndrome. The diagnosis depends on the associations and the results of surgical exploration. No specific therapy is available. Hormonal replacement is given as needed.

ADH Deficiency: Diabetes Insipidus

Etiology

Arginine vasopressin is also called ADH. Renal water output is dependent on the presence of a good concentration of ADH and a responsive distal nephron. Therefore, diabetes insipidus (DI) with excessive water loss may result from decreased responsiveness of the distal nephron to ADH (nephrogenic or vasopressin-resistant DI) or from decreased secretion of ADH (central DI).

Decreased Production of ADH

A decreased level of ADH despite increased serum osmolality occurs most commonly from organic disorders of the anterior hypothalamus, median eminence, or upper stalk (hypothalamic, neurogenic, central, or ADH-sensitive DI). Infrequently, functional suppression of ADH results from excessive ingestion of fluids (primary polydipsia or dipsogenic DI); this is associated with low serum osmolality.

Hypothalamic or Central DI

Hypothalamic or central DI may result from genetic or acquired disorders of the anterior hypothalamus, median eminence, or upper pituitary stalk. Genetic disorders are rare. Causes of acquired disorders include trauma (closed head trauma or neurosurgery); inflammatory or granulomatous disorders (sarcoidosis, tuberculosis, or histiocytosis X); primary neoplasms such as craniopharyngioma, germinoma, and optic glioma; and metastatic neoplasms primarily from the breast or lung. Idiopathic hypothalamic DI is probably the most common cause of the syndrome and may be an autoimmune disorder.

Dipsogenic DI

Dipsogenic DI may be idiopathic or associated with psychosis or, rarely, organic disorders of the anterior hypothalamus such as sarcoidosis or neoplasms.

Nephrogenic DI

Nephrogenic DI, or decreased responsiveness of the distal nephron to ADH, may also be caused by genetic or acquired disorders. The most common causes are chronic renal disease, electrolyte abnormalities (hypercalcemia or hypokalemia), and ADH-antagonist drugs such as lithium and demeclocycline.

Clinical Features

Polyuria and polydipsia, often with a preference for ice-cold water, are characteristic of patients with DI. Nocturia is usually present, and enuresis may be the presenting sign with children. An abrupt onset of symptoms usually points to central DI. Absence of nocturia, variable intensity or intermittency of symptoms, and a 24-hour urine output greater than 18 L suggest primary polydipsia.

DI leads to dehydration if the patient cannot compensate for the inability of the kidneys to concentrate urine and preserve body water by drinking more water. This may occur if the patient is unconscious for any reason, cannot obtain fluids, or has an impaired thirst mechanism. In such circumstances, extreme hyperosmolar dehydration and hypertonic encephalopathy may develop. Other clinical manifestations include those of DI and the etiologic disorder.

Endocrine Diagnosis

In patients with polyuria and dilute urine, the diagnosis of DI depends on the random measurement of plasma osmolality (serum sodium is a good surrogate) and urine osmolality levels under conditions of unrestricted fluid intake. The induction of plasma hyperosmolality (either by water deprivation or by administration of hypertonic saline) is used to assess the patient's ability to produce ADH and to respond to it. The patient's response can be assessed 1) indirectly by measurements of urine volume and osmolality before and after fluid restriction or ADH administration (or both) or 2) directly by measurements of plasma levels of ADH in addition to plasma and urine osmolalities.

Although the diagnosis of severe DI from any cause can be straightforward, the diagnosis is challenging when patients have partial DI. Moreover, prolonged periods of polyuria, regardless of the primary cause, may decrease the renal urine-concentrating ability (renal medullary washout), in effect adding a nephrogenic DI component to the basic disease process.

In a patient with polyuria and dilute urine, a random plasma osmolality greater than 295 mOsm/kg points to neurogenic or nephrogenic DI. These can be differentiated by the response to exogenous ADH. In an untreated patient with polyuria, a random plasma osmolality less than 280 mOsm/kg points to primary polydipsia.

Etiologic Diagnosis

Clinical evidence of hypothalamic-pituitary or systemic disorders is sought, and visual fields and anterior pituitary functions are evaluated. MRI is performed to look for structural abnormalities in the hypothalamic-pituitary region. The most common causes of central DI are idiopathic DI, trauma (accidental or neurosurgical), metastases from breast or lung cancer, and tumors in the hypothalamic area. Systemic diseases with hypothalamic or stalk involvement must be considered. Disorders involving the stalk may be congenital (ectopic neurohypophysis and Rathke cleft cyst), inflammatory (neurosarcoidosis, Langerhans cell histiocytosis, and lymphocytic hypophysitis), or neoplastic (craniopharyngioma, pituitary adenoma, metastatic disease, germinoma, and astrocytoma).

Therapy

Whenever possible, therapy for DI is directed at the cause. For mild central DI, free access to water may be all that is needed. Desmopressin is used for moderate to severe central DI, with the first aim being to ensure control of nocturnal polyuria and disturbed sleep. For nephrogenic DI, thiazides are the only treatment available.

KEY FACTS

- ✓ Hyperprolactinemia treatment—not indicated unless the patient has infertility, hypogonadism, socially embarrassing galactorrhea, or pituitary adenoma
- ✓ Pituitary apoplexy may be suggested by sudden-onset severe central headache with severe malaise, nausea, vomiting, and hypotension with or without visual disturbances
- ✓ Central DI—treat with desmopressin to control nocturnal polyuria
- ✓ Central DI—if the thirst mechanism is deranged, close monitoring of the blood pressure and sodium is indicated

---

ADH Excess: SIADH

Etiology

ADH excess, in the absence of a hyperosmolar stimulus, may be appropriate when it occurs in response to hypovolemia or hypotension and inappropriate when it occurs in the absence of a hypovolemic or hypotensive stimulus. SIADH can result from exogenous or endogenous disorders.

Exogenous ADH excess may result from the inappropriate administration of ADH (or its analogues such as desmopressin) or oxytocin. *Endogenous ADH excess* may originate from a eutopic hypothalamic or an ectopic extrahypothalamic source.

Eutopic ADH excess may be a consequence of 1) central nervous system or hypothalamic disorders (eg, traumatic, inflammatory, degenerative, vascular, or neoplastic disorders); 2) the use of agonist drugs that enhance ADH secretion or action (chlorpropamide, carbamazepine, vincristine,

vinblastine, cyclophosphamide, phenothiazines, monoamine oxidase inhibitors, tricyclic antidepressants, and clofibrate); or 3) neurogenic influences such as pain or nausea.

Ectopic extrahypothalamic ADH excess may result from 1) malignancies (cancers of the bronchus, pancreas, ureter, prostate, or bladder; lymphoma; leukemia; thymoma; or mesothelioma) or 2) benign pulmonary disorders (pneumonia, lung abscess, empyema or pneumothorax, tuberculosis, cystic fibrosis, and the use of positive-pressure ventilation).

Pathophysiology

Continued water intake and ADH hypersecretion in the absence of a hyperosmolar stimulus leads to increased renal water retention, hyponatremia, and hypoosmolality of body fluids with inappropriately concentrated urine. Homeostatic adjustments promote "renal escape" and natriuresis, including increased glomerular filtration rate, increased levels of atrial natriuretic hormones, and suppression of the renin-angiotensin-aldosterone axis. Natriuresis exacerbates plasma hypoosmolality, thus explaining the absence of edema.

Clinical Features

The clinical features of SIADH are a composite of the effects of the underlying disorder and those of the hyponatremic syndrome that depend on the degree and rapidity of its development. Patients with SIADH may be asymptomatic if the hyponatremia is mild or has developed gradually over weeks and months. When patients are symptomatic, the most frequent symptoms are lethargy, fatigue, ill health, anorexia, nausea and vomiting, headache, and irritability or confusion. Severe or rapidly developing hyponatremia can lead to a behavioral change, a change in the level of consciousness, or seizures.

Diagnosis

Appropriate ADH excess is associated with decreased cardiac output, renal failure, hepatic failure (hypervolemic), and dehydration (hyperosmolar and hypovolemic). SIADH is suspected in a patient with clinical euvolemia and hyponatremia. Hyperosmolar states and loss of intracellular water to the hyperosmolar extracellular fluid, as in hyperglycemic patients or patients who have received mannitol (plasma glucose, history of mannitol use, and increased plasma osmolality), should be excluded first. Those patients do not have hypoosmolality. True hyponatremia should then be confirmed. Now that sodium levels are measured with direct potentiometry ion-selective electrodes, so-called pseudohyponatremia from elevated triglycerides (severe) or protein (in monoclonal gammopathy) is not seen.

If hyponatremia and reduced serum osmolality have been documented in a patient with clinical euvolemia, thyroid function tests (free T4 and TSH) and cortisol measurements should be performed. These hormones are important for free water clearance. Hypothyroidism or cortisol deficiency (both from primary or hypothalamopituitary cause) can cause hyponatremia with hypoosmolality.

The main diagnostic challenge is to differentiate SIADH from subclinical hypovolemia. Urinary sodium concentration, serum creatinine or uric acid levels, plasma renin activity, and the aldosterone level are measured. In contrast to findings in SIADH, subclinical hypovolemia is associated with a urinary sodium concentration less than 20 mmol/L, increased serum creatinine and uric acid levels, and an increased plasma renin activity and plasma aldosterone level.

Therapy

Therapy for SIADH includes identifying and managing the underlying disorder. Restricting total water intake will control symptomatic hyponatremia (a good starting point is 800–1,000 mL of water daily, including water in food, drinks, and free water). Specific ADH antagonists, the vaptans, have become available (tolvaptan for oral use and conivaptan for intravenous use). These selective or nonselective vasopressin V2-receptor antagonists are currently indicated for the treatment of clinically significant hypervolemic and euvolemic hyponatremia (serum sodium ≤125 mmol/L with marked hyponatremia that is symptomatic and has resisted correction with fluid restriction). These drugs are used during hospitalization and with close monitoring of clinical status and serum sodium.

When acute neurologic sequelae are present, hypertonic saline can be given intravenously (200–300 mL of 5% saline over 3–4 hours). Serum sodium should be gradually increased (not to exceed 0.5 mmol/h or 12 mmol in 24 hours). Hypertonic saline should be given until the neurologic symptoms cease and a "safe" serum sodium level of 120 mmol/L is reached. Rapid correction of hyponatremia (eg, >12 mmol/L in 24 hours) can cause osmotic central pontine myelinolysis, which often is fatal.

18   Thyroid Disorders

MARIUS N. STAN, MD

Laboratory Assessment of Thyroid Function

Serum Thyrotropin

Current assays measure thyrotropin (previously called thyroid-stimulating hormone [TSH]) concentrations as low as 0.01 mIU/L, allowing differentiation between low-normal values and suppressed values. In patients with normal pituitary, thyrotropin levels are increased in primary hypothyroidism, during recovery from nonthyroid illness, and with thyroid hormone resistance. Thyrotropin levels are low in hyperthyroidism, in nonthyroidal illness, in the first trimester of pregnancy, and with the use of certain drugs (eg, somatostatin, dopamine, and glucocorticoids). Measurement of the thyrotropin level is the best single test of thyroid function in these patients.

In patients with pituitary disease, however, thyrotropin levels are unreliable since the values can be inappropriately normal in relation to thyroid hormone concentrations. Thus, thyrotropin levels may be normal or increased in patients with thyrotropin-producing tumors and normal or decreased in patients with central hypothyroidism.

Thyroxine

Free Thyroxine

Although the free thyroxine (T_4) concentration is frequently measured, the accuracy of the assays available for clinical use varies substantially. Serum free T_4 is decreased in hypothyroidism and the late phase of nonthyroidal illness and increased in hyperthyroidism, in the initial phase of nonthyroidal illness, and in patients with thyrotropin-producing pituitary tumors or thyroid hormone resistance.

Total Thyroxine

Measurement of the total T_4 concentration includes T_4 bound to thyroid hormone–binding proteins (99.98% of total T_4), unbound T_4, and free T_4. Therefore, conditions that affect the concentration of binding proteins (mainly thyroxine-binding globulin [TBG]) will affect total T_4 measurements. Androgens, anabolic steroids, glucocorticoids, chronic liver disease, niacin, and familial TBG deficiency decrease total TBG concentrations. Estrogens (including during pregnancy), acute hepatitis, and familial TBG excess increase TBG concentrations and, therefore, total T_4 concentrations.

Total Triiodothyronine

Similar to total T_4, the serum total triiodothyronine (T_3) concentration is decreased in hypothyroidism, in nonthyroidal illness, with the use of drugs that decrease the binding proteins, and with caloric deprivation. It is also decreased by drugs that inhibit the conversion of T_4 to T_3 (eg, propranolol, amiodarone, and glucocorticoids). Serum T_3 levels are increased in thyrotoxicosis and thyroid hormone resistance. Serum T_3 concentrations should be measured to establish or exclude the diagnosis of T_3 thyrotoxicosis in a patient who has a low thyrotropin level and a normal T_4 level.

Thyroid tests are used to diagnose subclinical thyroid disease. In subclinical hyperthyroidism, the thyrotropin level is suppressed, but T_3 and T_4 levels are normal. In subclinical hypothyroidism, the thyrotropin level is elevated, but T_3 and T_4 levels are normal (Table 18.1).

Thyroid Hormone–Binding Proteins

Measurement of thyroid hormone–binding proteins (TBG, transthyretin, and albumin) can be helpful when a discrepancy exists between total thyroid hormone concentrations and the results of other thyroid tests. The concentration of these proteins can be altered by medications (as described above), pregnancy, hepatitis, acute intermittent porphyria, terminal illness, hypothyroidism, and hyperthyroidism, or they can be abnormal because of an inherited condition (eg, TBG deficiency or excess). Similarly, their affinity for

Table 18.1 • Interpretation of Thyroid Function Test Results

Serum Concentration			
Thyrotropin	Free T$_4$	T$_3$	Diagnosis
Normal	Normal	Normal	Normal
High	Low	Normal or low	Primary hypothyroidism
High	Normal	Normal	Subclinical hypothyroidism
Low	High or normal	High	Hyperthyroidism
Low	Normal	Normal	Subclinical hyperthyroidism

Abbreviations: T$_3$, triiodothyronine; T$_4$, thyroxine.

T$_4$ and T$_3$ can be altered by medications (eg, increased by estrogens and decreased by androgens) or affected by inherited conditions.

Thyroid Scanning

Thyroid scanning displays the distribution of functioning thyroid tissue. It distinguishes between hyperthyroidism caused by Graves disease and toxic thyroid nodules, and it identifies ectopic thyroid tissue and metastatic disease in the follow-up of patients with differentiated thyroid cancer.

Radioactive Iodine Uptake

Results of the radioactive iodine uptake (RAIU) test represent the percentage of radioactive iodine retained for a specific time after it is administered (usually 24 hours). RAIU is indicated during the evaluation of hyperthyroidism to distinguish between low- and high-uptake states and to aid in dose calculations when radioactive iodine is used to treat Graves disease.

Serum Thyroglobulin

Thyroglobulin is used as a tumor marker in patients who have a differentiated thyroid carcinoma. It is also useful in the differential diagnosis of hyperthyroidism to distinguish between an endogenous hormone source (increased thyroglobulin) and an exogenous hormone source (suppressed thyroglobulin).

Thyrotropin Receptor Antibodies

Thyrotropin receptor antibodies (TRAbs) are a mixture of stimulating, inhibitory, and neutral antibodies. Some laboratories measure the stimulating fraction of TRAbs, called thyroid-stimulating immunoglobulins. They are markers of autoimmunity and are useful for diagnosing Graves disease in patients who cannot undergo RAIU testing (eg, pregnant women). In women with active Graves disease

or a history of it, an elevated TRAb level in the last trimester of pregnancy predicts an increased risk of neonatal hyperthyroidism.

Thyroglobulin and Thyroperoxidase Antibodies

Thyroglobulin and thyroperoxidase antibodies are used as markers of autoimmune thyroid disease. However, their absence does not exclude autoimmune thyroid disease. Conversely, they can also be found in healthy persons. High titers occur in more than 90% of patients with Hashimoto thyroiditis. When thyroglobulin antibodies are present, the measurement of thyroglobulin is unreliable for follow-up of thyroid malignancies.

Thyroid Ultrasonography

Ultrasonography is used for the anatomical assessment of thyroid nodules and goiter and for the follow-up of patients after thyroid cancer treatment.

KEY FACTS

- ✓ In pituitary disease, thyrotropin levels are unreliable (may appear normal in relation to thyroid hormone levels)
- ✓ Discrepancies between total thyroid hormone levels and other thyroid tests may be resolved by measuring thyroid hormone–binding protein levels
- ✓ Thyroid scanning—distinguishes between Graves disease and toxic thyroid nodules as cause of hyperthyroidism; also identifies ectopic thyroid tissue and metastatic disease in follow-up
- ✓ Thyroglobulin—tumor marker for differentiated thyroid carcinoma; also distinguishes between endogenous and exogenous hormone sources

Hyperthyroidism

Etiology

The etiology of primary thyroid disorders that cause hyperthyroidism can be divided into those characterized by increased production and release of T$_4$ (high RAIU) and those characterized by unregulated release of T$_4$ because of gland destruction (low RAIU) (Box 18.1).

The most common thyroid-related cause of hyperthyroidism in the United States is Graves disease. Other common causes are toxic nodular goiter and thyroiditis (lymphocytic or subacute). Exogenous hyperthyroidism is a common cause of nonthyroid hyperthyroidism, particularly in patients receiving combination T$_4$ and T$_3$ treatment.

Clinical Features

Most clinical features of hyperthyroidism reflect the effects of excess thyroid hormone. Typical symptoms and signs are listed in Box 18.2. Most patients with hyperthyroidism have a small, firm goiter.

Graves orbitopathy is specific for hyperthyroidism caused by Graves disease. Ocular manifestations include findings due to sympathetic overactivity from hyperthyroidism of any cause (retraction of the upper lid, stare, and lid lag) or findings unique to Graves orbitopathy (lid edema, conjunctival injection, chemosis, proptosis, and extraocular muscle weakness). Patients with Graves orbitopathy may complain of a gritty sensation in the eyes, excessive lacrimation, photophobia, and diplopia. Graves dermopathy can also develop in these patients, manifesting as an indurated, erythematous and thickened skin area, usually over the shins.

Elderly patients with hyperthyroidism may present with atypical findings that include apathy, weight loss, supraventricular tachyarrhythmia, and congestive heart failure. This

presentation is called *apathetic thyrotoxicosis.* Separately, gynecomastia may develop in younger men.

Diagnosis

The diagnosis of hyperthyroidism is biochemical: A low serum thyrotropin level alone is not diagnostic of hyperthyroidism because a low level can also be encountered in nonthyroid illness, glucocorticoid therapy, dopamine therapy, and secondary hypothyroidism.

Specific Causes

Graves Disease

Graves disease is characterized by hyperthyroidism with diffuse RAIU and the presence of TRAbs, which have a stimulatory effect on the thyrotropin receptor, causing the hyperthyroidism. The disease is more common in young women and causes the thyroid to be mildly enlarged and firm.

Graves orbitopathy and pretibial dermopathy are usually associated with Graves disease. TRAbs are the pathophysiologic link between them. Treating hyperthyroidism is an important first step in the management of these conditions. Both conditions tend to improve in response to hyperthyroidism treatment when it is initiated early in the disease process.

Painless Thyroiditis

Painless thyroiditis (also called postpartum thyroiditis or silent thyroiditis) is usually a self-limiting disease that occurs most commonly in the postpartum period and tends to recur with subsequent pregnancies. However, it can also occur unrelated to pregnancy and in males.

The classic presentation is a sequential triphasic pattern: 1) hyperthyroid phase, with suppressed thyrotropin, low RAIU, and increased levels of free T_4; 2) hypothyroid phase; 3) recovery phase, with normal thyroid function. This triphasic pattern may be abbreviated such that all 3 phases are not apparent in all patients.

Treatment is symptomatic. β-Blockers may be needed during the hyperthyroid phase, and temporary thyroid hormone replacement may be necessary during the hypothyroid phase. In some cases, the hypothyroidism may be permanent.

Antithyroid medication or radioactive iodine therapy is not indicated because the hyperthyroidism results from the release of preformed thyroid hormone, not from increased production.

Subacute Granulomatous Thyroiditis

Subacute granulomatous thyroiditis (also called de Quervain thyroiditis) is characterized by a painful, tender goiter. Patients often complain of fever, malaise, myalgia, and a history of upper respiratory tract infection. Transient hyperthyroidism (low RAIU) is often present at diagnosis and may be followed by transient hypothyroidism. The erythrocyte sedimentation rate is invariably increased.

Treatment is symptomatic. β-Blockers and thyroid hormone replacement are used as discussed for painless thyroiditis. Nonsteroidal anti-inflammatory drugs and corticosteroids are useful for pain. The response to corticosteroid therapy is dramatic, typically with relief of symptoms within 24 hours.

Multinodular Goiter

Toxic multinodular goiter occurs in patients with a long-standing nodular goiter, in which autonomous functioning nodules develop. The hyperthyroidism is usually mild, yet cardiovascular manifestations tend to dominate. The goiter is large, nodular, and asymmetric. In patients with retrosternal extension or a short neck, the thyroid may be difficult to palpate. Patients are at risk for exacerbation of symptoms from iodine-induced hyperthyroidism due to exposure to iodinated contrast media.

Toxic Thyroid Adenoma

Toxic thyroid nodules are follicular adenomas with autonomously increased thyroid hormone production. The nodule is solitary (usually >3 cm) and found in middle-aged women. It is easy to palpate and has a firm consistency. A radioisotope scan shows intense uptake in the nodule, with suppressed uptake in the rest of the gland.

Exogenous Hyperthyroidism

Exogenous hyperthyroidism can result from the use of T_4 or T_3 (or both). It should be suspected if thyrotoxic patients have low RAIU and no palpable goiter. Low serum levels of thyroglobulin help to differentiate this disorder from painless thyroiditis.

Therapy

Thionamides

Methimazole and propylthiouracil (PTU) can be used to treat hyperthyroidism due to increased production of thyroid hormone. They act by blocking thyroid hormone synthesis. Thionamides are used in Graves disease to control hyperthyroidism, with the hope that the disease will undergo spontaneous remission during therapy. Treatment is given for 12 to 18 months and then discontinued. The effect of thionamides is temporary, and hyperthyroidism often recurs after discontinuation. In about 50% of patients, the disease relapses within the first 12 months after treatment is stopped.

Potentially serious adverse effects include agranulocytosis and hepatitis. Agranulocytosis can develop abruptly, and its development seems to be dose related. Patients with agranulocytosis typically have fever and oropharyngeal infections (sore throat). Hepatitis is more common with PTU; therefore, methimazole is the drug of choice. The exceptions

favoring the use of PTU instead of methimazole are thyroid storm (PTU decreases T_3 levels faster because it inhibits the conversion of T_4 to T_3) and the first trimester of pregnancy (PTU is less teratogenic than methimazole).

Radioactive Iodine

Radioactive iodine therapy effectively ablates the thyroid gland. For high-RAIU hyperthyroidism, it is the most commonly used therapy in the United States. The goal of therapy is to render the patient hypothyroid, and the maximal effect is apparent within 2 to 3 months. Treatment of toxic multinodular goiter requires higher doses of radioactive iodine and often more than 1 course of treatment. Radioactive iodine therapy has not been associated with long-term risks, but pregnancy and breastfeeding are contraindications. Although radioactive iodine therapy can worsen the course of active Graves orbitopathy, that worsening can be avoided with the prophylactic use of glucocorticoids.

Surgery

Near-total or total thyroidectomy is used infrequently for the treatment of Graves disease or toxic multinodular goiter. If nodules appear suspicious with fine-needle aspiration (FNA), surgery should be strongly considered. Thyroid lobectomy is used for toxic thyroid adenoma. In addition, surgery is usually considered when *rapid* restoration of a euthyroid state is desired, such as when the patient is pregnant and large doses of thionamides are needed to control hyperthyroidism or when the patient has a large, compressive goiter. Damage to the recurrent laryngeal nerves or parathyroid glands is uncommon (<1%–2%) with experienced surgeons. To prevent thyroid storm and excessive bleeding from the overactive friable gland, the patient should be treated preoperatively with stable iodine solution in combination with antithyroid drug therapy and β-blockers. This approach should render the patient euthyroid or nearly euthyroid at surgery.

Supportive Therapy

Symptomatic patients should be given β-blockers to control adrenergic manifestations of hyperthyroidism while waiting for definitive therapy to take effect.

Thyroid Storm

Thyroid storm is a state of life-threatening hyperthyroidism with severe multisystem manifestations. It develops in patients who have acute illness superimposed on uncontrolled thyrotoxicosis and in patients who have a sudden increase in thyroid hormone levels from intraoperative thyroid manipulation or radiation-induced thyroiditis. Thyroid storm is usually characterized by delirium, fever, tachycardia, hypotension, vomiting, diarrhea, and, eventually, coma. Treatment should be initiated immediately in the intensive care unit. Antithyroid therapy with PTU is preferred. Iodine solution is added to inhibit the release of preformed thyroid hormone and to decrease peripheral conversion of T_4 to T_3. β-Blocker therapy, supportive therapy directed at systemic disturbances, and therapy directed at the precipitating event should be delivered in parallel.

KEY FACTS

✓ Primary thyroid disorders causing hyperthyroidism—high RAIU (increased T_4 production and release) or low RAIU (unregulated T_4 release from gland destruction)

✓ Graves disease—hyperthyroidism with diffuse RAIU; TRAbs stimulate thyrotropin receptors

✓ Thyroid storm—patients with acute illness and uncontrolled thyrotoxicosis or with suddenly increased thyroid hormone levels (from intraoperative thyroid manipulation or radiation-induced thyroiditis)

Key Definition

Thyroid storm: *life-threatening hyperthyroidism with severe multisystem manifestations.*

Hypothyroidism

Hypothyroidism can be primary (intrinsic thyroid disease) or secondary (hypothalamic-pituitary disease). Primary hypothyroidism accounts for more than 99% of all cases.

Etiology

The most common cause of hypothyroidism in the United States is Hashimoto thyroiditis, an autoimmune thyroid disease. It tends to cluster in families and is more common in women. Other causes of hypothyroidism include radioactive iodine treatment of hyperthyroidism, thyroidectomy, and radiotherapy for neck malignancies. Transient hypothyroidism may occur during the course of subacute granulomatous thyroiditis or painless thyroiditis.

Clinical Features

The clinical manifestation of hypothyroidism depends on the degree and duration of the deficiency. When symptoms are present, they are nonspecific (Box 18.3). Many patients are asymptomatic at presentation, with hypothyroidism having been diagnosed through routine screening.

Macrocytic anemia (due to pernicious anemia or autoimmune disease) or microcytic anemia (iron deficiency

---

Box 18.3 • Common Symptoms and Signs of Hypothyroidism

Symptoms
  Fatigue
  Cold intolerance
  Muscle cramps
  Mental slowing
  Constipation
Signs
  Coarse skin
  Dry hair
  Weight gain
  Periorbital puffiness
  Delayed ankle reflex

---

due to menorrhagia) may be present. Patients with prolonged increases in thyrotropin may experience galactorrhea (thyrotropin-releasing hormone stimulates prolactin secretion). Rarely, patients may have psychosis, deafness, or cerebellar ataxia (or any combination of these). Patients who have respiratory depression may also have central hypoventilation and apnea. Hyponatremia due to syndrome of inappropriate secretion of antidiuretic hormone may be present. Associated laboratory findings include hyperlipidemia and increased levels of aspartate aminotransferase, lactate dehydrogenase, or creatine kinase. When hypothyroidism is identified, another consideration is the possibility of associated endocrinopathies as part of a polyglandular autoimmune syndrome (Addison disease, type 1 diabetes mellitus, hypoparathyroidism, hypogonadism, or pernicious anemia). Hypothyroidism may also be associated with vitiligo and other autoimmune or connective tissue diseases.

Diagnosis

If nonthyroidal illness has been excluded, low T_4 and increased thyrotropin levels are diagnostic of overt primary hypothyroidism. Subclinical hypothyroidism is identified when the thyrotropin level is elevated but the T_4 level is normal. The decision to treat depends on the degree of thyrotropin elevation. Hashimoto thyroiditis is usually associated with a firm goiter and a high titer of antimicrosomal (thyroid peroxidase) antibodies. A low T_4 level and an inappropriately normal or low thyrotropin level indicate secondary hypothyroidism. Magnetic resonance imaging of the head should be performed in addition to pituitary function tests.

Therapy

Thyroid hormone replacement therapy is initiated with synthetic T_4 (levothyroxine). The goals of therapy are to normalize thyrotropin in primary hypothyroidism and to normalize T_4 in secondary hypothyroidism. Failure to normalize thyrotropin concentrations may indicate poor adherence to drug therapy, decreased absorption due to concomitant use of interfering medications (eg, sucralfate, calcium supplements, or ferrous sulfate), or gastrointestinal tract disease. Other possibilities include progressive thyroid disease, increased thyroid-binding proteins (as with pregnancy or estrogen use), and increased hormone clearance (eg, with phenytoin, carbamazepine or tyrosine-kinase inhibitors). Thyrotropin levels should be assessed annually or as indicated by the patient's symptoms.

Miscellaneous Circumstances

T_4 Replacement Therapy in Pregnancy

Most women with primary hypothyroidism require an increase in the dose of levothyroxine during pregnancy (average increase, 25%–30%). Women receiving T_4 replacement therapy should be counseled about the importance of ensuring adequate replacement *before* conception because of the importance of maternal thyroid hormone in fetal organogenesis and because of the multiple potential complications related to hypothyroidism for both mother and fetus, including first-trimester spontaneous abortion, preterm delivery, and perinatal morbidity and mortality. Thyrotropin levels should be assessed periodically during pregnancy, and the T_4 dose should be adjusted as necessary to maintain a normal thyrotropin.

T_4 Replacement Therapy in Patients With Cardiac Disease and in Elderly Patients

Replacement therapy for elderly patients and patients who have coronary artery disease should start at a low dose (25–50 mcg daily) and increase gradually until the thyrotropin level is normal. Hypothyroidism is not a contraindication for cardiac intervention, although the patient would have an increased risk of hyponatremia and other perioperative complications.

Subclinical Hypothyroidism

Subclinical hypothyroidism is a relatively common disorder, affecting 5% to 15% of elderly patients. The risk of progression to overt hypothyroidism increases with age, the presence of thyroid antibodies, and thyrotropin levels greater than 10 mIU/L. A trial of replacement therapy is indicated for symptomatic patients and for patients at risk of progressive disease.

Myxedema Coma

Myxedema coma is severe, life-threatening hypothyroidism. It occurs in patients who have severe, untreated hypothyroidism with a superimposed acute illness (eg, infection, surgery, or myocardial infarction), exposure to cold, or the use of sedatives or opiates. The onset is insidious, with progressive stupor culminating in coma. Seizures, hypothermia, hypotension, hypoventilation, hyponatremia, and hypoglycemia may be present. The mortality rate is high (20%–50%). Treatment should be initiated promptly in an intensive care unit with intravenous T_4 and supportive measures.

Key Definition

Myxedema coma: *life-threatening, untreated, severe hypothyroidism with superimposed acute illness, exposure to cold, or use of sedatives or opiates.*

Thyroid Nodules

Thyroid nodules are extremely common, and their frequency increases with age. They may be noticed by the patient, detected during a routine medical examination, or detected during neck imaging performed for other reasons. When nodules are identified, the primary concern is whether they are benign or malignant. At least 95% of palpable thyroid nodules are benign. The likelihood of malignancy increases with solitary nodules, older age, male sex, and a history of radiotherapy to the head and neck (especially during childhood).

Evaluation should begin with a thyrotropin measurement to determine whether the nodule functions autonomously. Malignancy is substantially less likely if the thyrotropin level is suppressed, in which case thyroid ultrasonography, a radioactive iodine scan and an RAIU test should be performed. A nontoxic nodule should be sampled by ultrasound-guided FNA if it is palpable or larger than 1 cm. Thyroid FNA has high sensitivity and specificity for excluding malignancy if performed and interpreted by experienced physicians. If the aspirate is benign, annual follow-up with palpation, thyroid ultrasonography, and thyrotropin measurement is adequate. A change in nodule size requires consideration of another biopsy. A nondiagnostic aspirate requires additional aspiration. If the aspirate is interpreted as suspicious or compatible with malignancy, surgical intervention is required. Compressive symptoms (dysphonia, dysphagia, and dyspnea) should prompt surgical intervention even if the nodule is benign.

Thyroid Cancer

Differentiated Thyroid Malignancies

Papillary Thyroid Carcinoma

Papillary thyroid carcinoma is the most common type of thyroid cancer (80%–90% of cases). It has a bimodal incidence distribution, with increased incidence in early adulthood and again in late adulthood. Dissemination is typically lymphatic. Lung and bone metastases may occur. Usually found as a thyroid nodule, papillary thyroid carcinoma may also manifest as cervical adenopathy or as an incidental finding in an excised thyroid gland.

Follicular Carcinoma

Follicular carcinoma is the diagnosis in 10% to 15% of thyroid cancer cases. It typically spreads hematogenously. The usual manifestation is a thyroid mass or metastases to the lungs, bones, or brain. Rarely, it causes thyrotoxicosis if the tumor burden is large.

Other Thyroid Cancers

Anaplastic Carcinoma

Anaplastic carcinoma typically manifests as a rapidly enlarging thyroid mass that causes pain and compressive local neck symptoms. It is highly undifferentiated, and the prognosis is extremely poor (median survival <3 months after diagnosis).

Medullary Thyroid Carcinoma

Medullary thyroid carcinoma is a neuroendocrine tumor that produces calcitonin. It is part of a familial syndrome in 25% of cases (multiple endocrine neoplasia type 2). It typically manifests as either a solitary nodule or a dominant nodule in a multinodular goiter, and it is frequently metastatic at diagnosis, with 50% of patients having lymph node involvement. Tumor production of hormonal substances can lead to diarrhea and facial flushing or Cushing syndrome. Because there are *RET* proto-oncogene mutations in the familial form, patients with medullary thyroid carcinoma should be offered genetic testing. Median survival is less than that for differentiated thyroid malignancies but significantly better than for anaplastic carcinoma.

Management of Thyroid Malignancy

Surgical excision is the therapy of choice for differentiated thyroid cancer and medullary thyroid carcinoma. Excision of anaplastic carcinoma may be undertaken as part of multimodality therapy or to palliate tracheal compression. Papillary cancer carries the best prognosis of all thyroid malignancies. Factors associated with a poorer prognosis include age older than 45 years at diagnosis, incomplete resection, extensive local invasion, large primary tumor, and presence of distant metastases. Cervical lymph node involvement does not affect the prognosis.

Patients at high risk for recurrence often undergo radioactive iodine therapy to ablate the thyroid remnant. Suppressive levothyroxine therapy is also pursued for these patients, with the target thyrotropin level less than 0.1 mIU/L. Patients at low risk for recurrence do not require thyroid remnant ablation and are treated with thyroid hormone replacement to maintain thyrotropin at the low end of the reference range (0.1–0.5 mIU/L). Patients should be reevaluated 3 to 6 months later and annually thereafter. Most differentiated thyroid malignancies synthesize and secrete thyroglobulin, which can be used as a marker of recurrent or persistent disease. Whole-body iodine scanning and neck ultrasonography are also used widely to follow patients after treatment of thyroid cancer. Recurrences are treated with excision or radioactive iodine, depending on location.

Miscellaneous Thyroid Disorders

Sick Euthyroid Syndrome

Patients with systemic illness frequently have abnormal thyroid function test results without identifiable intrinsic thyroid disease. The abnormalities resolve with recovery from the acute illness. Specific therapy is not required. The main challenge is to distinguish between nonthyroid illness and intrinsic thyroid or pituitary disease because the thyrotropin level may be normal or low initially but increase during recovery. Thyroid testing of inpatients should be avoided in the absence of specific features suggestive of thyroid disease (eg, goiter, extrathyroidal manifestations of Graves disease, hypopituitarism, or arrhythmias).

KEY FACTS

✓ Primary hypothyroidism therapy in pregnancy— usually need to increase levothyroxine dose by 25%–30%

✓ Palpable thyroid nodules—most (≥95%) are benign; increased malignancy risk with solitary nodules, older age, male sex, and head and neck radiotherapy (especially in childhood)

✓ Papillary thyroid carcinoma—most common thyroid cancer (80%–90%); bimodal distribution (younger adults and older adults)

✓ Sick euthyroid syndrome—avoid thyroid testing of inpatients who do not have features of thyroid disease (eg, goiter, Graves disease, hypopituitarism, or arrhythmias)

Amiodarone and the Thyroid

With its high iodine content, amiodarone causes thyroid dysfunction in about 15% of patients; amiodarone-associated thyroid dysfunction is more likely in patients with thyroid abnormalities. The most common abnormality in iodine-replete geographic areas is hypothyroidism. Hyperthyroidism may be caused by an increase in thyroid hormone production (type 1) or a destructive thyroiditis (type 2). Medical therapy is less effective than for other causes of hyperthyroidism; in some cases, thyroidectomy is needed. Periodic monitoring of thyroid function is essential for patients treated with amiodarone, particularly elderly patients.

Questions and Answers

Questions

Multiple Choice (choose the best answer)

III.1. New-onset atrial fibrillation is diagnosed in a 72-year-old man, and results of thyroid tests are found to be abnormal (thyrotropin <0.01 mIU/L and free thyroxine 2.3 ng/dL). Antiarrhythmic therapy is started, and the patient is referred to you. He reports palpitations and weight loss for 3 months in addition to redness, swelling, and pain over his eyes. His past medical history is clinically significant for hypertension, congestive heart failure, and ongoing nicotine dependence. On examination, his heart rate is irregular at 92 beats per minute, his blood pressure is 148/86 mm Hg, and his lungs are clear. The thyroid is nontender, about twice the normal size, and increased in consistency. He has bilateral exophthalmos with red and considerably swollen eyelids and injected conjunctivae. There is trace pitting edema of the lower extremities and an area of brownish thickening of the skin over the pretibial areas. What is the best management for the patient's thyroid dysfunction at this point?
a. Observation while the patient receives antiarrhythmic treatment and reevaluation in 6 weeks for possible hypothyroidism
b. Propylthiouracyl (PTU) treatment
c. Methimazole treatment
d. Total or near-total thyroidectomy
e. Radioactive iodine treatment

III.2. In January, a 64-year-old man had an increased alkaline phosphatase level on routine laboratory testing. On isoenzyme analysis, the bone fraction was high and the liver fraction was normal. He has lived in a nursing home for the past 3 years and is unable to ambulate because of a stroke. He does not complain of pain and has had no recent fractures. He has had more difficulty with his physical therapy during the winter and feels that he is weaker than he was 6 months ago. The creatinine level is within the reference range. Additional laboratory results include the following: calcium 9.1 mg/dL (reference range, 8.9–10.1 mg/dL), phosphorus 2.7 mg/dL (reference range, 2.5–4.5 mg/dL), and parathyroid hormone (PTH) 97 pg/mL (reference range, 15–65 pg/mL). Which of the following tests is most likely to establish the cause of the increased alkaline phosphatase level?
a. Parathyroid scanning
b. 1,25-Dihydroxyvitamin D concentration
c. 25-Hydroxyvitamin D_2 and D_3 concentration
d. Bone density measurement
e. Skeletal survey

III.3. A 55-year-old woman is in your office accompanied by her husband for follow-up examination after dismissal from her local emergency department for further evaluation of "reactive hypoglycemia." For years, she has had intermittent symptoms of diaphoresis and excessive hunger that does not resolve after eating. She remembers having a glucose tolerance test during which her glucose value decreased to about 60 mg/dL. She was advised to see a dietitian, eat regularly, and always have hard candy available to her to abort her symptoms. She has been experiencing more frequent symptoms and has gained some weight during the past year. She is otherwise healthy. She has no history of diabetes mellitus. She is currently not taking any medications. On the day of her evaluation in the emergency department, she was going about her usual activities in her home when she started experiencing the usual symptoms suspicious for hypoglycemia—diaphoresis and hunger. She recalls missing breakfast but does not recall any additional events until she was in the emergency department. Her husband recognized that she was not well and called the paramedics because he was worried that she was having a stroke. She was sweaty and could not respond to his questions. At the emergency department, several laboratory tests were done, and the patient was told her blood sugar level was low. She was given fluids and dextrose intravenously. She was dismissed and advised to have follow-up evaluation as an outpatient.

Reference ranges:

Glucose	70–140 mg/dL
C peptide	1.1–4.4 ng/mL
β-Hydroxybutyrate	<0.4 mmol/L

Which test results support abnormal endogenous insulin secretion as a cause for hypoglycemia?
a. Glucose 54 mg/dL, C peptide 0.6 ng/mL, β-hydroxybutyrate 4.9 mmol/L
b. Glucose 54 mg/dL, C peptide 0.6 ng/mL, β-hydroxybutyrate 0.2 mmol/L
c. Glucose 54 mg/dL, C peptide 0.6 ng/mL, β-hydroxybutyrate 0.2 mmol/L with negative sulfolnylurea screen
d. Glucose 54 mg/dL, C peptide 3.0 ng/mL, β-hydroxybutyrate 0.3 mmol/L
e. Glucose 54 mg/dL, C peptide 3.0 ng/mL, β-hydroxybutyrate 0.3 mmol/L with negative sulfonylurea screen

III.4. A 31-year-old married man presents with breast enlargement and tenderness of 6 months in duration. He reports normal sexual function and has 2 biologic children. He is not taking any medications, does not smoke or drink, and has not used any recreational drugs. Physical examination is unrevealing except for bilateral tender, symmetric gynecomastia. His secondary sex characteristics, external genitalia, and testicular size and consistency are all normal. Laboratory test results are normal for serum total and free testosterone, prolactin, thyrotropin, and dehydroepiandosterone sulfate (DHEA-S). His serum estradiol level is 78 pg/mL (reference range, 10–40 pg/mL), and his β-human chorionic gonadotropin (β-hCG) level is 50,000 IU/L (reference range, <1.4 IU/L). Which of the following tests is the most appropriate next step?

a. Ultrasonography of the testicles
b. Computed tomography of the adrenals
c. Magnetic resonance imaging of the pituitary
d. Mammography
e. Liver biopsy

III.5. A 26-year-old woman presents at 4 weeks postpartum with headaches, profound weakness, and nausea and vomiting. She had been breastfeeding. Results of her physical examination are unremarkable. Magnetic resonance imaging of the head shows a sellar mass with suprasellar extension but without chiasmal compression. Her serum sodium level is 125 mmol/L (reference range, 135–145 mmol/L), serum prolactin 72 ng/mL (reference range, 4.8–23.3 ng/mL), 8 am serum cortisol 3 mcg/dL (normal, 7–25 mcg/dL), and serum corticotropin 10 pg/mL (normal, 10–60 pg/mL). Her serum free thyroxine and thyrotropin levels are normal. Which of the following diagnoses is the most likely?

a. Primary adrenal insufficiency (Addison disease)
b. Prolactin-producing pituitary tumor
c. Nonfunctioning pituitary tumor
d. Pituitary apoplexy (Sheehan syndrome)
e. Lymphocytic hypophysitis

III.6. A 22-year-old woman presents with a 3-week history of tremors, palpitations, heat intolerance, and a 3.5-kg weight loss. She does not complain of any eye symptoms or rash. She denies use of any medications or nutritional supplements and has not undergone any imaging or surgical procedures in the past year. On examination, she is tachycardic (pulse 107 beats per minute) and has a tremor of her upper extremities, and her skin is moist.

Her thyroid is slightly enlarged and extremely tender. The thyrotropin level is 0.01 mIU/L (reference range, 0.4–4.2 mIU/L), free thyroxine level is 2.4 ng/dL (reference range, 0.9–1.7 ng/dL), and the radioiodine uptake was less than 1% at 24 hours. What is the best next step in management?

a. Begin treatment with a nonsteroidal anti-inflammatory drug (NSAID) or glucocorticoid.
b. Measure the serum thyroglobulin concentration.
c. Measure thyroid-stimulating immunoglobulins (TSI).
d. Give methimazole 20 mg daily.
e. Perform thyroid ultrasonography.

III.7. A 70-year-old man was hospitalized because of anterior chest pain. Vital signs were normal. Urgent coronary angiography led to angioplasty, which was successfully performed; the patient was discharged home 2 days later. During the next month, he experienced some nervousness, anxiety, and a 22-pound (10 kg) weight loss on his usual diet. His cardiologist has just determined that he had atrial fibrillation and prescribed a calcium channel blocker. Despite that treatment, you see him few days later in the emergency department with a ventricular rate of 130 beats per minute and shortness of breath. On examination, he is in no acute distress at rest but he is in atrial fibrillation with a rate 120 to 130 beats per minute. There are no tremors and no signs of Graves ophthalmopathy or dermopathy. His thyroid is low-lying, multinodular, nontender, and slightly enlarged. You learn of a long-standing history of nontoxic multinodular goiter. Because of the atrial fibrillation, thyroid tests were done and findings include a thyrotropin value of less than 0.01 mIU/L, free thyroxine 3.7 ng/dL, and negative thyroperoxidase antibodies. What is the most likely cause of this patient's thyrotoxicosis?

a. Lymphocytic thyroiditis
b. Autonomous thyroid nodule
c. Iodine-induced hyperthyroidism
d. Graves disease
e. Thyrotropin-producing pituitary adenoma

Answers

III.1. Answer c.

This patient has thyrotoxicosis with Graves ophthalmopathy and dermopathy, which are pathognomonic for Graves disease. Therefore, the possibility of thyroiditis is effectively excluded. The presence of moderate-to-severe ophthalmopathy in a smoker is a relative contraindication for the use of radioactive iodine, which might exacerbate the patient's eye condition, lead to a transient increase in thyroid hormone values, and not achieve euthyroidism for another 2 to 3 months. Surgery is also associated with additional risks in this patient who has several cardiac comorbidities. The safest and most effective treatment for him is an antithyroid drug; methimazole is the first choice, and PTU is a second-line drug because of its association with severe liver failure and death. PTU is still preferred in the first trimester of pregnancy and during thyroid storm.

III.2. Answer c.

The increased bone fraction of alkaline phosphatase is due to vitamin D deficiency and osteomalacia. Because it is winter and the patient resides in a nursing home, he has a high risk of vitamin D deficiency. Evaluate for nutritional vitamin D deficiency by measuring 25-hydroxyvitamin D_2 and D_3. Levels of the active form of vitamin D (1,25-dihydroxyvitamin D) are variable in patients with nutritional vitamin D deficiency. The low-normal serum calcium value indicates that the increased PTH level is secondary and not due to primary hyperparathyroidism. Parathyroid scanning is not useful in patients with secondary hyperparathyroidism. Although osteomalacia may cause low bone density, a bone density measurement will not establish the cause of an increased alkaline phosphatase level. A skeletal survey can identify the cause for this increase, such as an occult fracture, Paget disease of the bone, or metastatic bone lesions. However, none of these conditions would explain the secondary hyperparathyroidism.

III.3. Answer e.

The normal physiologic response to hypoglycemia is low insulin secretion with gradual development of ketosis. Endogenous insulin secretion is best determined by measuring not only insulin levels but also C peptide, the peptide cleaved from the insulin molecule after secretion, rendering it active. To ensure true excessive endogenous insulin secretion, the presence of insulin secretagogues must be ruled out as a potential explanation for hypoglycemia with increased or inappropriately normal insulin and C-peptide levels.

III.4. Answer a.

Gynecomastia is the most common disorder of the male breast and accounts for more than 80% of all male breast masses. It may result from a trivial cause or may be an early sign of a serious disorder. The basic mechanism of gynecomastia is relative estradiol excess, which can result from decreased androgen production or effect or from an increase in estrogen production or effect. In adults, the 2 most common causes of gynecomastia are drugs and alcohol-related liver disease. Less common causes include recovery from malnutrition or other serious chronic illness. Rare findings are hCG-producing tumors or adrenal or testicular tumors. In this patient, drugs and alcohol, gonadal failure, hyperthyroidism, and prolactin-producing pituitary tumor have been excluded. The patient has an hCG-producing tumor and increased estrogen production. Although the most common presentation of testicular tumors is a testicular enlargement or mass, small testicular tumors may often be occult. Of primary testicular tumors, 97% arise from seminiferous tubules (germ cell tumors), and about 3% arise from interstitial tissue. Germ cell tumors are the most common solid tumors in men between the ages of 15 and 34 years, occur primarily in white men, and are the main tumors that secrete hCG. Stimulation of Leydig cells by hCG results in an increased secretion of both estrogen and androgen. Testicular ultrasonography is the most appropriate step. A normal DHEA-S level excludes a diagnosis of an estrogen-producing adrenal tumor, a normal prolactin level excludes the diagnosis of a prolactin-producing pituitary tumor, and imaging studies of these glands is not warranted. Mammography is not required for evaluation of symmetric concentric gynecomastia; it is indicated for the evaluation of unilateral breast masses or when breast cancer is considered. Nothing in the presentation of this patient suggests occult liver disease or necessitates a liver biopsy.

III.5. Answer e.

Headaches, pituitary insufficiency, and magnetic resonance imaging findings consistent with a pituitary tumor in relationship to pregnancy should always lead to consideration of lymphocytic hypophysitis. Absence of a high corticotropin level excludes primary adrenal insufficiency. Pituitary tumors, whether prolactin-producing or nonfunctioning, are predominantly benign and slow growing, would have been present for sometime, and would in all likelihood have made the patient hypogonadotropic and infertile and therefore would not have their initial presentation in the postpartum state. Patients with Sheehan syndrome have a history of postpartum hemorrhage-induced hypotension or shock that requires blood transfusion, the signs and symptoms of hypopituitarism are usually recognized early after delivery, and there is loss of ability to breastfeed. Lymphocytic hypophysitis is therefore the most likely diagnosis.

III.6. Answer a.

This patient has symptoms and biochemical findings of thyrotoxicosis. The low iodine uptake and the neck tenderness confirm the diagnosis of subacute (painful) thyroiditis. The thyroid hormone levels are increased from the release of preformed hormone and not from excessive production, and therefore antithyroid medications are ineffective. Treatment is aimed at symptomatic relief. NSAIDs are often effective for mild-to-moderate disease, but glucocorticoids may be necessary for more severe or refractory pain. In view of the low iodine uptake and the absence of recent iodine load, this patient's condition is not consistent with Graves disease and thus TSI testing is not needed. Ultrasonography with color Doppler flow would be useful if the uptake were low in the setting of recent iodine load in order to distinguish thyroiditis from Graves disease, but it is not necessary for the diagnosis in this situation. Thyroglobulin is used in the setting of low-iodine-uptake thyrotoxicosis to distinguish between an endogenous and an exogenous source of thyroid hormone. Given the enlarged and tender thyroid, there is no reason to suspect factitious use of levothyroxine in this case.

III.7. Answer c.

This cause of hyperthyroidism can be easily overlooked and is likely more common than is realized. The presentation is usually that of apathetic hyperthyroidism, which can be masked even further by the use of β-blockers. The history of exposure to iodinated contrast agents a month earlier is a typical time frame for the development of thyrotoxicosis in persons with preexisting multinodular goiter. Treatment involves antithyroid drugs and supportive measures. The other choices can be excluded on clinical grounds. Lymphocytic thyroiditis is relatively rare in the elderly and is almost always associated with anti-thyroperoxidase antibodies, an absent finding in this case. This disorder can occur in patients with Graves disease with preexisting iodine insufficiency. However, the latter is rare in North America and the multinodular goiter also argues against Graves disease. An autonomous toxic nodule evolves slowly over many years rather than having the abrupt presentation described here, and the thyrotropin-producing adenoma can be excluded on the basis of the suppressed thyrotropin value.

Gastroenterology and Hepatology

Colonic Disorders

19

CONOR G. LOFTUS, MD

Inflammatory Bowel Disease

Inflammatory bowel disease refers to 2 disorders of unknown cause: ulcerative colitis and Crohn disease. Other possible causes of inflammation, especially infection, should be excluded before making the diagnosis of inflammatory bowel disease. The presence of chronic inflammation on biopsy is the key factor for making a diagnosis of inflammatory bowel disease.

Ulcerative colitis is mucosal inflammation involving only the colon. Crohn disease is transmural inflammation that can involve the gastrointestinal tract anywhere from the esophagus through the anus. The rectum is involved in about 95% of patients with ulcerative colitis and in only 50% of patients with Crohn disease. Ulcerative colitis is a continuous inflammatory process that extends from the anal verge to the more proximal colon (depending on the extent of the inflammation). Crohn disease is segmental inflammation in which inflamed areas alternate with virtually normal areas. Patients with ulcerative colitis usually present with frequent, bloody bowel movements with minimal abdominal pain, whereas patients with Crohn disease present with fewer bowel movements, less bleeding, and, more commonly, abdominal pain. Crohn disease is associated with intestinal fistulas, fistulas from the intestine to other organs, and perianal disease. Ulcerative colitis does not form fistulas, and perianal disease is uncommon. Strictures of the intestine are common with Crohn disease but rare in ulcerative colitis (when they are present, they suggest cancer).

Extraintestinal Manifestations

Arthritis occurs in 10% to 20% of patients with inflammatory bowel disease, usually as monarticular or pauciarticular involvement of large joints. Peripheral joint symptoms mirror bowel activity: Joint symptoms flare when colitis flares, and joint symptoms improve as colitis improves. When axial joint symptoms develop, such as those of ankylosing spondylitis (which has a relationship with HLA-B27) and sacroiliitis, they are usually progressive and do not improve when colitis improves.

Skin lesions occur in 10% of patients. The 3 lesions seen most commonly are erythema nodosum, pyoderma gangrenosum, and aphthous ulcers of the mouth. Erythema nodosum and aphthous ulcers usually improve with treatment of colitis, whereas pyoderma gangrenosum has an independent course. Severe, refractory skin disease is an indication for surgical treatment.

Eye lesions occur in 5% of patients. The lesion is usually episcleritis or uveitis (or both). Episcleritis usually mirrors inflammatory bowel disease activity, but uveitis does not. Patients with episcleritis typically present with a painless red eye, whereas those with uveitis often present with a painful red eye. Uveitis is an indication for emergent ophthalmologic evaluation.

Renal lithiasis occurs in 5% to 15% of patients. In Crohn disease with malabsorption, calcium oxalate stones occur. In ulcerative colitis, uric acid stones due to dehydration and loss of bicarbonate in the stool lead to acidic urine.

Liver disease occurs in 5% of patients. Primary sclerosing cholangitis is more common in ulcerative colitis than in Crohn disease. If the alkaline phosphatase level is increased in a patient with inflammatory bowel disease, the

Key Definitions

Inflammatory bowel disease: *inflammatory intestinal disease with an unknown cause; includes ulcerative colitis and Crohn disease.*

Ulcerative colitis: *mucosal inflammation that involves only the colon.*

Crohn disease: *transmural inflammation that can involve any portion of the gastrointestinal tract (from the esophagus through the anus).*

evaluation for primary sclerosing cholangitis may include ultrasonography, endoscopic retrograde cholangiopancreatography, and possibly liver biopsy.

Indications for Colonoscopy

Colonoscopy is indicated for evaluating the extent of the disease, performing biopsies, and evaluating strictures and filling defects. It is also indicated for differentiating Crohn disease from ulcerative colitis when they are otherwise indistinguishable. Another indication is monitoring with surveillance biopsies (typically, a total of 32 biopsies) for the development of dysplasia or cancer in patients who have had ulcerative colitis (involving colon proximal to the rectum) or Crohn colitis for more than 8 years. Patients who have ulcerative colitis limited to the rectum (ulcerative proctitis) are not at increased risk of dysplasia and colon cancer; they do not require surveillance colonoscopy.

Toxic Megacolon

In patients with active inflammation, avoid potential precipitants of toxic megacolon, such as opiates, anticholinergic agents, hypokalemia, and barium enema.

Treatment of Ulcerative Colitis

Sulfasalazine and other aminosalicylates can induce remission in 80% of patients with mild or moderate ulcerative colitis and are effective maintenance therapy for 50% to 75% of patients with ulcerative colitis. The active agent of sulfasalazine, 5-aminosalicylic acid (5-ASA), is bound to sulfapyridine (the vehicle). Colonic bacteria break the bond and release 5-ASA, which is not absorbed but stays in contact with the mucosa and exerts its anti-inflammatory action. The efficacy of 5-ASA may be related to its ability to inhibit the lipoxygenase pathway of arachidonic acid metabolism or to function as an oxygen free radical scavenger. It is effective in acute disease and in maintaining remission. The side effects include reversible sterility in men, malaise, nausea, pancreatitis, rashes, headaches, hemolysis, impaired folate absorption, hepatitis, aplastic anemia, and exacerbation of colitis. They are related to the sulfapyridine moiety and occur in 30% of patients who take sulfasalazine.

The 5-ASAs are a group of drugs that deliver 5-ASA to the intestine in various ways. They eliminate sulfa toxicity but are more expensive than sulfasalazine. Two of these drugs are mesalamine and olsalazine. Mesalamine can be given topically (Rowasa suppositories and Rowasa enema) or orally (Asacol, which is 5-ASA coated with an acrylic polymer that releases 5-ASA in the terminal ileum, and Pentasa, which has an ethylcellulose coating that releases 50% of the 5-ASA in the small bowel). Olsalazine consists of 2 molecules of 5-ASA conjugated with each other. Bacteria break the bond, releasing 5-ASA into the colon.

Aminosalicylates are used for mild to moderately active ulcerative colitis and for Crohn disease. Topical forms are useful for proctitis or left-sided colitis; systemic forms are used for pancolitis. Of the patients who do not tolerate sulfasalazine, 80% to 90% tolerate oral 5-ASA preparations. Side effects include hair loss, pancreatitis (often in patients in whom pancreatitis developed while they were taking sulfasalazine), reversible worsening of underlying renal disease, and exacerbation of colitis.

Topical corticosteroid preparations may be used for patients with active disease that is limited to the distal colon and is unresponsive to topical aminosalicylates. Oral corticosteroids should be added to the regimen for patients with more proximal disease if oral aminosalicylates do not control the attacks. Up to 50% of the dose can be absorbed. Oral preparations (prednisone 40 mg daily) are indicated in active pancolonic disease that is of moderate severity and is unresponsive to aminosalicylates. Prednisolone, the active metabolite, is the preferred form of drug for patients with cirrhosis (these patients may not be able to convert inactive prednisone to prednisolone). For patients who have a prompt response to oral corticosteroids, the dose may be tapered gradually at a rate not to exceed a 5-mg decrease in the total dose every 7 days. In severely ill patients, intravenous preparations should be given (methylprednisolone, 40–60 mg daily) for up to 7 to 10 days. If improvement occurs at that time, therapy should be converted to oral corticosteroids (40 mg daily). If improvement does not occur, infliximab (discussed in the Treatment of Crohn Disease subsection) may be considered for induction of remission. Additional biologic agents occasionally used in the treatment of patients with ulcerative colitis include adalimumab, golimumab, and vedolizumab. If there is no improvement, surgical intervention (colectomy) is required. Because corticosteroids are not thought to prevent relapse, they should not be prescribed after the patient has complete remission and is free of symptoms.

Total parenteral nutrition does not alter the clinical course of an ongoing attack. Indications for its use include severe dehydration and cachexia with marked fluid and nutrient deficits, excessive diarrhea that has not responded to standard therapy for ulcerative colitis, and debilitation in patients undergoing colectomy. Use of opiates (or their synthetic derivatives) and anticholinergic agents should be limited in ulcerative colitis because they can contribute to the development of toxic megacolon.

Surgical treatment is curative in ulcerative colitis. Indications for colectomy include severe intractable disease, acute life-threatening complications (perforation, hemorrhage, or toxic megacolon unresponsive to treatment), symptomatic colonic stricture, and suspected or documented colon cancer. Other indications are intractable moderate or severe colitis, refractory uveitis or pyoderma gangrenosum, growth retardation in pediatric patients, cancer prophylaxis, or inability to taper a regimen to low doses of corticosteroid (ie, <15 mg daily) over 2 to 3 months.

Treatment of Crohn Disease

The use of sulfasalazine is discussed above (see the Treatment of Ulcerative Colitis subsection). This drug is more effective for colonic disease than for small-bowel disease, although 5-ASA products designed to be released and activated in the small bowel may prove to be effective in the colon. Sulfasalazine does not have an additive effect or a steroid-sparing effect when given with corticosteroids, nor does it maintain remission in Crohn disease as it does in ulcerative colitis. None of the 5-ASA products are effective for the prophylaxis of Crohn disease.

The use of corticosteroids is discussed above (see the Treatment of Ulcerative Colitis subsection). Corticosteroids are the agents that are most effective at controlling an acute exacerbation of Crohn disease. They are the most useful drugs for treating acute small-bowel Crohn disease and for achieving rapid remission. Budesonide is favored for the treatment of mild to moderate small-bowel and proximal colonic Crohn disease since it has limited systemic toxicity owing to first-pass hepatic metabolism. Budesonide is ineffective for more distal colonic Crohn disease.

Azathioprine and 6-mercaptopurine (the active metabolite of azathioprine) have steroid-sparing effects. These immunomodulating medications are effective for maintaining remission but not for treating acute disease flares because they have a gradual onset of action (6–8 weeks). Their use should be reserved for patients who are taking corticosteroids for active disease and whose corticosteroid dose needs to be decreased (or a given dose needs to be maintained in the face of worsening disease activity).

Metronidazole (at a dose of 20 mg/kg) is effective for treating perianal Crohn disease. Six weeks may be needed for the therapeutic effect to become manifest. Recurrences are frequent when the drug dose is tapered or discontinued, leading to long-term therapy. It is less effective for colonic and small-bowel disease. Side effects include glossitis, metallic taste, vaginal and urethral burning sensation, neutropenia, dark urine, urticaria, disulfiram effect, and paresthesias.

Infliximab is a chimeric monoclonal antibody directed against tumor necrosis factor α. This intravenously administered anti-inflammatory agent is effective in treating moderately or severely active Crohn disease and ulcerative colitis that are refractory to conventional therapy and in treating fistulizing Crohn disease. Infliximab is a steroid-sparing agent that is effective in maintaining remission of Crohn disease. Infusion reactions (pruritus, dyspnea, or chest pain) may occur. The drug is associated with an increased risk of infection, including perianal abscesses, tuberculosis, and other respiratory infections. Rarely, subsequent infusions of infliximab may be associated with delayed hypersensitivity reactions. Additional monoclonal antibody–based therapeutic agents directed against tumor necrosis factor α include adalimumab and certolizumab pegol. Adalimumab and certolizumab are generally reserved for patients who no longer have a response to infliximab; these agents are administered by subcutaneous injection rather than intravenous infusion.

Additional biologic agents occasionally used in the treatment of patients with Crohn disease include natalizumab and vedolizumab.

Bowel rest per se does not have any role in achieving remission in Crohn disease. However, providing adequate nutritional support does help facilitate remission; any form of nutritional support is acceptable as long as the amount is adequate. Adequate nutrition can be essential in maintaining growth in children who have severe Crohn disease.

If a patient has Crohn disease during exploration for presumed appendicitis, the acute ileitis should be left alone (in many of these patients, chronic Crohn disease does not develop). Appendectomy can be performed if the cecum and appendix are free of disease. Of the patients with Crohn disease who have surgical treatment, 70% to 90% require reoperation within 15 years (many within the first 5 years after the initial operation). The anastomotic site is the most likely location for recurrence of disease. Indications for surgical treatment include intractable symptoms, acute life-threatening complications, obstruction, refractory fistulizing disease, abscess formation, and malignancy.

KEY FACTS

- ✓Extraintestinal manifestations of inflammatory bowel disease—
  - arthritis in 10%–20% of patients (usually monarticular or pauciarticular involvement of large joints)
  - when present, axial joint symptoms (eg, from ankylosing spondylitis or sacroiliitis) are usually progressive and do not improve when colitis improves
  - skin lesions in 10% of patients (eg, erythema nodosum, pyoderma gangrenosum, and aphthous ulcers of the mouth)
- ✓Colonoscopy for inflammatory bowel disease—
  - to evaluate extent of disease
  - to perform biopsies
  - to evaluate strictures and filling defects
- ✓Treatment of ulcerative colitis with sulfasalazine and other aminosalicylates—
  - can induce remission in 80% of patients with mild or moderate ulcerative colitis
  - effective maintenance therapy for 50%–75% of patients with ulcerative colitis
- ✓Treatment of Crohn disease—
  - Corticosteroids for acute exacerbation
  - Metronidazole (20 mg/kg) for perianal disease
- ✓Infliximab—
  - intravenous anti-inflammatory agent
  - effective in treating moderately or severely active Crohn disease and ulcerative colitis that are refractory to conventional therapy
  - effective in treating fistulizing Crohn disease

Gastrointestinal Tract Manifestations of AIDS

Gastrointestinal tract symptoms occur in 30% to 50% of North American and European patients who have AIDS and in nearly 90% of patients in developing countries. The gastrointestinal tract in patients with AIDS is predisposed to a spectrum of viral, bacterial, fungal, and protozoan pathogens. The most frequent gastrointestinal tract symptom is diarrhea, which is often chronic, associated with weight loss, and usually caused by 1 or more identifiable pathogens. Dysphagia, odynophagia, abdominal pain, and jaundice are less frequent, and gastrointestinal tract bleeding is rare. The goal of evaluation is to identify treatable causes of infection or symptoms. When no cause is identified, the condition may be idiopathic AIDS enteropathy or it may be caused by as yet unidentified pathogens.

Viral Pathogens

Cytomegalovirus

Cytomegalovirus is one of the most common and potentially serious opportunistic pathogens. It most commonly affects the colon and esophagus, although the entire gut, liver, biliary tract, and pancreas are susceptible. A patchy or diffuse colitis may progress to ischemic necrosis and perforation. Symptoms include watery diarrhea and fever and, less commonly, hematochezia and abdominal pain. Odynophagia may be present if the esophagus is involved. Diagnosis is based on biopsy specimens that show cytomegalic inclusion cells ("owl's eye" appearance) with surrounding inflammation. Treatment is ganciclovir 5 mg/kg twice daily for 14 to 21 days (Table 19.1). If the virus is resistant to ganciclovir, foscarnet should be used.

Herpes Simplex Virus

The 3 gastrointestinal tract manifestations of herpes simplex virus infection in patients with AIDS are perianal lesions (chronic cutaneous ulcers), proctitis, and esophagitis. As in cytomegaloviral infection, the organs most commonly affected are the colon and the esophagus. Symptoms include perianal lesions that are painful; proctitis that causes tenesmus, constipation, and inguinal lymphadenopathy; and esophagitis that causes odynophagia, with or without dysphagia. Diagnosis is based on the cytologic identification of intranuclear (Cowdry type A) inclusions in multinucleated cells and is confirmed with isolation of the virus from biopsies. Treatment is acyclovir given orally or intravenously (Table 19.1).

Adenovirus

Adenovirus affects the colon and reportedly causes watery, nonbloody diarrhea. Diagnosis is based on culture and biopsy. There is no treatment (Table 19.1).

Table 19.1 • Agents for Treating Gastrointestinal Tract Manifestations Caused by Various Pathogens in Patients With AIDS

Organism	Treatment
Viruses	
Cytomegalovirus	Ganciclovir
Herpes simplex virus	Acyclovir
Adenovirus	None
Bacteria	
Mycobacterium avium- intracellulare	Multidrug therapy: ethambutol, rifampin, and isoniazid
Salmonella	Amoxicillin, trimethoprim-sulfamethoxazole, or ciprofloxacin
Shigella flexneri	Trimethoprim-sulfamethoxazole, ampicillin, or ciprofloxacin
Campylobacter jejuni	Azithromycin or ciprofloxacin
Fungi	
Candida albicans	Nystatin, ketoconazole, fluconazole, or amphotericin B
Histoplasma capsulatum	Amphotericin B or itraconazole
Protozoa	
Cryptosporidium	Paromomycin
Cystoisospora belli	Trimethoprim-sulfamethoxazole
Microsporida	None
Entamoeba histolytica	Metronidazole
Giardia intestinalis	Metronidazole
Blastocystis hominis	None (not pathogenic)

Bacterial Pathogens

Mycobacterium avium-intracellulare

Mycobacterium avium-intracellulare causes infection of the gut in patients with disseminated disease. The small intestine is affected more commonly than the colon. Symptoms include fever, weight loss, diarrhea, abdominal pain, and malabsorption. Diagnosis is based on finding acid-fast organisms in the stool and tissue, with confirmation from culture of stool and biopsy specimens. Treatment is multidrug therapy with ethambutol, rifampin, and isoniazid (Table 19.1).

Other Bacteria

Other important bacteria include *Salmonella* ser Typhimurium, *Salmonella* ser Enteritidis, *Shigella flexneri*, and *Campylobacter jejuni*. AIDS patients with *Salmonella, S flexneri*, or *C jejuni* have a substantially higher incidence of intestinal infection, bacteremia, and prolonged or recurrent infections because of antibiotic resistance or compromised immune function, or both (Table 19.1).

Fungal Pathogens

Candida albicans

In patients with AIDS, *Candida albicans* causes locally invasive mucosal disease in the mouth and esophagus.

Disseminated candidiasis is rare because neutrophil function remains relatively intact. The presence of oral candidiasis in persons at risk of AIDS should alert the physician to possible infection with human immunodeficiency virus. If oral candidiasis is present, endoscopy is required to confirm esophageal involvement. The symptoms of odynophagia suggest esophageal involvement. Diagnosis is based on histologic examination showing hyphae, pseudohyphae, or yeast forms. However, endoscopy is not necessary for the initial evaluation of odynophagia in a patient who has AIDS and evidence of oral thrush. A trial of empirical antifungal therapy is reasonable. Treatment is with nystatin, ketoconazole, fluconazole, or amphotericin B (Table 19.1).

Histoplasma capsulatum

Histoplasma capsulatum causes an important opportunistic infection in AIDS patients who reside in areas where the organism is endemic. Colonic involvement is more common than small-bowel involvement. Symptoms include diarrhea, weight loss, fever, and abdominal pain. Diagnosis is established with culture. Colonoscopy may show inflammation and ulcerations, and histologic examination with Giemsa stain shows intracellular yeast-like *H capsulatum* within lamina propria macrophages. Treatment is with amphotericin B or itraconazole.

Protozoan Pathogens

Cryptosporidium

Cryptosporidium is among the most common enteric pathogens, occurring in 10% to 20% of patients who have AIDS and diarrhea in the United States and in 50% of those in developing countries. The organs affected are the small and large intestines and the biliary tree. Symptoms include voluminous watery diarrhea, severe abdominal cramps, weight loss, anorexia, malaise, and low-grade fever. Biliary tract obstruction has been reported. Diagnosis is based on microscopic identification of organisms in stool specimens with modified acid-fast staining or stains specific for *Cryptosporidium*. Organisms may also be identified in biopsy specimens or in duodenal fluid aspirates. Treatment is with paromomycin, which improves the diarrhea (Table 19.1).

Cystoisospora belli

Cystoisospora belli is the most common cause of diarrhea in developing countries. The small intestine is primarily affected, but the organisms can be identified throughout the gut and in other organs. Symptoms include watery diarrhea, cramping abdominal pain, weight loss, anorexia, malaise, and fever. Diagnosis is based on identifying oval oocysts in stool with a modified Kinyoun carbolfuchsin stain. Biopsy specimens from the small intestine may show organisms in the lumen or within cytoplasmic vacuoles in enterocytes. Although *C belli* oocysts resemble *Cryptosporidium* oocysts, *C belli* oocysts contain 2 sporoblasts. *Cryptosporidium* oocysts are small and round and contain 4 sporozoites. Treatment is with trimethoprim-sulfamethoxazole (Table 19.1).

Microsporida (*Enterocytozoon bieneusi*)

Organisms in the order Microsporida are emerging as important pathogens; they have been identified in up to 33% of AIDS patients who have diarrhea. The small intestine is affected, and symptoms include watery diarrhea with gradual weight loss but no fever or anorexia. Diagnosis is based on electron microscopic identification of round or oval meront (proliferative) and sporont (spore-forming) stages of Microsporida in the villous but not crypt epithelial cells of the duodenum and jejunum. There are reports of positive stool specimens with Giemsa staining. There is no known treatment (Table 19.1).

Other Protozoa

Other important protozoa include *Entamoeba histolytica*, *Giardia intestinalis* (formerly *Giardia lamblia*), and *Blastocystis hominis* (Table 19.1). The rates of symptomatic infection with *E histolytica*, *G intestinalis*, or *B hominis* are not markedly higher than in patients who do not have AIDS. In most patients with AIDS, *E histolytica* is a nonpathogenic commensal. Giardiasis may require prolonged treatment, as in other immunocompetent persons.

Diagnostic Evaluation of Patients With AIDS Who Have Diarrhea

When patients with AIDS have diarrhea, several studies should be performed, as listed in Box 19.1. If the results of studies listed in Box 19.1 do not yield a diagnosis, the

---

Box 19.1 • Diagnostic Studies for Evaluating Patients With AIDS Who Have Diarrhea

Initial studies

  Examination for stool leukocytes

  Stool cultures for *Salmonella* species, *Shigella flexneri*, and *Campylobacter jejuni* (≥3 specimens)

  Stool examination for ova and parasites (use of saline, iodine, trichrome, and acid-fast preparations)

  Stool assay for *Clostridium difficile* toxin

Additional studies

  Gastroscopy to inspect tissue, to aspirate luminal material, and to obtain biopsy specimens

  Examination of duodenal aspirate for parasites and culture

  Culture of duodenal biopsy specimens for cytomegalovirus and mycobacteria

  Colonoscopy to inspect tissue and to obtain biopsy specimens

  Culture of biopsy specimens for cytomegalovirus, adenovirus, mycobacteria, and herpes simplex virus

  Staining biopsy specimens with hematoxylin-eosin for protozoa and viral inclusion cells, with methenamine silver or Giemsa stain for fungi, and with the Fite method for mycobacteria

need for further evaluation is a matter of controversy. Most experts advocate empirical treatment with loperamide. Others recommend that biopsy specimens from the duodenum be examined with electron microscopy for Microsporida or from the colon for adenovirus. Empirical treatment with loperamide is favored because there is no treatment for either Microsporida or adenovirus.

Miscellaneous Infectious Causes of Colonic Disorders

Amebic Colitis

The colon is the usual initial site of amebic colitis. Symptoms vary from none to explosive bloody diarrhea with fever, tenesmus, and abdominal cramps. Proctoscopy shows discrete ulcers with undermined edges and normal adjacent mucosa. If exudate is present, it should be swabbed to make wet mounts to search for trophozoites. Indirect hemagglutination is useful for invasive disease. Radiography shows concentric narrowing of the cecum in 90% of patients. Amebic colitis is treated with metronidazole. The only pathogenic ameba in humans is *E histolytica*.

Tuberculosis

Patients with tuberculosis may present with diarrhea, a change in bowel habits, and rectal bleeding. The ileocecal area is the most commonly involved site. Radiography shows a contracted cecum and ascending colon and ulceration. Proctoscopy may show an ulcerating mass. Biopsy samples stained with Ziehl-Neelsen stain are positive for acid-fast bacilli. All cases are associated with pulmonary or miliary tuberculosis.

Streptococcus bovis Endocarditis

Streptococcus bovis endocarditis is associated with colonic disease (diverticulosis or cancer). The colon should be evaluated.

Pseudomembranous Enterocolitis

Pseudomembranous enterocolitis is a necrotizing inflammatory disease of the intestines characterized by the formation of a membranoid collection of exudate overlying a degenerating mucosa. Precipitating factors include colon obstruction, uremia, ischemia, intestinal surgery, and all antibiotics (except vancomycin).

Antibiotic Colitis

The symptoms of antibiotic colitis are fever, abdominal pain, and diarrhea (mucus and blood), which usually

occur 1 to 6 weeks after the initiation of antibiotic therapy. Sigmoidoscopy shows pseudomembranes and friability. Biopsy specimens show inflammation and microulceration with exudation. The condition usually remits, but it recurs in 15% of patients. Complications include perforation and megacolon. The pathogenesis begins with the antibiotic altering the colonic flora, resulting in an overgrowth of *C difficile*. The toxin produced by *C difficile* is cytotoxic, causing necrosis of the epithelium and exudation (pseudomembranes). Diagnosis is based on a stool toxin assay. Enzyme-linked immunosorbent assay (ELISA)-based stool testing has a sensitivity of 70% when a single stool sample is examined. The sensitivity increases to 90% when 2 stool samples are examined. Polymerase chain reaction (PCR)-based stool testing has a sensitivity of 95% when a single stool sample is examined. Proctoscopic findings may be normal or show classic pseudomembranes. The treatment is to discontinue the use of antibiotics and provide general supportive care (eg, fluids). Avoid the use of antimotility agents. Metronidazole (500 mg 3 times daily) is 80% effective and inexpensive and is recommended for patients with mild disease (leukocyte count $<15.0 \times 10^9$/L and normal serum creatinine). Vancomycin (125 mg 4 times daily) is recommended for patients with more severe

---

KEY FACTS

✓ Diagnostic studies for diarrhea in patients with AIDS—
  - stool examination: leukocytes, ova, and parasites
  - stool cultures: *Salmonella, Shigella*, and *Campylobacter*
  - stool assay: *Clostridium difficile* toxin
  - gastroscopy: inspect tissue, aspirate luminal material, and biopsy
  - duodenal aspirate: parasites and culture
  - culture of duodenal biopsy specimens: cytomegalovirus and mycobacteria
  - colonoscopy: inspect tissue and biopsy
  - culture of colonic biopsy specimens: cytomegalovirus, adenovirus, mycobacteria, and herpes simplex virus
  - staining of biopsy specimens: hematoxylin-eosin (protozoa and viral inclusion cells), methenamine silver or Giemsa (fungi), and Fite method (mycobacteria)

✓ Amebic colitis—colon is the usual initial site

✓ Colonic disease in patients with tuberculosis—
  - diarrhea, change in bowel habits, and rectal bleeding
  - ileocecal area is the most commonly involved site

✓ Antibiotic colitis—fever, abdominal pain, and diarrhea, usually 1–6 weeks after initiation of antibiotic therapy

disease (leukocyte count ≥15.0 × 10^9/L and elevated serum creatinine). For a first recurrence, the same antibiotic can be used or the drug can be switched. For multiple recurrences, add cholestyramine and prolong the course of treatment with antibiotics.

Radiation Colitis

Irradiation injury usually affects both the colon and the small bowel. Endothelial cells of the small submucosal arterioles are very radiosensitive and respond to large doses of irradiation by swelling, proliferating, and undergoing fibrinoid degeneration. The result is obliterative endarteritis.

Acute disease occurs during or immediately after irradiation; the mucosa fails to regenerate, and there is friability, hyperemia, and edema. *Subacute disease* occurs 2 to 12 months after irradiation. Obliterative endarteritis produces progressive inflammation and ulceration. *Chronic disease* consists of fistulas, abscesses, strictures, and bleeding from intestinal mucosal vessels. Predisposing factors include other diseases that produce microvascular insufficiency (eg, hypertension, diabetes mellitus, atherosclerosis, and heart failure) because they accelerate the development of vascular occlusion, total irradiation dose of 40 to 50 Gy, previous chemotherapy, adhesions, previous surgical procedure and pelvic inflammatory disease, and older age. The elderly are more susceptible. Radiography during acute disease shows fine serrations of the bowel, and radiography during chronic disease shows stricture of the rectum, which is involved most commonly. Endoscopy shows atrophic mucosa with telangiectatic vessels. Endoscopic coagulation is effective treatment for bleeding, but surgery may be required for fistulas, strictures, or abscesses.

Ischemia

Review of Vascular Anatomy

The *celiac trunk* supplies the stomach and duodenum. The *superior mesenteric artery* supplies the jejunum, ileum, and right colon. The *inferior mesenteric artery* supplies the left colon and rectum.

Acute Ischemia

The symptoms of acute ischemia are sudden and severe abdominal pain, vomiting, and diarrhea (with or without blood). Early in the course of ischemia, physical examination findings are normal despite complaints of severe abdominal pain. Risk factors include severe atherosclerosis, congestive heart failure, atrial fibrillation (source of emboli), hypotension, and oral contraceptives.

There are several syndromes. *Acute mesenteric ischemia* is due to embolic obstruction of the superior mesenteric artery in 80% of patients. Most emboli (95%) lodge in this artery because of laminar flow, vessel caliber, and the angle it takes off from the aorta. This syndrome may result in a loss of small bowel and produce short-bowel syndrome. Radiography shows ileus, small-bowel obstruction, and, later, gas in the portal vein. The treatment is embolectomy.

Ischemic colitis is due to a transient decrease in perfusion pressure with chronic, diffuse mesenteric vascular disease. This decrease occurs in severe dehydration or shock and results in ischemia of the gastrointestinal tract. It commonly involves areas of the colon between adjacent arteries (ie, "watershed areas") such as the splenic flexure and the rectosigmoid. Patients with this syndrome present with abdominal pain and rectal bleeding. The characteristic radiographic feature is thumbprinting of watershed areas. The treatment is supportive, with administration of intravenous fluids to maintain adequate tissue perfusion and consideration of antibiotics if clinically significant leukocytosis or fever is present. If the condition deteriorates, surgical resection may be necessary.

> ### Key Definition
>
> Ischemic colitis: *inflammation of the colon due to a transient decrease in perfusion pressure with chronic, diffuse mesenteric vascular disease.*

Nonocclusive ischemia is due to poor tissue perfusion caused by inadequate cardiac output. It can involve both small and large bowels. Its distribution does not conform to an area supplied by a major vessel. It occurs in patients with cardiac failure or anoxia and in patients who are in shock.

Chronic Mesenteric Ischemia (Intestinal Angina)

Chronic mesenteric ischemia is uncommon. Symptoms include postprandial pain and fear of eating, with secondary weight loss. At least 2 of 3 major splanchnic vessels must be occluded. Chronic mesenteric ischemia is associated with hypertension, diabetes mellitus, and atherosclerosis. An abdominal bruit is a clue to the diagnosis. Noninvasive imaging may be performed, including duplex ultrasonography or computed tomography or magnetic resonance angiography. The primary treatment options are angiography with possible stent placement or surgical revascularization.

Occlusion of the superior mesenteric vein accounts for approximately 10% of the cases of bowel ischemia. Risk factors include hypercoagulable states such as polycythemia vera, liver disease, pancreatic cancer, intra-abdominal abscess, and portal hypertension. Patients present with abdominal pain that gradually becomes severe. Diagnosis is based on noninvasive imaging studies such as duplex ultrasonography or computed tomography.

Irritable Bowel Syndrome

The term *irritable bowel syndrome* is used for symptoms that are presumed to arise from the small and large intestines. It refers to a well-recognized complex of symptoms resulting from interactions of the intestine, the psyche, and, possibly, luminal factors. Most patients have abdominal pain that is relieved with defecation or associated with a change in the frequency or consistency of the stool. Other associated symptoms include abdominal bloating and passage of excessive mucus with the stool.

Patients with irritable bowel syndrome usually have a long duration of symptoms, symptoms associated with situations of stress, and no weight loss, no intestinal bleeding, and no associated organic symptoms (eg, arthritis or fever). Irritable bowel syndrome is a diagnosis of exclusion: The diagnosis is confirmed by an appropriate medical evaluation that does not identify any organic illness. Always ask the patient whether symptoms are related to ingestion of dairy foods because lactase deficiency must be ruled out. Patients who have upper abdominal discomfort and bloating may require an ultrasonographic examination of the abdomen and esophagogastroduodenoscopy. Patients who have lower abdominal discomfort or a change in bowel habits may require stool studies, proctoscopic examination, or colonoscopy.

The treatment of irritable bowel syndrome is reassurance, stress reduction, and a high-fiber diet or the use of fiber supplements. The use of antispasmodics to control abdominal pain or antimotility agents to control diarrhea should be reserved for patients who do not have a response to a high-fiber diet.

Nontoxic Megacolon (Intestinal Pseudo-obstruction)

Acute pseudo-obstruction of the colon occurs postoperatively (after nonabdominal operations) and with spinal cord injury, sepsis, uremia, electrolyte imbalance, and drugs (narcotics, anticholinergics, and psychotropic agents). When the cecum diameter is more than 12 cm, the risk of perforation increases. Obstruction should be ruled out with a Hypaque enema. Treatment includes placement of a nasogastric tube, discontinuation of drug therapy, correction of metabolic abnormalities, and, if needed, neostigmine administration, colonoscopic decompression, or cecostomy.

Chronic pseudo-obstruction of the colon occurs with disorders that cause generalized intestinal pseudo-obstruction.

Congenital Megacolon

Congenital megacolon (Hirschsprung disease) occurs in 1 in 5,000 births. The incidence is increased with Down syndrome. Congenital megacolon usually becomes manifest in infancy; however, it can occur in adulthood. There is a variable length of aganglionic segment from the rectum to the proximal colon (usually confined to the rectum or rectosigmoid). The diagnosis is usually made at birth because of meconium ileus or obstipation. If the diagnosis is made when the patient is an adult, the patient usually has a history of chronic constipation. Radiography of the colon shows a characteristically narrowed distal segment and a dilated proximal colon. Rectal biopsy shows aganglionosis. Anorectal manometry shows loss of the anorectal inhibitory reflex. Treatment is with sphincter-saving operations.

Lower Gastrointestinal Tract Bleeding

The evaluation of acute rectal bleeding should begin with a digital rectal examination, anoscopy, and proctosigmoidoscopy. If a definitive diagnosis cannot be made, colonoscopy is necessary. The inability to cleanse the colon appropriately during active bleeding can make colonoscopy difficult to perform and interpret. Some advocate the use of nuclear scanning if the extent of bleeding is uncertain. If

---

KEY FACTS

✓ Vascular anatomy relevant for ischemia
- celiac trunk: stomach and duodenum
- superior mesenteric artery: jejunum, ileum, and right colon
- inferior mesenteric artery: left colon and rectum

✓ Acute ischemia—
- symptoms: sudden and severe abdominal pain, vomiting, and diarrhea (with or without blood)
- early in course: severe abdominal pain but normal physical examination findings
- risk factors: severe atherosclerosis, congestive heart failure, atrial fibrillation, hypotension, and oral contraceptives

✓ Nonocclusive ischemia—due to poor tissue perfusion caused by inadequate cardiac output

✓ Symptoms of irritable bowel syndrome—
- usually of long duration
- usually associated with stressful situations
- usually no weight loss, no intestinal bleeding, and no associated organic symptoms (eg, arthritis or fever)

✓ Treatment of irritable bowel syndrome—
- reassurance, stress reduction, and a high-fiber diet (or fiber supplements)
- if patients have no response to high-fiber diet, use antispasmodics (for abdominal pain) and antimotility agents (for diarrhea)

clinically significant active bleeding cannot be treated endoscopically, angiography may be necessary. Colonoscopy is not useful if bleeding in the lower gastrointestinal tract is torrential, but it may be of some benefit with a slower rate of bleeding. Colonoscopy is valuable for evaluating patients who have unexplained rectal bleeding and persistently positive findings on tests for occult blood in the stool. Important causes of lower gastrointestinal tract bleeding are listed in Box 19.2.

In the evaluation of lower gastrointestinal tract bleeding, stabilize the patient's condition, perform proctoscopy to rule out rectal outlet bleeding (due to hemorrhoids or anal fissure), and obtain a nasogastric tube aspirate or use esophagogastroduodenoscopy to rule out upper gastrointestinal tract bleeding. A radionuclide-tagged red blood cell scan may help determine whether bleeding is occurring, but it may not precisely localize the bleeding site. If bleeding stops or occurs at a slow rate, perform colonoscopy. If the patient is young, perform a Meckel scan. For persistent bleeding that is not amenable to endoscopic therapy, angiography may be used to localize the bleeding site; infusion of vasopressin or embolization may be useful. If colonoscopy shows bleeding, useful steps may include injection of epinephrine, electrocoagulation, or laser coagulation. If bleeding is massive or if marked bleeding continues, surgical management is necessary.

Angiodysplasia

Angiodysplasia is a common cause of lower gastrointestinal tract bleeding in elderly patients. Usually involving the cecum and ascending colon, angiodysplasia is associated with cardiac disease (especially aortic stenosis), advanced

---

Box 19.2 • Important Causes of Lower Gastrointestinal Tract Bleeding

Angiodysplasia—usually involves the right colon and small bowel; may respond to endoscopic treatment

Diverticular disease—usually bleeding without other symptoms

Inflammatory bowel disease (colitis)—in 5% of patients at presentation

Ischemic colitis—painful and bloody diarrhea

Cancer—rarely causes marked bleeding

Meckel diverticulum—the most common cause of lower gastrointestinal tract bleeding in young patients; it is usually painless

Internal hemorrhoids—painless with small volume of "outlet-type" bleeding

External hemorrhoids—pain with small volume of "outlet-type" bleeding

Anal fissure—very painful defecation associated with small volume of "outlet-type" bleeding and often coexisting with constipation

---

age, and chronic renal insufficiency. There are no associated skin or visceral lesions. Radiography of the colon is of no diagnostic value, but angiography localizes the extent of involvement. Colonoscopy may show lesions, and cautery application may be effective.

Diverticular Disease of the Colon

Definitions

Diverticula are acquired herniations of the mucosa and submucosa through the muscular layers of the colonic wall. **Diverticulosis** is the mere presence of uninflamed diverticula of the colon. **Diverticulitis** is the inflammation of 1 or more diverticula. The diagnosis and management of the complications of diverticular disease are outlined in Table 19.2.

Key Definitions

Diverticulosis: *presence of uninflamed diverticula of the colon.*

Diverticulitis: *inflammation of 1 or more diverticula of the colon.*

Diverticulitis

Microperforation or macroperforation of the diverticulum with subsequent peridiverticular inflammation is necessary to produce diverticulitis. The severity of the clinical symptoms depends on the extent of the inflammation. Free perforation is infrequent (diverticula are invested with longitudinal muscle and mesentery). Local perforations may dissect along the colonic wall and form intramural fistulas. The clinical presentation is left lower quadrant pain, fever, abdominal distention, change in bowel habits, and, occasionally, a palpable tender mass. Treatment includes resting the bowel or using a low-fiber diet and antibiotics and obtaining an early surgical consultation. Indications for surgical treatment include generalized peritonitis, an enlarging inflammatory mass, fistula formation, colonic obstruction, inability to rule out carcinoma in an area of stricture, or recurrent episodes of diverticulitis.

Colonic Polyps

Three types of epithelial polyps are benign: hyperplastic, hamartomatous, and inflammatory polyps. **Hyperplastic polyps** are metaplastic, completely differentiated glandular elements. **Hamartomatous polyps** are a mixture of normal tissues. **Inflammatory polyps** are an epithelial inflammatory reaction.

Table 19.2 • Diagnosis and Management of Complications of Diverticular Disease

Complication	Signs and Symptoms	Findings	Treatment
Diverticulitis	Pain, fever, and constipation or diarrhea (or both)	Palpable, tender colon Leukocytosis	Liquid diet (with or without antibiotics) or elective surgery
Pericolic abscess	Pain Fever (with or without tenderness) or pus in stools	Tender mass and guarding Leukocytosis Soft tissue mass on abdominal radiography or ultrasonography	Nothing by mouth Intravenous fluids Antibiotics Early surgical treatment with colostomy
Fistula	Depends on site: dysuria, pneumaturia, fecal discharge on skin or vagina	Depends on site: fistulogram and methylene blue dye injection	Antibiotics Clear liquids Colostomy Later, resection
Perforation	Sudden, severe pain Fever	Sepsis Leukocytosis Free air	Antibiotics Nothing by mouth Intravenous fluids Immediate surgical treatment
Liver abscess	Right upper quadrant pain Fever Weight loss	Tender liver, bowel, or mass Leukocytosis Increased serum alkaline phosphatase Lumbosacral scan (filling defect)	Antibiotics Surgical drainage Operation for bowel disease
Bleeding	Bright red or maroon blood or clots	Blood on rectal examination Sigmoidoscopy, colonoscopy, angiography	Conservative therapy Blood transfusion if needed, with or without operation

Key Definitions

Hyperplastic polyp: *metaplastic, completely differentiated glandular elements.*

Hamartomatous polyp: *mixture of normal tissues.*

Inflammatory polyp: *epithelial inflammatory reaction.*

The fourth type of epithelial polyp, *adenomatous polyps*, results from failed differentiation of glandular elements. Adenomatous polyps are the only neoplastic (premalignant) polyps. The types of adenomatous polyps are *tubular adenoma, mixed (tubulovillous) adenoma*, and *villous adenoma*. The risk of cancer with any adenomatous polyp depends on 2 features: size larger than 1 cm and the presence of villous elements. If a polyp is found on flexible sigmoidoscopy and biopsy shows a hyperplastic polyp, no further workup is needed. If biopsy shows an adenomatous polyp, colonoscopy should be performed to look for additional polyps and to perform polypectomy if necessary. Another type of polyp with neoplastic potential is the sessile serrated adenoma (mixed adenomatous and hyperplastic components).

Hereditary Polyposis Syndromes Associated With Risk of Cancer

Only the polyposis syndromes associated with adenomatous polyps carry a risk of cancer.

Familial Adenomatous Polyposis

Familial adenomatous polyposis (FAP) is characterized by adenomatous polyps of the colon. Colorectal carcinoma develops in more than 95% of patients, typically by age 40 years, if prophylactic colectomy is not performed. There are no extra-abdominal manifestations except for bilateral congenital hypertrophy of the retinal pigment epithelium. Diagnosis is based on family history and documentation of adenomatous polyps. Screening is indicated for all family members, and colectomy is indicated before malignancy develops. The inheritance is autosomal dominant; however, the phenotypic expression may vary considerably. The second most common malignancy in patients with FAP is cancer of the duodenum.

Gardner Syndrome

In Gardner syndrome, adenomatous polyps involve the colon, although rarely the terminal ileum and proximal small bowel are involved. Colorectal cancer develops in more than 95% of patients. Extraintestinal manifestations include congenital hypertrophy of the retinal pigment epithelium; osteomas of the mandible, skull, and long bones; supernumerary teeth; soft tissue tumors; thyroid and adrenal tumors; and epidermoid and sebaceous cysts. Screening is indicated for family members, and colectomy should be performed before malignancy develops. The inheritance is autosomal dominant.

Turcot Syndrome

In Turcot syndrome, adenomatous polyps of the colon are associated with malignant gliomas and other brain tumors. The inheritance is likely autosomal dominant but with variable penetrance.

Hereditary Polyposis Syndromes Not Associated With Risk of Cancer

In Peutz-Jeghers syndrome, hamartomas occur in the small intestine and, less commonly, in the stomach and colon. Pigmented lesions of the mouth, hands, and feet are associated with ovarian sex cord tumors and tumors of the proximal small bowel. The inheritance is autosomal dominant.

KEY FACTS

✓ Evaluation of acute rectal bleeding—
  - initially, digital rectal examination, anoscopy, and proctosigmoidoscopy
  - if definitive diagnosis is not possible, colonoscopy is necessary

✓ Angiodysplasia—common cause of lower gastrointestinal tract bleeding in elderly patients

✓ Clinical presentation of diverticulitis—left lower quadrant pain, fever, abdominal distention, change in bowel habits, and, occasionally, a palpable tender mass

✓ Familial adenomatous polyposis (FAP)—
  - adenomatous polyps of the colon
  - without prophylactic colectomy, 95% of patients have colorectal carcinoma (usually by age 40 years)

✓ Peutz-Jeghers syndrome—
  - hamartomas occur in small intestine (less commonly, in stomach and colon)
  - pigmented lesions of the mouth, hands, and feet (associated with ovarian sex cord tumors and proximal small bowel tumors)
  - autosomal dominant inheritance

20 Diarrhea, Malabsorption, and Small-Bowel Disorders

SETH R. SWEETSER, MD

Diarrhea

Diarrhea is a symptom or a sign, not a disease. As a symptom, it can manifest as 1 or more of the following: a decrease in consistency, an increase in fluidity, or an increase in number or volume of stools. A stool frequency of 3 or more times daily is considered abnormal; however, most people consider increased fluidity of stool as the essential characteristic of diarrhea. As a sign, diarrhea is an increase in stool weight or volume of more than 200 g or 200 mL per 24 hours for a person eating a Western diet. Although stool weight is often used in the objective definition, diarrhea should not be strictly defined by stool weight because the amount of dietary fiber influences the water content of the stool. Therefore, stool weight can vary considerably depending on fiber intake. In the United States, normal daily stool weight or volume is less than 200 g or 200 mL daily because of lower fiber intake (compared with up to 400 g or 400 mL daily in rural Africa).

Because diarrhea has multiple causes, its evaluation is often complex and time consuming. An understanding of the basic pathogenic mechanisms leading to diarrhea can help facilitate its evaluation and management.

The basic mechanism of all diarrheal diseases is incomplete absorption of fluid from luminal contents. Each day, approximately 10 L of fluid passes into the proximal small intestine (2 L from diet; 8 L from endogenous secretions). The small bowel absorbs most of the fluid (9 L), and the colon absorbs about 90% of the remaining 1 L, so that only about 1% of the original fluid entering the small intestine is excreted in the stool. A normal stool is approximately 75% water and 25% solids, with a normal fecal water output of 60 mL daily. An increase in fecal water output of only 100 mL is enough to cause increased stool fluidity or decreased stool consistency. This volume is approximately 1% of the fluid entering the proximal small intestine each day. Hence, malabsorption of only 1% of the fluid entering the intestine may be sufficient to cause diarrhea. Fortunately, the gut has considerable reserve absorptive capacity, with the small intestine having a maximal absorptive capacity of 12 L daily and the colon, 6 L daily.

Mechanisms of Diarrhea

Osmotic diarrhea occurs when a poorly absorbed substance remains in the intestinal lumen and causes water retention that maintains an intraluminal osmolality equal to that of body fluids (approximately 290 mOsm/kg). This occurs because, unlike the kidney, neither the small intestine nor the colon maintains an osmotic gradient. Osmotic diarrhea follows ingestion of an osmotically active substance and stops with fasting. Stool volume is less than 1 L daily, and the stool osmotic gap (SOG), calculated as follows, is greater than the sum of the measured concentrations of sodium (Na) and potassium (K) (the sum is doubled to account for their associated anions):

$$SOG = 290 \text{ mOsm/kg} - 2 \times (\text{Stool [Na]} + \text{Stool [K]}).$$

A normal stool osmotic gap is less than 50 mOsm/kg. However, with an osmotically active substance in the bowel, sodium and potassium levels will decrease (keeping stool osmotically neutral with the body). The calculated stool osmolality decreases, resulting in a gap (typically >100 mOsm/kg). Clinical causes of osmotic diarrhea include carbohydrate malabsorption, lactase deficiency, sorbitol-sweetened foods, saline cathartics, and magnesium-based antacids. In carbohydrate malabsorption (most commonly lactase deficiency), stool pH is often less than 6.0 because of colonic fermentation of the undigested sugars.

229

The term **secretory diarrhea** is used to indicate disordered intestinal epithelial electrolyte transport (ie, the intestine secretes electrolytes and fluid rather than absorbing them) even though secretory diarrhea is more commonly caused by reduced absorption than by net secretion. Stool volume is more than 1 L daily. The stool composition is predominantly extracellular fluid, so there is no stool osmotic gap. Secretory diarrhea persists despite fasting. Causes of secretory diarrhea include bacterial toxins, neuroendocrine tumors, surreptitious ingestion of laxative, bile acid diarrhea, and fatty acid diarrhea.

> ### Key Definition
>
> Secretory diarrhea: *intestine secretes electrolytes and fluid instead of absorbing them.*

A useful method to evaluate chronic watery diarrhea is to distinguish secretory diarrhea from osmotic diarrhea (Table 20.1) by measuring the concentrations of sodium and potassium in stool water (calculate the stool osmotic gap) and observing the patient's response to fasting.

Many disease processes cause diarrhea by more than 1 mechanism. For example, malabsorption in celiac disease has osmotic components (from carbohydrate malabsorption) and secretory components (unabsorbed fatty acids cause secretion in the colon).

In **exudative diarrhea**, abnormal membrane permeability allows serum proteins, blood, or mucus to be exuded into the bowel from sites of inflammation, ulceration, or infiltration. The volume of feces is small and the stools may be bloody. Examples include invasive bacterial pathogens (eg, *Shigella* and *Salmonella*) and inflammatory bowel disease.

In motility disorders, both *rapid transit* (inadequate time for chyme to contact the absorbing surface) and *delayed transit* (bacterial overgrowth) can cause diarrhea. Rapid transit occurs after gastrectomy or intestinal resection and with hyperthyroidism or carcinoid syndrome. Delayed transit occurs with structural defects (strictures, blind loops, and small-bowel diverticula) or with underlying illnesses that cause visceral neuropathy (diabetes mellitus) or myopathy (scleroderma), resulting in pseudo-obstruction.

> ### KEY FACTS
>
> ✓ Basic mechanism of diarrhea—incomplete absorption of fluid
> ✓ Osmotic diarrhea ends with fasting; secretory diarrhea does not
> ✓ Causes of osmotic diarrhea—carbohydrate malabsorption, lactase deficiency, sorbitol, saline cathartics, and magnesium-based antacids

> ### Key Definition
>
> Exudative diarrhea: *serum proteins, blood, or mucus are exuded into the bowel from sites of inflammation, ulceration, or infiltration.*

Clinical Approach to Diarrhea

Knowing the stool volume is potentially useful for distinguishing between diarrhea arising from the small bowel or ascending colon ("right-sided diarrhea") and diarrhea arising from the distal colon ("left-sided diarrhea") (Table 20.2). The distal left colon acts as a distensible reservoir that collects stool until defecation. With inflammation

Table 20.1 • Features Differentiating Osmotic Diarrhea From Secretory Diarrhea

Feature	Osmotic Diarrhea	Secretory Diarrhea
Daily stool volume, L	<1	>1
Effect of 48-h fasting	Diarrhea stops	Diarrhea continues
Fecal fluid analysis		
Osmolality, mOsm	290	290
([Na] + [K]) × 2[a], mEq/L	120	280
Solute gap[b]	>100	<50

Abbreviations: K, potassium; Na, sodium.
[a] Multiplied by 2 to account for anions.
[b] Calculated by subtracting ([Na] + [K]) × 2 from osmolality.
Adapted from Krejs GJ, Hendler RS, Fordtran JS. Diagnostic and pathophysiologic studies in patients with chronic diarrhea. In: Field M, Fordtran JS, Schultz SG, editors. Secretory diarrhea. Bethesda (MD): American Physiological Society; c1980. p. 141–51. Used with permission.

Table 20.2 • Features That Distinguish Right-Sided Diarrhea From Left-Sided Diarrhea

Feature	Right-Sided (Small-Bowel) Diarrhea	Left-Sided (Colonic) Diarrhea
Reservoir capacity	Intact	Decreased
Stool volume	Large	Small
Increase in number of stools	Modest	Large
Urgency	Absent	Present
Tenesmus	Absent	Present
Mucus	Absent	Present
Blood	Absent	Present

of the left colon, the reservoir becomes spastic and its ability to accommodate normal volumes of stool is impaired. As a result, left-sided diarrhea is characterized by frequent, small-volume stools and tenesmus with evidence of inflammation (blood or pus) in the stools. Proctosigmoidoscopic examination usually confirms mucosal inflammation.

Right-sided diarrhea is characterized by large-volume stools (due to normal distensibility of the rectum) and a modest increase in the number of stools. Symptoms attributed to inflammation of the rectosigmoid are absent, and proctoscopic examination findings are normal. Left-sided diarrhea usually suggests an exudative mechanism, whereas the mechanism for right-sided diarrhea is nonspecific.

Acute Diarrhea

Acute diarrhea is abrupt in onset and usually resolves in 3 to 10 days. It is self-limited, and the cause (often viral) usually is not found. No evaluation is necessary unless an invasive infection is suspected (eg, bloody stools, fever, travel history, or a common source outbreak). If these conditions exist, do not treat with antimotility agents. Begin the evaluation with stool studies for bacterial pathogens, ova, and parasites and proctosigmoidoscopy. Recognize the common situations that predispose to specific infections (see Noninvasive [Toxicogenic] Bacterial Diarrhea subsection).

Chronic Diarrhea

Chronic diarrhea is defined as diarrhea lasting longer than 4 weeks. The most common cause of chronic diarrhea is irritable bowel syndrome, but lactase deficiency should always be considered. Several features help differentiate organic diarrhea from functional diarrhea (Table 20.3).

Key Definitions

Acute diarrhea: *duration 3–10 days after abrupt onset.*

Chronic diarrhea: *duration >4 weeks.*

Physiology of Nutrient Absorption

The sites of nutrient, vitamin, and mineral absorption are the following: The duodenum absorbs iron, calcium, folate, water-soluble vitamins, and monosaccharides. The jejunum absorbs fatty acids, amino acids, monosaccharides, and water-soluble vitamins. The ileum absorbs monosaccharides, fatty acids, amino acids, fat-soluble vitamins (A, D, E, and K), vitamin B_{12}, and conjugated bile salts. The distal small bowel can adapt to absorb nutrients. The proximal small bowel cannot adapt to absorb vitamin B_{12} or bile salts.

Table 20.3 • Features That Distinguish Organic Diarrhea From Functional Diarrhea

Feature	Organic Diarrhea	Functional Diarrhea
Weight loss	Often present	Absent
Duration of illness	Variable (weeks to years)	Usually long (>6 mo)
Quantity of stool	Variable but usually large (>200 g in 24 h)	Usually small (<200 g in 24 h)
Blood in stool	May be present	Absent (unless from hemorrhoids)
Timing of diarrhea	No special pattern	Usually in the morning or after meals
Nocturnal symptoms	May be present	Absent
Fever, arthritis, skin lesions	May be present	Absent
Emotional stress	No relation to symptoms	Usually precedes or coincides with symptoms
Cramping abdominal pain	Often present	May be present

Adapted from Matseshe JW, Phillips SF. Chronic diarrhea: a practical approach. Med Clin North Am. 1978 Jan;62(1):141–54. Used with permission.

Fat absorption is the most complex process. Dietary fat consists mostly of long-chain triglycerides that must be digested by pancreatic lipase, which cleaves 2 of the 3 long-chain fatty acids from the glycerol backbone. The resultant free fatty acids and monoglycerides are solubilized by micelles for absorption. The fatty acids and monoglycerides are reesterified by intestinal epithelial cells into chylomicrons that are absorbed into the circulation via lymphatic vessels. Conversely, medium-chain triglycerides are absorbed directly into the portal venous system and do not require micellar solubilization.

Mechanisms of fat malabsorption are summarized in Table 20.4. Malabsorption should be suspected if the medical history suggests steatorrhea or if diarrhea occurs with weight loss (especially if intake is adequate), chronic diarrhea of indeterminate nature, or nutritional deficiency.

The causes of symptoms in malabsorption are summarized in Table 20.5, and various features that suggest specific malabsorption conditions are listed in Table 20.6.

The medical history, physical examination, or laboratory results may suggest a possible cause of diarrhea or malabsorption (Tables 20.7 and 20.8). For example, the medical history may include previous surgery (resulting in

Table 20.4 • Mechanisms of Fat Malabsorption

Alteration	Mechanism	Disease State
Defective digestion	Inadequate lipase	Pancreatic insufficiency
Impaired micelle formation	Duodenal bile salt concentration	Common duct obstruction or cholestasis
Impaired absorption	Small-bowel disease	Celiac disease, Whipple disease
Impaired chylomicron formation	Impaired β-globulin synthesis	Abetalipoproteinemia
Impaired lymphatic circulation	Lymphatic obstruction	Intestinal lymphangiectasia, intestinal lymphoma

short-bowel syndrome, dumping syndrome, blind loop syndrome, postvagotomy diarrhea, or ileal resection), irradiation, or systemic disease.

Diseases Causing Diarrhea

Osmotic Diarrhea

Lactose is normally split by the brush border enzyme lactase into glucose and galactose, which are absorbed in the small bowel. In lactase deficiency, lactose is not split in the small intestine but enters the colon, where it is fermented in the lumen by bacteria, forming lactic acid and liberating hydrogen. The result is diarrhea of low pH and increased intestinal motility. Several other disaccharidase deficiencies can also result in malabsorption of specific

Table 20.5 • Causes of Symptoms in Malabsorption

Extragastrointestinal Symptom	Cause
Muscle wasting, edema	Decreased protein absorption
Paresthesias, tetany	Decreased vitamin D and calcium absorption
Bone pain	Decreased calcium absorption
Muscle cramps	Weakness, excess potassium loss
Easy bruisability, petechiae	Decreased vitamin K absorption
Hyperkeratosis, night blindness	Decreased vitamin A absorption
Pallor	Decreased vitamin B_{12}, folate, or iron absorption
Glossitis, stomatitis, cheilosis	Decreased vitamin B_{12} or iron absorption
Acrodermatitis	Zinc deficiency

Table 20.6 • Features That Suggest Malabsorption Conditions

Feature	Condition
Diarrhea with iron deficiency anemia (evaluation for blood loss is negative)	Proximal small-bowel malabsorption (eg, celiac disease)
Diarrhea with metabolic bone disease	Proximal small-bowel malabsorption (from decreased calcium and protein levels)
Hypoproteinemia with normal fat absorption	Protein-losing enteropathy (with eosinophilia, eosinophilic gastroenteritis; with lymphopenia, intestinal lymphangiectasia)
Oil droplets (neutral fat) or muscle fibers (undigested protein) present in stool	Pancreatic insufficiency (maldigestion)
Normal serum levels (usually) of calcium, magnesium, and iron	Pancreatic insufficiency (serum levels of albumin may also be normal)
Howell-Jolly bodies (if there is no history of splenectomy) or dermatitis herpetiformis	Celiac disease
Fever, arthralgia, and neurologic symptoms	Whipple disease

carbohydrates; however, the most common disaccharidase deficiency involves lactase.

"Acquired" lactase deficiency (which is possibly genetic) is common in African Americans, Native Americans, and peoples of Asia and the Middle East. Diarrhea, abdominal cramps, and flatulence occur after ingestion of dairy products. The diarrhea improves with dietary changes. The pH of the stool is less than 6.0. In the lactose tolerance test, blood glucose levels increase less than 20 mg/dL after ingestion of lactose. Results of the hydrogen breath test may be abnormal. Jejunal biopsy results are normal (disaccharidase levels are decreased).

Table 20.7 • Patient History Features That May Suggest a Possible Cause of Diarrhea or Malabsorption

Feature	Suggested Cause
Age	Youth: lactase deficiency, inflammatory bowel disease, or sprue
Travel	Parasites or toxicogenic agents (exposure to contaminated food or water)
Drugs	Laxatives, antacids, antibiotics, colchicine, or lactulose
Family history	Celiac sprue, inflammatory bowel disease, polyposis coli, or lactase deficiency

Table 20.8 • Associated Signs and Symptoms of Systemic Illnesses Causing Diarrhea

Sign or Symptom	Diagnosis to be Considered
Arthritis	Ulcerative colitis, Crohn disease, Whipple disease, *Yersinia* infection
Marked weight loss	Malabsorption, inflammatory bowel disease, cancer, thyrotoxicosis
Eosinophilia	Eosinophilic gastroenteritis, parasitic disease
Lymphadenopathy	Lymphoma, Whipple disease
Neuropathy	Diabetic diarrhea, amyloidosis
Postural hypotension	Diabetic diarrhea, Addison disease, idiopathic orthostatic hypotension, autonomic dysfunction
Flushing	Malignant carcinoid syndrome
Proteinuria	Amyloidosis
Peptic ulcers	Zollinger-Ellison syndrome
Hyperpigmentation	Whipple disease, celiac disease, Addison disease, pancreatic cholera, eosinophilic gastroenteritis

Adapted from Fine KD. Diarrhea. In: Feldman M, Scharschmidt BF, Sleisenger MH, editors. Sleisenger & Fordtran's gastrointestinal and liver disease: pathophysiology, diagnosis, management. 6th ed. Vol. 1. Philadelphia (PA): WB Saunders Company; c1998. p. 128–52. Used with permission.

Transient lactose intolerance can occur whenever the intestinal mucosa is damaged, including simple viral gastroenteritis. In patients who eat a weight-reduction diet and drink diet soda or chew sugarless gum, osmotic diarrhea may develop from excessive ingestion of fructose or other artificial sweeteners.

KEY FACTS

- ✓ Acute diarrhea—self-limited; usually the cause is not identified
- ✓ Chronic diarrhea—commonly from irritable bowel syndrome or lactase deficiency
- ✓ Malabsorption—suspect with steatorrhea, diarrhea with weight loss, chronic diarrhea of indeterminate nature, or nutritional deficiency
- ✓ Any damage to the intestinal mucosa (eg, simple viral gastroenteritis) can cause transient lactose intolerance

Secretory Diarrhea

VIPoma

The **WDHA syndrome** (watery diarrhea, hypokalemia, and achlorhydria), also called Verner-Morrison syndrome or pancreatic cholera, is a massive diarrhea (5 L daily) with dehydration and hypokalemia. The patient may have

numerous endocrine tumors (with hypercalcemia or hyperglycemia). This diarrhea is associated with a non–beta islet cell tumor of the pancreas. Vasoactive intestinal polypeptide is the most common mediator; other mediators are prostaglandin, secretin, and calcitonin. VIPoma is diagnosed with a pancreatic scan or angiography and measurement of hormone levels. Treatment is with somatostatin or surgery.

> ### Key Definition
>
> WDHA syndrome: *watery diarrhea, hypokalemia, and achlorhydria.*

Carcinoid Syndrome

Carcinoid tumors arise from enterochromaffin cells of neural crest origin. About 90% of the tumors are in the terminal ileum. Features of carcinoid syndrome include episodic facial flushing (lasting up to 10 minutes), watery diarrhea, wheezing, right-sided valvular disease (endocardial fibrosis), and hepatomegaly. If the gut is normal, look for bronchial tumors or gonadal tumors. Dietary tryptophan is converted into serotonin (which causes diarrhea, abdominal cramps [intestinal hypermotility], nausea, and vomiting), histamine (responsible for flushing), and other chemicals (bradykinin and corticotropin). Persons with intestinal tumors are usually asymptomatic initially because the mediators have high first-pass clearance in the liver. Carcinoid syndrome arises when these mediators are released into the systemic bloodstream; this suggests that liver metastases or bronchial tumors are present. The diagnosis of carcinoid syndrome is made by finding increased urinary levels of 5-hydroxyindoleacetic acid and by performing liver biopsy. Treatment is with octreotide.

Laxative Abuse and Surreptitious Laxative Ingestion

Of the population older than 60 years, 15% to 30% admit that they take laxatives regularly. With the concealed ingestion of laxatives (surreptitious laxative ingestion), patients complain of diarrhea but do not admit that they take laxatives. In referral centers, this is a common cause of chronic watery diarrhea. Colonoscopy may show melanosis coli, which is a brown discoloration of the mucosa due to lipofuscin pigment accumulating in lamina propria macrophages. Melanosis coli is caused by anthraquinone laxatives (senna, cascara, and aloe). This benign condition is reversible with discontinuation of laxative use. A high degree of awareness is required to detect this condition. When surreptitious laxative ingestion is suspected, stool water can be analyzed for laxatives by chemical or chromatographic methods. Patients who ingest laxatives surreptitiously often have underlying emotional problems that should be addressed.

Bile Acid Malabsorption

Bile acid malabsorption is caused by ileal resection or disease. Diarrhea due to bile acid malabsorption may produce 2 clinical syndromes, each requiring a different treatment.

With a *limited resection* (≤100 cm of small intestine), malabsorbed bile acids enter the colon and stimulate secretion. Liver synthesis can compensate, so bile acid concentration in the upper small bowel is sufficient to achieve the critical micelle concentration and allow for normal fat absorption. The excess bile acids irritate the colon mucosa, causing a secretory diarrhea with minimal fat malabsorption. Treatment of the diarrhea is with cholestyramine, which binds excess bile acids.

With an *extensive resection* (>100 cm of small intestine), bile acid malabsorption is severe and enterohepatic circulation is interrupted. This limits synthesis, and the liver cannot compensate. Bile acid concentration is decreased in the upper small bowel, micelles cannot be formed, and fat malabsorption results. The malabsorbed fatty acids themselves stimulate secretion in the colon. Fat-soluble vitamins (A, D, E, and K) may be malabsorbed. Additionally, excess fatty acids bind intestinal calcium; this allows an increase in oxylate absorption, which increases the risk of oxylate renal stones. The treatment of this bile acid malabsorption is a low-fat diet (<50 g daily) rich in medium-chain triglycerides. Cholestyramine would further decrease the bile acid concentration and worsen the steatorrhea.

Bacterial Overgrowth

The proximal small intestine normally has low bacterial counts because it has several major defenses against excess small intestinal bacterial proliferation: intestinal peristalsis (the most important defense), gastric acid, and intestinal immunoglobulin (Ig)A. When these defenses are altered, bacterial overgrowth results. The mechanism of steatorrhea in bacterial overgrowth is the deconjugation of bile acids by bacteria that normally do not occur in the proximal intestine. Deconjugation of bile acids changes the ionization coefficient, and the deconjugated bile acids can then be passively absorbed in the proximal small bowel. Normally, conjugated bile acids are actively absorbed distally in the ileum. As a result, the critical micellar concentration is not reached, and mild steatorrhea results from the intraluminal deficiency of bile acids.

Clinical features of bacterial overgrowth are steatorrhea (typically >20 g daily), vitamin B_{12} malabsorption (macrocytic anemia), increased serum folate levels from bacterial production, and positive duodenal or jejunal cultures. Conditions associated with small intestinal bacterial overgrowth include postoperative conditions (blind loops, enteroenterostomy, or gastrojejunocolic fistula); structural abnormalities (diverticula, strictures, or fistulas); motility disorders (diabetes mellitus, scleroderma, or pseudo-obstruction); achlorhydria (atrophic gastritis or gastric resections; achlorhydria is corrected with antibiotics); and

impaired immunity. Two examples of impaired immunity are hypogammaglobulinemic sprue (in small-bowel biopsy specimens, no plasma cells are seen in the lamina propria and the villi are flat) and nodular lymphoid hyperplasia associated with IgA deficiency, which predisposes to *Giardia lamblia* infection.

KEY FACTS

✓ Diagnosis of carcinoid syndrome—based on liver biopsy findings and increased urinary levels of 5-hydroxyindoleacetic acid

✓ Causes of bile acid malabsorption—ileal resection or disease

✓ Limited resection of small intestine (≤100 cm)—malabsorbed bile acids enter the colon, stimulating secretion

✓ Extensive resection of small intestine (>100 cm)—severe bile acid malabsorption and interrupted enterohepatic circulation

✓ Bacterial overgrowth features—steatorrhea, vitamin B_{12} malabsorption, increased serum folate levels, and positive duodenal or jejunal cultures

---

Noninvasive (Toxicogenic) Bacterial Diarrhea

Toxicogenic bacterial diarrhea, characterized by watery stools without fecal leukocytes, is caused by several organisms (Table 20.9).

Staphylococcus aureus

Diarrhea caused by *S aureus* is of rapid onset and lasts for 24 hours. It is not accompanied by fever, vomiting, or cramps. The toxin is ingested with egg products, cream, and mayonnaise. Treatment is supportive.

Table 20.9 • Toxicogenic Causes of Bacterial Diarrhea

Organism	Onset, h	Mediated by Cyclic AMP	Fever	Intestinal Secretion
Staphylococcus aureus	1–6	+	−	+
Clostridium perfringens	8–12	−	±	+
Escherichia coli	12	+	+	+
Vibrio cholerae	12	+	Due to dehydration	++++
Bacillus cereus	1–6	+	−	+

Abbreviations: −, absence of feature; +, presence of feature (++++, strong presence); ±, feature may be present or absent; AMP, adenosine monophosphate.

Clostridium perfringens

The toxin of *C perfringens* (the "buffet pathogen") is ingested with precooked foods, usually beef and turkey, which have been kept warm under heating lamps in buffet lines. Heat-stable spores produce toxins. Although the bacteria are killed and the toxin is destroyed, the spores survive. When food is rewarmed, the spores germinate and produce toxin. The diarrhea is worse than the vomiting and is later in onset. It lasts 24 hours. Treatment is supportive.

Escherichia coli

The toxin of *E coli*, which causes traveler's diarrhea, is ingested with water and salads. It is a plasmid-mediated enterotoxin. Treatment is rehydration with correction of electrolyte imbalance and administration of ciprofloxacin, norfloxacin, or trimethoprim-sulfamethoxazole. This pathogen may be important in epidemic diarrhea of newborns.

Vibrio cholerae

The toxin of *V cholerae* is ingested with water. It is one of the few toxicogenic bacterial diarrhea illnesses in which antibiotics shorten the duration of the disease. Treatment is with tetracycline.

Bacillus cereus

Classically, the source of the *B cereus* toxin is fried rice in Asian restaurants. The toxin produces 2 syndromes: a rapid-onset syndrome that resembles *S aureus* infection and a slower-onset syndrome that resembles *C perfringens* infection. The diagnosis is typically made by clinical history but occasionally by isolating the organism from contaminated food. Treatment is supportive.

Other Toxicogenic Bacteria

Clostridium botulinum produces a neurotoxin that is ingested in improperly home-processed vegetables, fruits, and meats. It interferes with the release of acetylcholine from peripheral nerve endings. *Clostridium difficile* is discussed in the "Antibiotic Colitis" subsection of Chapter 19 ("Colonic Disorders").

Invasive Bacterial Diarrhea

Invasive bacterial diarrhea is characterized by fever, bloody stools, and fecal leukocytes. It is caused by several organisms (Table 20.10).

Shigella

Shigella infection is often acquired outside the United States. Bloody diarrhea is characteristic, and fever and bacteremia occur. Diagnosis is based on positive stool and blood cultures. Treatment is with ampicillin or a fluoroquinolone. Resistant strains are emerging for which chloramphenicol is an alternative. (Plasmids are responsible for antibiotic deactivation resistance.)

Table 20.10 • Causes of Invasive Bacterial Diarrhea

Organism	Fever	Bloody Diarrhea	Bacteremia	Antibiotic Effectiveness
Shigella	+	+	+	+
Salmonella	+	−	−	−
Vibrio parahaemolyticus	+	+	−	+[a]
Escherichia coli	+	+	−	−
Staphylococcus aureus (enterocolitis)	+	+	±	+
Yersinia enterocolitica	+	+	+	+
Campylobacter jejuni	+	+	±	+
Vibrio vulnificus	+	+	+	+

Abbreviations: −, absence of feature; +, presence of feature; ±, feature may be present or absent.
[a] Antibiotics are of questionable value, but erythromycin may be most effective.

Salmonella *(Non-Typhi)*

In the United States, *Salmonella typhimurium* is the most common agent. The organism is ingested with poultry. Fever and bloody diarrhea may be present. Diagnosis is based on a stool culture positive for *Salmonella*. Treatment is supportive. Severe symptoms should be treated with ciprofloxacin. Treating mild symptoms with other antibiotics may result in a prolonged carrier state.

Vibrio parahaemolyticus

The *V parahaemolyticus* toxin is ingested with undercooked shellfish. The infection is increasing in frequency in the United States (it is common in Japan). Fever and bloody diarrhea are the chief characteristics. Diagnosis is based on a stool culture positive for *Vibrio*. Antibiotics are of questionable value in treating this infection, but erythromycin may be most effective.

Escherichia coli

In the United States, enteroinvasive *E coli* is a rare cause of diarrhea. Enteroinvasive *E coli* affects the colon and causes abdominal pain with fever, bloody diarrhea, and profound toxicity (similar to *Shigella* infection). Shiga toxin–producing (also called enterohemorrhagic) *E coli* (serotype O157:H7) produces a cytotoxin that damages vascular endothelial cells. This serotype can cause sporadic or epidemic illness from contaminated hamburger and raw milk. Enterohemorrhagic *E coli* infection should be suspected when bloody diarrhea occurs after eating hamburger and when bloody diarrhea is complicated by hemolytic uremic syndrome or thrombotic thrombocytopenic purpura. Antibiotic treatment has not been effective and is not recommended because it may increase the risk of hemolytic uremic syndrome or thrombotic thrombocytopenic purpura from the rapid release of toxin during bacterial death.

Yersinia enterocolitica

A gram-negative rod, *Y enterocolitica* is hardy and can survive in cold temperatures. It grows on special cold-enriched medium. It is an invasive pathogen, with fecal-oral transmission in water and milk.

The spectrum of disease caused by *Y enterocolitica* includes acute and chronic enteritis. Acute enteritis is similar to shigellosis and usually lasts 1 to 3 weeks. It is characterized by fever, diarrhea, leukocytosis, and fecal leukocytes. Chronic enteritis occurs especially in children with diarrhea, failure to thrive, hypoalbuminemia, and hypokalemia. Other features are acute abdominal pain (mesenteric adenitis), right lower quadrant pain, tenderness, nausea, and vomiting. The disease mimics appendicitis or Crohn disease.

Extraintestinal manifestations are nonsuppurative arthritis and ankylosing spondylitis (associated with HLA-B27). Skin manifestations are erythema nodosum and erythema multiforme. Thyroid manifestations are Graves disease and Hashimoto disease. Multiple liver abscesses and granulomata are present.

Treatment is with aminoglycosides or trimethoprim-sulfamethoxazole. The bacteria are variably sensitive to tetracycline and chloramphenicol. β-Lactamases are frequently produced, making penicillin resistance common.

Campylobacter jejuni

The comma-shaped *C jejuni* organisms are motile, microaerophilic gram-negative bacilli. Transmission is linked to infected water, unpasteurized milk, poultry, sick dogs, and infected children. The incubation period is 2 to 4 days before invasion of the small bowel or colon. Infection results in the presence of blood and leukocytes in the stool. It may mimic granulomatous or idiopathic ulcerative colitis. It also may mimic small-bowel secretory diarrhea, with explosive, frequent watery diarrhea due to many *C jejuni* strains that produce a cholera-type toxin. The diarrhea usually lasts 3 to 5 days but may recur. Antibiotic treatment is with a macrolide antibiotic when severe, but treatment often is not needed. Postdiarrheal illnesses are hemolytic uremic syndrome and postinfectious arthritis.

Vibrio vulnificus

Noncholera *V vulnificus* organisms are extremely invasive and produce necrotizing vasculitis, gangrene, and shock. They are routinely isolated from seawater, zooplankton, and shellfish along the Gulf of Mexico and both coasts of the United States, especially in the summer. The 2 clinical syndromes are 1) wound infection, cellulitis, fasciitis, or myositis after exposure to seawater or cleaning shellfish

and 2) septicemia after the ingestion of raw shellfish (oysters). Patients at high risk of septicemia include those with liver disease, congestive heart failure, diabetes mellitus, renal failure, an immunosuppressive state, or hemochromatosis. Treatment is with tetracycline.

Aeromonas hydrophila

Infection with *A hydrophila* is a frequent cause of diarrhea after a person has been swimming in fresh or brackish water. The organisms produce several toxins. Treatment is with trimethoprim-sulfamethoxazole and tetracycline.

KEY FACTS

- ✓ Noninvasive (toxicogenic) bacterial diarrhea—watery stools without fecal leukocytes
- ✓ Invasive bacterial diarrhea—fever and bloody stools with fecal leukocytes
- ✓ Treatment of non-Typhi *Salmonella* diarrhea—supportive; for severe symptoms, ciprofloxacin (use of other antibiotics for mild symptoms may lead to carrier state)
- ✓ Treatment of enterohemorrhagic *E coli* diarrhea—antibiotics are not effective and may increase the risk of hemolytic uremic syndrome or thrombotic thrombocytopenic purpura (from rapid release of toxin as bacteria die)

Malabsorption Due to Diseases of the Small Intestine

Celiac Disease

Celiac disease, also known as gluten-sensitive enteropathy, is a multisystem disorder affecting approximately 1% of the population. It may affect multiple organ systems and have protean manifestations. Iron deficiency anemia is the most common clinical manifestation of celiac disease in adults. Gastrointestinal tract symptoms such as diarrhea are present in only approximately 50% of patients. Splenic atrophy may be a complication and cause an abnormal peripheral blood smear with Howell-Jolly bodies, which may be a clue to the diagnosis in 10% to 15% of patients. The pathognomonic skin manifestation is dermatitis herpetiformis.

The measurement of serum IgA tissue transglutaminase antibodies is the test of choice for noninvasive screening. If the results are positive, a small-bowel biopsy should be performed. False-negative results can occur in the IgA-based tests because about 5% of patients with celiac disease also have IgA deficiency. IgG-based testing or confirmation of normal total IgA levels should be performed with all sprue screening. If the result of the antibody testing is negative, another diagnosis should be considered. Small-bowel biopsy findings are not diagnostic. Diagnosis requires response to a gluten-free diet. If the patient has no response to the diet, the diet should be reviewed for inadvertent gluten ingestion. If symptoms recur after 10 to 15 years of successful dietary management, consider enteropathy-associated T-cell lymphoma, which is a characteristic complication of celiac disease, especially if there is associated abdominal pain and weight loss.

Tropical Sprue

In tropical sprue, diarrhea occurs 2 to 3 months after travel to the tropics. After 6 months, megaloblastic anemia develops because of folate deficiency and possible coexisting vitamin B_{12} deficiency. The pathogenesis is presumed to result from a type of bacterial overgrowth in the small bowel; however, the specific organism is somewhat controversial. Biopsies of the small bowel show villous atrophy, crypt hyperplasia, and an inflammatory infiltrate similar to findings in celiac disease. Treatment is with tetracycline (250 mg 4 times daily) and folate with or without vitamin B_{12}.

Whipple Disease

Whipple disease is a rare multisystem infectious disease that can involve the central nervous system (CNS), heart, kidneys, and small bowel. It occurs predominantly in middle-aged white men and is caused by chronic infection with the gram-positive bacillus *Tropheryma whipplei*. Diarrhea or steatorrhea is the most common presenting symptom. Arthritis is the most common extraintestinal symptom and affects the majority of patients. When Whipple disease involves the CNS, it causes oculomasticatory myorhythmia in 20% of patients. Oculomasticatory myorhythmia is pathognomonic and is characterized by continuous rhythmic jaw contractions that are synchronous with dissociated pendular vergence oscillations of the eyes.

In most patients with Whipple disease, the intestinal tract is involved regardless of the presence or absence of gastrointestinal tract symptoms. Thus, the primary diagnostic approach to a patient with clinically suspected Whipple disease is upper endoscopy with mucosal biopsy. Intestinal biopsy specimens show the characteristic finding of macrophages with periodic acid-Schiff (PAS)-staining particles that are *T whipplei* bacilli. Polymerase chain reaction assays may assist in detecting *T whipplei* DNA in the intestinal mucosa. Whipple disease should be suspected in patients who have recurrent arthritis, pigmentation, adenopathy, or CNS symptoms (dementia, myoclonus, ophthalmoplegia, visual disturbances, coma, or seizures). Treatment is with trimethoprim-sulfamethoxazole for 1 year.

Eosinophilic Gastroenteritis

Patients with eosinophilic gastroenteritis have a history of allergies (eg, asthma), food intolerances, and episodic symptoms of nausea, vomiting, abdominal pain, and diarrhea. Laboratory findings include peripheral eosinophilia, iron deficiency anemia, and steatorrhea or protein-losing enteropathy. Small-bowel radiographs show coarse folds and filling defects, and biopsy specimens show infiltration of the mucosa by eosinophils and, occasionally, the absence of villi. Parasitic infection should be ruled out. Treatment with corticosteroids produces a rapid response.

Systemic Mastocytosis

Systemic mastocytosis is a clonal proliferation of mast cells with activating mutations in the *c-kit* gene. It is characterized by mast cell infiltration of tissues, including those in the bone marrow, spleen, liver, and gastrointestinal tract. The characteristic dermatologic finding is urticaria pigmentosa. Typical symptoms include pruritus, flushing, tachycardia, asthma, and headache caused by the release of histamine from mast cells. Gastrointestinal tract manifestations include diarrhea and peptic ulcer disease. Symptoms may be provoked by heat; hence, bath pruritus (ie, itching after a hot bath) is a clue to the diagnosis. Treatment includes histamine receptor blockers, anticholinergics, cromoglycate, and glucocorticoids. Although the *c-kit* gene is mutated, the tyrosine kinase inhibitor, imatinib mesylate, is not an effective treatment.

Intestinal Lymphangiectasia

Intestinal lymphangiectasia is caused by lymphatic obstruction that results in dilatation of intestinal lymphatic channels with subsequent lacteal rupture and leakage of chylomicrons and protein-rich fluid into the intestine. The clinical features are edema (often unilateral leg edema), chylous peritoneal or pleural effusions, and steatorrhea or protein-losing enteropathy.

Laboratory findings include lymphocytopenia (average lymphocyte count, 0.6×10^9/L) due to enteric loss. Levels of all serum proteins, including immunoglobulins, are decreased. Small-bowel radiographs show edematous folds, and small-bowel biopsy specimens show dilated lacteals and lymphatics in the lamina propria that may contain lipid-laden macrophages. The same biopsy findings are seen in obstruction of mesenteric lymph nodes (lymphoma, Whipple disease, and Crohn disease) and obstruction of venous inflow to the heart (constrictive pericarditis and severe right heart failure). Diagnosis is based on abnormal small-bowel biopsy findings and enteric protein loss documented by finding increased α_1-antitrypsin levels in the stool.

Treatment is with a low-fat diet and medium-chain triglycerides (they enter the portal blood rather than the lymphatics). Occasionally, surgical excision of the involved segment is useful if the lesion is localized.

Amyloidosis

Amyloidosis is characterized by diffuse deposition of amorphous eosinophilic extracellular protein in the tissue. Gastrointestinal tract involvement can occur with AL amyloidosis, AA amyloidosis, and hereditary amyloidosis. The main sites of amyloid deposition are the walls of blood vessels and the mucous membranes and muscle layers of the intestine. Any portion of the gut may be involved. Amyloid damages tissues by infiltration (muscle and nerve infiltration causes motility disorders and malabsorption) and ischemia (obliteration of vessels causes ulceration and bleeding). Intestinal dysmotility can produce diarrhea, constipation, pseudo-obstruction, megacolon, and fecal incontinence. Clinical findings in patients who have amyloidosis include macroglossia, hepatomegaly, cardiomegaly, proteinuria, and peripheral neuropathy. Pinch (posttraumatic) purpura or periorbital purpura after proctoscopic examination may occur.

Small-bowel radiography shows symmetrical, sharply demarcated thickening of the plicae circulares. Histologic examination of duodenal biopsy specimens shows amyloid deposits in up to 100% of patients. It is the diagnostic test of choice when amyloid is suspected as a cause of gastrointestinal tract symptoms. Amyloid deposits may not be seen on routine histologic stains; Congo red staining is required. Subcutaneous fat pad aspirate stained with Congo red can be used to make the diagnosis in 80% of patients.

Miscellaneous Small-Bowel Disorders

Meckel Diverticulum

A Meckel diverticulum results from persistence of the vitelline duct, which is the communication between the intestine and the yolk sac. Persistence of the vitelline duct is the most frequent congenital abnormality of the small intestine and is an antimesenteric outpouching of the ileum usually occurring within 100 cm of the ileocecal valve. Because a Meckel diverticulum contains all layers of the intestinal wall, it is a true diverticulum. It may contain ectopic gastrointestinal tract mucosa, including gastric (most commonly), duodenal, biliary, colonic, or pancreatic tissue.

The most common manifestation is painless, maroon stools. Acid production by the ectopic gastric mucosa within the Meckel diverticulum causes peptic ulceration and bleeding. Other manifestations include intestinal obstruction due to intussusception or volvulus around the band that fixes the diverticulum to the bowel wall. Diverticulitis of a Meckel diverticulum can occur and mimic acute appendicitis.

The diagnostic test of choice is a Meckel scan (a technetium Tc 99m pertechnetate nuclear scan with mucous cells of gastric mucosa concentrating technetium), but false-positive and false-negative results can occur.

Aortoenteric Fistula

If a patient has a history of gastrointestinal tract bleeding and has had a previous aortic graft, immediate evaluation is required to rule out an aortoenteric fistula. Patients presenting with massive bleeding should not undergo endoscopy or arteriography. Emergency surgery is indicated.

Management of a smaller bleeding episode is more controversial, and urgent computed tomography or extended upper endoscopy has been suggested as a possible alternative to surgical exploration. If the presence of a graft fistula is confirmed (by air in the vessel wall on computed tomography or erosion of a graft into the intestinal lumen on endoscopy), emergent surgery is indicated.

KEY FACTS

✓ Celiac disease—Howell-Jolly bodies from splenic atrophy (in 10%–15% of patients)

✓ Complication of celiac disease—enteropathy-associated T-cell lymphoma (suspect with recurrence of celiac disease after several years of good dietary control)

✓ Diagnosis of Whipple disease—upper endoscopy with mucosal biopsy

✓ Amyloidosis—amyloid deposits in duodenal biopsy specimens

✓ Meckel diverticulum—painless, maroon stools; ectopic gastric mucosa in the diverticulum causes peptic ulceration and bleeding

✓ Aortoenteric fistula—consider this possibility immediately if the patient has a history of gastrointestinal tract bleeding and previous aortic graft

---

Chronic Intestinal Pseudo-obstruction

Pseudo-obstruction is a syndrome characterized by the clinical findings of mechanical bowel obstruction but without occlusion of the lumen. The 2 types are primary and secondary.

The primary type, also called *idiopathic pseudo-obstruction*, is a visceral myopathy or neuropathy. It is associated with recurrent attacks of nausea, vomiting, cramping abdominal pain, distention, and constipation, which are of variable frequency and duration. In familial causes, the patient has a positive family history and the condition is present when the patient is young. Esophageal motility is abnormal (achalasia) in most patients; occasionally, urinary tract motility is abnormal. Diarrhea or steatorrhea results from bacterial overgrowth. Upper gastrointestinal tract and small-bowel radiographs show dilatation of the bowel and slow transit (not mechanical obstruction).

Secondary pseudo-obstruction occurs in the presence of underlying systemic disease or precipitating causes (Box 20.1).

| **Box 20.1 • Causes of Secondary Pseudo-obstruction** |

Diseases involving intestinal smooth
    muscle: amyloidosis, scleroderma, systemic lupus
    erythematosus, myotonic dystrophy, and muscular
    dystrophy

Neurologic diseases: Parkinson disease, Hirschsprung
    disease, Chagas disease, and familial autonomic
    dysfunction

Endocrine disorders: hypoparathyroidism

Drugs: antiparkinsonian medications (levodopa),
    phenothiazines, tricyclic antidepressants, ganglionic
    blockers, clonidine, and narcotics

Approach to the Patient With Chronic Intestinal Pseudo-obstruction

If a patient has chronic intestinal pseudo-obstruction, first rule out a mechanical cause for the obstruction. Second, look for an underlying precipitating cause, such as metabolic abnormalities, medications, or an underlying associated disease. If a familial idiopathic cause is suspected, assess esophageal motility. Suspect scleroderma if intestinal radiography shows large-mouth diverticula of the small intestine. Suspect amyloidosis if the skin shows palpable purpura and if proteinuria and neuropathy are present.

21 | Esophageal and Gastric Disorders

AMY S. OXENTENKO, MD

Esophagus

Esophageal Function

The main functions of the esophagus are to transport food and prevent reflux. To transport food from the mouth to the stomach, the esophagus must work against a pressure gradient, with negative pressure in the chest and positive pressure in the abdomen. The lower esophageal sphincter (LES) helps to prevent reflux of gastric contents back into the esophagus.

The upper esophageal sphincter (UES), consisting of the cricopharyngeus muscle, and the muscle of the proximal one-third of the esophagus are striated muscle. A transition from skeletal to smooth muscle occurs in the midesophagus, with the distal one-third of the esophagus composed of smooth muscle under involuntary control. The LES is a zone of circular muscle located in the distal 2 to 3 cm of the esophagus.

Normal Motility

Immediately after a person swallows, the UES relaxes, allowing a food bolus to pass from the oropharynx into the esophagus. A peristaltic wave then passes through the body of the esophagus, and within 2 seconds after the swallow, the LES relaxes and remains so until the wave of peristalsis passes through it. The LES then contracts and maintains resting tone to prevent reflux. If the esophagus cannot perform its 2 main functions, symptoms of dysphagia or reflux may result.

Dysphagia

Dysphagia results from defective transport of food and is usually described as "difficulty swallowing" or "food sticking." Three causes of dysphagia must be distinguished: 1) oropharyngeal dysphagia (faulty transfer of a food or fluid bolus from the oropharynx into the esophagus); 2) mechanical dysphagia (structural abnormality of

the esophageal lumen); and 3) motor dysphagia (due to an underlying motility disorder).

Answers to 3 questions can help in making the diagnosis (Figure 21.1): 1) What types of food produce the dysphagia (solids or liquids or both)? 2) What is the time course of the dysphagia (intermittent or progressive)? 3) Is there associated heartburn? Esophagogastroduodenoscopy (EGD) is the test of choice for all patients with dysphagia unless features of oropharyngeal dysphagia are present (see below).

Oropharyngeal Dysphagia

Oropharyngeal dysphagia is the result of faulty transfer of a food bolus from the oropharynx into the esophagus and is most commonly caused by neuromuscular disorders and less commonly by proximal structural abnormalities (Box 21.1). In addition to having difficulty swallowing, patients with oropharyngeal dysphagia report coughing, choking, aspiration pneumonia, or nasal regurgitation with eating or drinking. The first test in the evaluation of oropharyngeal dysphagia is a video fluoroscopic swallowing test (also called a modified barium swallow). After oropharyngeal dysphagia is diagnosed, an evaluation to determine the underlying cause is needed; the diagnosis may be suggested by associated features, such as optic neuritis (with multiple sclerosis) or fatigability (with myasthenia gravis).

> **Key Definition**
>
> Oropharyngeal dysphagia: *faulty transfer of a food bolus from the oropharynx into the esophagus.*

Motor Dysphagia

Motor (or *motility*) *disorders* are characterized by dysphagia with both solids and liquids. These disorders may follow an intermittent or progressive course. The 3 important motor abnormalities of the esophagus are achalasia, scleroderma, and diffuse esophageal spasm.

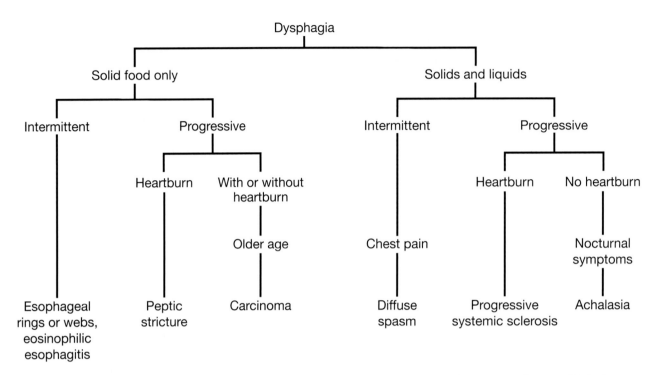

Figure 21.1 *Diagnostic Scheme for Dysphagia. The answers to 3 questions (see text) often suggest the most likely diagnosis.* (Adapted from MKSAP VI: part 1:44, 1982. American College of Physicians. Used with permission.)

Box 21.1 • Causes of Oropharyngeal Dysphagia

Muscular disorders

    Amyloidosis
    Dermatomyositis
    Hyperthyroidism
    Hypothyroidism
    Myasthenia gravis
    Myotonia dystrophica
    Oculopharyngeal myopathy
    Stiff man syndrome

Neurologic disorders

    Amyotrophic lateral sclerosis
    Multiple sclerosis
    Parkinson disease
    Polio
    Stroke
    Tabes dorsalis
    Tetanus

Structural causes

    Cervical osteophytes
    Cricopharyngeal dysfunction
    Esophageal webs
    Goiter
    Lymphadenopathy
    Zenker diverticulum

Achalasia

The term *achalasia* means failure to relax and results from degeneration of the myenteric plexus in the LES. Patients present with years of progressive dysphagia to both solids and liquids. Although these patients may have regurgitation of undigested and fermented food that never passed out of the esophagus (as evidenced by the presence of regurgitated food on their pillow after sleeping), heartburn is typically absent because the tonically contracted LES prevents acid from entering the esophagus. Chest radiography may show an air-fluid level within the esophagus in advanced cases. Barium esophagography typically shows a dilated esophagus with a pointed ("bird beak") tapering at the LES. The motility pattern in achalasia is characterized by 1) incomplete relaxation of the LES, 2) elevated resting tone of the LES, and 3) aperistalsis of the esophageal body. All patients with features of achalasia require an EGD because cancer infiltrating near the esophagogastric junction may have the same radiographic and manometric pattern of achalasia (termed *pseudoachalasia*). Patients with pseudoachalasia tend to be older, have more rapid onset of symptoms (months rather than years), and have more profound weight loss. Treatment of achalasia includes surgical methods (myotomy), injection of botulinum toxin into the LES, or pneumatic dilation. Healthy patients should be considered for a myotomy. Botulinum toxin injection into the LES decreases lower esophageal pressure for only 3 to 12 months and therefore should be considered for elderly patients and for patients with high surgical risk. In Brazil, the parasite *Trypanosoma cruzi* (which causes Chagas disease) produces a neurotoxin that destroys the myenteric plexus and leads to esophageal dilatation identical to that of achalasia.

Scleroderma

Esophageal involvement with *scleroderma* is associated with the CREST syndrome (calcinosis, Raynaud phenomenon, esophageal dysmotility, sclerodactyly, and telangiectasias). Patients have chronic, progressive dysphagia with both solids and liquids, along with severe heartburn and reflux. Barium swallow fluoroscopy may show a rigid esophagus and a widely patent LES. Although motility testing shows aperistalsis in the body of the esophagus similar to achalasia, the decreased LES tone in scleroderma distinguishes the 2 conditions.

Diffuse Esophageal Spasm

Patients with *diffuse esophageal spasm* usually present with chest pain, but they may have intermittent dysphagia with solids or liquids (or both); symptoms may be aggravated by stress, hot or cold liquids, and carbonated beverages. Imaging may show a corkscrew esophagus. Motility studies may demonstrate simultaneous contractions throughout the body of the esophagus during symptoms. A trial of acid suppression should be considered because acid reflux may precipitate esophageal spasm in some persons.

KEY FACTS

- ✓ Dysphagia has 3 causes—oropharyngeal, mechanical, and motor
- ✓ EGD—diagnostic test of choice for mechanical dysphagia or motor dysphagia
- ✓ Achalasia—EGD is required for ruling out pseudoachalasia (cancer near the esophagogastric junction)
- ✓ Scleroderma and achalasia—the body of the esophagus is aperistaltic in both conditions, but the LES tone is decreased in scleroderma

---

Mechanical Dysphagia

Dysphagia can result from compromise of the esophageal lumen to a diameter of less than 12 mm. This type of dysphagia usually begins with solid foods, but it may progress to involve liquids with further luminal narrowing. Depending on the cause, such as malignancy, weight loss may occur.

Peptic Strictures

A *peptic stricture* results from repeated esophageal reflux of acid. It is usually a short (<2 cm) narrowing in the distal esophagus immediately at or above the esophagogastric junction. Management includes esophageal dilation and long-term acid suppression; proton pump inhibitor (PPI) therapy after dilation of a peptic stricture has been proved to decrease recurrence.

Alkali-Induced Strictures

Alkali is more injurious to the esophagus than acid. *Alkali-induced strictures* can occur in patients after a total or partial gastrectomy or after lye ingestion. Inducing emesis after lye ingestion is contraindicated since the caustic substance can reinjure esophagus with subsequent exposure. Lye-induced strictures tend to be long (compared with peptic strictures). Repeated dilation or temporary stenting of the esophagus is often required after an alkali-induced stricture has occurred. Patients with lye-induced strictures have an increased incidence of squamous cell cancer of the esophagus.

Rings, Webs, and Diverticula

A *lower esophageal ring* (also called a Schatzki ring) is a constriction at the esophagogastric junction. The rings tend to cause intermittent solid food dysphagia or impaction, most notably with foods such as meat and bread (hence the name "steak house syndrome"). Esophageal dilation is the treatment of choice.

An *esophageal web* consists of a squamous membrane, which can be found throughout the esophagus, leading to dysphagia. If patients have an esophageal web with a proximal location, they can present with features of oropharyngeal dysphagia.

The *Plummer-Vinson syndrome* occurs in females who have iron-deficiency anemia, glossitis, and proximal esophageal webs. They have an increased risk of squamous cell carcinoma of the esophagus.

A *Zenker diverticulum*, an outpouching adjacent to the UES, results from increased tone within the UES. Patients present with dysphagia, regurgitation of small amounts of old food, and halitosis. Fullness in the neck may be apparent. Management includes resection of the diverticulum in combination with UES myotomy.

Eosinophilic Esophagitis

Patients with *eosinophilic esophagitis* present with intermittent solid food dysphagia and food impactions. This occurs most commonly in young men, but it may occur in all ages and in either sex. The patient may have a personal or family history of atopic conditions (eg, asthma, eczema, or seasonal allergies). Endoscopic findings may include concentric esophageal rings, furrows, or a featureless narrowed esophagus; some patients have normal findings. The diagnosis is established by finding more than 15 eosinophils per high-power field on midesophageal biopsies. Initial management is with a PPI trial, which may improve symptoms in a select number of patients with esophageal eosinophilia. For patients who have persistent symptoms despite acid suppression, swallowed, aerosolized corticosteroids are recommended. Recurrent symptoms are not uncommon after treatment. For children, elimination diets may be used. Severe tears can occur in untreated patients, so dilation of any associated strictures should be considered only after medical therapy has begun.

Esophageal Cancer

Squamous cell carcinomas of the esophagus are usually located in the proximal two-thirds of the esophagus, whereas tumors of the distal one-third are more commonly adenocarcinoma. The conditions that predispose to esophageal squamous cell carcinoma include achalasia, lye-induced stricture, Plummer-Vinson syndrome, human papillomavirus, tylosis, smoking, and alcohol consumption. Barrett esophagus is the most recognized risk factor for adenocarcinoma of the esophagus. In the United States, the majority of esophageal cancers are adenocarcinoma. Progressive dysphagia accompanied by weight loss is typical. The diagnosis is established by endoscopy with biopsy. After the diagnosis is confirmed, computed tomography of the chest and abdomen should be done to evaluate for metastatic disease. Endoscopic ultrasonography may be used to assess locoregional staging after distant metastases have been ruled out. The 5-year survival rate is only 7% to 15% since most patients have advanced disease at presentation.

Surgical resection is the treatment of choice for early-stage esophageal cancer. For patients with locally advanced disease or lymph node involvement, preoperative chemoradiotherapy may be considered, with restaging thereafter. For patients with extensive nodal or metastatic disease, palliative therapy can be offered, including chemotherapy, radiotherapy, and esophageal stenting.

Odynophagia

Odynophagia refers to painful swallowing. It results most commonly from inflammation (related to infection or medication) or spasm.

Key Definition

Odynophagia: *painful swallowing.*

Infections of the Esophagus

Patients with immunodeficiency disorders (eg, AIDS), diabetes mellitus, malignancies (especially lymphoma and leukemia), or esophageal motility disorders are susceptible to opportunistic infections of the esophagus and may present with odynophagia. The most important infections to recognize are those caused by *Candida albicans* (the most common cause), herpesvirus, or cytomegalovirus.

With candidal infection, endoscopy shows cottage cheese–like plaques adherent to the esophageal mucosa. The diagnosis is made by demonstrating pseudohyphae microscopically from brushings of the mucosa. Treatment is

with oral fluconazole for *Candida* esophagitis. For patients presenting with odynophagia who have evidence of thrush, therapy with oral fluconazole may be empirically started for presumed *Candida* esophagitis, reserving endoscopy for those in whom empirical therapy fails. If thrush is not present, patients should undergo endoscopy to establish a diagnosis unless there is a clear medication association.

If patients have herpesvirus infection, endoscopy may show multiple, small discrete ulcers, with biopsies from the edge of the ulcers revealing intranuclear inclusions and surrounding halos and multinucleated giant cells. Treatment is with acyclovir. In cytomegaloviral infection, endoscopy may show large, irregular ulcers, with biopsies from the ulcer base, showing "owl's eye" intranuclear inclusions and enlarged areas of cytoplasm. Treatment is with ganciclovir or foscarnet (in cases resistant to ganciclovir).

Medication-Induced Esophagitis

Patients with *medication-induced esophagitis* present with odynophagia (or, less frequently, dysphagia). Medication-induced esophagitis may occur if esophageal motility or anatomy is abnormal, but it occurs more frequently if medications are not taken with adequate fluids or if patients assume a supine position immediately after taking them. Medications commonly associated with esophagitis include tetracycline, doxycycline, quinidine, potassium supplements, bisphosphonates, ferrous sulfate, ascorbic acid, and nonsteroidal anti-inflammatory drugs. Stopping use of the medication for several days is often all that is needed, with clear instructions for administration if the medication is resumed. The use of these medications should be avoided if possible in patients with known esophageal strictures or dysphagia.

KEY FACTS

✓ Alkali causes more esophageal damage than acid

✓ Alkali-induced strictures—after gastrectomy (total or partial) or lye ingestion

✓ Eosinophilic esophagitis—intermittent solid food dysphagia and food impactions; midesophageal biopsy shows >15 eosinophils per high-power field

✓ Esophageal infections—most important ones are caused by *Candida albicans* (most common), herpesvirus, or cytomegalovirus

---

Gastroesophageal Reflux Disease

Reflux

Gastroesophageal reflux disease (GERD) is typically caused by inappropriate relaxation of the LES or by intragastric pressure that exceeds the LES pressure. Complications of reflux include esophagitis, bleeding, stricture formation, aspiration, Barrett esophagus, and adenocarcinoma of the esophagus.

Most patients with GERD describe classic heartburn or regurgitation. Atypical symptoms of GERD include noncardiac chest pain, asthma, chronic cough, hoarseness, and enamel defects. Reflux is the most common cause of noncardiac chest pain; however, it is imperative that cardiac status be evaluated before chest pain is attributed to reflux. Asthmatic patients with coexisting reflux should receive therapy for reflux because it may improve control of respiratory symptoms. Reflux should be considered in asthmatic patients who have postprandial or nocturnal wheezing.

Tests for Reflux

For patients with classic symptoms of reflux and heartburn with no alarm features (weight loss, anemia, dysphagia, odynophagia, or family history of cancer in the upper gastrointestinal tract), an empirical trial of PPI therapy is warranted. However, testing should be performed if patients have atypical features, symptoms refractory to a PPI trial, long-standing symptoms, or alarm features. The initial test in the evaluation of these symptoms should be an EGD. If esophagitis is present, reflux can be diagnosed with certainty. However, 40% of patients may have symptomatic reflux with no gross inflammation.

If an EGD does not show esophagitis or other features to support the diagnosis of reflux, a 24-hour ambulatory pH probe with impedance monitoring can be used to document esophageal acid exposure and symptom correlation. This allows a physiologic evaluation of reflux during daily activities. The test is valuable for patients who have had upper endoscopic results that are nondiagnostic (ie, no esophagitis is noted) and have ongoing or atypical features. Impedance technology, which has been added to standard 24-hour pH monitoring, allows the detection of non-acid reflux events that may be symptomatic and is useful in patients who have symptoms despite taking PPI therapy.

Barium esophagography is not useful in the evaluation of reflux, since reflux of barium occurs in 25% of controls. This test can be helpful in clarifying abnormal anatomical features (eg, paraesophageal hernia, intrathoracic stomach, and complicated strictures) but should not replace upper endoscopy.

Treatment of Reflux

The management of GERD is usually stepwise. Patients should be counseled on lifestyle modifications: The head of the patient's bed should be elevated 15 cm to keep the stomach lower than the esophagus, and patients should be advised to not eat for 3 hours before reclining, lose weight if overweight, avoid eating foods that personally trigger symptoms (eg, fatty foods, chocolate, peppermint, citrus juices, tomato products, and coffee), and avoid tobacco and alcohol. In addition, patients should avoid drugs that decrease LES pressure or delay gastric emptying (eg, anticholinergic agents, opioids, progesterone-containing agents, nitrates, and calcium channel blockers).

Medical therapy for reflux is graduated according to the degree of severity of the patient's symptoms. Over-the-counter antacids or H_2 receptor antagonists may be helpful for the patient who has occasional heartburn and reflux related to a triggering meal. PPIs (eg, omeprazole) are the most effective agents to relieve symptoms and promote mucosal healing. Long-term use of these agents is safe. Patients may take them once or twice daily, optimally 30 to 60 minutes before a meal. For patients with esophagitis, long-term PPI use is needed to allow for healing and prevent future complications such as a peptic stricture.

Antireflux surgery can be considered for younger patients who respond to PPI therapy but want to avoid lifelong medical treatment. Nissen fundoplication is the preferred operation. Those who do not respond to medical therapy are unlikely to have relief of symptoms after surgery. Those with dysphagia and bloating should avoid surgery, since both of these symptoms can occur or worsen after antireflux surgery. Patients with scleroderma should not have antireflux surgery because esophageal aperistalsis would lead to severe postoperative dysphagia.

Barrett Esophagus

Barrett esophagus is a complication of chronic GERD in which the normal esophageal squamous mucosa is replaced by intestinal metaplasia. Patients with Barrett esophagus are at increased risk of adenocarcinoma. Most experts recommend screening endoscopy for high-risk patients (obese white men older than 50 years) who have had chronic reflux for more than 5 years. If mucosal changes are seen endoscopically, biopsies are needed to confirm the diagnosis and to look for dysplasia. The surveillance frequency is based on the presence and degree of dysplasia found during the previous study. If high-grade dysplasia is identified and confirmed by 2 pathologists, the patient may elect to undergo an esophagectomy or be considered for ablative therapy, such as photodynamic therapy or endoscopic mucosal resection.

Noncardiac Chest Pain

All patients with chest pain should be thoroughly evaluated to rule out a potential cardiac cause before other diagnoses are considered. GERD is the most common cause of noncardiac chest pain, but esophageal pain may be due to a motor disorder (eg, spasm) or esophageal inflammation (eg, infection or injury). Esophageal spasm can closely mimic angina. EGD is used to rule out mucosal disease (eg, inflammation, neoplasm, or chemical injury). A 24-hour ambulatory pH probe with impedance can be used to document the presence of reflux and its correlation with chest pain. Therapy for noncardiac chest pain includes avoidance of precipitants. PPIs may be beneficial for patients with reflux. Sublingual nitroglycerin or calcium channel blockers are sometimes helpful in motor disorders. If appropriate, reassurance that cardiac disease is not present may be all that is necessary.

Other Esophageal Problems

Mallory-Weiss Tear

A **Mallory-Weiss tear** is a mucosal laceration at the esophagogastric junction. It accounts for about 10% of the cases of upper gastrointestinal tract bleeding; most patients have a history of retching or vomiting before the bleeding begins (eg, hyperemesis gravidarum, alcohol intoxication, or bulimia). The bleeding stops spontaneously in 90% of patients, but endoscopic hemostatic techniques can be used if needed.

Key Definition

Mallory-Weiss tear: *a mucosal laceration at the esophagogastric junction.*

Esophageal Perforation

Esophageal perforation most commonly occurs after dilation of a strictured area or with stenting of an esophageal cancer. Spontaneous perforation of the esophagus (Boerhaave syndrome) occurs after violent retching. The most common site of perforation is the left posterior aspect of the distal esophagus. If pleural fluid is present, it may have an increased concentration of amylase. The cervical esophagus may be perforated if a Zenker diverticulum is inadvertently intubated for an EGD or nasogastric tube placement.

KEY FACTS

✓ Causes of GERD—1) inappropriate LES relaxation or 2) intragastric pressure greater than LES pressure

✓ Complications of GERD—esophagitis, bleeding, stricture formation, aspiration, Barrett esophagus, and adenocarcinoma of the esophagus

✓ Empirical trial of PPI therapy—give to patients with classic symptoms of reflux and heartburn but no alarm features

✓ Antireflux surgery (Nissen fundoplication)—for younger patients who respond to PPI therapy and want to avoid lifelong medical treatment

---

Stomach and Duodenum

Peptic Ulcer Disease

Peptic ulcers are defects in the gastric or duodenal mucosa that result from an imbalance between acid and pepsin in the gastric juice and the host's protective mechanisms. Stimulators of acid production include acetylcholine, histamine, and gastrin. Inhibitors of gastric acid production include somatostatin and prostaglandin.

Peptic ulcers are categorized as being associated with 3 etiologic factors: 1) *Helicobacter pylori*; 2) nonsteroidal anti-inflammatory drugs (NSAIDs), including aspirin; or 3) miscellaneous causes. At least 90% of peptic ulcers are due to either *H pylori* or NSAIDs. Miscellaneous causes include gastrinomas (Zollinger-Ellison syndrome), Crohn disease, malignancy, drugs (cocaine), and viral infections (cytomegalovirus). There is no evidence that smoking or corticosteroids cause peptic ulcer disease (PUD), but either can result in decreased ulcer healing and increased complications.

Infection with *H pylori* causes more duodenal ulcers than gastric ulcers. Although NSAIDs tend to cause more gastric ulcers than duodenal ulcers, *H pylori* infection is still more likely to account for gastric ulcer disease in general.

Certain medical conditions may predispose to stress-induced peptic injury: ventilator use, underlying coagulopathy, significant burns, or central nervous system injury. Patients with these conditions should be considered candidates for prophylactic therapy.

Helicobacter pylori

The Organism

A gram-negative, spiral-shaped bacillus, *H pylori* is commonly acquired through oral ingestion and transmitted among persons living in close quarters. This fastidious organism resides and multiplies beneath and within the mucous layer of the gastric mucosa and produces several enzymes, such as urease, important for its survival and pathogenic effects.

Helicobacter pylori infection can lead to gastritis (acute to chronic), PUD, atrophic gastritis, mucosa-associated lymphoid tissue (MALT) lymphoma, or gastric malignancy.

Epidemiology

In the United States, *H pylori* has an age-related prevalence, occurring in 10% of the general population younger than 30 years and in 60% of persons older than 60 years. Overall, *H pylori* is more prevalent among blacks and Hispanics, poorer socioeconomic groups, and institutionalized persons. In developing countries, 50% of the population is infected by age 10 years and 70% by age 20, with 85% to 95% of the population infected overall. Evidence of person-to-person transmission exists.

Associated Diseases

Chronic Active Gastritis

The most common cause of chronic active gastritis is *H pylori* infection. The infection is predominantly an antral-based gastritis, although gastritis throughout the gastric body may be seen.

Duodenal Ulcer

In approximately 80% of patients with duodenal ulcers, *H pylori* is present. Among *H pylori*–positive patients with a duodenal ulcer who do not receive treatment targeted at the organism, most have ulcer relapse within 1 year. However, if the infection is successfully eradicated, the rate of relapse is extremely low.

Gastric Ulcer

In more than 50% of patients with gastric ulcers, *H pylori* is present. Eradication of the bacteria decreases the relapse rate of gastric ulcers.

Gastric Tumors

A known carcinogen as identified by the World Health Organization, *H pylori* is the leading cause of gastric malignancy in the world. The gastric cancer that results from *H pylori* infection is due to a progression from chronic gastritis to atrophic gastritis, to metaplasia, to dysplasia, and eventually to gastric adenocarcinoma.

MALT Lymphoma

MALT lymphoma of the stomach is a low-grade B-cell lymphoma. The majority of cases (90%) are related to *H pylori* infection. For early-stage disease, simple eradication of *H pylori* infection can induce complete or partial remission. For patients with more advanced disease, traditional lymphoma therapy is recommended.

Nonulcer Dyspepsia

Nonulcer dyspepsia is common, affecting about 20% of the US population. Among persons with nonulcer dyspepsia, up to 50% may be infected with *H pylori*; however, dyspepsia clinically improves with eradication therapy in only a small percentage of patients.

Diagnostic Tests for *H pylori* Infection

Various diagnostic tests are available for detecting the presence of *H pylori* infection. The choice of test is determined by the need for endoscopy, the use of certain medications, and cost (Table 21.1). For patients who need to be assessed for *H pylori* infection but do not require endoscopy, noninvasive evaluation with serologic antibody, stool antigen, or urea breath testing can be performed. The best noninvasive tests for determining eradication are the stool antigen test and the urea breath test.

Serology

Serologic testing is one of the most cost-effective, noninvasive ways to diagnose primary *H pylori* infection, and it is the 1 test for *H pylori* that is not affected by medications the patient may be taking. It is useful only in making the initial diagnosis, however, and should not be used for eradication testing.

Urea Breath Test

For the urea breath test, a radiolabeled dose of urea is given orally to the patient. If *H pylori* is present, the urease activity splits the urea, and radiolabeled carbon dioxide is exhaled.

Stool Antigen Test

The *H pylori* stool antigen test is simple and noninvasive. Unlike serologic testing, stool antigen testing does not depend on disease prevalence.

Rapid Urease Test

For the rapid urease test, a biopsy specimen taken during an EGD is impregnated into agar that contains urea and a pH indicator. As the urea is split by *H pylori*–produced urease, the pH of the medium changes the color of the agar. This test depends on bacterial urease: The more organisms present, the more rapidly the test produces positive results.

Histologic Examination

The *H pylori* organisms can be demonstrated with several specialized stains, including hematoxylin-eosin, Warthin-Starry, and immunostaining.

Table 21.1 • Tests for Detecting *Helicobacter pylori*

Test	Advantages	Disadvantages
Serology	Easy to perform Good negative predictive value Not affected by medications	Dependent on prevalence Indicates past infection only (not used for eradiation)
Stool antigen	Indicates active infection Useful for primary or eradiation testing	Stool collection Can be affected by antibiotics, acid suppression, or bismuth
Urea breath test	Indicates active infection Useful for primary or eradiation testing	Can be affected by antibiotics, acid suppression, or bismuth
Rapid urease test	Quick results	Expense of endoscopy Can be affected by antibiotics, acid suppression, or bismuth
Histology	Allows evaluation of histologic changes (dysplasia, etc)	Expense of endoscopy Dependent on expertise of pathologist

Treatment

With an *H pylori*–positive duodenal or gastric ulcer, the treatment goal is to heal the ulcer and eradicate the bacteria. All patients who are infected with *H pylori* should receive combination therapy. PPI-based triple therapy (usually in combination with amoxicillin and clarithromycin) for 10 to 14 days is the most commonly used initial therapy; metronidazole can be used in place of amoxicillin in patients who have a penicillin allergy. Because of emerging patterns of resistance to clarithromycin and metronidazole, these agents should be avoided if subsequent treatment is necessary and they were used as initial therapy. If the first course of therapy fails to eradicate the organism, quadruple therapy can be considered (PPI, metronidazole, bismuth, and tetracycline). Sequential therapy has also been used.

KEY FACTS

✓ Stress-induced peptic injury—consider prophylactic therapy with ventilator use, coagulopathy, significant burns, or central nervous system injury

✓ Prevalence of *H pylori* in the US general population—10% in persons younger than 30 years; 60% in persons older than 60 years

✓ Best noninvasive tests for determining eradication of *H pylori*—stool antigen test and urea breath test

---

NSAID-Induced Ulcers

NSAIDs inhibit gastroduodenal prostaglandin synthesis, which results in decreased secretion of mucus and bicarbonate, reduced mucosal blood flow, and stimulated acid production. NSAID-induced ulcers occur more commonly in the stomach (typically in the antrum) than in the duodenum.

The risk of PUD with NSAIDs is dose-dependent. Higher doses of NSAIDs or the combination of 2 or more NSAIDs (including low-dose aspirin) increases the risk of gastrointestinal tract injury. Selective cyclooxygenase 2 (COX-2) inhibition has been shown to decrease the rate of PUD and ulcer complications, such as bleeding, perforation, and pain. However, data suggest that even low-dose aspirin can reduce or eliminate any protective benefit of selective COX-2 drugs. For patients who require NSAID therapy, the lowest possible dose should be used and combination NSAID therapy avoided. The risk of PUD with NSAID initiation is maximal in the first month of treatment, and elderly patients and patients with a previous history of PUD are at highest risk.

The first step in the treatment of an NSAID-induced ulcer is to discontinue use of the drug if feasible. PPIs are most effective in healing and preventing ulcers and have few side effects. The synthetic prostaglandin agonist misoprostol decreases the incidence of NSAID-induced gastric ulcers; however, its usefulness is limited by the side effect of diarrhea and its role as an abortifacient (avoid using it in women of childbearing age).

Zollinger-Ellison Syndrome

Zollinger-Ellison syndrome is characterized by acid hypersecretion and the triad of peptic ulceration, esophagitis, and diarrhea (since excess acid inactivates pancreatic lipase) caused by a gastrin-producing tumor. The tumor usually is located in the "gastrinoma triangle," which includes the head of the pancreas, duodenal wall, and distal common bile duct. Two-thirds of gastrinomas are malignant and can metastasize. One-fourth of gastrinomas are related to multiple endocrine neoplasia type 1 (MEN-1) syndrome and are associated with pituitary adenomas and hyperparathyroidism.

Zollinger-Ellison syndrome should be considered in patients with *H pylori*–negative, NSAID-negative PUD, especially when there are multiple ulcers, ulcers in unusual locations (postbulbar duodenum), or refractory ulcers. Increased serum gastrin levels (>1,000 pg/mL) in patients who produce gastric acid are essentially diagnostic of gastrinoma. Increased serum gastrin levels may also be present in patients who are receiving PPI therapy (the most common reason) or who have atrophic gastritis (the next most common reason), pernicious anemia, postvagotomy states, or gastric outlet obstruction. Basal gastric acid output studies could be performed for patients who have increased levels of gastrin to see whether acid hypersecretion or achlorhydria is present. When the laboratory results are equivocal, a secretin test could be performed, if available; this test produces a paradoxical increase in the serum level of gastrin in patients with gastrinoma.

An octreotide scan (Octreoscan) can be used to localize a gastrinoma owing to the presence of somatostatin receptors. Endoscopic ultrasonography has been very successful in localizing gastrinomas because the pancreas and duodenal wall can be easily viewed with this test.

Since 50% of patients with gastrinomas have metastatic disease, curative surgery is not always feasible. Patients who are not candidates for surgery can receive high-dose acid suppression. Those with MEN-1 syndrome are usually not considered for surgical resection because of the multifocality of the disease.

Key Definition

Zollinger-Ellison syndrome: *acid hypersecretion with the triad of peptic ulceration, esophagitis, and diarrhea.*

Ulcer Diagnosis and Management

EGD is the best initial test to establish the diagnosis of PUD. At endoscopy, any active bleeding can be managed. Histologic evaluation can be performed if an ulcer has malignant features. If perforation is a concern, abdominal imaging should be the first test (endoscopy would be contraindicated).

A patient who has active bleeding from suspected ulcer disease needs to be hemodynamically stabilized before endoscopy is performed; endotracheal intubation may be required. PPI therapy should be initiated to stabilize clotting. Endoscopic therapy is selectively used according to stigmata of bleeding. All patients should be assessed for *H pylori* infection and NSAID use.

Angiography may be required for PUD if endoscopic therapy has failed to control active bleeding. Surgical intervention is infrequently needed for bleeding but would be considered if bleeding cannot be controlled angiographically. For perforation, urgent surgical consultation is necessary.

Chronic Gastritis

Chronic gastritis is most often caused by either *H pylori* infection or autoimmune gastritis. The most common cause of chronic gastritis is *H pylori* gastritis, which typically involves the antrum. Gastric ulcers and duodenal ulcers occur commonly, and the incidence of gastric adenocarcinoma is increased. *Helicobacter pylori*–related gastritis also predisposes to MALT lymphoma. If gastric biopsy results yield "chronic active gastritis," an evaluation for *H pylori* should ensue.

Autoimmune gastritis involves the body and fundus of the stomach (not the antrum). In a subset of patients, atrophic gastritis develops. Pernicious anemia with achlorhydria and megaloblastic anemia may result. Antiparietal cell or anti–intrinsic factor antibodies are found in more than 90% of these patients. Other autoimmune diseases are often present. The serum gastrin level may be markedly increased (given the lack of gastric acid to provide negative feedback) and may give rise to gastric carcinoid tumors, which usually follow an indolent course in these patients. Peptic ulcers do not typically develop in patients with autoimmune gastritis owing to achlorhydria, but the patients are at increased risk of intestinal metaplasia and gastric adenocarcinoma.

Gastric Cancer

In the 1940s, gastric cancer was the most common malignancy in the United States. Since then, the incidence in the United States has decreased dramatically. Currently, Japan has the highest mortality rate from gastric cancer. Known risk factors for gastric cancer are *H pylori* infection, autoimmune gastritis, and certain hereditary cancer syndromes. Known dietary risk factors include increased consumption of pickled foods, salted fish, processed meat, smoked foods, and products high in nitrates. The male to female ratio is as high as 2:1. Gastric cancer is more common in lower socioeconomic groups.

Clinical Aspects

Gastric cancer is often asymptomatic in the early stages, becoming symptomatic with advanced disease. The 2 types of gastric cancer are the intestinal type and the infiltrating type. The intestinal type of gastric cancer tends to appear as an ulcerated mass (similar to a cancer of the small or large intestine), with distinct borders and well-differentiated histology; patients often present with abdominal pain and iron-deficiency anemia. Gastric cancer that is in a diffuse or infiltrating form, also referred to as *linitis plastica*, often causes early satiety and weight loss because the stomach cannot stretch and accommodate food. The diffuse form tends to be poorly differentiated and is associated with signet ring cells and a very poor outcome. EGD is the initial test of choice to obtain a histologic diagnosis. After the diagnosis is established, computed tomography should be performed to evaluate for metastatic disease.

Treatment and Prognosis

For localized disease, resection with tumor-free margins often requires total gastrectomy. For disseminated disease, surgical treatment is necessary only for palliation. Response to chemotherapy is generally poor. Five-year survival is 90% if the tumor is confined to the mucosa and submucosa, 50% if the tumor is through the serosa, and 10% if the tumor involves regional lymph nodes.

Gastric Polyps

Gastric polyps are common and are typically found incidentally. There are 3 types of polyps: cystic fundic gland, hyperplastic, and adenomatous. *Cystic fundic gland polyps* are the most common gastric polyps and are not premalignant except in association with familial adenomatous polyposis (FAP). No additional therapy is needed unless FAP is known or suspected to be present. *Hyperplastic polyps* may occur with chronic gastritis, so patients should be tested for *H pylori*. Hyperplastic polyps rarely have malignant potential. *Adenomatous polyps* are deemed premalignant and need to be fully removed (like colon polyps).

The 3 types of carcinoid tumors may manifest as an incidentally noted gastric polyp: *Type 1 gastric carcinoids* are associated with autoimmune gastritis, whereas *type 2 gastric carcinoids* are associated with MEN-1 syndrome; both forms tend to follow an indolent course. *Type 3 gastric carcinoids* tend to be sporadic and behave aggressively.

Gastroduodenal Dysmotility Syndromes

Gastroparesis

Symptoms of delayed gastric emptying (ie, *gastroparesis*) may include nausea, vomiting, bloating, early satiety,

---

Box 21.2 • Conditions Causing Gastroparesis

Acute conditions

    Medication use (anticholinergic agents, opioids)
    Hyperglycemia
    Hypokalemia
    Pancreatitis
    Surgical procedures
    Trauma
    Viral infections

Chronic conditions

    Amyloidosis
    Diabetes mellitus
    Gastric dysrhythmias
    Pseudo-obstruction
    Scleroderma
    Vagotomy

---

anorexia, and weight loss. Diabetes mellitus is the most common cause of gastroparesis, which can occur with long-standing disease or with dramatic fluctuations in serum glucose levels. Other causes of gastroparesis exist (Box 21.2). After mechanical obstruction has been ruled out (usually with upper endoscopy), the test of choice to assess for gastroparesis is a 4-hour gastric scintigraphic study with a solid meal. Any medications known to alter gastric motility, namely opioids, need to be discontinued before testing.

Management of gastroparesis includes 1) dietary alterations, 2) antiemetic agents, and 3) prokinetic drugs, if needed. Metoclopramide is a dopamine antagonist and a cholinergic agonist that increases the rate and amplitude of antral contractions. It crosses the blood-brain barrier and can cause drowsiness and galactorrhea (from increased release of prolactin). The most feared complication of this medication is tardive dyskinesia, which can be irreversible. Erythromycin stimulates both cholinergic and motilin receptors, but because tachyphylaxis occurs with long-term use, it is most often used transiently in hospitalized patients.

KEY FACTS

✓ Risk of PUD increases with higher NSAID doses or with use of ≥2 NSAIDs

✓ Greatest risk of PUD from NSAIDs—during the first month of use, in elderly patients, and in patients with a previous history of PUD

✓ Diagnostic testing for gastroparesis—4-hour gastric scintigraphic study with a solid meal (after stopping opioids and after upper endoscopy to rule out mechanical obstruction)

Dumping Syndrome

Patients who have had prior resection of the gastric antrum and pylorus may be predisposed to *dumping syndrome*, which results from hyperosmolar substances rapidly exiting the stomach into the small bowel. Patients may complain of postprandial diarrhea, bloating, sweating, palpitations, and light-headedness. Symptoms can occur within 30 minutes after a meal (*early dumping*) or 1 to 3 hours after a meal (*late dumping*), which is associated with hypoglycemia and neuroglycopenic symptoms. Management includes having patients avoid hyperosmolar nutrient drinks, which aggravate symptoms; patients can modify their diets to include foods that delay gastric emptying (fats and proteins).

22 Hepatic Disorders[a]

WILLIAM SANCHEZ, MD AND JOHN J. POTERUCHA, MD

Interpretation of Abnormal Liver Test Results

The evaluation of patients who have abnormal liver test results includes many clinical factors: the patient's symptoms, age, risk factors for liver disease, personal or family history of liver disease, medications, and physical examination findings. A standard algorithm can aid in evaluating abnormal liver test results in an efficient, cost-effective manner.

Commonly Used Liver Tests

Aminotransferases

Aminotransferases are found in hepatocytes and "leak" out of liver cells within a few hours after liver cell injury. The aminotransferases are alanine aminotransferase (ALT) and aspartate aminotransferase (AST). ALT is more specific than AST for liver injury; however, markedly increased levels of muscle enzymes may also be associated with increases in both AST and ALT. Because ALT has a longer half-life, improvements in ALT lag behind improvements in AST.

Alkaline Phosphatase

Alkaline phosphatase is found not only on the hepatocyte but also in bone and placenta; thus, an isolated increase in serum alkaline phosphatase should prompt further testing to determine the origin of the elevation. This can be done either by determining alkaline phosphatase isoenzyme levels or by determining the level of γ-glutamyltransferase (GGT), a more specific hepatic enzyme. Other than to confirm the hepatic origin of an increased alkaline phosphatase level, GGT has little role in the diagnosis of diseases of the liver because its synthesis can be induced by many medications, thus reducing its specificity for clinically important liver disease.

Bilirubin

Indirect (unconjugated) bilirubin is the water-insoluble product of heme metabolism that is taken up by the hepatocyte and conjugated to make water-soluble direct bilirubin, which can then be excreted in the bile. Overproduction of bilirubin, such as during hemolysis or resorption of a hematoma, is characterized by indirect hyperbilirubinemia (<20% conjugated [direct] bilirubin). Hepatocyte dysfunction or impaired bile flow usually causes direct hyperbilirubinemia (usually >50% conjugated bilirubin). Conjugated bilirubin is water-soluble and may be excreted in the urine, resulting in darker urine; consequently, a lack of bilirubin pigments in the stool results in lighter stools.

Prothrombin Time and Albumin

Prothrombin time (PT), expressed as the international normalized ratio (INR), and serum albumin are markers of liver synthetic function. INR is a measure of the activity of coagulation factors II, V, VII, and X, which are synthesized in the liver. Because these factors are dependent on vitamin K for synthesis, vitamin K deficiency can also prolong INR. Vitamin K deficiency can result from antibiotic use associated with fasting, small-bowel mucosal disorders such as celiac disease, and severe cholestasis, with an inability to absorb fat-soluble vitamins. A simple way to distinguish between vitamin K deficiency and liver dysfunction in a

---

[a] Portions previously published in Poterucha JJ. Hepatitis. In: Bland KI, Büchler MW, Csendes A, Garden OJ, Sarr MG, Wong J, editors. General surgery: principles and international practice. 2nd ed. Vol 1. London (UK): Springer-Verlag; c2009. p. 921–32. Used with permission.

patient with a prolonged PT is to administer a 10-mg dose of oral vitamin K for 3 days or 10 mg of subcutaneous vitamin K. Vitamin K normalizes the PT within 48 hours in a vitamin K–deficient patient, but it has no effect on the PT in a patient with decreased liver synthetic function.

Because albumin has a half-life of 21 days, serum albumin does not decrease suddenly with liver dysfunction. However, serum albumin can decrease quickly with severe systemic illness such as bacteremia, likely from accelerated metabolism of albumin. A chronic decrease of albumin in a patient without liver disease should prompt a search for albumin in the urine.

Hepatocellular Disorders

Hepatocellular disorders primarily affect hepatocytes and are characterized predominantly by increases in aminotransferases. The disorders are best considered as acute (generally <3 months) or chronic. Common causes of marked acute increases in ALT are listed in Table 22.1.

Acute hepatitis may be accompanied by malaise, anorexia, abdominal pain, and jaundice. Acute hepatitis due to viruses or drugs generally produces markedly elevated aminotransferase levels (which are often thousands of units per liter); generally ALT is higher than AST. An ALT concentration greater than 5,000 U/L is usually caused by acetaminophen hepatotoxicity, hepatic ischemia (shock liver), or unusual viruses such as herpes simplex virus. Hepatic

ischemia typically occurs in patients with preexisting heart disease after an episode of hypotension. Aminotransferase levels are very high but decrease considerably within a few days. Transient bile duct obstruction, usually from a stone, can also cause aminotransferase elevations as high as 1,000 U/L, but they decrease within 24 to 48 hours. Pancreatitis with a transient increase in AST or ALT concentration suggests gallstone pancreatitis. Alcoholic hepatitis is characterized by more modest increases in aminotransferases (always <400 U/L and, at times, near the reference range) with an AST:ALT ratio greater than 2. Patients with alcoholic hepatitis often have a bilirubin level that is markedly elevated out of proportion to the aminotransferase elevations.

Diseases that produce a sustained (>3 months) increase in aminotransferase levels are in the category of *chronic hepatitis*. The increase (usually 2-fold to 5-fold) in aminotransferase levels is more modest than in acute hepatitis. Patients are usually asymptomatic but occasionally complain of fatigue and right upper quadrant pain. The differential diagnosis of chronic hepatitis is relatively lengthy; the more important and common causes are listed in Table 22.2.

KEY FACTS

✓ ALT—more specific than AST for liver injury (increased muscle enzyme levels may be associated with increased AST and ALT)

✓ Vitamin K deficiency—giving vitamin K normalizes the PT within 48 hours unless the patient has decreased liver synthetic function

✓ ALT >5,000 U/L—usually caused by acetaminophen hepatotoxicity, hepatic ischemia, or unusual viruses

✓ Transient increase in AST or ALT in a patient with pancreatitis suggests gallstone pancreatitis

✓ Alcoholic hepatitis—
  • modestly increased aminotransferases (<400 U/L and sometimes nearly normal)
  • AST:ALT ratio >2
  • bilirubin elevated out of proportion to aminotransferase elevations

Cholestatic Disorders

Diseases that predominantly affect the biliary system are called cholestatic diseases. They can affect the microscopic ducts (eg, primary biliary cirrhosis) or the large bile ducts (eg, pancreatic cancer causing obstruction of the common bile duct), or both (eg, primary sclerosing cholangitis). Generally, the predominant laboratory abnormality in these disorders is the alkaline phosphatase level. Although diseases that increase the bilirubin level are often referred to as cholestatic, severe hepatocellular injury (as in acute hepatitis) also produces hyperbilirubinemia because of hepatocellular dysfunction. The common causes of cholestasis are listed in Table 22.3.

Table 22.1 • Common Causes of a Marked Acute Increase in ALT

Disease	Clinical Clue	Diagnostic Test
Hepatitis A	Exposure history	IgM anti-HAV
Hepatitis B	Risk factors	HBsAg IgM anti-HBc
Drug-induced hepatitis	Compatible medication or timing	Improvement after withdrawal of the agent
Alcoholic hepatitis	History of alcohol excess AST:ALT >2 AST <400 U/L	Clinical improvement with abstinence
Hepatitic ischemia	History of hypotension and heart disease	Rapid improvement of aminotransferase levels
Acute biliary obstruction	Abdominal pain Fever ALT >3× reference range (specificity >95%, low sensitivity)	Cholangiography

Abbreviations: ALT, alanine aminotransferase; AST, aspartate aminotransferase; HAV, hepatitis A virus; anti-HBc, antibody to hepatitis B core antigen; HBsAg, hepatitis B surface antigen; Ig, immunoglobulin.

Table 22.2 • Common Causes of Chronic Hepatitis

Disease	Clinical Clue	Diagnostic Test
Hepatitis C	Risk factors	Anti-HCV HCV RNA
Hepatitis B	Risk factors	HBsAg
Nonalcoholic steatohepatitis	Obesity Diabetes mellitus Hyperlipidemia	Steatosis on liver imaging, liver biopsy
Alcoholic liver disease	History AST:ALT >2	Clinical liver biopsy
Autoimmune hepatitis	ALT 200–1,500 U/L Usually female Other autoimmune disease	Strongly positive antinuclear or anti– smooth muscle antibody (or both) Hypergammaglobulinemia Liver biopsy

Abbreviations: ALT, alanine aminotransferase; AST, aspartate aminotransferase; HBsAg, hepatitis B surface antigen; HCV, hepatitis C virus.

Jaundice

Jaundice is visibly evident hyperbilirubinemia, which occurs when the serum bilirubin concentration exceeds 2.5 mg/dL. Evaluation of a patient with jaundice is an important diagnostic skill (Figure 22.1). Conjugated hyperbilirubinemia must be distinguished from unconjugated hyperbilirubinemia. A common disorder that produces unconjugated hyperbilirubinemia is Gilbert syndrome, in which total bilirubin is generally less than 3.0 mg/dL and direct bilirubin is 0.3 mg/dL or less. The concentration of bilirubin is generally higher in the fasting state or in illness. A presumptive diagnosis of Gilbert syndrome can be made when an otherwise well person has unconjugated hyperbilirubinemia, normal hemoglobin (which excludes hemolysis), and normal liver enzymes (which exclude liver disease).

> **Key Definition**
>
> Jaundice: *visibly evident hyperbilirubinemia.*

Direct hyperbilirubinemia is a more common cause of jaundice than indirect hyperbilirubinemia. Patients with direct hyperbilirubinemia can be categorized as those with nonobstructive conditions and those with obstruction. Risk factors for viral hepatitis, a bilirubin concentration greater than 15 mg/dL, and persistently high aminotransferases suggest that the jaundice is from hepatocellular dysfunction. Abdominal pain, fever, or a palpable gallbladder (or a combination of these) suggests obstruction.

A sensitive, specific, and noninvasive test to exclude obstructive causes of cholestasis is hepatic ultrasonography.

Table 22.3 • Common Causes of Cholestasis

Disease	Clinical Clue	Diagnostic Test
Primary biliary cirrhosis	Middle-aged woman	Antimitochondrial antibody
Primary sclerosing cholangitis	Association with ulcerative colitis	Cholangiography (ERCP or MRCP)
Large bile duct obstruction	Jaundice or pain (or both)	Ultrasonography, ERCP, or MRCP
Drug-induced cholestasis	Compatible medication or timing	Improvement after withdrawal of the agent
Infiltrative disorder or malignancy	Other clinical features of malignancy, sarcoidosis, or amyloidosis	Ultrasonography Computed tomography Liver biopsy
Inflammation-associated cholestasis	Symptoms of underlying inflammatory state	Blood cultures Appropriate antibody tests

Abbreviations: ERCP, endoscopic retrograde cholangiopancreatography; MRCP, magnetic resonance cholangiopancreatography.

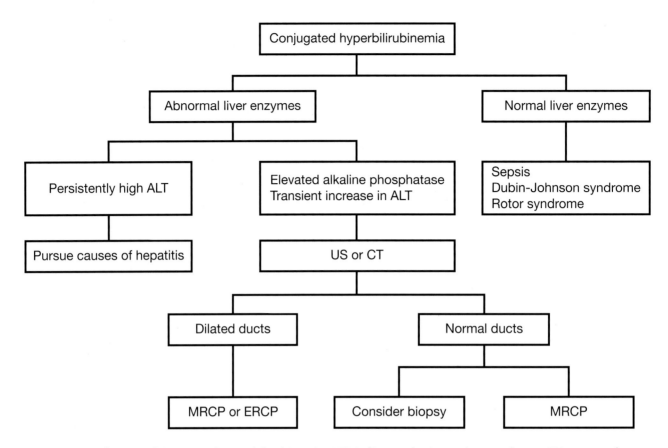

Figure 22.1 *Evaluation of Conjugated Hyperbilirubinemia. ALT indicates alanine aminotransferase; CT, computed tomography; ERCP, endoscopic retrograde cholangiopancreatography; MRCP, magnetic resonance cholangiopancreatography; US, ultrasonography.*
(Adapted from Poterucha JJ. Approach to the patient with abnormal liver tests and fulminant liver failure. In: Hauser SC, editor. Mayo Clinic gastroenterology and hepatology board review. 3rd ed. Rochester [MN]: Mayo Clinic Scientific Press and Florence [KY]: Informa Healthcare USA; c2008. p. 283–92. Used with permission of Mayo Foundation for Medical Education and Research.)

With diseases characterized by obstruction of a large bile duct, ultrasonography generally shows intrahepatic bile duct dilatation, especially if the bilirubin concentration is greater than 10 mg/dL and the patient has had jaundice for more than 2 weeks. Acute obstruction of a large bile duct, usually from a stone, may not allow time for the bile ducts to dilate. An important clue to the presence of an acute large-duct obstruction is a marked but transient increase in aminotransferases. If the clinical suspicion for obstruction of the bile duct is still strong despite negative ultrasonographic results, magnetic resonance cholangiography should be considered. Uncomplicated gallbladder disease, such as cholelithiasis with or without cholecystitis, does not cause jaundice or abnormal liver test results unless a common bile duct stone or sepsis is present.

Algorithms for Patients With Abnormal Liver Test Results

Algorithms for patients with abnormal liver test results are at best only guidelines and at worst misleading. The patient's clinical presentation should be considered when interpreting abnormal results. In general, patients with abnormal liver test results that are less than 3 times the normal value can be observed unless the patient is symptomatic or the albumin level, INR, or bilirubin concentration is abnormal. Persistent abnormalities should be evaluated. Algorithms for the management of patients with increased ALT or alkaline phosphatase are shown in Figures 22.2 and 22.3, respectively.

Specific Liver Diseases

Viral Hepatitis

Hepatitis A

Owing to vaccination and improvements in food handling, hepatitis A virus (HAV) is becoming an unusual cause of acute hepatitis in the United States. The disease generally is transmitted by the fecal-oral route and has an incubation period of 15 to 50 days. Major routes of transmission of HAV are ingestion of contaminated food or water and contact with an infected person. Persons at

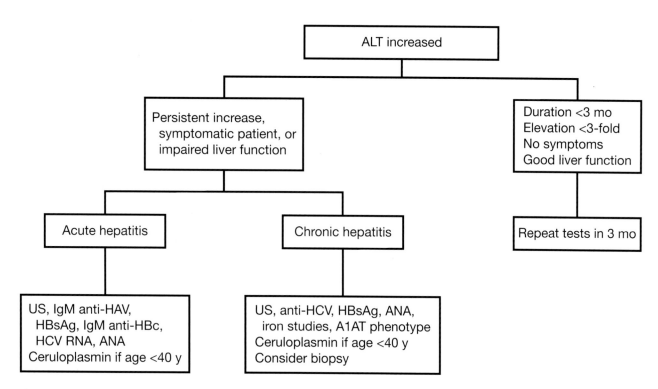

Figure 22.2 *Evaluation of Increased Levels of Alanine Aminotransferase (ALT). A1AT indicates* α$_1$*-antitrypsin; ANA, antinuclear antibody; anti-HAV, hepatitis A virus antibody; anti-HBc, antibody to hepatitis B core antigen; anti-HCV, hepatitis C virus antibody; HBsAg, hepatitis B surface antigen; HCV, hepatitis C virus; Ig, immunoglobulin; US, ultrasonography.*
(Adapted from Poterucha JJ. Approach to the patient with abnormal liver tests and fulminant liver failure. In: Hauser SC, editor. Mayo Clinic gastroenterology and hepatology board review. 3rd ed. Rochester [MN]: Mayo Clinic Scientific Press and Florence [KY]: Informa Healthcare USA; c2008. p. 283–92. Used with permission of Mayo Foundation for Medical Education and Research.)

highest risk of HAV infection are those living in or traveling to developing countries, children in day care centers, and homosexual men. Hepatitis caused by HAV is generally mild in children, who often have a subclinical or nonicteric illness. Infected adults are more ill and are usually icteric. The prognosis is excellent, although HAV can rarely cause acute liver failure. Chronic liver disease does not develop from HAV. Serum immunoglobulin (Ig) M anti-HAV is present during an acute illness and generally persists for 2 to 6 months. IgG anti-HAV appears slightly later, persists for life, and offers immunity from further infection.

Hepatitis B

Hepatitis B virus (HBV) is a DNA virus that is transmitted by exposure to blood or contaminated body fluids. In high-prevalence areas (eg, certain areas of Asia and Africa), HBV is acquired perinatally. High-risk groups in the United States include persons born in an area where HBV is endemic, injection drug users, and persons with multiple sexual contacts.

The clinical course of HBV infection varies. Symptoms of acute hepatitis (when present) are similar but generally more severe than those of HAV infection. Most acute infections in adults are subclinical, and even when symptomatic,

the disease resolves within 6 months with subsequent development of immunity. However, over 90% of those infected as neonates do not clear hepatitis B surface antigen (HBsAg) from the serum within 6 months and, thus, become chronically infected. These patients usually go through an immune-tolerant phase, characterized by normal ALT, positive hepatitis B e antigen (HBeAg), very high HBV DNA levels, and no fibrosis on liver biopsy. Treatment is not recommended. The natural history of chronic infection is illustrated in Figure 22.4.

The immune-tolerant phase evolves under immune pressure into the HBeAg-positive chronic hepatitis B phase, characterized by elevated ALT, the presence of HBeAg, high HBV DNA levels, and active inflammation and often fibrosis on liver biopsy. This phase leads to progressive liver damage, including cirrhosis and an increased risk of hepatocellular carcinoma. About 10% of patients per year become inactive carriers, a state characterized by a decrease in ALT, clearance of HBeAg, development of antibody to hepatitis B e antigen (anti-HBe) (seroconversion), and a decrease of HBV DNA. This inactive carrier state is not associated with progressive liver damage. About 60% of patients with chronic hepatitis B are in the inactive carrier phase. About one-third of inactive carriers have a recurrence of chronic hepatitis (HBeAg positive or negative), which is characterized by an

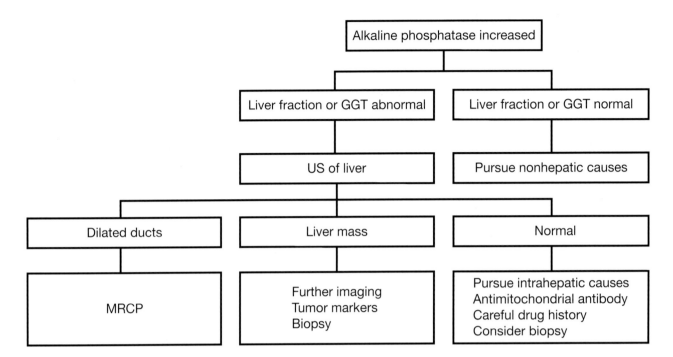

Figure 22.3 *Evaluation of Increased Levels of Alkaline Phosphatase. GGT indicates γ-glutamyltransferase; MRCP, magnetic resonance cholangiopancreatography; US, ultrasonography.*
(Adapted from Poterucha JJ. Approach to the patient with abnormal liver tests and fulminant liver failure. In: Hauser SC, editor. Mayo Clinic gastroenterology and hepatology board review. 3rd ed. Rochester [MN]: Mayo Clinic Scientific Press and Florence [KY]: Informa Healthcare USA; c2008. p. 283–92. Used with permission of Mayo Foundation for Medical Education and Research.)

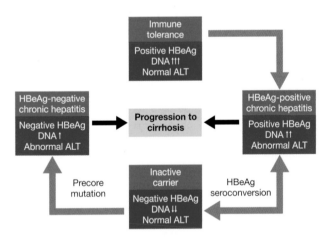

Figure 22.4 *Phases of Chronic Hepatitis B Virus Infection. Black arrows represent histopathologic changes; gray arrows represent changes in serologic markers between phases; thin arrows represent an increase or decrease in DNA level (↑, small increase; ↑↑, moderate increase; ↓↓, moderate decrease; ↑↑↑, large increase). ALT indicates alanine aminotransferase; HBeAg, hepatitis B e antigen.*
(Adapted from Pungpapong S, Kim WR, Poterucha JJ. Natural history of hepatitis B virus infection: an update for clinicians. Mayo Clin Proc. 2007 Aug;82[8]:967–75. Used with permission of Mayo Foundation for Medical Education and Research.)

abnormal ALT and an increased HBV DNA and is associated with progression of liver disease.

Patients with chronic hepatitis B and cirrhosis are at high risk for hepatocellular carcinoma (HCC), and liver ultrasonography should be performed every 6 to 12 months, especially for Asian men older than 40 years, Asian women older than 50 years, Africans older than 20 years, patients with a family history of HCC, and patients with persistent elevations of ALT and HBV DNA.

Patients with chronic hepatitis B, an abnormal ALT level, and high HBV DNA are candidates for therapy. Treatment options are compared and contrasted in Table 22.4. Treatment response is measured by the loss of HBeAg, the suppression of HBV DNA, and the appearance of anti-HBe (rarely, the loss of HBsAg). Peginterferon is considered for those with high serum aminotransferases, active hepatitis without evidence of cirrhosis on biopsy, and low serum levels of HBV DNA. The oral drugs are safer than peginterferon for patients with cirrhosis because flares of hepatitis and infectious complications are uncommon. Resistance is a concern with the oral agents; because of their low resistance rates, entecavir and tenofovir are the preferred oral drugs of choice for treatment.

A brief guide to the interpretation of serologic markers of hepatitis B is shown in Table 22.5. Viral markers in the

Table 22.4 • Agents for Treatment of Hepatitis B Virus

Feature	Peginterferon	Lamivudine	Adefovir	Entecavir	Telbivudine	Tenofovir
Treatment duration	12 mo	Indefinite	Indefinite	Indefinite	Indefinite	Indefinite
Side effects	Many	Minimal	Rarely renal	Minimal	Minimal	Minimal
Monthly charge, $	1,500–2,000	<500	1,000–1,499	500–999	500–999	500–999
Disease flare	Common	Rare	Rare	Rare	Rare	Rare
HBeAg seroconversion, %	27	20	12	21	22	20
Resistance	None	12%–15% yearly	1%–4% yearly	1%–2% yearly	22% at 2 y	None

Abbreviation: HBeAg, hepatitis B e antigen.

blood during a self-limited infection with HBV are shown in Figure 22.5. Note that IgM antibody to hepatitis B core antigen (anti-HBc) is nearly always present during acute hepatitis B.

Hepatitis B immune globulin should be given to household and sexual contacts of patients with acute hepatitis B. Infants should receive hepatitis B vaccine. The marker of immunity is hepatitis B surface antibody (anti-HBs). Because infected neonates are at high risk for chronic infection, all pregnant women should be tested for HBsAg. If a pregnant woman is HBsAg-positive, the infant should receive both hepatitis B immune globulin and hepatitis B vaccine. Some pregnant women with very high HBV DNA may be advised to undergo treatment with lamivudine or tenofovir during the third trimester. Patients who are HBsAg-positive and are receiving immunosuppressive therapy should also receive hepatitis B treatment, even if they do not meet the other recommendations for therapy.

Table 22.5 • Hepatitis B Serologic Markers

Test	Interpretation of Positive Results
Hepatitis B surface antigen (HBsAg)	Current infection
Antibody to hepatitis B surface (anti-HBs)	Immunity (immunization or resolved infection)
IgM antibody to hepatitis B core (IgM anti-HBc)	Usually recent infection; occasionally "reactivation" of chronic infection
IgG antibody to hepatitis B core (IgG anti-HBc)	Remote infection
Hepatitis B e antigen (HBeAg) or HBV DNA >10⁴ IU/mL	Active viral replication
Antibody to hepatitis B e (anti-HBe)	Remote infection

Abbreviations: HBV, hepatitis B virus; Ig, immunoglobulin.
Adapted from Poterucha JJ. Viral hepatitis. In: Hauser SC, editor. Mayo Clinic gastroenterology and hepatology board review. 5th ed. Rochester (MN): Mayo Clinic Scientific Press and New York (NY): Oxford University Press; c2015. p. 244–51. Used with permission of Mayo Foundation for Medical Education and Research.

KEY FACTS

✓ Presumptive diagnosis of Gilbert syndrome—
  • patient is well otherwise
  • unconjugated hyperbilirubinemia
  • normal hemoglobin
  • normal liver enzymes

✓ Hepatic ultrasonography—sensitive, specific, and noninvasive test for excluding obstructive causes of cholestasis

✓ HAV transmission—ingestion of contaminated food or water; contact with infected person

✓ HAV does not cause chronic liver disease

✓ Patients with chronic hepatitis B and cirrhosis— high risk for HCC (liver ultrasonography every 6–12 months for monitoring)

✓ Patients with chronic hepatitis B, abnormal ALT, and high HBV DNA should receive therapy

Hepatitis D

Hepatitis D virus (HDV), or delta agent, is a small RNA particle that requires the presence of HBsAg to cause infection. HDV infection can occur simultaneously with acute HBV infection (coinfection), or HDV may infect a patient with chronic hepatitis B (superinfection). Infection with HDV should be considered only for patients with HBsAg; diagnosis is based on HDV antibody (anti-HDV) seroconversion.

Hepatitis C

Hepatitis C virus (HCV), an RNA virus, is the most common chronic blood-borne infection in the United States. HCV has a role in 40% of all cases of chronic liver disease, and HCV infection is the most common indication for liver transplant. The most common risk factor is illicit drug use. Persons with a history of transfusion of blood products before 1992 (when routine testing of blood products for HCV was introduced) are also at considerable risk for infection with HCV. Sexual transmission of HCV occurs but seems to be inefficient. The risk of transmission of HCV

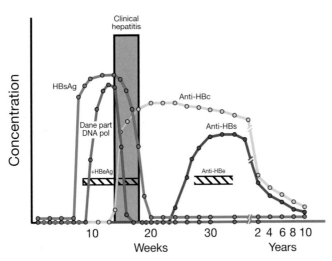

Figure 22.5 *Viral Markers in Blood During Self-limited Hepatitis B Virus Infection. Anti-HBc indicates hepatitis B core antibody; anti-HBe, hepatitis B e antibody; anti-HBs, hepatitis B surface antibody; HBeAg, hepatitis B e antigen; HBsAg, hepatitis B surface antigen; part, particle; pol, polymerase.*
(Adapted from Robinson WS. Biology of human hepatitis viruses. In: Zakim D, Boyer TD, editors. Hepatology: a textbook of liver disease. Vol 2. 2nd ed. Philadelphia [PA]: WB Saunders Company; c1990. p. 890–945. Used with permission.)

to health care workers by percutaneous (needlestick) exposure is also low—approximately 2% for a needlestick exposure to an infected patient.

Patients with HCV infection rarely present with acute hepatitis. The natural history of hepatitis C is summarized in Figure 22.6. In about 60% to 85% of persons who acquire hepatitis C, a chronic infection develops; after chronic infection is established, subsequent spontaneous loss of the virus is rare. Consequently, most patients with hepatitis C present with chronic hepatitis with mild to moderate increases in ALT. Some patients have fatigue or vague right upper quadrant pain. Patients may also receive medical attention because of complications of end-stage liver disease or, rarely, extrahepatic complications such as cryoglobulinemia or porphyria cutanea tarda. Because the majority of patients with hepatitis C are asymptomatic, treatment is generally aimed at preventing future complications of the disease. Patients with cirrhosis due to HCV generally have had HCV infection for more than 20 years.

Antibodies to HCV (anti-HCV) indicate exposure to the virus (current infection or previous infection with subsequent clearance) and are not protective. The presence of anti-HCV in a patient with an abnormal ALT and risk factors for hepatitis C is strongly suggestive of current HCV infection. Initial anti-HCV determination is with enzyme-linked

immunosorbent assay (ELISA). HCV infection is diagnosed by determining the presence of HCV RNA (Table 22.6). Levels of HCV RNA do not correlate with disease severity and are mainly used to stratify the response to therapy. Similarly, hepatitis C genotypes do not affect disease severity but do affect treatment response.

All patients with hepatitis C should be counseled on preventing liver damage, most notably through avoidance of alcohol. Most patients in the United States are infected with hepatitis C genotype 1. Therapy for hepatitis C has changed drastically in the recent past. Previously, peginterferon-based combination therapy required prolonged treatment (often 48 weeks) and was associated with a very high rate of adverse effects; a sustained virologic response was achieved in approximately 70% of treated patients. With the advent of potent, orally administered, direct-acting antiviral (DAA) agents, patients can now be treated with shorter courses (3–6 months) of oral medications with a low rate of adverse effects and sustained virologic response rates of more than 90%. If patients received peginterferon-based therapy that failed, or if they were unable to tolerate or were not candidates for peginterferon-based therapy, they are likely to be able to successfully undergo treatment with DAA agents. Treatment of hepatitis C continues to evolve, and new agents will likely continue to enter practice in the near future.

The risk of HCC complicating hepatitis C with cirrhosis is 1% to 4% per year. Surveillance with liver imaging every 6 to 12 months is advised for patients who are potential candidates for treatment with liver transplant, percutaneous ablation, transarterial chemoembolization, or radioembolization. Patients with HCV infection and decompensated cirrhosis should be considered for liver transplant.

Hepatitis E
Hepatitis E virus is an enterically transmitted RNA virus that causes acute hepatitis primarily in patients who have lived or traveled in areas where the virus is endemic (India, Pakistan, Mexico, and Southeast Asia); however, hepatitis E is increasingly diagnosed in patients who have not visited those areas. Clinically, hepatitis E resembles hepatitis A.

Other Viral Causes of Hepatitis
Epstein-Barr virus, cytomegalovirus, and herpesvirus may all cause hepatitis as part of a clinical syndrome. Infections with these agents are most serious in immunocompromised patients. Immunocompetent patients with infectious mononucleosis syndromes commonly have abnormal liver test results and mild increases in bilirubin, although clinically recognized jaundice is unusual. Herpes hepatitis generally occurs in immunosuppressed or pregnant patients and is characterized by fever, mental status changes, absence of jaundice, and AST and ALT greater than 5,000 U/L.

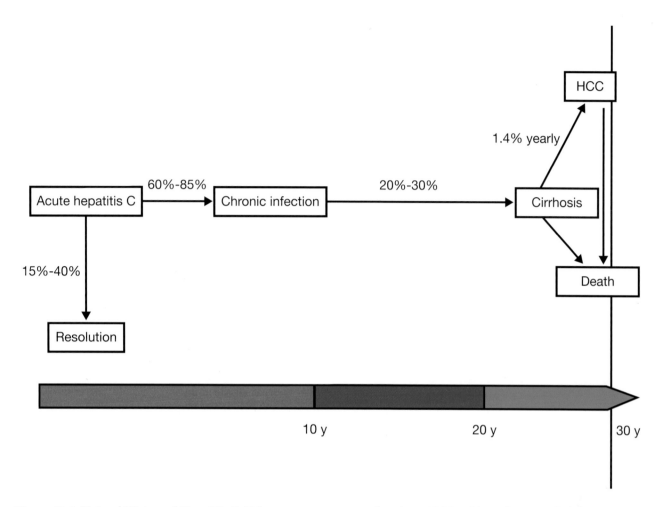

Figure 22.6 *Natural History of Hepatitis C. Values are percentages of patients. HCC indicates hepatocellular carcinoma.*
(Adapted from Poterucha JJ. Viral hepatitis. In: Hauser SC, editor. Mayo Clinic gastroenterology and hepatology board review. 5th ed. Rochester [MN]: Mayo Clinic Scientific Press and New York [NY]: Oxford University Press; c2015. p. 244–51. Used with permission of Mayo Foundation for Medical Education and Research.)

Autoimmune Hepatitis

Autoimmune hepatitis was previously called autoimmune chronic active hepatitis because the diagnosis required 3 to 6 months of abnormal liver enzyme test results. However, 40% of patients with autoimmune hepatitis present with

Table 22.6 • Interpretation of Anti-HCV Results

Anti-HCV by ELISA	Anti-HCV by RIBA	Interpretation
Positive	Negative	False-positive ELISA Patient does not have true antibody
Positive	Positive	Patient has antibody[a]
Positive	Indeterminate	Uncertain antibody status

Abbreviations: ELISA, enzyme-linked immunosorbent assay; anti-HCV, antibodies to hepatitis C virus; RIBA, recombinant immunoblot assay.

[a] Anti-HCV does not necessarily indicate current hepatitis C infection (see text).

clinical acute hepatitis. Autoimmune hepatitis can affect patients of any age, predominantly females. By definition, patients with autoimmune hepatitis should not have a history of drug-related hepatitis, HBV, HCV, or Wilson disease. Immunoserologic markers, such as antinuclear antibody (ANA), smooth muscle antibody, soluble liver antigen antibodies, or antibodies to liver-kidney microsomal (LKM) antigens, are usually detected. Patients with autoimmune hepatitis may have other autoimmune diseases, including Hashimoto thyroiditis. Aminotransferase levels are generally 4 to 20 times the reference range, and most patients have an increased gamma globulin. Corticosteroids (30–60 mg daily) produce improvement in most patients, and the improvement in liver test results and gamma globulin levels is often dramatic. Azathioprine is often used to allow the use of lower doses of prednisone. Immunosuppressive doses should be decreased to control symptoms and to maintain the serum aminotransferase values to less than 5 times the reference range. Even after an excellent response

KEY FACTS

✓ Hepatitis D—
  - requires HBsAg to replicate
  - can be transmitted with HBV (coinfection)
  - can develop in patients with chronic hepatitis B (superinfection)

✓ Major risk factors for acquiring hepatitis C infection—
  - injection drug use
  - transfusion of blood products before 1992

✓ Hepatitis C—rarely acute; usually HCV infection is chronic

✓ Treatment of hepatitis C—new DAA agents provide sustained virologic response rates >90% for most patients

✓ Autoimmune hepatitis—usually serum autoantibodies are present (eg, ANA and smooth muscle antibody) and IgG levels are increased

✓ Autoimmune hepatitis therapy—
  - corticosteroids help most patients
  - other immunosuppressants (eg, azathioprine) are used as steroid-sparing agents for maintenance therapy

to corticosteroids, relapse often occurs and the control of autoimmune hepatitis usually requires maintenance therapy.

Alcoholic Liver Disease

Alcoholic Hepatitis

Long-term, excessive use of alcohol (>20 g daily for women and >40 g daily for men) can produce advanced liver disease. Alcoholic hepatitis is characterized histologically by fatty change, degeneration and necrosis of hepatocytes (with or without Mallory bodies), and an inflammatory infiltrate of neutrophils. Almost all patients have fibrosis, and they may have cirrhosis. Clinically, patients with alcoholic hepatitis may be asymptomatic or icteric and critically ill. Common symptoms include anorexia, nausea, vomiting, abdominal pain, and weight loss. The most common sign is hepatomegaly, which may be accompanied by ascites, jaundice, fever, splenomegaly, and encephalopathy. AST is increased in 80% to 90% of patients, but it is almost always less than 400 U/L. The AST:ALT ratio is frequently greater than 2. Leukocytosis is commonly present, particularly in severely ill patients. Although the constellation of symptoms may mimic biliary disease, the clinical features are characteristic in an alcoholic patient. Because cholecystectomy carries a high morbidity among patients with alcoholic hepatitis, the clinical distinction is important.

Poor prognostic markers of alcoholic hepatitis include encephalopathy, spider angiomas, ascites, renal failure, prolonged PT, and a bilirubin concentration greater than 20 mg/dL.

Many patients have disease progression, particularly if alcohol intake is not curtailed. Corticosteroid therapy may be beneficial as an acute treatment of alcoholic hepatitis in patients with severe disease characterized by encephalopathy and a markedly prolonged PT. Pentoxifylline is a safe agent that has shown benefit in a single randomized controlled study. A *discriminant function* (DF) greater than 32 helps to identify patients with a poor prognosis:

$$DF = 4.6(PT_{patient} - PT_{control}) + Bilirubin \ (mg/dL).$$

Alcoholic Cirrhosis

Cirrhosis is defined histologically by septal fibrosis with nodular parenchymal regeneration. Only 60% of patients with alcoholic cirrhosis have signs or symptoms of liver disease, and most patients with alcoholic cirrhosis lack a clinical history of alcoholic hepatitis. Liver enzyme levels may be relatively normal in patients who have cirrhosis without alcoholic hepatitis. The prognosis for patients with alcoholic cirrhosis depends on whether they continue to consume alcohol and whether they have signs of chronic liver disease (jaundice, ascites, or gastrointestinal tract bleeding). For patients who do not have ascites, jaundice, or variceal bleeding and who abstain from alcohol, the 5-year survival rate is 89%; for patients who have any of those complications and continue to consume alcohol, it is 34%. Liver transplant is an option for patients with end-stage alcoholic liver disease if they show that they can maintain abstinence from alcohol. The outcome of liver transplant for alcoholic liver disease is similar to that of transplant for other indications.

Key Definition

Cirrhosis: *septal fibrosis with nodular parenchymal regeneration.*

Nonalcoholic Fatty Liver Disease

Nonalcoholic fatty liver disease (NAFLD) is a common cause of abnormal liver enzymes. A subset of NAFLD is nonalcoholic steatohepatitis (NASH), which is characterized histologically by fatty change and inflammation. Characteristically, patients with NAFLD have at least 1 of the following risk factors: obesity, hyperlipidemia, and diabetes mellitus. The aminotransferase levels are mildly abnormal, and alkaline phosphatase is increased in about one-third of patients. When advanced cirrhosis develops, fat may no longer be recognizable in liver tissue, and NASH most likely accounts for some cases of "cryptogenic" cirrhosis. The pathogenesis of NAFLD is unknown, and the effect of weight loss and control of hyperlipidemia and hyperglycemia is variable. In 10% of patients, NAFLD progresses to cirrhosis. The risk factors for more advanced disease are advanced age, marked obesity, and diabetes mellitus. Other than to control risk factors, there is no approved therapy for NAFLD. When patients have fat in the liver, other diseases that result in steatosis must be ruled out, including hepatitis C, celiac disease, Wilson disease, and alcoholic liver disease.

Aggressive treatment of obesity, hyperlipidemia, and diabetes is indicated for patients with NAFLD. The weight loss that occurs after bariatric surgery improves the histologic features of NAFLD. Vitamin E has been shown to improve liver test results and histologic features in patients with NAFLD. Use of agents such as pioglitazone and rosiglitazone has resulted in biochemical and histologic improvement but also in weight gain. For treatment of hyperlipidemia, the statin drugs are safe in patients with NAFLD. For patients with NAFLD who are given potentially hepatotoxic medications, liver enzymes should be monitored regularly, and use of the medications can continue as long as liver enzymes are less than 5-fold the reference value and liver function is preserved.

Chronic Cholestatic Liver Diseases

Primary Biliary Cirrhosis

Primary biliary cirrhosis (PBC) is a chronic, progressive, cholestatic liver disease that primarily affects middle-aged women. Its cause is unknown but appears to involve an immunologic disturbance resulting in small bile duct destruction. In many patients, the disease is identified by an asymptomatic increase in alkaline phosphatase. Common early symptoms are pruritus and fatigue. Patients may have Hashimoto thyroiditis or sicca complex. Biochemical features include increased alkaline phosphatase and IgM. When PBC is advanced, the concentration of bilirubin is high, the serum albumin is low, and PT is prolonged. Steatorrhea may occur because of progressive cholestasis. Fat-soluble vitamin deficiencies and metabolic bone disease are common.

Antimitochondrial antibodies are present in 90% to 95% of patients with PBC. The classic histologic lesion is granulomatous infiltration of septal bile ducts. Ursodiol treatment benefits patients who have this disease by improving survival and delaying the need for liver transplant. Cholestyramine and rifampin may be beneficial in the management of pruritus.

Primary Sclerosing Cholangitis

Primary sclerosing cholangitis (PSC) is a chronic cholestatic liver disease characterized by obliterative inflammatory fibrosis of extrahepatic and intrahepatic bile ducts. An immune mechanism has been implicated. Patients may have an asymptomatic increase in alkaline phosphatase or progressive fatigue, pruritus, and jaundice. Bacterial cholangitis may occur in patients who have dominant strictures or who have undergone instrumentation. Cholangiography,

with either endoscopic retrograde cholangiopancreatography (ERCP) or magnetic resonance cholangiopancreatography (MRCP), establishes the diagnosis of PSC, showing short strictures of bile ducts with intervening segments of normal or slightly dilated ducts. This cholangiographic appearance may be mimicked by human immunodeficiency virus (HIV)-associated cholangiopathy (due to cytomegalovirus or *Cryptosporidium*), ischemic cholangiopathy after intra-arterial infusion of fluorodeoxyuridine, and IgG4-associated cholangitis.

Among patients with PSC, 70% have ulcerative colitis (UC), which may antedate, accompany, or even follow the diagnosis of PSC. The treatment of UC has no effect on the development or clinical course of PSC. Patients with PSC are at higher risk for cholangiocarcinoma; its development may be manifested by rapid clinical deterioration, jaundice, weight loss, and abdominal pain. There is no effective medical therapy for PSC. Treatment of PSC is generally supportive, and many patients have progressive liver disease and

---

KEY FACTS

✓ Alcoholic liver disease—
- AST:ALT ratio typically 2:1
- AST and ALT nearly always <400 U/L

✓ Discriminant function in alcoholic hepatitis—
- $DF = 4.6(PT_{patient} - PT_{control}) + Bilirubin (mg/dL)$
- identifies patients who have severe hepatitis and may benefit from corticosteroid therapy

✓ NAFLD—
- risk factors: obesity, hyperlipidemia, and diabetes mellitus
- treatment centers on aggressive control of risk factors

✓ NAFLD—in some patients, NASH develops and may progress to cirrhosis, end-stage liver disease, and hepatocellular carcinoma

✓ PBC—
- typical presentation: fatigue, pruritus, and increased alkaline phosphatase levels in a middle-aged woman
- serum antimitochondrial antibody is present in 90%–95% of patients
- treatment with ursodiol improves survival

✓ PSC—
- strong association with UC, but PSC severity does not correlate with UC activity
- diagnosis: cholangiography with either ERCP or MRCP
- risk factor for bile duct cancer (cholangiocarcinoma)
- treatment: supportive, but many patients require liver transplant

require a liver transplant. Endoscopic balloon dilatation of bile duct strictures may offer palliation, especially in patients with recurrent cholangitis.

Hereditary Liver Diseases

Genetic Hemochromatosis

Genetic hemochromatosis is an autosomal recessively transmitted disorder characterized by iron overload. The physiologic defect appears to be an inappropriately high absorption of iron from the gastrointestinal tract. The *HFE* gene for genetic hemochromatosis has been identified. In the general population, the heterozygote frequency is 10%. Only homozygotes manifest progressive iron accumulation.

Patients often present with end-stage disease, although increased screening sensitivity is aiding in earlier diagnosis. The peak incidence of clinical presentation is between the ages of 40 and 60 years. Iron overload is manifested more often and earlier in men than in women because women are protected by the iron losses of menstruation and pregnancy. Although hemochromatosis is now usually diagnosed from screening iron test results, clinical features include arthropathy, hepatomegaly, skin pigmentation, diabetes mellitus, cardiac dysfunction, and hypogonadism. Hemochromatosis should be considered in patients presenting with symptoms or diseases such as arthritis, diabetes mellitus, cardiac arrhythmias, or sexual dysfunction.

Routine liver biochemistry studies generally show few abnormalities, and complications of portal hypertension are unusual. Transferrin saturation greater than 50% is the earliest biochemical iron abnormality in hemochromatosis. High serum ferritin levels indicate tissue iron overload in patients with hemochromatosis. Increased iron and ferritin may occur in other liver diseases, particularly advanced cirrhosis of any cause. Testing for mutations in the *HFE* gene is the standard method for diagnosing hemochromatosis. Of the patients with hemochromatosis, 80% to 90% are homozygous for C282Y. Heterozygotes for C282Y generally do not have the disease. Patients who are heterozygous for C282Y and heterozygous for H63D (compound heterozygosity) may have iron overload.

Liver biopsy in patients with abnormal iron tests is done only if patients are negative for C282Y or if there is a concern about cirrhosis. The knowledge of cirrhosis is important because of the increased risk of HCC. Generally, hepatic iron levels in hemochromatosis are greater than 10,000 mcg/g dry weight. A diagnostic algorithm is shown in Figure 22.7.

Patients with hemochromatosis should be treated with phlebotomy if the ferritin is high. Those with C282Y homozygosity and a normal ferritin can be observed every 2 to 3 years without treatment. The standard for phlebotomy is to remove 500 mL weekly to achieve a ferritin less than 50 mcg/L or iron saturation less than 50%. A maintenance program of 4 to 8 phlebotomies annually is then required. When initiated in the precirrhotic stage, removal of iron can render the liver normal and may improve cardiac function and control of diabetes. Treatment does not reverse arthropathy or hypogonadism, nor does it eliminate the increased risk (30%) of HCC if cirrhosis has already developed. All first-degree relatives of patients should be evaluated for hemochromatosis.

Wilson Disease

Wilson disease is an autosomal recessive disorder characterized by increased amounts of copper in tissues. The basic defect involves an inability of the liver to prepare copper for biliary excretion. The liver is chiefly involved in children and adolescents, whereas neuropsychiatric manifestations are more prominent in older patients. The Kayser-Fleischer ring is a brownish pigmented ring at the periphery of the cornea. It is not invariably present and is seen more commonly in patients with neurologic manifestations. Hepatic forms of Wilson disease include acute liver failure (often accompanied by hemolysis and renal failure), chronic hepatitis, steatohepatitis, and insidiously developing cirrhosis. The development of HCC is rare. Neurologic signs include tremor, rigidity, altered speech, and changes in personality. Fanconi syndrome and premature arthritis may occur.

Evidence of hemolysis (total bilirubin increased out of proportion to direct bilirubin), a low or normal alkaline phosphatase, and a low serum uric acid (due to uricosuria) suggest Wilson disease. The diagnosis is established on the basis of a low ceruloplasmin level and an increased urinary or hepatic concentration of copper. Ceruloplasmin levels may be misleading—they may be increased by inflammation or biliary obstruction and decreased by liver failure of any cause. High concentrations of copper in the liver are found in Wilson disease, although similarly high values can also occur in cholestatic syndromes. Genetic testing for Wilson disease is developing but is currently most reliable for screening among first-degree relatives when a specific mutation in the proband has been identified. Standard treatments for Wilson disease are penicillamine, which chelates and increases the urinary excretion of copper, and trientine. Zinc inhibits absorption of copper by the gastrointestinal tract and can be used as adjunctive therapy. All siblings of patients should be evaluated for Wilson disease. Liver transplant corrects the metabolic defect of the disease.

α_1-Antitrypsin Deficiency

α_1-Antitrypsin is synthesized in the liver. The gene is on chromosome 14. M is the common normal allele, and Z and S are abnormal alleles. Patients with the ZZ phenotype are at highest risk for liver disease. Inability to excrete the abnormally folded mutant protein results in intrahepatic accumulation of α_1-antitrypsin. Patients with α_1-antitrypsin deficiency may have a history of jaundice during the first 6 months of life. In later childhood or adulthood, cirrhosis may develop. Patients with α_1-antitrypsin–induced liver disease often lack clinically important lung disease, and

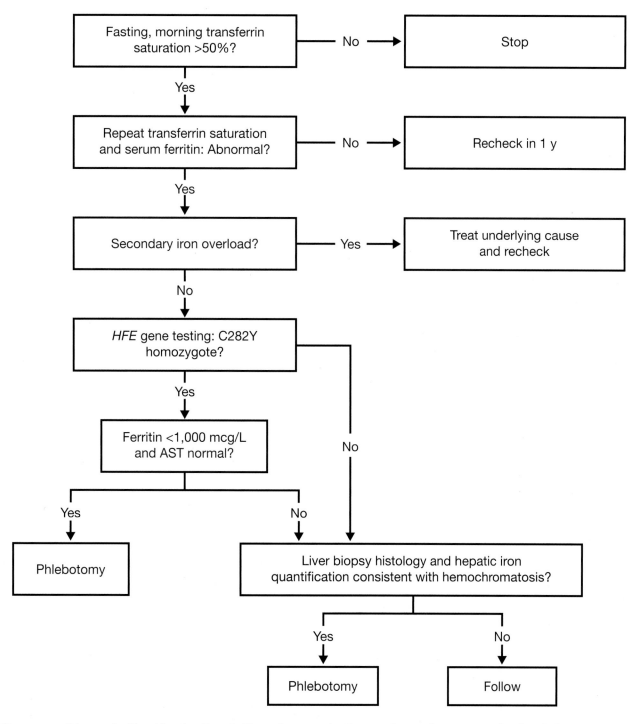

Figure 22.7 *Diagnostic Algorithm for Genetic Hemochromatosis. Causes of secondary iron overload include anemias with ineffective erythropoiesis, multiple blood transfusions, and oral or parenteral iron supplementation. AST indicates aspartate aminotransferase.*

(Adapted from Brandhagen DJ, Fairbanks VF, Batts KP, Thibodeau SN. Update on hereditary hemochromatosis and the *HFE* gene. Mayo Clin Proc. 1999 Sep;74[9]:917–21. Used with permission of Mayo Foundation for Medical Education and Research.)

infusions of α_1-antitrypsin do not protect against hepatic involvement. The prevalence of cirrhosis in patients with the MZ phenotype is likely increased, but the risk is small. HCC may complicate α_1-antitrypsin deficiency when cirrhosis is present, especially in males. α_1-Antitrypsin deficiency is diagnosed by determining the α_1-antitrypsin phenotype or genotype. The serum levels of α_1-antitrypsin may vary and be unreliable. Liver transplant corrects the metabolic defect and changes the recipient's phenotype to that of the donor.

Acute Liver Failure

Acute liver failure is hepatic failure that includes encephalopathy developing less than 8 weeks after the onset of jaundice in patients with no history of liver disease. The common causes are listed in Box 22.1. Acute liver failure due to acetaminophen hepatotoxicity or hepatitis A carries a better prognosis than acute liver failure due to other causes. Poor prognostic markers include a drug-induced cause (other than acetaminophen), older age, grade 3 or 4 encephalopathy, acidosis, and INR greater than 3.5. Treatment is supportive, and patients should be transferred to a medical center where liver transplant is available.

Drug-Induced Liver Injury

Drugs cause toxic effects in the liver in different ways, often mimicking liver disease from other causes. With the notable exception of acetaminophen hepatotoxicity, most drug-induced liver disorders are idiosyncratic and not dose-related. Drug-induced liver injury accounts for 2% of the cases of jaundice in hospitalized patients and 50% of the cases of acute liver failure. Consequently, all drugs that have been used by a patient presenting with liver disease must be identified.

Acetaminophen toxicity is the most common cause of acute liver failure. Toxicity may occur at relatively low doses (eg, 3 g daily) in alcoholics because alcohol induces hepatic microsomal cytochrome P450 enzymes, which metabolize acetaminophen to its toxic metabolite. Acetaminophen hepatotoxicity is characterized by aminotransferase values greater than 5,000 U/L and often by renal failure. *N*-acetylcysteine should be given to any patient with acute liver failure in whom acetaminophen toxicity is suspected. Valproic acid, tetracycline, and zidovudine may cause severe microvesicular steatosis associated with encephalopathy. Hepatotoxicity

due to amiodarone may have histologic features that mimic those of alcoholic hepatitis or NAFLD. Antituberculous agents that may cause acute hepatitis include isoniazid, rifampin, and ethambutol. Antibiotics are frequently associated with acute hepatitis. Amoxicillin-clavulanate is a relatively common cause of drug-induced liver injury and may result in prolonged cholestasis that can mimic obstruction of the large bile duct. Nitrofurantoin and minocycline can mimic autoimmune hepatitis. The chance of hepatotoxicity from lipid-lowering agents is extremely remote, even in patients with preexisting liver disease.

Liver Tumors

Hepatocellular Carcinoma

In the United States, 90% of HCC cases occur in patients with cirrhosis. The α-fetoprotein level is increased in only 50% of patients with HCC; however, an α-fetoprotein level greater than 400 ng/mL in a cirrhotic patient with a liver mass is essentially diagnostic of HCC. A lesion that enhances in the hepatic arterial phase with "washout" in the portal venous phase on computed tomography (CT) or magnetic resonance imaging (MRI) in a patient with cirrhosis is very suggestive of HCC, and biopsy is often not necessary for diagnosis. Common metastatic sites are lymph nodes, lung, bone, and brain. Liver transplant is an option for patients with 3 or fewer lesions (largest <3 cm) or a single lesion smaller than 5 cm. Transplant is advised particularly for patients with cirrhosis who may not tolerate resection because of poor liver reserve. Transarterial chemoembolization, radioembolization, and percutaneous ablative techniques, such as alcohol injection or radiofrequency ablation, may be useful as primary or neoadjuvant therapy.

Cholangiocarcinoma

The incidence of cholangiocarcinoma is increasing in the United States. Recognized risk factors are PSC, chronic biliary infection, and a history of choledochal cysts. Cholangiocarcinoma may be difficult to diagnose, especially in patients with PSC. For most patients, surgical resection is the treatment of choice, although resection is not possible in many patients. At some centers, liver transplant is considered in select patients with cholangiocarcinoma.

Adenoma

Adenomas are associated with the use of oral contraceptives or estrogen. Patients most commonly present with incidentally discovered liver mass lesions, although they can present with acute right upper quadrant pain and hemodynamic compromise because of bleeding. Avoidance of estrogens is advised for patients with hepatic adenomas.

Cavernous Hemangioma

Cavernous hemangioma is the most common benign tumor of the liver. CT or MRI with intravenous contrast is often diagnostic, demonstrating peripheral enhancement

---

Box 22.1 • Common Causes of Acute Liver Failure

Infective
  Hepatitis virus A, B, C (rare), D, and E
  Herpesvirus
Drug reactions and toxins
  Acetaminophen hepatotoxicity
  Idiosyncratic drug reaction
Vascular
  Ischemic hepatitis (shock liver)
  Acute Budd-Chiari syndrome
Metabolic
  Wilson disease
  Fatty liver of pregnancy
Miscellaneous
  Massive malignant infiltration
  Autoimmune hepatitis

of the lesion. Cavernous hemangiomas generally require no treatment and are not estrogen dependent.

Focal Nodular Hyperplasia

Focal nodular hyperplasia (FNH) is a benign liver lesion that is probably a reaction to aberrant arterial flow to the liver. These lesions are typically discovered incidentally, although large lesions that stretch the liver capsule may cause abdominal pain. Diagnosis can usually be made with imaging; the characteristic findings are intense vascular enhancement on the hepatic arterial phase and a central scar. Bleeding from FNH is rare and malignant transformation does not occur; therefore, resection is not necessary. Similar to cavernous hemangioma, FNH is not estrogen dependent.

Metastases

Metastases are more common than primary tumors of the liver. Frequent primary sites are the colon, stomach, breast, lung, and pancreas. Surgical resection of isolated colon cancer metastases has a limited effect on long-term survival.

KEY FACTS

✓ Genetic hemochromatosis—
  - autosomal recessive: *HFE* gene mutation C282Y is present in 80%–90% of affected patients
  - transferrin saturation >50%: earliest biochemical abnormality
  - high ferritin levels indicate tissue iron overload
  - treatment: phlebotomy to prevent cirrhosis and other end-organ complications

✓ Wilson disease—
  - rare autosomal recessive disorder
  - characterized by ineffective biliary excretion of copper
  - presentation: liver disease (more common in children and adolescents) or neuropsychiatric symptoms
  - Kayser-Fleischer ring: brown pigmented ring at periphery of cornea
  - diagnosis: low serum ceruloplasmin and high levels of copper in urine or liver
  - consider Wilson disease if patient has acute liver failure and hemolysis

- α_1-Antitrypsin deficiency—
  - patients with ZZ phenotype are at greatest risk for liver disease
  - α_1-antitrypsin infusions do not protect against liver damage (unlike in lung disease)

✓ Acetaminophen toxicity—typically, AST >5,000 U/L and ALT >5,000 U/L

✓ HCC—
  - in the United States, usually occurs with cirrhosis
  - serum α-fetoprotein level is often increased (>400 ng/mL strongly suggests HCC)

Complications of End-Stage Liver Disease

Most complications of cirrhosis are due to the development of portal hypertension. The mechanism of portal hypertension is related to increases in both portal vein blood flow and intrahepatic resistance to flow. Increased flow is related to splanchnic vasodilatation. Increased resistance is related to sinusoidal narrowing from fibrous tissue and regenerative nodules as well as to active vasoconstriction from alterations in production of endothelin and nitric oxide.

Ascites

The pathogenesis of ascites involves stimulation of the renin-angiotensin-aldosterone system, resulting in inappropriate renal sodium retention with expansion of plasma volume. Pleural effusion (*hepatic hydrothorax*) occurs in 6% of patients with cirrhosis and is right-sided in 67%. Edema usually follows ascites and is related to hypoalbuminemia and possibly to increased pressure on the inferior vena cava by the intra-abdominal fluid. The sudden onset of ascites should raise the possibility of hepatic venous outflow obstruction (Budd-Chiari syndrome).

Paracentesis is indicated at presentation to confirm the cause of ascites. Tests most useful for determining the cause of ascites are measurements of total protein and the serum-ascites albumin gradient (SAAG), which is calculated as

$$\text{SAAG} = [\text{Serum Albumin}] - [\text{Ascitic Fluid Albumin}].$$

A SAAG of 1.1 g/dL or more indicates portal hypertension. Ascites due to portal hypertension induced by congestive heart failure can be distinguished from cirrhotic ascites because congestive heart failure (and other conditions associated with hepatic venous outflow obstruction such as Budd-Chiari syndrome) usually has an ascitic fluid protein of 2.5 g/dL or more. Ascites from peritoneal carcinomatosis or tuberculosis generally has an ascitic fluid protein of 2.5 g/dL or more and a SAAG of less than 1.1 g/dL (Table 22.7).

Table 22.7 • Use of the Serum-Ascites Albumin Gradient (SAAG) and Ascites Protein to Determine the Cause of Ascites

SAAG, g/dL	Ascites Protein	
	<2.5 g/dL	≥2.5 g/dL
≥1.1	Portal hypertension due to cirrhosis	Portal hypertension due to hepatic venous outflow obstruction (including right heart failure)
<1.1	Nephrotic syndrome	Malignancy, tuberculosis

The treatment of ascites involves dietary sodium restriction and diuretics. Spironolactone (100–200 mg daily) and furosemide (20–40 mg daily) are usually used initially. The goal is to increase the concentration of urinary sodium and to allow the loss of 1 L of ascitic fluid (1 kg of body weight) per day. Paracentesis should be performed therapeutically in patients with tense ascites or with respiratory compromise from abdominal distention. Large-volume or even total paracentesis in combination with 6 to 8 g of albumin for each liter of ascitic fluid removed is safe and well tolerated. Refractory ascites is uncommon. Patients with cirrhotic ascites have a low concentration of urinary sodium (<10 mEq/mL on a random specimen) despite maximal diuretic therapy. Those who do not adhere to dietary sodium restriction excrete more than 80 mEq in 24 hours. For patients with refractory or resistant ascites, most physicians advocate therapeutic paracentesis as needed. A transjugular intrahepatic portosystemic shunt (TIPS) is effective in some patients with refractory ascites and is particularly useful for cirrhotic patients with pleural effusion as the main manifestation of fluid retention. Peritoneovenous shunts are complicated by disseminated intravascular coagulation and shunt malfunction and are rarely performed.

Spontaneous Bacterial Peritonitis

Spontaneous bacterial peritonitis (SBP) occurs in 10% to 20% of patients with cirrhosis who have ascites. SBP is a bacterial infection of ascitic fluid without an intra-abdominal source of infection. Fever, abdominal pain, and abdominal tenderness are classic symptoms; however, many patients have few or no symptoms. SBP should be considered in any patient with cirrhotic ascites, particularly if there has been clinical deterioration. For all patients presenting with ascites, diagnostic paracentesis is advisable as an initial step. Unless severe (INR >2.5 or platelets <10×10⁹/L), coagulopathy and thrombocytopenia are not contraindications for diagnostic paracentesis. A blood cell count and culture of ascitic fluid should be performed for all patients in whom SBP is being considered. Bedside inoculation of blood culture bottles with ascitic fluid increases the diagnostic yield of fluid cultures. SBP is more common in patients with large-volume ascites and in patients with a low ascitic fluid protein concentration (<1.0 g/dL). Also, blood from all patients with SBP should be cultured because almost 50% of these cultures are positive. Variants of SBP are listed in Table 22.8.

SBP and culture-negative neutrocytic ascites should be treated, usually with a third-generation cephalosporin. Albumin should also be given (1.5 g/kg on day 1 and 1 g/kg on day 3). Polymicrobial infection of ascitic fluid should prompt a search for an intra-abdominal focus of infection; SBP nearly always involves only 1 organism. Patients with a prior episode of SBP are at high risk for recurrence, and daily prophylactic therapy (usually with norfloxacin) is recommended.

Hepatorenal Syndrome

Hepatorenal syndrome is renal failure in the absence of underlying renal pathologic abnormalities in patients with portal hypertension. The differential diagnosis is given in Table 22.9. In cirrhotic patients presenting with renal insufficiency, hepatorenal syndrome is difficult to differentiate from prerenal azotemia; thus, a brief trial of volume expansion with albumin is indicated. Treatment is supportive, although vasoconstrictors such as midodrine or norepinephrine are used in patients with low blood pressure. After liver transplant, renal function usually improves, although this is confounded by the renal toxicity of the antirejection drugs tacrolimus and cyclosporine.

Key Definition

Hepatorenal syndrome: *renal failure and portal hypertension without renal pathologic abnormalities.*

Hepatic Encephalopathy

Hepatic encephalopathy is a reversible decrease in the level of consciousness of patients with severe liver disease. Disturbed consciousness, personality change, intellectual deterioration, and slowed speech are common manifestations. Patients often have asterixis (flapping tremor). The sudden development of hepatic encephalopathy in patients

---

Table 22.8 • Variants of Spontaneous Bacterial Peritonitis

| | Ascitic Fluid | | |
Condition	PMN Cell Count, cells/mL	Culture Results	Management
Spontaneous bacterial peritonitis	≥250	Positive	Antibiotics
Culture-negative neutrocytic ascites	≥250	Negative	Antibiotics
Bacterascites	<250	Positive	Treat if symptoms of infection are present; otherwise, repeat paracentesis for blood cell count and cultures

Abbreviation: PMN, polymorphonuclear.

Table 22.9 • Differential Diagnosis for Hepatorenal Syndrome

Variable	Prerenal Azotemia	Hepatorenal Syndrome	Acute Renal Failure
Urinary sodium concentration, mmol/L	<10	<10	>30
Urine to plasma creatinine ratio	>30	>30	<20
Urine osmolality	At least 100 mOsm > plasma osmolality	At least 100 mOsm > plasma osmolality	Equal to plasma osmolality
Urine sediment	Normal	Unremarkable	Casts, debris

Adapted from Arroyo V, Gines P, Guevara M, Rodes J. Renal dysfunction in cirrhosis: pathophysiology, clinical features and therapy. In: Boyer TD, Wright TL, Manns MP, Zakim D, editors. Zakim and Boyer's hepatology: a textbook of liver disease. 5th ed. Vol 1. Philadelphia (PA): Saunders/Elsevier; c2006. p. 423–52. Used with permission.

with stable cirrhosis should prompt a search for bleeding, infection (especially SBP), or electrolyte disturbances; however, simple precipitating events are increased dietary protein, constipation, or sedatives. Serum and arterial ammonia are usually increased but are not necessary for diagnosis. Lactulose decreases the nitrogenous compounds presented to the liver and is the first-line treatment of hepatic encephalopathy. Oral nonabsorbable antibiotics such as rifaximin or neomycin are given to patients who do not respond to or tolerate lactulose. Dietary protein restriction is advised only for patients with no response to medical therapy.

Variceal Hemorrhage

Esophageal varices are collateral vessels that develop because of portal hypertension. Varices also can occur in other parts of the gut. Most patients with cirrhosis who have varices do not hemorrhage, but mortality among patients with a first hemorrhage is 10% to 20%. For patients who have cirrhosis but have not had bleeding, endoscopy to assess for the presence of varices is advised. Patients with moderate-sized or large varices, especially if there are red marks on the varices, should be treated with a nonselective β-blocker (nadolol or propranolol) to prevent bleeding. Endoscopic variceal ligation is an alternative to nonselective β-blockers. An algorithm for the use of endoscopy to assess for esophageal varices is shown in Figure 22.8.

Bleeding from esophageal varices is generally massive. For patients with acute bleeding, early endoscopy is indicated for diagnosis and treatment. Endoscopic therapy consists of band ligation or, less commonly, sclerotherapy. Octreotide decreases portal venous pressure and may also be given for acute variceal bleeding. All patients with cirrhosis who are hospitalized for gastrointestinal tract bleeding should receive prophylactic antibiotics.

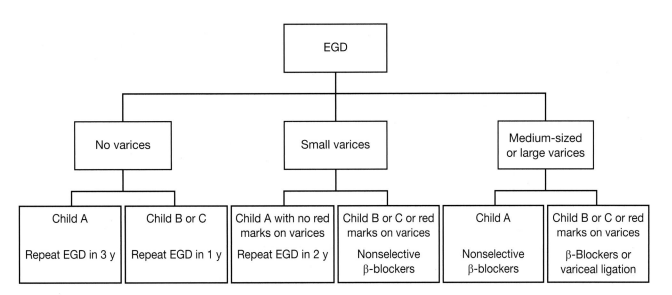

Figure 22.8 *Prophylaxis of Esophageal Variceal Bleeding in Patients With Cirrhosis. Child indicates Child-Pugh class (A, B, or C, in order of increasing severity of cirrhosis); EGD, esophagogastroduodenoscopy.*

Of the patients who bleed from esophageal varices, 80% to 100% have recurrent bleeding within 2 years after the first episode; therefore, secondary prophylaxis is advised. Oral propranolol or nadolol may be used alone to prevent rebleeding in patients with preserved liver function, although the most common recommendation is serial endoscopic variceal ligation in combination with β-blockers until the varices have been obliterated. TIPS is effective in controlling refractory variceal bleeding. The incidence of hepatic encephalopathy after TIPS is 10% to 40%, but this complication usually can be controlled with medical therapy. Patients bleeding from gastric varices are more likely to require TIPS than those bleeding from esophageal varices.

Patients with cirrhosis may also have gastrointestinal tract bleeding from portal hypertensive gastropathy. Bleeding from this lesion is usually gradual, and patients frequently present with iron deficiency anemia. Treatment is administration of nonselective β-blockers and iron. Any patient with bleeding from varices or portal hypertensive gastropathy should be considered for liver transplant.

Biliary Tract Disease

Gallstones and Cholecystitis

Gallstones can cause uncomplicated biliary pain, acute cholecystitis, common bile duct obstruction with cholangitis, and acute pancreatitis. Biliary pain is generally felt in the epigastrium or right upper quadrant and is usually severe and steady, lasting several hours. History is important; constant pain, food intolerance, and gaseousness are generally not features of biliary disease. Gallstones do not cause abnormal liver test results unless the common bile duct is obstructed or the patient has sepsis. Ultrasonography is 90% to 97% sensitive for detecting gallbladder stones. Cholecystitis may be suggested by gallbladder contraction, marked distention, surrounding fluid, or wall thickening. Ultrasonography also offers the opportunity to detect dilated bile ducts. If performed during an episode of pain, radionuclide biliary scanning is helpful in diagnosing cystic duct obstruction with cholecystitis. Positive test results are marked by nonvisualization of the gallbladder despite biliary excretion of radioisotope into the small intestine.

Gallstones require no therapy in asymptomatic patients, even in high-risk patients. Acalculous cholecystitis, probably precipitated by prolonged fasting and gallbladder ischemia, generally occurs only in patients hospitalized with critical illnesses. Clinical manifestations are fever and abdominal pain; liver test results may not be abnormal. Diagnosis is made with ultrasonography or radionuclide biliary scan. Patients with episodes of biliary colic or acute cholecystitis should have cholecystectomy. Patients with high surgical risk may undergo drainage with percutaneous cholecystostomy or an endoscopically placed nasocholecystic tube.

Many patients without gallstones have undergone cholecystectomy because a decrease in gallbladder ejection fraction was noted on radionuclide biliary scan. In most of these patients, pain does not resolve; therefore, a decreased gallbladder ejection fraction should be interpreted with caution since often the patient's symptoms are unrelated to the finding.

Bile Duct Stones

Most bile duct stones originate in the gallbladder, although a few patients, such as those with preexisting biliary disease (eg, PSC), have primary duct stones. CT and ultrasonography are relatively insensitive for common bile duct stones, and diagnosis generally requires MRCP, ERCP, or endoscopic ultrasonography. ERCP also offers therapeutic potential for patients with bile duct stones and is the test of choice when clinical suspicion is high. Patients with bile duct stones can have minimal or no symptoms, or they can have life-threatening cholangitis with abdominal pain, fever, and jaundice. Common bile duct stones should be removed; in nearly all patients, this can be accomplished with ERCP. The urgency of the procedure depends on the clinical presentation. Patients with minimal symptoms can have elective ERCP, but those with cholangitis and fever unresponsive to antibiotics should have urgent endoscopic treatment. Patients with gallbladder stones who have a sphincterotomy and clearance of their duct stones have only a 10% chance of having additional problems with their gallbladder stones; thus, cholecystectomy can be avoided in patients who are at high risk for complications with surgery.

Malignant Biliary Obstruction

Malignant biliary obstruction is usually the result of carcinoma of the head of the pancreas, bile duct cancer, or metastatic malignancy to hilar nodes. If the disease is unresectable, palliative endoscopic stenting is as effective as surgical bypass. Patients with malignant biliary obstruction and impending duodenal obstruction are usually considered for palliative surgery, although endoscopic techniques can be attempted by expert endoscopists.

Gallbladder Carcinoma

Gallbladder carcinoma has a strong association with a calcified gallbladder wall (ie, *porcelain gallbladder*); therefore, prophylactic cholecystectomy is advised. Most patients with gallbladder carcinoma present at an advanced stage and have a poor prognosis.

KEY FACTS

✓ SAAG—
- most useful for diagnosing cause of ascites
- SAAG >1.1 g/dL indicates portal hypertension

✓ Ascites treatment—dietary sodium restriction and diuretic therapy; paracentesis for tense ascites

✓ SBP—
- may occur with few or no symptoms
- polymorphonuclear cell count ≥250 cells/mL is diagnostic

✓ Esophageal varices—patients presenting with massive bleeding require resuscitation, endoscopic band ligation, octreotide infusion, and prophylactic antibiotics

✓ Gallstones do not cause abnormal liver test results unless common bile duct is obstructed or patient has sepsis

✓ Acalculous cholecystitis—
- usually only in patients hospitalized with critical illnesses
- manage with percutaneous cholecystostomy tube if patient has high surgical risk

✓ Bile duct stones—
- patients may have life-threatening cholangitis with abdominal pain, fever, and jaundice
- can usually be removed with ERCP

✓ Malignant biliary obstruction—
- usually results from carcinoma of the head of the pancreas
- treatment: palliative endoscopic stenting

23 Pancreatic Disorders

CONOR G. LOFTUS, MD

Classification of Pancreatitis

*A*cute pancreatitis is a reversible inflammation. The 2 varieties are interstitial pancreatitis and necrotizing pancreatitis. **Interstitial pancreatitis**, in which perfusion of the pancreas is intact, accounts for 80% of cases, with less than 1% mortality. **Necrotizing pancreatitis** is more severe and results when perfusion is compromised. It accounts for 20% of cases, with 10% mortality if sterile and 30% if infected.

> ### Key Definitions
>
> Interstitial pancreatitis: *acute pancreatitis in which perfusion of the pancreas is intact.*
>
> Necrotizing pancreatitis: *acute pancreatitis in which perfusion of the pancreas is compromised.*

Chronic pancreatitis is irreversible (ie, there is structural disease with endocrine or exocrine insufficiency). It is documented by pancreatic calcifications on abdominal radiography, parenchymal and ductal abnormalities on endoscopic ultrasonography (EUS), ductal abnormalities on endoscopic retrograde cholangiopancreatography (ERCP), scarring on pancreatic biopsy, endocrine insufficiency (diabetes mellitus), or exocrine insufficiency (malabsorption).

Acute Pancreatitis

In acute pancreatitis, activation of pancreatic enzymes causes autodigestion of the gland. The clinical features are abdominal pain, nausea and vomiting ("too sick to eat"), ileus, peritoneal signs, hypotension, and abdominal mass.

Etiologic Factors

Approximately 80% of acute pancreatitis episodes are due to either gallstones or alcohol ingestion. Significant increase (>3 times the upper limit of the reference range) in aspartate aminotransferase (AST) or alanine aminotransferase (ALT) in a patient with acute pancreatitis generally indicates that gallstones are the cause. The third most common cause is idiopathic (approximately 10% of cases).

The following drugs have been reported to cause pancreatitis: azathioprine, 6-mercaptopurine, L-asparaginase, hydrochlorothiazide diuretics, sulfonamides, sulfasalazine, tetracycline, furosemide, estrogens, valproic acid, pentamidine (both parenteral and aerosolized), and the antiretroviral drug didanosine. Evidence that the following drugs cause pancreatitis is less convincing: corticosteroids, nonsteroidal antiinflammatory drugs, methyldopa, procainamide, chlorthalidone, ethacrynic acid, phenformin, nitrofurantoin, enalapril, erythromycin, metronidazole, and non–sulfa-linked aminosalicylate derivatives such as 5-aminosalicylic acid and interleukin 2.

Other causes include hypertriglyceridemia, which may cause pancreatitis if the triglyceride level is greater than 1,000 mg/dL. Look for hyperlipoproteinemia types I, IV, and V and for associated oral contraceptive use. Hypertriglyceridemia may mask hyperamylasemia. Hypercalcemia may also cause pancreatitis; look for underlying multiple myeloma, hyperparathyroidism, or metastatic carcinoma. In immunocompetent patients, mumps and coxsackievirus cause acute pancreatitis. In AIDS patients, acute pancreatitis has been reported with cytomegalovirus infection. Pancreas divisum, or incomplete fusion of the dorsal and ventral pancreatic ducts, may predispose some people to acute pancreatitis, although this is a controversial matter.

Clinical Presentation

Pain may be mild to severe; it is usually sudden in onset and persistent. Typically, the pain is located in the upper abdomen and radiates to the back. Relief may be obtained by bending forward or sitting up. The ingestion of food or alcohol commonly exacerbates the pain. Patients without pain have a poor prognosis because they usually present with shock.

Fever, if present, is low grade, rarely exceeding 38.3°C in the absence of complications. A fever higher than 38.3°C suggests infection.

Most patients are *hypovolemic* because fluid accumulates in the abdomen.

Patients with pancreatitis may have a mild increase in the total bilirubin level, but they usually do not have clinical *jaundice*. When jaundice is present, it generally results from obstruction of the common bile duct by stones, compression by pseudocyst, or inflamed pancreatic tissue.

A wide range of *pulmonary manifestations* may occur. More than half of all patients with acute pancreatitis have some degree of hypoxemia, usually from pulmonary shunting. Patients often have atelectasis and may have pleural effusions.

Diagnosis

Serum Amylase

Determination of the serum level of amylase is the most useful test for diagnosing acute pancreatitis. The level of amylase increases 2 or 3 hours after an attack and remains increased for 3 or 4 days. The magnitude of the increase does not correlate with the clinical severity of the attack. Serum amylase levels may be normal in some patients (<10%) because of alcohol consumption or hypertriglyceridemia. A persistent increase suggests a complication such as pseudocyst, abscess, or ascites. Serum amylase is cleared by the kidney. The urinary amylase level remains elevated after the serum amylase level returns to normal. Isoenzyme identification may aid in distinguishing between salivary (ie, nonpancreatic) and pancreatic sources.

Serum lipase levels may help distinguish between pancreatic hyperamylasemia and an ectopic source (lung, ovarian, or esophageal carcinoma). Lipase levels are also increased for a longer time than amylase levels after acute pancreatitis.

Computed tomographic (CT) imaging of the abdomen may be useful. If the amylase level is mildly elevated and the patient has a history of vomiting but no signs of obstruction, consider performing esophagogastroduodenoscopy to rule out a penetrating ulcer.

Nonpancreatic Hyperamylasemia

Nonpancreatic hyperamylasemia may result from parotitis; renal failure; macroamylasemia; intestinal obstruction, infarction, or perforation; ruptured ectopic pregnancy; diabetic ketoacidosis; drugs (eg, morphine); burns; pregnancy; and neoplasm (lung, ovary, or esophagus).

Physical Findings

Physical findings in patients with acute pancreatitis include tachycardia, orthostasis, fat necrosis, and xanthelasmas of the skin. The Grey Turner sign (flank discoloration) and the Cullen sign (periumbilical discoloration) suggest retroperitoneal hemorrhage. The abdominal findings often are less impressive than the amount of pain the patient is experiencing.

Imaging Studies

A chest radiograph showing an isolated left pleural effusion strongly suggests pancreatitis; infiltrates may indicate aspiration pneumonia or acute respiratory distress syndrome. On an abdominal plain film, look for the sentinel loop sign (a dilated loop of bowel over the pancreatic area) and the colon cutoff sign (abrupt cutoff of gas in the transverse colon); pancreatic calcifications indicate chronic pancreatitis.

Ultrasonographic examination is the procedure of choice for helping to determine the cause of acute pancreatitis. Although ultrasonography gives information about the pancreas and is the best method for delineating gallstones, it is not a good method if the patient is obese.

CT is indicated for ruling out necrotizing pancreatitis in critically ill patients. CT scans are not required for patients with documented mild interstitial acute pancreatitis.

Endoscopic sphincterotomy is indicated when acute pancreatitis is associated with jaundice and cholangitis. ERCP has no role in the diagnosis of acute pancreatitis and should be avoided because it may cause infection.

Treatment

Supportive care is the backbone of treatment, along with monitoring for complications and treating them when they occur.

Fluids

Restore and maintain intravascular fluid volume; usually this can be accomplished with crystalloids and peripheral intravenous catheters. Monitor blood pressure, pulse, urine output, daily intake and output, and weight. Eliminate medications that may cause pancreatitis. The use of a nasogastric tube does not shorten the course or severity of pancreatitis, but it should be used for ileus or severe nausea and vomiting.

Analgesics

Common practice has been to use meperidine (75–125 mg intramuscularly every 3–4 hours) instead of morphine because meperidine purportedly causes less spasm of the sphincter of Oddi. Meperidine has potentially toxic metabolites, though, so it has been removed from many hospital formularies, and the in vivo link between meperidine and sphincter spasm is unclear. Standard methods of analgesia can generally be used with impunity. The efficacy of antisecretory drugs (eg, histamine$_2$ receptor antagonists, anticholinergic agents, somatostatin, and glucagon) has not been documented.

Nutrition

Patients with severe pancreatitis may require supplemental nutrition. This should be provided by means of a nasoenteric tube. Total parenteral nutrition is unnecessary in most cases of pancreatitis and should be considered only when enteral feeding has failed or is not feasible.

Antibiotics

Antibiotics are indicated in patients with necrotizing pancreatitis if infection is suspected (because of an otherwise unexplained fever and gas bubbles in areas of pancreatic necrosis on the CT scan).

Complications

A local complication is **pancreatic phlegmon**, a mass of inflamed pancreatic tissue. It may resolve. **Pseudocyst**, a fluid collection within a nonepithelial-lined cavity, should be suspected if the patient has persistent pain and persistent hyperamylasemia. In 50% to 80% of patients, this resolves within 6 weeks without intervention. A pancreatic abscess develops usually 2 to 4 weeks after the acute episode and causes fever (>38.3°C), persistent abdominal pain, and persistent hyperamylasemia. If a pancreatic abscess is not drained surgically, the mortality rate is virtually 100%. Give antibiotics that are effective for gram-negative and anaerobic organisms. Jaundice results from obstruction of the common bile duct. Pancreatic ascites results from disruption of the pancreatic duct or a leaking pseudocyst.

Key Definition

Pancreatic phlegmon: *a mass of inflamed pancreatic tissue that occurs as a local complication of acute pancreatitis.*

Key Definition

Pseudocyst: *a fluid collection within a nonepithelial-lined cavity.*

A well-recognized systemic complication of acute pancreatitis is acute respiratory distress syndrome. Circulating lecithinase probably splits fatty acids off lecithin, producing a faulty surfactant. Pleural effusion occurs in approximately 20% of patients with acute pancreatitis. Aspirate analysis shows a high amylase content. Fat necrosis may be due to increased levels of serum lipase.

Assessment of Severity

Most patients with acute pancreatitis recover without any sequelae. The overall mortality rate among patients with acute pancreatitis is 5% to 10%, and death is due most often to hypovolemia and shock, respiratory failure, pancreatic abscess, or systemic sepsis. Admission laboratory study results, including increased hematocrit and serum urea nitrogen, may be helpful in predicting which patients have severe pancreatitis. The Ranson criteria (Box 23.1) and the Acute Physiology and Chronic Health Evaluation (APACHE) criteria are reliable for predicting mortality in acute pancreatitis. Predicted mortality is calculated as follows: less than 3 Ranson criteria, 1%; 3 or 4 criteria, 15%; 5 or 6 criteria, 40%; and 7 or more criteria, more than 80%.

KEY FACTS

✓ Acute pancreatitis—
  - reversible inflammation
  - interstitial pancreatitis (perfusion is intact): 80% of cases (<1% mortality)
  - necrotizing pancreatitis (perfusion is compromised): 20% of cases but more severe (10% mortality if sterile; 30% mortality if infected)

✓ Chronic pancreatitis—irreversible (presence of structural disease with endocrine or exocrine insufficiency)

✓ Causes of acute pancreatitis—
  - gallstones or alcohol cause 80% of episodes
  - if gallstones, expect increased AST or ALT (>3 times upper limit of reference range)

✓ Diagnosis of acute pancreatitis—measurement of the serum level of amylase is the most useful test

✓ Physical findings in acute pancreatitis—retroperitoneal hemorrhage is suggested by the Grey Turner sign (flank discoloration) and the Cullen sign (periumbilical discoloration)

✓ Analgesics in acute pancreatitis—meperidine (75–125 mg intramuscularly every 3–4 hours) instead of morphine (meperidine causes less spasm of sphincter of Oddi)

✓ Assessment of severity of acute pancreatitis—results of admission laboratory studies, including increased hematocrit and serum urea nitrogen, may be helpful

---

Chronic Pancreatitis

Long-term alcohol use (≥10 years of heavy consumption) is the most common cause of chronic pancreatitis. Gallstones and hyperlipidemia usually do not cause chronic pancreatitis.

Box 23.1 • Ranson Criteria

At admission

Age >55 y
White blood cell count >15×10⁹/L
Serum glucose >200 mg/dL
Serum aspartate aminotransferase >250 U/L
Serum lactate dehydrogenase >350 U/L

At 48 h after admission

Pao_2 <60 mm Hg
Hematocrit decrease >10%
Serum albumin <3.2 g/dL
Serum urea nitrogen increase >5 mg/dL
Serum calcium <8 mg/dL
Estimated fluid sequestration >4 L

Adapted from Ranson JHC. Acute pancreatitis: surgical management. In: Go VLW, Gardner JD, Brooks FP, Lebenthal E, DiMagno EP, Scheele GA, editors. The exocrine pancreas: biology, pathobiology, and diseases. New York (NY): Raven Press; c1986. p. 503–11. Used with permission.

Hereditary pancreatitis is caused by a mutation in the cationic trypsinogen gene, which is inherited as an autosomal dominant trait with variable penetrance. Onset is usually before age 20, although 20% of patients present when they are older than 20. Hereditary pancreatitis is marked by recurring abdominal pain, positive family history, and pancreatic calcifications. It may increase the risk of pancreatic cancer.

Trauma with pancreatic ductal disruption causes chronic pancreatitis. Protein calorie malnutrition is the most common cause of chronic pancreatitis in Third World countries.

Triad of Chronic Pancreatitis

Patients with chronic pancreatitis present with abdominal pain. In addition, the triad of chronic pancreatitis consists of pancreatic calcifications, steatorrhea, and diabetes mellitus. Diffuse calcification of the pancreas is due to hereditary pancreatitis, alcoholic pancreatitis, or malnutrition. Local calcification is due to trauma, islet cell tumor, or hypercalcemia. By the time steatorrhea occurs, 90% of the pancreas has been destroyed and lipase output has decreased by 90%.

Diagnosis

Serum amylase and lipase levels may be normal, and stool fat may be normal. If malabsorption is present, stool fat is more than 10 g in 24 hours during a 48- to 72-hour stool collection while the patient is consuming a diet with 100 g of fat.

For the secretin-cholecystokinin (CCK) test of pancreatic function, secretin and CCK are injected intravenously and then the contents of the small bowel are aspirated and the concentration of pancreatic enzymes is determined.

CT shows calcifications, an irregular pancreatic contour, a dilated duct system, or pseudocysts. ERCP shows protein plugs, segmental duct dilatation, and alternating stenosis and dilatation, with obliteration of branches of the main duct. Endoscopic ultrasonography may show changes of chronic pancreatitis, including hyperechoic stranding, hyperechoic foci, and thickening of the pancreatic duct.

Pain

The mechanism for pain is not clearly defined; it may be due to ductular obstruction. One-third to one-half of patients have a decrease in pain after 5 years. The possibility of coexistent disease, such as peptic ulcer, should be considered. Complications of chronic pancreatitis (eg, biliary stricture, pancreatic ductal stricture, malignancy, and vascular thrombosis) should be excluded.

Abstinence from alcohol may relieve the pain. Analgesics, aspirin, or acetaminophen is used occasionally with the addition of codeine (narcotic addiction is a frequent complicating factor). Celiac plexus blocks relieve pain for 3 to 6 months, but long-term efficacy is less effective. A trial of pancreatic enzyme replacement for 1 to 2 months should be tried. Women with idiopathic chronic pancreatitis are most likely to have a response. Surgical treatment should be considered only if conservative measures have failed. Patients with a dilated pancreatic duct may have a favorable response to a longitudinal pancreaticojejunostomy (ie, the Puestow procedure).

Malabsorption

Patients have malabsorption not only of fat but also of essential fatty acids and fat-soluble vitamins. The goal of enzyme replacement is to maintain body weight. Diarrhea will not resolve. Enteric-coated or microsphere enzymes are designed to be released at an alkaline pH, thus avoiding degradation by stomach acid. The advantage is that they contain larger amounts of lipase. The disadvantages are that they are expensive and bioavailability is not always predictable.

Pancreatic Carcinoma

Pancreatic carcinoma is more common in men than in women. Patients usually present between the ages of 60 and 80 years. The 5-year survival rate is less than 2%. Risk factors include diabetes mellitus, chronic pancreatitis, hereditary pancreatitis, carcinogens, benzidine, cigarette smoking, and a high-fat diet. Patients with pancreatic carcinoma usually present late in the course of the disease.

They may have a vague prodrome of malaise, anorexia, and weight loss. Symptoms may be overlooked until pain or jaundice develop. Two signs associated with pancreatic cancer are the **Courvoisier sign** (painless jaundice with a palpable gallbladder) and the **Trousseau sign** (recurrent migratory thrombophlebitis). Recent-onset diabetes mellitus and nonbacterial (thrombotic) marantic endocarditis may be associated with pancreatic cancer.

Key Definitions

Courvoisier sign: *painless jaundice with a palpable gallbladder.*

Trousseau sign: *recurrent migratory thrombophlebitis.*

Routine laboratory blood analysis has limited usefulness. Patients may have increased levels of liver enzymes, amylase, and lipase or anemia, although this is variable. Tumor markers are also nonspecific. Abdominal ultrasonography and CT are each approximately 80% sensitive in localizing pancreatic masses. The "double duct" sign on CT scan is a classic feature with obstruction of the pancreatic ducts and the bile ducts. Either imaging method may be used in conjunction with fine-needle aspiration or biopsy to make a tissue diagnosis. If a mass in the pancreas is found and deemed resectable on CT scan, surgical consultation should be pursued as the next step (additional testing may not be necessary). ERCP and EUS are used if the abdominal ultrasonographic or CT results are inconclusive. ERCP and EUS each have a sensitivity greater than 90%. At ERCP, brushings and biopsies can be performed in an attempt to confirm the diagnosis.

Surgery is the only treatment that offers hope for cure; however, most lesions are not resectable. The criteria for resectability are a tumor smaller than 2 cm, the absence of lymph node invasion, and the absence of metastasis. Survival is the same with total pancreatectomy and with the Whipple procedure: 3-year survival, 33%; 5-year survival, 1%; and operative mortality, 5%.

Radiotherapy may have a role as a radiosensitizer in unresectable cancer. However, survival is unchanged. The results of chemotherapy have been disappointing, and studies have not consistently shown improved survival.

Cystic Fibrosis

Because patients with cystic fibrosis are living longer, internists should know the common intestinal complications of this disease. Exocrine pancreatic insufficiency (malabsorption) is the most important complication, and it is quite common (85%–90% of patients). Endocrine pancreatic insufficiency (diabetes mellitus) occurs in 20% to 30% of patients. Rectal prolapse occurs in 20% of patients, and a distal small-bowel obstruction from thick secretions occurs in 15% to 20%. Focal biliary cirrhosis develops in 20% of patients.

Pancreatic Endocrine Tumors

Zollinger-Ellison syndrome is a non–beta islet cell tumor of the pancreas that produces gastrin and causes gastric acid hypersecretion. This results in peptic ulcer disease (see Peptic Ulcer Disease subsection in Chapter 21, "Esophageal and Gastric Disorders").

Key Definition

Zollinger-Ellison syndrome: *a non–beta islet cell tumor of the pancreas that produces gastrin, causes hypersecretion of gastric acid, and results in peptic ulcer disease.*

Insulinoma is the most common islet cell tumor. It is a beta islet cell tumor that produces insulin and causes hypoglycemia. The diagnosis is based on finding increased fasting plasma levels of insulin and hypoglycemia. CT, EUS, or arteriography may be useful in localizing the tumor.

Glucagonoma is an alpha islet cell tumor that produces glucagon. Patients present with diabetes mellitus, weight loss, and a classic skin rash (migratory necrolytic erythema). The diagnosis is based on finding increased glucagon levels and on finding that the blood glucose level does not increase after an injection of glucagon.

Pancreatic cholera is a pancreatic tumor that produces vasoactive intestinal polypeptide (VIP), which causes watery diarrhea (see Secretory Diarrhea subsection in Chapter 20, "Diarrhea, Malabsorption, and Small-Bowel Disorders").

Somatostatinoma is a delta islet cell tumor that produces somatostatin, which inhibits insulin, gastrin, and pancreatic enzyme secretion. The result is diabetes mellitus and diarrhea. The diagnosis is based on finding increased plasma levels of somatostatin.

Octreotide is useful in treating pancreatic endocrine tumors except for somatostatinomas. Octreotide prevents the release of hormone and antagonizes hormonal effects on target organs.

KEY FACTS

✓ Most common cause of chronic pancreatitis—long-term alcohol use (≥10 years of heavy consumption)

✓ Presentation of patients with chronic pancreatitis—
- abdominal pain
- triad of chronic pancreatitis: pancreatic calcifications, steatorrhea, and diabetes mellitus

✓ Pancreatic carcinoma—
- 5-year survival rate <2%
- "double duct" sign on CT (from obstruction of the pancreatic ducts and bile ducts)

✓ Insulinoma—the most common islet cell tumor

✓ Pancreatic cholera—pancreatic tumor that produces VIP, which causes watery diarrhea

Questions and Answers

Questions

Multiple Choice (choose the best answer)

IV.1. A 52-year-old man presents for colon cancer screening. He is asymptomatic, and he states that he is not aware of any family member with a prior history of either colon cancer or colon polyps. The patient undergoes colonoscopy and is found to have the following polyps and histologic diagnoses: 2-mm cecal polyp and 4-mm transverse polyp (tubular adenomas, low-grade dysplasia), 6-mm sigmoid polyp (tubulovillous adenoma, low-grade dysplasia), and 3-mm rectal polyp (hyperplasia). If those 4 lesions were completely removed, what should you recommend for ongoing colon surveillance?
a. Colonoscopy in 1 year
b. Colonoscopy in 3 years
c. Colonoscopy in 5 years
d. Yearly fecal occult blood test and colonoscopy in 5 years
e. Computed tomographic colonography in 5 years

IV.2. While making rounds on the hospital service, your resident presents a 65-year-old man who was admitted through the emergency department with diarrhea for 3 days; the diarrhea was bloody for the past 2 days. He has remained hemodynamically stable overnight with intravenous hydration, and he is afebrile, but his diarrhea is no better. His laboratory test results are shown in Table IV.Q2.

Table IV Q2 •

Component	Yesterday	Today
White blood cell count, ×10⁹/L	18.0	19.5
Hemoglobin, g/dL	12.9	10.2
Platelet count, ×10⁹/L	198	110
Sodium, mmol/L	143	139
Potassium, mmol/L	4.0	3.6
Creatinine, mg/dL	1.1	1.5
Serum urea nitrogen, mg/dL	31	45
Aspartate aminotransferase, U/L	44	110
Alanine aminotransferase, U/L	32	31
Lactate dehydrogenase, U/L (reference range, 112–257 U/L)	230	450

Which of the following organisms is most likely?
a. *Shigella* species
b. Toxigenic *Escherichia coli*
c. Norwalk-like virus (*Norovirus*)
d. *Clostridium difficile*
e. *Escherichia coli* O157:H7

IV.3. A 35-year-old woman with ulcerative colitis of 5 years' duration presents with a red eye. She has no pain or headache, and her vision is normal. Her stools have been somewhat looser over recent weeks. She has been taking mesalamine at her usual dosage of 2.4 g daily, but she has missed doses occasionally. She recently quit smoking. What is the most likely cause of her red eye?
a. Uveitis
b. Giant cell arteritis
c. Episcleritis
d. Nicotine withdrawal and insomnia
e. Viral conjunctivitis

IV.4. A 33-year-old man presents with a history of 8 weeks of diarrhea and left lower quadrant discomfort. His diarrhea is described as 6 to 8 stools daily. The stools are bloody and very small in volume. He has frequent urgency. Stool cultures are negative for pathogens, and no parasites are seen. Many fecal leukocytes are found on stool analysis. Colonoscopy shows erythema and granularity extending from the anal verge to the midsigmoid colon (30 cm from the anal verge) and sparing the terminal ileum. Biopsy specimens from the involved rectosigmoid show chronic crypt architectural changes and mild acute inflammation. What therapy should you recommend next for this man?
a. Intravenous (IV) prednisone
b. Oral prednisone
c. Mesalamine enemas
d. Mesalamine suppositories
e. Corticosteroid enemas

IV.5. A 60-year-old woman presents with a 6-week history of diarrhea. She has had 6 to 8 large-volume watery stools daily. There has been no blood in the stool. She has not had fever or other systemic symptoms. Recently, she has not taken antibiotics or changed medication. Clinical examination findings are normal. Laboratory test results are unremarkable. Stool examination for fecal leukocytes is negative. On colonoscopy, the colon appears normal. On biopsy, a thickened subepithelial collagen band is apparent. What initial therapy should you recommend?
a. Oral prednisone
b. Bismuth subsalicylate
c. Budesonide
d. Ciprofloxacin
e. Metronidazole

IV.6. A 55-year-old woman presents to the emergency department with a 6-hour history of epigastric pain, nausea, and vomiting. She has a history of hypertension and hyperlipidemia. Her medications are aspirin 81 mg daily, lisinopril 10 mg daily, and simvastatin 20 mg daily. Her heart rate is 105 beats per minute, her blood pressure is 100/60 mm Hg, and her temperature is 36.4°C. On clinical examination, the patient has moderate epigastric tenderness and reduced bowel sounds. Laboratory test results include the following: hemoglobin 13 g/dL, white blood cell count 18×10⁹/L, amylase 2,563 U/L, lipase 5,637 U/L, aspartate aminotransferase (AST) 350 U/L, alanine aminotransferase (ALT) 250 U/L, and bilirubin 1.1 mg/dL. What should you recommend next?

    a. Computed tomographic (CT) scan of the abdomen with intravenous (IV) contrast medium

    b. Ultrasonography of the abdomen

    c. Emergent endoscopic retrograde cholangiopancreatography (ERCP)

    d. Plain abdominal radiography

    e. IV fluid, bowel rest, and observation

IV.7. A 50-year-old man presents to the emergency department with left lower abdominal pain. He has not had fever or a change in bowel habit. He is eating without difficulty. He has never had similar symptoms in the past. He has not undergone colon cancer screening. He has no comorbid conditions. On examination, he has mild tenderness in the left lower abdomen without peritoneal signs. The white blood cell count is 12.5×10⁹/L. Computed tomography (CT) shows changes consistent with diverticulitis without abscess. What should you recommend as the next step for this patient?

    a. Hospital admission, bowel rest, and intravenous antibiotics

    b. Outpatient antibiotics

    c. Colonoscopy

    d. Surgical consultation

    e. CT colonography

IV.8. A 32-year-old man presents for evaluation of difficulty swallowing. He has had intermittent symptoms for 3 years. He states that he has had problems with only solid foods. He reports having mild, periodic heartburn and reflux but no weight loss. He has made several trips to the emergency department when food remained stuck in his esophagus after a meal and he could not dislodge it on his own. He has undergone esophagogastroduodenoscopy (EGD) twice; findings were reported as normal. He has eczema that is well controlled with topical therapy; otherwise, he is healthy. Which of the following is the best next step?

    a. EGD with empirical dilation

    b. Reassurance alone

    c. EGD with esophageal biopsies

    d. Esophageal manometry

    e. Proton pump inhibitor (PPI) therapy

IV.9. A 52-year-old woman undergoes an evaluation for diarrhea. Laboratory evaluation shows the following: hemoglobin 9.8 g/dL, mean corpuscular volume 102 fL, positive tissue transglutaminase antibody, and serum gastrin 800 pg/mL. On esophagogastroduodenoscopy, pale, atrophic-appearing gastric mucosa is noted. Gastric biopsies show intestinal metaplasia, and small bowel biopsies are positive for celiac disease. Her diarrhea improves on a gluten-free diet. Which of the following is most likely to be diagnostically useful?

    a. Testing for the presence of antiparietal cell antibodies

    b. Secretin stimulation test

    c. Octreotide scan

    d. Testing for the presence of *Helicobacter pylori* stool antigen

    e. Recent use of proton pump inhibitor therapy

IV.10. A 63-year-old man undergoes esophagogastroduodenoscopy (EGD) and colonoscopy as part of an evaluation for mild iron deficiency anemia. He reports having no melena or hematochezia, and he has not lost weight. The only medication he takes is ibuprofen for intermittent joint aches, and he is otherwise healthy. His family history is unremarkable. The EGD showed multiple linear antral erosions and a 1.2-cm polyp in the body of the stomach. Biopsies from throughout the stomach showed a chemical gastritis, with no *Helicobacter pylori*, and biopsies of the polyp identified a tubular adenoma with low-grade dysplasia. Small bowel biopsy findings were normal. The colonoscopy showed only scattered sigmoid diverticula. Which of the following is the best next step?

    a. No further testing

    b. *Helicobacter pylori* stool antigen test

    c. Endoscopic ultrasonography

    d. EGD now with full removal of the polyp

    e. EGD in 1 year

IV.11. A 78-year-old man presents for evaluation of new swallowing problems. He states that for the past 3 months, food gets stuck when he swallows, although the food eventually passes spontaneously. He also notes difficulty swallowing liquids and senses fullness in his chest for a prolonged period after drinking any beverage. He reports regurgitation of fluid into the back of his throat. He has a 40–pack-year smoking history, and a long-standing history of reflux, which is well-controlled with proton pump inhibitor therapy as needed. He has lost 6.8 kg over the past few months. He had esophagogastroduodenoscopy (EGD) 1 year ago to screen for Barrett esophagus; results were negative. With his new symptoms, he now undergoes a barium esophagram, which shows a bird's beak narrowing at the distal esophagus; esophageal manometry shows an elevated pressure in the lower esophageal sphincter, which does not relax after a swallow, and aperistalsis. Which of the following is the best next step?

    a. Perform another EGD now.

    b. Inject botulinum toxin into the lower esophageal sphincter.

    c. Refer the patient to a surgeon for myotomy.

    d. Perform computed tomography of the chest.

    e. Test for anticentromere antibodies.

IV.12. A 49-year-old man presents with a 1-month history of diarrhea. He has approximately 10 watery bowel movements daily, and he has lost 4.5 kg while he has had diarrhea. Physical examination, complete blood cell count, and blood chemistry panel results are normal. A 72-hour stool collection shows 2,000 g of stool with 10 g of fat per 24 hours. Stool electrolyte concentrations are as follows: sodium 80 mmol/L and potassium 60 mmol/L. From these findings, what is the most likely cause of this patient's diarrhea?

    a. Whipple disease

    b. Vasoactive intestinal peptide tumor

    c. Celiac sprue

    d. Chronic pancreatitis

    e. Lactase deficiency

IV.13. A 40-year-old woman who has iron deficiency anemia began receiving oral iron therapy without response. She reports having no gastrointestinal tract symptoms or heavy menses. She has a normal appetite and reports no weight loss. There is no family history of colon cancer or inflammatory bowel disease. Fecal occult blood testing of the stool is negative. Which test should be performed next?

    a. Measurement of serum immunoglobulin (Ig)A and IgG tissue transglutaminase antibodies

    b. Upper endoscopy with small bowel biopsies

    c. Capsule endoscopy

    d. Small bowel follow-through

    e. Stool evaluation for ova and parasites

IV.14. A 45-year-old woman presents with abdominal discomfort and diarrhea. Almost every day, she has variable abdominal discomfort with up to 3 or 4 watery stools. She has associated abdominal bloating and flatulence. Eating and stress aggravate her symptoms, and her abdominal discomfort is relieved by defecation. She reports having no anorexia, weight loss, or blood in the stool. You suspect irritable bowel syndrome (IBS). Laboratory study results are normal for complete blood cell count, erythrocyte sedimentation rate, and C-reactive protein. Fecal leukocytes are present, but culture results for enteric pathogens and testing for *Clostridium difficile* are negative. Which intervention is appropriate at this time?

a. Loperamide

b. Rifaximin

c. Colonoscopy with biopsies

d. Reassurance and patient counseling

e. Stool-bulking agents

IV.15. A 33-year-old Asian woman receives a diagnosis of non-Hodgkin lymphoma, and chemotherapy is advised. She has a history of hepatitis B without complications. Her mother also had hepatitis B. On examination, the patient has cervical adenopathy consistent with lymphoma and no stigmata of chronic liver disease. Laboratory test results are as follows: platelet count 348×10^9/L, alanine aminotransferase 17 U/L, total bilirubin 0.6 mg/dL, hepatitis B surface antigen positive, hepatitis B e antigen (HBeAg) negative, antibody to HBeAg positive, immunoglobulin (Ig)G antibody to hepatitis B core antigen positive, and hepatitis B virus (HBV) DNA undetectable. Which of the following should you advise at this time?

a. Hepatitis B vaccination

b. Surveillance for hepatocellular carcinoma (HCC)

c. Lamivudine

d. Pegylated interferon

e. Nothing further at this time except chemotherapy

Answers

IV.1. Answer b.

Hyperplastic polyps do not infer an increased risk of colon cancer; therefore, the rectal lesion is of no clinical significance. The patient had 3 clinically significant polyps. Although each of these lesions was smaller than 1 cm, the interval to the next colonoscopy would be 3 years because there were 3 or more polyps and because 1 of the lesions had a villous component.

IV.2. Answer e.

This constellation of symptoms and laboratory findings is most suggestive of hemolytic uremic syndrome (HUS), a complication of infection with *E coli* O157:H7. This occurs more commonly in the elderly or very young, and the risk may be increased with the administration of antibiotic therapy. *Shigella* is also invasive and can cause bloody diarrhea, but it is not associated with HUS. Infections with the other listed organisms typically result in watery diarrhea.

IV.3. Answer c.

A patient with inflammatory bowel disease who has a red eye most likely has either episcleritis or uveitis. Uveitis is associated with pain in the eye. Episcleritis is typically painless. Patients with giant cell arteritis usually do not present with red eye, and they usually have a headache or vision loss.

IV.4. Answer c.

This man has chronic ulcerative proctosigmoiditis of mild to moderate severity. The initial treatment of this condition is topical therapy. Topical aminosalicylates are superior to topical corticosteroids for the induction of remission of ulcerative proctosigmoiditis. Treatment with suppositories for this patient would be inadequate (they are effective only for disease limited to the rectum, up to 10 cm from the anal verge). Treatment with corticosteroids, either oral or IV, would not be indicated in the initial management because this patient has mild to moderately active disease.

IV.5. Answer b.

The clinical presentation and the colonoscopic and histologic findings are typical of microscopic colitis (in this patient, collagenous colitis). Initial therapy for mild to moderate disease (3–6 bowel movements daily) is usually with an antidiarrheal such as loperamide hydrochloride or with bismuth subsalicylate. In more severe cases (>6 bowel movements daily), budesonide may be considered for initial therapy. Prednisone would be used only in patients with microscopic colitis that did not respond to the aforementioned therapies.

IV.6. Answer e.

The patient has acute pancreatitis as evidenced by the clinical presentation and the elevated levels of amylase and lipase. The cause is most likely gallstone disease (AST and ALT were moderately elevated). The most important initial step in the management of patients with acute pancreatitis is to ensure excellent hydration to optimize pancreatic perfusion and thereby decrease the risk of pancreatic necrosis. The patient does not have evidence of cholangitis (absence of fever, pain localizing to right upper quadrant, and jaundice), so there is no indication for emergent ERCP. CT scan of the abdomen with IV contrast medium may be indicated later in the clinical course to evaluate for pancreatic necrosis, but it is not indicated at initial presentation. Ultrasonography of the abdomen is a reasonable step but only after IV fluid resuscitation has been initiated.

IV.7. Answer b.

This patient is presenting with a first episode of uncomplicated diverticulitis. Since he is tolerating oral intake without difficulty, outpatient management may be pursued. If there were evidence of a complication (eg, abscess), or if the patient could not tolerate oral intake, hospitalization would be necessary. Since this is the patient's first episode of diverticulitis, and it is uncomplicated, surgery is not indicated. Colonoscopy is contraindicated with acute diverticulitis, but since this patient has not undergone colon cancer screening, it would be reasonable to perform colonoscopy 2 to 4 weeks after the acute symptoms have resolved.

IV.8. Answer c.

This patient has features highly suggestive of eosinophilic esophagitis (EE): intermittent solid food dysphagia, food impactions, and an underlying history of an atopic condition. Although endoscopic features can be very suggestive, normal EGD findings do not exclude EE. The diagnosis is established by obtaining midesophageal biopsies and finding 15 or more eosinophils per high-power field. Dilation of associated strictures may be necessary, but it should be done after treatment of EE because dilation increases the risk of severe esophageal tears or perforation. Reassurance alone without establishing the diagnosis of EE may result in recurrent food impactions and other complications. Esophageal manometry is useful to help clarify the diagnosis of achalasia, but it has no role in the evaluation of a patient with suspected EE. PPI therapy may control this patient's heartburn and reflux, and it is often first-line therapy for EE (even before fluticasone), but to empirically treat this patient without establishing a diagnosis would not be recommended.

IV.9. Answer a.

This patient most likely has autoimmune gastritis with associated achlorhydria, megaloblastic anemia, and secondary gastrin elevation because she has intestinal metaplasia of the stomach, no history of peptic ulcer disease, and another autoimmune condition. Antiparietal or anti–intrinsic factor antibodies are likely to be positive. Achlorhydria can lead to gastrin levels as high as those seen in Zollinger-Ellison syndrome. After the patient's celiac disease was treated, she did not have any clinical features suggestive of Zollinger-Ellison syndrome (diarrhea from fat malabsorption, peptic ulcer disease, or severe esophagitis), so additional testing with a secretin stimulation test or octreotide scan appears unnecessary. Although *H pylori* can cause intestinal metaplasia, it would be less likely because this patient has megaloblastic anemia and another autoimmune condition; *H pylori* can cause mild elevation of serum gastrin, but it would not be elevated to this degree. Proton pump inhibitor therapy can cause elevation of serum gastrin levels, but it would not explain the intestinal metaplasia.

IV.10. Answer d.

This patient has iron deficiency anemia that is likely due to the antral erosions that appear to have been induced by the nonsteroidal anti-inflammatory drug. However, he also has a gastric polyp that is a gastric adenoma; similar to colonic adenomas, gastric adenomas are deemed premalignant and require full endoscopic removal. The patient should have another EGD now with polypectomy since the polyp was simply biopsied and not fully removed during his previous EGD. To do no further testing would be inadequate because this polyp could continue to grow and progress to gastric cancer. Although gastric erosions can be caused by *H pylori*, this patient's histologic results were negative for *H pylori*, and he was not taking any medications that could lead to false-negative results for *H pylori* (proton pump inhibitor, antibiotics, etc); therefore, further testing for *H pylori* would not be needed. If the gastric polyp had been malignant, endoscopic ultrasonography would be needed to assess the depth of invasion and to complete locoregional staging, but that is not needed for an adenoma of this size. Waiting 1 year to repeat the EGD is not recommended because the polyp could continue to grow, progress to cancer, or cause bleeding, all of which could be prevented by removal now.

IV.11. Answer a.

This patient has clinical, radiographic, and manometric features consistent with achalasia; however, given his age, the rapid onset of his symptoms, and the weight loss, pseudoachalasia due to malignancy needs to be considered and ruled out. An EGD should be performed now to rule out esophageal or gastric cardia malignancy because his most recent EGD was 1 year ago (before the onset of his current symptoms), and an early lesion could have been missed. To refer this patient for any therapy targeted at achalasia, such as botulinum toxin injection into the lower esophageal sphincter or myotomy, would be premature until an EGD has been performed to rule out cancer. If a patient with clinical features of pseudoachalasia has negative findings on EGD, imaging of the chest may then be considered, especially with a smoking history. A pulmonary or mediastinal malignancy can infiltrate the lower esophageal sphincter complex and cause pseudoachalasia symptoms; however, this testing should not take place before another EGD is performed, allowing direct mucosal inspection. Anticentromere antibodies can be seen in CREST syndrome associated with scleroderma; similar to patients with achalasia, these patients may also have dysphagia to solids and liquids and are at increased risk for esophageal cancer. However, patients with esophageal involvement with scleroderma typically have a decreased lower esophageal sphincter tone, which is the opposite of what is seen in this patient.

IV.12. Answer b.

This patient's stool osmotic gap (290−2[80+60]) is less than 50 mmol/L, suggesting a secretory cause of diarrhea. Causes of secretory diarrhea include toxins from cholera and enterotoxigenic *Escherichia coli* and peptides produced from endocrine tumors (vasoactive intestinal peptide). The distinction between secretory and osmotic diarrhea helps in the differential diagnosis and evaluation of patients with chronic diarrhea. The 2 main methods to help distinguish between secretory and osmotic diarrhea are by calculating the stool osmotic gap and by assessing the response to fasting. Secretory diarrhea will not decrease substantially during a fast, whereas osmotic diarrhea will. The other answer choices (Whipple disease, celiac sprue, chronic pancreatitis, and lactase deficiency) are causes of osmotic diarrhea and are therefore incorrect.

IV.13. Answer b.

This woman has iron deficiency without evidence of gastrointestinal tract or menstrual blood loss, which suggests malabsorption of iron. The most common presentation of patients with celiac disease is iron deficiency anemia. Iron is mainly absorbed in the duodenum. Celiac disease preferentially affects the proximal small bowel, interfering with iron uptake. Therefore, upper endoscopy with small bowel biopsies should be performed to evaluate for celiac disease. A small bowel series or capsule endoscopy may suggest the diagnosis of celiac disease but does not provide tissue for diagnosis. Positive serologic testing (tissue transglutaminase antibodies) supports the diagnosis of celiac disease but, if results are negative, does not exclude the diagnosis for this patient who has a high pretest probability of celiac disease. In a patient with iron deficiency and no gastrointestinal tract symptoms, stool evaluation for ova and parasites would be low yield. Furthermore, a parasitic infection (eg, strongyloidiasis) would likely be detected on small bowel biopsy.

IV.14. Answer c.

This patient has signs and symptoms consistent with IBS. The only test required for patients who have typical diarrhea-predominant IBS symptoms and no alarm features is serologic testing for celiac disease. However, this patient has evidence of fecal leukocytes. This finding suggests colonic inflammation and warrants further investigation with colonoscopy and biopsy to evaluate for inflammatory bowel disease or microscopic colitis. Reassurance, antidiarrheals, and stool-bulking agents are therapies to consider for the patient with IBS. Rifaximin is a nonabsorbable antibiotic used to treat traveler's diarrhea, recurrent hepatic encephalopathy, and small intestinal bacterial overgrowth. Although rifaximin was recently found to alleviate IBS symptoms, it is not approved by the US Food and Drug Administration for this indication, and this patient with fecal leukocytes requires further evaluation with colonoscopy.

IV.15. Answer c.

Patients with hepatitis B who need immunosuppressive therapy are at risk for reactivation of disease and should receive hepatitis B treatment. An oral nucleoside or nucleotide analogue, such as lamivudine, is preferred because of the reliable antiviral effect and lack of toxicity. Ideally, hepatitis B treatment is started 2 weeks before initiation of chemotherapy and continued for several months after completion of the lymphoma treatment. Hepatitis B vaccination is not useful if the patient already has hepatitis B. Surveillance for HCC is advised for the following hepatitis B patients: patients who have cirrhosis, Asian women older than 50 years, Asian men older than 40 years, Africans older than 20 years, patients with a family history of HCC, and patients with persistently elevated liver test results and high HBV DNA levels. This patient does not meet any of those criteria.

Section V

General Internal Medicine

24 Clinical Epidemiology

SCOTT C. LITIN, MD AND JOHN B. BUNDRICK, MD

Interpretation of Diagnostic Tests

Diagnostic tests are tools that either increase or decrease the likelihood of disease. When a diagnostic test is applied to a population at risk for a particular disease, patients in the studied population can be assigned to 1 of 4 groups on the basis of disease status and the test result. Table 24.1 illustrates the concept.

By convention, the 4 groups are assigned the letters *a* for true positive (TP), *b* for false positive (FP), *c* for false negative (FN), and *d* for true negative (TN) (Table 24.2). On the basis of this table (called a *2×2 table*) several test characteristics can be defined.

Sensitivity

Sensitivity refers to a positive test result for a patient with the disease. The *TP rate* is the proportion of patients with the disease who have a positive test result:

$$\text{Sensitivity} = \frac{\text{TP}}{\text{TP} + \text{FN}}.$$

The 2×2 table definition of *sensitivity* is a/(a+c). The following rules are related to sensitivity:

1. If a test has 100% sensitivity, a negative test result rules *out* the disorder (mnemonic: *SN out*).

Table 24.1 • Four Outcomes of a Diagnostic Test

Outcome	Disease Status	Test Result
True positive	Present	Abnormal
False positive	Absent	Abnormal
False negative	Present	Normal
True negative	Absent	Normal

2. Screening tests are used to maximize sensitivity and avoid missing a person who has the disease.
3. Characteristics of a test are not affected by the prevalence of disease in the population.

Specificity

Specificity refers to a negative test result for a patient without the disease. The *TN rate* is the proportion of patients without the disease who have a negative test result:

$$\text{Specificity} = \frac{\text{TN}}{\text{TN} + \text{FP}}.$$

The 2×2 table definition of *specificity* is d/(b+d). The following rules are related to specificity:

1. If a test has 100% specificity, a positive test result rules *in* the disorder (mnemonic: *SP in*).
2. Confirmatory tests are used in follow-up to maximize specificity and avoid incorrectly labeling a healthy person as having disease.
3. Characteristics of a test are not affected by the prevalence of disease in the population.

Positive Predictive Value

When a patient's illness is evaluated by interpreting the result of a diagnostic test, the 2×2 table is read horizontally, not vertically. One really wants to know whether a patient with a positive test result actually has the disease; that is, how well the test result predicts a disease compared with the reference standard for that disease. Thus, in the 2×2 table, the horizontal rows for the diagnostic test result are of primary interest. Among all patients with a positive diagnostic test result (TP+FP), in what proportion, $\dfrac{\text{TP}}{\text{TP} + \text{FP}}$, has the diagnosis been predicted correctly or ruled in? This

285

Table 24.2 • 2×2 Table

		Target Disorder		
		Present	**Absent**	
Diagnostic Test Result	**Positive**	True positive a	False positive b	a+b
	Negative	c False negative	d True negative	c+d
		a+c	b+d	a+b+c+d

Prevalence = (a+c)/(a+b+c+d)
Test characteristics
  Sensitivity = a/(a+c)
  Specificity = d/(b+d)
Frequency-dependent properties
  Positive predictive value = a/(a+b)
  Negative predictive value = d/(c+d)

proportion is the **positive predictive value** (PPV): PPV is the proportion of patients who have the disease among all the patients who test positive for the disease. PPV provides information most useful in clinical practice. PPV is affected by the prevalence of the disease in the population. The 2×2 table definition of *PPV* is $\dfrac{TP}{TP + FP} = a/(a + b)$.

Negative Predictive Value

It is also important to know the percentage of patients with a negative test result (FN+TN) who actually do not have the disease. This proportion, $\dfrac{TN}{FN + TN}$, is the **negative predictive value** (NPV): NPV is the proportion of patients who do not have the disease of interest among all the patients who test negative for the disease. NPV is affected by the prevalence of disease in the population. The 2×2 table definition of *NPV* is $\dfrac{TN}{FN + TN} = d/(c + d)$.

Prevalence

Prevalence is defined as the proportion of persons with the disease in the population to whom the test has been applied. In terms of the 2×2 table, prevalence is written as follows:

$$\frac{TP + FN}{TP + FP + FN + TN} = \frac{a + c}{a + b + c + d}.$$

How to Construct a 2×2 Table

The sensitivity, specificity, and predictive values of normal and abnormal test results can be calculated with even a limited amount of information. For example, assume that a new diagnostic test is positive in 90% of patients who have the disease and is negative in 95% of patients who are disease-free. The prevalence of the disease in the population to which the test is applied is 10%. This provides the following information: sensitivity = 90%, specificity = 95%, and prevalence = 10%.

This test is now ready to be applied to a group of patients by filling in a 2×2 table (Table 24.3). The calculation is often easier if the test is applied to a large number of patients. For example, if it is applied to 1,000 patients, a+b+c+d=1,000.

Because the prevalence of the disease is 10%, 100 patients have the disease (0.1×1,000=100, or a+c=100). Of the patients, 90%, or 900, are disease-free (0.9×1,000=900, or b+d=900).

Sensitivity of 90% means that 90% of the 100 patients with disease have a positive test result (a = 0.9×100 = 90) and 10% have a negative result (c = 0.1×100 = 10).

Specificity of 95% means that 95% of the 900 patients who are disease-free have a negative test result (d = 0.95×900 = 855) and 5% have a positive test result (b = 0.05×900 = 45).

The 2×2 table in Table 24.3 shows that 135 patients (a+b) have a positive test result; however, only 90 of these 135 patients actually have the disease. Therefore, the PPV of a positive test is $\dfrac{a}{a+b} = \dfrac{90}{135} = 66.7\%$. That is, only two-thirds of all patients with a positive test result will actually have the disease. Similarly, one can determine that 865 patients (c+d) have a negative test result; 855 of these 865 patients are disease-free. Therefore, the NPV of the test is $\dfrac{d}{c+d} = \dfrac{855}{865} = 98.8\%$.

Clinicians should be able to perform these simple calculations. Clinical decision making by internists is more likely to depend on the PPV and NPV of test results for a given population than on the sensitivity or specificity of the test.

Table 24.3 • 2×2 Table for Test With 90% Sensitivity, 95% Specificity, and 10% Prevalence

		Disease Present	Disease Absent	
Diagnostic Test Result	**Positive**	90 a	b 45	135 a+b
	Negative	c 10	d 855	c+d 865
		a+c 100	b+d 900	a+b+c+d 1,000

Prevalence = (a+c)/(a+b+c+d) = 100/1,000 = 10%
Test characteristics
    Sensitivity = a/(a+c) = 90/100 = 90%
    Specificity = d/(b+d) = 855/900 = 95%
Frequency-dependent properties
    Positive predictive value = a/(a+b) = 90/135 = 66.7%
    Negative predictive value = d/(c+d) = 855/865 = 98.8%
Likelihood ratio (LR) for a positive test result:
    LR+ = Sensitivity/(1 − Specificity) = 90%/5% = 18
Likelihood ratio for a negative test result:
    LR− = (1 − Sensitivity)/Specificity = 10%/95% = 0.11
Pretest odds = Prevalence/(1 − Prevalence) = 10%/90% = 0.11
Posttest odds = Pretest odds × LR
Posttest probability = Posttest odds/(Posttest odds + 1)

KEY FACTS

✓ If a test has 100% sensitivity, a negative test rules *out* the disorder

✓ If a test has 100% specificity, a positive test rules *in* the disorder

✓ Prevalence—the proportion of persons with the disease in the population to whom the test has been applied

✓ Clinical decision making—more likely to depend on PPV and NPV of test results for a given population than on the test's sensitivity or specificity

---

For example, if the prevalence of the disease in the clinician's population is 2% instead of 10%, the PPV and NPV can be recalculated. The PPV of abnormal test results decreases to 26.9%, which is quite different from 66.7% (based on a prevalence of 10%), although the test's sensitivity (90%) and specificity (95%) have not changed (Table 24.4).

Use of Odds and Likelihood Ratios

Some physicians prefer interpreting diagnostic test results by using the likelihood ratio. This ratio takes properties of a diagnostic test (sensitivity and specificity) and makes them more helpful in clinical decision making. It helps the clinician determine the probability of disease in a specific patient after a diagnostic test has been performed.

The formula for a likelihood ratio for a positive test result (LR+) is

$$LR+ = \frac{\text{Positive Test in Disease}}{\text{Positive Test in No Disease}} = \frac{\text{Sensitivity}}{1 - \text{Specificity}}.$$

The formula for a likelihood ratio for a negative test result (LR−) is

$$LR- = \frac{\text{Negative Test in Disease}}{\text{Negative Test in No Disease}} = \frac{1 - \text{Sensitivity}}{\text{Specificity}}.$$

For example, if test A has a sensitivity of 95% and a specificity of 90%,

$$LR+ = \frac{\text{Sensitivity}}{1 - \text{Specificity}} = \frac{95}{10} = 9.5 \quad \text{and}$$

$$LR- = \frac{1 - \text{Sensitivity}}{\text{Specificity}} = \frac{5}{90} = 0.06.$$

However, if test B has a sensitivity of 20% and a specificity of 80%, then

$$LR+ = \frac{\text{Sensitivity}}{1 - \text{Specificity}} = \frac{20}{20} = 1 \quad \text{and}$$

Table 24.4 • 2×2 Table for Test With 90% Sensitivity, 95% Specificity, and 2% Prevalence

		Disease Present	Disease Absent	
Diagnostic Test Result	Positive	18 (a)	49 (b)	67 (a+b)
	Negative	2 (c)	931 (d)	933 (c+d)
		20 (a+c)	980 (b+d)	1,000 (a+b+c+d)

Prevalence = (a+c)/(a+b+c+d) = 20/1,000 = 2%
Test characteristics
 Sensitivity = a/(a+c) = 18/20 = 90%
 Specificity = d/(b+d) = 931/980 = 95%
Frequency-dependent properties
 Positive predictive value = a/(a+b) = 18/67 = 26.9%
 Negative predictive value = d/(c+d) = 931/933 = 99.8%

$$LR- = \frac{1-Sensitivity}{Specificity} = \frac{80}{80} = 1.$$

As a general rule, diagnostic tests with an LR+ greater than 10 or an LR− less than 0.1 have a greater influence on the posttest probability of disease (ie, they are better tests) than diagnostic tests with likelihood ratios between 10 and 0.1. In the 2 examples above, test A is more likely to rule in or rule out disease than test B.

Sample likelihood ratios are provided in the following example and in Table 24.5.

Example

A 40-year-old man is admitted to the hospital for pneumonia. He says that he consumes 2 six-packs of beer each week. On the basis of this history and your clinical judgment, you assume that he has a pretest probability of 20% for a diagnosis of alcoholism. You ask him questions from the CAGE (cut down, annoyed, guilty, eye-opener) questionnaire, and his responses are positive for all 4 questions. The LR+ for 3 or more CAGE questions is 250.

At this point, you have 2 choices. The first is to use a nomogram (Figure 24.1) and, with a straightedge, connect

Table 24.5 • Examples of Symptoms, Signs, and Tests and the Corresponding Likelihood Ratio (LR)

Target Disorder	Patient Population	Health Care Setting	Symptom, Sign, Test	No. of Signs or Symptoms	LR
Alcohol abuse or dependency	Patients admitted to orthopedic or medical services over 6-mo period	US teaching hospital	Yes to ≥3 questions on CAGE questionnaire		250
Sinusitis (by further investigation)	Patients with nasal complaints	US teaching hospital	Maxillary toothache, purulent nasal secretion, poor response to nasal decongestants, abnormal transillumination findings, or history of colored nasal discharge	≥4 3 2 1 0	6.4 2.6 1.1 0.5 0.1
Ascites	Male veteran patients	US veterans hospital	Presence of fluid wave (test done by internal medicine residents)		9.6

Abbreviation: CAGE, cut down, annoyed, guilty, eye-opener (screening questionnaire for potential alcoholism).

Data from Bush B, Shaw S, Cleary P, Delbanco TL, Aronson MD. Screening for alcohol abuse using the CAGE questionnaire. Am J Med. 1987 Feb;82(2):231–5; Williams JW Jr, Simel DL. Does this patient have sinusitis? Diagnosing acute sinusitis by history and physical examination. JAMA. 1993 Sep 8;270(10):1242–6; Williams JW Jr, Simel DL, Roberts L, Samsa GP. Clinical evaluation for sinusitis: making the diagnosis by history and physical examination. Ann Intern Med. 1992 Nov 1;117(9):705–10; Williams JW Jr, Simel DL. The rational clinical examination: does this patient have ascites? How to divine fluid in the abdomen. JAMA. 1992 May 20;267(19):2645–8; and Simel DL, Halvorsen RA Jr, Feussner JR. Quantitating bedside diagnosis: clinical evaluation of ascites. J Gen Intern Med. 1988 Sep–Oct;3(5):423–8.

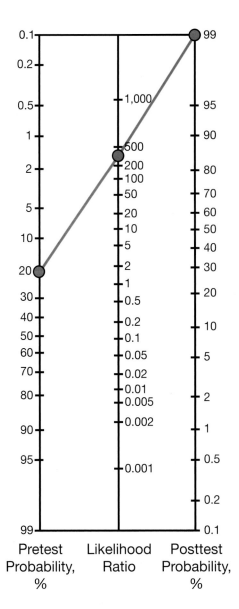

Figure 24.1 *Nomogram.*

$$\text{Odds} = \frac{\text{Probability}}{1\text{-Probability}} \quad \text{and}$$

$$\text{Probability} = \frac{\text{Odds}}{1+\text{Odds}}.$$

In the example, step 1 involves converting pretest probability to pretest odds. In this case, you estimated that the pretest probability of alcoholism is 20%. With the formulas above,

$$\text{Pretest Odds} = \frac{0.20}{1-0.20} = 0.25.$$

Therefore, 0.25 is the pretest odds of having the condition. Step 2 involves determining the posttest odds for a positive test result. This can be determined by multiplying the pretest odds (0.25) by the LR+ for 3 or more positive questions on the CAGE questionnaire (250): 0.25×250=62.5. Step 3 allows conversion of posttest odds to posttest probability by placing the numbers in the following formula:

$$\text{Posttest Probability} = \frac{\text{Odds}}{1+\text{Odds}} = \frac{62.5}{63.5} = 98.4\%.$$

In conclusion, the posttest probability for the diagnosis of alcoholism for this patient is 98.4%, which is close to the value obtained from the nomogram.

Interpretation of Therapeutic Results

Physicians often make treatment decisions on the basis of the results of randomized controlled trials (RCTs). To understand whether the results of such trials are impressive, the physician is required to translate these results into language understandable to both physicians and patients. This terminology can also be used to compare various therapies for the disease of interest. Several authors have coined terms and derived useful equations to help physicians make sense of RCTs concerned with therapy.

Relative Risk Reduction

The results of RCTs of anticoagulant therapy to prevent stroke in patients with atrial fibrillation have been published and summarized. In primary prevention studies, the average 1-year risk of stroke in the placebo group was 5%. Because no therapy was administered to that group, this can be called the *control event rate* (CER). In these studies of patients with atrial fibrillation treated with adjusted-dose warfarin (international normalized ratio [INR], 2.0–3.0), the approximate stroke risk was reduced to 2% per year. This can be called the *experimental event rate* (EER) because the patients received a particular therapy.

the pretest probability of 20% and the LR+ of 250 to the posttest probability. This shows that the posttest probability for a diagnosis of alcoholism is 99%.

The second option should be used when there is no nomogram for performing this simple calculation. Without a nomogram, the following steps must be done:

1. Convert the pretest probability to pretest odds.
2. Multiply the pretest odds by the likelihood ratio to obtain the posttest odds.
3. Convert the posttest odds to posttest probability.

Probability and odds can be converted somewhat interchangeably with the following formulas:

The traditional measure often used to report the difference between the treated and untreated groups is the *relative risk reduction* (RRR), which is calculated as $\frac{\text{CER} - \text{EER}}{\text{CER}}$. This measure relates the reduction in risk of the outcome event with the intervention to the baseline risk rate (ie, the CER). In this example, the RRR is $\frac{5\% - 2\%}{5\%} = 60\%$. Therefore, anticoagulant therapy reduced the yearly risk of a stroke in patients with atrial fibrillation by 60% compared with the baseline risk of a stroke with no therapy. However, the RRR often is not clinically helpful because the number itself does not provide information about the baseline risk rate (ie, the CER). For example, even if only a very small percentage of control patients (0.005%) and patients receiving anticoagulation (0.002%) experience stroke, the RRR is unchanged: $\frac{0.005\% - 0.002\%}{0.005\%} = 60\%$. Therefore, the RRR often is not useful to the clinician or patient, although a large RRR can be used to make a dramatic endorsement for therapy by proponents of that therapy.

- $\text{RRR} = \dfrac{\text{CER} - \text{EER}}{\text{CER}}$
- Often RRR is not clinically useful because it does not provide information about the baseline risk rate.

Absolute Risk Reduction

In the example above, it would be useful for the physician and patient to know the absolute difference in rates of stroke between the control group and the atrial fibrillation group given anticoagulants (CER–EER). This measure is called the *absolute risk reduction* (ARR). In the combined Stroke Prevention in Atrial Fibrillation (SPAF) trials, the ARR or (CER – EER) = (5% – 2%) = 3% per year.

- $\text{ARR} = (\text{CER} - \text{EER})$
- ARR is clinically more useful for interpreting therapeutic results.

Number Needed to Treat

The physician and patient often want to know the number of patients needed to treat (NNT) with a therapy to prevent 1 additional bad outcome. That number can be calculated as $\dfrac{1}{\text{ARR}}$. The NNT to prevent 1 stroke by using the adjusted dose of warfarin in patients with atrial fibrillation

would be $\dfrac{1}{0.03} = \dfrac{1}{3\%} = 33$. Therefore, the NNT would be 33 patients; that is, 33 patients would need to be treated with warfarin (INR, 2.0–3.0) for 1 year to prevent 1 additional stroke.

- NNT identifies the number of patients who need to be treated with a therapy to prevent 1 additional bad outcome.
- $\text{NNT} = \dfrac{1}{\text{ARR}}$

Number Needed to Harm

Conversely, if the rate of adverse events caused by the experimental therapy is known and compared with the rate of adverse events in the placebo group, the number needed to harm (NNH) can be calculated. This useful number tells the physician how many treated patients it takes to produce 1 additional harmful event. In the SPAF trials, the average risk of intracranial hemorrhage for the group given warfarin was 0.3% per year, compared with 0.1% per year for the placebo group. Therefore, the NNH can be calculated as the reciprocal of the absolute risk increase (ARI). The ARI is calculated by subtracting the harm CER from the harm EER or, in this case, 0.3%–0.1%=0.2%. In this example, $\text{NNH} = \dfrac{1}{0.2\%} = \dfrac{1}{0.002} = 500$. Therefore, 500 patients would need to be treated with anticoagulant for 1 year to cause 1 additional intracranial hemorrhage, compared with the control group.

- NNH identifies how many treated patients are needed to produce 1 additional harmful event.
- $\text{NNH} = \dfrac{1}{\text{Harm EER} - \text{Harm CER}}$

KEY FACTS

✓ Diagnostic tests with LR+ greater than 10 or LR– less than 0.1 are better tests than those with likelihood ratios in between

✓ Number needed to treat—how many patients need to be treated with a therapy to prevent 1 additional bad outcome

✓ Number needed to harm—how many treated patients are needed to produce 1 additional harmful event

25 Complementary and Alternative Medicine

TONY Y. CHON, MD AND BRENT A. BAUER, MD

omplementary and alternative medicine (CAM) has many meanings, each derived in part from its context. From a physician perspective (ie, the biomedical model), CAM has often been defined as "those therapies utilized by patients but not taught in medical school." Traditionally, CAM has encompassed treatments such as acupuncture, herbs and dietary supplements, massage, and chiropractic. Yet, in recent decades, the explosive growth of research in this arena (largely sponsored by the National Institutes of Health [NIH] National Center for Complementary and Alternative Medicine, now the National Center for Complementary and Integrative Health) has led to a number of therapies increasingly being incorporated into conventional training and practice. For example, teaching a patient a mind-body practice (eg, meditation) to help control hypertension is combined with the use of medications, lifestyle modifications, etc. This growing integration of evidence-based CAM therapies and conventional medicine is increasingly being referred to as *integrative medicine*.

Key Definition

Integrative medicine: *the growing integration of evidence-based complementary and alternative medicine therapies and conventional medicine.*

Figure 25.1 reflects survey data from 2002 (N=31,044) and 2007 (N=23,393) and suggests that nearly 40% of adults in the United States use some aspect of CAM as part of their health care. However, surveys of specific patient populations (eg, those with cancer, chronic pain, fibromyalgia) suggest that CAM use may be 80% to 90% in these groups.

Natural products (ie, herbs and supplements) are the most popular CAM therapy (Figure 25.2). However, the popularity of deep breathing, meditation, massage, yoga,

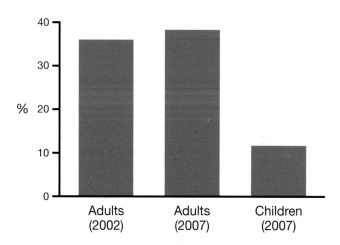

CAM Use by U.S. Adults and Children

Figure 25.1 Use of Complementary and Alternative Medicine by US Adults and Children.
(Adapted from Barnes PM, Bloom B, Nahin RL. Complementary and alternative medicine use among adults and children: United States, 2007. Natl Health Stat Report. 2008 Dec 10;[12]:1–23.)

progressive relaxation, and guided imagery also suggests that many patients are turning to CAM to help deal with stress.

Natural products deserve special attention because many can have toxic side effects and/or drug-herb interactions if not used thoughtfully and carefully.

Herbs and Dietary Supplements

The Dietary Supplement Health and Education Act (DSHEA) of 1994 defines a dietary supplement as "a product (other

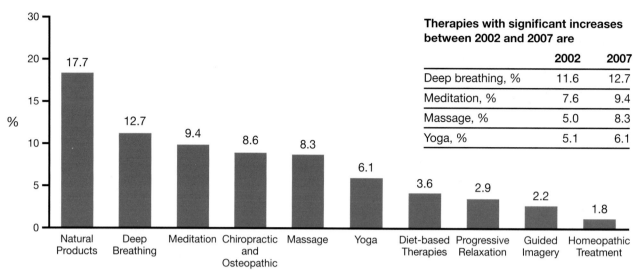

Figure 25.2 *Ten Most Common Complementary and Alternative Medicine Therapies Among Adults.*
(Adapted from Barnes PM, Bloom B, Nahin RL. Complementary and alternative medicine use among adults and children: United States, 2007. Natl Health Stat Report. 2008 Dec 10;[12]:1–23.)

than tobacco) that is intended to supplement the diet, which contains one or more of the following dietary ingredients: a vitamin, a mineral, an herb or other botanical, an amino acid, a dietary substance to supplement the diet by increasing the total daily intake, or a concentrate, metabolite, constituent, extract, or combinations of these ingredients." Table 25.1 describes common herbs and dietary supplements, their potential uses, and their potential adverse reactions. St John's wort is a commonly used herb and is associated with several potentially significant drug interactions (Table 25.2).

Table 25.1 • Common Herbs and Dietary Supplements

Herb or Dietary Supplement	Potential Uses	Description	Potential Adverse Reactions	Key Points
Black cohosh	Menopausal symptoms	Also called black snakeroot and bugbane. May have effects similar to estrogen	Gastrointestinal discomfort. May cause liver damage	Should not be used longer than 6 mo. Should not be taken during pregnancy
Echinacea	Cold and flu symptoms	Purported to boost the immune system	May cause allergic reactions	No clear evidence to support efficacy
Garlic	Hypertension, heart disease, hypercholesterolemia	May decrease low-density lipoprotein cholesterol	Breath and body odor, abdominal discomfort. May reduce blood clotting ability	May increase risk of bleeding in persons taking anticoagulant medications
Ginger	Nausea from pregnancy, motion sickness, and chemotherapy	Also available as powder, tablet, extract, tincture, and oil	High doses can cause abdominal discomfort. May increase risk of bleeding with anticoagulant medications	Not recommended for nausea during pregnancy with history of bleeding disorder or miscarriage
Ginkgo	Memory loss and dementia	Beneficial components believed to be flavonoids and terpenoids	May raise blood pressure with thiazide diuretics. May increase risk of bleeding	No clear evidence to support efficacy. Should be used cautiously when taking anticoagulant medications

Table 25.1 • (Continued)

Herb or Dietary Supplement	Potential Uses	Description	Potential Adverse Reactions	Key Points
Ginseng	Restore and enhance well-being	Used for allergies, asthma, fatigue, headaches, heart disease, many other conditions	May raise blood pressure in persons with hypertension	Should not exceed recommended daily doses Should not be used in persons with uncontrolled hypertension
Glucosamine and chondroitin sulfate	Osteoarthritis	Natural compounds found in cartilage	Generally well tolerated No known drug interactions	Research results are mixed
Omega-3 fatty acids (fish oil)	Cardiovascular health including hypertriglyceridemia	Contain both DHA and EPA Dietary sources include freshwater fish; flaxseed, walnut, canola, and soybean oils	Gastrointestinal discomfort, fishy odor May increase bleeding risk at high doses (>3 g daily)	May reduce triglycerides 20%–50% at dose of 2–4 g daily May lower risk of another heart attack, stroke, or death
S-Adenosyl methionine (SAMe)	Depression, osteoarthritis	Occurs naturally in the human body; not found in food Helps to produce and regulate hormones and cell functioning	Generally well tolerated Gas, nausea, diarrhea, and headaches at higher doses	Holds promise in depression and osteoarthritis; long-term benefits and risks unknown May interact with tricyclic antidepressants
Saw palmetto	Prostatic hyperplasia	Has also been used as sedative and antiseptic	Generally well tolerated	Research results are mixed
Soy	Menopausal symptoms, hypercholesterolemia, osteoporosis, heart disease	Active ingredients include isoflavones, weak forms of estrogen (phytoestrogen)	Generally well tolerated Potential allergy to soy May interact with monoamine oxidase inhibitor antidepressants	Research results are mixed
St John's wort	Depression, anxiety, insomnia	Flowers and leaves contain active ingredients (eg, hyperforin)	Generally well tolerated Some active compounds do not mix well with certain prescription drugs[a]	Several studies support for treatment of mild to moderate depression Potential significant drug interactions[a]

Abbreviations: DHA, docosahexaenoic acid; EPA, eicosapentaenoic acid.
[a] Potential significant interactions with St John's wort are listed in Table 25.2.

Table 25.2 • Potential Significant Drug Interactions With St John's Wort

Drug	Interactions
Warfarin	Increased breakdown of warfarin leading to increased risk of clotting
Oral contraceptive pills (OCPs)	Increased breakdown of OCPs leading to increased risk of pregnancy
Cyclosporine	Increased breakdown of cyclosporine leading to increased risk of transplant rejection
Digoxin	Increased breakdown of digoxin leading to decreased medication effectiveness
Human immunodeficiency virus protease inhibitors	Increased breakdown of protease inhibitors leading to decreased medication effectiveness
Anticonvulsants (carbamazepine, phenytoin)	Increased breakdown of anticonvulsants leading to increased risk of seizures
Selective serotonin reuptake inhibitors	Increased serotonin levels leading to serotonin syndrome

The passage of the DSHEA allowed supplements to be sold with suggested dosages, while at the same time specifically exempting manufacturers from having to demonstrate safety or efficacy of their products. As a result, herbal sales exploded in the United States in the past 20 years. However, the quality and purity of many products on US shelves were often poor, due in part to relatively limited oversight of the market by the US Food and Drug Administration. The good manufacturing practice guidelines passed in 2010 now mandate that all supplements manufactured or sold in the United States must contain what the label states, and nothing else. Coupled with these developments was a dramatic growth in the quality and quantity of clinical trials on supplements. Physicians can now focus on helping patients make informed decisions about the role of specific supplements in regard to their individual health needs.

KEY FACTS

✓ CAM therapies are used by nearly 40% of US adults and up to 90% of specific patient populations; natural products are most popular

✓ St John's wort can interfere with metabolism of many medications (eg, oral contraceptives, cyclosporine)

✓ SAMe may be useful for osteoarthritis and depression; fish oil for hypertriglyceridemia

✓ Ginkgo—ineffective in more recent large-scale trials

✓ Herbs and supplements that may increase risk of bleeding (and may need to be discontinued before surgery): garlic, ginger, ginseng, feverfew, fish oil, vitamin E

Box 25.1 • Traditional Chinese Medicine

Unique paradigm of medicine originated in China thousands of years ago

Paradigm helps to define how to diagnose and treat illness

Focus is on balance, harmony, the mind-body-spirit connection, and interactions with the outside world

Treatments include qi gong, acupuncture, tai chi, massage therapy, food therapy, physical manipulation, and herbal medicine

Limited evidence is available to recommend as a whole medical system

Herbal medications have potential risks, including interactions with prescription medications and contamination of herbal preparations

---

Box 25.2 • Ayurveda

Unique paradigm of medicine originated in India thousands of years ago

Paradigm is based on the theory that everything in the universe is interconnected and all forms of life consist of combinations of 5 energy elements: ether, wind, fire, water, and earth

These elements exist in 3 energetic patterns called *doshas*

When the elements and *doshas* are in balance, the person is healthy; when unbalanced, the body is weakened and susceptible to illness

Treatments include herbs, certain foods, therapeutic massage, fasting, yoga, and meditation

Limited evidence is available to recommend ayurvedic medicine as a whole medical system

Some ayurvedic supplements have been found to contain lead, mercury, arsenic, or other contaminants

Alternative Medical Systems

Alternative medical systems include traditional Chinese medicine, Ayurveda, and homeopathy. The major features of each are summarized in Boxes 25.1 through 25.3.

Manual Therapies

Manual therapies include chiropractic and massage therapy. The major features of each are summarized in Boxes 25.4 and 25.5.

KEY FACTS

✓ Herbal products from China may be contaminated with heavy metals or pesticides or adulterated with pharmaceuticals

✓ Ayurvedic preparations may contain toxic lead compounds

✓ Most homeopathic products are so diluted that they don't pose a risk unless used to the exclusion of proven conventional therapies

✓ Chiropractic—as effective as conventional treatment of acute low back pain in recent studies

✓ Aggressive cervical spine manipulation may cause vertebral artery dissection with resulting stroke

---

Mind-Body Medicine

According to the NIH, mind-body medicine focuses on the interactions among the mind, body, and behavior and

Box 25.3 • Homeopathy

Homeopathy is a whole medical system used for wellness and for prevention and treatment of many diseases

System is based on the concept "like cures like," in which a substance that causes the symptoms of a disease in healthy people can cure similar symptoms in patients who are sick

Practitioners provide medications from natural sources that are serially diluted to levels that no longer have any biologic effect

Research on the overall effectiveness of homeopathy is limited

Risks are generally limited unless patients pursue homeopathy to the exclusion of more proven conventional therapies in the setting of a serious but treatable condition

on the powerful ways in which emotional, mental, social, spiritual, and behavioral factors can directly affect health. Its therapies focus on providing positive thoughts, emotions, and influences to help promote physical health and help heal the body. In short, mind-body medicine helps to harness the power of the mind. Therapies include meditation, hypnotherapy, guided imagery, deep breathing, and biofeedback.

Box 25.4 • Chiropractic

Chiropractic focuses on the relationship between the spine and nervous system and its functioning

Chiropractic treatment aims to decrease pain, restore balance, and improve function related to restricted movement in the spine

Chiropractors use their hands to apply a controlled, sudden force to correct structural alignment and assist the body in healing

Chiropractors also may use massage, ultrasound, stretching, and electrical muscle stimulation

Evidence shows that chiropractic manipulation can be effective in providing relief from uncomplicated mild to moderate low back pain

Chiropractic manipulation is contraindicated in people with the following conditions:

- Severe osteoporosis
- Previous spinal surgery
- Coagulopathy
- Vertebral instability
- Unstable spine lesions or malignant spinal tumors
- Atherosclerotic disease in the cervical vasculature
- Inflammatory arthritis (rheumatoid arthritis)

Box 25.5 • Massage Therapy

Massage therapy involves manipulation of soft tissue to promote relaxation, ease muscle tension, ease muscle soreness, and decrease stress and anxiety

There are many types of massage; common types include Swedish, sports, trigger point, and deep tissue massage

Massage may help to release endorphins, improve circulation, and boost the immune system

This therapy is considered generally safe but may not be appropriate in persons with the following conditions:

- Severe osteoporosis
- Open wounds after surgery
- Bleeding disorders (avoid vigorous massage)
- Burns
- Fractures
- Deep vein thrombosis

Energy Medicine

Energy medicine is based on the belief that imbalances in the energy field of the body result in illness. Its therapies focus on providing and restoring balance of energy to heal the body and promote health. Therapies include acupuncture, therapeutic touch, healing touch, Reiki, and qi gong. In general, treatment of pain by acupuncture has the most evidence and clinical experience to support its use.

Key Definition

Energy medicine: *CAM therapies that focus on providing and restoring balance of energy to heal the body and promote health.*

Acupuncture

This traditional Chinese medical technique involves the insertion of extremely thin, solid, metallic needles through the skin to various depths at strategic points on the body. Acupuncture aims to restore and maintain health through the stimulation of specific points on the body. No unifying mechanism of action has been identified. An NIH consensus panel in 1997 determined that there was sufficient evidence of efficacy to support the use of acupuncture for 1) postoperative and chemotherapy-related nausea and vomiting in adults and 2) postoperative dental pain. The panel also identified the following as conditions for which acupuncture can be an effective part of an overall treatment strategy: headache, menstrual cramps, tennis elbow,

KEY FACTS

✓ Massage therapy shown to be effective in reducing postsurgical pain and anxiety

✓ Research supports massage as cost-effective treatment for chronic low back pain

✓ Incorporating mind-body medicine into patient care may improve symptoms and promote healing

✓ Acupuncture—the only energy medicine therapy with evidence supporting efficacy

fibromyalgia, myofascial pain, osteoarthritis, and low back pain.

Acupuncture is safe when performed properly, has few adverse effects, and can be useful as a complement to other treatment methods. The most common adverse effects of acupuncture are soreness and mild bleeding or bruising at the needle sites.

26 Dermatology

CARILYN N. WIELAND, MD

General Dermatology

Skin Cancer

Nonmelanoma skin cancers (basal cell carcinoma, squamous cell carcinoma) are the most common malignancies in the United States. Both basal cell and squamous cell carcinomas commonly occur on sun-exposed skin areas. Basal cell carcinoma typically presents as a pearly papule, often with telangiectasias and ulceration (Figure 26.1). It is usually slow-growing and locally invasive but may invade vital structures, cause

considerable disfigurement, and rarely metastasize. In contrast, squamous cell carcinoma has a higher risk of metastases. Squamous cell carcinoma most often presents as a hyperkeratotic or ulcerated papule (Figure 26.2). The following settings pose a high risk of nonmelanoma skin cancer: immunosuppression, areas of irradiated skin, chronic inflammation, and scar. Squamous cell carcinoma is the most common skin cancer in solid organ transplant recipients and is more aggressive, with a risk of metastasis of approximately 8%.

Malignant Melanoma

The strongest risk factors for melanoma are a family history of melanoma, multiple benign or atypical nevi, and a previous melanoma. Additional risk factors include fair

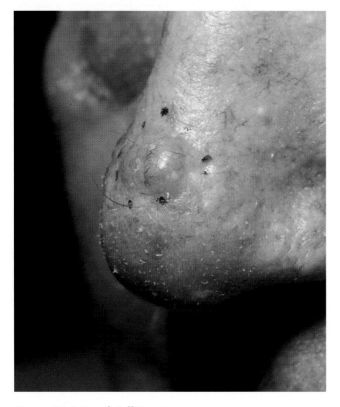

Figure 26.1 Basal Cell Carcinoma.

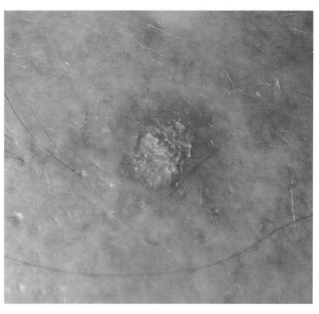

Figure 26.2 Squamous Cell Carcinoma.

skin, blond or red hair, sun sensitivity, freckling, intermittent sun exposure, blistering sunburns, immunosuppression, and tanning bed use. Inherited mutations in *CDKN2A* and *CDK4* genes, which have been documented in some families with melanoma, are associated with a 60% to 90% lifetime risk of melanoma. The familial atypical multiple mole melanoma syndrome is transmitted by an autosomal dominant gene.

The key to improved survival with malignant melanoma is early detection and diagnosis. A full skin examination is recommended for persons at risk, including an evaluation for *a*symmetry, *b*order irregularity, *c*olor variation, a *d*iameter more than 6 mm, and *e*volution (an **ABCDE evaluation**) (Figure 26.3). Changing or symptomatic moles or moles that stand out from other moles should be biopsied.

Table 26.1 • Survival in Malignant Melanoma, by Tumor Thickness[a]	
Tumor, mm	**5-Year Survival, %**
<1.0	95.3
1.01–2.00	89.0
2.01–4.00	78.7
>4.00	67.4

[a] No nodal or distant metastasis.

> ### Key Definition
>
> **ABCDE evaluation:** *evaluation for malignant melanoma, including *a*symmetry, *b*order irregularity, *c*olor variation, *d*iameter >6 mm, and *e*volution.*

Surgical management is recommended for treatment of the primary melanoma and consists of excision with tumor-free margins of 1 to 3 cm. Increase in thickness of a melanoma (Table 26.1), microscopic ulceration, and mitotic rate are all inversely correlated with survival. In cases with melanoma thickness (Breslow depth) greater than 0.75 mm or high mitotic activity, sentinel lymph node biopsy can also assist with staging and serve as a prognostic tool. Treatment options for metastatic melanoma include adjuvant high-dose interferon alfa-2b, targeted therapies such as BRAF inhibitors, and other immunomodulating therapies.

Cutaneous T-Cell Lymphoma

Cutaneous T-cell lymphoma is a non-Hodgkin lymphoma characterized by expansion of malignant T cells within the skin. The most common clinical presentations are mycosis fungoides and Sézary syndrome. Mycosis fungoides generally presents with discrete or coalescing patches, plaques, or nodules on the skin (Figure 26.4). Mycosis fungoides may progress to involve lymph nodes and viscera. Once extracutaneous involvement is recognized, the median duration of survival is about 2.5 years. The course of patients

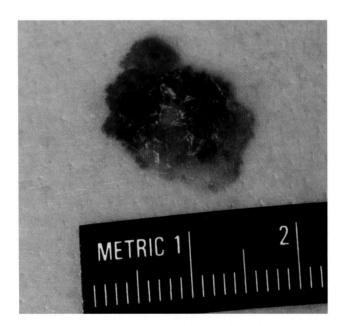

Figure 26.3 Malignant Melanoma.

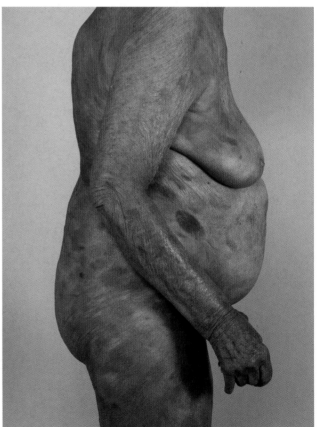

Figure 26.4 Mycosis Fungoides.

with patch- or plaque-stage cutaneous lesions, without extracutaneous disease, is less predictable, but the median duration of survival is approximately 12 years. Sézary syndrome, the more aggressive leukemic form of cutaneous T-cell lymphoma, is characterized by generalized erythroderma, keratoderma of the palms and soles, and a Sézary cell count of more than 1,000/mm³ in the peripheral blood. Most patients have severe pruritus.

Treatment of cutaneous T-cell lymphoma includes topical corticosteroids, topical nitrogen mustard, psoralen and UVA (PUVA), radiotherapy (electron beam, orthovoltage), and systemic chemotherapy. Extracorporeal photopheresis, interferons, retinoids, and monoclonal antibodies have also been used.

Psoriasis

Psoriasis is a chronic, inflammatory, multisystem disease that occurs in 2% of the US population. About a third of patients have a family history of psoriasis. Psoriasis commonly presents with discrete red plaques covered with a silvery scale. Patterns of psoriasis include psoriasis vulgaris, which presents with plaques involving the elbows, knees, and scalp (Figure 26.5). Guttate psoriasis is an acute form that often follows streptococcal pharyngitis and presents with small, scaly papules of psoriasis on the trunk and limbs. Other, less common, forms of psoriasis include pustular psoriasis, which may be localized to the hands and feet or may be generalized. Approximately 50% of patients with psoriasis have nail abnormalities, most commonly onycholysis, pitting, and oil spots. Lesions of psoriasis may occur at previous sites of trauma (koebnerization). Medications such as lithium, β-adrenergic blockers, and antimalarials and discontinuation of the use of systemic corticosteroids can precipitate or exacerbate psoriasis.

Psoriatic arthritis occurs in 5% to 8% of patients with skin psoriasis. An asymmetric oligoarthritis occurs in 70% of patients with psoriatic arthritis. This group includes patients with "sausage digits" and monarthritis. The second most common presentation is asymmetric arthritis clinically similar to rheumatoid arthritis, which occurs in 15% of patients

with psoriatic arthritis. Distal interphalangeal involvement, arthritis mutilans, and a spinal form of arthritis similar to ankylosing spondylitis each occurs in 5% of patients with psoriatic arthritis. Moderate to severe psoriasis has also been associated with obesity and cardiovascular disease.

The treatment of psoriasis includes topical corticosteroids, topical tar preparations, phototherapy, calcipotriene (a topical synthetic vitamin D analogue), and tazarotene (a topical retinoid). Systemic agents used in the treatment of resistant psoriasis include methotrexate, anti–tumor necrosis factor agents (infliximab, etanercept, and adalimumab), ustekinumab (directed against IL-12 and IL-23), acitretin, and cyclosporine. Systemic therapy should be considered if psoriasis involves a high percentage of cutaneous surface area or psoriatic arthritis is present, or both.

Atopic Dermatitis

Atopy is manifested by atopic dermatitis, asthma, and allergic rhinitis or conjunctivitis. Atopic dermatitis most often presents in infancy and childhood, but flares of dermatitis (or eczema) can occur at any age. Atopic dermatitis classically presents with erythema, lichenification, and crusting of the flexural areas (Figure 26.6).

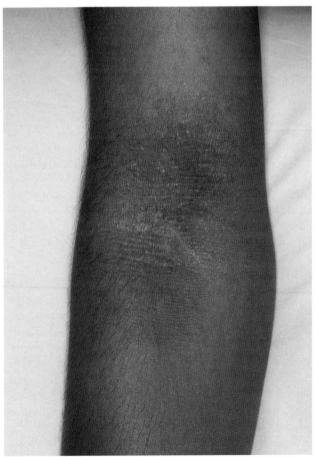

Figure 26.6 Atopic Dermatitis.

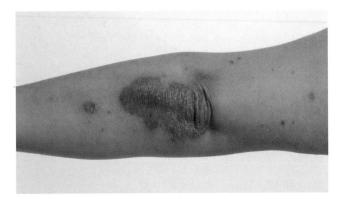

Figure 26.5 Psoriasis.

Disturbances in cell-mediated immunity lead to an increased incidence of bacterial and viral infections. Secondary colonization with *Staphylococcus aureus* presents as a weeping, crusting dermatitis (impetiginization). Eczema herpeticum is a secondary infection with the herpes simplex virus, which may be generalized.

Emollients and topical corticosteroids have been the mainstays of treatment in atopic dermatitis.

Allergic Contact Dermatitis

Allergic contact dermatitis is a form of localized or generalized dermatitis that results from exposure to an antigen. This is a type IV hypersensitivity reaction (delayed, cell-mediated). One must consider the anatomical location of the cutaneous lesions and environmental exposure to allergens, including occupational, household, and recreational contactants, to define the cause of the contact dermatitis. Workers in certain occupations (eg, health care workers, hair stylists) with persistent exposure to antigens over time are at greater risk for contact dermatitis.

Testing to identify specific contact allergens is performed with patch testing. Patch testing is performed by applying substances to a patient's back; each substance is placed under a small aluminum disk covered with adhesive tape. These are left on the patient's back for 48 hours, and the results are interpreted at 48 and 96 hours (since it is a delayed hypersensitivity reaction). Positive reactions occur often to the following antigens: nickel sulfate, neomycin sulfate, benzocaine, fragrances, thimerosal, paraphenylenediamine, and formaldehyde.

Nickel sulfate allergies are often associated with inexpensive jewelry, clothing snaps, and belt buckles (Figure 26.7). Neomycin sulfate and benzocaine are components of many topical antimicrobial and analgesic preparations. Thimerosal is a commonly used preservative in contact lens solutions. Paraphenylenediamine is present in hair dyes and other cosmetics; para-aminobenzoic acid in sunscreens is immunologically related to paraphenylenediamine. Formaldehyde is a common preservative in cosmetics and shampoos.

Acne Vulgaris

Acne occurs physiologically at puberty with varying degrees of severity but may persist into the second and third decades of life. The pathogenesis of acne is multifactorial; heredity, increase in sebaceous gland activity, hormonal influences, disturbances of keratinization, and bacterial infection have all been implicated. The primary lesions of acne are noninflammatory and include microcomedones, closed comedones (whiteheads), and open comedones (blackheads). The secondary or inflammatory lesions include papules and pustules, nodules, and cysts. Treatment options for acne are given in Table 26.2.

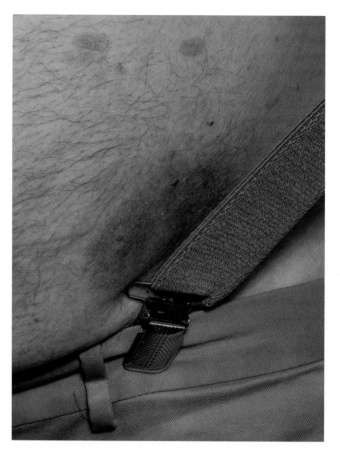

Figure 26.7 Allergic Contact Dermatitis.

Isotretinoin (13-*cis*-retinoic acid) is a synthetic vitamin A derivative used primarily for the treatment of severe nodulocystic acne vulgaris. The greatest risk associated with use of systemic retinoids is teratogenicity. Before isotretinoin is prescribed, female patients must be counseled on this adverse effect and use reliable contraception during therapy and for at least 1 month after use of the drug is discontinued. The systemic retinoids are associated with various cutaneous adverse effects, including xerosis (dry skin), dermatitis, and cheilitis. Potential laboratory abnormalities include hyperlipidemia, increased liver enzyme levels, and leukopenia. Skeletal hyperostosis may occur, particularly in association with long-term use. Concerns regarding depression, suicidal ideation, and inflammatory bowel disease are being studied.

Table 26.2 • Treatment of Acne Vulgaris

Type of Acne	Treatment
Comedonal	Topical tretinoin, benzoyl peroxide
Papular or pustular	Same as above, plus topical or systemic antibiotics
Cystic	Systemic antibiotics; if severe, isotretinoin

Autoimmune Bullous Diseases

Autoimmune bullous diseases are a diverse collection of conditions in which autoantibodies target various components of the skin, leading to varying clinical presentations. The diagnosis of autoimmune bullous disease can be aided by skin biopsy for direct immunofluorescence (which shows different patterns of antibody deposition in the skin) and serologic testing for autoantibodies.

Bullous pemphigoid (Figure 26.8) is the most common autoimmune blistering disease. The disease predominantly occurs in elderly patients and usually presents with large, tense bullae on an erythematous base with a predilection for flexural areas. Targeted antigens in bullous pemphigoid include basement membrane proteins, bullous pemphigoid antigen 1 (BP230), and bullous pemphigoid antigen 2 (BP180). Direct immunofluorescence testing shows a linear pattern at the basement membrane. Treatment of bullous pemphigoid includes topical and systemic corticosteroids, tetracyclines, and mycophenolate mofetil.

There are several other forms of pemphigoid. Cicatricial pemphigoid (or mucous membrane pemphigoid) is characterized by mucosal lesions, with limited or no cutaneous lesions. The disease predominantly affects oral and ocular mucous membranes. Often cyclophosphamide is used, particularly in patients with ocular involvement, because this condition can lead to blindness. Pemphigoid gestationis consists of intensely pruritic urticarial papules, plaques, or blisters, usually occurring in the latter half of pregnancy. The serum of approximately half of patients with herpes gestationis contains the HG factor, which is a complement-fixing IgG anti–basement membrane zone antibody.

Pemphigus vulgaris is typically characterized by oral lesions and more flaccid cutaneous bullae, since the autoantibodies affect more superficial components in the skin (intercellular proteins called desmogleins) (Figure 26.9). Direct immunofluorescence testing shows intercellular staining in the epidermis. Infliximab and high-dose corticosteroids generally are required to control pemphigus, but other, steroid-sparing immunosuppressive agents have been used.

Another variant of pemphigus is pemphigus foliaceus; its subsets include pemphigus erythematosus and fogo selvagem, an endemic form of pemphigus that occurs in South America. Pemphigus foliaceus may present with superficial scaling-crusting lesions of the head and neck area (in a seborrheic dermatitis-like pattern) or in a generalized distribution.

Dermatitis herpetiformis (Figure 26.10) is characterized by extremely pruritic, grouped vesicles occurring predominantly over the elbows, knees, buttocks, back of the neck and scalp, and lower part of the back, usually beginning in the third or fourth decade of life. Virtually all patients have some degree of gluten-sensitive enteropathy (celiac sprue), although it may be subclinical. This association is

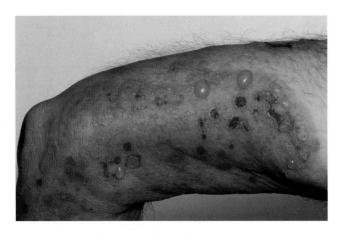

Figure 26.8 *Bullous Pemphigoid.*

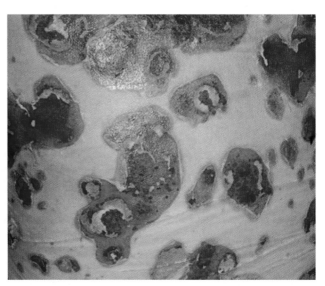

Figure 26.9 *Pemphigus Vulgaris.*

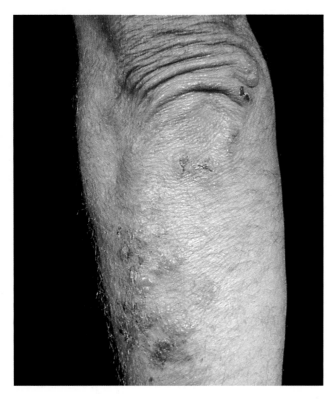

Figure 26.10 *Dermatitis Herpetiformis.*

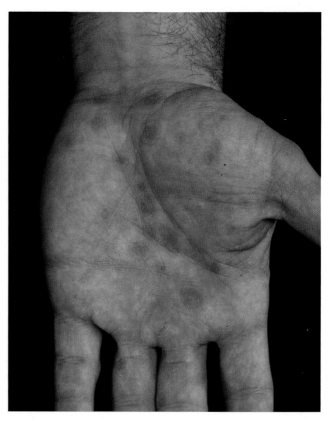

Figure 26.11 *Erythema Multiforme.*

important, since gluten-sensitive enteropathy is associated with an increased risk of small B-cell lymphoma, and only adherence to a gluten-free diet will affect this risk. Testing for tissue transglutaminase or endomysial antibodies is useful for both diagnosis and management of dermatitis herpetiformis, although these antibodies correlate with the degree of gluten-sensitive enteropathy rather than the skin lesions per se. The mainstays of treatment of dermatitis herpetiformis are dapsone and a gluten-free diet. Patients who strictly adhere to a gluten-free diet may have a decreased need for dapsone.

Linear IgA bullous dermatosis is characterized by vesicles or blisters on an erythematous base in a generalized distribution with a high rate of mucosal involvement. Drug-induced disease has occurred with vancomycin.

Erythema Multiforme

Erythema multiforme (Figure 26.11) is an acute, usually self-limited eruption of typically targetoid plaques. It often presents on the palms and lips. A subset of patients with erythema multiforme may have recurrent lesions. When erythema multiforme presents with mucosal as well as cutaneous lesions, it is referred to as Stevens-Johnson syndrome. Various etiologic factors have been implicated in erythema multiforme. The most commonly cited precipitating factor is viral infection, particularly herpes simplex virus. Herpes simplex virus infection is responsible for a considerable percentage of cases of recurrent erythema

multiforme. Other infectious agents that have been noted to cause erythema multiforme include *Mycoplasma pneumoniae* and *Yersinia enterocolitica*. Drugs have been reported to induce erythema multiforme, particularly sulfonamides, barbiturates, and anticonvulsants.

Lichen Planus

Lichen planus typically presents as polygonal, violaceous, flat-topped papules or plaques on the wrists and ankles (Figure 26.12). The lesions are very pruritic. A characteristic feature is fine, reticulated, whitish lines visible on top of the lesions, known as Wickham striae. Various forms of lichen planus can affect the oral mucosa, nails, or scalp. Oral lichen planus has been reported to be associated with hepatitis C.

Erythema Nodosum

Erythema nodosum (Figure 26.13) typically presents as tender, erythematous, subcutaneous nodules localized to the pretibial areas. The nodules may be acute and self-limited or chronic, lasting for months to years. The most common cause is streptococcal pharyngitis. Other infectious agents that have been implicated in the development of erythema nodosum include *Y enterocolitica*, *Coccidioides*, and *Histoplasma*. Drug-induced erythema

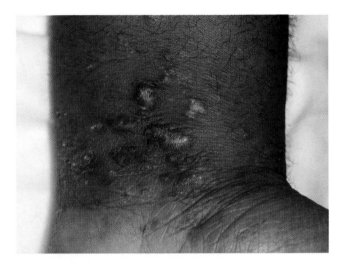

Figure 26.12 Lichen Planus.

nodosum most often is associated with oral contraceptives and sulfonamides. Other associations with erythema nodosum include sarcoidosis, inflammatory bowel disease, and Behçet syndrome.

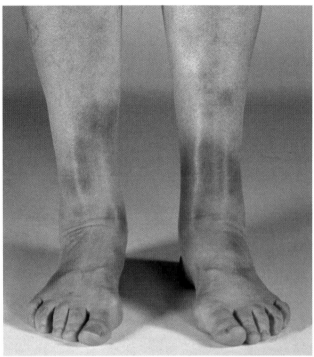

Figure 26.13 Erythema Nodosum.

KEY FACTS

✓ Bullous pemphigoid—most common autoimmune blistering disease, with large, tense bullae on erythematous base favoring flexural areas

✓ Pemphigus vulgaris—autoimmune blistering disease with oral lesions and more flaccid cutaneous bullae

✓ Dermatitis herpetiformis—very pruritic, grouped vesicles over elbows, knees, buttocks, back of neck and scalp, lower back; associated with gluten sensitivity

✓ Erythema multiforme most commonly caused by viral infection, particularly herpes simplex; also caused by other infectious agents, drugs

✓ Erythema nodosum most commonly caused by streptococcal pharyngitis; also caused by other infectious agents, drugs; associated with sarcoidosis, inflammatory bowel disease, Behçet syndrome

Drug Reactions

The morphologic spectrum of reactions that may be induced by medications is broad, and many different medications may produce a given cutaneous reaction. Types of cutaneous lesions induced by drugs include maculopapular eruptions, acne, folliculitis, necrotizing vasculitis, vesiculobullous lesions, erythema multiforme, erythema nodosum, fixed drug eruptions, lichenoid reactions, photosensitivity reactions, pigmentary changes, and hair loss. The most common types of clinical presentations (in descending order of frequency) are exanthematous or

morbilliform eruptions, urticaria or angioedema, fixed drug eruptions, and erythema multiforme. Stevens-Johnson syndrome, toxic epidermal necrolysis (diffuse skin sloughing), exfoliative erythroderma, and photosensitive eruptions are less common. Table 26.3 outlines the types of cutaneous reactions to drugs.

Exanthematous or morbilliform eruptions are the most common type of cutaneous drug reaction. This type of eruption usually begins within a week of onset of therapy, but it may occur more than 2 weeks after initiation of the therapy or up to 2 weeks after use of the drug has been discontinued. Ampicillin, penicillin, and cephalosporins are commonly associated with morbilliform eruptions. A fixed drug eruption is 1 or several lesions that recur at the same anatomical location on rechallenge with the medication. The genital and facial

Table 26.3 • Cutaneous Reactions to Drugs

Type of Skin Reaction	Cause
Urticarial	Aspirin, penicillin, blood products
Photoallergic	Sulfonamides, thiazides, griseofulvin, phenothiazines
Phototoxic	Tetracyclines
Slate-gray discoloration	Chlorpromazine
Slate-blue discoloration	Amiodarone
Yellow or blue-gray pigmentation	Antimalarials

areas are common sites of involvement. Phenolphthalein, barbiturates, salicylates, and oral contraceptives have been implicated in causing fixed drug eruptions. Lichenoid drug eruptions are morphologically similar to lichen planus (with violaceous papules of the skin) and most often have been associated with gold and antimalarial drugs, although various medications may induce this type of reaction.

Cutaneous Signs of Underlying Malignancy

Cutaneous metastasis occurs in 1% to 5% of patients with metastatic neoplasms. The types of neoplasms metastatic to the skin are lung, breast, kidney, gastrointestinal, melanoma, and ovary. Lesions usually present on the scalp, face, or trunk.

Paget disease of the nipple is an erythematous, scaly, or weeping eczematous eruption of the areola. Virtually all patients with Paget disease have an underlying ductal carcinoma of the breast. In contrast, extramammary Paget disease, a morphologically similar eruption that usually occurs in the anogenital region, is associated with underlying carcinoma in only about 50% of cases. Extramammary Paget disease may be associated with underlying cutaneous adnexal carcinoma or with underlying visceral carcinoma (particularly of the genitourinary or distal gastrointestinal tract).

Acanthosis nigricans (Figure 26.14) consists of velvety brown plaques of the intertriginous regions, particularly the axillae and groin. It most commonly occurs with obesity and insulin-resistant diabetes, but a sudden or diffuse presentation in an atypical clinical setting may be associated with adenocarcinoma of the gastrointestinal tract, particularly the stomach.

Pyoderma gangrenosum (Figure 26.15) consists of ulcers with undermined, inflammatory, violaceous borders that heal with cribriform scarring. The lesions are most

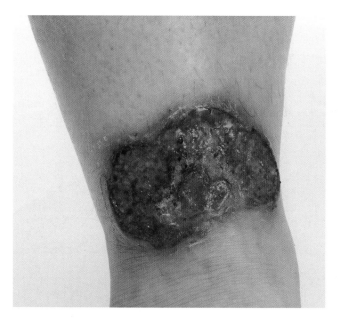

Figure 26.15 Pyoderma Gangrenosum.

commonly associated with inflammatory bowel disease or rheumatoid arthritis. The occurrence of the disease at sites of trauma (pathergy) is classic. Pyoderma gangrenosum may be associated with malignancy of the hematopoietic system, particularly leukemia.

The skin lesions of glucagonoma syndrome (necrolytic migratory erythema) (Figure 26.16) consist of erosions, crusting, and peeling involving the perineum and perioral areas, but they may be generalized. The syndrome also includes stomatitis, glossitis (beefy tongue), anemia, diarrhea, and weight loss. It is associated with an islet cell (α) tumor of the pancreas.

Gardner syndrome is a hereditary (autosomal dominant) form of colon polyposis. Cutaneous clinical features include soft-tissue tumors (dermoids, lipomas, and fibromas) and

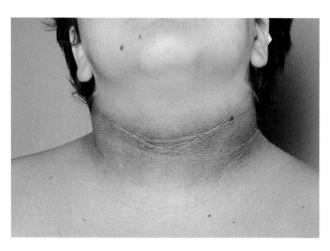

Figure 26.14 Acanthosis Nigricans.

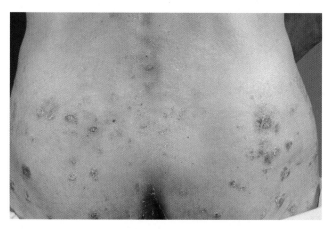

Figure 26.16 Glucagonoma Syndrome (Necrolytic Migratory Erythema).

sebaceous (epidermal inclusion) cysts of the face and scalp. There is a high incidence of colon carcinoma. Malignant tumors of other sites, including adrenal gland, ovary, and thyroid, have been associated with this syndrome.

Hirsutism may reflect androgen excess due to an adrenal or ovarian tumor, but hypertrichosis is an increase in hair unrelated to androgen excess, such as hypertrichosis lanuginosa acquisita (growth of soft downy hair). It has been associated with carcinoid tumor, adenocarcinoma of the breast, lymphoma, gastrointestinal tumors, and other types of neoplasms.

The skin lesions of Sweet syndrome (acute febrile neutrophilic dermatosis) consist of reddish plaques and nodules, most commonly located on the proximal aspects of the extremities and face (Figure 26.17). The syndrome is associated with leukemia, particularly acute myelocytic or acute myelomonocytic leukemia, although many other disease associations also have been noted.

Generalized pruritus is the presentation for many cutaneous and systemic disorders. Pruritus may be the presenting symptom in lymphoma.

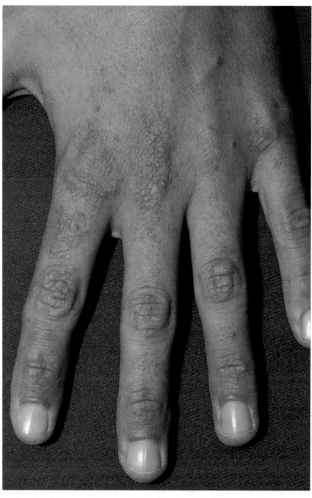

Figure 26.18 Dermatomyositis: Gottron Papules.

In dermatomyositis, the pathognomonic skin lesions are Gottron papules (Figure 26.18) involving the skin over the joints of the fingers, elbows, and knees. Poikilodermatous lesions or erythematous maculopapular eruptions may diffusely involve the face, particularly the periorbital area (heliotrope rash [Figure 26.19]), trunk, and extremities. The cutaneous lesions are photosensitive and pruritic. Dermatomyositis is characterized by proximal myositis. The disease is associated with an increased incidence of underlying malignancy, especially ovarian cancer.

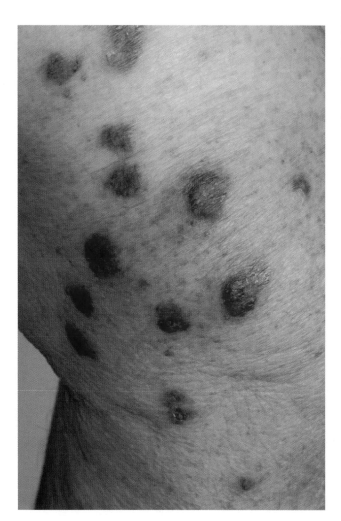

Figure 26.17 Sweet Syndrome.

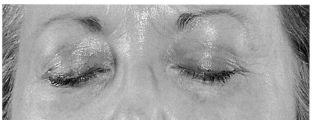

Figure 26.19 Dermatomyositis: Heliotrope Discoloration.

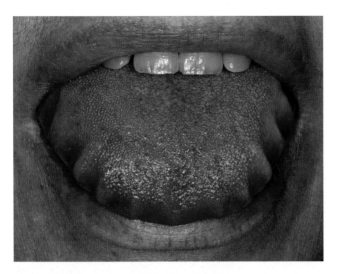

Figure 26.20 Amyloidosis: Macroglossia.

Amyloidosis may present clinically as macroglossia (Figure 26.20), waxy papules on the eyelids or nasolabial folds, pinch purpura, and postproctoscopic purpura (Figure 26.21). Amyloidosis may be associated with multiple myeloma.

Tylosis is a rare disorder characterized by palmar-plantar keratoderma associated with esophageal carcinoma. It has autosomal dominant inheritance.

KEY FACTS

✓ Exanthematous or morbilliform eruptions—most common type of cutaneous drug reaction

✓ Metastatic neoplasms (lung, breast, kidney, gastrointestinal, melanoma, and ovary) spread to skin in 1%–5% of patients

✓ Acanthosis nigricans most common with obesity and insulin-resistant diabetes; may be associated with gastrointestinal adenocarcinoma

✓ Pyoderma gangrenosum most common with inflammatory bowel disease and rheumatoid arthritis; may be associated with leukemia

✓ Dermatomyositis associated with increased incidence of underlying cancer, especially ovarian

---

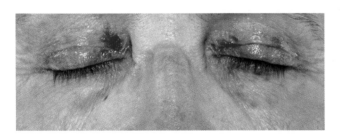

Figure 26.21 Amyloidosis: Postproctoscopic Purpura.

Dermatology: An Internist's Perspective

Pulmonary

The skin is involved in 15% to 35% of patients with sarcoidosis. Lesions may present as 1) lupus pernio (red swelling of the nose), 2) translucent papules around the eyes and nasolabial folds, 3) annular lesions with central atrophy, 4) nodules on the trunk and extremities, and 5) scar sarcoid (Figure 26.22). Acute sarcoidosis may present with a combination of erythema nodosum, bilateral hilar lymphadenopathy, fever, and arthralgias (Löfgren syndrome). Erythema nodosum is discussed in more detail earlier in this chapter.

In antineutrophil cytoplasmic autoantibody–associated granulomatous vasculitis, cutaneous involvement occurs in more than 50% of patients and is manifested by cutaneous infarction, ulceration, hemorrhagic bullae, purpuric papules, or urticaria. A skin biopsy may show hypersensitivity vasculitis or granulomatous vasculitis.

Churg-Strauss granulomatosis (allergic granulomatosis) is characterized by a combination of adult-onset asthma, peripheral eosinophilia, and pulmonary involvement with recurrent pneumonia or transient infiltrates. Skin lesions have been reported in up to 60% of patients and consist of palpable purpura, cutaneous infarcts, and subcutaneous nodules.

In relapsing polychondritis, there is episodic destructive inflammation of cartilage of the ears, nose, and upper airways. There may be associated arthritis and ocular

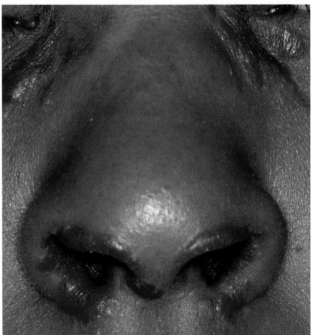

Figure 26.22 Sarcoidosis.

involvement. In the acute stage, the ears may be red, swollen, and tender. Later, they become soft and flabby. Nasal chondritis may lead to saddle-nose deformities. Relapsing polychondritis is mediated by antibodies to type II collagen.

Cardiovascular

Pseudoxanthoma elasticum may be transmitted by autosomal dominant or autosomal recessive inheritance. Yellow xanthoma-like papules ("plucked-chicken skin") occur on the neck, axillae, groin, and abdomen. Angioid streaks may occur in the fundus of the eye. Skin biopsy shows degeneration of elastic fibers. Systemic associations include stroke, myocardial infarction, peripheral vascular disease, and gastrointestinal hemorrhage.

Ehlers-Danlos syndrome includes 10 subgroups that vary in severity and systemic associations. Cutaneous findings are skin hyperextensibility with hypermobile joints and fish-mouth scars. Ehlers-Danlos syndrome is associated with angina, peripheral vascular disease, and gastrointestinal bleeding.

Erythema marginatum is one of the diagnostic criteria for acute rheumatic fever. This uncommon eruption occurs on the trunk and is characterized by erythematous plaques with rapidly mobile serpiginous borders.

Gastrointestinal

Osler-Weber-Rendu syndrome (hereditary hemorrhagic telangiectasia), an autosomal dominant disorder, is manifested by cutaneous and mucosal telangiectasias. Frequent nosebleeds and gastrointestinal bleeds may be a presenting feature. Pulmonary arteriovenous malformations and central nervous system angiomas are also features of this syndrome.

Acrodermatitis enteropathica is an inherited (autosomal recessive) or acquired disease characterized by zinc deficiency (failure of absorption or failure to supplement). The clinical features include angular cheilitis, a seborrheic dermatitis–like eruption, erosions, blisters, and pustules, with skin lesions particularly involving the face, hands, feet, and perineum. Alopecia and diarrhea are other features of this syndrome.

Peutz-Jeghers syndrome is an inherited (autosomal dominant) syndrome of intestinal polyposis. Patients have hamartomas, mostly involving the small bowel, and a slightly increased risk of carcinoma. Cutaneous lesions include macular pigmentation (freckles) of the lips, periungual skin, fingers, and toes and pigmentation of the oral mucosa.

Cutaneous Crohn disease may present as skin nodules with granulomatous histologic findings. Other manifestations include pyostomatitis vegetans (granulomatous inflammation of the gingivae), granulomatous cheilitis, oral aphthous ulceration, perianal skin tags, perianal fistulas, and peristomal pyoderma gangrenosum.

Dermatitis herpetiformis, pyoderma gangrenosum, Gardner syndrome, and glucagonoma syndrome are described earlier in this chapter.

Nephrologic

Partial lipodystrophy is associated with C3 deficiency and the nephrotic syndrome. Uremic pruritus is associated with end-stage renal disease and responds to UVB therapy.

Neurocutaneous

Fabry disease is an X-linked recessive disorder due to deficiency of the enzyme α-galactosidase A. The skin changes consist of numerous small vascular tumors (angiokeratomas) in a "bathing-suit" distribution that develop during childhood and adolescence. Corneal opacities are present in 90% of patients. Systemic manifestations include paresthesias and pain due to involved peripheral nerves, renal insufficiency, and vascular insufficiency of the coronary and central nervous system.

The clinical features of ataxia-telangiectasia include cutaneous and ocular telangiectasia, cerebellar ataxia, choreoathetosis, IgA deficiency, and recurrent pulmonary infections.

Tuberous sclerosis may be inherited in an autosomal dominant pattern (25%) or may occur sporadically (new mutation). Predominant cutaneous lesions include hypopigmented macules, adenoma sebaceum, subungual or periungual fibromas, and shagreen patch (connective tissue nevus) (Figure 26.23). This syndrome is associated with epilepsy (80%) and mental retardation (60%). Rhabdomyomas may occur in the heart in childhood. Angiomyolipomas occur in the kidneys in up to 80% of adults with this syndrome.

Neurofibromatosis (von Recklinghausen disease) (Figure 26.24) presents with the following skin findings: café au lait spots, axillary freckling (Crowe sign), neurofibromas, and Lisch nodules of the iris. Inheritance is autosomal dominant, and approximately 50% of cases are new mutations. The associated central nervous system tumors include acoustic neuromas, optic gliomas, and meningiomas. Other associated tumors include pheochromocytoma, neuroblastoma, and Wilms tumor. Café au lait spots and neurofibromas frequently occur in the absence of neurofibromatosis. The diagnostic criteria for neurofibromatosis are given in Box 26.1.

Sturge-Weber-Dimitri syndrome is characterized by capillary angioma (port-wine stain) in the distribution of the upper or middle branch of the trigeminal nerve. Associated meningeal angioma may be present in the same distribution. Intracranial tramline calcification, mental retardation, epilepsy, contralateral hemiparesis, and visual impairment may be associated.

KEY FACTS

✓ Up to 60% of patients with Churg-Strauss granulomatosis may have skin lesions (palpable purpura, cutaneous infarcts, subcutaneous nodules)

✓ Relapsing polychondritis—episodic inflammation destroying cartilage of ears, nose, upper airways

✓ Osler-Weber-Rendu syndrome—autosomal dominant disorder manifested by cutaneous and mucosal telangiectasias

✓ Skin changes of Fabry disease (X-linked recessive disorder due to α-galactosidase A deficiency)—numerous small vascular tumors in "bathing-suit" distribution

✓ Neurofibromatosis skin findings—café au lait spots, axillary freckling, neurofibromas, and Lisch nodules of iris

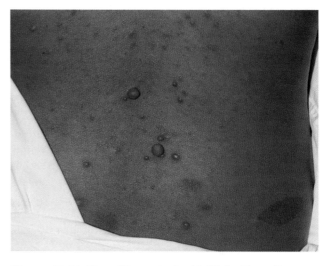

Figure 26.24 *Neurofibromatosis: Multiple Neurofibromas and Café au lait Macule.*

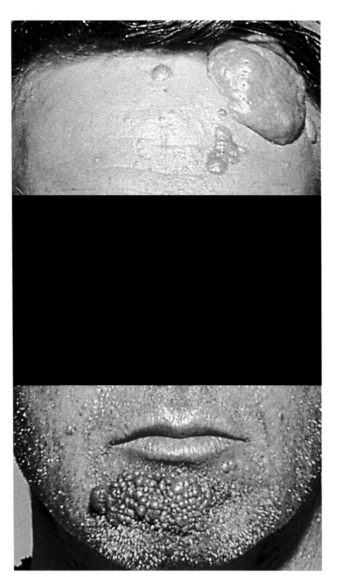

Figure 26.23 *Tuberous Sclerosis: Adenoma Sebaceum and Forehead Plaque.*

Rheumatologic

The skin manifestations of lupus erythematosus (LE) can be classified into acute cutaneous LE (malar rash, generalized photosensitive dermatitis, or bullous LE), subacute cutaneous LE (annular or papulosquamous variants), and chronic cutaneous LE (localized discoid LE, generalized discoid LE, lupus panniculitis, tumid lupus, or chilblain lupus).

Skin lesions are present in up to 85% of patients with acute systemic LE. A butterfly rash with erythema involving the nose and cheeks is characteristic. Erythematous papules and plaques also may occur on the dorsal aspect of the hands, with sparing of the skin overlying the interphalangeal and metacarpal phalangeal joints. Maculopapular erythema also may occur on sun-exposed areas.

Box 26.1 • Criteria for Diagnosis of Neurofibromatosis[a]

1. Six or more café au lait macules >0.5 cm in greatest diameter in prepubertal patients, or >1.5 cm in diameter in adults

2. Two or more neurofibromas of any type, or 1 plexiform neurofibroma

3. Freckling of skin in axillary or inguinal regions

4. Optic gliomas

5. Lisch nodules

6. Osseous lesion such as sphenoid dysplasia or thinning of long bone cortex with or without pseudarthrosis

7. First-degree relative with neurofibromatosis that meets the above diagnostic criteria

[a] Two or more criteria must be present for diagnosis.

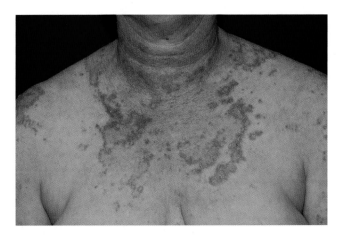

Figure 26.25 *Subacute Cutaneous Lupus Erythematosus.*

Subacute cutaneous LE (Figure 26.25) usually presents with generalized annular plaques often prominent on the upper part of the chest, back, and arms. Subacute cutaneous LE is characterized by the presence of anti-Ro (anti-SSA) antibodies in serum and photosensitivity. In the majority of cases, subacute cutaneous LE is not associated with systemic LE. Treatment is with photoprotection, topical corticosteroids, and hydroxychloroquine.

Discoid LE (Figure 26.26) is characterized by erythematous plaques with follicular hyperkeratosis and scale. It commonly affects the face, scalp, and ears and causes scarring. Although most patients with discoid LE lack manifestations of systemic LE, approximately 25% of patients with systemic LE have had cutaneous lesions of discoid LE at some point during the course of their illness. Circulating antinuclear antibodies are demonstrable in most patients with systemic LE and subacute cutaneous LE, but they are present in only a small percentage of patients with discoid LE.

The term *scleroderma* encompasses a wide spectrum of diseases ranging from generalized multisystem disease to localized cutaneous disease. The systemic end of the spectrum is represented by diffuse scleroderma and the CREST (*c*alcinosis cutis, *R*aynaud phenomenon, *e*sophageal involvement, *s*clerodactyly, and *t*elangiectasia) syndrome. The middle area of the spectrum is represented by eosinophilic fasciitis and linear scleroderma, which may have systemic involvement. Localized scleroderma (also known as morphea) may be a single plaque or may be multiple plaques in a generalized distribution.

Systemic scleroderma consists of diffuse sclerosis associated with smoothness and hardening of the skin, with masklike face and microstomia. Sclerodactyly, periungual telangiectasia, telangiectatic mats, hyperpigmentation, and cutaneous calcification may be observed. Esophageal, pulmonary, renal, and cardiac involvement may be associated with systemic scleroderma. The CREST syndrome (Figure 26.27) is associated with circulating anticentromere antibodies.

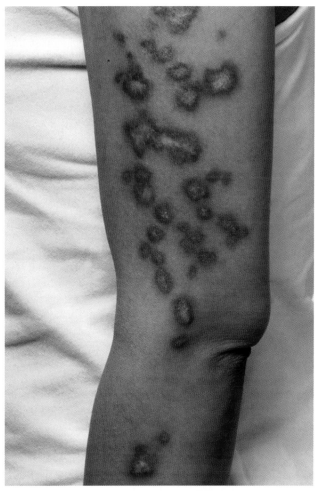

Figure 26.26 *Discoid Lupus Erythematosus.*

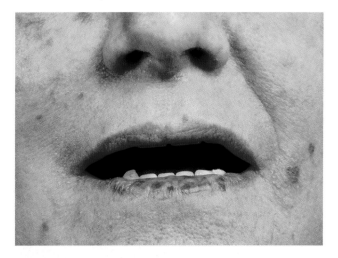

Figure 26.27 *Scleroderma: CREST (Calcinosis Cutis, Raynaud Phenomenon, Esophageal Involvement, Sclerodactyly, and Telangiectasia) Syndrome.*

Eosinophilic fasciitis manifests as tightly bound thickening of the skin and underlying soft tissues of the extremities. Other features include arthralgias, hypergammaglobulinemia, and peripheral blood eosinophilia.

Morphea manifests as discrete sclerotic plaques with a white, shiny center and erythematous or violaceous periphery (Figure 26.28). Localized or linear scleroderma may have various presentations depending on extent, location, and depth of sclerosis. Most lesions are characterized by sclerosis and atrophy associated with depression or "delling" of the soft tissue; underlying bone may be affected in linear scleroderma.

In rheumatoid arthritis, rheumatoid nodules may occur over the extensor surfaces of joints, most commonly on the dorsal aspects of the hands and elbows. Rheumatoid vasculitis with ulceration may occur in the setting of rheumatoid arthritis with a high circulating rheumatoid factor level.

Reactive arthritis consists of the triad of urethritis, conjunctivitis, and arthritis. The disease usually affects young men. Two-thirds of patients have skin lesions, namely, circinate balanitis (erythematous plaques of the penis) and keratoderma blennorrhagicum (pustular psoriasiform eruption of the palms and soles). Most patients test positive for HLA-B27.

Erythema migrans is an annular, sometimes urticarial, erythematous plaque presenting as a manifestation of Lyme disease. The plaque develops subsequent to a tick bite. The deer tick *Ixodes scapularis* contains the spirochete *Borrelia burgdorferi*, which is responsible for the syndrome. Only 25% of patients recall a tick bite. Other acute features of Lyme disease include fever, headaches, myalgias, arthralgias, and lymphadenopathy. Arthritis is a late complication of Lyme

Key Definition

Erythema migrans: *annular, sometimes urticarial, erythematous plaque presenting as a manifestation of Lyme disease.*

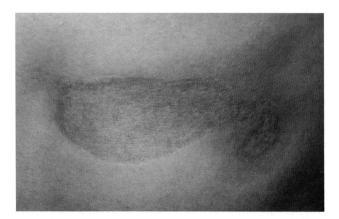

Figure 26.28 Morphea.

disease. Weeks or months after the initial illness, meningoencephalitis, peripheral neuropathy, myocarditis, atrioventricular node block, or destructive erosive arthritis may develop.

During the late stages of gout, tophi (urate deposits with surrounding inflammation) occur in the subcutaneous tissues. Improved methods of treatment account for the decrease in the incidence of tophaceous gout in recent years.

Dermatomyositis and psoriatic arthritis are reviewed earlier in this chapter.

Hematologic

Graft-versus-host disease (GVHD) most commonly occurs after bone marrow transplant and represents the constellation of skin lesions, diarrhea, and liver enzyme abnormalities. Acute GVHD begins 7 to 21 days after transplant, and the cutaneous abnormalities of acute GVHD include pruritus; numbness or pain of the palms and soles; an erythematous maculopapular eruption of the trunk, palms, and soles; and blisters that, when extensive, resemble toxic epidermal necrolysis. Chronic GVHD begins within months to 1 year after transplant and mainly affects skin and liver. Early chronic GVHD is characterized by a lichenoid reaction consisting of cutaneous and oral lesions that resemble lichen planus, with coalescing violaceous papules on the skin and white reticulated patches on the buccal mucosa. Late chronic GVHD is characterized by cutaneous sclerosis and scarring alopecia.

Mastocytosis (mast cell disease) can be divided into 4 groups, depending on the age at onset and the presence or absence of systemic involvement: 1) urticaria pigmentosa arising in infancy or adolescence without substantial systemic involvement, 2) urticaria pigmentosa in adults without substantial systemic involvement, 3) systemic mast cell disease, and 4) mast cell leukemia. The cutaneous lesions may be brown-to-red macules, papules, nodules, or plaques that urticate on stroking. Less commonly, the lesions may be bullous, erythrodermic, or telangiectatic. The systemic manifestations are due to histamine release and consist of flushing, tachycardia, and diarrhea.

Necrobiotic xanthogranuloma—indurated plaques with associated atrophy and telangiectasia with or without ulceration—may occur on the trunk or periorbital areas. Serum electrophoresis shows an IgG κ paraproteinemia or multiple myeloma.

Endocrinologic

Diabetes Mellitus

Several dermatologic disorders have been described in diabetes.

Necrobiosis lipoidica diabeticorum (Figure 26.29) classically occurs on the shins and presents as yellow-brown atrophic telangiectatic plaques that occasionally ulcerate. Two-thirds of patients with this skin disorder have diabetes mellitus.

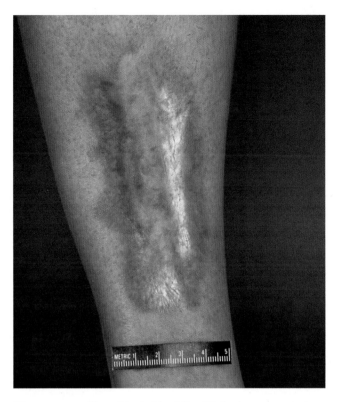

Figure 26.29 *Necrobiosis Lipoidica Diabeticorum.*

Granuloma annulare (Figure 26.30) is an asymptomatic eruption consisting of small, firm, flesh-colored or red papules in an annular configuration (less commonly nodular or generalized). The association with diabetes is disputed.

Rarely, patients with poorly controlled diabetes present with spontaneously occurring subepidermal blisters (bullosa diabeticorum) on the dorsal aspects of the hands and feet.

The stiff-hand syndrome has been reported in juvenile-onset type 1 diabetes mellitus. Patients have limited joint mobility and tight, waxy skin on the hands. There is an

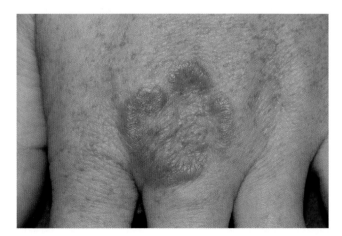

Figure 26.30 *Granuloma Annulare.*

increased risk of subsequent renal and retinal microvascular disease.

In scleredema, there is an insidious onset of thickening and stiffness of the skin on the upper part of the back and posterior aspect of the neck. The diabetes is often longstanding and poorly controlled.

Thyroid

Pretibial myxedema and thyroid acropachy (digital clubbing and swelling) are cutaneous associations of Graves disease.

KEY FACTS

✓ CREST syndrome—*c*alcinosis cutis, *R*aynaud phenomenon, *e*sophageal involvement, *s*clerodactyly, and *t*elangiectasia; associated with circulating anticentromere antibodies

✓ Reactive arthritis—triad of urethritis, conjunctivitis, and arthritis, usually in young men; two-thirds also have skin lesions

✓ Graft-versus-host disease—constellation of skin lesions, diarrhea, and liver enzyme abnormalities; most common after bone marrow transplant

✓ Mastocytosis can manifest as urticaria pigmentosa without substantial systemic involvement in children or adults

✓ Necrobiosis lipoidica diabeticorum—yellow-brown atrophic telangiectatic plaques on shins; two-thirds of patients have diabetes mellitus

---

Metabolic

The porphyrias are a group of inherited or acquired abnormalities of heme synthesis. Each type is associated with deficient activity of a particular enzyme. The porphyrias are usually divided into 3 types: erythropoietic, hepatic, and mixed.

Erythropoietic porphyria is a hereditary form (autosomal recessive) characterized by marked photosensitivity, blisters, scarring alopecia, hirsutism, red-stained teeth, hemolytic anemia, and splenomegaly. The skin lesions are severely mutilating. Onset is in infancy or early childhood.

Erythropoietic protoporphyria is an autosomal dominant syndrome that usually begins during childhood. It is characterized by variable degrees of photosensitivity and a marked itching, burning, or stinging sensation that occurs within minutes after sun exposure. It is associated with deficiency of ferrochelatase.

Porphyria cutanea tarda (Figure 26.31), one of the hepatic porphyrias, is the most common form of porphyria. It is an acquired or hereditary (autosomal dominant) disease associated with a defect in uroporphyrinogen decarboxylase. The disease may be precipitated by exposure to toxins

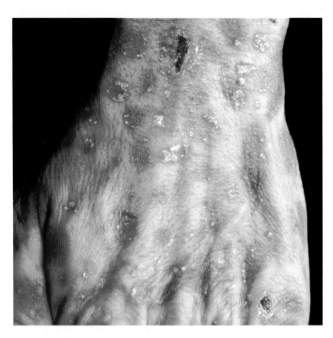

Figure 26.31 *Porphyria Cutanea Tarda.*

(such as chlorinated phenols or hexachlorobenzene), alcohol, estrogens, iron overload, underlying hemochromatosis, and infection with hepatitis C virus. Porphyria cutanea tarda usually presents in the third or fourth decade of life. Clinical manifestations include photosensitivity, skin fragility, erosions and blisters (particularly on dorsal surfaces of the hands), hyperpigmentation, milia, hypertrichosis, and facial suffusion. Sclerodermoid skin changes develop in some patients. The diagnosis is confirmed by the finding of increased porphyrin levels in the urine. Treatment includes phlebotomy or low-dose chloroquine.

Acute intermittent porphyria lacks skin lesions and is characterized by acute attacks of abdominal pain or neurologic symptoms.

Variegate porphyria (mixed porphyria) also follows autosomal dominant inheritance. Variegate porphyria is characterized by cutaneous abnormalities that are similar to those of porphyria cutanea tarda and by acute abdominal episodes, as in acute intermittent porphyria. Variegate porphyria tends to be precipitated by drugs such as barbiturates and sulfonamides.

Nail Clues to Systemic Disease

Onycholysis consists of distal and lateral separation of the nail plate from the nail bed. Onycholysis may be due to psoriasis, lichen planus, infection (such as *Candida* or *Pseudomonas*), a reaction to nail cosmetics, or a drug reaction. Drugs that have been noted to induce onycholysis include tetracycline and chlorpromazine. Association with thyroid disease (hyperthyroidism more than hypothyroidism) has also been noted.

Pitting is a common feature of psoriatic nails. Graph-like pits have been associated with alopecia areata.

Terry nails consist of whitening of the proximal or entire nail as a result of changes in the nail bed. This abnormality is associated with cirrhosis.

Muehrcke lines are white parallel bands associated with hypoalbuminemia.

Half-and-half nails (Lindsay nails) are nails in which the proximal half is white and the distal half is red. This abnormality may be associated with renal failure.

Yellow nails are associated with chronic edema, pulmonary disease, pleural effusion, chronic bronchitis, bronchiectasis, and lung carcinoma.

Beau lines are transverse grooves in the nail associated with high fever, chemotherapy, systemic disease, and drugs.

Koilonychia (spoon nails) is associated with iron deficiency anemia, but it also may be idiopathic, familial, or related to trauma.

Blue lunulae are associated with hepatolenticular degeneration (Wilson disease) and argyria.

Mees lines are white bands associated with arsenic exposure.

Cutaneous Manifestations of Human Immunodeficiency Virus Infection

Primary infection with human immunodeficiency virus (HIV) results in a flulike illness and an exanthem in 30% to 60% of patients. The exanthem may be morbilliform, vesicular, or pityriasis rosea–like. Oral ulceration and erosions, genital erosions, and erosive esophagitis also may occur at this stage. The acute exanthem and enanthem are self-limited and often go undiagnosed.

In the early stage of the disease, cutaneous manifestations include genital warts, genital herpes, psoriasis, seborrheic dermatitis, xerosis, and pruritic papular eruption. With symptomatic HIV infection (CD4 count of 200–400/mcL), both infections and inflammatory dermatoses occur more frequently. These include psoriasis, seborrheic dermatitis, oral hairy leukoplakia, candidiasis, herpes zoster, drug reactions, herpes simplex, tinea pedis, and onychomycosis.

As the CD4 count decreases to less than 200/mcL, patients may present with a disseminated fungal infection, recurrent or severe herpes zoster, persistent herpes simplex, bacillary angiomatosis, and molluscum contagiosum. Bacillary angiomatosis consists of 1 or more vascular papules or nodules caused by the gram-negative bacteria *Bartonella quintana* and *Bartonella henselae*. Eosinophilic folliculitis, a pruritic eruption primarily involving the head, neck, trunk, and proximal extremities, is characteristic of symptomatic HIV infection. Molluscum contagiosum, a common viral infection of otherwise healthy children, occurs in 10% to 20% of patients with HIV infection.

With advanced HIV infection (CD4 counts <50/mcL), overwhelming infection is characteristic. Infectious agents with skin manifestations include cytomegalovirus, *Cryptococcus, Acanthamoeba*, and extensive molluscum contagiosum. Oral hairy leukoplakia is caused by Epstein-Barr virus infection of the oral mucosa and usually occurs in patients with advanced HIV infection.

Epidemic Kaposi sarcoma usually presents as oval papules or plaques oriented along skin lines of the trunk, extremities, face, and mucosa. This presentation is in contrast to that of classic Kaposi sarcoma in elderly patients, which occurs predominantly on the distal lower extremities. Human herpesvirus 8 has been identified in tissue from patients with both epidemic and classic Kaposi sarcoma.

KEY FACTS

- ✓ Porphyria cutanea tarda—most common form of porphyria
- ✓ Pitting—nail feature often seen in patients with psoriasis
- ✓ Terry nails—whitening of proximal or entire nail due to changes in nail bed; associated with cirrhosis
- ✓ Primary HIV infection causes flulike illness and an exanthem in 30%–60% of patients
- ✓ Epidemic Kaposi sarcoma—oval papules or plaques along skin lines of trunk, extremities, face, and mucosa

27 Genetics

C. SCOTT COLLINS, MD AND CHRISTOPHER M. WITTICH, MD, PharmD

Chromosome Abnormalities

Chromosome abnormalities (Table 27.1) occur in 1 in 180 live births. One-third of these abnormalities are due to autosomal aneuploidy—an abnormal number of chromosomes. Risk factors for autosomal aneuploidy are maternal age 35 years or older and having had an affected child. The most common autosomal aneuploidy syndrome in term infants is Down syndrome.

Key Definition

Autosomal aneuploidy: *an abnormal number of chromosomes.*

Single Gene Defects

Single gene defects can be due to autosomal dominant, autosomal recessive, and X-linked recessive modes of inheritance. In autosomal dominant inheritance, 1 copy of the gene is sufficient for the trait to be expressed or for the disease to be present (ie, heterozygotes have the disease). There is a 50% chance that any child born to an affected person will inherit the abnormal gene. Penetrance varies in affected persons. In autosomal recessive inheritance, 1 copy of the abnormal gene is not sufficient to cause disease, and heterozygotes (carriers) are not clinically different from the general population. When 2 persons who are heterozygotes for a given gene defect mate, the children are at 25% risk of inheriting the abnormal gene from both parents and, thus, of having the disease.

X-linked recessive diseases are caused by defects located on the X chromosome. Female heterozygotes that have 1 abnormal gene on 1 X chromosome and 1 normal gene on the other X chromosome usually are clinically normal. Males who inherit the abnormal gene have no corresponding genetic loci on the Y chromosome and therefore are referred to as hemizygotes and are clinically affected. Any male child born to a heterozygous female is at 50% risk for having the disease; female children are at 50% risk for inheriting the gene and being carriers.

Table 27.1 • Genetic Disorders Caused by Chromosome Abnormalities

Disease/Genetic Abnormality	Features
Down syndrome/ Trisomy 21	Risk when maternal age ≥35 y Congenital heart defects (VSD and AV canal defects) Early-onset Alzheimer dementia Mild to moderate mental retardation Median survival, 60 y Increased risk of acute lymphocytic leukemia
Klinefelter syndrome/ 47,XXY	Tall, eunuchoid habitus Small testes Infertility Increased risk of germ cell tumors
Turner syndrome/ 45,X	Mentally normal Short stature, webbed neck Lack of secondary sex characteristics 30% risk of bicuspid aortic valve or aortic coarctation Increased risk of ascending aortic aneurysm May have Y chromosome material (eg, 45,X/46,XY mosaicism) and increased risk of gonadal cancer
Fragile X-linked syndrome/ Trinucleotide repeat (CGG) expansions on the X chromosome	May be physically normal or have a long, thin face, prominent jaw, large ears, and enlarged testes Mild to profound mental retardation

Abbreviations: AV, atrioventricular; VSD, ventricular septal defect.

Autosomal Dominant Defects

Table 27.2 lists important autosomal dominant conditions. *BRCA* mutations, hereditary spherocytosis, Huntington disease, low-density lipoprotein receptor deficiency (familial hypercholesterolemia), Lynch syndrome, multiple endocrine neoplasias types I, IIA, and IIB, polycystic kidney disease, and von Willebrand disease are other clinically important autosomal dominant conditions that are discussed in other chapters.

Key Definition

Osler-Weber-Rendu disease: *hereditary hemorrhagic telangiectasia.*

Table 27.2 • Selected Autosomal Dominant Genetic Disorders

Disease/Genetic Abnormality	Features
Ehlers-Danlos syndrome/Defect in gene coding for collagen. The defect varies by the syndrome subtype	Velvety textured, hyperextensible, and fragile skin Joints are hyperextensible and prone to dislocation Mitral valve prolapse occurs in many patients Most severe form results in tendency for arterial aneurysms and visceral organ rupture
Marfan syndrome/Defect in fibrillin-1 gene	Involves musculoskeletal, ocular, and cardiovascular systems Tall stature, scoliosis or kyphosis, and pectus deformities Dislocations of the lens occur in 50%–80% of patients; all patients should have ophthalmologic evaluation Cardiovascular manifestations include mitral valve prolapse and dilatation of the ascending aorta β-Adrenergic blockers might delay progressive aortic dilatation Surgical treatment is often successful for mitral and aortic regurgitation and aortic dissection About 20% of cases arise by new mutation
Myotonic dystrophy/Triplet repeat expansion in myotonin protein kinase gene	Most common form of muscular dystrophy in adults Diagnosis is based on clinical findings and a typical electromyographic pattern characterized by prolonged rhythmic discharges Genetic counseling is warranted for patients and family members Age at onset is usually in the second to third decade of life Myotonia, muscle atrophy and weakness, ptosis of eyelids, expressionless facies, and premature frontal baldness Testicular atrophy or menstrual irregularities, gastrointestinal symptoms Diabetes mellitus occurs in 6% of patients Cardiac disease occurs in two-thirds of patients, and sudden death may occur Sleep-related central and respiratory muscle hypoventilation are very common
Neurofibromatosis 1 and 2/Multiple different mutations have been identified	Neurofibromatosis 1 has markedly variable expression but very high penetrance Malignancy (often peripheral nerve sheath tumors) develops in approximately 10% of patients Characteristics of neurofibromatosis 2 are vestibular schwannomas, nervous system gliomas, and subcapsular cataracts
Osler-Weber-Rendu disease (hereditary hemorrhagic telangiectasia)/Multiple genetic defects have been identified	Characterized by abnormal blood vessel formation in the skin, mucous membranes, lungs, liver, and brain Arteriovenous malformations occur in larger organs Nosebleeds and gastrointestinal bleeding are common
Tuberous sclerosis complex/One gene defect that causes tuberous sclerosis is located on chromosome 9 (hamartin) and another on chromosome 16 (tuberin)	About 50% of cases arise by new mutation Characterized by nodules of the brain and retina, seizures, mental retardation in <50% of cases, depigmented "ash leaf " or "confetti" macules, facial angiofibromas, dental pits, subungual fibromas, and angiomyolipomas
Von Hippel-Lindau disease/The gene involved (*VHL*) is localized to chromosome 3p25–26. The normal gene has a key role in cellular response to hypoxia and acts as a tumor suppressor	Typical case: retinal, spinal cord, and cerebellar hemangioblastomas; cysts of kidneys, pancreas, and epididymis Renal cysts, hemangiomas, and benign adenomas are usually asymptomatic Retinal hemangioblastomas may be the earliest manifestation Periodic magnetic resonance imaging with gadolinium is recommended Renal cancer is a major cause of death

Table 27.3 • Selected Autosomal Recessive Genetic Disorders

Disease/Genetic Abnormality	Features
Friedreich ataxia/The gene involved (*FXN)* is localized to chromosome 9q13. The most frequent mechanism of mutation is expansion of a GAA trinucleotide repeat that results in abnormal accumulation of intramitochondrial iron	First sign of the disease is ataxic gait Mean age at onset is approximately 12 y Dysarthria, hypotonic muscle weakness, loss of vibration and position senses, and loss of deep tendon reflexes develop subsequently The major cause of death is cardiomyopathy
Gaucher disease/ Deficiency of the enzyme glucocerebrosidase results in lipid storage in the spleen, liver, bone marrow, and other organs	Frequent in Ashkenazi Jews May be asymptomatic or present in childhood or adulthood with hepatosplenomegaly, thrombocytopenia, anemia, degenerative bone disease, osteoporosis, or pulmonary disease Enzyme replacement and substrate reduction therapies are effective for nonneuronopathic Gaucher disease

Autosomal Recessive Defects

Table 27.3 lists important autosomal recessive conditions. α_1-Antitrypsin deficiency, cystic fibrosis, hemochromatosis, sickle cell anemia, the thalassemias, and Wilson disease are common autosomal recessive conditions that are discussed in other chapters.

X-Linked Recessive Defects

Table 27.4 lists 1 clinically important X-linked recessive condition. Hemophilia A and B are 2 other important X-linked recessive diseases that are discussed in other chapters.

Table 27.4 • Selected X-Linked Recessive Genetic Disorder

Disease/Genetic Abnormality	Features
Glucose-6-phosphate dehydrogenase (G6PD) deficiency/ Abnormally low G6PD levels	G6PD is important in red blood cell metabolism Most common human enzyme defect Patients may have hemolytic anemia due to infection, fava ingestion, medications including antimalarials (primaquine and chloroquine), sulfa drugs, and isoniazid Heinz bodies on peripheral smear Negative Coombs test

Mitochondrial Mutations

Mitochondrial disorders can arise as new mutations or be maternally inherited. Many mitochondrial enzymes, including most of the respiratory chain complex, are encoded by nuclear DNA and transported into the mitochondria. Mitochondrial DNA mutations cause Leber optic atrophy and the multisystem syndromes of mitochondrial myopathy, encephalopathy, episodes of lactic acidosis, and stroke (MELAS), myoclonic epilepsy with ragged red fibers (MERRF), and neuropathy, ataxia, and retinitis pigmentosa (NARP).

KEY FACTS

- ✓ The most common autosomal aneuploidy syndrome in term infants—Down syndrome
- ✓ Three modes of inheritance of single gene defects— autosomal dominant, autosomal recessive, and X-linked recessive
- ✓ Genetic disorders caused by chromosome abnormalities include Down, Klinefelter, Turner, and fragile X-linked syndromes
- ✓ Peripheral nerve sheath tumors can occur in neurofibromatosis 1; vestibular schwannomas, nervous system gliomas, and subcapsular cataracts characterize neurofibromatosis 2

28 Geriatrics

ERICKA E. TUNG, MD, MPH

Geriatric Assessment

The overarching goal of the geriatric assessment is to develop a holistic understanding of the older patient as a means to identify emerging problems and individual capabilities. This information guides treatment, care coordination, and evaluation of long-term care needs. Assessment of the older adult requires a multifaceted approach encompassing physical, cognitive, and psychosocial domains. The Comprehensive Geriatric Assessment takes this approach a step further and is *targeted* toward the frail older adult and involves an interdisciplinary team of geriatric care providers. Both the general assessment and the comprehensive assessment aim to enhance quality of life and optimize function. Given the time constraints placed on practicing physicians, a strategy of rapid screening of key geriatric domains, followed by a more in-depth assessment of worrisome areas, is an effective approach. The subsequent sections of this chapter describe the key components of the geriatric assessment.

Functional Status

An individual's capacity to perform tasks required of him or her by his or her environment carries important weight in the geriatric assessment. Functional status decline may be the harbinger of a previously undiagnosed medical condition or a manifestation of mismatch between the individual's needs and social support structure. Further, indicators of functional status are strong predictors of mortality, (re)hospitalization, and institutionalization. It is important to remember that an older person's functional state is dynamic; for example, illness or prolonged hospitalization may cause a dramatic decline in functional status.

Most validated functional status tools evaluate 3 tiers of activity: basic activities of daily living, the simplest activities required to remain independent; instrumental activities of daily living, the more complex activities required to maintain a household; and advanced activities of daily living, the activities required to thrive and interact within one's own community. Examples of the tasks in each tier are listed in Table 28.1.

Performance-based testing of mobility and function can be achieved by observing gait, balance, and transfers (Box 28.1). Among the diverse functional performance indicators, gait speed is recognized as a strong predictor of future disability and mortality and has been termed the "sixth vital sign" for older adults. One can measure gait speed by timing the patient as he or she walks a 4-m route (first as quickly as the patient can and then at his or her usual pace). A gait speed of 0.8 m/sec allows for independent community ambulation. Patients with speeds faster than 1.0 m/sec typically have healthier aging and life expectancy beyond the median for their age and sex. Finally, the clinician must integrate knowledge about the older patient's living environment,

Table 28.1 • Functional Status Assessment

Functional Status Tier	Tasks
Basic/self-care	Bathing
	Dressing
	Toileting/maintenance of continence
	Transferring from bed to chair
	Grooming
	Feeding oneself
Instrumental	Managing finances
	Taking medications
	Use of telephone
	Use of transportation
	Housework/laundry
	Meal preparation
	Shopping
Advanced	Participation at faith organization
	Volunteerism

Box 28.1 • Tests to Assess Gait, Balance, and Strength

Timed Up and Go Test
30-Second Chair Stand Test
Functional Reach Test
4-Stage Balance Test
Berg Balance Scale

---

goals of care, and current support structure with the results of the functional status assessment to determine whether additional support services are needed.

Falls

Between 30% and 40% of community-dwelling older adults fall each year; 1 in 10 falls will result in serious injury such as fracture or traumatic brain injury. Additionally, falls may lead to prolonged functional decline. Complications from falls are a leading cause of death from injury in this cohort. The increased frequency of falls among the elderly reflects a complex intersection between predisposing or intrinsic factors and precipitating or extrinsic risk factors. Predisposing factors can be normal age-related changes (eg, reduced depth perception, contrast sensitivity, lower extremity proprioceptive capacity) and disease-related changes (eg, dementia-related impulsivity, peripheral neuropathy due to diabetes mellitus). Precipitating factors include inappropriate choice of gait aid, environmental hazards, and risk-taking behaviors. Prevention of falls requires the clinician to consider an individual's specific risk factors for this common geriatric syndrome. Examples of independent risk factors for falls include a history of previous falls, balance impairment, muscle weakness, psychoactive medication use, and gait instability.

Screening for Falls

A recently updated guideline from the American Geriatrics Society and the British Geriatrics Society (AGS/BGS) suggests that all persons aged 65 years or older should be screened annually for falls. This guideline suggests that individuals who have fallen 2 or more times in the past year, present with fall-related injury, or report/display an unsteady gait should undergo assessment of their risk factors and corresponding risk factor mitigation.

Evaluation of Falls

Patients found to be at high risk for falls on the basis of the AGS/BGS risk stratification method should undergo a multidimensional assessment. The patient should be specifically asked about the circumstances surrounding the fall,

prodromal symptoms, and loss of consciousness. Loss of consciousness may suggest an acute cardiac or neurologic event. The high-risk patient should be assessed for known risk factors. The use of prescription and over-the-counter medications should be assessed. Psychotropic medications, including antidepressants, antipsychotics, and benzodiazepines, have been associated with increased risk of falls and hip fracture.

The physical examination should begin with measurement of orthostatic vital signs. As people age, baroreflex sensitivity declines, as manifested by decreased ability to increase heart rate in response to positional change. In addition, total body water declines with advancing age. Both physiologic changes can lead to orthostasis. The physical examination should include targeted cardiovascular, neurologic, and ophthalmologic examinations. A valid assessment of gait, balance, and strength is a necessary part of the physical examination. Frequently used tests are listed in Box 28.1.

Additional testing such as laboratory tests or Holter monitoring should only be performed when driven by the findings of the history and physical examination.

Treatment and Prevention of Future Falls

Evidence-based interventions for the treatment and prevention of future falls have been critically reviewed and incorporated into guidelines from the US Preventive Services Task Force and the AGS/BGS. Choice of targeted interventions is based on the findings of the assessment (Box 28.2).

KEY FACTS

✓ Geriatric assessment requires a multifaceted—physical, cognitive, and psychosocial—approach

✓ Gait speed is a strong predictor of future disability and death in older adults

✓ Precipitating factors in falls—wrong choice of gait aid, environmental hazards, risk-taking behaviors

✓ Psychotropic medications may increase the risk of falls and hip fracture

✓ Exercise therapy (focusing on strength and balance) and vitamin D supplementation are effective fall-prevention interventions

---

Cognitive Impairment
Mild Cognitive Impairment

A broad spectrum of neurocognitive changes occur commonly with aging, ranging from the occasional memory lapses that are common in people of all ages to overt dementia. Mild cognitive impairment (MCI) represents an intermediate stage between normal aging and dementia. The prevalence of MCI in population-based studies of adults

---

Box 28.2 • Treatment and Prevention of Falls in Community-Dwelling Older Adults

Exercise and physical therapy program focusing on balance and strength (eg, tai chi)

Vitamin D supplementation

Treatment of vision impairment. *First* cataract operation results in decreased rate of falls

Management of postural hypotension

Pacemaker placement in patients with carotid sinus hypersensitivity

Psychoactive medication reduction or elimination

Multifactorial interventions based on mitigation of an individual's fall-related risk factors. Such interventions can reduce falls for those at very high risk

---

Box 28.3 • Work-up of Dementia

Laboratory tests
  All patients:
    Thyroid-stimulating hormone
    Vitamin B_{12} level
  Based on clinical suspicion:
    Complete blood cell count
    Electrolytes
    Glucose
    Renal and liver function tests
    Testing for neurosyphilis, human immunodeficiency virus infection
    Erythrocyte sedimentation rate
Neuroimaging: most useful in younger patients and patients with rapid progression, focal neurologic deficits, symptoms of normal-pressure hydrocephalus, recent head trauma
    Noncontrast head computed tomography
    Magnetic resonance imaging

---

aged 65 years and older ranges from 10% to 20%. These individuals are at increased risk for progression to dementia (approximately 10% risk of progression per year), making it important for clinicians to recognize MCI and provide appropriate anticipatory guidance to patients and their loved ones.

MCI can manifest as 1 of 2 subtypes: amnestic MCI or nonamnestic MCI. The former is more likely to progress to Alzheimer disease (AD), whereas the latter may progress to non-AD dementia subtypes. Persons with MCI demonstrate noticeable changes in cognition that are not yet severe enough to negatively affect functional capacity. To date, no medications have been shown to decrease the rate of conversion to dementia. Randomized controlled trials examining the impact of cognitive rehabilitation for patients with MCI have demonstrated improvements in cognitive function.

Dementia

The general term *dementia* encompasses several disorders or subtypes of neurocognitive impairment that are progressive, are nonreversible, and have significant impact on the affected individual's function. These disturbances are not accounted for by another mental disorder or delirium. Dementia is a disease of later life, with at least 5% of the population older than 65 years and 35% to 50% older than 85 years having this geriatric syndrome. Cognitive domains that can be affected include learning and memory, language, executive function, complex attention, perceptual-motor function, and social cognition.

While there is insufficient evidence for universal screening, clinicians must consider case-finding measures when older patients present with memory concerns, nonadherence, functional decline, or new psychiatric symptoms. Clinicians must use collateral history from a

reliable informant, patient-provided history, and a standardized mental status examination (eg, Mini-Mental State Examination, Kokmen Short Test of Mental Status) when evaluating such symptoms. Reversible conditions such as depression, chronic alcohol use, medications, metabolic disorders, toxic agents, nutritional deficiencies, normal-pressure hydrocephalus, subdural hematoma, central nervous system (CNS) tumors, and CNS infections must be considered in the differential diagnosis of cognitive difficulties. Recommended laboratory and imaging studies are listed in Box 28.3.

The major subtypes of dementia are listed in Box 28.4, and the classic clinical features of each are described in the sections that follow.

Alzheimer Disease

AD is the most common form of dementia and is characterized by a progressive decline in cognitive functioning. Learning new tasks and information gradually becomes more difficult. Memory impairment begins with declarative memory (facts and recent events) and affects procedural and motor learning later in the course of illness. Both receptive and expressive language difficulties develop, in

---

Box 28.4 • Major Subtypes of Dementia

Alzheimer disease

Dementia with Lewy bodies

Parkinson disease dementia

Frontotemporal dementia

Vascular dementia

which the patient has difficulty naming familiar objects and understanding language. Advancing age is the most important risk factor for AD. Positive family history, Down syndrome, and apolipoprotein E4 genotype are also important risk factors; however, genotyping is not recommended for predictive risk assessment.

Microscopic findings include significant loss of neurons and loss of synaptic connections. The 2 neuropathologic hallmarks of AD are neuritic plaques and neurofibrillary tangles. Neuritic plaques represent extracellular deposits of protein containing amyloid. Neurofibrillary tangles are found inside neurons and are composed of paired helical filaments of hyperphosphorylated microtubule-associated tau protein. This intracellular deposition may cause cell death.

Dementia With Lewy Bodies

In addition to the cognitive features of dementia, patients with dementia with Lewy bodies (DLB) display parkinsonian signs with bradykinesia, extremity rigidity, and postural instability. Early in the syndrome, patients have difficulty maintaining attention and may show marked fluctuations in cognitive status. Absence of a resting tremor is common (unlike in Parkinson disease dementia). Detailed visual hallucinations and REM sleep behavior disorder are common with DLB. These patients may also have exquisite neuroleptic sensitivity and autonomic dysfunction.

Parkinson Disease Dementia

Dementia is common among patients with Parkinson disease. If Parkinson disease has been present for more than 1 year before the onset of cognitive symptoms, the diagnosis is more likely to be Parkinson disease dementia (PDD). Conversely, if the parkinsonian symptoms present at the same time as or shortly after the cognitive symptoms, the diagnosis of DLB is favored. Hallmarks of PDD include executive dysfunction and difficulty with visuospatial tasks. Memory deficits are also present, but less profound than in AD. The neuropsychiatric and sleep-related symptoms are similar to those with DLB.

Vascular Dementia

The memory impairment seen in vascular dementia can be due to either microvascular or macrovascular disease. The patient usually has a stepwise progression of cognitive impairment consistent with the multiple ischemic infarcts. Three main pathophysiologic causes of vascular dementia are possible, including large artery infarctions, small artery infarctions or lacunes, or chronic subcortical ischemia that occurs in the distribution of small arteries in the periventricular white matter. Cerebral amyloid angiopathy, a related condition, may cause cognitive impairment and is associated with lobar hemorrhage or infarctions.

The clinical presentation depends on which portion of the brain is affected by the ischemic insults; cognitive and neurologic impairments should correlate with the anatomical regions of ischemia. CNS imaging usually shows evidence of cortical or subcortical infarctions, ischemic changes, or leukoaraiosis. Modification of risk factors for cerebrovascular disease, such as hypertension, diabetes mellitus, and hyperlipidemia, is warranted. Antiplatelet therapy is usually given.

Frontotemporal Dementia

Frontotemporal dementia (FTD) is characterized by changes in personality and social behavior due to focal degeneration of the frontal and/or temporal lobes. Onset of FTD tends to be somewhat earlier than for AD, often in the 50s and 60s. Patients may exhibit disinhibition, language impairments, or hypersexual behavior. Memory impairment is often less profound than that seen in AD. Physical examination may reveal prominent frontal reflexes. Later in the course of illness, CNS imaging often reveals focal atrophy of the frontal and/or temporal lobes. One type of FTD is Pick disease, a rapidly progressive condition characterized pathologically by intraneuronal inclusion bodies known as Pick bodies. Management of the behavioral disturbance is the most challenging aspect of the treatment of this condition.

Treatment of Dementia

Nonpharmacologic treatment is paramount in all patients who have neurocognitive impairment. Important nonpharmacologic considerations are listed in Box 28.5.

Several factors must be considered before starting a medication in a patient with dementia, including renal clearance, potential for drug interactions, potential for adverse drug effects, and the individual's goals of care. Medications with anticholinergic activity can worsen cognitive function in patients with dementia.

Cognitive Enhancement Medications

Acetylcholinesterase inhibitors (donepezil, rivastigmine, tacrine, and galantamine) are approved by the US Food and Drug Administration (FDA) for the treatment of AD. Although acetylcholinesterase inhibitors are not considered disease-modifying drugs, they may transiently delay symptom progression and institutionalization.

Box 28.5 • Nonpharmacologic Treatment of Dementia

Cognitive rehabilitation

Supportive therapy

Physical exercise

Caregiver education and support

Environmental modification (eg, controlled amount of stimulation, routine schedule)

Safety enhancement (eg, fall prevention, driving assessment)

Anticipatory guidance and advance care planning

Improvement in abnormal behaviors associated with dementia may also occur with their use. Studies have demonstrated modest benefit for acetylcholinesterase inhibitors in DLB and PDD. The high prevalence of liver toxicity associated with tacrine has not been found with the other acetylcholinesterase inhibitors. Common adverse effects include nausea, vomiting, diarrhea, and anorexia.

Memantine, an *N*-methyl-D-aspartate antagonist, is FDA approved for the treatment of moderate to severe AD. This medication is postulated to have neuroprotective effects by reducing glutamate-mediated excitotoxicity. The most common adverse effects are dizziness, headache, and constipation. Increased confusion and hallucinations have been reported. This medication can be used as a single agent or in conjunction with an acetylcholinesterase inhibitor; however, a recent randomized controlled trial (Donepezil and Memantine in Moderate to Severe Alzheimer's Disease—the DOMINO-AD Trial) found that the addition of memantine to donepezil in moderate or severe AD was no better than donepezil alone. Evidence for cognitive enhancement medications in vascular dementia has been inconclusive.

Over-the-counter supplements such as *Ginkgo biloba* and nonsteroidal anti-inflammatory drugs are not supported by sufficient data to recommend their use in dementia. Data on the use of vitamin E have been mixed; however, this supplement may result in slower functional decline in patients with mild to moderate AD.

Treatment of Behavioral Dyscontrol

The neuropsychiatric symptoms associated with all subtypes of dementia are often more troublesome to patients and caregivers than the cognitive symptoms inherent to these conditions. Nonpharmacologic interventions are recommended as the first step. These interventions should be individualized and capitalize on the patient's preserved procedural memory. Pharmacologic therapy brings with it significant risk of adverse drug events and should be used only if the patient's distressing symptoms are refractory to nonpharmacologic interventions or are creating a dangerous situation. Antipsychotic agents are associated with increased risk of death, stroke, falls, and infections in this population.

Delirium

Delirium is an acute confusional state marked by inattention, fluctuating course, and abnormal level of consciousness. It is the prototypical geriatric syndrome and represents the final common pathway of the intersection between predisposing characteristics and precipitating factors (Figure 28.1). Delirium is one of the most common

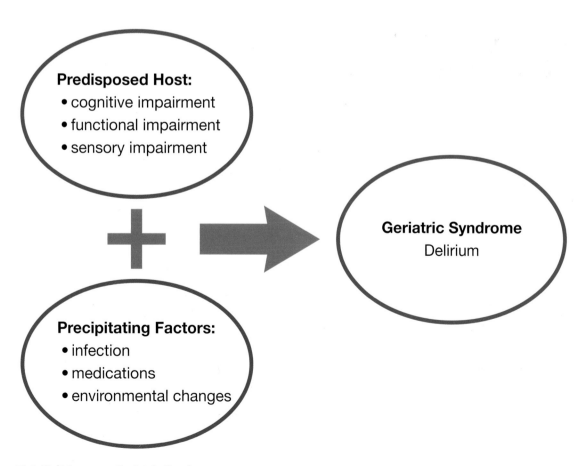

Figure 28.1 Delirium as a Geriatric Syndrome.

complications after surgery in older adults and may affect half of older adults undergoing hip fracture surgery and coronary artery bypass grafting. Baseline neurocognitive disorders are an important risk factor for delirium.

Key Definition

Delirium: *acute confusional state marked by inattention, fluctuating course, and abnormal level of consciousness.*

Delirium is a medical emergency, and clinicians must be attuned to its detection. The Confusion Assessment Method, a simple, widely used screening tool, is a helpful supplement to the clinician's careful history taking (from caregivers) and physical examination (Box 28.6). Laboratory evaluation can help to identify correctable precipitating factors. Choice of laboratory and imaging studies should be driven by clinical suspicion and may include a complete blood cell count, complete metabolic profile, liver enzyme tests, urinalysis, chest radiograph, electrocardiogram, and drug/toxin levels. Brain imaging, cerebrospinal fluid evaluation, and electroencephalography are needed only when there is a strong clinical suspicion of a primary neurologic cause. All medications should be reviewed, with particular attention to psychoactive medications.

Box 28.6 • Confusion Assessment Method Diagnostic Algorithm[a]

Feature 1: Acute change in mental status and fluctuating course

Is there evidence of an acute change in cognition from baseline?

Does the abnormal behavior fluctuate during the day?

Feature 2: Inattention

Does the patient have difficulty focusing attention (eg, easily distracted, difficulty keeping track of what is being said)?

Feature 3: Disorganized thinking

Is the patient's thinking disorganized or incoherent? Does the patient have rambling or irrelevant conversations or unpredictable switching from subject to subject?

Feature 4: Abnormal level of consciousness

Is the patient anything besides alert—hyperalert, lethargic, stuporous, or comatose?

[a] The diagnosis of delirium requires features 1 and 2 and either 3 or 4.

Adapted from Inouye SK, van Dyck CH, Alessi CA, Balkin S, Siegal AP, Horwitz RI. Clarifying confusion: the confusion assessment method: a new method for detection of delirium. Ann Intern Med. 1990 Dec 15;113(12):941–8. Used with permission.

Prevention is always the best strategy; concentrated efforts aimed at targeting risk factors, such as sleep disruption, immobility, sensory impairment, dehydration, and cognitive impairment, have been successful in reducing the incidence of delirium. Treatment is largely supportive and begins with mitigation of contributing factors. Examples include environmental simplification, removal of "tethers," optimization of sensory input, and regulation of sleep-wake cycle. Delirious patients are at risk for iatrogenic complications, so careful surveillance and preventive strategies are important. There are no FDA-approved medications to treat delirium, and pharmacologic therapies should be used cautiously because they may actually prolong the syndrome. Medications may be necessary to control frightening psychotic symptoms or dangerous behaviors.

Late-Life Depression

Late-life depression is especially common in patients receiving long-term care and those with multiple comorbidities. Older adults with depression are more likely than their younger counterparts to present with somatic symptoms such as pain or unexplained weight loss. This condition can be challenging to diagnose, as comorbid conditions and their associated treatments often result in overlap symptoms such as fatigue, memory impairment, and sleep disturbance. Screening for the presence of low mood and anhedonia is a recommended strategy, as these 2 symptoms are less likely to be confounded by medical illnesses. The Patient Health Questionnaire (PHQ-9) can be used for screening and for assessment of treatment response. The Geriatric Depression Scale is often used in this population because it offers yes/no responses and does not include somatic and sleep-related questions. It is useful for screening and diagnosis, but not for measuring response to treatment.

Although older patients attempt suicide less often than younger patients, they are more likely to complete suicide. White men aged 85 years and older have the highest risk of completed suicide. Clinicians should screen older patients for suicidality and intervene, when necessary, with collaborative care interventions.

Undernutrition

Normal aging results in predictable changes in body composition, including increased fat mass and decreases in bone mass, lean muscle mass, and water content. Normal aging is also associated with reduced ability to concentrate urine, reduced thirst perception, and impaired response to serum osmolarity, culminating in increased risk of dehydration.

Both undernutrition and obesity are common among older adults and increase the risk of morbidity, mortality, and functional decline. Unintended weight loss or poor intake may reflect underlying illness. Other than body mass index, anthropometric tools are often impractical for use in the ambulatory primary care setting. Laboratory markers that reflect undernutrition and have been correlated with increased mortality among the elderly include hypoalbuminemia and low serum levels of cholesterol. However, serum albumin lacks enough sensitivity and specificity to warrant routine use as a screening tool. Prealbumin has a shorter half-life and can be used to measure the effectiveness of nutritional interventions.

Advance Care Planning

Advance care planning is an established process for patients to communicate their preferences for medical care, should they ever lose their capacity to make medical decisions or articulate their wishes. Completion of an advance health care directive is an important element of this process and should be strongly encouraged.

The 2 main types of advance medical directives include durable power of attorney for health care, which designates a proxy decision maker for health-related decisions, and instructional directive or living will, which allows an individual to communicate his or her preferences for specific types of medical care in future states of health.

KEY FACTS

✓ If parkinsonian symptoms present at the same time as cognitive symptoms or shortly afterward, DLB is more likely than PDD

✓ Acetylcholinesterase inhibitors do not change AD's course but may slow its symptoms

✓ The Confusion Assessment Method—a helpful screening tool to supplement the history and physical examination in patients with acute mental status changes

✓ Pharmacologic therapies may actually prolong delirium; use with caution

✓ Advance directive documents are activated only if the patient loses decision-making capacity

Vision Loss

Vision impairment is defined as visual acuity of 20/40 or worse; **blindness** is defined as visual acuity of 20/200 or worse. Both increase with advancing age; more than 25% of people older than 85 years have significant visual impairment. The American Academy of Ophthalmology recommends a comprehensive eye examination every 1 to 2 years for older adults; however, the United States Preventive Services Task Force concluded that there is insufficient evidence to recommend for or against routine vision screening among asymptomatic older adults. New eye symptoms in an older adult should be thoroughly evaluated, as vision impairment is associated with decreased quality of life, falls, and motor vehicle crashes in this population.

Key Definitions

Vision impairment: *visual acuity of 20/40 or worse.*

Blindness: *visual acuity of 20/200 or worse.*

Worldwide, the 2 leading causes of visual impairment are refractive error and cataracts. The most common refractive error in older adults is increasing hyperopia (farsightedness) with age. Cataract extraction has consistently been a well-tolerated operation in the older population and has demonstrated improvements in important outcomes such as vision-related quality of life and fall rate. Providers should consider referring patients for cataract extraction when the visual deficits due to the cataract impair the patient's quality of life or limit the ophthalmologist's ability to monitor other ocular conditions, such as retinal disease.

There are 2 main types of age-related macular degeneration (AMD), a leading cause of irreversible blindness in the elderly. The dry form is usually of slower onset, while the wet form can result in more sudden central vision loss. Risk factors for AMD include advancing age, family history of AMD, and cardiovascular risk factors such as hypertension and cigarette smoking. (See Chapter 31, "Otolaryngology and Ophthalmology.")

Glaucoma is the second leading cause of irreversible blindness worldwide and the most common cause of blindness in African Americans. Increased intraocular pressure is an important risk factor for the optic nerve damage and visual field loss most commonly associated with this syndrome. Primary open-angle glaucoma characterized by blocked passage of aqueous humor is much more common and indolent than acute angle-closure glaucoma, which happens more suddenly and presents with a painful red eye and acute vision loss. Both are described in Chapter 31, "Otolaryngology and Ophthalmology."

Hearing Loss

Hearing loss is a common, underrecognized condition among older adults that profoundly affects quality of life. Hearing loss is typically multifactorial in older patients and may present atypically with social withdrawal or low mood. Although there is no consensus among professional specialty groups regarding *universal* screening,

Table 28.2 • Differentiating Sensorineural vs Conductive Hearing Loss

| Factor | Hearing Loss | |
	Sensorineural	Conductive
Anatomy	Cochlear/retrocochlear	External ear/middle ear
Sample causes	Drug-induced hearing loss Labyrinthitis	Cerumen impaction Cholesteatoma Otitis media
Weber test[a]	Lateralizes to better-hearing ear	Louder in affected ear
Rinne test[b]	Both bone and air conduction will be equally suppressed	Air-conducted sound will not be heard

[a] For Weber test, strike tuning fork and place gently against a midline structure of the skull (mid forehead or vertex). Normally, sound should be transmitted to both sides equally.

[b] For Rinne test, strike tuning fork and place on the mastoid bone. When the patient ceases to hear the vibration, move the tines close to the external auditory meatus to check air conduction. Normally, sound should persist via air conduction for an additional 30 to 60 seconds.

any person with subjective hearing loss or multiple risk factors for hearing loss should be evaluated by a medical provider. This evaluation should include a careful physical examination of the ear to evaluate for structural abnormality (eg, cerumen impaction or otitis) as well as a valid screening test. Options for testing include self-assessment questionnaires, office-based examination techniques (eg, whisper test), and handheld otoscopic tone generators. If an abnormality is identified with 1 of these 3 tests, the Weber and Rinne tests can then help the clinician elucidate the anatomical cause of the hearing loss (Table 28.2). When objective hearing loss is identified, patients should be offered referral for a formal audiologic evaluation. If the hearing loss occurs suddenly, oral corticosteroid therapy and urgent otolaryngologic referral should be considered. Sudden hearing loss may be due to an autoimmune cause.

Numerous hearing aid options exist. Patients and their providers must decide on factors and hearing aid features that best meet their needs. Patients that cannot or choose not to use a hearing aid can benefit from assistive listening devices such as personal handheld amplifiers. Providers must also counsel hearing-impaired patients about the utility of adaptive equipment and future avoidance of ototoxic medications (eg, aminoglycosides, vancomycin, loop diuretics, salicylates, erythromycin).

Surgical management is often required for mechanical problems that have led to conductive loss. Cochlear implants can be very effective for older adults with severe, bilateral, sensorineural hearing loss that has been refractory to hearing aids. Cochlear implants function by bypassing the damaged cochlear hair cells and providing direct electrical stimulation to the auditory nerve fibers of the cochlea. These signals are then sent to the auditory system of the brain. Patients must be motivated, fit for general anesthesia, and capable of participation in postimplant rehabilitation.

Pressure Ulcers

Pressure ulcers are most common among older adults who are hospitalized or receiving long-term care services; they cause significant morbidity among frail older adults. Compression of the skin overlying bony prominences such as the sacrum, greater trochanter, and calcaneus is most common, but pressure ulcers can also result from poorly fitting appliances such as splints and casts. Prevention of pressure ulcers is of paramount importance and begins with identification of patients at risk. Assessment should occur longitudinally, and identified risk factors should be coupled to appropriate preventive strategies. The 2 most commonly used tools to identify patients at risk for pressure ulcers are the Norton scale and the Braden scale. The Norton scale requires the clinician to assess 5 main domains to calculate the risk score: physical condition, mental condition, physical activity, mobility, and continence. The Braden scale includes assessment of sensation, moisture exposure, physical activity, mobility, nutrition, exposure to friction, and sheering. Preventive strategies for pressure ulcers are listed in Box 28.7.

Box 28.7 • Preventive Strategies for Pressure Ulcers

Frequently reposition bed-bound individuals. A 2-h minimum interval between assisted turnings is recommended

Do not elevate the head of the bed more than 30° to prevent friction-induced injury

Choose the appropriate support surface on the basis of patient characteristics

Minimize exposure to excess moisture

Ensure optimal protein intake

Avoid excessive dryness/scaling with the use of lotions containing fatty acids

> ### Box 28.8 • General Treatment Strategies for Pressure Ulcers
>
> Relieve pressure over the ulcer with appropriate positioning and support surfaces
>
> Débride nonviable tissue
>
> Optimize the wound environment (prevent wound maceration and avoid friction and shearing forces) to promote the formation of granulation tissue
>
> Manage other conditions (malnutrition or infection when present) that may delay wound healing
>
> Manage pain

Pressure ulcers can be classified into 1 of 6 groups. Ulcers covered with eschar or slough are not stageable until the eschar or slough is removed.

Stage I: Nonblanchable erythema of intact skin. There may be associated edema.

Stage II: Partial-thickness skin loss of the dermis. The ulcer is superficial and may present as a blister or shallow crater with a red wound bed.

Stage III: Full-thickness tissue loss with damage or necrosis of subcutaneous tissue. The damage may extend to the fascia. The ulcer is a deep crater.

Stage IV: Full-thickness skin loss with exposed muscle, bone, or tendons. Sinus tracts may be present.

Unstageable/unclassified: Full-thickness skin or tissue loss—depth unknown. Full-thickness tissue loss in which the actual depth of the ulcer is obscured by slough (yellow, tan exudate) or eschar (brown, black). These are typically stage III or IV. Stable (no sign of infection) eschar on the heels should not be removed.

Suspected deep tissue injury—depth unknown. The skin over a bony prominence appears purple or maroon. There may be an associated blood-filled blister. Deep tissue injury may progress rapidly despite optimal treatment.

Treatment of pressure ulcers depends on the depth and extent of the wound (Box 28.8).

Urinary Incontinence

Urinary incontinence is common among older adults, affecting at least 15% of those living independently and about 50% of those in nursing homes. Important complications include urinary tract infection, skin breakdown, social isolation, and depression. Urinary incontinence affects caregiver burden and remains a significant reason for nursing home placement.

Evaluation of Incontinence

The evaluation of urinary incontinence includes a thorough medical history, physical examination, and several selected laboratory tests. The history should include urine volume, duration of symptoms, precipitating factors, whether symptoms of obstruction exist (low urinary force of stream, sensation of incomplete bladder emptying, and hesitancy), and functional status. Also, symptoms of neurologic disease, associated disease states, menstrual status and parity, and medications taken should be documented. Medications that may worsen incontinence include diuretics, cholinesterase inhibitors, calcium channel antagonists, narcotic analgesics, sedative-hypnotics, and oral estrogen.

Red flag symptoms such as sudden development of incontinence, pelvic pain, or hematuria require prompt work-up.

Physical examination of the abdomen should evaluate bladder distention and possible abdominal masses. Examination of the pelvis should include a pelvic examination, rectal examination, and neurologic evaluation (with testing of sacral cord function).

Work-up should always include a urinalysis. Patients should also complete a voiding diary that records fluid intake, types of fluids ingested, and voiding (both continent and incontinent). A postvoid residual bladder volume test can be performed to rule out retention in those with long-standing diabetes, prostatic enlargement, recurrent infection, or pelvic organ prolapse.

Urodynamic studies are occasionally indicated to establish the diagnosis of incontinence when the patient has a medically confusing history or more than 1 type of urinary incontinence (mixed incontinence). Urodynamic studies consist of multiple components, including cystometry, which measures bladder volume and pressure and can be used to detect uninhibited detrusor muscle contractions, lack of bladder contractions, and bladder sensation; uroflow, which measures urinary flow rate; and pressure flow studies, which determine whether poor flow is due to detrusor weakness or obstruction.

Types of Incontinence

Several mechanisms contribute to urinary incontinence and can be categorized as urge incontinence, stress incontinence, mixed urge/stress incontinence, and overflow incontinence. Patients are said to have functional incontinence if they have a condition such as cognitive impairment or difficulty with ambulation that limits their ability to reach the toilet. Features of each type and treatment options are described in Table 28.3.

Urinary Tract Infections

Urinary tract infections are one of the most common bacterial infections of older adults. Functional impairment, incomplete emptying of the bladder, urinary instrumentation, and catheterization all predispose the elderly to urinary tract infection. Among community-dwelling women, the

Table 28.3 • Types of Urinary Incontinence

Type	Cause	Symptoms	Treatment Options
Urge incontinence	Detrusor overactivity	Urgency, frequency, nocturia. Loss of small to moderate amounts of urine	Behavioral: bladder training (timed voiding to reduce bladder volume plus urge suppression), elimination of bladder irritants, prompted voiding for cognitively impaired patients, pelvic muscle exercises Pharmacologic: antimuscarinic medications Surgical: intradetrusor botulinum toxin injection, sacral nerve stimulation
Stress incontinence	Urinary outlet incompetence from intrinsic urethral sphincter insufficiency or bladder hypermobility	Loss of small amounts of urine associated with transient increases in intra-abdominal pressure (eg, cough, sneeze, laugh)	Behavioral: pelvic floor muscle exercises, weight loss Devices: vaginal cones, urethral plugs, continence pessaries Pharmacologic: duloxetine Surgical: urethral sling, tension-free vaginal tape, bladder suspension, injection of periurethral bulking agents
Overflow incontinence	Urinary outlet obstruction or detrusor underactivity	Difficulty emptying bladder, low urine flow, straining to void, urinary dribbling	Treatment depends on cause of obstruction Surgical: relief of bladder outlet obstruction (TURP) Pharmacologic: α-adrenergic antagonists Indwelling or intermittent bladder catheterization

Abbreviation: TURP, transurethral resection of prostate.

most common pathogens are *Escherichia coli, Klebsiella pneumoniae, Proteus mirabilis,* and *Enterococcus faecalis.* Rates of antibiotic resistance are on the rise, including that for fluoroquinolone-resistant *E coli.*

Asymptomatic bacteriuria becomes more common with age; 6% to 16% of women in the community and 25% to 54% of women in nursing homes are affected. Asymptomatic bacteriuria is a colonization state and should not be treated, as this practice can lead to selection of resistant organisms and potential for adverse drug events.

Only symptomatic patients should be evaluated with urinalysis and urine culture. Symptoms specific for urinary tract infection, such as acute dysuria, new or worsening urgency, increase in frequency, new incontinence, suprapubic or costovertebral pain, or fever, should prompt the clinician to consider urine studies. Repeated urine testing to assess for cure is not indicated. See Chapter 46, "Sexually Transmitted, Urinary Tract, and Gastrointestinal Tract Infections," for information on treatment of urinary tract infection.

Sexual Function and Sexuality

Multiple physical and psychosocial changes that occur with aging can result in changes in the desire and capacity of older adults for sexual activity. With age, men require more direct stimulation to achieve and sustain erections, experience prolonged refractory periods (in some men, it can be days before they are able to have sexual activity again), and are more likely to have testosterone deficiency compared to their younger counterparts. Postmenopausal women experience vaginal atrophy with an associated decrease in lubrication, have a decline in sexual desire, and may also require more direct stimulation. Coexisting aging-related changes such as pelvic organ prolapse, osteoarthritis, and incontinence are important factors affecting sexual function. Lack of an available partner is an important social barrier. Although there is some decline in the frequency of intercourse among older adults, 50% to 80% continue to be sexually active and report high rates of sexual satisfaction. Clinicians need to be aware that older adults are at risk for sexually transmitted illnesses and continue to counsel them about preventive strategies.

Medications

Aging has an impact on the 4 principal pharmacokinetic functions. Drug *absorption* may take longer, but the extent of drug absorption is not affected with normal aging. Changes in body composition, including increased adipose tissue and decreased total body water and lean body mass, affect drug *distribution.* For example, lipophilic medications such as diazepam may have a much larger volume of distribution and more prolonged effect. Hepatic *metabolism* of medications decreases with age

"Start low and go slow"

Minimize overprescribing by frequently reviewing the patient's medication list

Encourage patients to bring all medications to office visits

Consider medication adverse effects or adverse drug events as a cause of new symptoms as a result of altered pharmacokinetics and pharmacodynamics with aging

Avoid prescribing potentially inappropriate medications. Clinical tools such as the 2012 American Geriatrics Society Beers Criteria can help in identifying high-risk medications

and disease-related decrease in hepatic perfusion. Finally, drug *elimination* decreases with reductions in renal function. The serum level of creatinine is a poor measure of renal function in the elderly and tends to underestimate the degree of renal insufficiency. Because lean body mass decreases with advancing age, less creatinine is produced. Thus, an elderly patient who has as much as a 30% reduction in renal function may have a normal serum level of creatinine.

Adverse drug events are common in the elderly patients and are a potentially preventable cause of hospital admissions. The most common culprits include warfarin, oral antiplatelet medications, insulin, and oral hypoglycemic medications. A number of established prescribing principles should be considered when caring for older patients (Box 28.9).

KEY FACTS

✓ Hearing loss in older patients—typically multifactorial; may present with social withdrawal or low mood

✓ Poorly fitting appliances (eg, splints, casts) can cause pressure ulcers

✓ Urinalysis should always be part of the work-up for incontinence; patients should keep a voiding diary

✓ Bladder training and avoidance of dietary bladder irritants are effective nonpharmacologic therapies for urge incontinence

✓ Asymptomatic bacteriuria is a colonization state and should not be treated

29 Medical Ethics[a]

KEITH M. SWETZ, MD, MA AND C. CHRISTOPHER HOOK, MD

Medicine is first and foremost a relationship—a coming together of a patient, who is ill or has specific needs, and a physician, whose goal is to help the patient. The physician-patient relationship is a *fiduciary* relationship; physicians have knowledge, skills, and privileges that patients do not have. In turn, patients trust that physicians act in their patients' best interests.

Medical ethics consists of a set of principles and systematic methods that guide physicians on how they ought to act in their relationships with patients and others and how to resolve moral problems that arise in the care of patients. These principles and methods are based on moral values shared by both the lay society (which may vary from culture to culture) and the medical profession. Advances in medical science and the ever-changing social and legal milieu result in dynamic changes, challenges, and ethical dilemmas in medical practice.

An *ethical dilemma* is a predicament caused by conflicting moral principles in which there is no clear course to resolve a problem (ie, credible evidence exists both for and against a certain action).

Principles of Medical Ethics

A widely used framework for medical ethics is principalism, which delineates 4 principles that encompass most clinical ethical concerns. These principles (in no specific order) are 1) **beneficence**—the duty to do good; 2) **nonmaleficence**—the duty to prevent harm; 3) **respect for patient autonomy**—the duty to respect persons and their rights of self-determination; and 4) **justice**—the duty to treat patients fairly (free of bias and based on medical need).

The principles are *prima facie*, that is, the rule is valid in most situations, but the priority of each principle may change on a case-by-case basis. In clinical practice these principles can be at odds with each other. For example, a beneficent physician may recommend an intervention with minimal risks of harm. However, the patient may exert his or her autonomy and decline the procedure.

Although beneficence is a primary motivating ethical principle for most physicians, the other principles contextualize and inform our orientation to accomplish the good (Figure 29.1).

Key Definitions

Beneficence: *duty to do good.*

Nonmaleficence: *duty to prevent; "first, do no harm."*

Respect for patient autonomy: *duty to respect persons and their right of self-determination.*

Justice: *duty to treat patients fairly, without bias, within available health care constraints.*

Beneficence

Beneficence is acting to benefit patients by preserving life, restoring health, relieving suffering, and restoring or maintaining function. The physician is obligated to pursue the good, or benefit, of the patient, as that benefit is defined by the patient in the context of his or her goals, beliefs, and values, not by the physician. This principle may be viewed on several levels of benefit, including how an intervention may 1) biomedically or physiologically benefit a patient, 2) personally benefit the patient (eg, waiting for family to

[a] Portions previously published in Mueller PS, Hook CC, Fleming KC. Ethical issues in geriatrics: a guide for clinicians. Mayo Clin Proc. 2004 Apr;79(4):554–62. Used with permission of Mayo Foundation for Medical Education and Research.

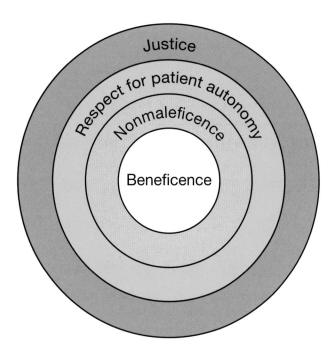

Figure 29.1 *The 4 Principles of Medical Ethics.*

arrive before withdrawing a ventilator), or 3) ultimately benefit the patient (ie, in respect to a patient's belief system or world view).

Nonmaleficence

Nonmaleficence closely couples with beneficence and requires that physicians should minimize harm or risk of harm to patients. This principle has roots in the Hippocratic corpus: "as to diseases, help, but at least do no harm." This principle also addresses unprofessional behavior, such as verbal, physical, and sexual abuse of patients or uninformed and undisclosed interventions or experimentation on patients. Practical examples are listed in Box 29.1.

Respect for Patient Autonomy

The word *autonomy* derives from the Greek words *auto* ("self") and *nomos* ("rule"). The principle of respect for patient autonomy is the concept that persons have the right to establish, pursue, and maintain their values and goals (the right to self-determination). For patients to be fully autonomous, an ideal that no one can fully achieve, they must 1) be informed (see "Informed Consent and Exceptions" section), 2) have liberty (be free from coercion or duress and have the opportunity to influence the course of their life and medical treatment), and 3) have decision-making capacity. Notably, decision-making capacity is not the same as the legal term *competence*. **Decision-making capacity** is a physician's clinical determination of a patient's ability to understand his or her situation and make appropriate

---

Box 29.1 • Practical Applications of Nonmaleficence in Clinical Practice

Nonabandonment—an ethical obligation to provide ongoing medical care once the patient and physician mutually concur to enter into an alliance

Nonabandonment is closely related to the principles of beneficence and nonmaleficence and is fundamental to the long-term physician-patient relationship

Patient nonadherence, in terms of taking medications or following a physician's instructions, is not grounds for abandonment

A physician should strive to respond to a patient's needs over time but should not trespass his or her own values in the process

Conflict of interest—an ethical obligation to refrain from activities that are not in patients' best interests

Such conflicts may unduly influence physicians' practices (eg, prescribing, ordering of tests, or therapeutic recommendations)

For example, accepting a gift from a representative of a pharmaceutical company constitutes a conflict of interest if the physician accepting the gift writes prescriptions for drugs manufactured by that company

Physician impairment—according to the American Medical Association, the impaired physician is one who is "unable to practice medicine with reasonable skill and safety to patients because of physical or mental illness, including deteriorations through the aging process, or loss of motor skill, or excessive use or abuse of drugs including alcohol"

Impairment is distinct from competence, which specifically concerns the physician's knowledge and skills to adequately perform his or her duties as a physician. Impairment and incompetence both may compromise patient care and safety

Physicians have a moral, professional, and legal obligation to report impaired and incompetent colleagues to the appropriate authority. Specifics of reporting vary by state, but all states have a reporting requirement

Typical authorities to contact include the institutional chief of staff or impairment program, local or state medical society impairment programs, or the state licensing body. Reporting the behavior of a colleague must be based on objective evidence rather than supposition

Double effect—pursuing beneficence may lead to unintended injury or death. Use of palliative sedation and analgesia for terminally ill patients is discussed more fully in Chapter 32, "Palliative Care"

---

decisions for treatment. **Competence** is the legal determination and status that an individual has the right to make life-affecting decisions (not only health-related decisions but also, for example, financial decisions).

In clinical practice, the lack of decisional capability should be proved, not presumed. Confusion, disorientation, psychosis, and other cognitive changes caused by diseases, metabolic disturbances, and medical interventions can affect decision-making ability. Decisionally capable patients have the right to refuse all medical interventions, even at the risk of death (Box 29.2).

KEY FACTS

✓ Principalism is a widely used framework for medical ethics

✓ Four principles that encompass most clinical ethical concerns—beneficence, nonmaleficence, respect for patient autonomy, and justice

✓ Physicians are ethically obligated to avoid activities not in patients' best interests

✓ Physician impairment—due to physical or mental illness, loss of motor skill, or drug use or abuse; distinct from incompetence

✓ Pursuing beneficence may have a double effect, leading to unintended injury or death

The ethical principle of respect for patient autonomy and numerous court decisions, from the Quinlan (1976) and Cruzan (1990) cases to the Schiavo (2005) case and others, established a patient's right to refuse

Box 29.2 • Clinical Standards to Assess Decision-making Capacity

The patient can make and communicate a choice

The patient understands the medical situation and prognosis, the nature of the recommended care, available alternative options, and the risks, benefits, and consequences of each

The patient's decisions are stable over time

The decision is consistent with the patient's values and goals

The decision is not due to delusions or altered mental status

medical treatment, even if death inevitably follows such refusals.

Promoting and Preserving Patient Autonomy

Physicians commonly care for patients who lack or lose decision-making capacity. To preserve their autonomy, patients who lose capacity nonetheless may express their wishes through 2 means: advance directives and surrogate decision makers. These means are discussed, along with futility and demands for nonbeneficial interventions, in Chapter 32, "Palliative Care."

Informed Consent and Exceptions

A derivative of the principle of respect for patient autonomy (and nonmaleficence) is informed consent (and refusal): the voluntary acceptance (or refusal) of physician recommendations by decisionally capable patients, or their surrogates, who have been provided sufficient information regarding the risks, benefits, and alternatives of the proposed interventions. There are 3 required elements of informed consent: 1) patient decision-making capacity, 2) patient voluntariness, and 3) receipt of accurate and sufficient information from which to make a decision. The amount of information shared with the patient should be guided not only by what the physician believes is adequate (professional practice standard) but also by that which the average, prudent person would need in order to make an appropriate decision (reasonable person standard). Discussion of available alternatives to the proposed treatment, including doing nothing, should be included.

In shared decision making, the physician should present the patient with recommendations that the patient can accept or reject. Simply laying out a menu of choices before the patient may lead to confusion or the perception by the patient that the physician is unconcerned with his or her welfare. If the patient refuses the recommended treatment and chooses one of the alternatives, the physician should respect the patient's choice. The final plan should reflect an agreement between a well-informed patient and a well-informed, sympathetic, and unbiased physician.

In rare exceptions, the physician can treat a patient without informed consent (eg, in an emotionally unstable patient who requires urgent treatment, when informing the patient of the details may produce further problems). The principle of implied consent is invoked when true informed consent is not possible because the patient (or surrogate) is unable to express a decision regarding treatment. This situation often occurs in emergencies in which physicians are compelled to provide immediate, medically necessary therapy, without which harm would result. Implied consent and duty to assist a person in urgent need of care have been legally accepted (eg, Good Samaritan laws) and provide the physician a legal defense against battery (although not negligence).

Truth Telling and Therapeutic Privilege

The physician must provide decisionally capable patients with truthful information to assist them in making informed medical decisions. Without the receipt of sufficient, accurate, and true information, patients cannot make autonomous decisions. Occasionally, the physician may withhold part or all of the truth if he or she believes that telling the truth is highly likely to cause considerable injury, a concept known as *therapeutic privilege*. The decision for intentional nondisclosure must be fully recorded in the medical record. Although invoking therapeutic privilege may be ethically justified in some circumstances, legal protection for less-than-full disclosure is not guaranteed.

Some decisionally capable patients may forgo complete disclosure, referring the receipt of information and decision making to others. Waiver of complete disclosure may occur by individual preference or in the context of cultural norms. Regardless, this preference should be respected as the patient's autonomous choice.

Medical Errors

Errors committed in the course of treatment require full, honest disclosure, because patients deserve to know the truth about what has happened. Frank disclosure helps to preserve and/or restore trust in the physician-patient relationship. Physicians often fear that if they disclose errors they will be sued, but the opposite is more often true. Patients are more likely to pursue legal action if they suspect something has gone awry, or subsequently discover the error, but were not told. Studies have shown that many patients sue physicians primarily to discover the truth.

Confidentiality

Privacy is integral to respect persons and to protect an individual's autonomy. Confidentiality respects the right to privacy and provides the patient with security to keep sensitive, personal information within the realm of the physician-patient relationship. The physician is ethically and legally obliged to maintain a patient's medical information in strict confidence, a tradition dating back to the Hippocratic Oath. Ensuring confidentiality encourages complete communication of all relevant information that may affect the patient's health.

However, the obligation to protect patients may be overridden when serious bodily harm to the patient or others may result if reasonable steps are not taken. In some instances, a patient's data must be shared with public health care agencies. Examples include certain infectious diseases, physical abuse, gunshot wounds, and other concerns to the public health and welfare. There is state-to-state variability in reporting requirements, and physicians should be aware of local statutes.

Conscientious Objection

Another conflict between patient and physician (and other health care providers) occurs when the patient requests an intervention that may be legally sanctioned, but is morally unacceptable to the physician. In this situation, the ethical issue centers on moral acceptability of the intervention and not on efficacy. An objector may believe so strongly against the intervention that he or she considers the intervention as commission of evil.

Historically, dating back to the Hippocratic Oath, medical ethics has recognized that physicians, in their obligations to protect life, may conscientiously object to acts involving the deliberate taking of human life. Many states have conscience laws protecting health care providers from being forced to be complicit in acts that would violate their conscience.

What constitutes an issue of conscience? In medicine, the issue of objection must regard a specific act. Claims of conscience regard acts, not persons. Claims of conscience that intrinsically involve discrimination against a given individual (eg, race, color, sexual preference, nationality, religion) are not legitimate and violate the principle of justice (see "Justice" section). Furthermore, the conscientious objector is restricted to forgoing participation only in the specific objectionable act, not in providing the rest of the patient's care. To do otherwise would be an act of abandonment. For example, a physician may refuse to participate in performing an abortion (including providing anesthesia and those actions directly and immediately involved in the act), but a physician may not decline postoperative care of a patient who might experience complications of the procedure.

Although the conscientious objector has the right to decline participation in the requested intervention, he or she should not berate or obstruct the patient in receiving that intervention from others. Health care organizations may legitimately expect the physician to refer the patient to another provider, or at least to institutional resources that can assist the patient in securing legally sanctioned interventions, such as a patient affairs office or an administrator.

KEY FACTS

✓ Decision-making capacity, determined by the physician, should not be confused with competence, a legal determination

✓ A patient's decision-making capacity needs to be assessed; incapacity should not be presumed

✓ Informed consent has 3 required elements—patient decision-making capacity, patient voluntariness, and accurate and sufficient information

✓ If a patient requests an intervention that a physician finds morally objectionable, the physician can refuse that intervention but not abandon the patient or other care

Justice

The principle of justice expresses that every patient deserves and must be fairly provided optimal care as warranted by the underlying medical condition and within the constraints of available resources. The identification of optimal medical care should be based on the patient's medical need and the perceived medical benefit to the patient. The patient's social status, ability to pay, or perceived social worth should not dictate the quality or quantity of medical care. The physician's clear-cut responsibility is to the patient's well-being (beneficence). Physicians should not make decisions about individual patient care based on larger societal needs, because the bedside is not the place for general policy decisions. Nevertheless, physicians should be conscious of larger societal needs and should be leaders in developing fair policies to regulate the allocation of scarce or costly resources, but these endeavors should take place away from the bedside and an individual physician-patient relationship.

Ethics, Law, and Death

Definition of Death

Death is the irreversible cessation of circulatory and respiratory function or the irreversible cessation of all functions of the entire brain, including the brainstem. Clinical criteria (at times supported by electroencephalographic testing or assessment of cerebral perfusion) permit the reliable diagnosis of brain death.

> ### Key Definition
>
> Death: *irreversible cessation of circulatory and respiratory function, or irreversible cessation of all functions of entire brain, including brainstem.*

The family should be informed of brain death but should not be asked to decide whether medical therapy should be continued. One exception is when the patient's surrogate (or the patient, via an advance directive) permits certain decisions, such as organ donation, in the case of brain death.

Once it is ascertained that the patient is "brain dead" and that no further therapy can be offered, the primary physician, preferably after consultation with another physician involved in the patient's care, may withdraw supportive measures. This approach is accepted throughout the United States, with the exception of some states, which have modified their definition-of-death statutes to allow a religious exemption for groups (such as Orthodox Jews) that do not accept brain death as a valid criterion for death. In these states, continued care may be requested of the caregivers until circulatory and respiratory function collapses.

Physician-Assisted Death

All 4 principles of medical ethics have an impact on the issue of physician aid in dying (previously referred to as physician-assisted suicide) and euthanasia. Historically, the medical profession has taken a strong stand against physicians directly killing patients, but this prohibition has been challenged on the basis of patient autonomy, beneficence or compassion, and other grounds. The American Medical Association, the American College of Physicians, and other large professional medical groups have maintained a stance against physician aid in dying and euthanasia.

In 1997, the US Supreme Court ruled that states may maintain laws prohibiting euthanasia and physician aid in dying but may also pass laws allowing these practices. Although the Court did not find a right to physician-assisted death, it emphasized the patient's right to adequate, aggressive pain control, even if it might shorten the patient's life. In 1997, the people of Oregon reiterated their support for physician aid in dying by reapproving a referendum first passed in 1994 legalizing physician aid in dying but prohibiting euthanasia. The Oregon law requires that the patient 1) have a terminal condition, 2) be decisionally capable, 3) have initiated 2 verbal requests and 1 written request for a prescription for a lethal overdose, 4) undergo a second-opinion consultation, 5) receive appropriate psychiatric intervention if perceived to be depressed, and 6) undergo a 15-day waiting period after the request has been made to allow the patient to change his or her mind. Similar decisions have been made in Washington State, Montana, and Vermont. At the time of publication, physician aid in dying is illegal in the 46 other states and euthanasia is illegal throughout the United States.

Regardless of one's position on physician aid in dying and euthanasia, physicians are obligated to address the underlying concerns that lead patients and physicians to believe that physician aid in dying and euthanasia are necessary. Physicians should be acquainted with appropriate means of pain management and palliative care and treat patients' distressing symptoms.

30 | Men's Health[a]

THOMAS J. BECKMAN, MD

Benign Prostatic Hyperplasia

Benign prostatic hyperplasia (BPH) is common among older men. The prostate is the size of a walnut (20 cm³) in men younger than 30 years and gradually increases in size, leading to BPH in most men older than 60 years. BPH results from epithelial and stromal cell growth in the prostate, which in turn causes urinary outflow resistance. Over time, this resistance leads to detrusor muscle dysfunction, urinary retention, and lower urinary tract symptoms (LUTS), such as urgency, frequency, and nocturia. There is evidence that BPH progresses when left untreated. This progression is manifested as worsening prostate symptom scores (see "History and Physical Examination" section), decreasing urinary flow rates, and increased risk of acute urinary retention. Other complications of BPH include urinary tract infections, obstructive nephropathy, and recurrent hematuria.

Diagnosing BPH is challenging because prostate size correlates poorly with LUTS and numerous conditions other than BPH cause LUTS (Table 30.1). Nonetheless, assessing symptom severity, identifying prostatic enlargement on digital rectal examination (DRE), and documenting decreased urinary flow rates with increased postvoid residual volumes yield accurate diagnoses in most cases.

> ### Key Definition
>
> Benign prostatic hyperplasia: *urinary outflow resistance that results from epithelial and stromal cell growth in the prostate.*

History and Physical Examination

When obtaining a history, consider the patient's age. Because prostate size increases with age, LUTS are most likely due to BPH in men older than 50 years and most likely due to other conditions in men younger than 40 years. Reviewing medications is also essential because many medications cause LUTS by affecting detrusor muscle and urinary sphincter function: 1) anticholinergic and antimuscarinic medications decrease detrusor muscle tone, 2) sympathomimetic medications increase urethral sphincter tone, and 3) diuretics increase urinary frequency (Table 30.1). Additionally, over-the-counter cold medications may cause LUTS by various mechanisms. When older men with subclinical BPH simply discontinue taking new medications, LUTS often resolve. Finally, a focused review of systems should identify fever, hematuria (indicating urothelial malignancy), urethral instrumentation or sexually transmitted diseases (suggesting the possibility of urethral stricture), sleep disturbances, patterns of fluid intake, and use of alcohol and caffeine.

The American Urological Association International Prostate Symptom Score (AUA/IPSS) is an objective measure of LUTS associated with BPH. The AUA/IPSS aids in diagnosing BPH and following the progression of BPH over time (Figure 30.1). Numerous studies have shown the reliability and validity of the AUA/IPSS. The AUA/IPSS questionnaire asks 7 questions about the following symptoms: frequency, nocturia, weak stream, hesitancy, intermittency, incomplete bladder emptying, and urgency. Each question is answered on a 5-point scale. When the responses to the 7 questions are summed, a score of 0 to 7 represents mild symptoms of BPH, 8 to 19 represents moderate symptoms, and 20 to 35 represents severe symptoms.

[a] Portions previously published in Beckman TJ, Mynderse LA. Evaluation and medical management of benign prostatic hyperplasia. Mayo Clin Proc. 2005 Oct;80(10):1356–62. Errata in: Mayo Clin Proc. 2005 Nov;80(11):1533; and Beckman TJ, Abu-Lebdeh HS, Mynderse LA. Evaluation and medical management of erectile dysfunction. Mayo Clin Proc. 2006 Mar;81(3):385–90. Used with permission of Mayo Foundation for Medical Education and Research

Table 30.1 • Differential Diagnosis for Lower Urinary Tract Symptoms

Category	Examples	Comments
Malignant	Adenocarcinoma of the prostate Transitional cell carcinoma of the bladder Squamous cell carcinoma of the penis	Men should be offered PSA testing in conjunction with DRE With microhematuria on urinalysis, consider urothelial malignancy
Infectious	Cystitis Prostatitis Sexually transmitted diseases (eg, chlamydial infection, gonorrhea)	Urinalysis and urinary Gram stain are useful in evaluating for cystitis Prostatic massage specimens (VB3) assist in diagnosis of prostatitis Sexually transmitted diseases may cause LUTS from urethral scarring and stricture
Neurologic	Spinal cord injury Cauda equina syndrome Stroke Parkinsonism Diabetic autonomic neuropathy Multiple sclerosis Alzheimer disease	Primary mechanisms for neurologic causes of LUTS are detrusor weakness or uninhibited detrusor contractions (or both) Alzheimer disease can cause functional urinary incontinence
Medical	Poorly controlled diabetes mellitus Diabetes insipidus Congestive heart failure Hypercalcemia Obstructive sleep apnea	Medical conditions associated with urinary frequency are often overlooked causes of LUTS
Iatrogenic	Prostatectomy Cystectomy Traumatic urethrocystoscopic procedures Radiation cystitis	Surgery sometimes causes neurologic impairment Traumatic urethrocystoscopic procedures can cause scarring and urethral strictures
Anatomical	BPH Ureteral and bladder stones	Hematuria may be seen on urinalysis Consider urinary cytologic, cystoscopic, and renal imaging studies
Behavioral	Polydipsia Excessive alcohol or caffeine consumption	Consider assessing serum sodium level Voiding diary may provide useful information about fluid intake
Pharmacologic	Diuretics (eg, furosemide, hydrochlorothiazide) Sympathomimetics (eg, ephedrine, dextroamphetamine) Anticholinergics (eg, oxybutynin, amantadine) Antimuscarinics (eg, diphenhydramine, amitriptyline) Over-the-counter decongestants	Diuretics increase urinary frequency Sympathomimetic medications increase urethral resistance Anticholinergic and antimuscarinic medications decrease detrusor contractility Over-the-counter medications may cause LUTS by various mechanisms
Other	Overactive bladder	UDS can help distinguish BPH from isolated detrusor dysfunction

Abbreviations: BPH, benign prostatic hyperplasia; DRE, digital rectal examination; LUTS, lower urinary tract symptoms; PSA, prostate-specific antigen; UDS, urodynamic studies; VB3, voiding bottle 3 (postprostatic massage) urine specimen.

Adapted from Beckman TJ, Mynderse LA. Evaluation and medical management of benign prostatic hyperplasia. Mayo Clin Proc. 2005 Oct;80(10):1356–62. Erratum in: Mayo Clin Proc. 2005 Nov;80(11):1533. Used with permission of Mayo Foundation for Medical Education and Research.

Patients with LUTS should be evaluated for neurologic deficits, especially if the patients have a history or presenting symptoms that suggest a neurologic disorder. In such cases, useful findings include saddle anesthesia, decreased rectal sphincter tone, absent cremasteric reflex, or lower extremity neurologic abnormalities. On examination of the abdomen, masses resulting from a renal tumor, hydronephrosis, or bladder distention may be detected. The penis should be examined for pathologic changes. DRE findings most consistent with BPH are symmetrical enlargement and firm consistency, often likened to the thenar muscle or the

tip of the nose. In contrast, findings consistent with adenocarcinoma of the prostate are prostate asymmetry, induration, and nodularity, often likened to the consistency of a knuckle or the forehead.

Evaluation

A specimen for urinalysis should be obtained routinely when evaluating men who have LUTS. Urinalysis findings may include pyuria and bacteriuria, which suggest infection; hematuria, which suggests inflammation or urothelial

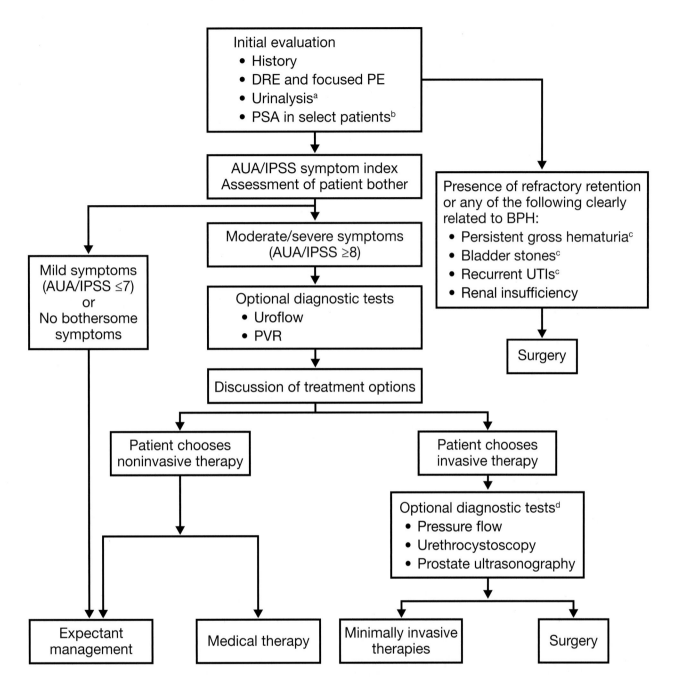

Figure 30.1 *A Treatment Algorithm for Benign Prostatic Hyperplasia (BPH). Treatment decisions are based partly on patient symptom severity as determined with the American Urological Association International Prostate Symptom Score (AUA/IPSS). DRE indicates digital rectal examination; PE, physical examination; PSA, prostate-specific antigen; PVR, postvoid residual urine; UTI, urinary tract infection.*

[a] In patients with clinically significant prostatic bleeding, a course of a 5α-reductase inhibitor may be used. If bleeding persists, tissue ablative surgery is indicated.

[b] Patients with at least a 10-year life expectancy for whom knowledge of the presence of prostate cancer would change management or patients for whom the PSA measurement may change the management of voiding symptoms.

[c] After exhausting other therapeutic options.

[d] Some diagnostic tests are used in predicting response to therapy. Pressure-flow studies are most useful in men before surgery.

(Adapted from AUA Practice Guidelines Committee. AUA guideline on management of benign prostatic hyperplasia [2003]. Chapter 1. Diagnosis and treatment recommendations. J Urol. 2003 Aug;170[2 Pt 1]:530–47. Used with permission.)

malignancy; and active urine sediment, which suggests a possible postobstructive nephropathy.

Optional studies include measuring serum creatinine and prostate-specific antigen (PSA) concentrations. The PSA measurement is optional because the results do not help discriminate BPH from adenocarcinoma of the prostate. Nevertheless, because LUTS may indicate prostate cancer, it is appropriate to routinely offer PSA testing. Although there is conflicting evidence regarding the utility of screening for prostate cancer with PSA, screening for prostate cancer with DRE and PSA may be appropriate for men aged 50 to 75 years, depending on the patient's preference after engaging in shared decision making with his physician.

Methods for interpreting serum PSA levels are listed in Box 30.1.

A uroflow study with ultrasonographic measurement of residual urine volume is an objective, noninvasive way to evaluate men presenting with LUTS. An accurate study requires urine volumes of at least 150 mL. Men with BPH often have peak flow rates less than 15 mL/s and increased residual urine volume (Figure 30.2). Notably, men with detrusor dysfunction also have abnormal results. Consequently, as with any test, interpreting the results of uroflow studies depends on the pretest probability of disease. If the pretest probability of BPH is high, an abnormal test result is useful for confirming the diagnosis. But if the pretest probability is intermediate, an abnormal uroflow result is less useful. In such cases, patients may need to undergo complete urodynamic studies to further distinguish BPH from other causes of LUTS.

Medical Management of BPH

Although this chapter focuses on the medical management of BPH, clinicians should recognize the indications for urologic referral and consideration of invasive therapy. These indications are moderate or severe symptoms, persistent

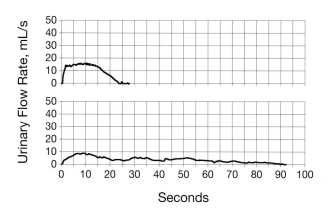

Figure 30.2 *Uroflow Tracings. Top, Uroflow tracing from a young, asymptomatic man. Note the parabolic flow curve and peak flow rate greater than 15 mL/s. Bottom, Uroflow tracing from an elderly man with benign prostatic hyperplasia. Note the prolonged voiding time and peak flow rate less than 10 mL/s. This patient's ultrasonographically measured residual urine volume was 100 mL.*
(Adapted from Beckman TJ, Mynderse LA. Evaluation and medical management of benign prostatic hyperplasia. Mayo Clin Proc. 2005 Oct;80[10]:1356–62. Erratum in: Mayo Clin Proc. 2005 Nov;80[11]:1533. Used with permission of Mayo Foundation for Medical Education and Research.)

gross hematuria, urinary retention, renal insufficiency due to BPH, recurrent urinary tract infections, and bladder calculi.

Expectant management is reasonable for patients with mild or moderate symptoms. These patients are monitored at least yearly or when new symptoms arise. In addition, these patients may be advised to practice scheduled voiding (every 3 hours during the day), to avoid excess evening fluid intake, and to be aware of potential adverse effects of over-the-counter decongestants.

Nearly all patients presenting with BPH are candidates for medical therapy. Moreover, medical therapy has replaced interventional therapy as the most common treatment of BPH. Prescription medications available for treating BPH are α_1-adrenergic antagonists (eg, tamsulosin) and 5α-reductase inhibitors (eg, finasteride).

The α_1-adrenergic antagonist medications work on the dynamic component of bladder outlet obstruction by decreasing prostatic smooth muscle tone. They are the first line of medical therapy for most men with BPH. Although all α_1-adrenergic antagonist medications are equally efficacious in treating BPH, terazosin and doxazosin are more likely to cause adverse effects (mainly orthostatic hypotension) than other medications in this class. Other common adverse effects of α_1-adrenergic antagonists include dizziness, hypotension, edema, palpitations, erectile dysfunction (ED), and fatigue.

The second class of prescription medications for treating BPH, the 5α-reductase inhibitors, act on the static

---

Box 30.1 • Methods for Interpreting Serum Prostate-Specfic Antigen Levels

Cutoff value. The traditional cutoff is 4 ng/mL

Age-adjusted values. Age-adjusted normal limits are commonly used because prostate volume increases with age

Ratio of free prostate-specific antigen (PSA) to total PSA. The level of free (unbound) PSA is lower in men with adenocarcinoma of the prostate; therefore, a low ratio of free PSA to total PSA is more consistent with prostate adenocarcinoma than with benign prostatic hyperplasia

PSA velocity. A rapidly increasing PSA value is more suggestive of carcinoma than benign prostatic hyperplasia; in particular, an annual PSA velocity greater than 0.75 ng/mL is considered abnormal

(anatomical) component of bladder outlet obstruction. These medications decrease the conversion of testosterone to dihydrotestosterone in the prostate, thereby limiting prostate growth. Two commonly prescribed 5α-reductase inhibitors are finasteride and dutasteride.

The following points about finasteride are important: it is most useful in men with severe BPH and large prostates (>40 cm³), it may need to be taken for more than 6 months before an optimal drug effect is apparent, and it can significantly decrease serum PSA. For this reason, experts recommend correcting the serum PSA value in men taking finasteride by multiplying the value by 2. Adverse effects with finasteride are uncommon. The most frequent adverse effects are related to sexual dysfunction and include decreased libido, ejaculatory dysfunction, and ED. Finally, evidence supports the use of α₁-adrenergic antagonists in combination with 5α-reductase inhibitors in men with inadequate responses to either drug alone.

Herbal medications used to treat BPH include derivatives from African star grass, African plum tree bark, rye grass pollens, stinging nettle, and cactus flower. The most commonly used alternative treatment of BPH is saw palmetto (*Serenoa repens*). Many mechanisms for saw palmetto have been entertained, yet none are proven. Saw palmetto is considered safe, and studies including randomized trials and a meta-analysis have shown that it compares favorably with finasteride and that, compared with placebo, saw palmetto improves flow and decreases symptoms.

KEY FACTS

- ✓ In men with BPH, prostate size on examination correlates poorly with LUTS
- ✓ In men presenting with LUTS, the test that should always be considered is urinalysis with microscopy
- ✓ Refer men with BPH to a urologist for possible invasive therapy if they have moderate or severe symptoms, persistent gross hematuria, urinary retention, renal insufficiency due to BPH, recurrent urinary tract infections, or bladder calculi
- ✓ Nearly all patients with BPH are candidates for medical therapy—α₁-adrenergic antagonist medications are considered first-line therapy

Erectile Dysfunction

Male sexual dysfunction includes ED, decreased libido, anatomical abnormalities (eg, Peyronie disease), and ejaculatory dysfunction. **ED**, defined as the inability to achieve erections firm enough for vaginal penetration, affects millions of men in the United States. The Massachusetts Male Aging Study showed that the prevalence of ED increased by age: approximately 50% of men experienced ED at age 50 years, and nearly 70% at age 70.

Key Definition

Erectile dysfunction: *the inability to achieve erections firm enough for vaginal penetration.*

KEY FACTS

- ✓ Risk factors for ED and cardiovascular disease are nearly identical; risk of ED is lower in men who are physically active and have normal BMI
- ✓ Patients should be instructed to take PDE-5 inhibitors on an empty stomach at least 1 hour before sexual activity
- ✓ Men who can achieve 5–6 METs on cardiac stress testing without evidence of ischemia likely can safely engage in sexual activity and take PDE-5 inhibitors
- ✓ Testosterone replacement has not been shown to improve erectile function in men with normal serum testosterone levels

Erectile physiology includes hormonal, vascular, psychological, neurologic, and cellular components. Testosterone is primarily responsible for maintaining sexual desire (libido), and hypogonadism is sometimes associated with ED. Other hormonal causes of ED include hyperthyroidism and prolactinomas. The penile blood supply begins at the internal pudendal artery, which branches into the penile artery, ultimately giving rise to the cavernous, dorsal, and bulbourethral arteries. Psychogenic erections, triggered by fantasy or visual stimulation, are mediated by sympathetic input from the thoracolumbar chain (T11 through L2). Reflex erections are caused by tactile stimulation and are mediated by the parasympathetic nervous system (S2 through S4). Overall, parasympathetic signals are responsible for erection, and sympathetic signals are responsible for ejaculation.

Sexual arousal and parasympathetic signals to the penis initiate intracellular changes necessary for erection (Figure 30.3). Endothelial cells release nitric oxide, which in turn increases the level of cyclic guanosine monophosphate (cGMP). Increased levels of cGMP cause relaxation of arterial and cavernosal smooth muscle and increased penile blood flow. As the intracavernosal pressure increases, penile emissary veins are compressed, thus restricting venous return from the penis. The combination of increased arterial flow and decreased venous return results in erection. This process is reversed by the activity of cGMP phosphodiesterase (PDE) type 5 (PDE-5), which breaks down cGMP, resulting in cessation of erection.

Although ED is generally not an indicator of serious diseases, it is strongly associated with cardiovascular risk factors. In fact, the Health Professionals Follow-up Study showed that

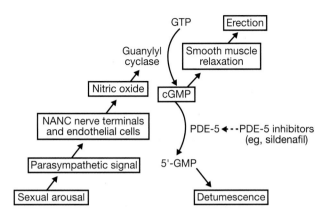

Figure 30.3 Mechanism for Penile Erection and the Molecular Activity of Phosphodiesterase Type 5 (PDE-5) Inhibitor Medications. cGMP indicates cyclic guanosine monophosphate; GMP, guanosine monophosphate; GTP, guanosine triphosphate; NANC, nonadrenergic noncholinergic. (Adapted from Beckman TJ, Abu-Lebdeh HS, Mynderse LA. Evaluation and medical management of erectile dysfunction. Mayo Clin Proc. 2006 Mar;81[3]:385–90. Used with permission of Mayo Foundation for Medical Education and Research.)

risk factors for ED and cardiovascular disease were nearly identical and that physically active men had a 30% lower risk of ED than inactive men. Therefore, men with diabetes mellitus, hypertension, and coronary artery disease are at increased risk for ED. Not surprisingly, randomized controlled trial data show that erectile function significantly improves in obese men who lose weight through diet and exercise.

Evaluating Patients Who Have ED

History and Physical Examination

Certain questions should be asked routinely when taking a history from patients who have ED (Table 30.2). Especially important are questions about common ED risk factors, such as cardiovascular disease, smoking, diabetes mellitus, hypertension, hyperlipidemia, prescription medications, alcohol use, recreational drug use, and mood disorders. In addition, validated questionnaires, such as the International Index of Erectile Function, are useful for monitoring patients' responses to ED treatments.

A complete multisystem examination may identify indicators of cardiovascular disease (eg, obesity, hypertension, femoral arterial bruits), endocrinopathies (eg, visual field defects, thyromegaly, gynecomastia), or neurologic abnormalities (eg, decreased sphincter tone, absent bulbocavernosus reflex, saddle anesthesia). The penis should be palpated in the stretched position to detect fibrous plaques consistent with Peyronie disease, which may be present on the dorsum and base of the penis. The testicles should be evaluated for masses (indicating malignancy) and decreased size and soft consistency (indicating hypogonadism). Finally, examining

patients with ED is often a good opportunity to screen for prostate cancer and to assess for benign glandular enlargement.

Laboratory Testing

Although disease-specific testing is favored, serum testosterone levels are often measured in a men's health practice. If a patient is hypogonadal, serum prolactin and luteinizing hormone levels should be assessed. If the prolactin level is elevated or the luteinizing hormone level is not elevated, magnetic resonance imaging of the brain should be used to rule out a pituitary adenoma. Additional useful testing that pertains to ED risk factors includes measuring the levels of fasting glucose, fasting lipids, and thyrotropin.

Medical Management of ED

PDE-5 Inhibitors

PDE-5 inhibitor medications are the first line of therapy for most men with ED. PDE-5 inhibitors have revolutionized the treatment of ED since the introduction of sildenafil in 1998, and experts have observed that these medications have considerably affected (both positively and negatively) the sexual culture of older people. There were initial concerns about cardiovascular risks associated with PDE-5 inhibitors, but studies have shown that these medications are generally safe, even in patients with stable coronary artery disease who are not taking nitrate therapy.

Three commonly prescribed PDE-5 inhibitor medications are sildenafil (Viagra), vardenafil (Levitra), and tadalafil (Cialis). These medications inhibit cGMP PDE-5, thereby increasing cGMP levels and shifting the physiologic balance in favor of erection (Figure 30.3). In the absence of comparative clinical trials and meta-analyses, it appears that each of these medications is equally efficacious. Tadalafil has a longer half-life than sildenafil or vardenafil, which affords more spontaneity to tadalafil users (up to 36 hours). Patients should be instructed to take PDE-5 inhibitors at least 1 hour before sexual activity on an empty stomach. Patients should also realize that PDE-5 inhibitors will not cause erections in the absence of sexual arousal (unlike intraurethral alprostadil and penile injection therapy).

The PDE-5 inhibitors have several common adverse effects due to the presence of PDE throughout the body: headache, flushing, gastric upset, diarrhea, nasal congestion, and lightheadedness. A unique reaction to sildenafil is blue-tinged vision, which is probably related to the activity of sildenafil on PDE type 6 (PDE-6) in the retina. This reaction resolves with discontinuation of therapy. It is noteworthy that some varieties of retinitis pigmentosa have a PDE-6 gene defect. Consequently, patients with retinitis pigmentosa should not receive medications from the PDE-5 inhibitor class.

A contraindication to the use of PDE-5 inhibitors is nitrate therapy. Indeed, patients treated for acute coronary syndromes should not receive nitrate therapy within 24 hours of

Table 30.2 • Questions to Ask When Taking a History From Patients With Erectile Dysfunction

Question	Comment
Do you have difficulty achieving erections or difficulty with orgasms and ejaculation?	Sexual dysfunction includes various diagnoses, so it is important to determine whether the patient's primary complaint is ED
How often do you achieve erections? Are your erections firm enough for vaginal penetration?	Often patients are not satisfied with the quality of their erections, yet if patients can achieve erections adequately firm for vaginal penetration most of the time, their complaints are not classically defined as ED
Did your ED occur suddenly? Do you have nocturnal erections? Do you feel anxious or depressed? Do you and your partner have a satisfactory relationship?	The sudden onset of ED and the persistence of nocturnal erections indicate an inorganic (psychogenic) cause; in such cases, physicians should explore the psychosocial context of the patient's sexual history, such as whether the patient feels anxious or depressed or whether the patient is experiencing interpersonal relationship difficulties
Do you have a desire to engage in sexual activity?	Decreased sexual desire may indicate hypogonadism; if patients are not interested in sexual activity, serum testosterone levels should be assessed and mood disorders should be considered
Do you have penile curvature or pain with erections?	A positive response to this question may indicate Peyronie disease, which is sometimes detected on physical examination; identifying Peyronie disease is important because it precludes intraurethral alprostadil and penile injection therapy
Can you engage in vigorous physical activity without chest pain or unusual dyspnea?	PDE-5 inhibitor medications will be considered in most patients, and sexual activity is associated with cardiovascular stress; hence, a history should be obtained to identify undiagnosed ischemic heart disease or to assess the stability of known ischemic heart disease
What medications are you taking?	Numerous medications are associated with ED, especially antihypertensives and psychotropics; medications inhibiting cytochrome P-450 (eg, ritonavir) should be identified because they increase plasma levels of PDE-5 inhibitor medications; an absolute contraindication to PDE-5 inhibitors is the concurrent use of nitrates (eg, isosorbide mononitrate); combining PDE-5 inhibitors with α_1-adrenergic antagonists can cause hypotension
How much alcohol do you consume? Do you use illegal drugs?	Substance abuse, including alcoholism, is commonly overlooked as a cause of ED
Which ED treatments have you already tried?	Knowing which medications patients have tried will help physicians decide the next therapeutic plan
Do you have a history of diseases involving your heart, blood vessels, nervous system, or hormones?	Common risk factors for ED should be identified
Do you have a history of hypertension, hyperlipidemia, diabetes mellitus, or tobacco abuse?	
Do you have a history of penile trauma or genitourinary surgery?	
Do you ride a bicycle regularly?	Prolonged, frequent bicycle riding can cause excessive pudendal pressure, leading to ED

Abbreviations: ED, erectile dysfunction; PDE-5, phosphodiesterase type 5.

Adapted from Beckman TJ, Abu-Lebdeh HS, Mynderse LA. Evaluation and medical management of erectile dysfunction. Mayo Clin Proc. 2006 Mar;81(3):385–90. Used with permission of Mayo Foundation for Medical Education and Research.

taking sildenafil or vardenafil and within 48 hours of taking tadalafil. Physicians should also be cautious about prescribing PDE-5 inhibitors for patients with poorly controlled blood pressure or multidrug antihypertensive regimens. In patients with known or suspected ischemic heart disease, cardiac stress testing is useful for stratifying the risk of PDE-5 inhibitor therapy; patients who achieve 5 to 6 metabolic equivalent tasks without ischemia probably have a low risk of complications from engaging in sexual activity.

Treatment options for patients who have not had a response to PDE-5 inhibitors or who cannot take PDE-5 inhibitors include intraurethral alprostadil and penile injection therapy. These are generally more effective than PDE-5 inhibitors, but their obvious drawback is inconvenience. Contraindications for these treatments include blood cell dyscrasias (eg, sickle cell disease, leukemia, multiple myeloma) and penile deformity, especially Peyronie disease. Anticoagulation is an additional contraindication to penile injection therapy. There is inadequate information on the safety of using PDE-5 inhibitors in combination with injection therapy, and hence, their coadministration is not advised.

Intraurethral Alprostadil

Intraurethral alprostadil (commercially available as MUSE [Medicated Urethral System for Erection]) is effective in men of all ages who have ED from various causes. Intraurethral alprostadil is inserted into the urethral meatus at the tip of the penis with an applicator. Patients should be instructed on the application technique. Additionally, owing to the risk of syncope, administration of the first dose should be supervised by a health care provider. The most common adverse effect is urethral and genital burning, and hypotension can occur. As for all medical ED treatments, patients are educated about priapism, and they are instructed to go to an emergency department if they have erections for more than 4 hours.

Intracavernosal Penile Injections

Intracavernosal penile injection, an efficacious and generally safe therapy, is the most effective medical treatment of ED. In practice, a triple-therapy combination of alprostadil, papaverine, and phentolamine is usually used. These medications increase penile blood flow. Specifically, alprostadil and papaverine cause relaxation of cavernosal smooth muscle and penile blood vessels, and phentolamine antagonizes α-adrenoreceptors. Although many patients are hesitant to attempt penile injection, this method is associated with minimal discomfort.

Testosterone

Various hormonal therapies, including testosterone, were once widely used to treat ED. The penile nitric oxide pathway is testosterone dependent, and for this reason, screening for low serum testosterone levels is necessary in men who have no response to medical therapy with sildenafil or whose presentation suggests hypogonadism. Hypogonadism is diagnosed by the presence of hypogonadal symptoms (eg, decreased libido, cognitive decline, generalized muscle weakness) and by morning fasting total testosterone levels less than 200 ng/dL on at least 2 separate occasions. In hypogonadal men, PDE-5 inhibitor therapy in combination with testosterone is often effective. Testosterone replacement alone increases sexual interest, nocturnal erections, and frequency of sexual intercourse. Nevertheless, testosterone replacement has not been shown to improve erectile function in men with normal serum testosterone levels.

Testosterone is available by injection, skin patch, topical gel, or buccal oral tablets. Testosterone therapy is associated with potential risks. For example, prolonged use of high-dose, orally active 17α-alkyl androgens (eg, methyltestosterone) is associated with hepatic neoplasms, fulminant hepatitis, and cholestatic jaundice. Other risks of exogenous testosterone therapy include gynecomastia, alterations in the lipid profile (mainly decreased high-density lipoprotein cholesterol), erythropoietin-mediated polycythemia, edema, sleep apnea, hypertension, infertility (through suppression of spermatogenesis), and BPH. Exogenous testosterone also increases the risk of prostate carcinoma. Although testosterone replacement may not cause prostate carcinoma, it could stimulate the growth of existing occult prostate cancer. For this reason, all men should have screening for prostate cancer with DRE and serum PSA before using exogenous testosterone.

The goal of testosterone replacement is to increase serum testosterone levels to the low or middle portion of the reference range. A recommended treatment is to apply topical testosterone, 1% gel at a starting dose of 5 g daily, to the shoulders, upper parts of the arms, or abdomen. A total testosterone level may be reassessed as soon as 14 days after starting treatment. The patient's therapeutic response and testosterone level are reassessed at 3 months, and decisions are then made about whether to continue using testosterone and whether to adjust the dose.

Although patients who have serum testosterone levels in the normal range as a result of testosterone replacement therapy should not be at risk for adverse effects, monitoring patients during testosterone therapy is essential. Baseline determinations include whether the patient has a history of prostate cancer, BPH, obstructive sleep apnea, liver disease, hypertension, or hyperlipidemia. Baseline testing includes a complete blood cell count and levels of serum PSA, lipids, and liver transaminases. PSA levels and prostate-related symptoms should be assessed at 6 months and then annually, and patients with elevated or increasing PSA levels should not be treated with testosterone. The hematocrit and levels of lipids should be monitored biannually for the first 18 months and annually thereafter; the testosterone dose should be decreased or therapy discontinued if hematocrit values are greater than 50%. Finally, patient response to therapy and adverse effects are monitored quarterly during the first year of treatment.

Nonmedical Treatments

Other ED treatments include topical vacuum pump devices and surgically inserted inflatable penile implants. Penile pumps work by creating a vacuum around the penis, thus drawing blood into the penis. When the penis is engorged with blood, an elastic ring is placed over the base of the penis and the pump is removed. Importantly, patients should use vacuum pump devices with vacuum limiters, which prevent negative pressure injury to the penis. Penile implants are generally not offered unless patients have no response to medical treatments, including maximal-strength injection therapy.

31 Otolaryngology and Ophthalmology

NERISSA M. COLLINS, MD

Otolaryngology

Otitis Externa

Acute Otitis Externa

Acute otitis externa, also known as swimmer's ear, is an infection of the external auditory canal. A moist environment, eczematous dermatitis, repeated insertion of foreign bodies (eg, cotton swabs), and psoriasis can predispose to otitis externa. Most patients present with otalgia and otorrhea. On examination, the tympanic membrane appears normal, but the external auditory canal is erythematous, often with exudate. Typical examination findings include pain with pressure on the tragus and with traction of the pinna. Management of otitis externa includes avoidance of excessive water exposure and application of topical antibiotics and corticosteroids.

Malignant Otitis Externa

Malignant otitis externa is a feared complication of acute otitis externa in diabetic patients and other immunocompromised patients. It is typically caused by *Pseudomonas aeruginosa*. The infection can penetrate the cartilaginous structures of the ear canal into the temporal bone, where it causes osteomyelitis. Patients present with severe pain, fever, and possibly cranial neuropathies. On examination, granulation tissue is often present in the external auditory canal. The condition requires emergent care with intravenous antibiotics and sometimes surgical débridement of the skull base osteomyelitis.

Pharyngitis

Most cases of pharyngitis are viral. The goal is to identify patients with group A streptococcal (GAS) pharyngitis and to treat them to prevent rheumatic fever. With the Centor clinical prediction criteria for the diagnosis of GAS pharyngitis, 1 point is assigned for each of the following: fever, anterior cervical lymphadenopathy, tonsillar exudates, absence of cough.

With the modified Centor criteria, a point is added if the patient is younger than 18 years and subtracted if the patient is older than 44 years. Patients who have no more than 1 Centor criterion have a low probability of GAS pharyngitis and should be observed. Most guidelines suggest rapid streptococcal antigen testing and treating with antibiotics only if test results are positive and 2 or 3 criteria are present. If all 4 criteria are present, empirical antibiotic therapy is indicated. Recommended first-line agents include penicillin or amoxicillin for 10 days. In patients with a nonanaphylactic allergy to penicillin, a first-generation cephalosporin for 10 days, clindamycin or clarithromycin for 10 days, or azithromycin for 5 days can be used.

Ophthalmology

Red Eye

The red eye is a common ocular complaint. While the majority of causes are benign, the clinician should be able to recognize the syndromes on examination to determine when an emergent referral to an ophthalmologist is indicated.

Subconjunctival Hemorrhage

Subconjunctival hemorrhage (Figure 31.1) is typically unilateral and painless. It may follow trauma, coughing, straining, or emesis. Subconjunctival bleeding also occurs in patients with uncontrolled arterial hypertension, in patients who are receiving anticoagulants or antiplatelet agents, and in patients with intrinsic disorders of coagulation. It resolves spontaneously and requires only reassurance.

Conjunctivitis

Conjunctivitis can result from allergic, viral, and bacterial causes. Patients with allergic conjunctivitis present with

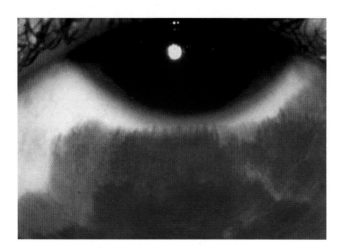

Figure 31.1 Subconjunctival Hemorrhage. The sharply de-marcated hemorrhage prevents visualization of underlying structures. There is no inflammation in contiguous areas. This disorder does not affect vision and almost always clears spontaneously.
(Adapted from Leibowitz HM. The red eye. N Engl J Med. 2000 Aug 3;343[5]:345–51. Used with permission.)

bilaterally red, itchy eyes with excessive tearing. Other allergic symptoms, such as sneezing and nasal conges-tion, typically accompany the eye symptoms. Systemic or topical antihistamines are usually effective for managing symptoms.

Viral conjunctivitis causes bilateral ocular redness, irri-tation, and excessive tearing. Preauricular lymphadenopa-thy may be present. Viral conjunctivitis is usually caused by an adenovirus and is highly contagious. It is a self-limited condition, and no antimicrobials are warranted.

Patients with bacterial conjunctivitis usually present with acute unilateral redness, irritation, and discharge. The infection warrants topical antibacterial therapy. Failure to resolve within 7 to 10 days should prompt consultation with an ophthalmologist. Chlamydial and gonorrheal con-junctivitis should be suspected in high-risk patients.

KEY FACTS

✓ Predisposing factors for otitis externa—moist environment, eczematous dermatitis, foreign bodies (eg, cotton swabs), psoriasis

✓ Malignant otitis externa calls for emergent care—intravenous antibiotics and sometimes surgical débridement

✓ For GAS pharyngitis, penicillin and amoxicillin are the recommended first-line agents

✓ Usual presenting symptoms of bacterial conjunctivitis—acute unilateral redness, irritation, and discharge

---

Blepharitis

A **hordeolum**, or **stye**, is an infectious, painful, erythema-tous, localized nodule of the eyelid. An external hordeo-lum is caused by a blockage and subsequent infection of the glands of the eyelid. An internal hordeolum is caused by infection of the meibomian glands. *Staphylococcus aureus* is responsible for the majority of these infections. Although most of the lesions drain spontaneously, some require incision and drainage by an ophthalmologist. Application of warm compresses may assist in spontane-ous drainage. Antibiotics are not generally required unless the infection has spread beyond the nodule.

Key Definition

Hordeolum, *or* stye: *an infectious, painful, erythematous, localized nodule of the eyelid.*

A chalazion is a more chronic, rarely painful, and always internal noninfectious eyelid disorder. It is caused by gran-ulomatous inflammation in the meibomian glands. It may be removed if bothersome or large.

Episcleritis

Patients with episcleritis (Figure 31.2) present with sec-torial injection of the episcleral vessels. Most cases are idiopathic, but sometimes there is an associated dis-ease. Typically, the diseases associated with episcleritis are the same as those associated with scleritis. The con-dition is usually self-limited, and an oral nonsteroidal

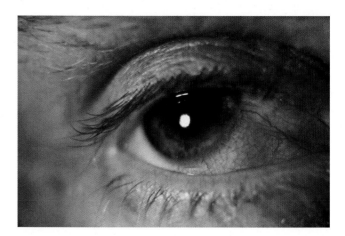

Figure 31.2 Episcleritis. Segmental bright-red injection. Distinguished from conjunctivitis by absence of discharge.
(Adapted from McDonald FS. Mayo Clinic images in internal medicine: self-assessment for board exam review. Rochester [MN]: Mayo Clinic Scientific Press and Boca Raton [FL]: CRC Press; c2004. p. 123. Used with permission of Mayo Foundation for Medical Education and Research.)

anti-inflammatory medication is usually sufficient to relieve symptoms.

Scleritis

Scleritis manifests as an intense, deep pain in the eye caused by scleral inflammation. The pain worsens with movement of the eye and may be referred to the ipsilateral temple. On examination, the scleral vessels are dilated and the eye appears red. Many patients with scleritis have an associated systemic disorder, such as polyarteritis nodosa, systemic lupus erythematosus, granulomatosis with polyangiitis, seronegative spondyloarthropathies (eg, ankylosing spondylitis), and rheumatoid arthritis. Successful therapy requires treatment with topical corticosteroids, cycloplegics, and systemic therapy for any underlying disease.

Iritis

Iritis, also called acute anterior uveitis (Figure 31.3), is inflammation of the iris and ciliary body. Patients typically present with erythema, photophobia, pain, and blurred vision. Disorders associated with iritis include autoimmune diseases. Patients with HLA-B27 are at an increased risk of iritis. The diagnosis requires a slit-lamp examination, and immediate referral to an ophthalmologist is necessary.

> ### Key Definition
>
> Iritis: *inflammation of the iris and ciliary body. Also called acute anterior ureitis.*

Angle-Closure Glaucoma

The development of acute angle-closure glaucoma (Figure 31.4) is a medical emergency. Patients with angle-closure glaucoma present with abrupt ocular pain, headache, visual blurring, and often nausea. Frequently, there is diffuse redness of the eye, and the cornea is hazy. It is more common in the elderly. Patients with angle-closure glaucoma should be immediately referred to an ophthalmologist.

Glaucoma

Glaucoma is a form of optic neuropathy caused by elevated intraocular pressure. Risk factors for open-angle glaucoma include age, being African American, and having diabetes mellitus. The majority of patients with glaucoma are treated with ocular hypotensive drops. Patients who cannot tolerate topical medications or those whose glaucoma progresses despite treatment are candidates for surgical therapies, such as laser trabeculoplasty.

Age-Related Macular Degeneration

Age-related macular degeneration (AMD) is a common cause of visual impairment in older adults. Women and

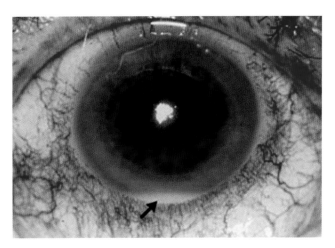

Figure 31.3 *Acute Anterior Uveitis. The pupil is constricted, irregular, and poorly reactive to light. Conjunctival hyperemia is most pronounced adjacent to the limbus. A hypopyon is present (arrow). This disorder can cause loss of vision and warrants immediate referral to an ophthalmologist.*
(Adapted from Leibowitz HM. The red eye. N Engl J Med. 2000 Aug 3;343[5]:345–51. Used with permission.)

cigarette smokers are at higher risk for AMD. There are 2 forms of the disease: dry AMD is characterized by soft drusen and pigmentary changes, whereas wet AMD is characterized by exudative and choroidal neovascular changes. Patients with dry AMD typically present with more gradual loss of central vision, central scotoma, visual distortion, and color changes. In wet AMD, the

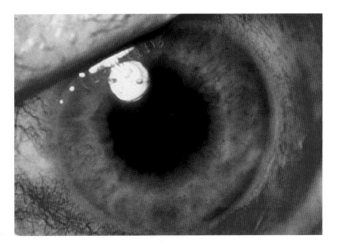

Figure 31.4 *Angle-Closure Glaucoma. The pupil is moderately dilated and unreactive to light. Corneal edema causes the iris markings to appear less sharp than those of the unaffected eye. Prompt, aggressive treatment of this disorder is necessary to prevent optic atrophy.*
(Adapted from Leibowitz HM. The red eye. N Engl J Med. 2000 Aug 3;343[5]:345–51. Used with permission.)

changes often occur more abruptly. Treatment options for AMD are limited; however, on the basis of the results of the Age-Related Eye Disease Study trials, patients with either dry or wet AMD should consider treatment with a supplement containing vitamin C, vitamin E, lutein, zeaxanthin, zinc, and copper. In addition, certain patients with wet AMD may benefit from specific therapies, such as intravitreous injection of vascular endothelial growth factor inhibitor, thermal laser photocoagulation, or photodynamic therapy.

KEY FACTS

✓ Scleritis is often associated with polyarteritis nodosa, systemic lupus erythematosus, granulomatosis with polyangiitis, seronegative spondyloarthropathies, and rheumatoid arthritis

✓ Acute angle-closure glaucoma is a medical emergency

✓ Risk factors for open-angle glaucoma—age, African American, diabetes mellitus

✓ AMD is more likely in women and cigarette smokers

32 Palliative Care[a]

JACOB J. STRAND, MD AND KEITH M. SWETZ, MD, MA

Pain Management in Patients With Serious Illness

Cancer-related pain affects up to 60% of patients receiving cancer-directed therapies and between 70% and 90% of those patients with advanced-stage cancers. However, pain is a common symptom in many patients with serious illnesses other than cancer. Patients with chronic obstructive pulmonary disease, heart failure, end-stage renal disease requiring hemodialysis, and a variety of neurodegenerative disorders experience pain from their conditions. Pain in these conditions is often underrecognized and undertreated, which can lead to functional impairment and suboptimal quality of life.

Barriers to optimal pain management include inadequate pain assessment by health care professionals, clinician reluctance to use opioids and inadequate knowledge about safely using them, and public fear of misuse of opioids.

General Principles

For pain related to a serious illness, reversible causes should be sought and treated as indicated by the history, physical examination findings, results of pertinent imaging studies, and patient goals. For most patients with pain due to a serious illness, such as cancer-related pain, opioid therapy will be required.

Oral medications remain the most common forms of opioids used to treat cancer-related pain. The opioids commonly prescribed in clinical practice (eg, morphine, oxycodone) are not systemically absorbed via the buccal mucosa in appreciable concentrations and thus will take 30 to 60 minutes to reach peak effect. Lipophilic drugs, such

as methadone, fentanyl, and ketamine, have improved transmucosal (buccal or sublingual) absorption, but their use typically requires the input of a palliative care or anesthesia pain specialist and will not be discussed in further detail.

When rapid analgesia is required because of severe pain or limitations of the oral route, parenteral medications should be used. Intravenous opioids reach peak effect in 5 to 15 minutes, and subcutaneous opioids in 20 to 30 minutes. Intramuscular administration of opioids is strongly discouraged because of pain from the injection and erratic drug absorption.

Patient Evaluation

Evaluation of a patient in pain should include the following components: 1) detailed history regarding onset, quality, severity, and location of pain; exacerbating and relieving factors; and associated symptoms; 2) comprehensive physical examination, including neurologic assessment; and 3) diagnostic studies guided by the history and physical examination findings. Administration of analgesia should not be delayed while awaiting results of diagnostic studies or other tests.

Pain Treatment

Treatment of pain in patients with serious illness involves a 3-tiered approach as suggested by the World Health Organization (Box 32.1). Figures 32.1 and 32.2 present algorithms for treatment of severe cancer pain (pain score of 7–10 on 0–10 scale) with intravenous opioids; mild to moderate cancer pain (pain score of 4–6 on 0–10 scale) with oral opioids.

---

[a] Portions previously published in Mueller PS, Hook CC, Hayes DL. Ethical analysis of withdrawal of pacemaker or implantable cardioverter-defibrillator support at the end of life. Mayo Clin Proc. 2003 Aug;78(8):959–63. Used with permission of Mayo Foundation for Medical Education and Research.

Box 32.1 • Three-Tiered Approach to Pain Treatment Suggested by the World Health Organization

Step 1. Mild pain

　Acetaminophen
　Nonsteroidal anti-inflammatory drugs
　Nonopioid adjuvants (eg, neuropathic agents, topical analgesics)

Step 2. Moderate pain

　Add a short-acting opioid to step 1 therapies

　　Oxycodone immediate release
　　Morphine immediate release
　　Hydromorphone

　Avoid opioid-acetaminophen combinations (not recommended because of acetaminophen's dose limitations)

　Avoid codeine products (not recommended because of their variable pharmacokinetics and metabolism)

Step 3. Severe pain

　For severe pain or inadequate pain relief with steps 1 and 2, titrate a short-acting opioid combined with a long-acting opioid, such as:

　　Morphine extended release
　　Oxycodone extended release
　　Fentanyl transdermal patch

　Refer patients with escalating doses or adverse effects to a palliative medicine or anesthesia pain specialist

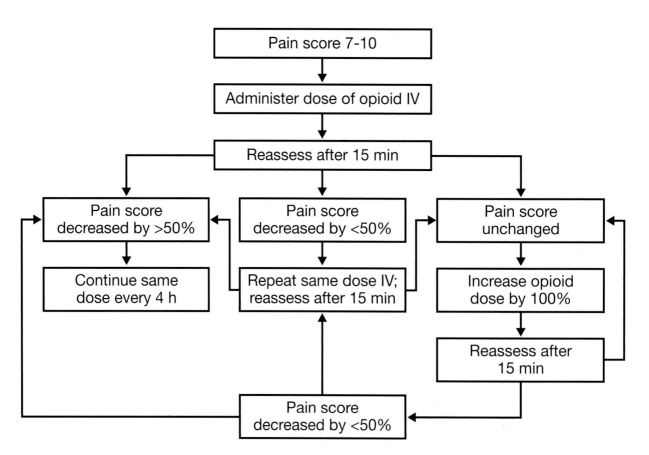

Figure 32.1 *Algorithm for Treatment of Severe Cancer Pain With Intravenous Opioids. Dose of opioid should be determined by patient's level of tolerance and previous use. IV indicates intravenously.*

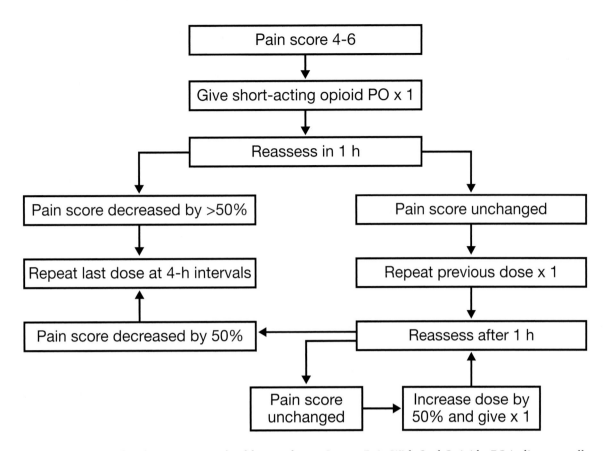

Figure 32.2 *Algorithm for Treatment of Mild to Moderate Cancer Pain With Oral Opioids. PO indicates orally.*

Basic Opioid Management: Pearls

Initial medication selection should be based on patient-specific factors as well as availability. Patients with substantial renal impairment should avoid morphine products, given the possibility of rapid accumulation of metabolites that can lead to neurotoxicity.

For opioid-naïve patients, treatment should be started with low doses of short-acting opioids (eg, morphine, oxycodone, hydromorphone), with close monitoring for efficacy and adverse effects (Table 32.1).

For patients already taking opioids, the total amount of opioid taken in the preceding 24 hours should be

calculated. An immediate-release form of opioid equivalent to 10% to 15% of the 24-hour total dose should be administered as the initial dose.

When therapy is being rotated between opioids, validated equivalency charts should be used (Table 32.2).

For patients requiring long-acting opioids for basal analgesia, the patient's total 24-hour use of short-acting opioids should be calculated. A basal agent is often started at 25% to 50% of the 24-hour total.

Adverse Effects of Opioids

Adverse effects of opioids include sedation, nausea, constipation, respiratory depression, and myoclonus. Appropriate use of opioids in patients with a serious

Table 32.1 • Starting Doses for Opioid-Naïve Patients

Opioid	Dose
Oral	
Oxycodone	2.5–5 mg
Morphine	5–7.5 mg
Hydromorphone	2 mg
Intravenous	
Morphine	2–4 mg
Hydromorphone	0.4 mg
Fentanyl	25 mcg

Table 32.2 • Opioid Equivalencies

Opioid	PO	IV/SQ
Morphine	30 mg	10 mg
Oxycodone	20 mg	NA
Hydromorphone	7.5 mg	1.5 mg
Fentanyl	NA	100 mcg

Abbreviations: IV, intravenous; NA, not available; PO, oral; SQ, subcutaneous.

illness should not lead to respiratory depression. While an excessive dose of opioids or other patient factors can cause overdose and respiratory depression, respiratory depression is typically preceded by sedation. Somnolent patients with reduced respiratory rate require close monitoring, dose reduction or discontinuation, and review of concurrently used medications (eg, benzodiazepines) and may require opioid-reversal agents, such as naloxone.

Tolerance to opioid-associated sedation and nausea typically develops within a few days. For persistent nausea, opioid rotation and antidopaminergic antiemetics (eg, prochlorperazine, haloperidol, metoclopramide) are commonly used. For opioid-associated constipation, colonic stimulants (eg, senna, bisacodyl) and osmotic agents (eg, polyethylene glycol, lactulose) are first-line agents. Fiber and bulking agents should be avoided in opioid-induced constipation unless promotility agents are being used concurrently.

KEY FACTS

✓ Up to 60% of patients receiving therapy for cancer have cancer-related pain

✓ Physician barriers to optimal pain management—inadequate pain assessment, inadequate knowledge about safe opioid use, and reluctance to use them

✓ Opioids are most commonly used in the oral form to treat mild-moderate cancer-related pain

✓ Avoid morphine in patients with marked renal impairment—metabolites can accumulate rapidly, leading to neurotoxicity

---

Principles of Palliative Care

Palliative care aims to reduce the pain and symptoms of patients with serious illness while working to improve quality of life for patients and families. There is a focus on delineating a patient's goals, values, and preferences while attempting to match their medical care with these goals. Early integration of palliative care in a number of illnesses (eg, cancer, heart failure) has been found to improve quality of life, reduce psychological comorbidity, and enhance patient and caregiver satisfaction with care. Subspecialty palliative care can be used for complex symptom management and difficult communication encounters. All patients facing a serious illness can be candidates for palliative care, regardless of their current treatments, and this involvement has been associated with improved quality of life and, in some cases, improved survival.

Ethical Care at the End of Life

Goals of Care

Clinicians should communicate with their patients to ensure that the medical plan of care meets the patient's goals,

---

Box 32.2 • Keys to Effective Goals-of-Care Conversations

Require appropriate context and a basis of prognostic awareness on the part of the patient

Should happen early, when the patient is not struggling with acute illness

Should continue on an iterative basis as the patient's goals and medical situation change

Focus on goals, preferences, and values, not a menu of treatments or procedures

Require guidance and recommendations from clinicians

Involve surrogate decision makers when possible

---

values, and preferences whenever possible. Such conversations allow patients to be engaged in decision making to the degree they are able and promotes patient autonomy. Keys to effective goals-of-care conversations are listed in Box 32.2.

Patients Lacking Decision-Making Capacity

The Patient Self-Determination Act was passed in 1991 to ensure that patients are informed of their rights to accept or refuse medical interventions and to create and execute an advance directive. This act requires that hospitals, nursing homes, hospices, managed care organizations, and home health care agencies provide this information to patients at the time of admission or enrollment.

An **advance directive** is a document in which a person either states choices for medical treatments or designates an individual who should make treatment choices when the patient does not possess decision-making capacity. The term also can apply to oral statements from the patient to caregivers, given at a time when the patient was decisionally capable. Oral statements to a physician regarding a patient's desires should be recorded in the medical record at the time of the communication. Advance directives may take various forms, listed in Box 32.3.

Box 32.3 • Various Forms of Advance Directives

Living will

Durable power of attorney for health care (DPAHC)

A document appointing a health care surrogate (in jurisdictions that do not formally recognize a DPAHC)

Disease or treatment-specific directive

Health care directive that combines elements of the living will and the DPAHC

Advance Directives: Pearls

Laws concerning advance directives vary from jurisdiction to jurisdiction, and physicians should be familiar with their local statutes.

A traditional living will requires that the patient be terminally ill and lack decision-making capacity to be acted upon. It provides guidance to surrogate decision makers regarding goals and preferences for or against medical treatments. If a patient is unable to make decisions but is not terminally ill (definition may vary by jurisdiction), or if the living will contains vague language, it may have limited effectiveness in aiding complex medical decision making.

The **durable power of attorney for health care** is a document that simply designates a surrogate decision maker should the patient lose decision-making capacity. It is often combined with a living will that provides information to a patient's surrogate decision makers about a patient's preference for or against certain forms of therapy. Effective advance directives focus on a patient's goals, identify when a patient's quality of life may not be acceptable to him or her, and provide information about end-of-life preferences.

A treatment-specific medical care directive is useful for patients who have specific desires never to receive certain forms of therapy. For instance, a Jehovah's Witness may use this directive to state a refusal for blood or blood products.

> ### Key Definition
>
> Advance directive: *a document in which a person either states choices for medical treatments (a living will) or designates an individual who should make treatment choices when the patient does not possess decision-making capacity (durable power of attorney for health care).*

> ### Key Definition
>
> Durable power of attorney for health care: *a document that legally designates a surrogate decision maker should the patient lose decision-making capacity.*

Surrogate Decision Making

A surrogate is a person who represents the patient's interests and previously expressed wishes, should the patient be unable or unwilling to do so for himself or herself. The surrogate is optimally designated by the patient before he or she loses decisional capacity. There are 3 broad types of surrogates: 1) an individual designated in a durable power of attorney for health care to speak on the patient's behalf, 2) the patient's family or the court, and 3) a moral surrogate (usually a family member) who best knows the patient and has the patient's interests at heart.

In the absence of an explicit directive, the surrogate should decide to the best of his or her ability, based on the patient's beliefs and values. Applying choices that the patient would make if he or she were able to speak for himself or herself (not what the surrogate would choose) is referred to as substituted judgment. In some circumstances, the surrogate may not have engaged in adequate communication with the patient to be able to project how the patient would decide. In these circumstances, the surrogate's and clinician's obligations are to try to decide in the patient's best interest (best interest standard).

Patients may also delegate decision making to a surrogate, even while still possessing decisional capacity. This situation arises in certain cultural contexts in which decision-making authority is given to a certain member of the family or to a community leader. It is respectful of the patient's autonomy to accept his or her delegation of decision making to another.

Situations may arise in which a surrogate's decisions or instructions to physicians conflict with a patient's previously expressed directive or with those of other family members. Because the physician's primary responsibility is to the patient, the physician should determine as best as possible what the patient would choose for himself or herself. When the physician is unable to resolve the conflict, it may be helpful to involve an independent third-party arbitrator, such as ethics consultants or legal counsel. Once it has been established what the patient would want, it is the obligation of the treating physician(s) to comply with those wishes, even if surrogates disagree. Only if clear evidence can be provided that the advance directive does not reflect what the patient really desired can the directive be overruled.

Withholding and Withdrawing Life-Sustaining Treatments

Transitioning from full therapeutic efforts against illness to comfort care for patients approaching death can be difficult. Nevertheless, compassionate, ongoing care for patients at the end of life is critical. Carrying out patients' requests to withhold or withdraw unwanted medical treatments is legal and ethical and is not the same as physician-aid in dying, previously termed physician-assisted suicide) or euthanasia. In physician-aid in dying, the patient personally terminates his or her life by using an external means provided by a clinician (eg, lethal prescription). In euthanasia, the clinician directly terminates the patient's life (eg, lethal injection). In physician-aid in

Table 32.3 • Options at the End of Life: How Do They Differ?

	Life-Sustaining Treatment		Palliative Sedation and Analgesia	Physician Aid in Dying	Euthanasia
	Withhold	**Withdraw**			
Cause of death	Underlying disease	Underlying disease	Underlying disease[a]	Intervention prescribed by physician and used by patient	Intervention used by physician
Intent/goal of intervention	Avoid burdensome intervention	Remove burdensome intervention	Relieve symptoms	Termination of patient's life	Termination of patient's life
Legal?	Yes[b]	Yes[b]	Yes	No[c]	No

[a] Palliative sedation and analgesia may hasten death ("double effect").

[b] Several states limit the power of surrogate decision makers regarding life-sustaining treatment.

[c] Legal only in Oregon, Washington, Vermont, and Montana (at the time of publication).

dying and euthanasia, a new intervention is introduced (eg, drug), whose sole intent is the patient's death. In contrast, when a patient dies after an intervention is withheld or withdrawn, the underlying disease remains the cause of death (Table 32.3). The intent is freedom from interventions that are perceived as burdensome.

The right to refuse medical treatments is not a "right to die," as it has been frequently described, but rather a "right to be left alone," or a "freedom from unwanted touching." Notably, there is no ethical or legal distinction between withholding treatment in the first place and withdrawing a treatment once begun. The right of a decisionally capable person to refuse artificial hydration and nutrition was upheld by the US Supreme Court), but a surrogate decision maker's right to refuse treatment for decisionally incapable persons may have restrictions in some states. Some states require "clear and convincing evidence" that withdrawal or withholding of life-sustaining treatment would be the patient's desire. The value of each medical therapy (risk:benefit ratio) should be assessed for each patient. When appropriate, the withholding or withdrawal of life support is best accomplished with input from more than 1 experienced clinician. These topics, along with other ethical considerations, are discussed in Chapter 29, "Medical Ethics."

Do-Not-Resuscitate Orders

Do-not-resuscitate (DNR) orders affect administration of cardiopulmonary resuscitation (CPR) only; other therapeutic options should not be influenced by the DNR order. A DNR order can be compatible with maximal forms of treatment (eg, elective intubation, elective cardioversion, surgery). Every person whose medical history is unclear or

unavailable should receive CPR in the event of cardiopulmonary arrest.

Futility or Demands for Nonbeneficial Interventions

Patients have the right to refuse any and all medical therapies, but the principle of respect for autonomy does not give patients, or their surrogates, the right to demand treatments. Such concerns can arise when patients or families request treatments that have little chance of resulting in survival or meaningful recovery, or if a clinician feels compelled to consider unilaterally withholding or withdrawing medical interventions. Conflict between patient autonomy and the professional judgment, moral autonomy, and integrity of the caregivers can occur, and as moral agents, physicians should not be forced to violate their ethical beliefs.

KEY FACTS

✓ Palliative care is appropriate for all patients with serious illness and may improve survival for some

✓ Withholding or withdrawing treatments at the patient's request is not morally the same as physician-aid in dying

✓ DNR orders apply only to CPR, not to other therapeutic options

✓ Although patients can refuse any and all therapies, patient autonomy should not be interpreted as a right to any and all medical therapies/interventions. Clinicians are not obligated to provide medically inappropriate care and have an ethical responsibility to be an active participant in shared-decision making with patients. Clinicians are under no obligation to grant all requests demanded by patients

Preoperative Evaluation[a]

33

KARNA K. SUNDSTED, MD AND KAREN F. MAUCK, MD, MSC

Risks of Anesthesia and Surgery

Mortality associated with anesthesia and surgery has decreased markedly in the past several decades. Today the overall mortality is 1:250,000 even though more complex surgical procedures are performed on sicker patients. The American Society of Anesthesiologists (ASA) classification, with broadly defined categories, is used to estimate overall risk of mortality within 48 hours postoperatively (Table 33.1).

Neuraxial anesthesia and general anesthesia are not associated with significantly different outcomes for mortality and cardiac events. The type of operation performed is also an important determinant of cardiovascular morbidity and mortality. However, the importance of comorbid disease in determining surgical risk may outweigh the nature of the procedure or the type of anesthesia in predicting outcome.

Cardiac Risk Assessment and Risk Reduction Strategies

Coronary artery disease is a frequent cause of perioperative cardiac mortality and morbidity after noncardiac surgery. Perioperative myocardial infarction (MI) occurs in approximately 1% of general surgical procedures and in up to 3.2% of vascular surgical procedures. Among patients who have a perioperative MI, the hospital mortality rate is 15% to 25%, and those who survive to dismissal from the hospital have an increased risk of another MI and cardiovascular death for 1 year postoperatively. Perioperative death attributed to cardiac causes is less prevalent and occurs in 1% to 2% of all surgical procedures.

Cardiac Risk Assessment

A stepwise approach is used for perioperative cardiac assessment as outlined in the "ACC/AHA 2014 Guideline on Perioperative Cardiovascular Evaluation and Management of Patients Undergoing Noncardiac Surgery" (Figure 33.1). This guideline presents a framework for determining which patients are candidates for further testing on the basis of a risk estimate that incorporates both patient-related and surgery-related risk factors.

There are patient-specific factors and surgery-specific factors that contribute to cardiac risk. The patient-specific risk factors are clinical predictors (including the patient's relevant clinical history) and the patient's functional status. The surgery-specific risks are most often related to urgency, duration, and type of surgery.

> ### KEY FACTS
>
> ✓ Overall mortality associated with anesthesia and surgery is 1:250,000
>
> ✓ Neuraxial anesthesia has no advantage over general anesthesia in terms of mortality and cardiac events
>
> ✓ Frequency of perioperative myocardial infarction— about 1% for general surgery and up to 3.2% for vascular surgery
>
> ✓ Cardiac risk assessment includes patient-specific factors (clinical predictors and functional status) and surgery-specific factors (urgency, duration, and type)

The ACC/AHA guideline focuses on estimating perioperative risk of a major adverse cardiac event by stratifying patients into either a low (<1%) or moderate/high (>1%) risk

---

[a] Portions previously published in Mauck KF, Litin SC. Clinical pearls in perioperative medicine. Mayo Clin Proc. 2009 Jun;84(6):546–50. Used with permission of Mayo Foundation for Medical Education and Research.

Table 33.1 • American Society of Anesthesiologists Classification of Anesthetic Mortality Within 48 Hours Postoperatively

Class	Physical Status	Mortality at 48 h
I	Healthy person younger than 80 y	0.07%
II	Mild systemic disease	0.24%
III	Severe but not incapacitating systemic disease	1.4%
IV	Incapacitating systemic disease that is a constant threat to life	7.5%
V	Moribund patient not expected to survive 24 h, regardless of surgery	8.1%
E	Suffix added to any class to indicate emergency procedure	Doubles risk

Adapted from Smith T, Pinnock C, Lin T, Jones R. Fundamentals of anaesthesia. 3rd ed. Cambridge (UK): Cambridge University Press; c2009. Used with permission.

group on the basis of combined patient and surgical characteristics. This stratification scheme does not apply to patients who require emergency surgery or who have active cardiac conditions, including acute coronary syndrome, symptomatic heart failure, symptomatic valvular disease, or arrhythmias.

Clinical predictors of increased perioperative MI, heart failure, and death include both active cardiac conditions and clinical risk factors (Boxes 33.1 and 33.2). The surgery-specific cardiac risk of noncardiac surgery is related to 2 important factors: 1) the type of surgery itself, which may identify a patient with a greater likelihood of underlying heart disease (eg, vascular surgery), and 2) the degree of hemodynamic cardiac stress associated with the surgery. Certain operations may be associated with, for example, pain, blood loss, and profound alterations in heart rate, blood pressure, and vascular volume. Types of procedures and their surgery-specific risks of cardiac death and nonfatal MI are outlined in Table 33.2.

Functional capacity (Table 33.3) is estimated from the patient's history and is expressed in **metabolic equivalent tasks** (METs). One MET is a unit of sitting or resting oxygen uptake per kilogram of body weight per minute.

Key Definition

Metabolic equivalent task: *1 MET is a unit of sitting or resting oxygen uptake per kilogram of body weight per minute.*

Cardiac Risk Reduction Strategies

Evidence suggests that surgical or percutaneous intervention is rarely necessary simply to decrease the surgical risk unless the intervention is indicated irrespective of the preoperative context. Because percutaneous or surgical intervention is also associated with risk of adverse cardiac outcomes, a morbidity and mortality advantage has not been shown for most patients when these interventions are performed before noncardiac surgery. The exception, however, is patients who would have been referred for intervention irrespective of the preoperative context. In general, preoperative revascularization is beneficial in patients who have any of the following: 1) clinically significant

Figure 33.1 Stepwise Approach to Perioperative Cardiac Assessment. Footnote a indicates that recommendations for patients with symptomatic heart failure, valvular heart disease, or arrhythmias are discussed in sections 2.2, 2.4, and 2.5, respectively, of the article cited below; footnote b, clinical practice guidelines (CPGs) for ST-segment elevation myocardial infarction (STEMI) and for unstable angina/non-STEMI are listed in Table 2 of the article cited below. Class indicates class of recommendation: Class I, the benefit is much greater than the risk (the procedure should be performed); Class IIa, the benefit is greater than the risk (it is reasonable to perform the procedure); Class IIb, the benefit may be greater than or the same as the risk (the procedure may be considered); Class III:NB, no benefit (the procedure is not helpful). ACS indicates acute coronary syndrome; CAD, coronary artery disease; GDMT, guideline-directed medical therapy; MACE, major adverse cardiac event; MET, metabolic equivalent task.

(Adapted from Fleisher LA, Fleischmann KE, Auerbach AD, Barnason SA, Beckman JA, Bozkurt B, et al. 2014 ACC/AHA guideline on perioperative cardiovascular evaluation and management of patients undergoing noncardiac surgery: executive summary: a report of the American College of Cardiology/American Heart Association Task Force on Practice Guidelines. Circulation. 2014 Dec 9;130[24]:2215–45. Epub 2014 Aug 1 and Fleisher LA, Fleischmann KE, Auerbach AD, Barnason SA, Beckman JA, Bozkurt B, et al; American College of Cardiology; American Heart Association. 2014 ACC/AHA guideline on perioperative cardiovascular evaluation and management of patients undergoing noncardiac surgery: a report of the American College of Cardiology/American Heart Association Task Force on practice guidelines. J Am Coll Cardiol. 2014 Dec 9;64[22]:e77–137. Epub 2014 Aug 1. Used with permission.)

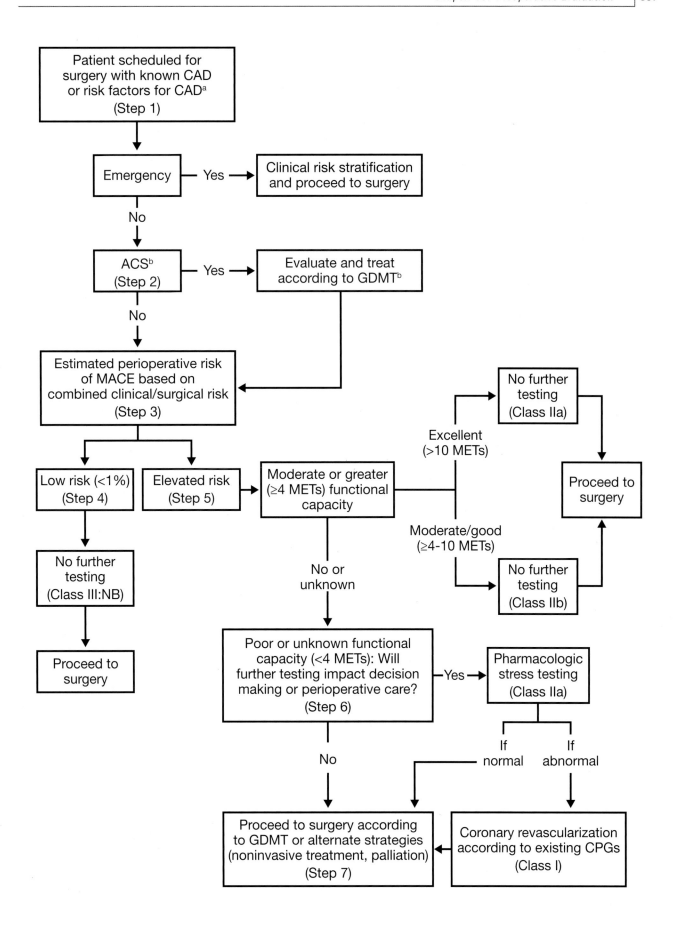

Box 33.1 • Active Cardiac Conditions

Active Cardiac Conditions

Heart failure

Symptoms: dyspnea, orthopnea, paroxysmal nocturnal dyspnea

Physical examination findings: peripheral edema, jugular venous distention, rales, third heart sound

Imaging findings: chest radiograph demonstrating pulmonary edema or pulmonary vascular redistribution

Valvular heart disease

Clinically suspected moderate or severe valvular stenosis or regurgitation if no echocardiography within the last year or substantial change in clinical status or physical examination findings

Arrhythmias

High-grade atrioventricular block

Supraventricular arrhythmias if clinically unstable condition or uncontrolled ventricular rate

Ventricular arrhythmias associated with structural heart disease, hemodynamic compromise, or inherited electrical disorders

Acute Coronary Syndromes

Unstable angina

Non–ST-segment myocardial infarction
ST-segment myocardial infarction

Data from Fleisher LA, Fleischmann KE, Auerbach AD, Barnason SA, Beckman JA, Bozkurt B, et al. 2014 ACC/AHA guideline on perioperative cardiovascular evaluation and management of patients undergoing noncardiac surgery: executive summary: a report of the American College of Cardiology/American Heart Association Task Force on Practice Guidelines. Circulation. 2014 Dec 9;130(24):2215–45. Epub 2014 Aug 1 and Fleisher LA, Fleischmann KE, Auerbach AD, Barnason SA, Beckman JA, Bozkurt B, et al; American College of Cardiology; American Heart Association. 2014 ACC/AHA guideline on perioperative cardiovascular evaluation and management of patients undergoing noncardiac surgery: a report of the American College of Cardiology/American Heart Association Task Force on practice guidelines. J Am Coll Cardiol. 2014 Dec 9;64(22):e77–137. Epub 2014 Aug 1.

Box 33.2 • Revised Cardiac Risk Index (RCRI) and American College of Surgeons National Surgical Quality Improvement Program (NSQIP) Database

RCRI[a]

High-risk surgery (intraperitoneal, intrathoracic, or suprainguinal vascular)

History of ischemic heart disease

History of compensated or prior heart failure

History of cerebrovascular disease

Diabetes on insulin

Renal insufficiency (creatinine level >2.0 mg/dL)

NSQIP[b]

Type of surgery

Dependent functional status

Abnormal creatinine level (>1.5 mg/dL)

American Society of Anesthesiologists score

Increased age

[a] RCRI points and risk of major adverse cardiac event: 0, 0.4%; 1, 1.0%; 2, 2.4%; 3 or greater, 5.4%.

[b] Calculator is available at http://www.surgicalriskcalculator.com/miorcardiacarrest.

Data from Lee TH, Marcantonio ER, Mangione CM, Thomas EJ, Polanczyk CA, Cook EF, et al. Derivation and prospective validation of a simple index for prediction of cardiac risk of major noncardiac surgery. Circulation. 1999 Sep 7;100(10):1043–9 and Gupta PK, Gupta H, Sundaram A, Kaushik M, Fang X, Miller WJ, et al. Development and validation of a risk calculator for prediction of cardiac risk after surgery. Circulation. 2011 Jul 26;124(4):381–7. Epub 2011 Jul 5.

---

left main coronary artery disease; 2) 3-vessel disease; 3) 2-vessel disease with proximal involvement of the left anterior descending coronary artery; 4) coronary artery stenosis and either an ejection fraction less than 50% or demonstrable ischemia on noninvasive testing; 5) high-risk, unstable angina or non–ST-segment elevation MI; 6) acute ST-segment elevation MI.

The expected timing of the planned surgical procedure also needs to be considered when deciding on the type of revascularization procedure. Surgery performed within 30 days of coronary artery bypass graft surgery is associated with an increased risk of postoperative cardiac complications. Percutaneous interventions with angioplasty alone or in conjunction with stent placement also require an appropriate course of dual antiplatelet therapy during vessel injury healing and reendothelialization.

β-Blockers have been reported to decrease the risk of perioperative cardiac complications in patients who are at risk, although the subject is controversial because of more recent data showing mixed results. The current recommendations for perioperative beta-blockade, based on the 2014 ACC/AHA guideline, are summarized in Box 33.3.

Patients With Coronary Stents

The "ACC/AHA 2014 Guideline on Perioperative Cardiovascular Evaluation and Management of Patients Undergoing Noncardiac Surgery" also recommends an approach to patients who have had coronary stent placement in the past. Premature discontinuation of dual antiplatelet therapy markedly increases the risk of catastrophic stent thrombosis and death or MI.

To decrease the risk of adverse cardiac outcomes and death, elective and nonurgent surgery should be postponed for at least 14 days after balloon angioplasty, 30 days after bare metal stent placement, and 365 days after drug-eluting stent placement. Elective noncardiac surgery after implantation

Table 33.2 • Cardiac Risk Stratification According to Surgical Procedure Type

Reported Cardiac Risk[a]	Procedure
High—often >5%	Emergent major operations, particularly in the elderly Aortic and other major vascular procedures Peripheral vascular procedures Anticipated prolonged surgical procedures associated with large fluid shifts or blood loss (or both)
Intermediate—generally <5%	Carotid endarterectomy Head and neck operations Intraperitoneal and intrathoracic procedures Orthopedic procedures Prostate operations
Low—generally <1%[b]	Endoscopic procedures Superficial procedures Cataract extraction Breast operation

[a] Combined incidence of cardiac death and nonfatal myocardial infarction.
[b] Further preoperative cardiac testing is not generally required.

Adapted from Fleisher LA, Beckman JA, Brown KA, Calkins H, Chaikof E, Fleischmann KE, et al. ACC/AHA 2007 guidelines on perioperative cardiovascular evaluation and care for noncardiac surgery: a report of the American College of Cardiology/American Heart Association Task Force on Practice Guidelines (Writing Committee to Revise the 2002 Guidelines on Perioperative Cardiovascular Evaluation for Noncardiac Surgery): developed in collaboration with the American Society of Echocardiography, American Society of Nuclear Cardiology, Heart Rhythm Society, Society of Cardiovascular Anesthesiologists, Society for Cardiovascular Angiography and Interventions, Society for Vascular Medicine and Biology, and Society for Vascular Surgery. Circulation. 2007 Oct 23;116(17):e418–99. Epub 2007 Sep 27. Errata in: Circulation. 2008 Aug 26;118(9): e143–4. Circulation. 2008 Feb 5;117(5):e154 and Fleisher LA, Beckman JA, Brown KA, Calkins H, Chaikof E, Fleischmann KE, et al. ACC/AHA 2007 guidelines on perioperative cardiovascular evaluation and care for noncardiac surgery: a report of the American College of Cardiology/American Heart Association Task Force on Practice Guidelines (Writing Committee to Revise the 2002 Guidelines on Perioperative Cardiovascular Evaluation for Noncardiac Surgery). J Am Coll Cardiol. 2007 Oct 23;50(17):e159–242. Used with permission.

Table 33.3 • Estimated Functional Capacity Requirements for Various Activities

Requirement	Activity
1 MET	Can you take care of yourself? Eat, dress, or use the toilet? Walk indoors around the house? Walk a block or 2 on level ground at 2–3 mph (3.2–4.8 kph)? Do light work around the house like dusting or washing dishes?
4 METs	Climb a flight of stairs or walk up a hill? Walk on level ground at 4 mph (6.4 kph)? Run a short distance? Do heavy work around the house like scrubbing floors or lifting or moving heavy furniture? Participate in moderate recreational activities such as golf, bowling, dancing, doubles tennis, or throwing a baseball or football?
>10 METs	Participate in strenuous sports such as swimming, singles tennis, football, basketball, or skiing?

Abbreviations: kph, kilometers per hour; MET, metabolic equivalent task; mph, miles per hour.

Adapted from Eagle KA, Brundage BH, Chaitman BR, Ewy GA, Fleisher LA, Hertzer NR, et al. Guidelines for perioperative cardiovascular evaluation for noncardiac surgery. Report of the American College of Cardiology/American Heart Association Task Force on Practice Guidelines (Committee on Perioperative Cardiovascular Evaluation for Noncardiac Surgery). Circulation. 1996 Mar 15;93(6):1278–317 and Eagle KA, Brundage BH, Chaitman BR, Ewy GA, Fleisher LA, Hertzer NR, et al. Guidelines for perioperative cardiovascular evaluation for noncardiac surgery. Report of the American College of Cardiology/American Heart Association Task Force on Practice Guidelines (Committee on Perioperative Cardiovascular Evaluation for Noncardiac Surgery). J Am Coll Cardiol. 1996 Mar 15;27(4):910–48. Used with permission.

Box 33.3 • Recommendations for Perioperative Beta-Blockade

Beta-blockade should not be started on the day of surgery

In patients already taking a β-blocker, the drug should be continued without interruption perioperatively

For patients with intermediate- or high-risk myocardial ischemia on preoperative testing, it may be reasonable to begin beta-blockade perioperatively

For patients with 3 or more Revised Cardiac Risk Index risk factors, it may be reasonable to begin beta-blockade perioperatively

In patients in whom a β-blocker is to be started prior to surgery, the drug should be started early enough to assess tolerability, preferably 2–7 days prior to surgery

of a drug-eluting stent may be considered after 180 days if the risk of further delay is greater than the expected risks of ischemia and stent thrombosis. After the recommended time frame for dual antiplatelet therapy has passed, aspirin should be continued perioperatively unless the risk of bleeding outweighs the increased risk of cardiac events.

If urgent or emergent surgery is needed within the window for required dual antiplatelet therapy, a difficult choice has to be made. The generally accepted policy is to stop antiplatelet therapy 7 to 10 days before a surgical or endoscopic procedure because of the possibility of excessive bleeding. However, premature discontinuation of antiplatelet therapy markedly increases the risk of stent thrombosis, a catastrophic event that frequently leads to MI or death. Premature discontinuation of antiplatelet therapy results in a perioperative cardiac death rate that is increased 5 to 10 times, with an average incidence of death of about 30%. The case-fatality rate is 45% for patients in whom stent thrombosis develops. This obviously puts internists, surgeons, and patients in a difficult situation, and a thorough discussion of risks and benefits is required, including discussion of a potentially catastrophic outcome should stent thrombosis occur while antiplatelet therapy is interrupted.

Pulmonary Risk Assessment and Risk Reduction Strategies

Pulmonary complications (respiratory failure, atelectasis, and pneumonia) are as common as cardiac complications in patients undergoing noncardiothoracic surgery, with rates varying between 1.2% and 10.9% depending on ASA class. These complications account for an increase in hospital length of stay and in perioperative morbidity and mortality.

Pulmonary Risk Assessment

Data demonstrate an association between obstructive sleep apnea (OSA) and adverse perioperative outcomes, including acute respiratory failure, desaturation, and cardiac events. Previously, OSA was shown to be associated with an increase in the number of unplanned intensive care unit transfers and in hospital length of stay. Patients should be screened for OSA preoperatively, and if increased risk is identified, the patient should be monitored with continuous pulse oximetry postoperatively. Alternatively, the patient may be referred to a sleep specialist for further evaluation and treatment preoperatively if time permits. All patients with OSA should be instructed to bring their continuous positive airway pressure device to the hospital.

Although it seems intuitive that obesity, asthma, and restrictive lung disease would be associated with an increased incidence of perioperative pulmonary complications, there is not good evidence that this is the case. Clinical studies have not shown an increased risk of postoperative pulmonary complications in obese patients, even if they are morbidly obese. Patients with mild or moderate asthma have not been shown to have increased risk, nor have patients with chronic restrictive lung disease or restrictive physiologic characteristics (neuromuscular disease or chest wall deformities). Patients who are taking inhaled medications should be instructed to continue using them in the perioperative period.

A risk calculator for postoperative respiratory failure is available (Chest. 2011 Nov;140[5]:1207–15). The calculator identifies 5 factors that contribute to the risk of respiratory failure postoperatively: 1) type of surgery, 2) emergency case, 3) ASA class, 4) preoperative sepsis, and 5) dependent functional status. Although it does not take into account several important factors, such as postoperative medications and presence of comorbidities such as OSA, the calculator provides clinicians with a predictive tool, which may aid in early identification and intervention for postoperative pulmonary issues.

Risk Reduction Strategies

All patients who are identified as having an increased risk of postoperative pulmonary complications should receive both of the following interventions postoperatively: 1) deep breathing exercises or incentive spirometry (positive airway pressure for patients unable to perform these); 2) selective use of a nasogastric tube (as needed for postoperative nausea and vomiting, inability to tolerate oral intake, or symptomatic abdominal distention). 3) For patients with suspected OSA, continuous postoperative pulse oximetry or apnea monitoring, or both, is recommended. Continuous positive airway pressure or bilevel positive airway pressure may be used if apnea is identified. Aspiration precautions should be implemented as appropriate.

Table 33.4 • Application of Caprini Risk Score in Nonorthopedic Surgery Patients

Risk of DVT	Caprini Score	Recommended VTE Prophylaxis
Very low (<0.5%)	0	Early ambulation
Low (~1.5%)	1–2	IPC
Moderate (~3%)	3–4	LMWH, LDUH (3 times daily), or mechanical prophylaxis, preferably with IPC
High (~6%)	>5	LMWH or LDUH (3 times daily) in addition to mechanical prophylaxis
Cancer		Extend for 4 wk

Abbreviations: DVT, deep vein thrombosis; IPC, intermittent pneumatic compression; LDUH, low-dose unfractionated heparin; LMWH, low-molecular-weight heparin; VTE, venous thromboembolic disease.

Data from Gould MK, Garcia DA, Wren SM, Karanicolas PJ, Arcelus JI, Heit JA, et al; American College of Chest Physicians. Prevention of VTE in nonorthopedic surgical patients: Antithrombotic Therapy and Prevention of Thrombosis, 9th ed: American College of Chest Physicians Evidence-Based Clinical Practice Guidelines. Chest. 2012 Feb;141(2 Suppl):e227S–77S. Erratum in: Chest. 2012 May;141(5):1369.

Each Risk Factor Represents 1 Point

☐ Age 41-60 y
☐ Swollen legs (current)
☐ Varicose veings
☐ Obesity (BMI >25)
☐ Minor surgery planned
☐ Sepsis (<1 mo)
☐ Serious lung disease, including pneumonia (<1 mo)
☐ Oral contraceptives or hormone replacement therapy
☐ Pregnancy or postpartum (<1 mo)
☐ History of unexplained stillborn infant, recurrent spontaneous abortion (≥3), premature birth with toxemia or growth-restricted infant
☐ Other risk factors _____

☐ Acute myocardial infarction
☐ Congestive heart failure (<1 mo)
☐ Medical patient currently at bed rest
☐ History of inflammatory bowel disease
☐ History of prior major surgery (<1 mo)
☐ Abnormal pulmonary function (COPD)

Subtotal:

Each Risk Factor Represents 5 Points

☐ Stroke (<1 mo)
☐ Elective major lower extremity arthroplasty
☐ Hip, pelvis, or leg fracture (<1 mo)
☐ Acute spinal cord injury (paralysis) (<1 mo)
☐ Multiple trauma (<1 mo)

Subtotal:

Each Risk Factor Represents 2 Points

☐ Age 61-74 y
☐ Arthroscopic surgery
☐ Malignancy (present or previous)
☐ Laparoscopic surgery (>45 min)
☐ Patient confined to bed (>72 h)
☐ Immobilizing plaster cast (<1 mo)

☐ Central venous access
☐ Major surgery (>45 min)

Subtotal:

Each Risk Factor Represents 3 Points

☐ Age ≥75 y
☐ History of DVT/PE
☐ Positive factor V Leiden
☐ Elevated serum homocysteine
☐ Heparin-induced thrombocytopenia (HIT) (Do not use heparin or any low-molecular-weight heparin)
☐ Elevated anticardiolipin antibodies
☐ Other congenital or acquired thrombophilia

☐ Family history of thrombosis*
☐ Positive prothrombin 20210A
☐ Positive lupus anticoagulant

If yes: Type _____
*most frequently missed risk factor

Subtotal:

Total Risk Factor Score:

Figure 33.2 *Caprini Risk Score. BMI indicates body mass index calculated as weight in kilograms divided by height in meters squared; COPD, chronic obstructive pulmonary disease; DVT, deep vein thrombosis; PE, pulmonary embolism.*
(Adapted from Caprini JA. Thrombosis risk assessment as a guide to quality patient care. Dis Mon. 2005 Feb-Mar;51[2–3]:70–8. Used with permission.)
Abbreviations: kph, kilometers per hour; MET, metabolic equivalent task; mph, miles per hour.
Adapted from Eagle KA, Brundage BH, Chaitman BR, Ewy GA, Fleisher LA, Hertzer NR, et al. Guidelines for perioperative cardiovascular evaluation for noncardiac surgery. Report of the American College of Cardiology/American Heart Association Task Force on Practice Guidelines (Committee on Perioperative Cardiovascular Evaluation for Noncardiac Surgery). Circulation. 1996 Mar 15;93(6):1278–317 and Eagle KA, Brundage BH, Chaitman BR, Ewy GA, Fleisher LA, Hertzer NR, et al. Guidelines for perioperative cardiovascular evaluation for noncardiac surgery. Report of the American College of Cardiology/American Heart Association Task Force on Practice Guidelines (Committee on Perioperative Cardiovascular Evaluation for Noncardiac Surgery). J Am Coll Cardiol. 1996 Mar 15;27(4):910–48. Used with permission.

Box 33.4 • Pearls on VTE Prophylaxis

Inferior vena cava filters and periodic surveillance with venous compression ultrasonography should not be used for primary VTE monitoring and prevention

Patients undergoing an operation for hip or knee replacement, hip fracture, or cancer are at particularly high risk for VTE. In these patient populations, prophylaxis is more aggressive and data suggest that prophylaxis should continue after hospital dismissal (up to 35 days)

Renal impairment should be considered when deciding on doses of low-molecular-weight heparin, fondaparinux, and other antithrombotic drugs that are renally excreted, particularly for elderly patients and those at high risk for bleeding. Many of these drugs are contraindicated in patients receiving dialysis

In all patients undergoing neuraxial anesthesia or analgesia, special caution is needed when using anticoagulants for DVT prophylaxis—it may be best to wait until the catheter is removed

Some patients should continue a prolonged course of DVT prophylaxis well after hospital dismissal. Patients undergoing major surgery for cancer require 4–6 weeks of prophylaxis postoperatively

For general and intra-abdominal or pelvic surgical patients at high VTE risk (Caprini score >5) for whom heparin is contraindicated or unavailable and who are not at high risk for major bleeding, low-dose aspirin or fondaparinux is preferred to no prophylaxis

For patients at high risk for VTE for whom anticoagulation is contraindicated because of increased bleeding risk, mechanical prophylaxis, preferably with intermittent pneumatic compression, is recommended

Abbreviations: DVT, deep vein thrombosis; VTE, venous thromboembolism.

Table 33.5 • Preoperative Testing

Test	Indication
Coagulation studies	Medical conditions associated with impaired hemostasis (eg, liver disease, malnutrition) Anticoagulant therapy History or examination findings suggesting an underlying coagulation disorder (eg, excessive bleeding with previous procedures)
Complete blood cell count	History of anemia or disease known to cause anemia (eg, chronic kidney disease) Surgical procedure associated with substantial blood loss Signs or symptoms of infection Disease or medication known to affect platelet or white blood cell count (eg, myeloproliferative disorder)
Creatinine	Consider in all patients older than 50 y History of disease that may affect creatinine (eg, chronic kidney disease, hypertension, heart failure, diabetes) Medication known to affect creatinine (eg, diuretics, angiotensin-converting enzyme inhibitors)
Fasting blood glucose	Rarely indicated, except in patients who are at very high risk for diabetes, are taking corticosteroids, or have signs/symptoms of undiagnosed diabetes
Hemoglobin A$_{1c}$	All patients with diabetes
Electrolytes	All patients with history of renal dysfunction Medication known to affect electrolytes (eg, digoxin, diuretics, antihypertensives) Disease known to affect electrolytes (eg, heart failure, liver disease)
Liver function tests	Rarely needed History of liver disease for which results may affect decision to proceed with surgery
Urinalysis	Urologic procedures Procedures to implant prosthetic materials (eg, joint arthroplasty)
Electrocardiography	Cardiovascular signs or symptoms Known coronary artery disease, symptomatic valvular disease, peripheral arterial disease, cerebrovascular disease, known structural heart disease High-risk procedure Intermediate-risk procedure and at least 1 clinical risk factor (Revised Cardiac Risk Index) Not indicated in patients undergoing low-risk procedures
Chest radiography	Pulmonary signs or symptoms
Pulmonary function tests	Rarely indicated Reasonable to test if patient has history of underlying pulmonary disease (eg, chronic obstructive pulmonary disease) and function does not appear to be at baseline

Venous Thromboembolic Prophylaxis

Although all surgical patients are at increased risk for venous thromboembolic (VTE) disease, certain patients form a high-risk subset, including those who are elderly and those who have prolonged anesthesia, previous VTE, hereditary disorders of thrombosis, prolonged immobilization or paralysis, malignancy, obesity, varicosities, or pharmacologic estrogen use. The American College of Chest Physicians released the ninth edition of its antithrombotic therapy and prevention of thrombosis guidelines, which include updated guidelines on prevention of VTE in both orthopedic and nonorthopedic surgery patients. For nonorthopedic surgery patients, the new guidelines include application of the updated **Caprini Risk Score** (Table 33.4 and Figure 33.2). This offers an individualized VTE prophylaxis strategy based on patient comorbidities and risk of deep vein thrombosis. In orthopedic surgery patients, the new guidelines recommend use of both intermittent pneumatic compression devices and an antithrombotic agent, with extension of thromboprophylaxis for at least 10 to 14 days and optimally 35 days. Low-molecular-weight heparin is the agent of choice (Box 33.4).

Key Definition

Caprini Risk Score: *A scoring system that offers an individualized prophylaxis strategy for venous thromboembolic disease based on patient comorbidities and risk of deep vein thrombosis.*

Perioperative Medical Comorbidities

Liver, adrenal, or thyroid disease requires special consideration perioperatively. Patients with compensated liver disease are often able to proceed with surgery. However, those with severe liver disease and its complications are at increased risk. The Model for End-Stage Liver Disease (MELD) score and the Child-Turcotte-Pugh (CTP) classification should be used to risk-stratify patients. Those with CTP class C and MELD score greater than 15 are considered to be at high risk and are generally advised to avoid elective surgery; they are often referred for transplant evaluation prior to consideration for elective surgery. Intermediate-risk patients should be referred to a hepatologist to optimize management of complications before consideration for surgery. Patients with hypothyroidism can generally proceed to surgery with continuation of levothyroxine therapy. It is important that the thyroid-stimulating hormone

level be checked within 6 months of surgery. Although guidelines vary on the specific corticosteroid dose and duration that place patients at risk for perioperative adrenal insufficiency, high-risk patients should be given stress doses of corticosteroids perioperatively, and intermediate-risk patients may be tested with morning cortisol measurement or cosyntropin stimulation test prior to surgery to determine the need for perioperative coverage.

Preoperative Testing Guidelines

Results of routine laboratory and diagnostic tests often have little effect on perioperative management and can result in increased costs and unnecessary surgical delay. Therefore, routine preoperative testing should not be obtained. Rather, testing should be directed by specific indications and by the history and physical examination findings (Table 33.5). There are no data on how long previous laboratory results may be applied to the preoperative evaluation. The ASA task force suggests that results obtained within 6 months of surgery are acceptable if the medical history has not changed appreciably.

KEY FACTS

✓ The only patients who need surgical or percutaneous intervention to reduce cardiac risk before surgery are those who would have been referred regardless

✓ Surgery within 30 days of coronary artery bypass grafting is associated with an increased risk of postoperative cardiac complications

✓ Postpone elective and nonurgent surgery after stent placement—30 days for bare metal stents and 365 days for drug-eluting stents

✓ After balloon angioplasty, postpone elective and nonurgent surgery for at least 14 days

---

KEY FACTS

✓ Patients are as likely to have pulmonary complications as cardiac complications when undergoing noncardiothoracic surgery

✓ All patients at risk for postoperative pulmonary complications require deep breathing exercises or incentive spirometry

✓ Risk of venous thromboembolism is increased in all patients undergoing surgery

✓ Patients with liver, adrenal, or thyroid disease need special consideration before surgery

✓ Preoperative laboratory and diagnostic testing should not be routine; it may not alter management and may increase costs and delay surgery

34 Preventive Medicine

AMY T. WANG, MD AND KAREN F. MAUCK, MD, MSc

Key Concepts in Preventive Medicine

Types of Prevention

Preventive medicine focuses on preventing disease and keeping patients healthy. There are 3 levels of prevention:

1. *Primary prevention:* preventing disease before it occurs (eg, immunization to prevent disease, use of condoms to prevent sexually transmitted diseases) (Box 34.1).
2. *Secondary prevention:* detecting preclinical disease to start early treatment for better outcomes (eg, cancer screening, treating hypertension to prevent cardiovascular disease) (Box 34.2).
3. *Tertiary prevention:* improving outcomes (quality of life, disease progression) in known disease (eg, use of aspirin after myocardial infarction to decrease recurrence, rehabilitation after a stroke).

Key Definition

Secondary prevention: *detecting preclinical disease to start early treatment for better outcomes.*

Bias

For screening tests to be used and interpreted effectively, sources of bias must be considered.

1. *Volunteer bias,* a type of selection bias, occurs when the trial population used to study a screening test is not representative of the target population to be screened. This happens when study participants who volunteer for or comply with screening tests tend to be healthier than those who do not.

Box 34.1 • Routine Counseling Recommendations

Stop tobacco use

Reduce harmful alcohol use

Dental health: Visit dental care provider regularly; brush and floss daily

Skin health: Use sunscreen

Physical activity: Participate in moderate-intensity physical activity for ≥150 min weekly and muscle-strengthening exercises at least twice weekly

Healthful dietary choices: Limit intake of saturated fats and processed foods, and increase intake of vegetables, fruits, whole grains, and unsaturated fats

Injury prevention

Use safety belt in vehicles
Use helmet with motorcycles, all-terrain vehicles, and bicycles
Practice home safety measures, including use of smoke detectors, setting water heaters to less than 120°F, and weapon safety

Chemoprophylaxis

Women of childbearing age should take a multivitamin with folic acid daily
Weigh risks and benefits of aspirin for primary prevention of cardiovascular events in adults at increased risk for coronary artery disease

Healthful aging

Use routine inquiry and simple tests to screen for vision and hearing loss
Evaluate for polypharmacy, fall risk, home safety, and elder abuse
Discuss advance directives

---

2. *Lead-time bias* occurs when screened patients appear to live longer than unscreened patients because the time between early detection and clinical presentation of disease (lead time) is wrongly included in survival estimates.

365

Box 34.2 • Routine Screening Recommendations for Asymptomatic Disease

Abdominal aortic aneurysm: a 1-time abdominal ultrasonographic examination is recommended for men aged 65–75 y who have ever smoked (>100 cigarettes)

Alcoholism: screen for alcohol use and dependence

Chlamydia infection: screening for all sexually active women 25 y or younger and others at increased risk

Depression: screen in practices with systems to support effective management

Diabetes mellitus, gestational: screening with glucose tolerance testing is recommended during pregnancy after 24 weeks' gestation

Diabetes mellitus, type 2: screening is recommended for adults with hypertension

HIV infection: voluntary HIV testing should be offered to all adults

Hypertension: blood pressure screening at least every 2 y for all adults

Lipid disorders: routine screening is recommended every 5 y starting at age 35 for men and age 45 for women; if individuals have risk factors for coronary artery disease, start at age 20

Obesity: BMI calculation periodically

Osteoporosis: bone mineral density testing for women 65 y or older and for high-risk women younger than 65

Sexually transmitted diseases other than *Chlamydia* and HIV infections: screening for syphilis or gonorrhea (or both) in high-risk persons (consider local prevalence)

Tuberculosis: screening with TST or IGRA in high-risk groups

Abbreviations: BMI, body mass index; HIV, human immunodeficiency virus; IGRA, interferon-γ release assay; TST, tuberculin skin test.

Box 34.3 • Features of an Ideal Screening Test

Features of the disease

　Be common

　Cause significant morbidity and mortality

　Have a long preclinical phase (providing time to give early treatment)

　Have an effective and acceptable treatment that is readily available

Features of the test

　Be safe, acceptable, and easy to perform

　Be highly sensitive and/or have a complementary, highly specific confirmatory test

　Have an acceptable rate of false-positive results

　Be inexpensive

Features of the patient

　Be at risk for the specific condition

　Have access to testing

　Have adequate life expectancy and quality of life

　Be likely to follow through with additional testing and treatment

3. *Length-time bias* occurs most often in observational studies because indolent disease is much more likely to be detected by a screening test than is aggressive, rapidly progressive disease. Therefore, individuals with screening-detected disease live longer than those with symptomatic presentation of disease because of the nature of the disease rather than because of the screening test itself. An extreme example of this is overdiagnosis, which occurs when an indolent, nonprogressive, or regressive disease that would have never affected a person's life is detected.

Features of an Ideal Screening Test

A useful screening test should have the features outlined in Box 34.3.

Routine Screening for Adults

All adults should be evaluated with a thorough history and physical examination including a detailed review of systems, allergy and immunization history, use of medication (prescription, over-the-counter, herbal medicine, and supplements), social history, and family history.

Healthy lifestyle and behavioral counseling

Recommendations for routine lifestyle and behavioral counseling are outlined in Box 34.1.

Chronic disease screening

Recommendations for screening adults for chronic disease are outlined in Box 34.2.

Cancer Screening

Although efforts in cancer prevention, screening, and treatment have improved cancer mortality, cancer remains the second leading cause of death in the United States.

Lung Cancer

Lung cancer is the second most common cancer and the leading cause of cancer death among men and women in the United States. The 5-year survival rate is 17.4%.

Screening Recommendations

Individuals at high risk for lung cancer are defined as adults aged 55 to 80 years with a 30 pack-year smoking history (current or former smokers who have quit within the past 15 years). The US Preventive Services Task Force (USPSTF) recommends annual low-dose chest computed tomography for lung cancer screening in high-risk patients. Screening should be stopped if a health problem develops that substantially limits the patient's life expectancy or ability or willingness to have curative lung surgery.

Key Definition

Individuals at high risk for lung cancer: *adults aged 55 to 80 years with a 30 pack-year smoking history (current or former smokers who have quit within the past 15 years).*

For asymptomatic average-risk individuals, no screening for lung cancer is currently recommended.

Lung Cancer Prevention

Smoking is the leading preventable cause of cancer in the United States and a leading cause of heart disease and stroke. Smoking causes 85% of all lung cancers. Smoking cessation decreases the risk of lung cancer in a former smoker by 20% to 90%. Physician advice to stop smoking, use of nicotine cessation aids and medications, and referral to smoking cessation programs have been shown to be helpful in smoking cessation. Population-based strategies, such as cigarette taxes and smoking restrictions in public places, have also been effective.

Breast Cancer

Breast cancer is the most commonly diagnosed cancer in women and the second leading cause of cancer death in women in the United States. The lifetime risk is estimated at 1 in 8 women. The estimated 5-year survival rate is 89.4%.

Screening Recommendations

Timing of initiation and frequency of breast cancer screening is a controversial topic. The USPSTF guidelines (December 2009; update in progress though proposed recommendations are comparable) are summarized as follows:

1. For women aged 40 to 49 years, the age to start screening mammography should be an individualized decision that takes into account patient context, benefits, and risks.
2. For women aged 50 to 74, biennial screening mammography is recommended.
3. For women aged 75 or older, there is insufficient evidence to assess the benefits and harms of screening mammography.
4. There is insufficient evidence to recommend clinical breast examination.
5. The recommendation is against breast self-examination because studies have found more imaging and biopsies in women in the self-examination group compared to controls.

The American College of Physicians, the American Academy of Family Physicians, and the Institute for Clinical Systems Improvement have adopted similar guidelines.

Other organizations, such as the American Cancer Society, the American College of Radiology, and the American College of Obstetricians and Gynecologists, recommend annual mammography starting at age 40. Many of these organizations also recommend yearly clinical breast examinations and breast awareness, encouraging women to know how their breasts normally look and feel.

Benefits of Screening Mammography

Screening mammography is associated with an overall relative risk reduction of 19% in breast cancer mortality (about 15% for women in their 40s, 16% for women in their 50s, and 32% for women in their 60s). Absolute risk varies according to a woman's baseline risk; estimates can be found in Table 34.1.

Table 34.1 • Benefits of Regular Screening Mammography Over 10 Years

Age Group, y	Relative Risk (95% CI) With Screening Mammography	Absolute Risk Reduction With Screening Mammography	Breast Cancer Deaths Averted, No./10,000 Women	NNI to Avoid 1 Breast Cancer Death
40s	0.85 (0.75–0.96)	0.0005	5	1,904
50s	0.86 (0.75–0.99)	0.0007	10	1,339
60s	0.68 (0.54–0.87)	0.0027	42	377

Abbreviation: NNI, number needed to invite to screen.

Potential Harms of Screening Mammography

Part of the controversy stems from potential harms associated with screening mammography: false-positive results and overdiagnosis. Screening mammography has a high false-positive rate, which leads to further testing (additional imaging with or without biopsies) and may lead to increased anxiety that may persist even after a woman learns that she does not have breast cancer. More than half of women undergoing screening over a 10-year period will have a false-positive result. False-positives are more common in younger women and in women without previous mammograms. The other main harm from screening is overdiagnosis, which is detection by screening of a breast cancer that if left undetected, would not have affected a woman's life, leading to further harms from overtreatment. It is estimated that 10% to 30% of screening-detected breast cancers represent overdiagnosis.

KEY FACTS

✓ Screened patients appear to live longer than unscreened patients if survival estimates wrongly include the time between early detection and clinical presentation (lead-time bias)

✓ Diagnosis of a disease that progresses too slowly to ever affect a person's life is overdiagnosis (length-time bias)

✓ USPSTF recommendation for lung cancer screening in high-risk patients—annual low-dose chest computed tomography

✓ Potential harms of screening mammography—false-positive results and overdiagnosis

---

Individuals at Increased Risk for Breast Cancer

The most significant risk factors for breast cancer include family history (first-degree relatives with breast or ovarian cancer, multiple relatives with breast or ovarian cancer on 1 side of the family, premenopausal or male breast cancer; several screening tools are available to help identify potential inherited syndromes) and personal history of atypical hyperplasia or lobular carcinoma in situ. If the family history is suggestive of a harmful mutation, the patient should be referred for genetic counseling to discuss the pros and cons of BRCA testing. If any of these risk factors are present, the examining physician should perform or refer the patient for a formal breast cancer risk assessment. Women with a 20% or greater lifetime risk of breast cancer (as determined with models largely dependent on family history) qualify for annual screening breast magnetic resonance imaging in addition to routine screening mammography, according to American Cancer Society guidelines. Both the USPSTF and the American Society of Clinical Oncology recommend discussing breast cancer risk-reducing medications such as raloxifene and tamoxifen with women who have a 5-year risk of 1.66% or more based on the Gail model.

High breast density is another common risk factor for breast cancer and affects up to 50% of women. Twenty-four states have now passed legislation requiring mandatory breast density notification for women receiving mammograms. High breast density decreases sensitivity of a mammogram but also independently increases breast cancer risk beyond that of masking alone. Digital mammography has been shown to be better than film mammography in women with high breast density. Although supplemental screening tests are available in some areas, currently supplemental screening is not routinely recommended for women with high breast density without additional risk factors.

Colorectal Cancer

Colorectal cancer (CRC) is the second leading cause of cancer death and the fourth most commonly diagnosed cancer in the United States. The 5-year survival rate is 64.9% overall and 90.1% for localized colon and rectal cancer. Most colorectal tumors are thought to develop from adenomatous polyps over a period of 10 years. The risk of a polyp becoming malignant is increased by the following features: size greater than 10 mm, presence of high-grade dysplasia, villous or tubulovillous morphology, and having 3 or more polyps.

Screening Recommendations

Multiple options are recommended by the USPSTF for CRC screening of average-risk adults (those with no known risk factors other than age) starting at age 50:

1. Colonoscopy every 10 years
2. Flexible sigmoidoscopy every 5 years (case-control data: 60%–80% decrease in CRC mortality; 60%–70% sensitivity compared with colonoscopy) with interval stool testing every 3 years
3. Fecal occult blood test (FOBT) or fecal immunochemical test annually (randomized controlled trial data for FOBT: 15%–33% decrease in CRC mortality; 37%–79% sensitivity)

The American Cancer Society, the US Multi-society Task Force on Colorectal Cancer, the American College of Radiology guidelines and the American College of Gastroenterology give 2 further options:

4. Double-contrast barium enema every 5 years (sensitivity, 48%–75%)
5. Computed tomography colonography every 5 years (sensitivity, 86%–92% depending on size of polyp)

These groups also give preference to cancer prevention tests (tests 1, 2, 4, and 5, which can detect adenomas in addition to cancer) vs cancer detection tests (3). Colonoscopy is the preferred screening test of the American College of Gastroenterology.

Individuals at Increased Risk for Colorectal Cancer

An algorithm for CRC screening, based on age and risk factors for CRC, is shown in Figure 34.1. The following are special cases:

1. Family history of hereditary syndromes with a high risk of colon cancer, such as familial adenomatous polyposis and hereditary nonpolyposis CRC: recommendations vary according to the syndrome and counseling for genetic testing.
2. Family history of colon polyps or colon cancer in a first-degree relative or in 2 second-degree relatives: colonoscopy at age 40 or 10 years before the youngest case in the immediate family (whichever is first) and then every 5 years.
3. Inflammatory bowel disease: colonoscopy 8 years after diagnosis if pancolitis (12–15 years if left-sided colitis) and then every 1 to 2 years.

Prostate Cancer

Prostate cancer is the leading cancer diagnosis among men and the second most common cause of cancer death among men, accounting for 10% of male cancer deaths annually in the United States. The 5-year survival rate is 98.9%. Reviews of autopsy series have identified prostate cancer in 46% of men in their 50s, 70% of men in their 60s, and 83% of men in their 70s who died of other causes. The lifetime risk of prostate cancer is estimated at 1 in 6 men.

Screening Recommendations

Due to the very small potential for benefit and a much greater chance of harms related to prostate cancer screening and subsequent treatment, the USPSTF recommends against prostate-specific antigen screening for prostate cancer. These harms not only relate to screening itself (biopsies and complications from biopsies, including bleeding, infection, and lasting anxiety), but more importantly to overdiagnosis and overtreatment of prostate cancer (sexual dysfunction, urinary incontinence, radiation-induced bowel dysfunction, and complications of surgery, including a small chance of premature death). Other organizations, including the American College of Physicians, the American Cancer Society, and the American Urological Association, recommend shared decision making for

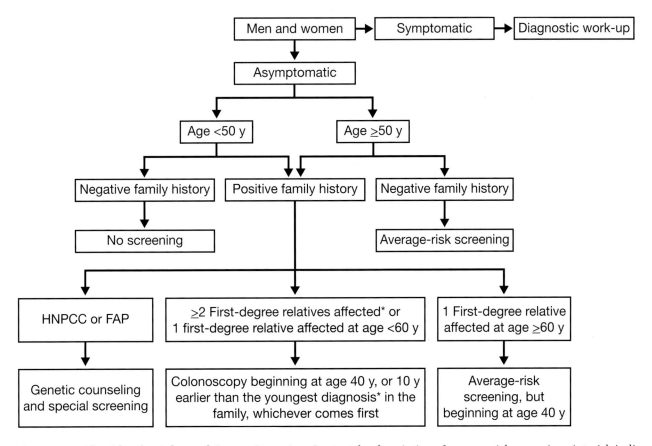

Figure 34.1 *Algorithm for Colorectal Cancer Screening. See text for description of average-risk screening. Asterisk indicates either colorectal cancer or adenomatous polyp. FAP indicates familial adenomatous polyposis; HNPCC, hereditary nonpolyposis colorectal cancer.*

(Adapted from Winawer S, Fletcher R, Rex D, Bond J, Burt R, Ferrucci J, et al. Colorectal cancer screening and surveillance: clinical guidelines and rationale—update based on new evidence. Gastroenterology. 2003 Feb;124[2]:544–60. Used with permission.)

men starting from age 50 to 69 years (age ranges vary by organization).

Individuals at Increased Risk for Prostate Cancer

Organizations including the American College of Physicians and American Cancer Society recommend starting discussions at an earlier age for men at increased risk for prostate cancer. Significant risk factors include known or suspected *BRCA1* or *BRCA2* mutations, a first-degree relative with prostate cancer before age 65, or being African American.

Cervical Cancer

Cervical cancer screening has proved to be very effective, contributing to decreases in cervical cancer incidence and mortality of approximately 50% since the 1980s; currently the 5-year survival rate is 67.8%. Despite this success, racial and socioeconomic disparities in the burden of cervical cancer persist, with disproportionately higher rates of cervical cancer death in the underserved US population and in developing countries. Human papillomavirus (HPV) infection is essential to the development of cervical cancer. HPV types 16 and 18 are thought to be responsible for approximately 70% of cervical cancer cases.

Screening Tests

1. Cytology (Pap smear): Sensitivity is 68% to 80%; specificity, 75% to 95%. The adequacy of the cervical sample affects the test's accuracy. There is no clinically important difference between conventional cytology and liquid-based cytology, except that HPV testing, if desired, can be done on the same preparation.
2. HPV testing: Some studies have shown improved sensitivity with HPV testing alone and in conjunction with a Pap smear.

Screening Recommendations

The USPSTF recommends screening women aged 21 to 65 years with cytology (Pap smear) every 3 years. Women aged 30 to 65 who want less-frequent screening can be screened with cytology and HPV testing every 5 years, although they should be aware of higher rates of false-positives and the possibility of additional testing with this strategy.

The USPSTF recommends against screening for cervical cancer with HPV testing, alone or in combination with cytology, in women younger than 30 years because of high prevalence of HPV, higher likelihood of regression of precancerous lesions, and low incidence of cervical cancer in this age group. The task force also recommends against screening in women who have had hysterectomy for benign reasons and in women older than 65 who have had adequate prior screening and are not at high risk for cervical cancer.

KEY FACTS

- ✓ Prostate cancer can be found in more than 80% of men in their 70s who died of other causes
- ✓ Harms from prostate cancer overdiagnosis and overtreatment—sexual dysfunction, urinary incontinence, radiation-induced bowel dysfunction, and complications of surgery
- ✓ USPSTF recommendations for cervical cancer screening—women aged 21 to 65, cytology (Pap smear) every 3 years; women aged 30 to 65 who want less-frequent screening, cytology and HPV testing every 5 years
- ✓ USPSTF recommends against HPV testing in women younger than 30
- ✓ Cervical cancer screening can be stopped after hysterectomy for benign reasons and after age 65 if prior screening was adequate and risk is not high

---

Immunizations

Immunization is one of the greatest successes of modern medicine for improving morbidity and mortality.

Key Concepts

Types of Immunity

1. *Active immunity:* Antigen is presented to the host, which produces an immune response that lasts for years.
2. *Passive immunity:* Large amounts of preformed antibodies prevent or diminish the effect of infection (eg, tetanus immune globulin, hepatitis B immune globulin); immune response lasts for months.

Types of Vaccines

Live virus vaccines are generally contraindicated in pregnant women and in people who are severely immunocompromised or who are receiving immunosuppressive therapy, such as high-dose corticosteroids. Human immunodeficiency virus (HIV)–infected persons who are immunocompetent (CD4 count >200 cells/μL) and persons with some types of leukemia in remission for at least 3 months may be vaccinated with certain live vaccines. Individuals with chronic lymphocytic leukemia, even if in remission, should not receive live virus vaccines. Examples of live virus vaccines include measles-mumps-rubella (MMR), varicella virus, and smallpox.

Inactivated vaccines are generally safe in pregnant women in whom they are indicated and in immunocompromised persons. The response may be decreased in immunocompromised persons.

In general, if vaccination series are interrupted, they should be resumed as soon as possible but do not have to be restarted in most cases.

Advisory Committee on Immunization Practices (ACIP) Recommendations Summary

The schedule for recommended adult immunizations is summarized in Figure 34.2.

Influenza Vaccination

Annual influenza vaccination is recommended for all adults.

Intranasally administered live, attenuated influenza vaccine (FluMist) is an option only for healthy, nonpregnant adults without egg allergy through age 49 years.

If a person can eat scrambled eggs without a reaction, inactivated influenza vaccine (IIV) can be administered routinely. If a person has an egg allergy causing hives only, recombinant influenza vaccine (RIV) is egg-free and can be administered routinely to persons aged 18 to 49, *or* IIV can be given with observation for at least 30 minutes after vaccination. For persons with other reactions (respiratory distress, angioedema, etc), RIV can be given to those aged 18 to 49, *or* IIV can be administered by a physician who has expertise in management of allergic conditions, with observation for at least 30 minutes after vaccination.

Tetanus-Diphtheria (Td) and Tetanus-Diphtheria-Acellular Pertussis (Tdap) Vaccination

The primary vaccination series should be completed in early childhood: the first tetanus-containing vaccine is given, the second vaccination occurs 1 to 2 months later, and the third occurs 6 to 12 months after the second. Adults with an unknown or incomplete primary vaccination history should begin or complete the series.

A single dose of Tdap vaccine is recommended for all previously unvaccinated adults regardless of when they last received a tetanus-containing vaccine, and a Td booster should be administered every 10 years thereafter.

Pregnant women should receive a dose of Tdap vaccine during each pregnancy, preferably between 27 and 36 weeks' gestation, regardless of timing of previous Tdap or Td vaccination.

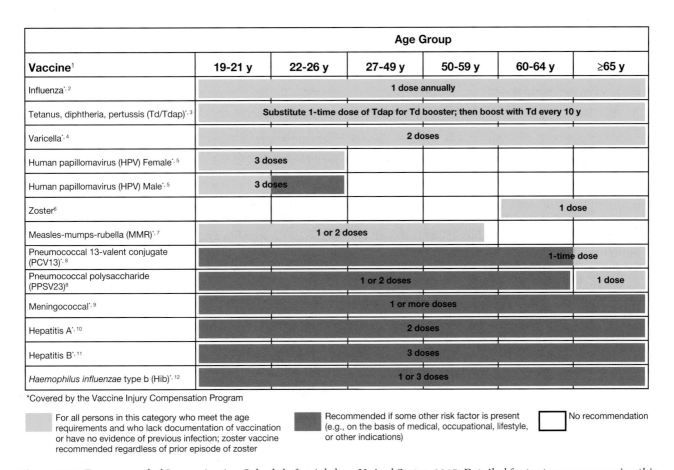

*Covered by the Vaccine Injury Compensation Program

Figure 34.2 *Recommended Immunization Schedule for Adults—United States, 2015. Detailed footnotes accompanying this figure are published at http://www.cdc.gov/vaccines/schedules/downloads/adult/adult-schedule.pdf.*

(Adapted from Centers for Disease Control and Prevention. Recommended immunization schedule for adults—United States, 2015 [Internet]. Atlanta [GA]; [cited 2015 Sep 23]. Available from: http://www.cdc.gov/vaccines/schedules/downloads/adult/adult-schedule.pdf.)

Recommendations for vaccination after an injury are as follows:

1. If the primary vaccination status is complete and the wound is clean and minor, no further vaccination is needed.
2. If the primary vaccination status is complete and the wound is contaminated, give Td booster if >5 years since the last booster.
3. If the primary vaccination status is unknown or incomplete, give both Td and TIG.

Varicella Vaccination

Healthy persons without evidence of immunity (laboratory evidence of immunity or confirmation of disease, birth in the United States before 1980 [not considered evidence of immunity for health care workers, pregnant women, immunocompromised persons], or diagnosis or verification of a history of varicella or herpes zoster by a health care provider) should receive varicella vaccination. Two doses should be given 4 to 8 weeks apart. If more than 8 weeks have passed since the first dose, the second dose can be given at any time.

Pregnant women without evidence of varicella immunity should be vaccinated in the immediate postpartum period. Women of childbearing age should wait 1 month after receiving the varicella vaccine to become pregnant.

Herpes Zoster Vaccination

All persons 60 years or older should be vaccinated against herpes zoster unless there is a contraindication (severe immunodeficiency). Zoster vaccine can be given regardless of past history of varicella or zoster infection, though not during an active shingles episode. The US Food and Drug Administration has approved the vaccine for persons aged 50 to 59, but the ACIP does not recommend its use in this age group, given that the effect of the vaccine generally wanes 5 years after vaccination; thus, individuals will not be protected when their risk of herpes zoster and associated complications is the greatest.

MMR Vaccination

Adults born after 1956 who do not have a medical contraindication should be vaccinated if they do not have documentation of at least 1 dose of MMR vaccine, physician-documented disease, or an immune titer. Adults who have never been vaccinated should receive 2 doses given at least 1 month apart. If an unvaccinated person is exposed to measles, vaccine should be given within 72 hours, or immune globulin should be given within 6 days if the person is not a candidate for vaccination.

Rubella immunity should be documented for women of childbearing age. If a nonpregnant woman is not immune to rubella, she should be vaccinated. If a pregnant woman is not immune to rubella, she should be vaccinated in the immediate postpartum period.

Pneumococcal Vaccination

There are 2 types of pneumococcal vaccine: the pneumococcal polysaccharide vaccine (PPSV23) with 23 pneumococcal subtypes and the pneumococcal conjugate vaccine (PCV13) with 13 subtypes.

Adults aged 65 years or older should receive PCV13 followed by PPSV23 6 to 12 months later. Adults aged 19 years or older with immunocompromising conditions, functional or anatomic asplenia, cerebrospinal fluid leaks, or cochlear implants should also receive PCV13 first, followed by a dose of PPSV23 at least 8 weeks later (Table 34.2). PCV13 and PPSV23 should not be given together owing to increased risk of injection site reaction and the minimum acceptable interval of 8 weeks between the 2 vaccinations.

1. For those previously vaccinated with PPSV23, give PCV13 at least 1 year after the most recent PPSV23 dose.
2. For those who require a second PPSV23 dose and have not received PCV13, give PCV13; the second PPSV23 dose should be given at least 6 to 12 months after PCV13 *and* at least 5 years after the most recent dose of PPSV23.

Adults aged 19 years or older with chronic cardiovascular or pulmonary disease (including asthma and smokers), diabetes mellitus, alcoholism, or chronic liver disease should receive a dose of PPSV23 and do not require revaccination after 5 years. At age 65, they should receive PCV13 followed by PPSV23 6 to 12 months later.

HPV Vaccination

HPV is responsible for nearly all cases of cervical cancer. The HPV vaccine is available as a bivalent vaccine (HPV2) against HPV 16 and 18 to prevent cervical cancer in females and as a quadrivalent vaccine (HPV4) against HPV 6, 11, 16, and 18 for prevention of cervical, vulvar, and vaginal cancers and precancerous lesions in females and anal cancers and genital warts in both males and females.

Routine vaccination is recommended at age 11 or 12 years with HPV4 or HPV2 for females and with HPV4 for males. Vaccination can also be given from age 9 through 26 years. Both vaccines are given on a 3-dose schedule. The second dose should be given 1 to 2 months after the first dose, then the third dose 6 months after the first dose.

Meningococcal Vaccination

Adults with asplenia or complement component deficiencies, military recruits, and those traveling to or residing in countries where meningococcal disease is common should

Table 34.2 • Medical Conditions or Other Indications for Administration of PCV13, and Indications for PPSV23 Administration and Revaccination for Adults 19 Years or Older

Risk Group	Underlying Medical Condition	PCV13 Recommended	PPSV23[a] Recommended	Revaccination at 5 y After 1st Dose
Immunocompetent persons	Chronic heart disease[b]		✓	
	Chronic lung disease[c]		✓	
	Diabetes mellitus		✓	
	CSF leaks	✓	✓	
	Cochlear implants	✓	✓	
	Alcoholism		✓	
	Chronic liver disease		✓	
	Cigarette smoking		✓	
Persons with functional or anatomic asplenia	Sickle cell disease/other hemoglobinopathies	✓	✓	✓
	Congenital or acquired asplenia	✓	✓	✓
Immunocompromised persons	Congenital or acquired immunodeficiencies[d]	✓	✓	✓
	HIV infection	✓	✓	✓
	Chronic renal failure	✓	✓	✓
	Nephrotic syndrome	✓	✓	✓
	Leukemia	✓	✓	✓
	Lymphoma	✓	✓	✓
	Hodgkin disease	✓	✓	✓
	Generalized malignancy	✓	✓	✓
	Iatrogenic immunosuppression[e]	✓	✓	✓
	Solid-organ transplant	✓	✓	✓
	Multiple myeloma	✓	✓	✓

Abbreviations: CSF, cerebrospinal fluid; HIV, human immunodeficiency virus; PPSV23, pneumococcal polysaccharide vaccine; PVC13, pneumococcal 13-valent conjugate vaccine.

[a] All adults 65 years of age or older should receive a dose of PPSV23, regardless of previous history of vaccination with pneumococcal vaccine.

[b] Including congestive heart failure and cardiomyopathies.

[c] Including chronic obstructive pulmonary disease, emphysema, and asthma.

[d] Includes B- (humoral) or T-lymphocyte deficiency, complement deficiencies (particularly C1, C2, C3, and C4 deficiencies), and phagocytic disorders (excluding chronic granulomatous disease).

[e] Diseases requiring treatment with immunosuppressive drugs, including long-term systemic corticosteroid therapy, and radiation therapy.

Adapted from Centers for Disease Control and Prevention. PCV$_{13}$ (pneumococcal conjugate) vaccine: recommendations, scenarios and Q&As for healthcare professionals about PCV$_{13}$ for adults [Internet]. Atlanta (GA); [updated 2015 Sep 3; cited 2015 Sep 23]. Available from: http://www.cdc.gov/vaccines/vpd-vac/pneumo/vac-PCV13-adults.htm.

be vaccinated. First-year college students up to age 21 years who are living in dormitories should be vaccinated if they have not received a dose after turning 16. There are 2 types of meningococcal vaccines. The 2-dose meningococcal conjugate vaccine should be given 2 months apart for those who need vaccination and are between ages 2 and 55, while the polysaccharide vaccine is preferred for adults aged 55 and older. Adults who remain at high risk should receive a booster every 5 years.

Hepatitis A Vaccination

Adults traveling to countries with high rates of hepatitis A virus infection, persons with chronic liver disease and those receiving clotting factor concentrates, injection drug users, and men who have sex with men should be vaccinated. A protective antibody level is induced within 4 weeks after hepatitis A vaccination. Revaccination is recommended at 6 to 12 months for long-lasting immunity.

Hepatitis B Vaccination

Efforts are being directed toward universal infant vaccination and catch-up vaccination for children and adolescents. Adult vaccination (3-dose series: initial dose, second dose 1 month after initial dose, and third dose 2 months after second dose) is recommended for high-risk groups, including the following:

1. Adults with high-risk behavior (persons with multiple sexual partners, persons with sexually transmitted diseases, men who have sex with men, and injection drug users)

2. Household and sexual contacts of persons with chronic hepatitis B virus infection
3. Health care personnel with exposure to blood or body fluids
4. Adults with end-stage renal disease (including those on dialysis), chronic liver disease, or HIV and adults with diabetes mellitus who are younger than 60 years
5. Travelers planning extended stays in endemic areas
6. Adults in the following settings: sexually transmitted disease treatment facilities, hemodialysis facilities, correctional facilities, and institutions for the developmentally disabled

Haemophilus Influenzae Type b (Hib) Vaccination

Persons with asplenia or sickle cell disease should receive 1 dose. Hib vaccination should be given 14 or more days prior to elective splenectomy. A 3-dose regimen is recommended for recipients of hematopoietic stem cell transplants.

Rabies Vaccination

Preexposure vaccination (3 doses) is recommended for veterinarians, animal handlers, and laboratory personnel working with rabies virus. Vaccination may be considered for travelers to hyperendemic areas staying at least 1 month and for persons whose activities involve exposure to potentially rabid animals.

Postexposure prophylaxis requirements are as follows:

1. Persons with preexposure vaccination require 1 immediate dose of rabies vaccine and a second dose 3 days later.

2. Unimmunized persons require rabies immune globulin and 4 doses of rabies vaccine.

KEY FACTS

- ✓ Live virus vaccines are generally contraindicated—but inactivated vaccines are generally safe—in pregnant women and immunocompromised persons
- ✓ Tdap vaccine in pregnancy—give a dose during each pregnancy, preferably between 27 and 36 weeks
- ✓ Herpes zoster vaccine—recommended for all persons 60 years or older regardless of past history of varicella or zoster infection
- ✓ Pneumococcal vaccine recommendation for adults aged 65 or older—PCV13 followed in 6 to 12 months by PPSV23
- ✓ HPV vaccine recommended routinely at age 11 or 12 (HPV4 or HPV2 for girls, HPV4 for boys); can also be given from age 9 through 26
- ✓ Hib vaccination prior to elective splenectomy—give at least 14 days prior to operation

---

Vaccines for Potential Bioterrorism Agents

Currently, routine vaccination against smallpox, anthrax, and plague is not recommended. Enough live smallpox vaccine has been stockpiled to vaccinate everyone in the United States, and a smallpox response plan has been developed in case of emergency. Anthrax and plague vaccines are recommended only for certain high-risk individuals, including laboratory personnel working directly with *Bacillus anthracis* or *Yersinia pestis*, respectively.

35 Quality Improvement and Patient Safety[a]

JORDAN M. KAUTZ, MD AND CHRISTOPHER M. WITTICH, MD, PharmD

Quality Improvement

Quality improvement, broadly interpreted, refers to any formal approach taken to understand and better the performance of a system. Quality improvement, conversationally, more often is taken to mean those methodologies or tools appropriated from industry and applied to health care. The genesis of the quality movement in health care is often traced to 2 landmark Institute of Medicine reports. "To Err is Human" cast a magnifying glass on safety gaps in care delivery, implicating preventable medical errors in the death of nearly 100,000 hospitalized patients annually. "Crossing the Quality Chasm" further indicted the entire care delivery system for failing its aim to provide consistent, high-quality care to all people, care that is safe, timely, efficient, effective, equitable, and patient-centered. Both publications called urgently to reengineer systems to achieve improvements. W. Edwards Deming's System of Profound Knowledge described 4 components underpinning improvement: appreciation of a system, understanding of variation, theory of knowledge, and psychology. An appreciation, however superficial, of these complex interdependencies underlies the application of process improvement methods and tools increasingly regarded as requisite learning for any health care professional.

Quality Improvement Methods

Many health care organizations today subscribe less to a single approach in favor of a blended framework, such as the Model for Improvement, promoted by organizations such as the Institute for Healthcare Improvement. The model poses 3 questions (What are we trying to accomplish? How will we know that a change is an improvement? What changes can we make that will result in improvement?), then uses the PDSA (Plan, Do, Study, Act) cycle to test, refine, and spread the most promising change ideas. However, 3 approaches are here singled out, both for their historical import and for the fact that their respective emphases are germane to some of the most relevant and frequently encountered problems in health care.

Lean is a term first coined to describe the Toyota Production System during the early 1990s. The core idea is to maximize customer value while minimizing waste. Waiting is the most common waste patients encounter. One example where Lean may be deployed is operating rooms to improve turnover time between cases.

Six Sigma is a set of tools and techniques developed by Motorola, Inc. The core idea is to remove defects and variation at the process level. The name refers to 6 SDs about the mean, which represents 3.4 defects per 1 million opportunities. One example where Six Sigma may be applicable is in intensive care units to address glycemic control.

PDSA cycles grew out of Bell Labs and the experience of Deming in post-war industrial Japan. Primary features of the method include use of iterative cycles, prediction-based

Key Definition

Quality improvement: *systematic and continuous actions that lead to measurable improvement in health care services and the health status of targeted patient groups.*

---

[a] Recommended patient safety strategies previously published in Shekelle PG, Pronovost PJ, Wachter RM, McDonald KM, Schoelles K, Dy SM, et al. The top patient safety strategies that can be encouraged for adoption now. Ann Intern Med. 2013 Mar 5;158(5 Pt 2):365–8. Used with permission.

testing of change, initial small-scale testing, and use of data over time to refine interventions.

Quality Improvement Tools

Important at the outset of any improvement effort is a well-conceived aim statement, which should include the specific patient population affected, the specific health care problem addressed, a quantitative measure of the baseline level of performance, and a quantitative goal (how much) and explicit timeline (by when) for the improvement effort. Experience from other industries and quality improvement experts indicate that applying some or all of the following tools, often regarded as foundational, can solve the majority of operational problems.

Flowchart

Flowcharts are diagrams that use graphic symbols to depict the nature and flow of the steps in a process. Process maps can include diagrams such as a swimlane, SIPOC (Suppliers, Inputs, Process, Outputs, Controls) diagram, or value stream map (Figure 35.1).

Pareto Chart

Pareto charts (Figure 35.2) are a specialized bar chart arranged in descending order of frequency. The objective is to identify the vital few from the trivial many, elsewhere stated as the 80–20 rule: 80% of the problem is attributable to 20% of the causes.

Check Sheet

Check sheets are simple forms used to observe a process and to collect quantitative and qualitative data in real time. They should clearly articulate a data collection plan and operational definitions. They can be used to monitor adherence to hand hygiene or to strict isolation.

Histogram

Histograms are charts that group numeric data into bins, displaying the bins as segmented columns, depicting the distribution of a data set: how often values fall into ranges. Large data sets can be succinctly summarized graphically.

> **Key Definition**
>
> Histogram: *chart that groups numeric data into bins, displaying the bins as segmented columns, depicting the distribution of a data set.*

Scatter Plot

Scatter plots are used to study and identify the possible relationship between 2 variables. The stronger the relationship, the more the diagram resembles a straight line. Correlation does not mean causation, as a confounder may influence both variables.

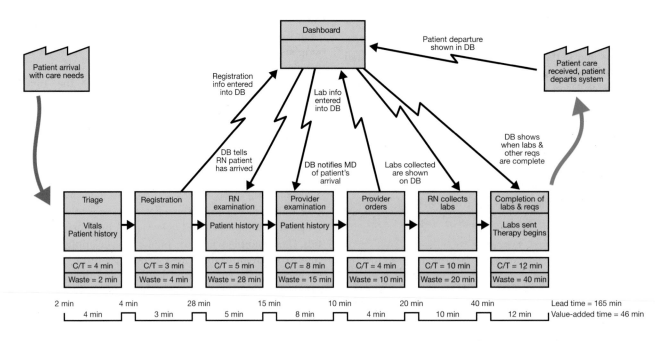

Figure 35.1 *Value Stream Map. C/T indicates cycle time; DB, dashboard; info, information; lab, laboratory test result; MD, physician; reqs, requisitions; RN, registered nurse.*

(Adapted from Dickson EW, Singh S, Cheung DS, Wyatt CC, Nugent AS. Application of lean manufacturing techniques in the Emergency Department. J Emerg Med. 2009 Aug;37[2]:177–82. Epub 2008 Aug 23. Used with permission.)

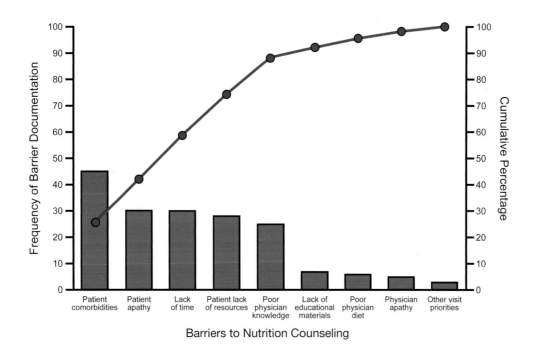

Figure 35.2 *Pareto Chart.*

(Adapted from Fluker SA, Whalen U, Schneider J, Cantey P, Bussey-Jones J, Brady D, et al. Incorporating performance improvement methods into a needs assessment: experience with a nutrition and exercise curriculum. J Gen Intern Med. 2010 Sep;25[Suppl 4]:S627–33. Used with permission.)

Cause-and-Effect Diagram

A cause-and-effect diagram (Figure 35.3) is a quality improvement tool that organizes root causes of a problem. These diagrams are also known as fish bone diagrams owing to their visual appearance or Ishikawa diagrams after the man who popularized their use.

Control Chart

Control charts (Figure 35.4), or statistical process control, are useful for understanding performance of and changes

in a process over time. The chart includes a line representing the mean in the center and lines representing the upper and lower control limits based on 3 SDs on either side of the mean. These are determined by the data. The chart may also include 2 additional lines—specification limits—which are dictated by customer requirements.

For example, an anticoagulation clinic may have a process by which, for a population, the mean International Normalized Ratio is 2.5 and 3 SDs plus/minus 1.1. The upper and lower control limits would be 3.6 and 1.4,

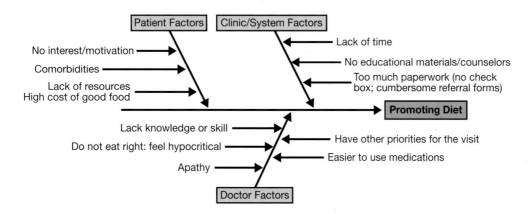

Figure 35.3 Cause-and-Effect (Fish Bone) Diagram.

(Adapted from Fluker SA, Whalen U, Schneider J, Cantey P, Bussey-Jones J, Brady D, et al. Incorporating performance improvement methods into a needs assessment: experience with a nutrition and exercise curriculum. J Gen Intern Med 2010 Sep;25[Suppl 4]:S627–33. Used with permission.)

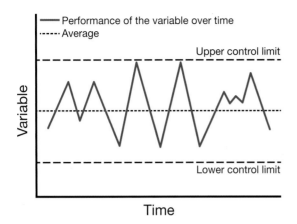

Figure 35.4 *Control Chart.*
(Adapted from Varkey P, Reller MK, Resar RK. Basics of quality improvement in health care. Mayo Clin Proc. 2007 Jun;82[6]:735–9. Used with permission of Mayo Foundation for Medical Education and Research.)

respectively, but the upper and lower specification limits (in this case, the therapeutic window) would be 3.0 and 2.0, respectively.

A process is said to be stable when it is in statistical control, or exhibiting only common cause variation (ie, all data points lie within 3 SDs of either side of the mean). Numerous rules exist to analyze special cause variation. A different approach can be taken toward improvement depending on the type of variation in the process.

Patient Safety

Quality improvement and patient safety are complementary but not synonymous: safety is but 1 dimension of quality care, and quality improvement but 1 behavior of safe care. First, do no harm is 1 of the fundamental precepts of biomedicine; if individuals do not intend harm, how does it nonetheless occur? James Reason proposed what has come to be known as the Swiss Cheese Model. Although successive layers of defense, barriers, and safeguards ("slice") lie between causes and accidents, active failures and latent conditions ("holes"), if aligned, can and will result in harm. This perspective again places blame more squarely on the shoulders of the system, but hardly exonerates the individual. Indeed, understanding human factors—the interactions among humans and other elements of the system—is critical to improving safety by constructing systems wherein it is easier for individuals to do the right thing and harder to do the wrong thing. Again,

such an approach has been robustly employed in other industries, such as aviation and nuclear power. Such high-reliability organizations display the following characteristics: preoccupation with failure, commitment to resilience, and a culture of safety.

KEY FACTS

✓ Three quality improvement methods germane to health care—Lean, Six Sigma, and PDSA cycles

✓ Quality improvement tools—flowchart, Pareto chart, check sheet, histogram, scatter plot, cause-and-effect diagram, and control chart

✓ Check sheets are simple forms with uses such as monitoring adherence to hand hygiene or strict isolation

✓ Quality improvement and patient safety complement each other but are not the same

✓ Patient safety can be improved by constructing systems that make it easier for individuals to do the right thing and harder to do the wrong thing

Selected Topics

Recent scholarship has helped identify a broad array of patient safety strategies for which sufficient evidence exists for widespread adoption and implementation: preoperative and anesthesia checklists to prevent operative and postoperative events; bundles that include checklists to prevent central line–associated bloodstream infections; interventions to reduce urinary catheter use, including catheter reminders, stop orders, or nurse-initiated removal protocols; bundles that include head-of-bed elevation, sedation vacations, oral care, and subglottic suctioning endotracheal tubes to prevent ventilator-associated pneumonia; hand hygiene; the do-not-use list for hazardous abbreviations; multicomponent interventions to reduce pressure ulcers; barrier precautions to prevent health care–associated infections; use of real-time ultrasonography for central line placement; and interventions to improve prophylaxis for venous thromboembolism.

Several major national safety initiatives target certain harmful events and call for increased efforts to eliminate them. In addition to those just mentioned, emphasis has been placed on rapid response teams; evidence-based care for heart failure, myocardial infarction, and pneumonia; adverse drug events, including judicious use of high-risk medications (eg, anticoagulants, narcotics); errors related to handoffs and communication; and wrong-site surgery.

36

Women's Health

NICOLE P. SANDHU, MD, PHD; LYNNE T. SHUSTER, MD; AND AMY T. WANG, MD

Menstruation and Menopause

Menstruation

The menstrual cycle is composed of the follicular (proliferative), periovulatory, and luteal (secretory) phases. At periovulation, the mature follicle triggers a surge in luteinizing hormone (LH) level, causing ovum release and stimulating the residual ovarian follicle to transform into a corpus luteum. Circulating estrogen and progestin levels increase. A thickened, enriched endometrium develops owing to progestin secretion from the corpus luteum. Without fertilization, the corpus luteum atrophies, estrogen and progestin levels decline, follicle-stimulating hormone (FSH) release is stimulated, and the endometrium sloughs (menstruation). FSH then initiates follicle maturation, increasing estrogen production and endometrial growth. The duration of menstruation averages 4 to 6 days. The average menstrual cycle lasts 24 to 35 days, but about 20% of women have irregular cycles. Women at extremes of body mass index often have longer mean cycle lengths. Women within 5 to 7 years after menarche and 10 years before menopause have greater cycle variability.

Premenstrual Syndrome

Premenstrual syndrome (PMS) is the cyclic occurrence of symptoms a week prior to menses that interfere with social and economic function and are relieved within a few days after menstruation. Symptoms include irritable mood, abdominal bloating, breast tenderness, back pain, headache, appetite changes, fatigue, and difficulty concentrating. Premenstrual dysphoric disorder (PDD) differs in that emotional symptoms predominate in severity over physical symptoms. PDD may include markedly depressed mood, anxiety, anger or emotional lability, lethargy, difficulty concentrating, insomnia or hypersomnia, and a sense of being out of control. Symptoms occur during the last week of the luteal phase and resolve within a few days of menstruation. To meet the diagnostic criteria for PDD, symptoms must markedly interfere with work, school, or usual social activities and relationships with others.

Reducing caffeine, salt, sugar, and alcohol intake and eating small, frequent meals with complex carbohydrates may help some women with mild to moderate premenstrual symptoms and PMS. Exercise, stress reduction, and relaxation techniques can also be helpful, as can supplementation with calcium carbonate, vitamin B_6, or magnesium. Nonsteroidal anti-inflammatory drugs (NSAIDs) and oral contraceptives are effective for physical symptoms of PMS. Selective serotonin reuptake inhibitors are the treatment of choice for emotional symptoms. They may be prescribed continuously or cyclically (luteal phase).

Abnormal Uterine Bleeding (in Women of Reproductive Age)

Bleeding that is excessive or outside the normal cyclic bleeding pattern is called abnormal uterine bleeding (Box 36.1). The terms *menorrhagia, metrorrhagia,* and *oligomenorrhea* have been replaced by *heavy menstrual bleeding* (ovulatory heavy bleeding), *intermenstrual bleeding* (bleeding in between regular menses), and *ovulatory dysfunction* (irregular nonovulatory bleeding).

Etiology of uterine bleeding is classified with the mnemonic PALM COEIN. PALM (polyp, adenomyosis, leiomyoma, malignancy and hyperplasia) represents structural causes of bleeding, while COEIN (coagulopathy, ovulatory dysfunction, endometrial, iatrogenic, and not yet classified) represents nonstructural causes.

The history should include date of last period; timing, duration, and amount of bleeding; bleeding pattern; associated pain; evidence of ovulatory cycling (regular menses, cyclic symptoms); contraceptive history; weight changes;

Box 36.1 • Possible Causes of Abnormal Uterine Bleeding

Pregnancy

Anovulation or oligo-ovulation

Fibroids

Polyps, endometrial or endocervical

Adenomyosis

Endometriosis

Infection, including pelvic inflammatory disease

Endometrial hyperplasia

Endometrial carcinoma

Coagulation disorders

Hyperprolactinemia

Liver disease

Thyroid dysfunction

Obesity

Anorexia

Rapid fluctuations in weight

Corticosteroids

Hormonal contraceptives

Tamoxifen

medications; substance abuse; and impact of bleeding on quality of life. History suggestive of an underlying bleeding disorder should be elicited, especially in adolescents.

Physical examination includes pelvic, breast, and thyroid examinations and assessment of body habitus and hair distribution. Uterine source of bleeding should be verified whenever possible. Mucosal lesions should be noted and evaluated appropriately. Obese women can have irregular, anovulatory bleeding due to increased circulating estrogen (from androgen conversion in adipose tissue). Underweight patients may have ovulatory dysfunction as a result of hypothalamic dysfunction. Hirsutism suggests polycystic ovary syndrome. Vaginal atrophy and cervical lesions can cause postcoital spotting or bleeding. Pregnancy and ectopic pregnancy must be considered when evaluating abnormal uterine bleeding.

Laboratory assessment includes pregnancy testing, a complete blood cell count, and if ovulatory dysfunction is present, thyrotropin (thyroid-stimulating hormone) and prolactin levels. Cervical cancer screening should be up-to-date. Testing for gonorrhea and chlamydial infection should be done in patients who are at high risk, have purulent discharge, or have tenderness on pelvic examination. For women aged 45 years or older, endometrial sampling is recommended as first-line testing. In women younger than 45 years, endometrial cancer is related to endometrial proliferation in the absence of withdrawal bleeding. Thus, endometrial sampling is indicated in women younger than 45 years who have persistent anovulation, did not respond to medical management, or are at high risk for endometrial cancer. Transvaginal ultrasonography is useful in evaluating for structural abnormalities suspected from physical examination and in women who continue to have symptoms despite treatment. Using transvaginal ultrasonography to measure endometrial thickness can be an alternative to endometrial sampling in postmenopausal women but not in premenopausal women, as endometrial thickness varies through the menstrual cycle.

When possible, treatment is directed at the underlying cause, including medical conditions, such as polycystic ovarian syndrome, hypothyroidism, hyperprolactinemia, and chronic endometritis, and structural abnormalities, such as endometrial polyps and submucosal fibroids, which can be resected with hysteroscopy. Pharmacologic therapy can be given to control bleeding and restore quality of life. Estrogen-progestin contraceptives, oral progestin, and a levonorgestrel-releasing intrauterine device (IUD) are effective first-line therapies. NSAIDs and tranexamic acid can be used in patients who have contraindications to hormonal therapies. In women who are trying to conceive in the near future, oral progestin is preferred; NSAIDs can also be used but should be stopped on conception because of increased risk of congenital anomalies and miscarriage. Definitive therapy with endometrial ablation or hysterectomy is an option for those who have completed childbearing and want to avoid medication or IUDs.

KEY FACTS

✓ Emotional symptoms predominate in premenstrual dysphoric disorder; physical symptoms in premenstrual syndrome

✓ Nonsteroidal anti-inflammatory drugs and oral contraceptives are effective for physical symptoms of premenstrual syndrome; selective serotonin reuptake inhibitors for emotional symptoms

✓ PALM COEIN mnemonic for abnormal uterine bleeding—PALM (polyp, adenomyosis, leiomyoma, malignancy and hyperplasia) represents structural causes; COEIN (coagulopathy, ovulatory dysfunction, endometrial, iatrogenic, and not yet classified) represents nonstructural causes

✓ Endometrial sampling is needed to evaluate abnormal uterine bleeding in women aged 45 years or older

✓ First-line therapies for abnormal uterine bleeding— estrogen-progestin contraceptives, oral progestin, or levonorgestrel-releasing intrauterine device

Contraception and Infertility

Contraception

Contraceptive methods include hormonal (oral, transdermal, vaginal, intrauterine, intradermal implant, and intramuscular injection), barrier, chemical, and physiologic

Table 36.1 • Contraception Options

Contraceptive Method	Adverse Effects/Risks	Benefits
Combined hormonal contraceptives (pill, patch, vaginal ring)	Increased risk of DVT, MI, CVA, HTN, hepatic adenoma; nausea, headaches, spotting, mastalgia, mood changes	Reduced risk of dysmenorrhea, heavy menstrual bleeding, anemia, ovarian and endometrial cancers, acne
Progestin-only pill	Unpredictable spotting, bleeding	Can use when estrogen is contraindicated (HTN, CV disease, breast cancer, clotting). Does not interfere with lactation
Depo-progestin	Menstrual changes, weight gain, headache, delayed return to ovulation	Lactation not disturbed; convenience
Progesterone implant	Delayed return to ovulation	Convenience
IUD (copper or levonorgestrel)	Spotting, cramping, back pain	Convenience
Condom	Requires planning ahead; may decrease sensation	Protects against STIs
Diaphragm	Requires planning ahead; must be left in place for 6–8 h after sexual intercourse; requires spermicide	Avoids hormone-related adverse effects
Female sterilization (tubal ligation)	Surgical complications, increased risk of ectopic pregnancy, regret	Convenience
Male sterilization (vasectomy)	Surgical complications	More effective and fewer complications than female sterilization
Fertility awareness–based methods	Pregnancy risk 9%–19%; takes time to learn; requires abstaining from sexual intercourse or using barrier method during fertile window	Learning biomarkers of fertility can help a committed couple plan pregnancy or avoid pregnancy

Abbreviations: CV, cardiovascular; CVA, cerebrovascular accident; DVT, deep vein thrombosis; HTN, hypertension; IUD, intrauterine device; MI, myocardial infarction; STI, sexually transmitted infection.

approaches. None are 100% effective, and all carry some degree of risk (Table 36.1).

Factors to consider include efficacy, convenience, duration of action, reversibility and time to return of fertility, effect on uterine bleeding, risk of adverse events, affordability, and protection against sexually transmitted infections. Balancing the advantages and disadvantages of each method guides individual decisions. Methods consistent with a woman's values and lifestyle are most likely to be successful. Effective contraceptive use requires education and counseling regarding appropriate use.

Hormonal contraceptives may include estrogen plus a progestogen or a progestogen alone. They come in various forms, including a transdermal patch and a vaginal ring; the most common form is the combination estrogen-progestogen pill. Estrogen prevents ovulation by suppressing FSH and LH and contributing to corpus luteum degeneration. Progestogens inhibit ovulation by suppressing the midcycle LH and FSH peak; they also thicken cervical mucus and alter tubal motility, interfering with sperm transport, and lead to an atrophic endometrium, interfering with fertilized ovum implantation.

Combination estrogen-progestogen pills are highly effective (97%–99%) when used *correctly*; the failure rate is about 3 per 1,000 in the first year of use. However, with *typical* use, the failure rate is estimated to be 8%. Noncontraceptive benefits include menstrual cycle regularity; maintenance of bone mineral density; reduced risk of endometrial and ovarian cancer; and frequent use in treating acne, hirsutism, symptomatic leiomyomas, and endometriosis. Common adverse effects include breakthrough bleeding (more common with missed pills or low-dose estrogen), bloating, and breast tenderness. Estrogen-containing oral contraceptives are thrombogenic, but the absolute risk of venous thromboembolism is low. Increasing age and obesity are also associated with an increased risk. Women older than 35 years who smoke cigarettes have a relative contraindication to combination oral contraceptives because of an increased risk of myocardial infarction and stroke (Box 36.2). Combination oral contraceptives are also contraindicated in women with a history of migraine with aura and in women with uncontrolled hypertension. Progestogen-only pills should be considered in women with migraine headaches, hypertension, diabetes mellitus, personal or family history of thromboembolism, cardiac or cerebrovascular disease, or hypertriglyceridemia and in women older than 35 years who smoke.

KEY FACTS

✓ As typically used, combination oral contraceptives fail in approximately 8% of patients

✓ Noncontraceptive benefits of oral contraceptives— menstrual cycle regularity, maintenance of bone mineral density, reduced risk of endometrial and ovarian cancer, and treatment of other conditions

✓ Common adverse effects of oral contraceptives— breakthrough bleeding, bloating, and breast tenderness

✓ Consider progestogen-only pills in women smokers older than 35 years

Women seeking longer-acting contraception also have several options. Depot medroxyprogesterone acetate injections can be given either intramuscularly or subcutaneously every 3 months. Several forms of long-term progestin-only contraception are available as implants in the upper arm (etonogestrel and levonorgestrel) or as an IUD; these last for 3 to 5 years, depending on the type and formulation. Copper IUDs are another option for women who have contraindications to hormone use and can be left in place for 10 years.

Infertility

Infertility is the inability to conceive after 1 year of intercourse without contraception and may be due to male or female factors, or both. The cause may be difficult to identify. Declining oocyte quality with advanced age is a major cause of infertility. Other common causes of female infertility are ovulatory disorders (eg, polycystic ovary syndrome, hypothyroidism, hyperprolactinemia, eating disorders, extreme stress), endometriosis, pelvic adhesions, and tubal abnormalities.

Key Definition

Infertility: *the inability to conceive after 1 year of intercourse without contraception; may be due to male or female factors, or both.*

Evaluation includes the history (duration of infertility; prior evaluation or interventions; menstrual history; sexual history; lifestyle factors, including exercise, diet, stress, smoking, and substance abuse; medical and surgical history), partner semen analysis, documentation of ovulation through history and midluteal serum progesterone level, assessment of ovarian reserve (day 3 serum FSH and estradiol levels), assessment of fallopian tube patency and the uterus with hysterosalpingography, and exclusion of endocrinologic causes by measurement of prolactin and thyroid function.

Medical Issues of Pregnancy

Preconception Counseling and Prenatal Care

Prenatal care is associated with improved pregnancy outcomes. Lifestyle factors (diet, exercise, and avoidance of tobacco, alcohol, and illicit drug use) should be addressed. Adequate folic acid supplementation before conception decreases the risk of neural tube defects. Alcohol use during pregnancy is associated with early spontaneous abortion, placental abruption, and fetal alcohol syndrome and is the third leading cause of intellectual disability. Smoking is associated with low birth weight, perinatal death, infertility, spontaneous abortion, ectopic pregnancy, placenta previa and placental abruption, and sudden infant death syndrome. Caffeine intake of 1 to 2 cups of coffee or other caffeinated beverage daily is not associated with miscarriage or birth defects.

Immunizations and Pregnancy

Live vaccines should be avoided during pregnancy, but certain inactivated vaccines should be routinely administered during pregnancy, including the tetanus-diphtheria-acellular pertussis vaccine (Tdap), which is recommended for all pregnant women during 27 to 36 weeks of gestation for each pregnancy, and the inactivated influenza vaccine during influenza season (Box 36.3).

Medical Care During Pregnancy

Hypertension complicates up to 10% of pregnancies and is an important cause of maternal and fetal morbidity and death.

Box 36.2 • Contraindications to Use of Estrogen-Containing Oral Contraceptives

Absolute contraindications

History of deep vein thrombosis or pulmonary embolism, unless defined nonhormonal cause
History of arterial thromboembolism
Active liver disease
Cardiovascular disease such as congestive heart failure, myocardial infarction or coronary artery disease, atrial fibrillation, mitral stenosis, mechanical heart valve
Systemic diseases that affect the vascular system (such as systemic lupus erythematosus, diabetes mellitus with retinopathy or nephropathy)
Cigarette smoking by women >35 y
Uncontrolled hypertension
History of breast cancer
Undiagnosed amenorrhea

Relative contraindications

Classic migraine
Hypertriglyceridemia
Depression

Box 36.3 • Vaccinations and Pregnancy

Inactivated vaccines

Hepatitis A: Vaccinate if at high risk for disease

Hepatitis B: Vaccinate if at risk

Human papillomavirus: Not recommended during pregnancy

Before or after pregnancy, vaccinate through age 26 y

Influenza: Vaccinate with inactivated flu vaccine all women who will be pregnant during the influenza season. *Avoid administration of nasal flu vaccine (FluMist), a live attenuated viral vaccine, during pregnancy*

Meningococcus: Administer if indicated. Vaccine should be administered to women at increased risk, such as those who are asplenic due to terminal complement component deficiencies, first-year college students living in a dormitory, military recruits, and persons traveling to countries in which meningococcal disease is hyperendemic

Pneumococcus: Administer if indicated. Vaccine should be administered to women at increased risk, such as those who are asplenic and those with diabetes mellitus, cardiopulmonary or chronic kidney disease, or chronic liver disease

Toxoid vaccines

Td plus acellular pertussis (Tdap): Administer during each pregnancy, ideally between 27 and 36 weeks of gestation; if missed, give in the immediate postpartum period

Live attenuated vaccines: Avoid during pregnancy

Influenza nasal vaccine (FluMist)

MMR: Avoid conception for 4 wk after MMR vaccination

Varicella: Avoid conception for 4 wk after varicella vaccination

Abbreviations: MMR, measles, mumps, and rubella; Td, tetanus/diphtheria.

Pregnancy creates a thrombogenic state, yet thromboembolism is uncommon during pregnancy. However, women with hereditary thrombophilias are at high risk for thrombosis during pregnancy, with potentially serious complications. Low-molecular-weight heparin is the preferred treatment for thromboembolism during pregnancy or for prevention in high-risk women. Warfarin is teratogenic and increases the risk of spontaneous abortion and should be avoided during pregnancy.

Maternal hypothyroidism is associated with infertility, miscarriage, stillbirth, placental abruption, preeclampsia, and motor and intellectual disability in the infant. Thyrotropin (thyroid-stimulating hormone) should be measured early in pregnancy, and women taking thyroid hormone should be monitored regularly. About 20% require a dose increase. Hyperthyroidism occurs in only about 0.2% of pregnancies. Symptoms and signs may overlap with normal findings in pregnancy, and low weight gain may be the only clue. Poorly controlled hyperthyroidism may lead to spontaneous abortion, premature delivery, preeclampsia, congestive heart failure, and low birth weight. Propylthiouracil is the treatment of choice during pregnancy to prevent fetal goiter and hypothyroidism. In many women, the dose of propylthiouracil can be tapered or discontinued in the last trimester. Radioiodine is absolutely contraindicated during pregnancy and lactation. Surgery should not be considered unless hyperthyroidism is refractory to medical therapy.

Diseases of the Uterus and Adnexa

Endometriosis

Endometriosis is the presence of endometrial glands and stroma outside the endometrial cavity and uterine wall. The most common sites (in decreasing frequency) are the ovaries, cul-de-sac, broad and uterosacral ligaments, uterus, fallopian tubes, sigmoid colon, appendix, and round ligaments. The most common symptom is pain, which may manifest as pelvic pain, chronic dyspareunia or dysmenorrhea, or cyclic bowel or bladder symptoms. Endometriosis is found in 20% to 40% of infertile women and in up to 65% of women with chronic pelvic pain. Physical examination findings may be normal. Localized tenderness in the cul-de-sac or uterosacral ligaments suggests endometriosis. Pelvic ultrasonography findings may be suggestive of the diagnosis, but definitive diagnosis requires direct visualization and biopsy of endometriosis, ideally laparoscopically.

Key Definition

Endometriosis: *the presence of endometrial glands and stroma outside the endometrial cavity and uterine wall.*

Treatment is directed at symptom relief (Table 36.2) and depends on symptom severity, disease extent and location, desire for pregnancy, patient age, and prior treatment response. Empirical medical therapy with an NSAID, oral contraceptive, or gonadotropin-releasing hormone agonist is reasonable when endometriosis is suspected prior to definitive surgical diagnosis. If this fails, a diagnostic laparoscopy is often done, during which ablation and excision of implants and adhesions can be performed. Postoperative medical suppressive therapy has been shown to decrease recurrence. Definitive surgical therapy involves hysterectomy and oophorectomy. The surgical approach depends on the severity of symptoms, the age of the patient, and the desire for fertility.

Table 36.2 • Treatment Options for Endometriosis

Symptom	Treatment Options	Impact on Endometriotic Implants	Adverse Effects
Mild pelvic pain	Analgesics (eg, NSAIDs)	Do not reduce endometriotic implants	Minimal
	Oral contraceptives	Evidence conflicts on whether therapy reduces implant size or inhibits progression of disease	Minimal
Moderate to severe pain Pain that does not respond to analgesics or oral contraceptives	GnRH agonist (eg, leuprolide, nafarelin, goserelin)	Reduces size of endometriotic implants	Menopausal symptoms, bone loss FDA approval for no more than 6 mo of continuous use Combination with progestins or low-dose estrogen-progestin therapy minimizes adverse effects and allows prolonged use
	Progestins (oral or depot medroxyprogesterone acetate)	Evidence unclear as to effect on implant size or inhibition of disease progression	Weight gain, irregular uterine bleeding, mood changes
	Danazol	Reduces size of endometriotic implants	Weight gain, muscle cramps, decreased breast size, acne, hirsutism, lipid changes, hot flushes, mood changes
Severe pain Pain unresponsive to medical management Advanced disease Large or symptomatic endometrioma	Surgery	Reduces size of endometriotic implants and adhesions	May lead to development of postsurgical adhesions

Abbreviations: FDA, US Food and Drug Administration; GnRH, gonadotropin-releasing hormone; NSAID, nonsteroidal anti-inflammatory drug.

KEY FACTS

✓ Tdap vaccine is recommended at 27 to 36 weeks' gestation during each pregnancy

✓ The treatment of choice for hyperthyroidism during pregnancy is propylthiouracil

✓ Endometriosis most commonly causes pain, manifested as pelvic pain, chronic dyspareunia or dysmenorrhea, or cyclic bowel or bladder symptoms

✓ Factors to consider in choosing treatment of endometriosis—symptom severity, disease extent and location, desire for pregnancy, patient age

Uterine Fibroids

Uterine leiomyomas (fibroids or myomas) are benign monoclonal tumors that arise from the smooth muscle of the myometrium. They are the most common female pelvic tumors, occurring in 50% to 80% of women, and are most prevalent during the reproductive years, usually regressing after menopause. Approximately 25% are symptomatic. Fibroid-related symptoms are grouped into 3 categories: menstrual (eg, dysmenorrhea, heavy menstrual bleeding), bulk-related (eg, pelvic pain, pelvic pressure, urinary frequency, constipation, dyspareunia), and reproductive dysfunction (eg, recurrent miscarriage, obstetric complications).

Key Definition

Uterine leiomyomas (fibroids or myomas): *benign monoclonal tumors that arise from the smooth muscle of the myometrium.*

Fibroids are suggested by an enlarged, irregularly shaped, firm, nontender uterus on pelvic examination. Transvaginal ultrasonography should be done if the diagnosis is uncertain; fibroids appear as symmetric, well-defined, hypoechoic, heterogeneous masses. Hysteroscopy may be used, particularly if myomectomy is planned. Annual pelvic examination should be done; further evaluation is warranted if symptoms change or uterine size increases. Routine surveillance imaging is not recommended.

Treatment is necessary only if fibroids are symptomatic. A trial of medical therapy before surgical therapy is appropriate for symptomatic fibroids (anemia, heavy bleeding, or pain). Gonadotropin-releasing hormone agonists (eg, leuprolide) cause amenorrhea and reduce uterine size in most cases. The levonorgestrel IUD may reduce menstrual blood loss and uterine size. Surgical treatment is indicated when symptoms persist despite medical treatment, when infertility or recurrent pregnancy loss is related to fibroids, or when malignancy is suspected. Surgery should be considered in a postmenopausal woman with a new or enlarging pelvic mass to exclude uterine sarcoma.

Surgical options include myomectomy (if there is no suspicion of malignancy) or hysterectomy. Myomectomy involves removal of the fibroids with uterine conservation and preserves childbearing potential. Less invasive options when childbearing is complete and there is no suspicion of malignancy include endometrial ablation, myolysis, uterine artery embolization, and magnetic resonance–guided focused ultrasound ablation.

Cervical Cancer Screening

Cervical cancer screening is covered in Chapter 34: Preventive Medicine. Additional evaluation and treatment based on cervical cytologic findings depend on the abnormality. Up-to-date consensus guidelines and algorithms for managing abnormal results of cervical cancer screening tests can be found online through the American Society of Colposcopy and Cervical Pathology (http://www.asccp.org/Portals/9/docs/ASCCP%20Management%20Guidelines_August%202014.pdf).

Vulvar Skin Disorders

Vulvar itching, burning, and pain are common symptoms and may be acute or chronic. Common causes of vulvar pruritus (Box 36.4) include vulvovaginal candidiasis, contact dermatitis, lichen sclerosus, lichen simplex chronicus, neoplastic conditions (eg, vulvar intraepithelial neoplasia, squamous cell carcinoma, Paget disease of the vulva), or vulvar manifestations of systemic disease (eg, Crohn disease). Vulvodynia is pain at the vaginal opening often described as burning, stinging, rawness, or soreness, with or without pruritus. Typically, there are no visible vulvar skin changes and cotton swab testing reproduces pain. Contact dermatitis may be acute (blisters, itching, and weeping) or chronic (redness, burning, and swelling). Physical findings range from mild erythema and scaling to intense erythema, fissures, erosions, and ulcers. Treatment is removal of the offending irritant or allergen and topical corticosteroid ointments.

Lichen simplex chronicus may present with persistent intense itching, typically with scaling and lichenified plaques that result from chronic rubbing or scratching. If the condition is long-standing, vulvar skin may appear thickened and leathery, with areas of hyperpigmentation or hypopigmentation.

Lichen sclerosus has the following features: thinned, whitened, and crinkling skin; porcelain-white papules and

---

Box 36.4 • Conditions Commonly Associated With Vulvar Itching

Acute

  Contact dermatitis
  Infections: fungal, trichomoniasis, molluscum, scabies

Chronic

  Dermatoses: contact dermatitis, lichen sclerosus, lichen planus, lichen simplex chronicus, psoriasis, genital atrophy
  Neoplasia: vulvar intraepithelial neoplasia, vulvar cancer, Paget disease
  Vulvar manifestations of systemic disease: eg, Crohn disease

Adapted from ACOG Practice Bulletin No. 93: diagnosis and management of vulvar skin disorders. Obstet Gynecol. 2008 May;111(5):1243–53. Used with permission.

---

plaques; areas of ecchymoses or purpura; and possible agglutination of tissues with fusion of the labia minora and phimosis of the clitoral hood. Biopsy should be done to confirm the diagnosis before initiation of topical corticosteroid treatment (typically clobetasol) and to rule out squamous cell carcinoma.

Lichen planus is an inflammatory disorder with mucous membrane findings ranging from white irregular lines to deep, painful, erythematous erosions and scarring resulting in vaginal obliteration. As with lichen sclerosus, biopsy is recommended to confirm the diagnosis and rule out cancer. Treatment options include topical and systemic corticosteroid, topical and oral cyclosporine, topical tacrolimus, and intramuscular triamcinolone. Lichen planus is chronic and tends to be treatment-resistant.

The common symptoms of vulvovaginal atrophy are vulvar irritation and dryness. On examination, there is loss of labial and vulvar fullness, urethral and vaginal mucosal pallor, and dryness. Diagnosis is based on physical examination findings and is confirmed by an increased vaginal pH (6.0–7.5). Treatment is with topical estrogen (cream, tablet, or vaginal ring).

Perimenopause

Perimenopause typically lasts several years and is characterized by erratic hormone levels and irregular menstrual periods. Symptoms such as hot flushes, vaginal dryness, and sleep disturbances are common, as are anovulatory cycles, which contribute to irregular menstrual bleeding. Despite reduced fertility, pregnancy is possible until menopause (either 12 months of no menstrual periods or FSH levels consistently >30 mIU/mL).

> ## Box 36.5 • Menopause-Related Terms
>
> **Natural/spontaneous menopause:** the final menstrual period, confirmed after 12 consecutive mo of amenorrhea with no obvious pathologic cause
>
> **Induced menopause:** permanent cessation of menstruation after bilateral oophorectomy or iatrogenic ablation of ovarian function
>
> **Perimenopause or menopausal transition:** span of time when menstrual cycle changes and endocrine changes occur a few years before and 12 mo after the final menstrual period, resulting from natural menopause
>
> **Premature menopause:** menopause reached at or before age 40 y
>
> **Premature ovarian failure:** ovarian insufficiency occurring before age 40 y and leading to permanent or transient amenorrhea
>
> **Early menopause:** natural or induced menopause occurring at or before age 45 y

Menstrual changes may include lighter or heavier bleeding, irregular bleeding duration, or skipped periods. Certain bleeding patterns warrant evaluation: very heavy flow, especially with clots; bleeding lasting more than 7 days; bleeding intervals less than 21 days; intermenstrual spotting or bleeding; and postcoital bleeding.

The decision about when to stop oral contraceptives or switch to postmenopausal hormone therapy is not straightforward. Clinical signs of menopause are masked by use of hormonal contraceptives. FSH levels are labile in perimenopause, and unless they are consistently higher than 30 mIU/mL, menopause is not confirmed. Hormonal contraceptives may lower FSH levels, confounding interpretation. FSH testing after a contraceptive pill–free interval of 1 to 2 months, while alternative contraception is being used, can help to establish menopause, if needed.

Terms related to menopause are defined in Box 36.5.

Menopause

Menopause is the permanent cessation of menses occurring when ovarian follicles are depleted. Natural menopause, a clinical diagnosis, is confirmed when a woman has no menses for 12 months, typically occurring between ages 42 and 58 years (average, 51 years). It often occurs earlier in smokers and nulliparous women. Menopause may also be induced by surgery, chemotherapy, or pelvic irradiation.

The hallmark symptom of menopause is hot flushes (also called hot flashes) (abrupt onset of warmth and red skin blotching involving the chest, face, and neck) often associated with transient anxiety, palpitations, and profuse sweating. Most menopausal women have hot flashes; 10% to 15% report that they are frequent or severe. Hot flashes often begin more than 2 years before menopause and usually peak within 2 to 3 years after menopause, but they continue in some women for many years after menopause. Frequency, duration, and intensity vary. Hot flashes coincide with declining estrogen levels, but they are not due to hypoestrogenism. The mechanism is attributed to dysfunction of the thermoregulatory center in the hypothalamus.

Other postmenopausal symptoms include vaginal dryness and irritation, urinary urgency and frequency, dyspareunia, changes in sexual function, mood swings, and cognitive function changes. Menopausal symptoms tend to be more intense after surgically induced menopause than natural menopause.

When hot flashes occur in a healthy woman of typical menopausal age, no diagnostic testing is necessary. However, if the clinical scenario is atypical, testing for an increased FSH level may be helpful. In the setting of an atypical clinical scenario and normal premenopausal FSH and estradiol levels, other causes of hot flashes should be considered (eg, thyroid dysfunction, infection, carcinoid syndrome, pheochromocytoma, autoimmune disorders, mast cell disorders, malignancies).

Postmenopausal Bleeding

In postmenopausal women with bleeding not caused by vaginal or endometrial atrophy or cervical lesions, endometrial cancer must be excluded, unless the patient is using cycling hormonal therapy. Transvaginal ultrasonography or endometrial biopsy should be considered. If endometrial thickness is more than 5 mm on ultrasonography, there are other endometrial abnormalities (eg, a focal lesion), or bleeding is persistent, biopsy is indicated. Once malignancy is excluded, reassurance is usually sufficient.

Hormone Therapy

Estrogen is the most effective treatment of hot flushes and other menopausal symptoms, but it is associated with potential risks (Box 36.6). Postmenopausal hormone therapy is appropriate only for women with moderate to severe symptoms of menopause interfering with quality of life or activities of daily living. It should be prescribed at the lowest dose that relieves symptoms and for the shortest duration needed for treatment goals. It is not indicated to treat osteopenia or osteoporosis in most women. In women with an intact uterus, unopposed estrogen increases the risk of uterine dysplasia and malignancy, and thus a cyclic progestogen must be used; women must be made aware that cyclic bleeding will occur in this setting.

Breast Conditions

Evaluation of the Palpable Breast Mass

Breast lumps are common and usually benign. Benign characteristics are insufficient to exclude cancer; if clinical suspicion is high, negative findings even on mammography and ultrasonography do not definitively exclude cancer.

History should include location, duration, behavior related to menstrual cycle, associated pain, skin or nipple changes (eg, discharge, excoriation), trauma, and changes prior to evaluation. Risk factors should be considered, but a lack of defined risk factors does not exclude the possibility of cancer. Physical examination should include visual inspection for asymmetry, puckering, dimpling, nipple lesions or retraction, erythema, and peau d'orange. Palpation should include tissue from the clavicle to the inframammary area and from the sternum to the midaxillary line. The axillary, cervical, and supraclavicular nodal regions should be included.

Initial imaging evaluation includes diagnostic mammography and ultrasonography in women aged 30 years or older and ultrasonography in women younger than 30 years. Symptomatic simple cysts can be aspirated. Nonbloody fluid does not require cytologic evaluation. A complex cyst should be aspirated to confirm complete resolution of the cyst.

Tissue evaluation options are fine-needle aspiration (FNA), core needle biopsy (CNB), and excisional biopsy. FNA is inexpensive and can be done in an office setting, but the sensitivity and specificity are highly variable. A negative FNA result does not exclude cancer, particularly when clinical or imaging suspicion is high. CNB provides enough tissue for histologic diagnosis and is often done with imaging guidance; it has higher sensitivity and better specimen quality than FNA. Concordance between CNB and excisional biopsy exceeds 90%. Excisional biopsy is reserved for cases in which FNA and CNB are technically unfeasible or when the findings on FNA or CNB are discordant with the physical examination or imaging findings. CNB or excisional biopsy should be done when FNA shows atypical cells. Excisional biopsy should be done when CNB shows atypical hyperplasia (to exclude malignancy).

Mammographic features of malignancy include soft tissue masses or clustered microcalcifications. The most specific mammographic feature of malignancy is a spiculated mass. Calcifications that are large and diffuse or scattered are usually benign, whereas those described as clustered punctate, fine pleomorphic, or fine linear branching suggest malignancy.

KEY FACTS

- ✓ Fibroids need treatment only if they cause symptoms
- ✓ Before starting topical corticosteroid therapy, confirm the diagnosis of lichen sclerosus with vulvar biopsy
- ✓ Prescribe postmenopausal hormone therapy at the lowest dose and for the shortest time needed to reach treatment goals
- ✓ If breast calcifications on mammography are large and diffuse or scattered, they are usually benign; if clustered punctate, fine pleomorphic, or fine linear branching, usually malignant

Breast Pain

Breast pain (mastalgia) is classified as cyclic, noncyclic, or extramammary. Cyclic mastalgia occurs in premenopausal women. The pain begins in the luteal phase (2 weeks prior to menses) and resolves or substantially improves with menstruation. Pain is usually diffuse, bilateral, and concentrated in the upper outer aspect of the breasts, but it may be more severe in one breast.

Noncyclic mastalgia is not associated with the menstrual cycle; it can affect premenopausal and postmenopausal women. The cause is often elusive, but it may be due to pregnancy, duct dilatation, cysts, fibroadenomas, injury, prior breast surgery, infection, or exogenous estrogen. Breast pain alone is due to cancer in less than 10% of cases, and less than 1% of women with breast pain and normal results on clinical examination and breast imaging have cancer. The evaluation of focal breast pain should include history and clinical examination, age-appropriate mammography, and ultrasonography. Ultrasonography alone should be used in women younger than 30 years who present with focal pain. In women whose history is consistent with cyclic pain and in whom results of clinical examination are negative, reassurance and pain management, depending on severity, are usually sufficient.

For persistent or moderate to severe pain, initial treatment strategies include a well-fitted support brassiere (including nighttime use), heat and/or cold packs, gentle massage, dietary changes (eg, reduced intake of caffeine, sodium, and dietary fat), relaxation techniques, and exercise. Over-the-counter analgesics may be effective. Eliminating or adjusting exogenous estrogen doses may alleviate breast pain. Other hormonal agents may be effective in patients with severe cyclic breast pain unresponsive to conservative measures. Danazol is the only US Food and Drug Administration–approved medication for mastalgia; adverse androgenic effects limit its utility.

Nipple Discharge

Nipple discharge is common in reproductive-aged women and is usually benign. Nipple discharge can be classified as due to ductal lesions or galactorrhea (discharge of milk or milklike secretions 6 months or more postpartum in a nonbreastfeeding woman). Galactorrhea presents as spontaneous, milky discharge from multiple ducts of both breasts as a result of increased serum prolactin. Evaluation and treatment of galactorrhea due to hyperprolactinemia are discussed in Chapter 17, "Pituitary Disorders." Treatment is offered only if the patient is bothered by the discharge, is unable to conceive, or has evidence of hypogonadism or low bone density.

Nipple discharge not due to galactorrhea may be benign or caused by ductal lesions, including malignancy. Benign nipple discharge typically is bilateral, nonbloody, and multiductal, but it may be unilateral. Green, gray, or blue discharge is typical of fibrocystic breast change. Brown or yellow discharge is also usually benign. Clear (watery) discharge is usually benign, but malignancy must be excluded. Pathologic discharge (which may be due to malignancy) is typically unilateral, uniductal, and spontaneous. It is typically bloody, serosanguineous, or, sometimes, watery or clear. The most common cause of bloody nipple discharge is a benign intraductal papilloma, followed by ductal ectasia (ductal dilatation with or without inflammation) and

---

Box 36.7 • Factors That Increase the Likelihood of Cancer Associated With Nipple Discharge

Associated palpable mass

Age >40 y

Grossly bloody, guaiac-positive, serosanguineous, or watery or clear discharge

Unilateral

Spontaneous

Persistent

Single duct

---

carcinoma. Factors associated with an increased likelihood of cancer are detailed in Box 36.7.

Mammography and ultrasonography should be done for all nonlactating women with nipple discharge older than 30 years and ultrasound alone in women younger than 30 years, unless discharge is clearly due to fibrocystic change. Galactography and ductoscopy are not routinely used in the evaluation of nipple discharge.

Patients with nipple discharge that is neither pathologic nor galactorrhea and with normal diagnostic breast imaging results can be reassured and observed. Patients with pathologic discharge that can be clinically localized to 1 duct should be considered for surgical duct excision, even when imaging results are negative. Figure 36.1 is a suggested algorithm for the evaluation of spontaneous nipple discharge.

Benign Breast Disease

Simple cysts are the most common cause of discrete benign breast lumps and occur most often between ages 35 and 50 years. Fibroadenomas are the most common solid benign masses; the median age at diagnosis of fibroadenomas is 30 years, but they may also occur in postmenopausal women. There are many other histologic classifications of benign breast disease. The main significance lies in whether they confer an increased risk of breast cancer. Patients at significantly increased risk should be counseled about appropriate screening and risk reduction options. The magnitude of risk varies depending on the histologic classification. The classification is detailed in Box 36.8.

Depression and Anxiety in Women

The lifetime prevalence of depression is higher in women than men, and the peak age at onset is lower (33 to 45 years in women vs >55 years in men). Women are less likely to commit suicide but twice as likely to attempt suicide, and white women are twice as likely as African American women to commit suicide. There is no sex difference for bipolar disorder.

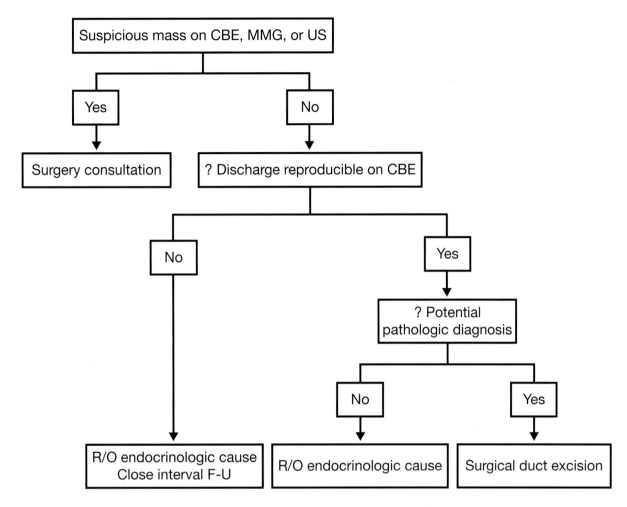

Figure 36.1 *Algorithm for Evaluation of Spontaneous Nipple Discharge. CBE indicates clinical breast examination; F-U, follow-up; MMG, mammography; R/O, rule out; US, ultrasonography.*

The risk of depressive symptoms and clinical depression increases during perimenopause, whether natural or surgically induced. Postmenopausal estrogen may improve mild depressive symptoms, but it is not sufficient for treatment of clinical depression.

Postpartum depression affects 10% to 15% of women and develops in the first month after childbirth. It is often unrecognized. Risk factors include prior major or postpartum depression, depression during pregnancy, unmarried status, or unplanned pregnancy. It is essential to evaluate thyroid function in postpartum women with depressive symptoms because of overlap in presentation. Psychosis can occur in women with postpartum depression and usually requires acute hospitalization.

Anxiety disorders that are more prevalent in women include panic disorder, agoraphobia, social phobia, generalized anxiety disorder, and posttraumatic stress disorder. An anxiety disorder may underlie persistent somatic complaints. If nonpharmacologic measures are inadequate, combined medication and cognitive behavioral therapy should be offered.

Box 36.8 • Categories of Benign Breast Disease

Nonproliferative breast lesions (RR, 1.27)

    Duct ectasia
    Fibroadenoma without proliferative epithelial changes
    Fibrosis
    Mastitis
    Mild hyperplasia without atypia
    Cysts
    Simple apocrine metaplasia
    Squamous metaplasia

Proliferative breast lesions without atypia (RR, 1.88)

    Fibroadenoma with proliferative epithelial changes
    Moderate or florid hyperplasia without atypia
    Sclerosing adenosis
    Papilloma
    Radial scar

Atypia (RR, 4.24)

    Atypical ductal hyperplasia
    Atypical lobular hyperplasia

Abbreviation: RR, relative risk.

The risks and benefits of pharmacologic therapy need to be considered in pregnant or nursing women. Tricyclic antidepressants and some selective serotonin reuptake inhibitors are relatively safe, although there are isolated adverse reports of infants exposed to these agents through breast milk.

Intimate Partner Violence

Intimate partner violence is intentional controlling or violent behavior. Controlling behavior may include physical or emotional abuse, sexual assault, economic control, or social isolation of the victim. In 95% of reported cases, a man is the perpetrator and a woman is the victim. At least 1 in 3 US women is assaulted by a partner during her lifetime. Female victims most often present for care indirectly related to abuse injuries. Battered women use health services 6 to 8 times more than nonbattered women and have an increased incidence of headaches, sexually transmitted diseases, irritable bowel syndrome, depression, and anxiety. Suggestive aspects of the history include depression, chronic pain syndromes, gastrointestinal complaints, an overprotective partner, injuries during pregnancy, frequent visits for injuries, and a history of childhood abuse. All women should be asked about intimate partner violence. Routine prenatal screening for intimate partner violence is particularly important because abuse occurs in 1 of 6 pregnancies and often begins or escalates in early pregnancy.

Suggestive physical examination findings include injuries incompatible with the history, multiple injuries in various healing stages, injuries suggestive of a defensive posture (eg, ulnar fractures), and pattern injuries (eg, burns, choking or bite marks, wrist or ankle abrasions).

Documentation in the medical record is essential and may provide evidence to help the victim separate from the perpetrator. If the victim consents, injury photographs should be obtained. Physical evidence should be preserved.

Victims need treatment of injuries, support, safety assessment, and referral to appropriate resources to prevent further abuse. A safety assessment by a victim's advocate, social worker, or law enforcement personnel is critical. When these persons are not available, a trained physician or nurse should perform a safety assessment. Immediate psychiatric referral should be arranged for patients expressing suicidal or homicidal intentions. The assessment must include inquiries regarding children in the home, and any child abuse must be reported to child abuse authorities. Some jurisdictions require reporting to the child abuse authorities any intimate partner violence in a home where children reside. Because intimate partner violence homicides are more likely to occur immediately after separation, ensuring the safety of the victim during separation is critical.

Sexual Assault

Sexual assault is any sexual act performed without consent. Most cases are unreported, and about half of victims have some acquaintance with their attacker. A sexual assault victim should be evaluated by a trained sexual assault nurse examiner. Evidence can be collected up to 120 hours after the assault. In certain cases, treatment to prevent sexually transmitted infections (gonorrhea/chlamydia, hepatitis B, human immunodeficiency virus) and pregnancy may be offered.

Key Definition

Sexual assault: *any sexual act performed without consent.*

KEY FACTS

✓ Initial therapies for mastalgia—a well-fitted support brassiere, heat and/or cold packs, gentle massage, dietary changes, relaxation techniques, and exercise

✓ Benign nipple discharge—typically bilateral, nonbloody, and multiductal

✓ Pathologic nipple discharge—typically unilateral, uniductal, and spontaneous, and bloody, serosanguineous, or, sometimes, watery or clear

✓ Document intimate partner violence in the medical record; may provide evidence to help victim separate from perpetrator

Questions and Answers

Questions

Multiple Choice (choose the best answer)

V.1. A patient presents with recurrent episodes of the skin findings shown in Figure V.Q1. What is the most likely infectious association?
   a. Herpes simplex virus
   b. *Pseudomonas*
   c. Dermatophyte
   d. *Borrelia burgdorferi*
   e. *Mycobacterium marinum*

V.2. An 86-year-old man has an itchy, new rash. At the nursing home where he lives, the rash has been treated with different antihistamines and topical corticosteroids without response. A clinic visit is arranged. On examination he has red papules and excoriations on the hands, groin, and axillae (Figure V.Q2). He has nodular areas on his scrotum. What diagnosis should you consider?
   a. Chronic idiopathic urticaria
   b. Urticarial vasculitis
   c. Bullous pemphigoid
   d. Pemphigus vulgaris
   e. Scabies

V.3. A 26-year-old woman presents with a facial rash that first appeared last summer and returned during her recent trip to Arizona. Initially, she says that she feels well, but then she describes fatigue and malaise. She has a family history of rheumatoid arthritis. On examination, she is afebrile and she has no active synovitis. Both cheeks are erythematous and have small papules (Figure V.Q3). There are no other concerning signs on examination. What is the diagnosis?
   a. Malar rash of lupus
   b. Seborrheic dermatitis
   c. Allergic contact dermatitis
   d. Rosacea
   e. Acne vulgaris

V.4. A 49-year-old woman presents with a persistent, pruritic, red rash on her face, chest, elbows, knees, and hands. The rash began last summer and is unresponsive to topical corticosteroids. Her past medical history is significant for asthma and migraines. For the past month, she has been having more problems with shortness of breath and headaches. Some of her skin findings are shown in Figure V.Q4. She has mild wheezing. Neurologic examination findings are normal. Laboratory test results are positive for antinuclear antibody and normal for the complete blood cell count, liver function tests, and renal function tests. What other laboratory testing would be most important?

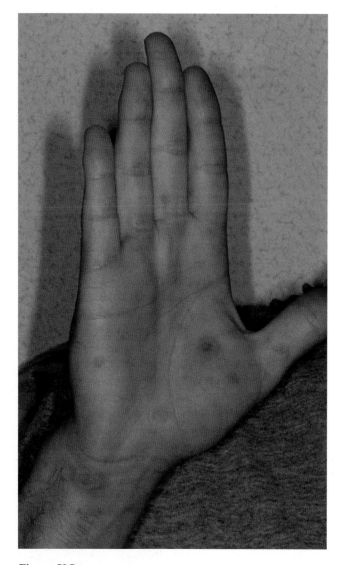

Figure V.Q1

(Adapted from Drage LA, Bundrick JB, Litin SC. Clinical pearls in dermatology. Mayo Clin Proc. 2012 Jul;87[7]:695–9. Used with permission of Mayo Foundation for Medical Education and Research.)

391

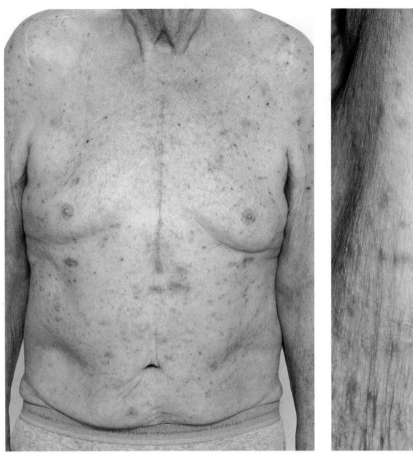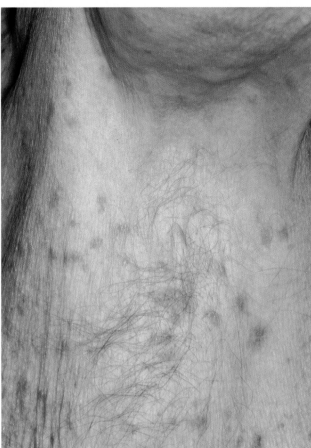

Figures V.Q2

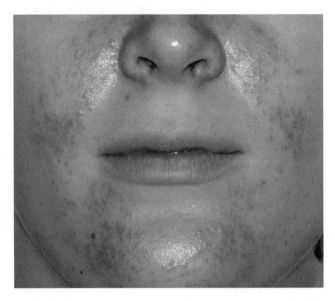

Figure V.Q3

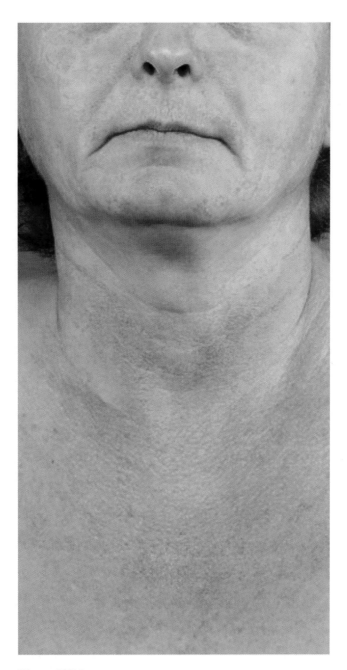

Figure V.Q4

a. Chest radiography and mammography
b. Patch testing
c. Lupus serologies
d. Tissue transglutaminase testing
e. Light testing

V.5. Which of the following vaccinations should *not* be administered during pregnancy?
a. Human papillomavirus (HPV)
b. Meningococcus
c. Pneumococcus
d. Hepatitis A
e. Tetanus-diphtheria (Td)

V.6. A healthy 37-year-old woman presents to your office for further evaluation of vaginal symptoms. She reports that for the past 3 months she has had persistent vaginal irritation, with itching and burning and a somewhat thick discharge. She has normal menses. She has been in a monogamous relationship with the same partner for the past 15 years. She uses oral contraceptives. She appears mildly uncomfortable but otherwise well. Her examination is significant for vulvar erythema without any lesions; she has a mildly thick discharge. The speculum examination shows normal findings, but she is uncomfortable during it and during the bimanual examination. A Papanicolaou test is performed. The pH of the vagina is 4.3. The whiff test is negative. Microscopy shows only a moderate number of large rods, and Gram staining shows gram-positive rods. Culture results are negative for *Trichomonas vaginalis*. What is the most likely diagnosis?
a. Vaginal candidiasis
b. Trichomoniasis
c. Contact dermatitis
d. Bacterial vaginosis

V.7. Your clinic has access to magnetic resonance imaging (MRI) technology. You are evaluating a patient who has a diabetic foot infection. There is no exposed bone. You are concerned that he has not responded well to antibiotic treatment, and you determine that his current pretest likelihood of having underlying osteomyelitis is 50%. Recently, you read an article that evaluated the role of MRI in diagnosing foot osteomyelitis. The sensitivity of this test is 90%, and the specificity is 85% (compared with bone biopsy as the referenced standard). If you use MRI for this patient, and it is positive for osteomyelitis, what is the likelihood that he indeed will have osteomyelitis on bone biopsy?

a. 94%
b. 89%
c. 86%
d. 50%
e. 11%

V.8. Refer to the information in question V.10. If the magnetic resonance imaging (MRI) findings were negative, what is the likelihood that this patient would *not* have osteomyelitis?

a. 94%
b. 89%
c. 86%
d. 50%
e. 11%

V.9. You have recently read about a randomized controlled trial that compared the efficacy of warfarin (international normalized ratio 2.0–3.0) with that of aspirin (325 mg) in stroke prevention in a subset of elderly patients (75 years or older) who had atrial fibrillation. The patients were followed for 3 years. The final results showed that the chance of major stroke, intracranial hemorrhage, or systemic embolism was 5% among patients treated with warfarin and 10% among patients treated with aspirin. For the group treated with warfarin compared with the group treated with aspirin, what is the absolute risk reduction (ARR) of a major event at 3 years?

a. 5%
b. 10%
c. 20%
d. 50%
e. 100%

V.10. You serve on the sentinel event review committee at your hospital. An event occurred in which a patient received an overdose of heparin. Your committee completes a root cause analysis and finds that the error resulted from a gap in physician knowledge about heparin dosing, the lack of an institutional consensus on heparin dosing, and a cumbersome order entry system. From the root cause analysis, which of the following interventions is most likely to have a sustained effect?

a. An online education module on heparin dosing
b. Distribution of a heparin dosing pocket card
c. A heparin order set

d. A new institutional policy on heparin dosing
e. A physician education conference on heparin dosing

V.11. An 83-year-old woman comes to your office with a 2-day history of a red left eye associated with dull, achy pain and tears. She denies having any trauma or visual problems. On examination, she has clear tears and a focal area of redness in the medial sclera. What would you recommend for control of her symptoms?

a. Acetaminophen and avoiding contact with others until the symptoms resolve
b. Aspirin and reassurance
c. Urgent referral to ophthalmology
d. Gentamicin eyedrops for 7 to 10 days
e. Corticosteroid eyedrops for 1 week

V.12. A 42-year-old kindergarten teacher presents to your office with a 2-week history of an upper respiratory illness. She initially noted a low-grade fever, achiness, sinus congestion with clear discharge, and cough, which improved over 10 days but then seemed to recur with a vengeance. Now she has a severe sore throat, enlarged glands, and fever. She does not have a cough or shortness of breath. On examination, she has a fever (39°C), tonsillar exudate, and cervical adenopathy, and she appears ill and uncomfortable. Abdominal examination findings are unremarkable. Which of the following is most appropriate?

a. Mononucleosis spot test
b. Throat culture and Gram stain
c. Rapid streptococcal antigen test
d. Empirical penicillin V for 10 days
e. Chest radiograph

V.13. Whch features could potentially distinguish between acute angle-closure glaucoma and acute anterior uveitis?

a. Circumcorneal injection
b. Blurry vision
c. Hypopyon
d. Pain
e. Unilateral presentation of symptoms

V.14. Mr. Smith is an 86-year-old man hospitalized with respiratory failure due to congestive heart failure pneumonia. His consciousness is waxing and waning, and he cannot make medical decisions. His 3 children are struggling with making decisions about his care. Of the following statement and questions, which one would best help the children make decisions for their father?

a. "What would you like us to do for your father?"
b. "If your father were able to speak for himself, what decisions would he make?"
c. "Would you like to speak with a social worker or chaplain?"
d. "Since your father doesn't have an advance directive, it is impossible to know his wishes. Thus, you should make decisions based on what is in his best interest."
e. "You should have the court appoint a guardian to make decisions for your father."

Answers

V.1. Answer a.

Patients who have erythema multiforme present with target lesions that are often located on the palms and soles but may occur as generalized eruptions. Drugs such as sulfonamides, barbiturates, and anticonvulsants are commonly associated with development of erythema multiforme, but recurrent lesions are most often linked to a herpes simplex infection. Although the skin signs of an active herpes simplex infection may be apparent, the outbreak may be subclinical. Discontinuing use of any culprit drugs and a trial of acyclovir or other appropriate antiviral would be suitable in cases of recurrent erythema multiforme.

V.2. Answer e.

Scabies is caused by infestation with the mite *Sarcoptes scabiei* var *hominis*. Infection occurs as a result of direct skin-to-skin contact; fomite transmission is uncommon. It causes epidemics in schools, hospitals, and nursing homes. The rash results from a hypersensitivity reaction to the mite protein. The main complaint is pruritus, especially at night. Clinical features include inflammatory, excoriated papules in the web spaces of the hands and feet, axillae, groin, and wrists and the areolae and submammary sites of women. Nodules or thickened areas in the scrotum are also helpful clues. The pathognomonic finding is a burrow, commonly located on finger webs. Identification of mites on a scabies preparation is diagnostic. In immunocompromised patients, a highly contagious form of scabies may appear as a generalized scaling eruption (ie, crusted scabies, formerly called Norwegian scabies). Treatment of classic scabies includes the topical application of permethrin; oral ivermectin may be used to treat crusted scabies.

V.3. Answer d.

Not all malar rashes result from lupus. Rosacea is a common facial rash with red papules and small pustules on a base of erythema and telangiectasia. It commonly affects the central facial area. Sun, vasodilators, caffeine, and hot or spicy foods may trigger flares. It may be associated with eye findings, but otherwise it has no systemic associations. Mild rosacea is treated with topical metronidazole, use of sunscreens, and avoidance of triggering factors. Anti-inflammatory antibiotics, such as tetracycline, are used in more severe cases. Rhinophyma can be treated with laser and other surgical methods.

V.4. Answer a.

Dermatomyositis is an inflammatory myositis with distinctive skin findings. Skin signs of dermatomyositis may include heliotrope rash, Gottron papules, photosensitivity, Gottron sign (erythema over the extensor surfaces of the finger joints, knees, and elbows), periorbital edema, scalp erythema and pruritus, violaceous erythema of sun-exposed or extensor surfaces, periungual erythema and telangiectasia, cuticle hypertrophy, generalized pruritus, shawl sign, and holster sign. Patients may present with skin findings but without clinical weakness or muscle enzyme abnormalities (amyopathic dermatomyositis or dermatomyositis sine myositis). Dermatomyositis may be a skin sign of internal malignancy with a significantly higher risk of lung, breast, or ovarian cancer. A workup for underlying malignancy should be pursued.

V.5. Answer a.

The HPV vaccine is an inactivated viral vaccine that is likely safe (pregnancy category B), but it has not been studied well in this population, and current guidelines recommend against its use during pregnancy. Women inadvertently vaccinated during pregnancy should have their exposure to the vaccine reported to the Vaccine in Pregnancy Registry. The other vaccines listed as answer choices are known to be safe during pregnancy. Hepatitis A, pneumococcal, and meningococcal vaccines should be administered to pregnant women who are considered to be at high risk rather than to all pregnant women. Td should be administered to pregnant women whose latest booster was 10 or more years earlier or who have a deep or dirty wound.

V.6. Answer c.

Although the sensitivity of the whiff test is relatively low, this patient's vaginal pH is normal, effectively excluding bacterial vaginosis. Large rod-shaped bacilli in the vaginal secretions represent normal vaginal flora (lactobacilli) and are not indicative of infection. No motile species are noted on microscopy, so *Trichomonas* is unlikely and the negative culture results confirm the absence of *Trichomonas*. The patient should eliminate potential irritants (eg, laundry detergent, douching, vulvar sprays, fragranced cleansers) and be reassessed if her symptoms do not resolve.

V.7. Answer c.

A 2×2 table must be constructed to determine the positive predictive value for MRI among patients who have a pretest probability of 50% in an evaluation for foot osteomyelitis. As determined from Table V.A7, the correct answer is $\frac{a}{a+b}$ or 90/105 = 86%.

V.8. Answer b.

The negative predictive value of the MRI is $\frac{d}{c+d}$ or 85/95 = 89%.

V.9. Answer a.

You are asked to determine the ARR in a randomized controlled trial that showed that the anticoagulant therapy group had an experimental event rate (EER) of 5%. The aspirin group had a control event rate (CER) of 10%. The formula for ARR is CER − EER. In this trial, ARR = 10% − 5% = 5% over 3 years.

Table V.A7 ·

Diagnostic Test Result		Disease Present		Disease Absent			
	Positive	90	a	b	15	a+b	105
	Negative	10	c	d	85	c+d	95
			a+c	b+d		a+b+c+d	
		100			100		200

V.10. Answer c.

Quality improvement interventions have a hierarchy for sustainability. Education tools, such as online modules, conferences, pocket cards, and signs, tend to have a positive initial effect, but this effect is not lasting. Although an institutional consensus or policy may be a good idea, it is difficult to implement and develop consistent adherence. In this question, the order set is most likely to provide a sustained improvement. If it is integrated into a computerized order entry system, it will prompt physicians about correct dosing and thus decrease the risk of human error.

V.11. Answer b.

This patient has episcleritis, which is a self-limited, possibly autoimmune-mediated inflammation of the episcleral vessels. Although vision is unaffected and tearing may be minimal, rapid-onset redness associated with achy pain and tenderness is evident. In this scenario, one would also want to rule out the possibility of temporal arteritis, although it does not manifest with eye symptoms. If symptoms persist or recur, the patient should be referred to an ophthalmologist.

V.12. Answer d.

On the basis of the Centor criteria (fever, tonsillar exudates, tender anterior cervical lymphadenopathy, and lack of cough), this patient has a high probability of group A β-hemolytic streptococcal (GABHS) pharyngitis. Guidelines from the Infectious Diseases Society of America recommend rapid streptococcal antigen testing for adults with suspected GABHS infection (ie, 2 Centor criteria) and no testing or treatment for those at low risk (0 or 1 Centor criterion). Patients at high risk (3 or 4 Centor criteria) should receive empirical antibiotic therapy.

V.13. Answer c.

Both acute angle-closure glaucoma and acute anterior uveitis are emergent processes associated with rapid onset, circumcorneal injection, pain, and unilateral manifestation. Acute angle-closure glaucoma is associated with a tense affected eye on palpation in an older patient; acute anterior uveitis usually manifests in a young or middle-aged adult and is associated with the presence of inflammatory cells and protein in the anterior chamber of the eye. This collection of pus (hypopyon) may occasionally be observed in severe cases of acute anterior uveitis.

V.14. Answer b.

For the patient who lacks decision-making capacity, the surrogate decision maker should not make decisions based on the surrogate's values and preferences. Rather, the surrogate has ethical and legal obligations to make decisions that are based on the patient's health care preferences, values, and goals, if known (substituted judgment). To facilitate substituted judgment, clinicians should ask surrogates questions such as, "If your father could wake up for 15 minutes and understand his condition fully, and then had to return to it, what would he tell you to do?" If these preferences, values, and goals are not known, the surrogate should make decisions based on what is in the best interests of the patient. Clinicians should not defer these conversations to others (eg, social workers, chaplains). A court-appointed guardian is usually not needed for this situation.

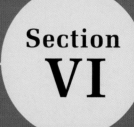

Section
VI

Hematology

Benign Hematologic Disorders

37

NASEEMA GANGAT, MBBS

Anemias

Evaluation of Anemia

Anemia is a reduction in the mass of healthy circulating red blood cells (RBCs). It results from 1 of 3 mechanisms: 1) inadequate production of RBCs by the bone marrow (ie, marrow failure, intrinsic RBC synthetic defects, or lack of essential RBC components such as vitamins); 2) blood loss; or 3) premature destruction of RBCs (ie, hemolysis). After a complete history and physical examination, the mean corpuscular volume (MCV) is used to classify anemia as microcytic, macrocytic, or normocytic.

Microcytic Anemias

Microcytic anemia indicates the presence of small RBCs (MCV <80 fL). The most common forms of anemia are microcytic (Tables 37.1 and 37.2). The causes of hypochromic microcytic anemias can be remembered with the mnemonic *TAILS* (thalassemia, anemia of chronic disease, iron deficiency, lead poisoning, and sideroblastic anemia).

A complete blood cell count and iron parameters (serum iron, total iron-binding capacity, transferrin saturation, and ferritin) aid in making a diagnosis (Table 37.2). Blood loss should be considered in all patients with microcytic anemia. Investigating the gastrointestinal tract (the most common site of occult blood loss) is essential in the workup for microcytic anemia.

Iron Deficiency

Iron deficiency is the most common cause of anemia in the world and is especially common among menstruating or pregnant women and the elderly (Figure 37.1). Mechanisms of iron deficiency include 1) blood loss, 2) increased requirements (as in pregnancy), and 3) decreased absorption, including partial gastrectomy and malabsorption syndromes (eg, celiac disease).

Blood loss includes gastrointestinal tract disorders (eg, ulcers, malignancy, telangiectasia, arteriovenous malformations, hiatal hernia, and long-distance runner's anemia); respiratory disorders (eg, malignancy and pulmonary hemosiderosis); menstruation; phlebotomy (eg, blood donation, diagnostic phlebotomy, treatment of polycythemia vera or hemochromatosis, and self-inflicted or factitious injury); trauma; and surgery.

Patients may have a normal MCV if they have early iron deficiency or if they have a condition that causes macrocytosis (eg, iron deficiency in combination with folate deficiency).

The serum ferritin test is the most useful initial test for iron deficiency. A ferritin level less than 15 mcg/L almost always indicates iron deficiency. Ferritin is an acute phase reactant, and the level is increased in inflammatory states. Thus, patients with these conditions may have iron deficiency even if the ferritin level is normal or increased. An elevated soluble transferrin receptor (sTfR) measurement, which is not an acute phase reactant, also signifies iron deficiency.

Oral iron replacement therapy is the treatment of choice for iron deficiency. Gastric acid is required for optimal iron absorption. Reticulocytosis is seen in 4 to 7 days after initiating oral iron replacement therapy, improvement in anemia in 3 to 4 weeks, and correction of anemia in 6 weeks. Continue iron replacement therapy for another 6 months to replenish iron reserves.

Indications for intravenous iron therapy include hemodialysis (with recombinant erythropoietin) and inability to tolerate or absorb iron orally.

Table 37.1 • Typical Features of Uncomplicated Microcytic Anemias (Decreased MCV)

Variable	Type of Anemia	
	Thalassemia	Iron Deficiency
RBC count, ×10^{12}/L	≥5.0	<5.0
RBC distribution width, %	<16	≥16

Abbreviations: MCV, mean corpuscular volume; RBC, red blood cell.

Table 37.2 • Comparison of the Most Common Hypochromic Microcytic Anemias

Disease State	MCV	Red Blood Cell Count	TIBC	Transferrin Saturation	Serum Ferritin	Marrow Iron
Iron deficiency anemia	Decreased	Decreased	Increased	Low	Low	Absent
Anemia of chronic disease	Normal or decreased	Decreased	Normal or low	Normal or increased	Normal or increased	Normal or increased
Thalassemia minor	Decreased	Usually increased	Normal	Normal	Normal or increased	Normal

Abbreviations: MCV, mean corpuscular volume; TIBC, total iron-binding capacity.

Adapted from Savage RA. Cost-effective laboratory diagnosis of microcytic anemias of complex origin. ASCP check sample H84–10(H-153). Used with permission.

Thalassemias

The thalassemias are common single-gene disorders. β-Thalassemia results when β-globin chains are decreased or absent in relation to α-globin. In α-thalassemia, the converse is true: Excess β-globin chains precipitate as tetramers called *hemoglobin H*. Genetic counseling is indicated after the diagnosis of α- or β-thalassemia has been established.

β-Thalassemia

Point mutations result in β-thalassemia of varying severity. Clinically, β-thalassemia is categorized as follows:

1. *β-Thalassemia trait*—microcytosis and either normal hemoglobin or mild anemia

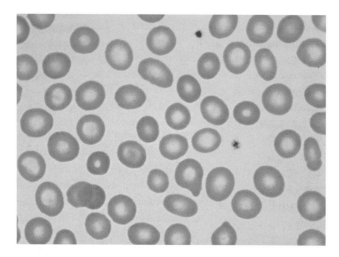

Figure 37.1 Hypochromic Microcytic Anemia. The erythrocytes are small with increased central pallor and assorted aberrations in size (anisocytosis) and shape (poikilocytosis). This pattern is characteristic of iron deficiency rather than thalassemia; in thalassemia, red blood cells are small but more uniform. If a mature lymphocyte is available for reference, the diameter of a normal erythrocyte (7 μm) should be similar to the diameter of the nucleus of the lymphocyte (peripheral blood smear; Wright-Giemsa).
(Courtesy of Curtis A. Hanson, MD, Mayo Clinic, Rochester, Minnesota. Used with permission.)

2. *β-Thalassemia intermedia*—microcytosis and moderate anemia without long-term transfusion dependence
3. *β-Thalassemia major* (also known as Cooley anemia)—profound anemia and lifelong transfusion dependence

In β-thalassemia, the hemoglobin A_2 level is elevated (Figure 37.2). However, if the patient has iron deficiency, the hemoglobin A_2 level may be normal.

α-Thalassemia

Normally, a person has 4 α-globin genes but only 2 β-chain loci. α-Thalassemia is classified as follows:

1. *α-Thalassemia minor* (*α-thalassemia trait*)—absence of 1 or 2 of the 4 α-globin genes (patients are asymptomatic, usually with a low-normal MCV and normal hemoglobin)
2. *Hemoglobin H disease*—absence of 3 α-globin genes (patients have chronic hemolytic anemia of moderate severity and may benefit from splenectomy if hemolysis becomes problematic)
3. Absence of all 4 α-globin genes is not compatible with life and results in stillbirth (hydrops fetalis).

KEY FACTS

✓ Microcytic anemia—most common form of anemia
✓ TAILS—mnemonic for causes of hypochromic microcytic anemia (thalassemia, anemia of chronic disease, iron deficiency, lead poisoning, and sideroblastic anemia)
✓ Early iron deficiency or macrocytosis—MCV may be normal
✓ Best initial test for iron deficiency—serum ferritin (<15 mcg/L)
✓ Therapy for iron deficiency is oral iron—
  • requires gastric acid for best absorption
  • in 4–7 days: reticulocytosis
  • in 3–4 weeks: improvement in anemia
  • in 6 weeks: correction of anemia (continue iron for 6 more months to replenish reserves)

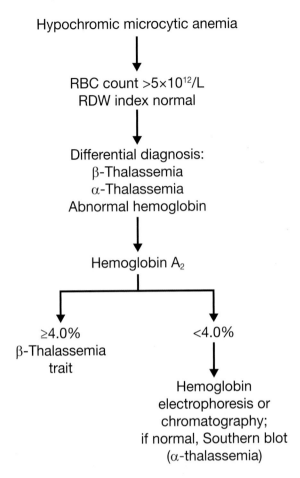

Hypochromic microcytic anemia

↓

RBC count >5×10^{12}/L
RDW index normal

↓

Differential diagnosis:
β-Thalassemia
α-Thalassemia
Abnormal hemoglobin

↓

Hemoglobin A$_2$

≥4.0%
β-Thalassemia
trait

<4.0%

Hemoglobin
electrophoresis or
chromatography;
if normal, Southern blot
(α-thalassemia)

Figure 37.2 Algorithm for Approach to Diagnosis of Hypochromic Microcytic Anemia With an Increased Total Red Blood Cell (RBC) Count and a Normal RBC Distribution Width (RDW) Index.
(Adapted from Savage RA. Cost-effective laboratory diagnosis of microcytic anemias of complex origin. ASCP check sample H84–10[H-153]. Used with permission.)

Macrocytic Anemias

Macrocytic anemia indicates the presence of large RBCs (MCV >100 fL). The differential diagnosis of macrocytic anemias includes vitamin B$_{12}$ deficiency, folate deficiency, drugs, liver disease, alcohol abuse, hypothyroidism, heavy tobacco use, myelodysplasia or other primary bone marrow disorders, cold agglutinin disease (artifactual clumping of cells in an automated counter), and reticulocytosis (reticulocytes are larger than mature RBCs). A laboratory approach to macrocytic anemias is outlined in Figure 37.3. An MCV greater than 115 fL almost always indicates a deficiency of either vitamin B$_{12}$ or folate or an artifact due to RBC agglutination. Common drug-related causes of macrocytosis are chemotherapy drugs that inhibit purine or pyrimidine synthesis (eg, azathioprine and 5-fluorouracil), deoxyribonucleotide synthesis

(hydroxyurea and cytarabine), or dihydrofolate reductase (methotrexate).

Vitamin B$_{12}$ Deficiency

Vitamin B$_{12}$ (cobalamin) is present mainly in animal products. Hydrochloric acid is necessary to free cobalamin from food. Free cobalamin is immediately bound by R-binders, which protect cobalamin from the acidic gastric environment. As the complex passes into the duodenum, pancreatic proteases facilitate release of the R-binders. The free cobalamin then combines with intrinsic factor and is absorbed in the terminal ileum.

Vitamin B$_{12}$ deficiency due to inadequate dietary intake is very rare (seen usually in strict vegetarians). Causes of vitamin B$_{12}$ deficiency include pernicious anemia (defective production of intrinsic factor, due to anti–intrinsic factor or anti–parietal cell antibodies), atrophic gastritis, total or partial gastrectomy, ileal resection or Crohn disease involving the ileum, bacterial overgrowth syndromes, infection with *Diphyllobothrium latum*, and pancreatic insufficiency. Prolonged metformin use has also been more recently described as a cause of vitamin B$_{12}$ deficiency.

The symptoms and signs of vitamin B$_{12}$ deficiency include a beefy and atrophic tongue, diarrhea, and neurologic signs (eg, paresthesias, gait disturbance, mental status changes ["B$_{12}$ madness"], vibratory/position sense impairment [dorsal column "dropout"], the absence of ankle reflexes, and extensor plantar responses).

The MCV is increased, and hypersegmented neutrophils are usually present (Figure 37.4). As in folate deficiency, serum homocysteine levels are increased; however, unlike in folate deficiency, serum and urinary levels of methylmalonic acid are also increased. A serum vitamin B$_{12}$ level less than 200 ng/L strongly suggests vitamin B$_{12}$ deficiency. Vitamin B$_{12}$ levels of 200 to 400 ng/L (borderline or low-normal range) can also indicate deficiency; if clinical suspicion is high, methylmalonic acid levels can help establish the diagnosis. When present, an abnormal intrinsic factor antibody confirms pernicious anemia as the cause of vitamin B$_{12}$ deficiency.

Vitamin B$_{12}$ deficiency, including pernicious anemia, is treated with oral or intramuscular vitamin B$_{12}$. Lifelong maintenance treatment is required.

Folate Deficiency

In contrast to anemia caused by vitamin B$_{12}$ deficiency, macrocytic anemia caused by folate deficiency develops quickly (ie, within months) in patients with inadequate dietary intake of folic acid. Folate is present in green leafy vegetables, and many foods are fortified with folate in most Western countries. It is absorbed in the duodenum and proximal jejunum. Mechanisms of folate deficiency include 1) increased requirements (eg, pregnancy and hemolytic anemia); 2) poor folate intake (eg, alcoholism and malnutrition); 3) poor absorption (eg, celiac disease, bariatric surgery,

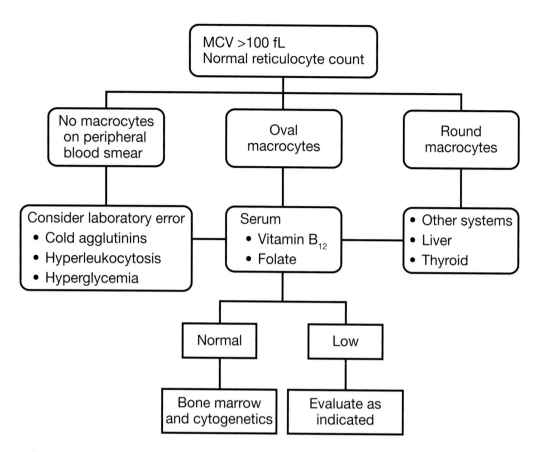

Figure 37.3 *Laboratory Approach to Macrocytic Anemias. MCV indicates mean corpuscular volume.*
(Adapted from Colon-Otero G, Menke D, Hook CC. A practical approach to the differential diagnosis and evaluation of the adult patient with macrocytic anemia. Med Clin North Am. 1992 May;76[3]:581–97. Used with permission.)

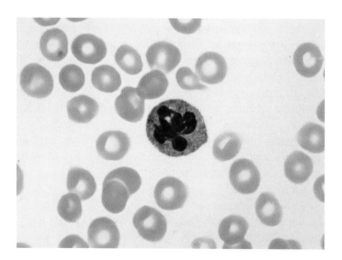

Figure 37.4 *Hypersegmented Neutrophil. Polymorphonuclear leukocytes with 5 or more nuclear lobes are characteristic of vitamin B$_{12}$ or folate deficiency and are not typically seen in other causes of macrocytic anemia (peripheral blood smear; Wright-Giemsa).*

and drugs that interfere with absorption, such as phenytoin, phenobarbital, and primidone); and 4) interference with the recycling of folate from liver stores to tissue (eg, alcohol).

The possibility of coexistent vitamin B$_{12}$ or iron deficiency should be considered if the response to replacement folate therapy is not optimal. Folate helps convert homocysteine to methionine; thus, folate deficiency leads to an increased homocysteine level. In contrast to vitamin B$_{12}$ deficiency, in folate deficiency the level of methylmalonic acid is normal.

Normocytic Anemias

Normocytic anemia is defined as anemia with an MCV of 80 to 100 fL. The differential diagnosis includes mixed nutritional deficiency (eg, concomitant folate and iron deficiency), erythropoietic failure (aplastic anemia and pure RBC aplasia), marrow replacement (malignancy and fibrosis), kidney disease with lack of erythropoietin production, hemolysis, acute hemorrhage, chemotherapy, anemia of acute disease, and anemia of chronic disease (ACD) (eg, infections, neoplasia, rheumatoid arthritis, and other inflammatory rheumatologic conditions).

Anemia of Chronic Disease

ACD is usually moderate (ie, hemoglobin 9–11 g/dL), MCV is normal or modestly decreased, and the reticulocyte count is low. ACD is sometimes called anemia of chronic inflammation, since it results from the inhibitory effects of inflammatory cytokines on the bone marrow. A peptide produced by the liver, hepcidin, is elevated in ACD. Hepcidin sequesters iron and decreases iron absorption. As a consequence, serum iron levels are low in ACD, but unlike in iron deficiency, total iron-binding capacity is normal or low and ferritin is usually normal or elevated (Table 37.2).

Early in the evaluation of patients with suspected ACD, it is important to exclude hemolysis and gastrointestinal tract blood loss. No single blood test confirms ACD, but diagnosis is probable if 1) inflammatory markers are present; 2) results of iron studies are typical (ie, normal total iron-binding capacity, normal or increased serum ferritin, and normal or increased transferrin saturation); 3) another cause for the normocytic anemia is not apparent; and 4) the clinical setting is appropriate. The sTfR concentration is normal in ACD in contrast to iron deficiency anemia, in which sTfR is usually elevated. Patients with ACD do not benefit from iron therapy.

Sideroblastic Anemias

The sideroblastic anemias are characterized by microcytic, normocytic, or macrocytic anemia and ring sideroblasts in the bone marrow (Figure 37.5), which are abnormal erythroid precursors ineffective at heme synthesis and are often seen in myelodysplastic syndromes. Reactive causes include alcohol, zinc toxicity, and drugs such as isoniazid and pyrazinamide. Several forms of congenital sideroblastic anemia respond to vitamin B$_6$ (pyridoxine) therapy.

Aplastic Anemia

Aplastic anemia is a rare disorder characterized by pancytopenia, bone marrow hypocellularity, and absence of another disorder that would explain the hypocellularity (eg, myelodysplastic syndrome, T-cell clonal disorders, or other congenital bone marrow failure syndromes). Acquired aplastic anemia is often idiopathic. Common causes include drugs (eg, chloramphenicol, sulfonamides, gold, and benzene), toxins, radiation, infections (eg, from hepatitis A virus, Epstein-Barr virus [EBV], cytomegalovirus, human immunodeficiency virus [HIV], and human parvovirus B19), and autoimmune marrow suppression. The criteria for severe

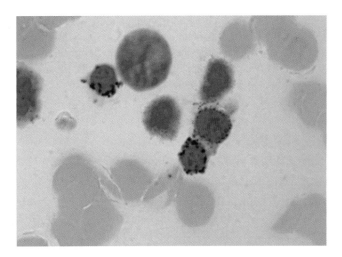

Figure 37.5 Ring Sideroblasts. Seen on iron staining of a bone marrow aspirate, ring sideroblasts can be reactive, congenital, or part of a myelodysplastic syndrome or other clonal myeloid disorder (bone marrow aspirate; iron stain with potassium ferrocyanide and nuclear fast red counterstain). (Courtesy of Curtis A. Hanson, MD, Mayo Clinic, Rochester, Minnesota. Used with permission.)

aplastic anemia include less than 25% of expected marrow cellularity and 2 of the following: 1) neutrophil count less than 0.5×10⁹/L; 2) platelet count less than 20×10⁹/L; and 3) a corrected reticulocyte count less than 1%.

Allogeneic hematopoietic stem cell transplant is the therapy of choice for patients with an identical twin, for patients younger than 20 years, or for high-risk patients between the ages of 20 and 40 who have an HLA match. For patients older than 40, the treatment of choice is antithymocyte globulin in combination with corticosteroids and cyclosporine. Without treatment, 80% of patients who have severe aplastic anemia die within 2 years after receiving the diagnosis.

Sickle Cell Disorders

Classification and Pathophysiology

The sickle cell disorders include sickle cell anemia (homozygous hemoglobin S), sickle cell trait (heterozygous hemoglobin S), and compound states (hemoglobin S with thalassemia or other hemoglobinopathies).

Sickle cell disorders occur in persons of sub-Saharan African descent: Approximately 1 of every 8 African Americans carries 1 copy of the sickle cell gene, and sickle cell disease occurs in 1 of 500. Hemoglobin S substitutes valine for glutamic acid at the sixth position of the β chain. Deoxygenated hemoglobin S distorts the cell into a sickle shape and injures the cell membrane (Figure 37.6). Sickling is inhibited by hemoglobin F; therefore, symptoms are not apparent until after 6 months of age. Acute chest syndrome is the leading cause of death (25% of deaths) in sickle cell anemia; clinical features include fever, chest pain, tachypnea, leukocytosis, and pulmonary infiltrates. Infection is usually caused by pneumococci, *Mycoplasma, Haemophilus, Salmonella,* or *Escherichia coli.* Aplastic crises are often associated with human parvovirus B19 infection. Osteomyelitis is caused by *Salmonella, Staphylococcus,* or *pneumococci.* Acute and chronic complications of sickle cell anemia are summarized in Box 37.1.

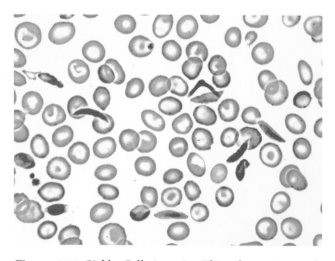

Figure 37.6 *Sickle Cell Anemia. This photomicrograph shows several irreversibly sickled cells. Abundant target cells indicate hyposplenism from autoinfarction of the spleen. Liver disease due to transfusional hemosiderosis was also a contributing factor to these target cells (peripheral blood smear; Wright-Giemsa).*

Box 37.1 • Complications and Treatment of Sickle Cell Anemia

Acute complications

    Vasoocclusive episodes
    Acute chest syndrome
    Dactylitis
    Splenic sequestration
    Stroke
    Aplastic crisis
    Infection
    Acute cholecystitis
    Priapism
    Renal papillary necrosis

Chronic complications

    Hemolytic anemia
    Growth retardation
    Pulmonary hypertension
    Folate deficiency
    Retinopathy
    Chronic renal insufficiency
    Accelerated cardiovascular disease
    Transfusional hemochromatosis
    Nonhealing skin ulcers
    Osteopenia
    Avascular necrosis

Treatment

    Pain crises: gentle hydration and pain control
    Stroke, acute chest syndrome, priapism, progressive retinopathy: exchange transfusion with goal hemoglobin S <30%

Laboratory findings include severe anemia (hemoglobin, 5.5–9.5 g/dL), sickled cells, ovalocytes, target cells, basophilic stippling, polychromatophilia, reticulocytosis (3%–12%), and hyposplenia with Howell-Jolly bodies (Figure 37.7). A persistent increase in the white blood cell count to 12×10^9/L to 15×10^9/L (in the absence of infection) with eosinophilia is characteristic. Evidence of chronic hemolysis may be present. Routine diagnostic tests include the sickle solubility test, electrophoresis, and chromatography.

Treatment

Sickle cell crises can be prevented by avoiding infection, fever, dehydration, acidosis, hypoxemia, cold, and high altitude. Most patients with sickle cell disease undergo autosplenectomy through recurrent infarction by age 5. Immunizations for encapsulated organisms, penicillin prophylaxis, and folate supplementation are indicated. Treatment of complications is summarized in Box 37.1.

Treatment with hydroxyurea decreases the frequency of painful vasoocclusive crises (by about 50%) and acute chest syndrome and the number of transfusions and

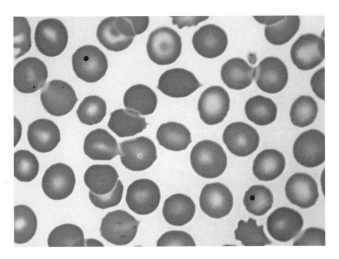

Figure 37.7 *Howell-Jolly Bodies. These small, round blue inclusions are seen with Wright-Giemsa or a comparable stain. They are characteristic of hyposplenism due to splenectomy or to a functionally defective spleen. Howell-Jolly bodies should not be confused with Heinz bodies, which require a special Heinz body preparation to observe and are not seen on a conventional peripheral smear (peripheral blood smear; Wright-Giemsa).*

hospitalizations. It is indicated for patients who have had severe complications such as acute chest syndrome and frequent, painful crises.

Hematopoietic stem cell transplant with marrow or umbilical cord blood from HLA-identical siblings may be curative. Indications for transplant include stroke and recurrent acute chest syndrome.

Sickle Cell Trait and Compound States

Sickle cell trait (heterozygous hemoglobin S) is not associated with anemia, RBC abnormalities, increased risk of infections, or increased mortality. Sickle cell trait is associated with hematuria due to renal papillary necrosis, splenic infarction at high altitude (>3,000 m), hyposthenuria, pyelonephritis in pregnancy, and pulmonary embolism. Compound states such as sickle cell–hemoglobin C disease and hemoglobin S/β-thalassemia are generally milder than sickle cell disease, depending on the hemoglobin concentrations.

Hemolytic Anemias

Hemolysis is the premature destruction of RBCs. If hemolytic anemia is suspected, the first step is to confirm the presence of hemolysis. Hemolytic anemias are characterized by increased RBC destruction and increased RBC production (Box 37.2).

Peripheral smear findings such as the following can assist in making a diagnosis:

> **Box 37.2 • Characterization of Hemolytic Anemia**
>
> Increased red blood cell (RBC) destruction
>
>   Increased indirect bilirubin level (>8 mg/dL suggests concomitant liver disease)
>
>   Increased lactate dehydrogenase level
>
>   Decreased haptoglobin level (haptoglobin, a scavenger of free hemoglobin, may be transiently decreased after transfusion or hemodialysis)
>
> Increased RBC production
>
>   Elevated reticulocyte count
>
>   Marrow erythroid hyperplasia

- *Spherocytes* (Figure 37.8)—hereditary spherocytosis, alcohol abuse, autoimmune hemolytic anemia
- *Basophilic stippling*—lead poisoning, β-thalassemia, arsenic poisoning
- *Hypochromia*—thalassemia, sideroblastic anemia, lead poisoning
- *Target cells* (Figure 37.9)—thalassemia, liver disease, postsplenectomy
- *Agglutination* (Figure 37.10)—cold agglutinin disease
- *Stomatocytes*—acute alcoholism, artifact
- *Spur cells* (*acanthocytes*) (Figure 37.11)—chronic severe liver disease, abetalipoproteinemia, malabsorption
- *Burr cells* (*echinocytes*) (Figure 37.12)—uremia, but disappearing with hemodialysis
- *Heinz bodies*—glucose-6-phosphate dehydrogenase (G6PD) deficiency (seen with supravital stain)

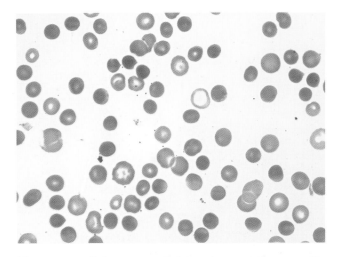

Figure 37.8 *Spherocytes. Spherocytes are the smooth, small, and spheroidal darkly stained cells with minimal or no central pallor. They are most commonly seen in hereditary spherocytosis or autoimmune hemolytic anemia (peripheral blood smear; Wright-Giemsa).*

(Courtesy of Curtis A. Hanson, MD, Mayo Clinic, Rochester, Minnesota. Used with permission.)

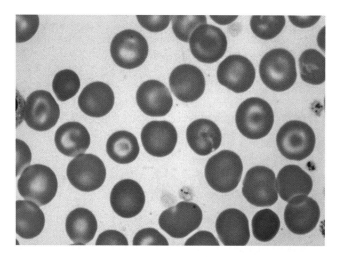

Figure 37.9 *Target Cells. Target cells are the red blood cells with a broad diameter and dark center with a pale surrounding halo. They are most commonly seen in hemoglobin C disease, thalassemia, and liver disease and after splenectomy (peripheral blood smear; Wright-Giemsa).*
(Courtesy of Curtis A. Hanson, MD, Mayo Clinic, Rochester, Minnesota. Used with permission.)

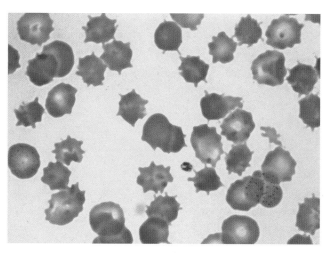

Figure 37.11 *Spur Cells (Acanthocytes). Note the thin, thorny, or fingerlike projections. Spur cells are characteristic of advanced liver disease and must be distinguished from burr cells (echinocytes) (Figure 37.12) (peripheral blood smear; Wright-Giemsa).*
(Courtesy of Curtis A. Hanson, MD, Mayo Clinic, Rochester, Minnesota. Used with permission.)

- *Howell-Jolly bodies* (Figure 37.7)—hyposplenism
- *Polychromasia* (Figure 37.13)—reticulocytosis
- *Intraerythrocytic parasitic inclusions* (Figure 37.14)—malaria, babesiosis

Hemolytic anemias may result from factors that are intrinsic or extrinsic to the RBC and may be direct Coombs-negative or direct Coombs-positive (Figure 37.15). A positive direct Coombs test, also called the direct antiglobulin test (DAT), indicates the presence of complement component C3 or immunoglobulin (Ig) G (or both) on the surface of RBCs. Notably, an aplastic crisis may occur in chronic hemolytic anemia and usually results from folate deficiency or parvovirus infection.

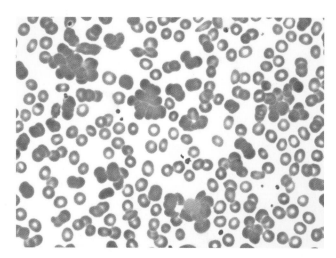

Figure 37.10 *Agglutination. The random clumping of red blood cells most commonly indicates cold agglutinin disease or laboratory artifact. It is important to distinguish agglutination from rouleaux (Figure 37.16) (peripheral blood smear; Wright-Giemsa).*

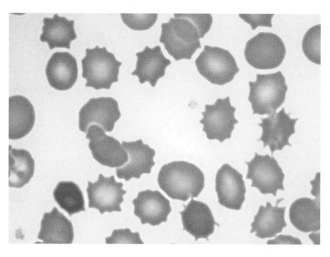

Figure 37.12 *Burr Cells (Echinocytes). Burr cell projections are much smaller and more uniform in size than spur cell projections. Burr cells are characteristic of uremia, and the membrane abnormality is reversible with hemodialysis (peripheral blood smear; Wright-Giemsa).*

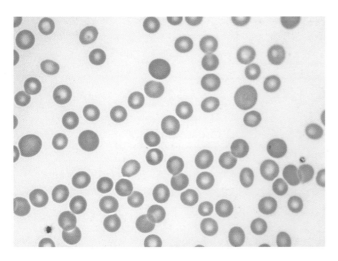

Figure 37.13 *Polychromasia. The larger cells are reticulocytes. These are often seen in high numbers during recovery from blood loss or hemolysis (peripheral blood smear; Wright-Giemsa).*

Intravascular Hemolysis Compared With Extravascular Hemolysis

In **intravascular hemolysis**, RBCs are destroyed while circulating within blood vessels. Their destruction releases free hemoglobin into the bloodstream, leading to hemoglobinemia, hemoglobinuria, and hemosiderinuria, all of which occur exclusively with intravascular hemolysis. Hemosiderinuria indicates that desquamated renal tubular cells absorbed free hemoglobin days to weeks earlier. Causes of intravascular hemolysis include transfusion reactions from ABO blood group antibodies, microangiopathic hemolytic anemia, paroxysmal nocturnal hemoglobinuria, paroxysmal cold hemoglobinuria, cold agglutinin syndrome, immune-complex drug-induced hemolytic anemia,

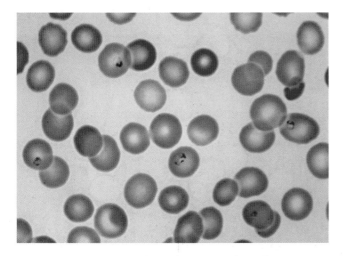

Figure *37.14* *Intraerythrocytic Ring-Shaped Parasites of Babesiosis. Malaria is the other common disease with an intraerythrocytic parasite (peripheral blood smear; Wright-Giemsa).*

infections (including falciparum malaria and clostridial sepsis), and G6PD deficiency. All other forms of hemolysis are primarily **extravascular hemolysis**, in which the RBCs are lysed in the macrophages of the spleen and liver.

Key Definitions

Hemolysis: *premature destruction of RBCs.*

Intravascular hemolysis: *destruction of RBCs circulating within blood vessels.*

Extravascular hemolysis: *destruction of RBCs in macrophages of spleen and liver.*

Autoimmune Hemolytic Anemia

Mechanisms of Drug-Induced Hemolytic Anemia

There are 3 distinct mechanisms of drug-induced hemolytic anemia. In the *autoantibody mechanism*, methyldopa may form autoantibodies that can induce hemolysis. Direct Coombs test results are positive in 3 to 6 months. Discontinuing the use of methyldopa usually leads to a rapid reversal in hemolysis.

In the *drug adsorption mechanism*, the use of high doses of penicillins or cephalosporins for more than 7 days may lead to immunohemolytic anemia due to antibodies formed against the drug–RBC membrane antigen complex. In 3% of patients, the direct Coombs test is positive.

In the *immune complex mechanism*, exposure to quinidine may cause an antidrug antibody to form and create an immune complex, which is adsorbed on the RBCs and may activate complement. The direct Coombs test is positive because of the complement on the RBC surface.

Cold Agglutinin Syndrome (Primary Cold Agglutinin Disease)

Cold agglutinin syndrome is characterized by chronic hemolytic anemia, agglutination, and a positive direct Coombs test (anti–complement component C3). IgM autoantibodies are reactive at temperatures below 37°C. The cause is most commonly idiopathic but can also be secondary to infection (most commonly from *Mycoplasma pneumoniae* or EBV) or malignancy (B-cell lymphoma, chronic lymphocytic leukemia, multiple myeloma, and Waldenström macroglobulinemia). Clinical signs and symptoms relate to small-vessel occlusion, including acrocyanosis of the fingers, toes, ears, and tip of the nose.

The peripheral blood smear shows RBC agglutination that disappears if prepared at 37°C (Figure 37.10). Agglutinated RBCs clump together, spuriously elevating the MCV. Therapy includes avoidance of the cold. In severe cases, rituximab and cytotoxic agents are used. Agglutination should not be confused with rouleaux, in which RBCs stack in a linear pattern (Figure 37.16).

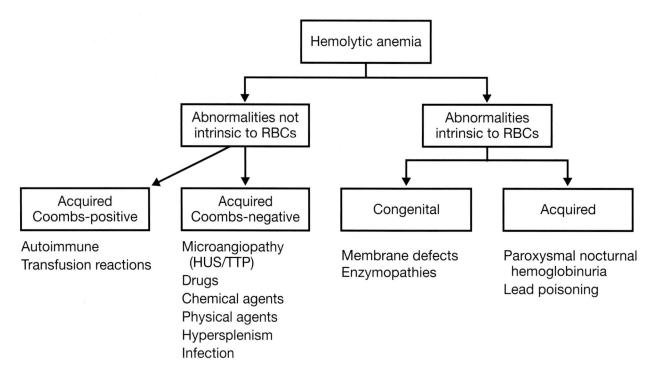

Figure 37.15 *Differential Diagnosis of Hemolytic Anemia. HUS indicates hemolytic uremic syndrome; RBC, red blood cell; TTP, thrombotic thrombocytopenic purpura.*

Warm Agglutinin Autoimmune Hemolytic Anemia

Warm agglutinins are IgG antibodies that bind to RBCs at physiologic temperatures rather than primarily in the cold. The direct Coombs test is positive for both IgG and complement component C3. Associated causes include autoimmune disorders (systemic lupus erythematosus), lymphoproliferative

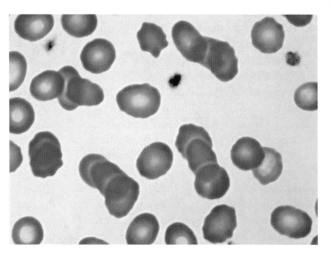

Figure 37.16 *Rouleaux. Stacking of red blood cells in a linear pattern distinguishes rouleaux from agglutination (Figure 37.10). Rouleaux are most commonly associated with hypergammaglobulinemia, especially in human immunodeficiency virus infection or monoclonal plasma cell disorders (peripheral blood smear; Wright-Giemsa).*
(Courtesy of Curtis A. Hanson, MD, Mayo Clinic, Rochester, Minnesota. Used with permission.)

disorders (chronic lymphocytic leukemia), drugs, and transfusion. The first general principle in the treatment of warm agglutinin autoimmune hemolytic anemia is to treat the underlying disease (if one can be identified) and to discontinue the use of drugs that have been implicated in hemolysis.

Paroxysmal Cold Hemoglobinuria (Complement-Mediated Lysis)

Paroxysmal cold hemoglobinuria is the least common cause of autoimmune hemolytic anemias. A positive Donath-Landsteiner test is diagnostic; it detects an IgG antibody

---

KEY FACTS

✓ Acute chest syndrome—
  - leading cause of death in sickle cell anemia
  - clinical features: fever, chest pain, tachypnea, leukocytosis, and pulmonary infiltrates

✓ Sickle cell anemia therapy—immunizations for encapsulated organisms, penicillin prophylaxis, and folate supplementation

✓ Increased RBC destruction in hemolytic anemia—increased indirect bilirubin and lactate dehydrogenase; decreased haptoglobin

✓ Hemosiderinuria—evidence that desquamated renal tubular cells absorbed free hemoglobin days to weeks earlier

✓ Cold agglutinin syndrome—idiopathic (usually) or secondary to infection (*Mycoplasma pneumonia* or EBV) or malignancy

that binds to RBCs at low temperatures, causing hemolysis. Paroxysmal cold hemoglobinuria is often idiopathic and can be associated with syphilis, mononucleosis, mycoplasma, and childhood exanthems. The condition usually resolves after the infection clears.

Coombs-Negative Hemolytic Anemia

The differential diagnosis of Coombs-negative hemolytic anemia is broad and includes hereditary RBC disorders such as enzymopathies (eg, G6PD deficiency and pyruvate kinase deficiency), hemoglobinopathies, and membrane disorders; paroxysmal nocturnal hemoglobinuria; Wilson disease; and microangiopathic conditions, including thrombotic thrombocytopenic purpura (TTP). Rarely, warm agglutinin autoimmune hemolytic anemia is Coombs-negative owing to low antibody titers.

G6PD Deficiency

G6PD deficiency, a sex-linked disorder, is the most common RBC enzyme deficiency. It causes decreased levels of glutathione (an antioxidant), making RBCs more sensitive to oxidative damage by infections, toxins (eg, naphthalene in mothballs), and drugs. G6PD deficiency confers some protection against falciparum malaria.

Hemolysis does not usually occur in the steady state but occurs with infections, diabetic ketoacidosis, ingestion of fava beans (seen only in G6PD Mediterranean), and drugs. Drugs that commonly cause hemolysis include antimalarial agents (eg, primaquine and chloroquine), dapsone, sulfonamides, nitrofurantoin, high-dose aspirin, probenecid, and nitrites.

Abnormal laboratory findings include intravascular hemolysis, methemoglobinemia, and methemalbuminemia (specific for intravascular hemolysis due to enzymopathy). Supravital staining for Heinz bodies is a good screening test, but their absence does not rule out the diagnosis. The G6PD assay is the definitive test but should not be done during acute hemolysis. Therapy includes treating the underlying infection and withdrawing use of the offending drug.

Hereditary Spherocytosis

Hereditary spherocytosis is typically an autosomal dominant disorder, but it can be autosomal recessive or sporadic. It is caused by an underlying defect in the RBC cytoskeleton because of a partial gene deficiency (eg, in ankyrin or spectrin). Features include jaundice, splenomegaly, negative direct Coombs test, spherocytes, and increased osmotic fragility. The osmotic fragility test is almost always abnormal and is the most reliable diagnostic test. Pigment gallstones are present in most patients by age 50. Treatment is splenectomy after the first decade of life for moderate or severe hemolysis, which invariably reduces hemolysis. Asymptomatic adults may be observed if the hemoglobin concentration is greater than 11 g/dL and the reticulocyte count is less than 6%.

Paroxysmal Nocturnal Hemoglobinuria

Paroxysmal nocturnal hemoglobinuria (PNH) is an acquired, clonal, stem cell disorder. Blood cells are unusually sensitive to activated complement and are lysed, primarily at night when plasma is more acidotic from sleep-related physiology (eg, relative hypoxia).

A mutation in the *PIGA* gene causes cells in PNH to have a decrease or absence of glycosylphosphatidylinositol (GPI)-linked proteins, including CD14, CD55, and CD59. Clinically, PNH is characterized by chronic intravascular hemolytic anemia, pancytopenia, and venous thrombosis of the portal system, brain, and extremities. Budd-Chiari syndrome (hepatic vein thrombosis) is the main cause of death. In up to 10% of patients, myelodysplasia or acute myeloid leukemia develops. The most useful assay for diagnosis of PNH is flow cytometry to establish the absence of the GPI-linked antigens. Up to 60% of patients respond to prednisone; eculizumab is a complement (C5) monoclonal antibody that can be used for long-term therapy for hemolysis in PNH.

Thrombotic Microangiopathies: Differential Diagnosis

In microangiopathic hemolytic anemia, RBCs are fragmented and deformed by fibrin deposits in the peripheral blood (Figure 37.17). Direct Coombs testing is negative. The associated disorders, characterized by widespread microvascular thrombosis leading to end-organ injury, include TTP, hemolytic uremic syndrome (HUS), malignant hypertension, pulmonary hypertension, acute glomerulonephritis, renal allograft rejection, obstetric catastrophes, HELLP syndrome (hemolysis, elevated liver function tests, and low platelet count), disseminated intravascular coagulopathy, collagen vascular diseases (scleroderma), vascular malformations including Kasabach-Merritt syndrome (giant hemangiomas that trap platelets), viral infections (HIV), bacterial infections (*E coli* O157:H7), drug-induced disorders (eg, mitomycin C, quinine, ticlopidine, tacrolimus, cisplatin, and cyclosporine), bone marrow transplant, and solid organ transplant.

Thrombotic Thrombocytopenic Purpura

The features of TTP include the pentad of microangiopathic hemolytic anemia, thrombocytopenia, neurologic signs (headache, coma, mental changes, paresis, seizure, aphasia, syncope, visual symptoms, dysarthria, vertigo, agitation, confusion, and delirium), fever, and kidney abnormalities (abnormal urinary sediment and elevated creatinine level). Most patients do not manifest all 5 features. The primary criteria are thrombocytopenia and microangiopathy, and these are sufficient to establish the diagnosis. The anemia is normochromic normocytic, with microangiopathic hemolytic features (Figure 37.17). Direct Coombs test results are negative. Results of coagulation studies are normal, in contrast to abnormal results in disseminated intravascular coagulopathy. The cause of TTP is unknown

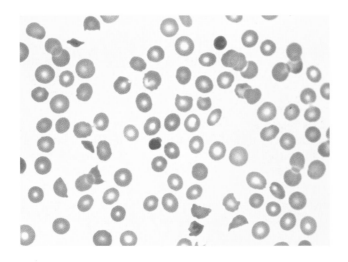

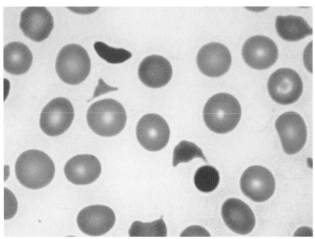

Figure 37.17 Schistocytes. A and B, Fragmented red blood cells are shaped like helmets, triangles, or kites. These are characteristic of any microangiopathic hemolytic process (peripheral blood smear; Wright-Giemsa).
(Courtesy of Curtis A. Hanson, MD, Mayo Clinic, Rochester, Minnesota. Used with permission.)

in more than 90% of patients; however, it is associated with pregnancy, use of oral contraceptives, HIV infection, cancer, bone marrow transplant, certain chemotherapy drugs (especially mitomycin C and bleomycin), and other drugs (eg, crack cocaine, ticlopidine, and cyclosporine).

Patients with TTP are deficient in the von Willebrand factor–cleaving protease ADAMTS13. Even when ADAMTS13 assays are available, results can take days to return; thus, the assay is not useful for initial treatment decisions.

Without treatment, more than 90% of patients die of multiorgan failure, but with treatment, 70% to 80% survive the disease and have few or no sequelae. The treatment of choice is plasma exchange. Relapses are also managed with plasma exchange. The management of refractory TTP includes rituximab, splenectomy, vincristine, or intravenous high-dose γ-globulin. Platelet transfusion should be used only when required for an invasive procedure since it can exacerbate the disease.

Hemolytic Uremic Syndrome

HUS is characterized by microangiopathic hemolytic anemia, thrombocytopenia, and acute kidney injury. Fever and neurologic signs are usually not present. It is associated with infections (*E coli* O157:H7 and *Shigella dysenteriae*), pregnancy, bone marrow transplant, chemotherapy, and immunosuppressive medications such as cyclosporine. HUS is usually not associated with a decrease in ADAMTS13 activity. Management of HUS is supportive. In adults, treatment with plasma exchange is indicated, but the response is variable.

KEY FACTS

✓ G6PD deficiency—drugs that cause hemolysis include antimalarial agents, dapsone, sulfonamides, nitrofurantoin, high-dose aspirin, probenecid, and nitrites

✓ Hereditary spherocytosis—abnormal osmotic fragility test

✓ Paroxysmal nocturnal hemoglobinuria—activated complement lyses sensitive blood cells primarily during sleep (more acidotic)

✓ TTP pentad of features—
  - microangiopathic hemolytic anemia
  - thrombocytopenia
  - neurologic signs
  - fever
  - kidney abnormalities

Transfusion Reactions

The primary cause of major transfusion reactions and transfusion-related deaths is medical error, which includes bypassed safeguards, similar patient names, and verbal or faxed communications. The major transfusion reactions include acute hemolytic transfusion reactions, transfusions associated with anti-IgA antibodies, transfusion-related acute lung injury (TRALI), acute respiratory distress syndrome (ARDS), delayed hemolytic transfusion reactions, febrile transfusion reactions, urticarial (allergic) transfusion reactions, and circulatory overload (Table 37.3).

Acute Hemolytic Transfusion Reactions

Acute hemolytic transfusion reactions are the most life-threatening transfusion reactions and occur within minutes to hours. The recipient's RBC antibodies (usually IgM) react against the donor's RBCs and cause complement-mediated hemolysis. The most common cause is human error,

Table 37.3 • Risks of Complications From Transfusions in the United States

Complication	Risk Per Units of Transfused Blood
Minor allergic reaction	3/100
Circulatory overload	Variable
Febrile, nonhemolytic	3/100
Delayed hemolytic transfusion reaction	1/4,000
TRALI	1/10,000
Acute hemolytic transfusion reaction	$1/2.5 \times 10^4$ to $1/1.0 \times 10^6$
HIV infection	$1/2.1 \times 10^6$
Hepatitis B virus infection	$1/2.0 \times 10^5$
Hepatitis C virus infection	$1/1.9 \times 10^5$
HTLV type I or II infection	$1/2.0 \times 10^5$
West Nile virus infection	Unknown
Bacterial infections	$1/2,000$ to $1/5.0 \times 10^5$
IgA-related anaphylaxis	$1/1.0 \times 10^5$
Graft-vs-host disease	Rare
Immunosuppression	Unknown
Posttransfusion purpura	Rare
Prion infection	Unknown

Abbreviations: HIV, human immunodeficiency virus; HTLV, human T-cell leukemia virus; Ig, immunoglobulin; TRALI, transfusion-related acute lung injury.

especially when blood is released emergently. The mortality rate is about 20%; of the fatal transfusion reactions, 85% involve ABO incompatibility. ABO compatibility is illustrated in Table 37.4. Other, nonclerical causes include antibodies not detected before transfusion, such as Kell, Duffy (Fy^a), and Kidd (Jk^a). Clinically, patients experience pain at the intravenous site, a sense of impending doom, back pain, abdominal pain, fever, chills, chest pain, hypotension, nausea, flushing, and dyspnea. Direct Coombs testing is positive in most cases.

Complications include oliguria, acute kidney injury, and disseminated intravascular coagulation. Treatment includes immediate termination of the transfusion, vigorous administration of fluids, and furosemide to increase renal cortical blood flow.

Allergic Transfusion Reactions

Allergic transfusion reactions are a complication in 3% of transfusions and are caused by a recipient's antibody against foreign-donor serum proteins. Transfusion reactions can also be associated with anti-IgA antibodies. These include anaphylactic reactions, which occur most commonly in patients with IgA deficiency who may have circulating complement-binding anti-IgA antibodies that react with donor IgA. Clinical features are similar to those of an acute hemolytic transfusion reaction. Treatment includes stopping the transfusion and giving antihistamines and conventional antianaphylactic drugs. Transfusion protocols for patients include use of washed RBCs and IgA-deficient plasma.

Transfusion-Related Acute Lung Injury

Transfusion-associated ARDS or TRALI results from an interaction between the recipient's leukocytes and donor antileukocyte antibodies. TRALI often is unrecognized and ranks third among causes of transfusion-related deaths. It is characterized by acute respiratory distress during transfusion or within 6 hours after completion of transfusion, hypotension, bilateral pulmonary infiltrates, normal or low pulmonary capillary wedge pressure, no evidence of circulatory overload, and fever. With appropriate supportive care, recovery is rapid, occurring in 24 to 48 hours.

Delayed Hemolytic Transfusion Reactions

Delayed hemolytic transfusion reactions (occurring in 1 in 4,000 transfusions) occur because of the inability to detect clinically significant recipient antibodies before transfusion. They usually occur 5 to 10 days after transfusion and are less dangerous than an acute hemolytic reaction. The recipient's plasma contains antibody before transfusion

Table 37.4 • Blood Product Compatibility in the ABO System[a]

	Acceptable Donor ABO Groups		
Recipient ABO Group	Packed Red Blood Cells	Platelets and Fresh Frozen Plasma	Whole Blood (Rarely Used)
O	O	AB, A, B, or O	O
A	A or O	A or AB	A
B	B or O	B or AB	B
AB	AB, A, B, or O	AB	AB

[a] Natural alloimmunization against A and B antigens occurs in people lacking these antigens. Upon transfusion of ABO-incompatible blood, preformed antibodies serve as hemagglutinins, resulting in life-threatening acute hemolysis and complement activation. Hemagglutinins are found primarily in plasma; platelets are considered similar to plasma products with respect to ABO compatibility.

because of a previous transfusion or previous pregnancy. There is evidence of hemolysis, and direct Coombs testing is positive. One-third of the patients are asymptomatic, and the reactions are detected by the recurrence of laboratory-detected anemia without clear cause; other patients present with symptoms of anemia, chills, jaundice, and fever. Management consists of monitoring hemoglobin concentration and renal output and avoiding the use of units with the offending antigen in the future.

Febrile Transfusion Reactions

Febrile transfusion reactions are characterized by chills, fever, flushing, headache, tachycardia, myalgias, and arthralgias. They usually begin about 1 hour after the transfusion starts and last for 8 to 10 hours. They occur in 1% of all transfusions. Causes include cytokines from leukocytes and platelets against donor antigens and antiserum protein antibodies. Treatment consists of stopping the transfusion to evaluate the patient; initially, a febrile reaction cannot be distinguished from a hemolytic transfusion reaction. Preventive methods include leukoreduction.

Circulatory Overload

Circulatory overload may cause tightness in the chest, dry cough, and acute edema. It occurs in patients who already have an increased intravascular volume or decreased cardiac reserve, with symptoms generally developing within several hours after transfusion. Management includes slowing the transfusion to 100 mL/h, placing the patient in the sitting position, and giving diuretics.

Posttransfusion Purpura

Posttransfusion purpura is a rare syndrome in which the recipient makes antiplatelet antibodies, which cause an abrupt onset of severe thrombocytopenia 5 to 10 days after blood transfusion. Most cases involve patients who lack human platelet antigen 1a and who have an antibody from a previous pregnancy or transfusion.

Infection

Pathogen transmission may occur with transfusions. These risks and other risks of transfusion are summarized in Table 37.3.

Porphyria

The porphyrias are enzyme disorders that are autosomal dominant with low disease penetrance, except for congenital erythropoietic porphyria (which is autosomal recessive)

Table 37.5 • Comparison of Porphyrias

Porphyria Cutanea Tarda	Acute Intermittent Porphyria	Porphyria Variegata
Features		
Most common type of porphyria Iron overload Skin lesions on light-exposed areas Hypertrichosis (usually mild) Increased uroporphyrins in urine No neuropathic features	Increased urinary δ-aminolevulinic acid and porphobilinogen during acute symptomatic episodes, with normal levels between episodes Neurologic symptoms: abdominal pain of 3–5 days' duration without anatomical cause, focal neurologic problems such as polyneuropathy and motor paresis, psychiatric problems with hallucinations, confusion, psychosis, seizures Decreased porphobilinogen deaminase activity Normal protoporphyrin and coproporphyrin in stool	Clinically: photosensitivity, abdominal pain, neurologic symptoms similar to those in acute intermittent porphyria Increased protoporphyrin and coproporphyrin in stool
Associations		
Alcoholic liver disease, chronic hepatitis C, hemochromatosis Estrogens: females; males treated for prostatic carcinoma Hexachlorobenzene	Drugs can precipitate crises (eg, sulfonamides, barbiturates, alcohol) Menstrual cycle can exacerbate symptoms Infection or surgery can precipitate crisis Inadequate nutrition can precipitate crisis	Common in South Africa (due to founder effect), Holland
Treatment		
Phlebotomy to remove iron Chloroquine Low-dose antimalarials	Avoid prolonged fasting and crash diets Large amounts of carbohydrate (400 g daily) Intravenous hematin Luteinizing hormone–releasing hormone agonists for suppression of hormonal fluctuation	Same as for acute intermittent porphyria

and porphyria cutanea tarda (which may be acquired and is associated with hepatitis C and hemochromatosis). Most persons remain biochemically and clinically normal throughout most of their lives. Clinical expression is linked to environmental and acquired factors.

Disease manifestations depend on the type of excess porphyrin intermediate. With an excess of the earlier precursor molecules (δ-aminolevulinic acid and porphobilinogen), the clinical manifestations are neuropsychiatric, including autonomic dysfunction (abdominal pain, vomiting, constipation, tachycardia, and hypertension), psychiatric symptoms, fever, leukocytosis, and paresthesias. If the excess is in the later intermediates (uroporphyrins, coproporphyrins, and protoporphyrins), the manifestations are cutaneous (photosensitivity, blister formation, facial hypertrichosis, and hyperpigmentation). An excess of both early and late porphyrins results in both neuropsychiatric and cutaneous manifestations.

Porphobilinogen production and excretion are increased during marked symptoms caused by the 3 neuropathic porphyrias, which include acute intermittent porphyria, hereditary coproporphyria, and porphyria variegata. Hereditary coproporphyria and porphyria variegata are characterized by an accumulation of coproporphyrinogen/ coproporphyrin or protoporphyrinogen/protoporphyrin and a concomitant increase in δ-aminolevulinic acid and porphobilinogen. In the acute porphyrias, determine the 24-hour urinary porphobilinogen level during an attack. Patients with acute intermittent porphyria lack skin lesions. It is important to check fecal porphyrins in protoporphyria, porphyria variegata, and coproporphyria. An elevated coproporphyrin level alone, therefore, does not support a diagnosis of porphyria. The porphyrias are compared in Table 37.5.

KEY FACTS

- ✓ Acute hemolytic transfusion reactions—usually from human error, especially with emergent release of blood
- ✓ TRALI—acute respiratory distress during transfusion or ≤6 hours after transfusion
- ✓ TRALI—hypotension, bilateral pulmonary infiltrates, normal or low pulmonary capillary wedge pressure, no evidence of circulatory overload, and fever
- ✓ Acute porphyrias—determine 24-hour urinary porphobilinogen level during attack

38 Hemostatic Disorders[a]

RAJIV K. PRUTHI, MBBS

Functions of the Coagulation System

The 2 essential functions of the coagulation system (maintaining hemostasis and preventing and limiting thrombosis) are served by the procoagulant and anticoagulant components. Vascular injury results in activation of the phases of hemostasis, including vasospasm, platelet plug formation (platelet activation, adhesion, and aggregation), and fibrin clot formation (by activation of coagulation factors in the procoagulant system). The anticoagulant system controls excessive clot formation, while the fibrinolytic system breaks down and remodels blood clots.

Evaluation for a Bleeding Disorder

Bleeding disorders consist of clotting factor deficiencies or inhibitors, vascular bleeding disorders, and platelet disorders (quantitative and qualitative). Each of these is broadly classified into congenital disorders and acquired disorders.

The best screening tool to evaluate for a bleeding disorder is a thorough clinical evaluation (personal and family hemostatic history and physical examination). The presence of a bleeding disorder may be suggested from inquiry into the presence and age at onset of spontaneous bleeding (eg, epistaxis, easy bruising, or joint bleeding), unusual or unexpected posttraumatic or surgical bleeding (including dental extractions), and family history. A thorough clinical evaluation should also include review of medications and coexisting medical problems to identify clinical risk factors for thrombosis.

Laboratory Testing to Evaluate a Bleeding Patient

To evaluate a bleeding patient, tests should include a complete blood cell count (CBC), prothrombin time (PT), activated partial thromboplastin time (aPTT), and fibrinogen. Additional testing that may not be generally available includes assays for von Willebrand disease (vWD), coagulation factor assays, factor XIII (FXIII) assays, and platelet function tests.

PT (International Normalized Ratio)

The PT assesses the extrinsic and final common pathways of the procoagulant cascade (Figure 38.1). Prolonged PT is caused by deficiencies or inhibitors of clotting factors. The PT is mainly useful as a monitoring test for warfarin anticoagulation and as an initial screening test for patients who have bleeding symptoms. The international normalized ratio reduces interlaboratory variation of the PT and is calculated and reported by the laboratory. Preoperative patients do not need routine PT testing.

Activated Partial Thromboplastin Time

The aPTT assesses the intrinsic and final common pathways of the procoagulant cascade (Figure 38.1); deficiencies or inhibitors of clotting factors within the intrinsic and final common pathways result in prolongation of the aPTT. The aPTT is commonly used to monitor unfractionated heparin (UFH) therapy and direct thrombin inhibitor therapy (eg, argatroban and lepirudin) and as an initial screening test for the presence of lupus anticoagulant or for patients who have bleeding symptoms.

---

[a] Portions previously published in Pruthi RK. A practical approach to genetic testing for von Willebrand disease. Mayo Clin Proc. 2006 May;81(5):679–91; and Kamal AH, Tefferi A, Pruthi RK. How to interpret and pursue an abnormal prothrombin time, activated partial thromboplastin time, and bleeding time in adults. Mayo Clin Proc. 2007 Jul;82(7):864–73. Used with permission of Mayo Foundation for Medical Education and Research.

Intrinsic   **Extrinsic**

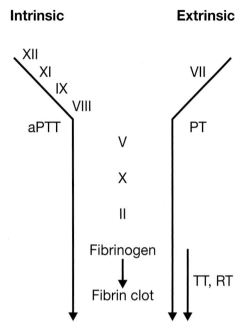

Figure 38.1 Coagulation Cascade. aPTT indicates activated partial thromboplastin time; PT, prothrombin time; RT, reptilase time; TT, thrombin time.

Bleeding Time

Use of the bleeding time (BT) test has been discontinued in many hospitals. A review of multiple studies led to the following conclusions: 1) If a patient does not have a clinical history of a bleeding disorder, BT is not a useful predictor of risk of hemorrhage with surgical procedures; 2) normal BT does not exclude the possibility of excessive hemorrhage with invasive procedures; and 3) BT cannot reliably identify patients exposed to aspirin or nonsteroidal anti-inflammatory drugs.

Approach to a Prolonged PT or aPTT

When a patient has a prolonged PT or aPTT, first exclude artifactual causes (eg, elevated hematocrit; nonfasting, lipemic sample; or heparin contamination of the specimen). Second, perform a mixing study in a 1:1 ratio with normal pooled plasma. If the clotting time corrects (ie, the aPTT normalizes), a coagulation factor deficiency is implied, and follow-up factor assays are then performed. If the aPTT is inhibited (ie, the aPTT shortens but does not normalize), the implication is that an inhibitor is present. The inhibitors may be medications (eg, heparins and direct thrombin inhibitors), specific factor inhibitors (eg, factor VIII [FVIII] or factor V inhibitors), or nonspecific inhibitors (eg, lupus anticoagulants). Appropriate follow-up testing typically leads to the diagnosis of the underlying cause of the prolongation of the PT and aPTT.

> **Box 38.1 • Disorders Not Detected With the PT and aPTT**
>
> Qualitative platelet defects (requires specialized platelet function testing)
>
> von Willebrand disease (requires assays for von Willebrand factor)
>
> Factor XIII deficiency (requires specialized factor XIII screening or functional assays)
>
> Deficiency of antiplasmin and plasminogen activator inhibitor 1 (requires specific assays)
>
> Abbreviations: aPTT, activated partial thromboplastin time; PT, prothrombin time.

> **KEY FACTS**
>
> ✓ Essential functions of coagulation system—maintaining hemostasis (procoagulant component) and limiting thrombosis (anticoagulant component)
>
> ✓ Screening for a bleeding disorder—thorough clinical evaluation is the best tool
>
> ✓ PT—assesses extrinsic and final common pathways of the procoagulant cascade
>
> ✓ aPTT—assesses intrinsic and final common pathways of the procoagulant cascade

Bleeding Disorders Not Detected With PT and aPTT

Several disorders are not detected with the PT and aPTT (Box 38.1).

Congenital Plasmatic Bleeding Disorders (Factor Deficiencies)

Of the congenital plasmatic bleeding disorders, vWD is the most common. Others include hemophilia A, hemophilia B, and hemophilia C. Other factor deficiency states are rare (Table 38.1). All clotting factors are produced by the liver except von Willebrand factor (vWF), which is produced by vascular endothelial cells and megakaryocytes.

von Willebrand Disease

Definition and Classification
vWD is a deficiency or dysfunction of vWF. It is classified according to whether the defect is quantitative (types 1 and 3) or qualitative (types 2A, 2B, 2M, and 2N).

> **Key Definition**
>
> von Willebrand disease: *deficiency or dysfunction of vWF.*

Table 38.1 • Congenital Bleeding Disorders

Congenital Disorder	Deficient Factor	PT	aPTT	Prevalence	Mode of Inheritance
Hemophilia A	Factor VIII	NL	Prol	1:5,000[a]	X-linked recessive
Hemophilia B	Factor IX	NL	Prol	1:30,000[a]	X-linked recessive
Hemophilia C	Factor XI	NL	Prol	Up to 4%[b]	Autosomal recessive
von Willebrand disease	von Willebrand factor	NL	NL or Prol	Up to 1%	Autosomal dominant or recessive
Factor VII deficiency	Factor VII	Prol	NL	1:500,000	Autosomal recessive
Rare coagulation factor deficiencies					
Factor V	Factor V	Prol	Prol	1:1 million	Autosomal recessive
Factor II	Factor II	Prol	NL or Prol	Rare	Autosomal recessive
Factor X	Factor X	Prol	NL or Prol	1:500,000	Autosomal recessive
Factor XIII	Factor XIII	NL	NL	Rare	Autosomal recessive
Combined factors VIII and V	Factors VIII and V	Prol	Prol	Rare	Autosomal recessive

Abbreviations: aPTT, activated partial thromboplastin time; NL, normal; Prol, prolonged; PT, prothrombin time.

[a] Live male births.

[b] Among Ashkenazi Jews.

Biochemistry and Function of vWF

Endothelial cells and platelets store vWF. After secretion, the ultra-large-molecular-weight multimers of vWF, the most hemostatically active, are cleaved into multimers of smaller size by a protease, ADAMTS13 (a disintegrin and metalloprotease with thrombospondin type 1 motif, 13).

vWF mediates platelet adhesion and aggregation. It acts as a carrier protein for FVIII, protecting it from proteolytic inactivation.

Clinical Features

Patients who have mild vWD may be asymptomatic and bleed only when challenged with trauma or minor surgery (eg, dental extraction) or major surgery.

Patients who have severe vWD may have spontaneous bleeding. Spontaneous bleeding is typically mucocutaneous (bruising, epistaxis, hematuria, or gastrointestinal tract hemorrhage); in type III vWD, bleeding occurs in joints and soft tissue. Bleeding may be exacerbated by the use of aspirin or nonsteroidal analgesics.

Laboratory Testing

Laboratory testing includes testing for vWF antigen, vWF activity, and FVIII activity (Box 38.2). If initial results are abnormal, vWF multimer analyses are performed to determine the subtype of vWD (Box 38.3).

Variables Affecting vWF Levels

Healthy people with blood group O have vWF levels that are 25% to 30% lower than in people with blood groups A, B, or AB and thus may receive a misdiagnosis of vWD. Therefore, ABO typing should be part of the initial testing.

Acquired defects of vWF (ie, *acquired von Willebrand syndrome*) may occur in patients with aortic

Box 38.2 • Stepwise Approach to Assessment for von Willebrand Disease (vWD)

1. Bleeding history
2. Complete blood cell count
3. vWD profile testing

   vWF:Ag
   RCoF
   VIII:c

4. ABO blood group
5. Optional tests if initial data suggest vWD

   vWF multimers
   vWF:CBA
   vWF:VIIIB
   RIPA

6. Genetic tests if indicated

Abbreviations: Ag, antigen; CBA, collagen-binding assay; VIIIB, factor VIII binding assay; VIII:c, factor VIII coagulant activity; RCoF, ristocetin cofactor; RIPA, ristocetin-induced platelet aggregation; vWF, von Willebrand factor.

Box 38.3 • Subtypes of von Willebrand Disease

Type 1—mild to moderate reduction in the level and activity of vWF:Ag

Type 2—disproportionate reduction in the activity of the vWF function, called the *ristocetin cofactor* (RCoF), compared with vWF:Ag

Type 3—absence of vWF

Abbreviations: vWF, von Willebrand factor; vWF:Ag, von Willebrand factor antigen.

stenosis, myeloproliferative disorders, and monoclonal protein disorders. The syndrome mimics congenital type 2 vWD.

Short-term physical exertion, inflammation, malignancy, hyperthyroidism, estrogens, and pregnancy increase vWF levels to normal and may mask a diagnosis of vWD. Hypothyroidism is associated with decreased vWF levels.

Type 2B vWD is associated with thrombocytopenia. Type 2N vWD results from mutations in the FVIII binding domain of vWF. This subtype may be mistaken for mild hemophilia A.

Inheritance of vWD

Type 1 vWD is inherited as an autosomal dominant trait with variable penetrance. Types 2A, 2B, and 2M vWD are inherited as autosomal dominant traits. Type 3 vWD and type 2N (Normandy) vWD are inherited as autosomal recessive traits.

Management

The goals for managing vWD include preventing and treating hemorrhage (Box 38.4). When a diagnosis of vWD has been established, a desmopressin acetate (DDAVP) treatment trial should be performed for patients with types 1, 2A, or 2M vWD. Intravenous infusion of 0.3 mcg/kg body weight releases vWF from its storage sites; levels should be measured 60 minutes after infusion. Desmopressin is generally not helpful if patients have type 2B vWD because the release of endogenous vWF worsens thrombocytopenia. Patients with type 3 vWD have no response to desmopressin and should not undergo a desmopressin trial. Desmopressin is indicated for prevention or treatment of minor bleeding, for minor procedures such as dental extraction, and for the management of menorrhagia in women with vWD. An intranasal formulation of desmopressin is also available. For patients who have no response to desmopressin and for those in whom it is contraindicated, administration of purified plasma-derived vWF concentrates is the therapy of choice.

Hemophilia A and Hemophilia B

Hemophilia A and hemophilia B are clinically indistinguishable, X-linked recessive bleeding disorders. Hemophilia A is due to a deficiency in blood coagulation FVIII, and hemophilia B is due to a deficiency in factor IX (FIX). Hemophilia is classified according to levels of FVIII and FIX as severe (<1%), moderate (1%–5%), or mild (>5%–40%).

Clinical Features

Patients who have *mild hemophilia* seldom experience spontaneous hemorrhage but will bleed after trauma or surgery; rarely, they may not receive a diagnosis of hemophilia until adulthood. Patients who have *moderate hemophilia* experience spontaneous bleeding infrequently but typically bleed after minor trauma and surgery.

Patients who have *severe hemophilia* frequently experience spontaneous bleeding, including hemarthrosis, soft tissue hematomas, and intracranial hemorrhage, in addition to minor hemorrhage such as epistaxis and ecchymoses. Regular prophylactic administration of vWF concentrates to patients with severe disease has reduced the frequency and associated chronic complications related to bleeding.

Management

At the initial diagnosis of mild or moderate hemophilia A, as with vWD, a desmopressin trial is performed; FVIII levels are checked before infusion and 1 hour after infusion. For patients who have hemophilia A and respond to desmopressin, administer desmopressin for *minor* hemorrhage or for prophylaxis and treatment of minor surgical hemorrhage. Use recombinant or plasma-derived FVIII concentrates as therapy for *major* hemorrhages and as prophylaxis for major surgery.

Desmopressin is not used for hemophilia B; instead, recombinant or plasma-derived FIX concentrates are used.

Complications of Treatment

Transfusion-transmitted viral infections occur (eg, viral hepatitis and human immunodeficiency virus [HIV] infection), although with contemporary clotting factor manufacturing processes and the introduction of recombinant factors, these are rare. *Recurrent hemarthrosis* (in severe hemophilia and in patients who have FVIII or FIX inhibitors) leads to premature degenerative joint disease. *Development of FVIII and FIX inhibitors* is the most

---

Box 38.4 • Management of von Willebrand Disease

General measures

  Provide patient education
  Recommend a medical condition identification tag
  Generate treatment guidelines for managing bleeding
  Refer to a comprehensive hemophilia treatment
    center for periodic follow-up

Specific measures

  Administer desmopressin
  Administer adjunctive ε-aminocaproic acid or vWF
    concentrates preoperatively to prevent bleeding or
    to manage bleeding
  Administer vWF concentrates

Abbreviation: vWF, von Willebrand factor.

serious complication. Standard FVIII and FIX concentrates are ineffective, and bypassing agents (eg, recombinant factor VIIa or activated prothrombin complex concentrates) are required for management of surgical bleeding and hemorrhage.

Factor VII Deficiency

Factor VII deficiency is typically a mild bleeding disorder that is usually detected with a preoperative prolonged PT. Factor VII levels as low as 10% of the reference value may be undetected for many years. Bleeding symptoms are similar to those of hemophilia. Recombinant factor VIIa is the treatment of choice for preventing and treating hemorrhage; however, fresh frozen plasma is also an option.

Factor XI Deficiency (Hemophilia C)

Factor XI (FXI) deficiency is a rare autosomal recessive disorder that is prevalent among Ashkenazi Jews. It is a mild bleeding disorder; patients usually present after surgery or trauma or after starting therapy with antiplatelet agents or anticoagulants.

Bleeding symptoms do not correlate well with FXI levels (ie, patients with mild deficiencies may have significant bleeding symptoms, whereas patients with more severe deficiencies may remain asymptomatic until after surgery or initiation of an anticoagulant or antiplatelet agent).

Fresh frozen plasma is the treatment of choice for prevention and treatment of hemorrhage. FXI concentrates are being studied in clinical trials.

FXIII Deficiency

FXIII deficiency has an autosomal recessive inheritance pattern. Severe FXIII deficiency is characterized by clinically significant bleeding but normal results from screening tests (PT and aPTT). Other characteristics include umbilical cord bleeding, delayed wound healing, delayed hemorrhage, and recurrent pregnancy loss. Cryoprecipitate and FXIII concentrates are the treatment of choice for prevention and treatment of hemorrhage.

Factor Deficiencies That Prolong the aPTT But Do Not Result in Hemorrhage

Deficiencies of factor XII, high-molecular-weight kininogen, and prekallikrein can result in a marked prolongation of the aPTT, yet even severe deficiencies are not risk factors for hemorrhage. Their roles in hemostasis are being defined.

KEY FACTS

✓ Mild vWD—patients may be asymptomatic and bleed only with trauma or surgery

✓ Severe vWD—patients may bleed spontaneously (typically bruising, epistaxis, hematuria, or gastrointestinal tract hemorrhage)

✓ Hemophilia A and hemophilia B—
  • clinically indistinguishable
  • X-linked recessive bleeding disorders

✓ Factor VII deficiency—
  • typically mild bleeding disorder
  • usually detected with a preoperative prolonged PT

✓ Factor XI deficiency—
  • rare autosomal recessive mild bleeding disorder
  • prevalent among Ashkenazi Jews

✓ Factor XIII deficiency—
  • autosomal recessive inheritance
  • if severe, characterized by clinically significant bleeding but normal PT and aPTT results

---

Acquired Bleeding Disorders

Acquired bleeding disorders can result from decreased production of coagulation factors by the liver (as in liver disease), increased consumption of coagulation factors (as in disseminated intravascular coagulation [DIC] and fibrinolysis), or the development of inhibitors against coagulation factors (Table 38.2).

Liver Disease

Since most coagulation factors (except vWF) are produced in the liver, hepatocellular damage and liver failure lead to decreased production of clotting factors and a bleeding tendency.

Table 38.2 • Causes of Acquired Coagulation Factor Deficiencies

Cause of Deficiency	Deficient Factor
Warfarin	Vitamin K–dependent factors
Decreased nutritional intake or malabsorption	Vitamin K–dependent factors
Liver failure	Multiple factors
Amyloid	Factor X
Myeloproliferative disease	Factor V
Acquired von Willebrand syndrome	von Willebrand factor and factor VIII
Disseminated intravascular coagulation	Multiple factors

Supportive management includes replenishment of the deficient coagulation factors with fresh frozen plasma (cryoprecipitate is a more concentrated form for fibrinogen and FXIII) until the liver recovers or is replaced by a transplanted liver.

Disseminated Intravascular Coagulation

DIC is a dynamic process with various causes that result in microvascular thrombosis and consumption of clotting factors (Box 38.5).

Clinical Features

DIC should be suspected in a patient presenting with underlying conditions known to predispose to DIC (Box 38.5). Most patients present with a new onset of bleeding; occasionally, patients present with thrombosis or both bleeding and thrombosis.

Bleeding manifestations include bleeding from surgical wounds and venipuncture sites, ecchymoses, petechiae, hematomas, vaginal bleeding, or hemorrhage from the gastrointestinal tract or genitourinary system.

Thrombotic manifestations occur less frequently than bleeding and include necrotic skin lesions, venous thromboembolism (deep vein thrombosis and pulmonary embolism), and acute arterial occlusions (stroke and myocardial infarction).

Pathophysiology

An understanding of the pathophysiology of DIC helps with understanding laboratory testing and management. The underlying disease (Box 38.5) stimulates the procoagulant system, generating thrombin and resulting in consumption of coagulation factors and platelets. The fibrinolytic system also is activated, converting plasminogen to plasmin. Plasmin prevents stabilization of fibrin clots (resulting in circulating fibrin monomers) and degrades existing fibrin clots and fibrinogen-releasing cleavage products called D-dimers. The circulating fibrin monomers are soluble and thus form weak clots.

Laboratory Testing

Laboratory findings in suspected DIC vary, and no single laboratory test is diagnostic. Clinical findings need to be interpreted along with laboratory data. Typical laboratory findings in DIC include thrombocytopenia, prolonged PT and aPTT, low levels of fibrinogen due to consumption, and increased levels of D-dimers and soluble fibrin monomer complexes.

Management

Principles of DIC management include identifying and treating underlying disease while managing the coagulopathy.

Blood Component Replacement Therapy

Observation may be reasonable for patients who have low-grade compensated DIC with mild coagulopathy and no bleeding. However, for patients who have symptomatic hemorrhage or abnormal laboratory results and for those at risk for bleeding, therapy includes transfusion of blood components (Box 38.6).

Ancillary Therapies

Although *UFH* inhibits thrombin and interrupts the cycle of consumptive coagulopathy, it is also associated with hemorrhage, including intracranial hemorrhage. Thus, in patients with acute DIC, heparin usually has a limited role, if any (except with acute DIC associated with promyelocytic leukemia), but it may have a role in chronic DIC as seen with solid tumors, the retained dead fetus syndrome, aortic aneurysm, and giant hemangiomas. *Recombinant activated protein C* improves mortality among patients with severe sepsis. *Antithrombin concentrate* has not been shown to improve mortality among patients with DIC. *Fibrinolysis inhibitors*, such as ε-aminocaproic acid or tranexamic acid, are generally contraindicated in DIC.

Acquired von Willebrand Syndrome

Acquired von Willebrand syndrome is an acquired quantitative or qualitative abnormality of vWF that is associated with monoclonal protein disorders, myeloproliferative disease, hypothyroidism, and other malignancies. Occasionally no underlying disease is found. Management consists of infusion of vWF concentrates to prevent and treat hemorrhage; desmopressin is seldom effective.

> ### Key Definition
>
> Acquired von Willebrand syndrome: *an acquired quantitative or qualitative abnormality of vWF associated with monoclonal protein disorders, myeloproliferative disease, hypothyroidism, and other malignancies.*

Acquired (Autoimmune) Hemophilia

In acquired (autoimmune) hemophilia, the development of FVIII inhibitors in previously healthy people results in a potentially life-threatening bleeding disorder. Management consists of maintaining hemostasis with special factor concentrates (activated prothrombin complex concentrates or recombinant factor VIIa) and immunosuppression (glucocorticoids, cytotoxic chemotherapy, and anti-CD20 antibody [rituximab]).

> ### KEY FACTS
>
> ✓ Hepatocellular damage and liver failure—
> - decreased production of clotting factors (most are produced in the liver)
> - bleeding tendency
>
> ✓ DIC—suspect if patient presents with condition known to predispose to DIC
>
> ✓ Acquired (autoimmune) hemophilia—development of FVIII inhibitors in a previously healthy person causes a potentially life-threatening bleeding disorder

Platelet Disorders

Platelets are produced in the bone marrow and, after circulating for 7 to 10 days, are destroyed in the reticuloendothelial system. Thrombocytopenia is most commonly acquired and poses a risk of bleeding. It commonly occurs as a result of decreased production or accelerated destruction. When thrombocytopenia occurs for the first time, the diagnosis of pseudothrombocytopenia should be excluded with examination of a peripheral blood smear. Rarely, thrombocytopenia is congenital.

Pseudothrombocytopenia

Pseudothrombocytopenia is due to EDTA-induced platelet clumping; platelets range from 50×10^9/L to 100×10^9/L. The CBC should be repeated with a blood sample collected in a citrate tube to prevent clumping. A peripheral blood smear (Figure 38.2) is useful to detect clumping.

After exclusion of pseudothrombocytopenia, other causes are broadly classified as accelerated platelet destruction, decreased platelet production, or splenic sequestration (careful physical examination for splenomegaly will help exclude this possibility) (Box 38.7). Potentially serious causes of thrombocytopenia should be excluded, including heparin-induced thrombocytopenia (HIT), thrombotic thrombocytopenic purpura, and the HELLP syndrome (hemolysis, elevated liver enzymes, and low platelet count) occurring in pregnancy.

Abnormally large platelets (Figure 38.3) are seen in immune thrombocytopenia, clonal myeloid disorders (eg, essential thrombocythemia), and congenital disorders of platelet synthesis and function (eg, conditions associated with mutations of the *MYH9* gene [eg, May-Hegglin anomaly] and Bernard-Soulier syndrome).

Thrombocytopenia Due to Increased Platelet Destruction

Autoimmune Thrombocytopenic Purpura

Autoimmune thrombocytopenic purpura, formerly called idiopathic thrombocytopenic purpura, is an autoimmune disease characterized by thrombocytopenia, usually with a normal white blood cell count and hemoglobin concentration (Table 38.3).

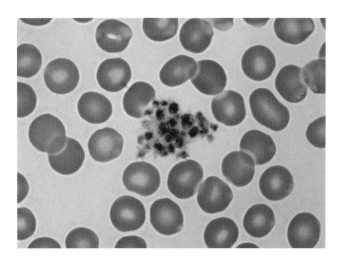

Figure 38.2 *Platelet Clumping (Agglutination). Agglutination is a cause of artifactual thrombocytopenia. Drawing the blood in a citrate tube rather than an EDTA-anticoagulated tube usually eliminates this in vitro phenomenon (Wright-Giemsa).* (Courtesy of Curtis A. Hanson, MD, Mayo Clinic, Rochester, Minnesota. Used with permission.)

Box 38.7 • Causes of Thrombocytopenia

Pseudothrombocytopenia

Dilutional

  Massive transfusion
  Pregnancy

Increased destruction

  Immune

    Autoimmune
    Idiopathic
    Secondary (drug-induced and connective tissue
      diseases)

  Nonimmune

    Consumptive (DIC)
    Sepsis

Decreased production

  Bone marrow failure syndromes

    Primary: anaplastic anemia
    Secondary: metastatic disease, hematologic
      malignancies

  Nutritional

    Vitamin B_{12} and folate deficiency

  Infections

    Viral (HIV infection, CMV infection, viral
      hepatitis)

Abbreviations: CMV, cytomegalovirus; DIC,
  disseminated intravascular coagulation; HIV, human
  immunodeficiency virus.

Table 38.3 • Autoimmune Thrombocytopenic Purpura

Characteristic	Acute	Chronic
Presentation	Abrupt onset of petechiae, purpura, mucosal bleeding	Insidious petechiae, menorrhagia
Usual age	Children (2–6 y)	Adults (20–40 y)
Female to male ratio	1:1	3:1
Antecedent infection	Common (85%) Typically an upper respiratory tract infection	Uncommon
Platelet count, ×10⁹/L	<20	30–80
Duration	2–6 wk	Months to years
Spontaneous remission	80% within 6 mo	Uncommon, fluctuates

Adapted from Liel MS, Recht M, Calverley DC. Thrombocytopenia
caused by immunologic platelet destruction. In: Greer JP, Arber DA,
Glader B, List AF, Means RT Jr, Paraskevas F, Rodgers GM, editors.
13th ed. Wintrobe's clinical hematology. Philadelphia (PA): Lippincott
Williams & Wilkins; c2014. p. 1061–76. Used with permission.

The diagnosis of autoimmune thrombocytopenic purpura is a diagnosis of exclusion (Box 38.8).

Clinical Manifestations

In adults, autoimmune thrombocytopenic purpura is often diagnosed from an incidental finding on routine CBC or from an initial presentation with bleeding (eg, petechiae and purpura, mucous membrane hemorrhage, and cerebromeningeal bleeding). Up to 60% of adults progress to a chronic state of autoimmune thrombocytopenic purpura. Only 10% of patients have splenomegaly. If splenomegaly is present, one should think of other causes.

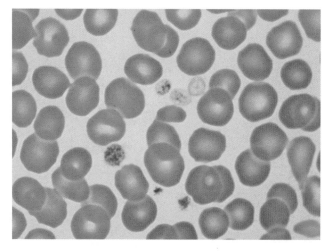

Figure 38.3 *Giant Platelets. Giant platelets may be associated with congenital platelet synthesis disorders, acquired clonal myeloid disorders, or immune thrombocytopenia (Wright-Giemsa).*

(Courtesy of Curtis A. Hanson, MD, Mayo Clinic, Rochester, Minnesota. Used with permission.)

Box 38.8 • Diagnosis of Autoimmune Thrombocytopenic Purpura

Examine a peripheral blood smear to exclude microangiopathy.

In mild to moderate thrombocytopenia, exclude congenital causes for thrombocytopenia, such as type 2B von Willebrand disease and other macrothrombocytopenia, which are typically associated with a lifelong personal and family history of bleeding and bruising.

Evaluate for heavy alcohol use and drugs associated with thrombocytopenia.

Test for human immunodeficiency virus infection and hepatitis C in patients with risk factors.

Laboratory Findings

In most patients, the platelet count is less than 50×10^9/L; in 30%, it is less than 10×10^9/L (spontaneous bleeding may occur at this level). The mean platelet volume is increased. Antibodies to specific platelet-membrane glycoproteins, usually the glycoprotein IIb/IIIa complex, and platelet-associated immunoglobulin G can be detected in most patients but are not necessary for diagnosis or treatment.

In patients older than 60 years, a bone marrow examination is appropriate to rule out another disorder causing thrombocytopenia (eg, a myelodysplastic syndrome or lymphoma). Bone marrow examination in autoimmune thrombocytopenic purpura shows a normal to increased number of megakaryocytes.

Treatment

The American Society of Hematology guidelines for treatment are shown in Box 38.9.

Splenectomy, the treatment of choice for steroid-refractory autoimmune thrombocytopenic purpura, removes the predominant site of antibody production and platelet destruction; the likelihood of remission is 75%, with about 60% of patients remaining in long-term remission. Pneumococcal, meningococcal, and *Haemophilus influenzae* vaccines should be administered 2 weeks before splenectomy. The absence of Howell-Jolly bodies on a post-splenectomy peripheral blood smear suggests the presence of an accessory spleen, and accessory splenectomy can result in remission. Pulsed dexamethasone (40 mg daily for 4 sequential days, every 28 days, for 12 months) is an option for the treatment of resistant autoimmune thrombocytopenic

purpura or disease relapse. Other agents used in refractory cases include azathioprine, cyclophosphamide, colchicine, cyclosporine, rituximab, vincristine, vinblastine, anti-Rh_0(D) immune globulin, danazol, and immunoadsorption apheresis on staphylococcal protein A columns.

Novel agents approved for use in patients with corticosteroid-refractory autoimmune thrombocytopenic purpura include oral (eltrombopag) and parenteral (romiplostim) thrombopoietin receptor agonists.

Drug-Induced Thrombocytopenia

Drug-induced thrombocytopenia is caused by direct marrow toxicity or by haptens bound to a carrier protein. Common drugs include heparin, quinidine, quinine, valproic acid, gold, trimethoprim-sulfamethoxazole, amphotericin B, carbamazepine, chlorothiazide, chlorpropamide, procainamide, rifampin, and vancomycin. Glycoprotein IIb/IIIa antagonists have also been implicated. Heparin causes one of the most lethal drug-induced thrombocytopenias, HIT.

Drug-induced thrombocytopenia subsides in 4 to 14 days after use of the drug is discontinued—except for gold-induced thrombocytopenia, which may take much longer. In contrast, viral-induced thrombocytopenia resolves in 2 weeks to 3 months.

Heparin-Induced Thrombocytopenia

Type I HIT is a benign, nonimmune-mediated thrombocytopenia that occurs in association with UFH, typically in the first 4 days of heparin therapy. *Type II HIT* is a more serious, immune-mediated thrombocytopenia.

The incidence of HIT is 1% to 8% with UFH; the incidence is lower with low-molecular-weight heparin. HIT can develop at any dose of heparin, including low-dose prophylaxis for venous thrombosis postoperatively. The onset of thrombocytopenia varies (Box 38.10).

The platelet count decreases 50% from baseline (ie, from before heparin administration). Thrombosis may or may not occur and may be venous (more commonly) or arterial. Laboratory testing includes functional assays (serotonin release assay) and antigen assays (heparin-dependent antibody against platelet factor 4).

Immunoglobulin G antibodies to platelet factor 4–heparin complexes result in platelet activation, generation

---

Box 38.9 • American Society of Hematology Guidelines for Treatment of Autoimmune Thrombocytopenic Purpura

Patients with platelet counts $\geq50\times10^9$/L do not routinely require treatment.

Patients with platelet counts between 30×10^9/L and 50×10^9/L should be treated if they have mucous membrane bleeding or risk factors for bleeding, including hypertension, peptic ulcer disease, and a vigorous lifestyle.

Patients with platelet counts $<30\times10^9$/L (with or without bleeding) should be treated.

Prednisone is the mainstay of initial treatment; initially, 70% of patients respond, with a 40% chance of long-term remission (prednisone 1 mg/kg daily for up to 1 month; then a tapering schedule).

If bleeding is severe, treat with intravenous immunoglobulin (1 g/kg daily for 2 days) and platelets; high-dose intravenous corticosteroids can also be considered (eg, methylprednisolone, 1 g daily for 2–3 consecutive days; initial response rate, 80%).

Box 38.10 • Onset of Thrombocytopenia in Heparin-Induced Thrombocytopenia

Typical: 4–14 days after initiating heparin administration

Rapid: <4 days in patients with recent (≤3 months) heparin exposure

Delayed: 2–3 weeks after discontinuation of heparin administration

---

Box 38.11 • Rare Complications of Heparin-Induced Thrombocytopenia

Warfarin-induced venous gangrene with limb damage

Acute platelet activation syndromes (fevers, chills, or transient amnesia) 5–30 minutes after an intravenous bolus of heparin

Painful, necrotic skin lesions at the site of the heparin injection

---

of thrombin, and a high risk of thrombosis. Rare complications are listed in Box 38.11.

Anticoagulant management involves administering a parenteral direct thrombin inhibitor (bivalirudin or argatroban) (Box 38.12). Argatroban is the treatment of choice for patients with renal insufficiency because of its hepatic elimination; in contrast, for patients with hepatic failure, bivalidrudin (which is renally excreted) is an option (lepirudin is no longer marketed).

Chemotherapy-Associated Thrombocytopenia

The threshold for platelet transfusion is 10×10^9/L unless other risk factors for bleeding (eg, fever or mucosal lesion) are present. Interleukin 11 (oprelvekin) is modestly effective but is associated with fluid retention and atrial dysrhythmias. Pharmacologic agents stimulating the thrombopoietin receptor have been approved for clinical use.

Thrombocytopenia Due to Decreased Platelet Production

Thrombocytopenia caused by decreased platelet production typically occurs as the result of disorders affecting the bone marrow. These can be broadly classified as shown in

---

Box 38.12 • *Do*'s and *Don't*s of HIT

Do promptly stop all use of heparin (UFH and LMWH), including line flushes and heparin-impregnated catheters, if HIT is clinically suspected

Do administer a DTI (eg, lepirudin, bivalirudin, or argatroban)

Do record heparin as an allergy for patients with HIT

Do not switch to LMWH; the antibody has high cross-reactivity with an LMWH–platelet factor 4 complex

Do not administer warfarin until the platelet count increases to $100,000–150,000 \times 10^9$/L

Do not administer warfarin

Abbreviations: DTI, direct thrombin inhibitor; HIT, heparin-induced thrombocytopenia; LMWH, low-molecular-weight heparin; UFH, unfractionated heparin.

Box 38.13 • Disorders That Decrease Platelet Production in the Bone Marrow

Primary marrow or metastatic malignancy (eg, solid tumor, leukemia or lymphoma)

Infections (eg, human immunodeficiency virus infection, cytomegalovirus infection, sepsis, or viral hepatitis)

Inflammatory or autoimmune states (eg, connective tissue diseases such as systemic lupus erythematosus and rheumatoid arthritis)

Nutritional deficiencies (eg, vitamin B_{12} or folate deficiencies)

Bone marrow failure states (eg, myelodysplastic syndrome or aplastic anemia)

Box 38.13. Management consists of identifying and treating the underlying disease.

Congenital Platelet Disorders

Congenital abnormalities of the platelet receptor glycoproteins lead to platelet dysfunction and thrombocytopenia. Lifelong mucocutaneous bleeding and postoperative bleeding are typical. Platelet transfusions are used for prevention and treatment of hemorrhage. A risk of frequent transfusions is platelet alloimmunization. Diagnosis is based on platelet function testing (Box 38.14).

Thrombocytopenia in Pregnancy

Mild thrombocytopenia (platelets $>70 \times 10^9$/L) occurs in 6% to 8% of pregnant women at term and in 25% of

---

Box 38.14 • Diagnosis of Congenital Platelet Disorders

Bernard-Soulier syndrome

Due to abnormalities in the glycoprotein Ib/IX complex receptor

Characterized by large platelets

Platelet aggregation is decreased with ristocetin but normal with adenosine diphosphate, epinephrine, collagen, and arachidonate

Glanzmann thrombasthenia

Due to abnormalities in the glycoprotein IIb/IIIa complex

Platelet aggregation is normal with ristocetin but decreased with adenosine diphosphate, epinephrine, collagen, and arachidonate

Wiskott-Aldrich syndrome

Associated with small platelets

KEY FACTS

✓ Pseudothrombocytopenia—caused by EDTA-induced platelet clumping

✓ Autoimmune thrombocytopenic purpura—usually leukocyte count and hemoglobin concentration are normal

✓ Splenectomy—treatment of choice for steroid-refractory autoimmune thrombocytopenic purpura

✓ Drug-induced thrombocytopenia—caused by direct marrow toxicity or by haptens bound to a carrier protein

✓ Type I HIT—

- benign, nonimmune-mediated thrombocytopenia
- occurs with use of UFH, typically in first 4 days of heparin therapy

✓ Type II HIT—serious, immune-mediated thrombocytopenia

✓ Thrombocytopenia in pregnancy—

- mild (platelets $>70 \times 10^9$/L)
- occurs in 6%–8% of pregnant women at term
- occurs in 25% of women with preeclampsia

women with preeclampsia. The most common causes of thrombocytopenia in pregnancy are physiologic gestational thrombocytopenia and nonphysiologic benign gestational thrombocytopenia, which account for 75% of cases. No treatment is required. Platelet counts generally recover within 72 hours after delivery without adverse maternal or fetal outcomes. The diagnosis is one of exclusion.

Other common causes include preeclampsia (including the HELLP syndrome), idiopathic autoimmune thrombocytopenia (or autoimmune thrombocytopenic purpura), DIC, acute fatty liver of pregnancy, HIV infection, antiphospholipid antibodies, drugs (quinine, quinidine, cocaine, and heparin), nutritional deficiency, and thrombotic thrombocytopenic purpura. The primary treatment of the HELLP syndrome is stabilization of the patient's condition and delivery of the fetus.

39 Malignant Hematologic Disorders

CARRIE A. THOMPSON, MD

The hematologic neoplasms include the following:

1. Lymphoproliferative disorders—chronic lymphocytic leukemia (CLL) (Box 39.1), hairy cell leukemia (HCL), large granular lymphocyte (LGL) leukemia (Box 39.2), Hodgkin lymphoma (Box 39.3), and non-Hodgkin lymphoma (NHL)
2. Plasma cell disorders—multiple myeloma, Waldenström macroglobulinemia, light chain amyloidosis, and plasmacytoma
3. Acute leukemias—acute myeloid leukemia (AML) and acute lymphocytic leukemia (ALL)
4. Chronic myeloid neoplasms—myelodysplastic syndromes (MDSs), chronic myeloid leukemia (CML), and myeloproliferative neoplasms

Lymphoproliferative Disorders

The risk of lymphoproliferative disorders is increased for immunocompromised patients, including those receiving immunosuppressive medications for autoimmune diseases or solid organ transplant (Box 39.4) and those with human immunodeficiency virus (HIV) infection.

Chronic Lymphocytic Leukemia

CLL is a clonal disorder of mature lymphocytes (Figure 39.1) that is primarily seen in older patients (median age, 65–70 years). Median survival is about 10 years.

The diagnosis of CLL requires a B-lymphocyte count of more than 5.0×10^9/L; a smaller B-cell clone is also considered CLL if accompanied by lymphadenopathy, splenomegaly, marrow infiltration, or cytopenias attributable to CLL. A small B-cell clone may be detected incidentally by flow cytometry in about 5% of patients

---

Box 39.1 • WHO Classification of the Mature B-Cell Neoplasms (2008)

Chronic lymphocytic leukemia/small lymphocytic lymphoma

B-cell prolymphocytic leukemia

Splenic marginal zone lymphoma

Hairy cell leukemia

Splenic lymphoma/leukemia, unclassifiable[a]

    Splenic diffuse red pulp small B-cell lymphoma[a]
    Hairy cell leukemia-variant[a]

Lymphoplasmacytic lymphoma

Waldenström macroglobulinemia

Heavy chain diseases

    Alpha heavy chain disease
    Gamma heavy chain disease
    Mu heavy chain disease

Plasma cell myeloma

Solitary plasmacytoma of bone

Extraosseous plasmacytoma

Extranodal marginal zone lymphoma of mucosa-associated lymphoid tissue (MALT lymphoma)

Nodal marginal zone lymphoma

Pediatric nodal marginal zone lymphoma[a]

Follicular lymphoma

Pediatric follicular lymphoma[a]

Primary cutaneous follicle center lymphoma

Mantle cell lymphoma

DLBCL, NOS

    T-cell/histiocyte-rich large B-cell lymphoma
    Primary DLBCL of the central nervous system
    Primary cutaneous DLBCL, leg type
    EBV-positive DLBCL of the elderly[a]

DLBCL associated with chronic inflammation

Lymphomatoid granulomatosis

(Continued on next page)

Primary mediastinal (thymic) large B-cell lymphoma

Intravascular large B-cell lymphoma

ALK-positive large B-cell lymphoma

Plasmablastic lymphoma

Large B-cell lymphoma arising in HHV8-associated multicentric Castleman disease

Primary effusion lymphoma

Burkitt lymphoma

B-cell lymphoma, unclassifiable, with features intermediate between diffuse large B-cell lymphoma and Burkitt lymphoma

B-cell lymphoma, unclassifiable, with features intermediate between diffuse large B-cell lymphoma and classical Hodgkin lymphoma

Abbreviations: ALK, anaplastic lymphoma kinase; DLBCL, diffuse large B-cell lymphoma; EBV, Epstein-Barr virus; HHV8, human herpesvirus 8; NOS, not otherwise specified; WHO, World Health Organization.

[a] Provisional entities for which the WHO Working Group felt there was insufficient evidence to recognize as distinct diseases at this time.

Adapted from Jaffe ES, Harris NL, Stein H, Isaacson PG. Classification of lymphoid neoplasms: the microscope as a tool for disease discovery. Blood. 2008 Dec 1;112(12):4384–99. Used with permission.

Peripheral T-cell lymphoma, NOS

Angioimmunoblastic T-cell lymphoma

Anaplastic large cell lymphoma, ALK-positive

Anaplastic large cell lymphoma, ALK-negative

Abbreviations: ALK, anaplastic lymphoma kinase; EBV, Epstein-Barr virus; NK, natural killer; NOS, not otherwise specified; WHO, World Health Organization.

[a] Provisional entities for which the WHO Working Group felt there was insufficient evidence to recognize as distinct diseases at this time.

Adapted from Jaffe ES, Harris NL, Stein H, Isaacson PG. Classification of lymphoid neoplasms: the microscope as a tool for disease discovery. Blood. 2008 Dec 1;112(12):4384–99. Used with permission.

Box 39.2 • WHO Classification of the Mature T-Cell and NK-Cell Neoplasms (2008)

T-cell prolymphocytic leukemia

T-cell large granular lymphocytic leukemia

Chronic lymphoproliferative disorder of NK cells[a]

Aggressive NK cell leukemia

Systemic EBV-positive T-cell lymphoproliferative disease of childhood

Hydroa vacciniforme–like lymphoma

Adult T-cell leukemia/lymphoma

Extranodal NK/T-cell lymphoma, nasal type

Enteropathy-associated T-cell lymphoma

Hepatosplenic T-cell lymphoma

Subcutaneous panniculitis-like T-cell lymphoma

Mycosis fungoides

Sézary syndrome

Primary cutaneous CD30+ T-cell lymphoproliferative disorders

Lymphomatoid papulosis
Primary cutaneous anaplastic large cell lymphoma

Primary cutaneous γ-δ T-cell lymphoma

Primary cutaneous CD8+ aggressive epidermotropic cytotoxic T-cell lymphoma[a]

Primary cutaneous CD4+ small/medium T-cell lymphoma[a]

older than 60 years without accompanying cytopenias, adenopathy, or splenomegaly; these patients have monoclonal B-cell lymphocytosis (MBL) and should be observed.

The peripheral blood smear in CLL classically shows *smudge cells*, which are lymphocytes that break apart during slide processing (Figure 39.1). Interphase fluorescence in situ hybridization (FISH) testing identifies the characteristic CLL immunophenotype: clonal light-chain expression, CD5+ (also expressed in mantle cell lymphoma), CD19+, CD23+, and CD20+. The 2 widely used staging classifications are outlined in Tables 39.1 and 39.2.

Recurrent infections are a common complication, in part because of hypogammaglobulinemia. Prophylactic γ-globulin may reduce infection rates and should be considered for patients with recurrent serious infections. About 5% of patients have autoimmune hematologic complications, including hemolytic anemia, thrombocytopenia, and pure red cell aplasia. Patients with CLL also are at increased risk for second malignancies, including evolution to a more

Box 39.3 • WHO Classification of Hodgkin Lymphoma (2008)

Nodular lymphocyte-predominant Hodgkin lymphoma

Classical Hodgkin lymphoma

Nodular sclerosis classical Hodgkin lymphoma
Lymphocyte-rich classical Hodgkin lymphoma
Mixed cellularity classical Hodgkin lymphoma
Lymphocyte-depleted classical Hodgkin lymphoma

Abbreviation: WHO, World Health Organization.

Adapted from Jaffe ES, Harris NL, Stein H, Isaacson PG. Classification of lymphoid neoplasms: the microscope as a tool for disease discovery. Blood. 2008 Dec 1;112(12):4384–99. Used with permission.

Table 39.1 • Staging of Chronic Lymphocytic Leukemia: Rai Classification

Stage	Characteristics	Median Survival Time, mo
0	Peripheral lymphocytosis ($>15\times10^9$/L), bone marrow lymphocytosis (>40%)	>150
I	Lymphocytosis, lymphadenopathy	101
II	Lymphocytosis, splenomegaly	71
III	Lymphocytosis, anemia (hemoglobin <11 g/dL), excluding AIHA	19
IV	Lymphocytosis, thrombocytopenia	19

Abbreviation: AIHA, autoimmune hemolytic anemia.

Data from Rai KR, Sawitsky A, Cronkite EP, Chanana AD, Levy RN, Pasternack BS. Clinical staging of chronic lymphocytic leukemia. Blood. 1975 Aug;46(2):219–34.

aggressive B-cell malignancy (ie, *Richter transformation*), skin cancer, and solid organ malignancies. If CLL patients have fever, exclude infection and transformation to diffuse large B-cell lymphoma (DLBCL) before attributing the fever to progressive CLL.

For patients with early-stage CLL, the standard practice is observation. Treatment indications include cytopenias, progressive adenopathy or splenomegaly, constitutional symptoms, or rapid lymphocyte doubling time. Chemotherapy in combination with immunotherapy, including a purine analogue (fludarabine or pentostatin) in combination with rituximab (an anti-CD20 monoclonal antibody), is the initial treatment of choice for most patients. The major adverse effects of chemoimmunotherapy are myelosuppression and immunosuppression, which predispose the patient to infection.

Hairy Cell Leukemia

HCL is a rare mature B-cell neoplasm characterized by an insidious onset of cytopenias and the presence of cells with "hairy" cytoplasmic projections. The male to female ratio is 4:1 (Figure 39.2).

The symptoms are related to cytopenias, infections, and splenomegaly. The bone marrow often yields a "dry tap" (ie, no liquid marrow is obtained); core biopsy specimens are hypercellular, with diffuse infiltration by neoplastic cells and fibrosis. With treatment, most patients live for

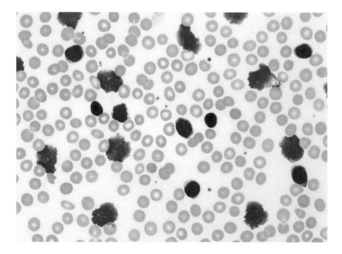

Figure 39.1 *Chronic Lymphocytic Leukemia. Many small and mature lymphocytes have nuclei approximately the same size as red blood cells. Smudge cells are also characteristic of this disorder (peripheral blood smear; Wright-Giemsa).*

(Courtesy of Curtis A. Hanson, MD, Mayo Clinic, Rochester, Minnesota. Used with permission.)

Table 39.2 • Staging of Chronic Lymphocytic Leukemia: International Workshop on Chronic Lymphocytic Leukemia Classification

Clinical Stage	Features
A	No anemia or thrombocytopenia and <3 areas of lymphoid enlargement (spleen, liver, and lymph nodes in cervical, axillary, and inguinal regions)
B	No anemia or thrombocytopenia, but ≥3 involved areas of lymphoid enlargement
C	Anemia (hemoglobin <10 g/dL) or thrombocytopenia (or both)

Adapted from International Workshop on CLL. Chronic lymphocytic leukaemia: proposals for a revised prognostic staging system. Br J Haematol. 1981 Jul;48(3):365–7. Used with permission.

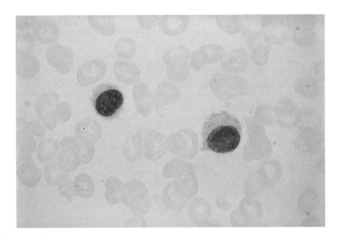

Figure 39.2 Hairy Cell Leukemia. These mature lympho-cytes have eccentrically placed nuclei, pale cytoplasm, and characteristic projections (bone marrow aspirate smear; Wright-Giemsa).

more than 10 years. HCL causes immunosuppression and increases the risk of infection. Atypical mycobacterial infections are a classic association.

LGL Leukemia

LGLs are cytotoxic T cells or natural killer cells (Figure 39.3), and clonal expansion of LGLs is called LGL leukemia. T-cell LGL leukemia is associated with neutropenia, splenomegaly, and anemia. It occurs most commonly in older patients (median age, 60 years). Up to one-third of T-cell LGL leukemia patients have rheumatoid arthritis, and there is overlap with Felty syndrome (ie, triad of neutropenia, rheumatoid arthritis, and splenomegaly). The diagnosis is suggested by flow cytometry and can be confirmed by T-cell receptor gene rearrangement studies.

T-cell LGL leukemia is a chronic disorder that requires treatment only if symptoms are present. Immunosuppressive therapy with methotrexate, cyclophosphamide, or cyclosporine is often effective.

Hodgkin Lymphoma

Treatment of Hodgkin lymphoma is a major success of modern cancer therapy. With treatment, more than 80% of patients with Hodgkin lymphoma are now cured.

The age at presentation has a bimodal distribution, with the first peak at a median age of 25 years and the second peak after age 60 years. Patients with Hodgkin lymphoma usually present with locally limited disease. The typical finding at presentation is lymphadenopathy; less common presentations include pruritus, cytopenias, and pain in involved lymph nodes after alcohol consumption.

The diagnosis of Hodgkin lymphoma is based on the presence of Reed-Sternberg cells, which typically have 2 or more nuclei with prominent nucleoli that give the cells the appearance of owl eyes (Figure 39.4).

Disease stage is the principal factor in selecting treatment (Table 39.3). The disease is routinely staged with use of computed tomography of the chest, abdomen, and pelvis and positron emission tomography. Currently, the treatment of choice for localized disease (stages IA and IIA) is a short course of combination chemotherapy with ABVD (doxorubicin [Adriamycin], bleomycin, vinblastine, and dacarbazine) and low doses of radiotherapy. Most patients with localized disease are cured. The treatment of choice for advanced disease is combination chemotherapy; cure rates are up to 65%. Autologous stem cell transplant is considered for relapses after chemotherapy.

Late complications of Hodgkin lymphoma therapy are substantial. They include infertility, premature menopause, hypothyroidism, cardiomyopathy, coronary artery disease,

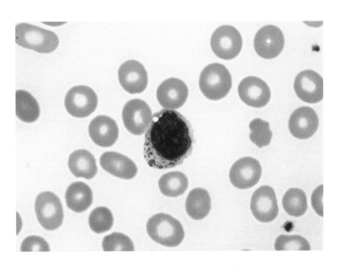

Figure 39.3 Large Granular Lymphocyte. The pale blue cy-toplasm contains azurophilic granules (peripheral blood smear; Wright-Giemsa).

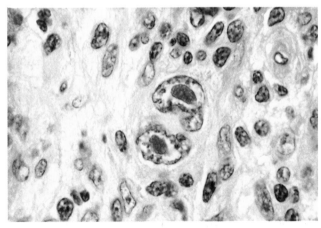

Figure 39.4 Hodgkin Lymphoma. A Reed-Sternberg cell, the large binuclear cell, is present (bone marrow biopsy section; hematoxylin-eosin).

(Courtesy of Curtis A. Hanson, MD, Mayo Clinic, Rochester, Minnesota. Used with permission.)

Table 39.3 • Cotswold Staging Classification of Hodgkin Lymphoma

Classification	Description
Stage I	Involvement of a single lymph node region or lymphoid structure
Stage II	Involvement of ≥2 lymph node regions on the same side of the diaphragm (the mediastinum is considered a single site, whereas hilar lymph nodes are considered bilaterally)
Stage III	Involvement of lymph node regions or structures on both sides of the diaphragm
Stage III-1	With or without involvement of splenic, hilar, celiac, or portal nodes
Stage III-2	With involvement of para-aortic, iliac, and mesenteric nodes
Stage IV	Involvement of ≥1 extranodal sites in addition to a site for which the *E* designation has been used
Designations Applicable to Any Disease Stage	
A	No symptoms
B	Fevers (>38°C), drenching night sweats, unexplained loss of >10% of body weight within the preceding 6 mo
X	Bulky disease (widening of the mediastinum by more than one-third or the presence of a nodal mass with a maximal dimension >10 cm)
E	Involvement of a single extranodal site that is contiguous or proximal to the known nodal site
CS	Clinical stage
PS	Pathologic stage (as determined by laparotomy)

Adapted from Lister TA, Crowther D. Staging for Hodgkin's disease. Semin Oncol. 1990 Dec;17(6):696–703. Used with permission.

pulmonary fibrosis, and secondary malignancies. Potential secondary malignancies include AML, MDS, non-Hodgkin lymphoma, and solid tumors (eg, breast, lung, and thyroid cancer, if those areas are included in the irradiated field).

KEY FACTS

✓ Risk of lymphoproliferative disorders—increased for immunocompromised patients, such as those infected with HIV or receiving immunosuppressive agents for autoimmune diseases or solid organ transplant

✓ Peripheral blood smear in CLL—smudge cells (lymphocytes that break apart during slide processing)

✓ CLL—increases the risk of second malignancies (eg, more aggressive B-cell malignancy, skin cancer, and solid organ malignancies)

✓ Hodgkin lymphoma—
• cure rate >80%
• typical presentation: lymphadenopathy
• less common presentations: pruritus, cytopenias, pain in lymph nodes after alcohol consumption

✓ Late complications of Hodgkin lymphoma therapy—
• infertility, premature menopause, hypothyroidism
• cardiomyopathy, coronary artery disease
• pulmonary fibrosis
• secondary malignancies: AML, MDS, non-Hodgkin lymphoma, and solid tumors (in areas included in the irradiated field)

Non-Hodgkin Lymphomas

NHL is a diverse group of lymphoproliferative disorders. The Ann Arbor Staging System, which is very similar to the staging system for Hodgkin lymphoma in Table 39.3, has traditionally been used for NHL.

Low-Grade (Indolent) Lymphomas

Low-grade (indolent) lymphomas may remain in a chronic phase for many years or transform into aggressive lymphomas. Patients with follicular lymphoma, the most common type of indolent lymphoma, often have a t(14;18) translocation resulting in amplification of the antiapoptotic *BCL2* gene.

Low-grade NHLs are not curable unless they are stage I disease, which can sometimes be cured with radiotherapy. At diagnosis, most patients have stage III or IV disease, which is not curable; however, median survival is 8 years. Observation is an option for asymptomatic patients with no evidence of bulky disease. Treatment is indicated for patients with symptoms, bulky disease, cytopenias, or progressive disease. Many therapeutic regimens exist, including bendamustine with rituximab, CVP (cyclophosphamide, vincristine, and prednisone) with rituximab; rituximab alone; R-CHOP (rituximab, cyclophosphamide, hydroxydaunomycin [Adriamycin], vincristine [Oncovin], and prednisone); and fludarabine.

Gastric mucosa–associated lymphoid tissue (MALT) lymphomas are associated with *Helicobacter pylori* infections. Up to 70% of patients respond to a regimen of antibiotics in combination with a proton pump inhibitor. If this is unsuccessful, chemotherapy or irradiation is typically administered.

Aggressive Lymphomas

In contrast to low-grade lymphomas, aggressive lymphomas are potentially curable, but the duration of survival is short if the patient does not have remission. Patients typically present with symptomatic disease, including *B* symptoms (as in Table 39.3: fevers, drenching night sweats, and weight loss).

The most common aggressive lymphoma is diffuse large B-cell lymphoma. Standard therapy is R-CHOP chemotherapy. For patients with aggressive lymphoma that relapses after complete remission, autologous stem cell transplant is the standard therapy. The International Prognostic Factor Index uses age, lactate dehydrogenase level, performance status scores, disease stage, and extranodal involvement to predict survival of patients who have DLBCL. Five-year survival ranges from 26% to 73%, depending on risk factors.

Mantle cell lymphoma is characterized by a CD5⁺ and CD20⁺ immunophenotype and a t(11;14) translocation, with overexpression of the cyclin D1 oncogene. Patients may present with gastrointestinal tract involvement (ie, *lymphomatous polyposis*). Unlike other aggressive lymphomas, mantle cell lymphoma is not curable.

Very aggressive lymphomas, such as Burkitt lymphoma and lymphoblastic lymphoma, are treated with regimens similar to those used for ALL. These subtypes carry a high risk of central nervous system involvement and tumor lysis syndrome.

Plasma Cell Disorders (Monoclonal Gammopathies)

The plasma cell disorders (monoclonal gammopathies) are characterized by clonal proliferation of plasma cells, usually associated with the presence of monoclonal immunoglobulins (M proteins) in the serum or urine (or both).

Monoclonal Gammopathies of Undetermined Significance

In monoclonal gammopathies of undetermined significance (MGUS), the most common form of dysproteinemia, the serum M-protein level is low (typically <3 g/dL) and the bone marrow has less than 10% plasma cells. The serum creatinine, calcium, and hemoglobin levels are within the reference ranges, and the urine has either no M protein or only a small amount. Osteolytic bone lesions are absent, and patients are usually asymptomatic.

MGUS is common—an M protein is present in the serum of 5% of persons older than 70 years. MGUS progresses to a malignant monoclonal gammopathy at an annual rate of about 1%. Patients with MGUS should be observed.

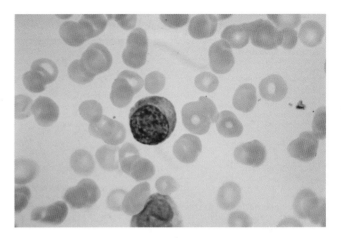

Figure 39.5 *Plasma Cell. The round nucleus is eccentrically placed; the copious, dark blue cytoplasm has a characteristic pale-staining area adjacent to the nucleus (bone marrow aspirate smear; Wright-Giemsa).*

Multiple Myeloma

The median age at onset of multiple myeloma is 65 years. It is more common in men and in African Americans. By definition, patients must have 10% or more clonal plasma cells in the bone marrow (Figure 39.5), an M protein in the serum or urine, and signs of end-organ damage that are thought to be related to the plasma cell proliferative disorder (mnemonic, *CRAB*: calcium [ie, hypercalcemia], renal failure, anemia, and bone lesions [osteolytic]). The presence of more than 10% clonal plasma cells in the bone marrow without end-organ damage or symptoms is called "smoldering" multiple myeloma.

Clinical features of multiple myeloma include fatigue, bone pain, anemia, renal insufficiency, hypercalcemia, and spinal cord compression. A peripheral blood smear may show rouleaux.

The median survival has improved with newer treatments. The International Staging System for Multiple Myeloma is useful for prognostication, with median survival ranging from 29 to 62 months (Table 39.4).

Therapy for fit patients involves "induction" of a response with dexamethasone in combination with lenalidomide, thalidomide, or bortezomib followed by autologous stem cell transplant. For patients who are older or who have poor performance status, melphalan is used in combination with prednisone, often with thalidomide or bortezomib. Palliative radiotherapy is effective in managing bone pain. Bisphosphonate therapy delays the onset of skeletal-related events and reduces bone pain. The most worrisome side effect of bisphosphonate therapy is osteonecrosis of the jaw.

KEY FACTS

✓ Gastric MALT lymphoma—
  • associated with *H pylori* infection
  • therapy: antibiotics with proton pump inhibitor (70% response rate)

✓ Diffuse large B-cell lymphoma—
  • most common aggressive lymphoma
  • R-CHOP chemotherapy

✓ MGUS—
  • progression to malignant monoclonal gammopathy (annual rate 1%)
  • observe

✓ *CRAB* (mnemonic for multiple myeloma)—
  • calcium (ie, hypercalcemia)
  • renal failure
  • anemia
  • bone lesions (osteolytic)

Waldenström Macroglobulinemia

Waldenström macroglobulinemia is characterized by an immunoglobulin M paraprotein, clonal lymphoplasmacytic cells in the bone marrow, and anemia, hyperviscosity, lymphadenopathy, or hepatosplenomegaly. Bence Jones proteinuria may be present, and hyperviscosity syndrome occurs in 15%.

Hyperviscosity syndrome is characterized by fatigue, dizziness, blurred vision, bleeding, sausage-shaped retinal veins, and papilledema. The initial treatment of hyperviscosity is plasmapheresis followed by chemotherapy. Active drugs include rituximab, alkylating agents, and purine nucleoside analogues such as fludarabine.

Amyloidosis

The **amyloidoses** (Box 39.5) comprise a group of diseases that are characterized by extracellular deposition of insoluble fibrillar proteins that stain with Congo red.

Key Definition

Amyloidoses: *diseases characterized by extracellular deposition of insoluble fibrillary proteins that stain with Congo red.*

The amyloid fibrils in AL amyloidosis are fragments of immunoglobulin light chains. The bone marrow usually has less than 20% plasma cells, and there are no lytic bone lesions. Initial biopsies should include fat aspiration of the abdominal wall (80% positive) and bone marrow biopsy (50% positive).

Patients with AL amyloidosis may present with fatigue, weight loss, hepatomegaly, macroglossia, renal insufficiency, nephrotic syndrome, congestive heart failure, orthostatic hypotension, carpal tunnel syndrome, or peripheral neuropathy. When patients have cardiac involvement, electrocardiography may show low voltage or Q waves. The echocardiogram is abnormal in 60%, with concentrically thickened ventricles or a thickened intraventricular septum and sometimes a speckled appearance. Peripheral neuropathy is often associated with autonomic failure, as manifested by diarrhea, pseudo-obstruction of the bowel, or orthostatic syncope.

For AL amyloidosis, treatment with melphalan and dexamethasone is modestly effective. Autologous stem cell transplant provides benefit in carefully selected patients. The median survival for all patients with AL amyloidosis is 13 months.

Table 39.4 • International Staging System for Multiple Myeloma

Stage	Serum β$_2$-Microglobulin, mg/L	Serum Albumin, g/dL	Median Survival, mo
I	<3.5	≥3.5	62
II	3.5–5.5	<3.5	44
III	>5.5	...	29

Adapted from Greipp PR, San Miguel J, Durie BG, Crowley JJ, Barlogie B, Blade J, et al. International staging system for multiple myeloma. J Clin Oncol. 2005 May 20;23(15):3412–20. Epub 2005 Apr 4. Erratum in: J Clin Oncol. 2005 Sep 1;23(25):6281. Harousseau, Jean-Luc [corrected to Avet-Loiseau, Hervé]. Used with permission.

Box 39.5 • Classification of Amyloidoses

Primary amyloidosis (AL amyloidosis)—accounts for 90% of amyloidosis in the United States

Secondary amyloidosis (AA amyloidosis)—caused by chronic infections (eg, osteomyelitis) or autoimmune disease

Familial amyloidosis—associated with mutations in transthyretin or other proteins

Senile amyloidosis—associated with aging

Localized amyloidosis—involves the skin, bladder, or other organs

Hemodialysis-associated amyloidosis—characterized by deposits of β$_2$-microglobulin

Treatment of AA amyloidosis involves correcting the underlying disease. Liver transplant may be valuable in familial cases in which an amyloidogenic protein is made by the liver.

Acute Leukemias

Acute leukemia is defined by the presence of at least 20% blast cells in the bone marrow. If the cells exhibit myeloid differentiation, the diagnosis is **AML**; if the cells have lymphoid markers, the diagnosis is **ALL**.

> ### Key Definitions
>
> Acute leukemia: *presence of ≥20% blast cells in the bone marrow.*
>
> Acute myeloid leukemia: *acute leukemia with myeloid differentiation.*
>
> Acute lymphocytic leukemia: *acute leukemia with lymphoid markers.*

Acute Myeloid Leukemia

The cause of AML is unknown in most cases, but there are many associations: previous myeloproliferative neoplasm or MDSs; exposure to radiation or benzene; prior chemotherapy; and congenital disorders such as Down syndrome, Fanconi syndrome, and ataxia-telangiectasia.

The median age of patients with AML (Figure 39.6) is about 65 years. Patients may present with nonspecific symptoms, such as fatigue and headache, or cytopenias.

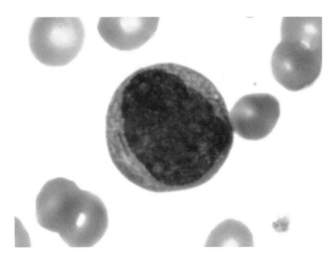

Figure 39.6 Acute Myeloid Leukemia. Blast cells are large and have an open, granular nuclear chromatin, often with 1 or more nucleoli. The presence of an Auer rod means that the blast is myeloid rather than lymphoid (bone marrow aspirate smear; Wright-Giemsa).

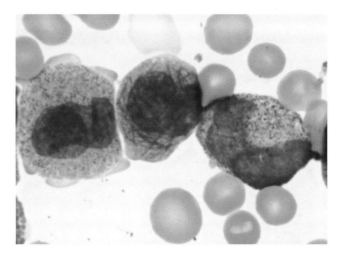

Figure 39.7 Leukemic Cells in Acute Promyelocytic Leukemia (AML-M3). Abundant cytoplasmic granules and Auer rods are present (bone marrow aspirate smear; Wright-Giemsa).
(Courtesy of Curtis A. Hanson, MD, Mayo Clinic, Rochester, Minnesota. Used with permission.)

For patients who present with extreme leukocytosis (leukocyte count >80×10⁹/L) and acute leukemia, the initial complication of most concern is cerebral hemorrhage due to leukostasis. Emergency treatment includes leukapheresis followed by treatment of the specific type of leukemia. Patients with acute promyelocytic leukemia (AML-M3) (Figure 39.7) typically have a t(15;17) translocation and often present with disseminated intravascular coagulation.

Treatment of AML is divided into 1) induction therapy (cytarabine and an anthracycline agent) and 2) consolidation therapy (high-dose cytarabine). Relapse occurs eventually in most patients with AML. In patients with relapsed AML, reinduction of remission is followed by hematopoietic stem cell transplant. The 5-year survival for younger patients with a good cytogenetic profile is 60%, but for patients who have a poor cytogenetic profile or who are older, the 5-year survival is less than 10%.

All-*trans*retinoic acid (ATRA) is the treatment of choice in AML-M3 with the t(15;17) translocation. Induction chemotherapy is with ATRA and an anthracycline-based program, followed by consolidation therapy. Maintenance therapy includes ATRA for 1 to 2 years.

Acute Lymphocytic Leukemia

ALL is most common in children; their complete remission rates are greater than 90%. In adults, however, ALL is less common and outcomes are much poorer. Remission rates in adults are up to 75%, but relapse occurs in most patients.

Bone pain, lymphadenopathy, splenomegaly, and hepatomegaly are more common in ALL than in AML.

All patients receive intensive chemotherapy with intrathecal therapy because of the risk of relapse in the central nervous system. Allogeneic transplant is recommended for patients with adverse risk factors.

KEY FACTS

✓ Waldenström macroglobulinemia—
- immunoglobulin M paraprotein
- clonal lymphoplasmacytic cells in bone marrow
- anemia, hyperviscosity, lymphadenopathy, or hepatosplenomegaly

✓ AL amyloidosis—
- fatigue, weight loss, macroglossia
- hepatomegaly
- renal insufficiency, nephrotic syndrome
- congestive heart failure, orthostatic hypotension
- carpal tunnel syndrome, peripheral neuropathy

✓ AL amyloidosis with cardiac involvement—
- electrocardiogram: low voltage or Q waves
- echocardiogram (abnormal in 60%): concentrically thickened ventricles or thickened intraventricular septum and sometimes a speckled appearance

✓ Acute leukemia with extreme leukocytosis—cerebral hemorrhage may result from leukostasis (treat with leukapheresis and treat specific leukemia)

✓ AML-M3—
- usually t(15;17) (treat with ATRA)
- often disseminated intravascular coagulation

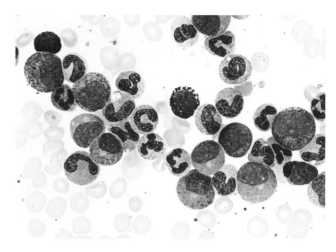

Figure 39.8 *Chronic Myeloid Leukemia. Normal-appearing myeloid cells show all stages of maturation, with a decreased number of erythropoietic cells and 1 basophil precursor in the center (bone marrow aspirate smear; Wright-Giemsa).* (Courtesy of Curtis A. Hanson, MD, Mayo Clinic, Rochester, Minnesota. Used with permission.)

Chronic Myeloid Disorders

Chronic myeloid disorders include MDS, CML, and myeloproliferative neoplasms. Patients with these disorders, in contrast to AML, have less than 20% blast cells in the bone marrow. Chronic myeloid disorders can, however, evolve into AML.

Myelodysplastic Syndromes

MDSs are heterogeneous and share 3 common features: peripheral blood cytopenia, abnormal "dysplastic" bone marrow morphology, and a tendency to evolve to AML. Transformation to acute leukemia occurs in about 25% to 30% of patients. Infection is the most common cause of death, followed by complications of AML progression and hemorrhage.

Clonal karyotypic abnormalities are common. Patients with del(5q) MDS have a favorable prognosis and respond well to lenalidomide treatment. The standard of care for most patients is supportive. Those who are eligible should be considered for allogeneic bone marrow transplant.

Chronic Myeloid Leukemia

CML constitutes 20% of all leukemias. The Philadelphia chromosome, t(9;22), is the hallmark of this disease. The molecular equivalent of the Philadelphia chromosome is the abnormal *BCR-ABL* fusion (Figure 39.8).

Symptoms include malaise, dyspnea, anorexia, fever, night sweats, weight loss, abdominal fullness, gout, and priapism. Splenomegaly is present in 85% of patients.

Characteristic laboratory findings include leukocytosis. Leukocyte counts of 100×10⁹/L are common, but leukapheresis is not usually required since the leukocytes are mature and do not cause leukostasis. Granulocytes in all stages of maturation are present in peripheral blood smears, with basophilia and eosinophilia and a characteristic *myelocyte bulge* (ie, increased numbers of myelocytes in relation to other stages of granulocyte differentiation).

Standard treatment is a tyrosine kinase inhibitor, such as imatinib, which inhibits the *BCR-ABL* fusion. Patients who are resistant to tyrosine kinase inhibitors may be eligible for allogeneic stem cell transplant.

Philadelphia Chromosome–Negative Myeloproliferative Neoplasms

The classic myeloproliferative neoplasms include polycythemia vera, primary myelofibrosis, and essential thrombocythemia. Their characteristic features are listed in Table 39.5. These disorders may progress to AML, which is usually refractory to therapy. Each of these disorders carries a risk of thrombosis and hemorrhage.

Activating mutations involving JAK2 tyrosine kinase are present in almost all patients with polycythemia vera and in about half of those with primary myelofibrosis or essential thrombocythemia.

Table 39.5 • Characteristic Features of Chronic Myeloproliferative Neoplasms

Characteristic	Polycythemia Vera	Primary Myelofibrosis	Essential Thrombocythemia	Chronic Myeloid Leukemia
Increased erythrocyte mass	Yes	No	No	No
Myelofibrosis	Later	Yes	Rare	Later
Leukocytosis	Variable	Variable	Variable	Yes
Thrombocytosis	Variable	Variable	Yes	Variable
BCR-ABL oncogene	No	No	No	Yes
JAK2 V617F mutation	>95%	50%	50%	Never

Primary Myelofibrosis, Postpolycythemic Myelofibrosis, and Postthrombocythemic Myelofibrosis

Splenomegaly occurs in virtually all patients with myelofibrosis and is a hallmark of primary myelofibrosis. Other features are a leukoerythroblastic peripheral blood smear, including nucleated red blood cells and dacrocytes (teardrop cells), and hypercellular marrow with increased fibrosis (Figure 39.9).

Foci of extramedullary hematopoiesis can occur in any area of the body but are most common in the spleen, liver, lung and pleural space, skin, eye, and central nervous system. The median survival is 3 to 5 years.

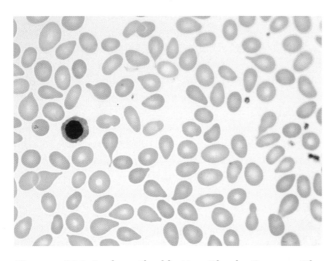

Figure 39.9 Leukoerythroblastic Blood Smear. The teardrop-shaped erythrocytes (dacrocytes) and nucleated red blood cell are characteristic of marrow fibrosis, whether due to primary myelofibrosis or a reactive cause (peripheral blood smear; Wright-Giemsa).

Asymptomatic patients should be observed. Medical therapy for anemia includes transfusion with packed red blood cells, androgens, or erythropoietin. Some patients respond to thalidomide or lenalidomide.

Essential Thrombocythemia

Essential thrombocythemia is a clonal hematologic disorder in which patients present with thrombocytosis and sometimes leukocytosis. Patients may be asymptomatic, or they may have thrombosis or hemorrhage. Life expectancy is relatively long (>10 years). The risk of acute leukemic transformation is less than 5% at 15 years.

Diagnostic features of essential thrombocythemia include a sustained platelet count greater than 450×10^9/L, megakaryocytic hyperplasia in the bone marrow, and absence of the Philadelphia chromosome. It may be challenging to distinguish essential thrombocythemia from reactive thrombocytosis or iron deficiency.

Treatment depends on the clinical situation. All patients who can tolerate aspirin should receive low-dose aspirin. Platelet apheresis should be used only for emergent management of acute bleeding or thrombosis and is not indicated from the platelet count alone. Cytoreductive therapy is recommended for patients with acute thrombosis or a previous history of thrombosis and for patients older than 60 years. Young asymptomatic patients may be observed.

Polycythemia Vera

Polycythemia vera is a myeloproliferative disorder that results from activating mutations involving JAK2 tyrosine kinase. Clinical features include postbathing pruritus, fatigue, erythromelalgia, and headache. More than 50% of patients have leukocytosis and thrombocytosis in addition to erythrocytosis. Polycythemia vera should be considered in the evaluation of an idiopathic thrombosis, especially in an atypical site such as an abdominal vessel or a dural sinus in the brain.

Bone marrow findings in polycythemia vera typically include trilineage hyperplasia. Erythropoietin levels are low or low normal.

The mainstay of therapy for all patients with polycythemia vera is phlebotomy, with the goal of maintaining the hematocrit at less than 45%. Low-dose aspirin therapy is indicated for all patients who do not have a contraindication. For patients who are older than 60 or who have had prior thrombosis, cytoreductive therapy is indicated.

KEY FACTS

✓ CML—
- 20% of all leukemias
- hallmark: Philadelphia chromosome, t(9;22)
- treatment: tyrosine kinase inhibitor (eg, imatinib), which inhibits *BCR-ABL* fusion

✓ Activating mutations involving JAK2 tyrosine kinase—
- in nearly 100% of patients with polycythemia vera
- in 50% of patients with primary myelofibrosis or essential thrombocythemia

✓ Polycythemia vera—a consideration in idiopathic thrombosis, especially in atypical site (eg, abdominal vessel or dural sinus in brain)

40 Thrombotic Disorders

RAJIV K. PRUTHI, MBBS

Thrombophilia: The Hypercoagulable States

Thrombophilia refers to the tendency for thromboembolism (ie, having risk factors for thromboembolism), which may be inherited or acquired (Box 40.1). The presence of increasing numbers of risk factors further increases the risk of venous thromboembolism (VTE). Antiphospholipid antibodies (lupus anticoagulant, anticardiolipin antibodies, and anti–β_2-glycoprotein I antibodies) and hyperhomocysteinemia are risk factors not only for VTE but also for arterial thrombosis.

Key Definition

Thrombophilia: *tendency for thromboembolism (ie, having inherited or acquired risk factors for thromboembolism).*

Epidemiology

VTE (which consists of deep vein thrombosis [DVT] and pulmonary embolism [PE]) affects 1 in 1,000 people; this increases to 1 in 100 among those older than 70 years in the western hemisphere. VTE is a major cause of morbidity, and the annual mortality rate of 50,000 is higher than that for breast cancer.

Thrombophilic defects can be broadly classified into abnormalities of the procoagulant system and abnormalities of the anticoagulant system.

Defects in the Procoagulant System

Inherited Risk Factors for VTE

Factor V Leiden

The most common inherited defect is activated protein C (APC) resistance due to the factor V Leiden (FVL) mutation

Box 40.1 • Inherited and Acquired Thrombophilia

Inherited thrombophilia

  Activated protein C resistance due to factor V Leiden mutation

  Prothrombin G20210A mutation

  Anticoagulant deficiencies: antithrombin, protein C, protein S

  Selected dysfibrinogenemia

Acquired thrombophilia

  Lupus anticoagulant or antiphospholipid antibody syndrome

  Pregnancy

  Immobilization (trauma, postoperative state)

  Estrogens (oral contraceptives, hormone replacement therapy)

  Solid organ malignancy

  Myeloproliferative diseases

  Paroxysmal nocturnal hemoglobinuria

  Prolonged travel

  Obesity

  Age

Mixed risk factors

  Hyperhomocysteinemia

  Elevated levels of factors VIII, IX, and XI

(R506Q). This causes activated factor V to be resistant to inactivation by APC. The condition is common among white people but rare among people of Asian or African ancestry.

Laboratory testing consists of performing the APC resistance assay and, if the results are abnormal, follow-up DNA-based testing for FVL to determine whether the person is heterozygous or homozygous (Box 40.2).

Prothrombin G20210A

The second most common defect is the prothrombin G20210A mutation, which results in an elevated plasma

Box 40.2 • FVL Mutation Prevalence and Risk of VTE

Prevalence of heterozygous mutation

In the healthy white population, 5%-7%
Among persons with VTE, 20%-50%

Risk of VTE

For heterozygotes, relative risk is increased 2- to 4-fold (absolute annual risk is about 0.45%)
For homozygotes, relative risk is increased 80-fold
Compared to oral contraceptive users without FVL, FVL carriers taking estrogen-containing oral contraceptives have a relative risk of VTE that is increased up to 30-fold (absolute annual risk is about 0.3%)

Abbreviations: FVL, factor V Leiden; VTE, venous thromboembolism.

prothrombin level. The heterozygous mutation has a prevalence of approximately 3% in the healthy white population and 6% to 18% among persons with VTE. Heterozygotes have an approximately 2-fold increased risk of VTE. These defects are common among white people and rare among people of Asian or African ancestry. Laboratory testing consists of DNA-based testing for the presence or absence of the mutation.

Other Risk Factors for VTE

Additional abnormalities of procoagulant proteins that confer an increased risk of VTE include increased levels of factors VIII, IX, and XI. Currently, there is no established cutoff for this increased risk and there is no known genetic basis for these abnormalities. Although abnormalities of fibrinogen (dysfibrinogenemias) generally pose a bleeding risk, rare variants pose a risk of venous or arterial thrombosis rather than hemorrhage.

Defects in the Anticoagulant System

Congenital deficiencies of the anticoagulants antithrombin, protein C, and protein S confer an increased risk of VTE. In the majority of patients, VTE develops by 50 years of age.

Acquired Risk Factors for VTE

Patients with antiphospholipid antibodies (lupus anticoagulant, anticardiolipin antibodies, and anti–β_2-glycoprotein I antibodies) have a serious risk of both venous thrombosis and arterial thrombosis. Antiphospholipid antibody syndrome is characterized by clinical and laboratory criteria

that include 1) vascular thrombosis (venous or arterial) or recurrent miscarriage, or both, and 2) the presence and persistence (on subsequent testing after 12 weeks) of lupus anticoagulant or medium to high titers of anticardiolipin or anti–β_2-glycoprotein I antibody.

If testing of asymptomatic patients shows the presence of antiphospholipid antibodies, empirical anticoagulant therapy is not recommended. However, such patients should receive VTE prophylaxis in the appropriate high-risk clinical situations. Patients with vascular thrombosis and persistent antiphospholipid antibodies should be treated with long-term therapeutic anticoagulation, and women with recurrent fetal loss benefit from heparin (unfractionated heparin [UFH] or low-molecular-weight heparin [LMWH]) in combination with aspirin during pregnancy to prevent recurrent fetal loss.

Other acquired risk factors for VTE include immobilization (hospitalization, paralysis, etc), orthopedic or general surgery, cancer and chemotherapy, and estrogen-containing drugs, which pose a considerable risk of VTE. When any of these risk factors is combined with an underlying inherited risk factor (eg, FVL), the chances of symptomatic VTE increase significantly.

Mixed Inherited and Acquired Risk Factors for VTE

Hyperhomocysteinemia is a risk factor for VTE; certain genetic determinants (eg, *MTHFR* gene mutations) may predispose persons to hyperhomocysteinemia when compounded by acquired determinants (eg, dietary deficiencies of folate and vitamins B$_6$ and B$_{12}$). However, in the absence of hyperhomocysteinemia, routine testing for the *MTHFR* gene mutation is not advised.

VTE as a Multifactorial Disease

Patients with inherited risk factors have a baseline increased risk. Symptomatic VTE develops when inherited risk factors are present in combination with acquired risk factors, such as pregnancy, estrogen use, or surgery.

Prevention of VTE

All hospitalized medical, surgical, and trauma patients should be assessed for the risk of VTE and given appropriate VTE prophylaxis (Box 40.3). The risk of VTE must be balanced against the risk of hemorrhage and the presence of contraindications to anticoagulation (Table 40.1). Although the benefits of mechanical and pharmacologic prophylaxis have been shown, only 30% of patients at risk receive prophylaxis. The risk of VTE in surgical patients varies with the site of surgery, surgical technique, duration of the procedure, type of anesthesia, complications (infection, shock, etc), and degree of immobilization.

Box 40.3 • Suggested Strategies for VTE Prophylaxis

1. Education and early ambulation—Educate all patients about the signs and symptoms of VTE and the role of prophylaxis. Encourage patients to ambulate as early and as often as feasible.

2. Low-risk patients—Focus on education and early ambulation.

3. Moderate- or high-risk patients—Same as for low-risk patients, with the additions of elastic graded compression stockings (below knee), intermittent pneumatic compression if immobilized, and pharmacologic prophylaxis (UFH and LMWH are equivalent).

4. Very high-risk patients—Same as for moderate- or high-risk patients but with the following differences: UFH is not recommended; LMWH, fondaparinux, and adjusted-dose warfarin are used to keep the INR between 2.0 and 3.0; and extended out-of-hospital prophylaxis may be needed.

5. Patients with a previous history of VTE or thrombophilia—Same strategies as for very high-risk patients.

Abbreviations: INR, international normalized ratio; LMWH, low-molecular-weight heparin; UFH, unfractionated heparin; VTE, venous thromboembolism.

High-risk surgical procedures include open abdominal or urologic surgery, neurosurgery, gynecologic surgery, and orthopedic surgery of the lower extremities (joint replacement and hip fracture repair). In addition, patient-related risk factors include intensive care unit admission, age, cardiac dysfunction, acute myocardial infarction, congestive heart failure, cancer and its treatment, paralysis, prolonged immobility, prior VTE, obesity, varicose veins, central venous catheters, inflammatory bowel disease, lobar pneumonia, nephrotic syndrome, pregnancy, and estrogen use.

KEY FACTS

✓ Antiphospholipid antibodies and hyperhomocysteinemia—risk factors for both VTE and arterial thrombosis

✓ Relative risk of VTE for oral contraceptive users— up to 30-fold higher for FVL carriers (vs users without FVL)

✓ Relative risk of VTE for FVL homozygotes—80-fold higher

✓ VTE prevention—assess VTE risk for all hospitalized medical, surgical, and trauma patients and give appropriate prophylaxis

Evaluation for VTE

Upon radiologic testing, more than 75% of ambulatory patients who present with symptoms worrisome for VTE are found not to have the disease. Thus, a sensitive and specific strategy to reduce excess radiologic imaging studies without compromising patient safety is required. A history of the presence or absence of acquired risk factors for VTE should be obtained. Considerations in the clinical evaluation include patient and family history of VTE, pregnancy, recurrent miscarriage, estrogen use, recent trauma, surgery, hospitalization, malignancy, and travel. A physical examination should include evaluation for venous stasis and for detection of an underlying malignancy. The most critical initial component of the examination is to determine the presence or absence of venous limb gangrene (ie, **phlegmasia cerulea dolens**), in which severe obstruction of extremity venous drainage leads

Key Definition

Phlegmasia cerulea dolens: *venous limb gangrene from severe obstruction of venous drainage in the extremity, leading to congestion and eventual obstruction of arterial inflow.*

Table 40.1 • VTE Risk Factors and Incidence

Level of Risk	Surgery	Additional Risk Factors	Incidence, %			
			CVT	Proximal DVT	Clinical PE	Fatal PE
Low	Minor	None	2	0.4	0.2	0.002
Moderate	Minor	Yes	10–20	2–4	1–2	0.1–0.4
High	Major	Yes	20–40	4–8	2–4	0.4–1.0
Very high	Major (hip or knee arthroplasty, hip fracture, major trauma, spinal cord injury)	Prior VTE, active malignancy	40–80	10–20	4–10	0.2–0.5

Abbreviations: CVT, calf vein thrombosis; DVT, deep vein thrombosis; PE, pulmonary embolism; VTE, venous thromboembolism.

Table 40.2 • Wells Model for Predicting Clinical Pretest Probability of Deep Vein Thrombosis

Clinical Variable	Points[a]
Active cancer	1
Paralysis or recent limb casting	1
Recent immobility for >3 d	1
Local vein tenderness	1
Limb swelling	1
Unilateral calf swelling >3 cm	1
Pitting edema	1
Collateral superficial vein	1
Alternative diagnoses likely	−2

[a] Pretest probability of deep vein thrombosis according to total score: ≥3 points, high; 1 or 2 points, moderate; <1 point, low.

to congestion and eventual obstruction of arterial inflow. If venous limb gangrene is present, thrombolytic therapy, fasciotomy, or thrombectomy may be indicated.

Clinical findings alone, although important, are poor predictors of the presence or severity of VTE, and objective diagnostic testing may eventually be required. Initial steps, however, consist of estimating the clinical pretest probability of VTE and using the D-dimer assay with further diagnostic testing as indicated.

Step 1: Determine the Clinical Pretest Probability

The Wells model (Table 40.2) categorizes the pretest probability of DVT as high (≥3 points), moderate (1 or 2 points), or low (<1 point). A similar model applied to PE (Table 40.3) stratifies patients according to whether PE is less likely (≤4) or more likely (>4). For patients in the low-risk category, determining the level of D-dimer (a breakdown product from cross-linked stabilized fibrin clots) is recommended. The result helps to determine whether further imaging studies are probably needed.

Table 40.3 • Wells Model for Predicting Clinical Pretest Probability of Pulmonary Embolism

Clinical Variable	Points[a]
Clinical signs and symptoms of DVT	3
Alternative diagnoses less likely	3
Heart rate >100 beats per minute	1.5
Immobilization or surgery in previous 4 wk	1.5
Previous DVT or pulmonary embolism	1.5
Hemoptysis	1
Malignancy	1

Abbreviation: DVT, deep vein thrombosis.

[a] Pretest probability of pulmonary embolism according to total score: ≤4 points, less likely; >4 points, more likely.

Step 2: Determine the D-Dimer Level

For ambulatory outpatients, a D-dimer level within the reference range has a high negative predictive value for DVT; thus, additional imaging tests to exclude VTE are unnecessary. High levels have a low positive predictive value for PE and so should be used only in conjunction with the clinical pretest probability assessment. (Advanced age and pregnancy are associated with increased levels.) The D-dimer test should be used only for ambulatory outpatients. It should not be used to exclude VTE in hospitalized patients; in patients with malignancy or recent trauma, surgery, or hemorrhage; or in patients with an intermediate or high clinical probability of VTE. It is appropriate for these patients to proceed directly to imaging studies.

Diagnostic Approach for DVT

For patients with a low clinical pretest probability and normal D-dimer results, DVT is effectively ruled out and no radiologic imaging is needed unless new or progressive symptoms occur. With this approach, VTE subsequently develops in less than 1% of patients.

For patients with a moderate or high clinical pretest probability, diagnostic imaging studies should be performed (eg, duplex ultrasonography with compression). If the imaging study results are negative, checking the D-dimer level is reasonable. If the level is elevated, further imaging studies are indicated.

Compression ultrasonography, the most commonly used noninvasive test, has a diagnostic accuracy of 90% to 95% in detecting iliac and femoral DVT. Serial compression ultrasonography is recommended for high-risk patients because it has a 15% detection rate for DVT after an initial negative study. Magnetic resonance imaging has a high sensitivity and specificity for the diagnosis of pelvic DVT.

Diagnostic Approach for PE

PE should be considered in patients with dyspnea, pleuritic chest pain, and tachypnea. Hemodynamic stability should be assessed. Alternative therapies such as thrombolytic therapy or surgical thrombectomy may be indicated. Physical examination, electrocardiography, chest radiography, blood gas abnormalities, troponin levels, B-type natriuretic peptide (BNP) level, and increased plasma D-dimer level have low specificity and sensitivity for the diagnosis of PE, but when the results are considered together, they may be helpful.

BNP and the N-terminal fragment of the BNP precursor (NT-proBNP) are specific markers of ventricular stress and have a strong correlation with right ventricular dysfunction in patients with PE. Patients who have PE and high levels of BNP are at higher risk of in-hospital adverse events (odds ratio, 6.8) and 30-day all-cause mortality (odds ratio, 7.6). Chest radiographic findings may be normal and electrocardiographic findings nonspecific.

Both the PaO_2 and the alveolar-arterial gradient in the partial pressure of oxygen (PAO_2-PaO_2) may be normal in 15% to 20% of patients. The PAO_2-PaO_2 shows a linear correlation with the severity of PE, but a normal PAO_2-PaO_2 does not exclude PE. Most patients with acute PE are hypocapnic.

Ventilation-perfusion scanning is used less commonly in the diagnosis of acute PE and is generally reserved for patients with renal insufficiency or allergy to contrast agents. A "high-probability" lung scan has a sensitivity of 41% and a specificity of 97% (90% probability of PE). A "low-probability" lung scan excludes the diagnosis of PE in more than 85% of patients. An "intermediate-probability" lung scan is associated with PE in 21% to 30%. Therefore, an intermediate-probability lung scan usually requires additional study. A negative or normal perfusion-only scan (excluding a ventilation scan) rules out PE with a very high probability.

Computed tomographic (CT) angiography permits ultrafast scanning of pulmonary arteries during contrast injection. Sensitivity and specificity rates greater than 95% have been reported. Spiral CT has the greatest sensitivity in the diagnosis of PE in the main, lobar, or segmental arteries. Ventilation-perfusion scanning is preferred for patients who may have chronic thromboembolic disease owing to the distal nature of the thrombotic material. Magnetic resonance imaging may have the advantage of detecting both DVT and PE. Dysfunction of the right ventricle (frequently seen in submassive, massive, and recurrent PE) can be detected with transthoracic Doppler echocardiography. Echocardiography is not necessary for all PE patients, especially those with normal BNP levels; however, it is extremely useful for the clinically unstable patient.

Pulmonary angiography is the gold standard but has been largely replaced by CT angiography. It should be performed within 24 to 48 hours after the diagnosis has been considered. After pulmonary angiography, major complications occur in 1% of patients, and minor complications in 2%; mortality from the procedure is 0.5%.

Patients with PE should be hospitalized for at least 24 hours to assess clinical stability. Selected asymptomatic, clinically stable patients may be treated as outpatients with LMWH and warfarin as described above.

Thrombophilia Testing

For patients who have VTE after a temporary risk factor (eg, recent surgery, immobilization, or pregnancy) and do not have a family history of VTE, thrombophilia testing is not recommended. In other subgroups of patients, it is reasonable to consider thrombophilia testing with the recognition that selected assays are affected by acute thrombotic events, heparin, and warfarin. Testing should be considered if results will affect long-term management of anticoagulation. Thrombophilia testing can be performed before initiation of anticoagulation or after completion of anticoagulation appropriate for a thrombotic event if certain caveats are recognized and appropriate follow-up testing is performed.

DNA-based testing (eg, FVL and prothrombin G20210A mutation) is not affected by acute thrombosis, heparin anticoagulation, or warfarin. However, the optimal time for thrombophilia testing is 4 to 6 weeks after completion of anticoagulation.

Thrombophilia does not alter acute management of VTE except in 2 circumstances. If the baseline activated partial thromboplastin time (aPTT) is prolonged in association with lupus anticoagulants, consider monitoring of UFH complex, use of the heparin assay (anti-Xa levels), or use of LMWH (which requires no monitoring). With congenital deficiency of protein C or protein S, the risk of warfarin skin necrosis increases, especially if heparin therapy (with UFH or LMWH) is prematurely discontinued (see Treatment of VTE subsection). For thrombophilic conditions that impart a high risk of recurrence, a longer duration of anticoagulation is needed.

Idiopathic DVT, particularly when recurrent, may indicate the presence of neoplasm in 10% to 20% of patients.

For patients with objectively confirmed VTE, initial laboratory testing should include a complete blood cell count (and, if abnormal, a blood smear), serum tests of liver and kidney function, baseline prothrombin time and aPTT (before initiation of anticoagulants), and urinalysis. Testing should also include age-appropriate cancer screening. Additional investigations (eg, radiologic studies) should be reserved for further investigation of abnormal initial history, examination, and laboratory findings and patient risk factors (eg, smoking).

KEY FACTS

✓ VTE evaluation—
- first, determine clinical pretest probability
- second, determine D-dimer level

✓ D-dimer test to exclude VTE—
- use for ambulatory outpatients only
- do not use in patients who are hospitalized; who have malignancy or recent trauma, surgery, or hemorrhage; or who have intermediate or high clinical probability of VTE

✓ Serial compression ultrasonography for DVT diagnosis—recommended for high-risk patients (15% DVT detection rate after initial negative study)

✓ Thrombophilia testing—
- not recommended if patient has a temporary risk factor (eg, recent surgery, immobilization, or pregnancy) and does not have a family history of VTE
- consider performing if results would affect long-term management of anticoagulation

Treatment of VTE

Initial Management of VTE

The aims of initial therapy for VTE include preventing extension or embolization of the thrombus and reducing postphlebitic syndrome. Patients who are hemodynamically unstable should be hospitalized. For most hemodynamically stable patients, however, outpatient anticoagulation is reasonable. After contraindications to anticoagulation have been excluded, several options for acute and long-term anticoagulation are available depending on the oral anticoagulant agent chosen.

For patients who will be managed with warfarin, initiate therapeutic doses of either intravenous UFH or subcutaneous LMWH, and simultaneously initiate oral warfarin therapy. UFH is monitored with aPTT or heparin levels (anti-Xa assay); LMWH does not need monitoring, but the international normalized ratio (INR) is used to assess warfarin effect. Continue therapy with both agents for at least 5 days or until the INR is in the therapeutic range (ie, 2–3) for at least 48 hours before discontinuing the UFH or LMWH.

For patients who will be managed with oral direct-acting anticoagulants, such as direct thrombin inhibitors (DTIs) (eg, dabigatran), after a period of UFH or LMWH, transition to the oral DTI.

For patients who will be managed with oral direct factor Xa inhibitors (eg, rivaroxaban), initial UFH or LMWH is not required.

Use of knee-high compression stockings has been shown to reduce the incidence of postphlebitic syndrome.

Calf Vein Thrombosis

Patients with asymptomatic calf vein thrombosis can be observed if they are willing and able to return for follow-up compression ultrasonography to document stability or progression of the clot. If patients have symptomatic or progressive calf vein thrombosis, anticoagulation should be initiated.

Proximal DVT

Management of proximal DVT should be as described above in the Initial Management of VTE subsection.

Pulmonary Embolism

PE is the cause of death in 5% to 15% of hospitalized patients. Poor prognostic factors include age older than 70 years, cancer, congestive heart failure, chronic obstructive pulmonary disease, systolic arterial hypotension, tachypnea, and right ventricular hypokinesis. PE is detected in 25% to 30% of routine autopsies. Antemortem diagnosis is made in less than 30%, owing to the variable and nonspecific presentation of patients with PE.

Etiology

The most common cause of PE is DVT of the lower extremities. In approximately 45% of patients with femoral and iliac DVT, emboli move to the lungs. Other sources of emboli include thrombi in the upper extremities, right ventricle, and indwelling catheters. The congenital and acquired risk factors for PE are listed in Box 40.1. The incidence of DVT in various clinical circumstances is listed in Table 40.1.

Thrombolytic Therapy

For patients with massive PE or PE with hemodynamic instability, thrombolytic therapy is recommended. The use of thrombolytics in submassive, hemodynamically stable PE is controversial. Ideally, thrombolytic agents should be administered within 24 hours after PE. After thrombolytic therapy, heparin infusion is begun or resumed if the aPTT is less than 80 seconds. The risk of intracranial bleeding in patients who have PE treated with thrombolytic drugs is about 1%.

Inferior Vena Cava Interruption

Inferior vena cava interruption is indicated in the following situations: anticoagulant therapy is contraindicated, complications result from anticoagulant therapy, anticoagulant therapy fails, a predisposition to bleeding is present, chronic recurrent PE and secondary pulmonary hypertension occur, or surgical pulmonary thromboendarterectomy has been performed or is intended to be performed. After the filter has been inserted, anticoagulant therapy is aimed at preventing DVT at the insertion site, inferior vena cava thrombosis, cephalad propagation of a clot from an occluded filter, and propagation or recurrence of lower extremity DVT. PE occurs in 2.5% of patients despite inferior vena cava interruption.

Long-term Management of VTE (Secondary Prophylaxis)

The aim of long-term therapy for VTE is secondary prevention or reducing the risk of recurrence. After an initial 3 months of anticoagulation, a decision should be made on the duration of anticoagulation (Table 40.4). Continuation of warfarin anticoagulation should be balanced with the risk of hemorrhage. For patients receiving warfarin, the INR is monitored every 4 to 6 weeks. For patients receiving the direct-acting anticoagulants, monitoring is not needed. Long-term outcomes have been shown to be superior when VTE is managed in anticoagulation clinics and with home INR devices.

Table 40.4 • Duration of Anticoagulation for Long-term Management of VTE

Clinical Situation	Duration of Anticoagulation
VTE from temporary risk factor (eg, surgery or pregnancy)	Discontinue anticoagulation at 3 mo
VTE from persistent risk factor	Continue oral agent (warfarin or direct-acting anticoagulants) for extended duration
DVT without risk factors (idiopathic)	Additional 3 mo of warfarin for secondary prophylaxis
Recurrent DVT	Extended secondary prophylaxis
PE—hemodynamically significant or idiopathic	Long-term treatment with warfarin
VTE with underlying thrombophilia (eg, from lupus anticoagulant or deficiency of protein C, protein S, or antithrombin)	Long-term treatment with warfarin
VTE in patients who are compound heterozygous for factor V Leiden and prothrombin G20210A mutation	Long-term treatment with warfarin

Abbreviations: DVT, deep vein thrombosis; PE, pulmonary embolism; VTE, venous thromboembolism.

KEY FACTS

✓ Initial management of VTE—
- if oral direct-acting anticoagulants (eg, DTIs) will be used, transition to oral DTI after use of UFH or LMWH
- if oral direct factor Xa inhibitors (eg, rivaroxaban) will be used, initial use of UFH or LMWH is not necessary

✓ Thrombolytic therapy—recommended for patients with massive PE or PE with hemodynamic instability

✓ Indications for inferior vena cava interruption—
- anticoagulant therapy is contraindicated, results in complications, or fails
- patient has predisposition to bleeding or has chronic recurrent PE and secondary pulmonary hypertension
- surgical pulmonary thromboendarterectomy has been or will be performed

✓ Long-term management of VTE—
- discontinue anticoagulation if risk factor is temporary (eg, surgery or pregnancy)
- give warfarin for 3 more months for idiopathic DVT
- provide extended secondary prophylaxis for recurrent DVT
- give long-term warfarin for hemodynamically significant or idiopathic PE, for VTE with thrombophilia, and for compound heterozygote for FVL and prothrombin G20210A mutation

Questions and Answers

Questions

Multiple Choice (choose the best answer)

VI.1. A 67-year-old man is evaluated for exertional dyspnea. He recalls that 3 years ago he was told he had anemia. In reviewing his records, you note that at that time his hemoglobin level was 9.5 g/dL and his hematocrit was 33% with an increased mean corpuscular volume (MCV); the remainder of his complete blood cell count was normal. On physical examination, he had conjunctival pallor, normal heart and lung findings, no lymphadenopathy, no hepatomegaly or splenomegaly, and no petechiae or ecchymoses. Diagnostic testing results are shown in Table VI.Q1.

Table VI.Q1 •

Component	Finding
Hemoglobin, g/dL	7.5
Hematocrit, %	23
Mean corpuscular volume, fL	110 (reference range, 86–98)
Leukocyte count, ×10⁹/L	2.1
Neutrophils, %	20
Lymphocytes, %	70
Monocytes, %	6
Basophils, %	3
Eosinophils, %	1
Platelet count, ×10⁹/L	64
Reticulocyte count, % of erythrocytes	0.3 (reference range, 0.5–1.5)
Absolute reticulocyte count, ×10⁹/L	10.0 (reference range, 29.5–87.3)
Peripheral blood film	Dimorphic erythrocyte population with pronounced macrocytes
Lactate dehydrogenase, U/L	150 (reference range, 140–280)

Which of the following is the most likely explanation for these findings?
a. Acute myeloid leukemia (AML)
b. Vitamin B_{12} deficiency

c. Hemolytic anemia
d. Myelodysplastic syndrome (MDS)
e. Primary myelofibrosis

VI.2. A 45-year-old woman is admitted to the surgical service with severe arterial insufficiency of the right second toe. She has no prior medical history and takes no medications. Physical examination findings are normal except for mild splenomegaly and signs of early gangrene in the right second toe. All pulses are full and equal throughout. Diagnostic testing results are shown in Table VI.Q2.

Table VI.Q2 •

Component	Finding
Hemoglobin, g/dL	13.2
Hematocrit, %	39
Leukocyte count, ×10⁹/L	15.5
Segmented neutrophils, %	78
Band cells, %	4
Lymphocytes, %	20
Monocytes, %	5
Basophils, %	2
Eosinophils, %	1
Platelet count, ×10⁹/L	1,300
Mean corpuscular volume, fL	88
Erythrocyte sedimentation rate, mm/h	28
Leukocyte alkaline phosphatase score	110 (reference range, 13–130)
Serum ferritin	Within reference range
Serum iron	Within reference range
Serum total iron-binding capacity	Within reference range
Peripheral blood film	Increased large platelets with some clustering; leukocytes and erythrocytes are unremarkable
Bone marrow aspiration and biopsy	Increased cellularity with increased and atypical megakaryocytes in clusters; reticulin staining is normal
Chromosomal analysis	Normal female karyotype (46XY)

Which of the following is the most likely diagnosis?
a. Essential thrombocythemia
b. Vasculitis
c. Philadelphia chromosome–negative chronic myeloid leukemia (CML)
d. Primary myelofibrosis (PMF)

VI.3. A 70-year-old man presents with weakness of his right arm and leg. His symptoms began yesterday and are now resolved. He also reports a 6-month history of recurrent headaches and fatigue. He is a nonsmoker. His medical history is significant for high blood pressure. His blood pressure is 167/88 mm Hg, his oxygen saturation is 93% with room air, his face is plethoric, and a right carotid bruit is heard. Other findings on physical examination are normal. Diagnostic testing results are shown in Table VI.Q3.

Table VI.Q3 •

Component	Finding
Hemoglobin, g/dL	20.5
Hematocrit, %	58
Mean corpuscular volume, fL	88
Leukocyte count, ×10⁹/L	12.5
Neutrophils, %	83
Lymphocytes, %	12
Monocytes, %	3
Basophils, %	2
Platelet count, ×10⁹/L	600
Erythropoietin, mIU/mL	<2 (reference range, 0–19)

Carotid ultrasonography shows a 30% stenotic lesion in the right carotid. The patient is hospitalized and begins antiplatelet therapy. Which of the following should you order next?
a. *JAK2* V617F mutation testing
b. Fluorescence in situ hybridization (FISH) for *BCR-ABL* testing
c. Arterial blood gas analysis
d. Bone marrow aspiration and biopsy

VI.4. A 16-year-old female patient presents with menorrhagia. She attained menarche at 13 years of age and has had heavy periods since then. She experienced epistaxis as a child, but it has resolved. Her family history is notable for a maternal aunt who was a "bleeder" and for her mother who experienced menorrhagia. The patient has been told that she is iron deficient. Physical examination findings are normal. Laboratory test results (and reference ranges) are as follows: prothrombin time (PT), 10 seconds (8.3–10.8 seconds); activated partial thromboplastin time (aPTT), 33 seconds (23–33 seconds); and fibrinogen, 250 mg/dL. Which of the following tests should be ordered to evaluate this patient's bleeding?
a. Bleeding time
b. Electron microscopy of the patient's platelets
c. Platelet aggregation studies
d. von Willebrand factor testing
e. Platelet function analysis

VI.5. A 62-year-old man underwent right total knee replacement 8 days ago. Swelling has developed in his right lower extremity, and Doppler ultrasonography confirms the presence of a right superficial femoral vein thrombosis. His current medications include oxycodone and subcutaneous unfractionated heparin. Results of preoperative tests, including a complete blood cell count and liver and kidney function, were normal. Other

laboratory data include the following: hemoglobin 12.2 g/dL, leukocyte count 8.5×10⁹/L, and platelet count 60×10⁹/L. In addition to stopping the use of subcutaneous heparin, what is the next most appropriate step in management of this patient?
a. Start low-molecular-weight heparin therapy.
b. Start intravenous therapeutic doses of heparin.
c. Start direct thrombin inhibitor therapy.
d. Start aspirin therapy.

VI.6. A 22-year-old woman is brought to the emergency department after having 1 witnessed tonic-clonic seizure. She had appeared confused for the preceding few hours. On examination, she is febrile and appears slightly confused; otherwise, neurologic and physical examination findings are normal. Laboratory test results are shown in Table VI.Q6, and the peripheral blood smear is shown in Figure VI.Q6.
What is the most appropriate next step in management?
a. Red blood cell transfusion
b. Platelet transfusion
c. Gamma globulin administration
d. Plasma exchange

Table VI.Q6 •

Component	Finding	Reference Range
Hemoglobin, g/dL	8	12–15
Platelet count, ×10⁹/L	50	150–450
Leukocyte count, ×10⁹/L	8	3.5–10.0
Creatinine, mg/dL	2.5	0.8–1.3

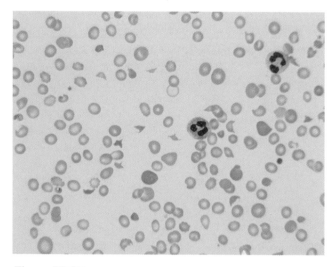

Figure VI.Q6

VI.7. At her annual physical examination, an asymptomatic 68-year-old woman has lymphocytosis (32×10⁹/L) with a normal hemoglobin level and platelet count. On examination, she has 1-cm lymphadenopathy in the cervical region and no palpable liver or spleen enlargement. A peripheral blood smear shows identically appearing mature lymphcytes with smudge cells. Flow cytometry of the peripheral blood lymphocytes shows a monoclonal B population with dim expression of λ light chain and CD20 that is positive for expression of CD5, CD19, and CD23. Which of the following is the best next step in her management?

a. Combination chemoimmunotherapy

b. Chlorambucil therapy

c. Allogeneic peripheral blood stem cell transplant

d. Combination monoclonal antibody therapy

e. Active monitoring for disease progression and complications

VI.8. An 80-year-old man is admitted to the hospital after falling on an icy sidewalk and fracturing his hip. He undergoes open reduction and internal fixation of the fracture. At surgery, there does not appear to be any bone disease at the fracture site. The patient was previously asymptomatic. Physical examination findings are otherwise unremarkable. Serum protein electrophoresis and immunofixation show an immunoglobulin (Ig)M κ monoclonal protein (0.3 g/dL). The complete blood cell count and serum creatinine levels are normal. Skeletal survey shows no additional bone defects. Which of the following statements is true for this patient?

a. He has multiple myeloma and requires treatment.

b. He has a lower risk of a clinically significant lymphocytic or plasma cell malignancy than patients with an IgG monoclonal protein.

c. He requires a radioisotope bone scan to evaluate his bone integrity.

d. He requires regular follow-up and serial measurements of his monoclonal protein level.

e. He has a 10% annual risk of multiple myeloma.

VI.9. A 55-year-old man presented to his primary care physician for evaluation of fatigue. He was previously healthy with the exception of chronic musculoskeletal low back pain, for which he occasionally takes non-steroidal anti-inflammatory drugs. On examination, he is pale. Complete blood cell count results are as follows: hemoglobin 8.3 g/dL, mean corpuscular volume 73 fL, leukocyte count 6.9×10^9/L, and platelet count 398×10^9/L. Results of the fecal occult blood test are positive. During upper and lower endoscopy, a 1.2×2.5-cm ulcerative lesion is noted in the lesser curvature of the stomach. The lesion is biopsied and identified as a MALT lymphoma. Which of the following is characteristic of MALT lymphoma?

a. Most cases are treated with anthracycline-based chemotherapy.

b. It is caused by chronic stimulation with *Chlamydophila psittaci*.

c. Radiotherapy is necessary in most cases.

d. It frequently undergoes transformation to a large-cell lymphoma.

e. The combination of amoxicillin, omeprazole, and clarithromycin is the most appropriate first-line treatment.

VI.10. A 73-year-old woman presented to the emergency department with new-onset back pain, confusion, and constipation over the past week. Her past medical history is significant only for hypertension. On examination, she is slightly pale with slow cognition and point tenderness over the lumbar spine. Plain films of the lumbar spine show osteolytic lesions in L2, L3, and L5. Laboratory values are as follows: hemoglobin 9.3 g/dL, leukocyte count 4.6×10^9/L with a normal differential count, platelet count 230×10^9/L, creatinine 1.6 mg/dL, total calcium 13.1 mg/dL, albumin 3.6 g/dL, and total protein 9.1 g/dL. What is the most likely diagnosis?

a. Metastatic breast cancer

b. Hydrochlorothiazide use

c. Multiple myeloma

d. Primary hyperparathyroidism

e. Milk alkali syndrome

Answers

VI.1. Answer d.

Patients with MDS most commonly present with isolated macrocytic anemia. MDS can evolve to include pancytopenia over several years; the typical peripheral smear findings include a dimorphic erythrocyte population (microcytes and oval macrocytes) with an overall prominent macrocytosis and MCV around 110 fL. The chronicity of MDS—in particular, anemia preceding the diagnosis of pancytopenia by several years—is in contrast to the typically acute manifestation of AML, which is therefore an unlikely possibility in this patient. Primary myelofibrosis, a myeloproliferative neoplasm, causes fibrosis in the bone marrow, resulting in extramedullary hematopoiesis and significant splenomegaly, and typically does not cause a macrocytic anemia. Vitamin B_{12} deficiency can cause a megaloblastic anemia and manifest with slowly evolving macrocytic anemia and eventually pancytopenia, but the peripheral smear would not show a dimorphic erythrocyte population.

VI.2. Answer a.

Extreme thrombocytosis may be reactive and occur with severe iron deficiency or inflammatory states (with elevated erythrocyte sedimentation rates) or after splenectomy; patients are typically asymptomatic. Clonal thrombocytosis is related to a myeloproliferative neoplasm, which usually causes splenomegaly. Typical bone marrow findings include a hypercellular bone marrow with increased atypical megakaryocytes in clusters. Essential thrombocythemia may cause extreme thrombocytosis (platelet count >1,000×10⁹/L); however, it can also occur less commonly with polycythemia rubra vera (typically with erythrocytosis), the cellular phase of PMF, or rarely CML. The normal karyotype makes CML much less likely since it typically manifests with the Philadelphia chromosome t(9;22). Increased reticulin fibrosis would have be seen on the bone marrow biopsy if the patient had PMF.

VI.3. Answer a.

Polycythemia may be secondary, as with erythropoietin-mediated causes such as chronic hypoxia, living at high altitude, and high oxygen affinity hemoglobinopathies. Polycythemia vera is a myeloproliferative neoplasm, and patients can present with arterial thrombosis secondary to hyperviscosity from the increased concentration of erythrocytes. The low erythropoietin rules out erythropoietin-mediated causes, leaving the presumptive diagnosis of polycythemia vera. With *JAK2* V617F mutation testing of peripheral blood, results are positive for approximately 90% of patients who have polycythemia vera. FISH for *BCR-ABL* testing would screen for chronic myeloid leukemia; patients with chronic myeloid leukemia do not present with polycythemia. Although bone marrow aspiration and biopsy would be helpful, it is not immediately necessary and could be considered later.

VI.4. Answer d.

The most common inherited bleeding disorder is von Willebrand disease. Typically, the PT and aPTT are normal in von Willebrand disease, and specific assays are required for diagnosis. The bleeding time test, considered to be a screening test, has a very low sensitivity and specificity for diagnosis of bleeding disorders; moreover, it is probably not

available in many institutions. Platelet electron microscopy is not indicated without initial platelet aggregation studies; however, platelet function defects are extremely rare and are detected with platelet aggregation studies. One should test for von Willebrand disease before embarking on platelet function testing. Platelet function analysis is considered to be a screening test for platelet function or drug effect, and it is not indicated in this situation.

VI.5. Answer c.

The timing and degree of thrombocytopenia are consistent with immune-mediated heparin-induced thrombocytopenia type II. Unfractioned heparin and low-molecular-weight heparin are contraindicated. Aspirin would not be the sole management agent for established thrombosis. The most appropriate step is to start a direct thrombin inhibitor.

VI.6. Answer d.

Plasma exchange is the treatment of choice for thrombotic thrombocytopenic purpura (TTP). Although red blood cell transfusion may be indicated, it does not address the underlying pathogenesis of TTP. Platelets are thought to be contraindicated in TTP because of the theoretical possibility of worsening the TTP. Gamma globulin is ineffective in increasing the platelet count in TTP.

VI.7. Answer e.

Chronic lymphocytic leukemia (CLL) is a clonal lymphoproliferative disorder of mature lymphocytes. The clinical diagnosis requires a B-lymphocyte count of more than 5×10⁹/L. Peripheral blood smears typically show smudge cells, which are lymphocytes that have broken during processing of the slide. The clinical course of CLL is chronic in most patients. For those with early-stage disease, standard practice is to withhold treatment until the disease is active or progressive. However, patients need to be monitored for disease progression, autoimmune complications, infections, and second cancers.

VI.8. Answer d.

This patient has monoclonal gammopathy of undetermined significance (MGUS), the most common dysproteinemia. In MGUS, the M protein level is typically less than 3 g/dL, the bone marrow has less than 10% plasma cells, and the hemoglobin, creatinine, calcium, and bone radiographs are normal. The risk of progression to a lymphocytic or plasma cell malignancy is about 1% per year. Patients with an IgM or IgA monoclonal protein are at higher risk of progression than those with an IgG protein. Patients with MGUS need to be observed.

VI.9. Answer e.

With combination antibiotic therapy, 70% of gastric MALT lymphomas are cured. In cases refractory to antibiotics, tumors may carry the t(11;18) translocation, and involved field radiotherapy is effective. Combination chemotherapy is reserved for advanced disease. The majority of cases are associated with *Helicobacter pylori* infection.

VI.10. Answer c.

This patient has multiple myeloma with evidence of end-organ damage from the plasma cell proliferative disorder (hypercalcemia, renal failure, anemia, and osteolytic bone lesions). The other answer choices are possible causes of hypercalcemia, but only multiple myeloma accounts for all the presenting symptoms, including the elevated level of total protein.

Section VII

Infectious Diseases

Central Nervous System Infections

41

PRITISH K. TOSH, MD AND M. RIZWAN SOHAIL, MD

Bacterial Meningitis

Acute bacterial meningitis is an infectious disease emergency. The incidence of bacterial meningitis is estimated to be 3.0 cases per 100,000 person-years, and its overall case fatality rate is 25% in adults. Common predisposing conditions for community-acquired meningitis include acute otitis media, altered immune states, alcoholism, pneumonia, diabetes mellitus, sinusitis, and a cerebrospinal fluid (CSF) leak. Risk factors for death among adults with community-acquired meningitis include age 60 years or older, altered mental status at presentation, pneumococcal cause, and occurrence of seizures within 24 hours of symptom onset. In two-thirds of patients, classic features of fever and nuchal rigidity are present.

The organisms most commonly causing community-acquired meningitis in adults are *Streptococcus pneumoniae* (38%), *Neisseria meningitidis* (14%), *Listeria monocytogenes* (11%), streptococci (7%), *Staphylococcus aureus* (5%), *Haemophilus influenzae* (4%), and gram-negative bacilli (4%).

Indications for computed tomography before lumbar puncture in cases of suspected meningitis include age greater than 60 years, immunocompromise, new-onset seizures, papilledema, altered consciousness, and focal neurologic deficits. Laboratory and radiographic testing should not delay commencement of empirical antimicrobial therapy.

Typical CSF characteristics in bacterial meningitis include a white blood cell count of 1,000 to 5,000/mcL and a glucose value less than 40 mg/dL or CSF to serum glucose ratio of less than 0.4. The differential blood cell count is likely to show a predominance of neutrophils. Gram stain is positive in 60% to 90% of the cases. Countercurrent immunoelectrophoresis or latex agglutination tests may provide results in 15 minutes and are useful for the detection of *H influenzae* type B; *S pneumoniae; N meningitidis* types A, B, C, and Y; *Escherichia coli* K1; and group B streptococci in the absence of a positive Gram stain. CSF cultures are positive in 70% to 85% of bacterial meningitis cases. Blood cultures may be helpful in establishing the diagnosis and should be routinely performed in all instances where bacterial meningitis is suspected.

Management of suspected community-acquired bacterial meningitis is outlined in Figure 41.1; recommendations for antimicrobial therapy are listed in Table 41.1. Causative organisms, affected age-groups, and predisposing factors in bacterial meningitis are listed in Table 41.2, and empirical treatment in various age-groups and patient groups is outlined in Table 41.3.

Treatment guidelines from the Infectious Diseases Society of America suggest a role for dexamethasone use in the early treatment of suspected pneumococcal meningitis in adults and *H influenzae* type B meningitis in children. Of note, corticosteroids are beneficial when administered either concurrently or before antimicrobial therapy. When it is subsequently determined that the patient does not have pneumococcal meningitis, dexamethasone therapy should be discontinued.

KEY FACTS

✓ Acute bacterial meningitis is an infectious disease emergency

✓ In adults, the most common cause of community-acquired meningitis is *Streptococcus pneumoniae*

✓ Computed tomography before lumbar puncture is indicated in the case of suspected meningitis with the following characteristics: patient age >60 years, immunocompromise, new-onset seizures, papilledema, altered consciousness, or focal neurologic deficits

✓ Typical characteristics of CSF in bacterial meningitis include cell count of 1,000–5,000/mcL and glucose level <40 mg/dL

✓ In bacterial meningitis, the differential blood cell count is likely to show a high proportion of neutrophils

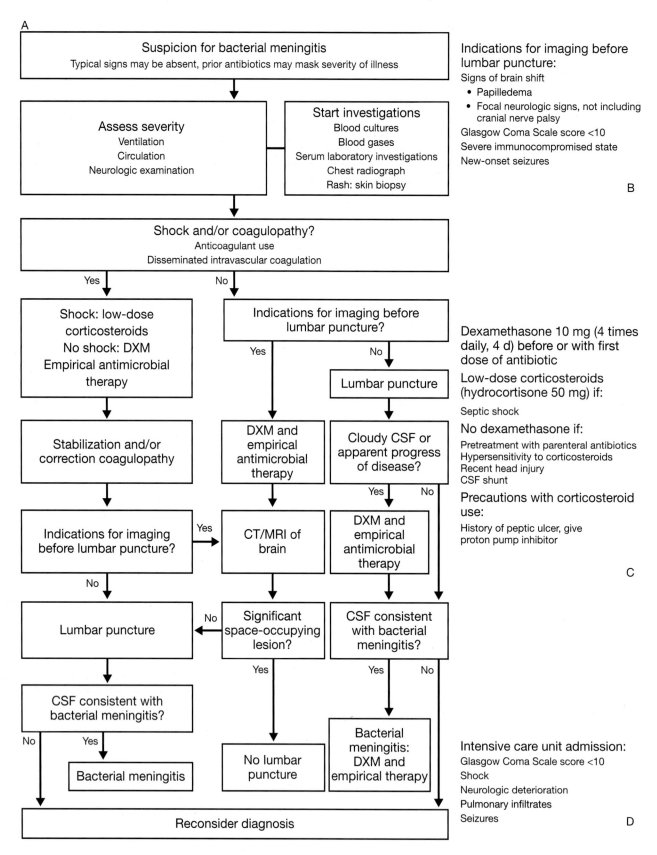

Figure 41.1 *Algorithm for Management of Suspected Community-Acquired Bacterial Meningitis. A, Algorithm for initial treatment of adults with bacterial meningitis. B, Indications for performing imaging before lumbar puncture. C, Recommendations for adjunctive dexamethasone therapy in adults with bacterial meningitis. D, Criteria for admission of patients with bacterial meningitis to the intensive care unit. CSF indicates cerebrospinal fluid; CT, computed tomography; DXM, dexamethasone; MRI, magnetic resonance imaging.*

(Adapted from van de Beek D, de Gans J, Tunkel AR, Wijdicks EFM. Community-acquired bacterial meningitis in adults. N Engl J Med. 2006 Jan 5;[Suppl Appendix]354[1]:44–53. Used with permission.)

Table 41.1 • Recommendations for Antimicrobial Therapy in Adults With Community-Acquired Bacterial Meningitis

Empirical Therapy		
Predisposing Factor	**Common Bacterial Pathogen**	**Antimicrobial Therapy**
Age, y		
16–50	Neisseria meningitidis, Streptococcus pneumoniae	Vancomycin plus a third-generation cephalosporin[a,b]
>50	S pneumoniae, N meningitidis, Listeria monocytogenes	Vancomycin plus a third-generation cephalosporin plus ampicillin[b,c]
With risk factor present[d]	S pneumoniae, L monocytogenes, Haemophilus influenzae	Vancomycin plus a third-generation cephalosporin plus ampicillin[b,c]

Specific Antimicrobial Therapy		
Microorganism, Susceptibility	**Standard Therapy**	**Alternative Therapy**
S pneumoniae		
Penicillin MIC		
<0.1 mg/L	Penicillin G or ampicillin	Third-generation cephalosporin,[b] chloramphenicol
0.1–1.0 mg/L	Third-generation cephalosporin[b]	Cefepime, meropenem
≥2.0 mg/L	Vancomycin plus a third-generation cephalosporin[b,e]	Fluoroquinolone[f]
Cefotaxime or ceftriaxone MIC		
≥1.0 mg/L	Vancomycin plus a third-generation cephalosporin[b,g]	Fluoroquinolone[f]
N meningitidis		
Penicillin MIC		
<0.1 mg/L	Penicillin G or ampicillin	Third-generation cephalosporin,[b] chloramphenicol
0.1–1.0 mg/L	Third-generation cephalosporin[b]	Chloramphenicol, fluoroquinolone, meropenem
L monocytogenes	Penicillin G or ampicillin[h]	Trimethoprim-sulfamethoxazole, meropenem
Group B streptococcus	Penicillin G or ampicillin[h]	Third-generation cephalosporin[b]
Escherichia coli and other Enterobacteriaceae	Third-generation cephalosporin[b]	Aztreonam, fluoroquinolone, meropenem, trimethoprim-sulfamethoxazole, ampicillin
Pseudomonas aeruginosa	Ceftazidime or cefepime[h]	Aztreonam,[h] ciprofloxacin,[h] meropenem[h]
H influenzae		
β-Lactamase negative	Ampicillin	Third-generation cephalosporin,[b] cefepime, chloramphenicol, fluoroquinolone
β-Lactamase positive	Third-generation cephalosporin[b]	Cefepime, chloramphenicol, fluoroquinolone
Chemoprophylaxis[i] for N meningitidis	Rifampicin (rifampin), ceftriaxone, ciprofloxacin, azithromycin	

Abbreviation: MIC, minimal inhibitory concentration.

[a] Only in areas with very low rate of penicillin resistance (<1%) should monotherapy with penicillin be considered, although many experts recommend combination therapy for all patients until results of in vitro susceptibility testing are known.

[b] Cefotaxime or ceftriaxone.

[c] Only in areas with very low rates of penicillin resistance and cephalosporin resistance should combination therapy of amoxicillin (ampicillin) and a third-generation cephalosporin be considered.

[d] Alcoholism, altered immune status.

[e] Consider addition of rifampicin (rifampin) when dexamethasone is given.

[f] Gatifloxacin or moxifloxacin; no clinical data on use in patients with bacterial meningitis.

[g] Consider addition of rifampicin (rifampin) when the MIC of ceftriaxone is ≥2 mg/L.

[h] Consider addition of an aminoglycoside.

[i] Prophylaxis is indicated for persons in close contact (defined as those with intimate contact, which covers those eating and sleeping in the same dwelling and those having close social and kissing contacts) or health care workers who perform mouth-to-mouth resuscitation, endotracheal intubation, or endotracheal tube management. Patients with meningococcal meningitis who receive monotherapy with penicillin or amoxicillin (ampicillin) should also receive chemoprophylaxis because carriage is not reliably eradicated by these drugs.

Note: The duration of therapy for patients with bacterial meningitis has often been based more on tradition than on evidence-based data and needs to be individualized on the basis of the patient's response. In general, antimicrobial therapy is given for 7 days for meningitis caused by N meningitidis and H influenzae, 10 to 14 days for S pneumoniae, and at least 21 days for L monocytogenes.

Adapted from van de Beek D, de Gans J, Tunkel AR, Wijdicks EFM. Community-acquired bacterial meningitis in adults. N Engl J Med. 2006 Jan 5;354(1):44–53. Used with permission.

Table 41.2 • Organisms Involved, Affected Age-groups, and Predisposing Factors in Bacterial Meningitis

Organism	Risk Group	Comment	Predisposing Factors
Streptococcus pneumoniae	Any age, but often advanced age	Most common cause of recurrent meningitis in adults	Cerebrospinal fluid leak, alcoholism, splenectomy, functional asplenia, multiple myeloma, hypogammaglobulinemia, Hodgkin disease, HIV infection
Neisseria meningitidis	Infants to 40 y	Petechial rash common Epidemics in closed populations	Terminal component complement deficiency
Haemophilus influenzae, type B	Infant to 6 y	Significant decrease in incidence since licensure of *H influenzae* B vaccine	Hypogammaglobulinemia in adults, HIV infection, splenectomy, functional asplenia
Escherichia coli, group B streptococci	Neonates		Maternal colonization
Gram-negative bacilli	Any age	*Staphylococcus aureus* and coagulase-negative staphylococci also common after neurosurgical procedure	Neurosurgical procedures; bacteremia due to urinary tract infection, pneumonia, and other conditions; *Strongyloides* hyperinfection syndrome
Listeria monocytogenes	Neonates; immunosuppressed persons		

Abbreviation: HIV, human immunodeficiency virus.

Meningococcus

Neisseria meningitidis is a gram-negative diplococcus that is carried in the nasopharynx of otherwise healthy persons. Because of widespread use of *H influenzae* vaccination in children, *N meningitidis* has emerged as a leading cause of bacterial meningitis in children and young adults. Most sporadic cases (95%–97%) are caused by serogroups B, C, and Y, whereas A and C strains are usually observed in epidemics. Risk factors for meningococcal infection include

host and environmental factors. Host characteristics include terminal complement component (C5-C9) deficiency, which increases infection rates but is associated with low mortality rates. The organism is spread through airborne droplets from asymptomatic pharyngeal carriers. Risk factors include a preceding viral respiratory infection; crowding in a household, barracks, or dormitory; chronic medical illnesses; corticosteroid use; and active or passive smoking. Travel to the "meningitis belt" of north central Africa or to the Hajj in Saudi Arabia is a risk factor for meningococcal

Table 41.3 • Empirical Therapy for Bacterial Meningitis

Age-group/Patient Group	Common Pathogens	Antimicrobial Therapy
Age		
0–4 wk	Group B streptococci, *Escherichia coli, Listeria monocytogenes, Klebsiella pneumoniae, Enterococcus* spp, *Salmonella* spp	Ampicillin plus cefotaxime or ampicillin plus an aminoglycoside
1–23 mo	Group B streptococci, *E coli, L monocytogenes, Haemophilus influenzae, Streptococcus pneumoniae, Neisseria meningitidis*	Vancomycin plus cefotaxime or ceftriaxone
2–50 y	*N meningitidis, S pneumoniae*	Vancomycin plus cefotaxime or ceftriaxone
>50 y	*S pneumoniae, L monocytogenes*, aerobic gram-negative bacilli	Vancomycin plus either cefotaxime or ceftriaxone plus ampicillin (cephalosporins have **no** activity against *Listeria*)
Basilar skull fracture	*S pneumoniae, H influenzae*, group A β-hemolytic streptococci	Vancomycin plus cefotaxime or ceftriaxone
Postneurosurgery	Coagulase-negative staphylococci, *Staphylococcus aureus*, aerobic gram-negative bacilli (including *Pseudomonas aeruginosa*)	Vancomycin plus cefepime or ceftazidime or meropenem

Adapted from Tunkel AR, Hartman BJ, Kaplan SL, Kaufman BA, Roos KL, Scheld WM, et al. Practice guidelines for the management of bacterial meningitis. Clin Infect Dis. 2004 Nov 1;39(9):1267–84. Epub 2004 Oct 6. Used with permission.

meningitis, and vaccination is recommended before travel to these areas.

Neisseria meningitidis infection often begins with a mild upper respiratory tract illness that may disseminate into the bloodstream, leading to a petechial rash that often occurs around the same time as fever and meningeal signs. The diagnosis can be made by visualizing the small gram-negative diplococci on a CSF Gram stain. Treatment is with penicillin G when the minimum inhibitory concentration is less than 0.1 mcg/mL; otherwise, high-dose ceftriaxone or cefotaxime treatment is preferred (Table 41.1). Recommended treatment duration is 7 days for meningococcal meningitis.

Persons in close contact of the index case (eg, hospital workers with direct exposure to respiratory secretions during intubation, roommates, persons in the same household, daycare center members, persons exposed to the patient's oral secretions) should be offered chemoprophylaxis within 24 hours of exposure. For adults, ciprofloxacin (500 mg, oral, single dose), ceftriaxone (250 mg, intramuscularly, single dose), or rifampin (600 mg, oral, twice daily for 2 days) are recommended. Rare cases of ciprofloxacin-resistant *N meningitidis* have been reported. Because penicillin does not eliminate the carrier state, the index patient may require a prophylaxis regimen for its eradication. Immunization of certain populations (eg, military recruits, college students living in dormitories, Hajj pilgrims, patients with terminal complement component deficiencies or asplenia) is also recommended. Two meningococcal vaccines are currently available for serogroups A, C, Y, and W-135: the older polysaccharide vaccine (Menomune [Sanofi Pasteur Inc]) and a newer conjugate vaccine (Menactra [Sanofi Pasteur Inc], meningococcal vaccine [MCV4]) that offers longer protection. The MCV4 vaccine is now recommended as part of the routine vaccine series in children.

KEY FACTS

✓ *Neisseria meningitidis* infection often begins with a mild upper respiratory tract illness, which may disseminate into the bloodstream and leads to a petechial rash that often occurs around the same time as fever and meningeal signs

✓ Meningococcal immunization is recommended for military recruits; college students living in dormitories; pilgrims from Hajj, Saudi Arabia; and patients with terminal complement component deficiency or asplenia

---

Pneumococcus

Streptococcus pneumoniae is the most common cause of bacterial meningitis in adults (Figure 41.2), including those with recurrent meningitis due to CSF leaks. Meningitis due to susceptible strain of *S pneumoniae* can still be treated

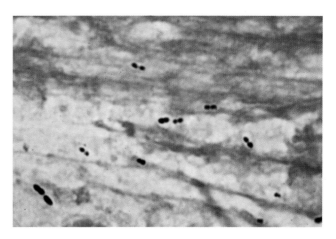

Figure 41.2 Streptococcus pneumoniae *in Sputum (Gram Stain).*

successfully with high-dose penicillin G. However, given the spread of penicillin-resistant strains, bacterial meningitis should be empirically treated with high-dose cefotaxime or ceftriaxone in combination with vancomycin while awaiting the susceptibility results (Table 41.1). Adjunctive treatment with dexamethasone has been shown to be beneficial when started at the same time as or before the first dose of antibiotic. The recommended treatment duration for pneumococcal meningitis is 10 to 14 days.

Haemophilus influenzae

Widespread use of the vaccine against *H influenzae* B has dramatically reduced the incidence of this invasive disease in children. Infections caused by *H influenzae* include pneumonia, meningitis, epiglottitis, sinusitis, otitis media, and primary bacteremia. The organism is also associated with infectious exacerbations of chronic obstructive pulmonary disease. Chronic lung disease, pregnancy, human immunodeficiency virus infection, hypogammaglobulinemia, splenectomy, and malignancy are risk factors for invasive disease.

Infection with *H influenzae* is now an uncommon cause of meningitis in adults, although it can occur with hypogammaglobulinemia, asplenia, or CSF leak. Third-generation cephalosporins (cefotaxime or ceftriaxone) are the drugs of choice for treatment of *H influenzae* meningitis. The recommended treatment duration is 7 days.

Listeria

Listeria monocytogenes is a small, motile, gram-positive rod. Meningitis and bacteremia are the most common presentation of *Listeria* infection. Elderly persons, neonates, pregnant women, and immunocompromised persons (eg, persons taking corticosteroids) are at highest risk for invasive disease due to *Listeria*. Epidemics have been associated with consumption of contaminated dairy products and some ready-to-eat foods, such as hot dogs and luncheon meats. Diarrhea is usually a feature of epidemic listeriosis. *Listeria* meningitis is often subacute. The organism may be difficult to visualize and CSF Gram stain is positive in only 25% to 30% of the cases.

Penicillin and ampicillin are the most effective agents against *Listeria*. Ampicillin coverage for *Listeria* should always be included for bacterial meningitis in patients older than 50 years or who are immunosuppressed, because *Listeria* is always resistant to cephalosporins. Combination therapy with an aminoglycoside is often recommended for treatment of severe disease. Trimethoprim-sulfamethoxazole is an effective alternative for the penicillin-allergic patient. Recommended treatment duration for *Listeria* meningitis is 3 weeks.

Group B β-Hemolytic Streptococci: *Streptococcus agalactiae*

This organism, a frequent part of the normal flora of the genital and gastrointestinal tracts, is an important cause of postpartum maternal and neonatal infections. It also is an important cause of bacteremia and metastatic infection in elderly adults, especially nursing home residents and those with chronic underlying diseases, such as diabetes. In this latter population, the mortality rate is as high as 38%. The penicillins are the treatment of choice for infections caused by *Streptococcus agalactiae*. Meningitis, which most commonly occurs in neonates, is best treated with penicillin (or ampicillin) plus gentamicin. Prepartum vaginal culture for group B streptococcus may identify persons at highest risk for infection and allow eradication of the organism before delivery.

Aseptic Meningitis and Encephalitis

Aseptic meningitis syndrome is characterized by an acute onset of meningeal symptoms, fever, CSF pleocytosis (usually lymphocytic), and negative CSF bacterial cultures. Noninfectious causes include medications, such as nonsteroidal anti-inflammatory drugs and trimethoprim-sulfamethoxazole; chemical meningitis; and neoplastic meningitis. Often, this syndrome is a meningoencephalitis due to viruses, which may be differentiated by an accurate exposure history and seasonality (Table 41.4).

CSF analysis should always be performed in cases of suspected meningoencephalitis. Cultures for bacteria and fungi and polymerase chain reaction (PCR) assays for herpes simplex virus (HSV), Epstein-Barr virus, varicella zoster virus, the enteroviruses, and *Mycobacterium tuberculosis* may be helpful. CSF and serum antigen tests for *Cryptococcus neoformans* and urine antigen tests for *Histoplasma* or *Blastomyces* may be useful in the appropriate clinical

Table 41.4 • Epidemiologic Clues to Infectious Causes of Acute Aseptic Meningitis and Meningoencephalitis

Season, Exposure, and Risk Factors	Pathogens
Late summer or fall	Enteroviruses
Winter	Mumps
Rodent urine	Lymphocytic choriomeningitis virus
Mosquito bites	Eastern and Western Equine viruses, West Nile virus, St. Louis virus, La Crosse virus
Ticks	*Borrelia burgdorferi, Ehrlichia,* or *Anaplasma* infection, Rocky Mountain spotted fever
Risk factors for sexually transmitted infections	Herpes simplex virus or human immunodeficiency virus
Immunocompromise	*Cryptococcus neoformans*
Travel to endemic area	Histoplasmosis, blastomycosis, coccidioidomycosis, Japanese encephalitis virus, yellow fever, rabies, tickborne encephalitis

setting. *Treponema pallidum* (syphilis) and *Borrelia burgdorferi* (Lyme disease) infections can be detected with the CSF Venereal Disease Research Laboratory (VDRL) test and serum *B burgdorferi*–specific antibody test. For patients in whom there is a clinical suspicion of HSV encephalitis but negative results on initial CSF PCR for HSV, repeat testing in 1 to 3 days may yield positive results.

Besides CSF testing, blood tests may be helpful for establishing a cause of encephalitis. Serologic testing for human immunodeficiency virus, Epstein-Barr virus, and *Mycoplasma pneumoniae* may be useful. Depending on the patient's epidemiologic exposure, additional serologic tests on serum samples may be indicated (Table 41.4).

Imaging may be helpful for establishing a cause of encephalitis. Magnetic resonance imaging may be helpful for localizing findings in specific infections such as HSV encephalitis (which localizes to the temporal lobes) (Figure 41.3). Electroencephalography can be helpful for identifying patients with nonconvulsive seizure activity who are confused, obtunded, or comatose. It shows characteristic periodic, lateralized epileptiform discharges in HSV encephalitis.

Empirical therapy for encephalitis should always include intravenous high-dose acyclovir and antibiotics (to cover the possibility of bacterial meningitis), including doxycycline when risk factors for *Rickettsia* or *Ehrlichia* infection are present. After an etiologic agent is identified, therapy should be targeted to that pathogen and the use of other antimicrobial agents should be discontinued. Recommended treatment duration for HSV encephalitis is 14 to 21 days.

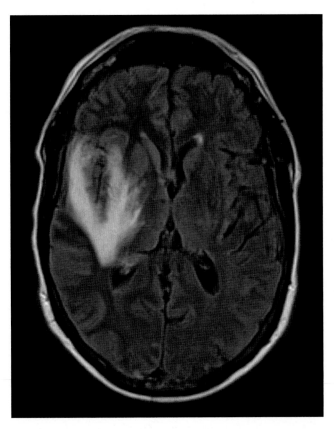

Figure 41.3 *Herpes Simplex Virus Encephalitis Localized in the Temporal Lobe, Seen With Magnetic Resonance Imaging.*
(Adapted from Knipe H, Gaillard F, et al. Herpes simplex encephalitis [Internet]. Radiopaedia.org. c2015 Dr Frank Gaillard [cited 2015 Jul 9]. Available from: http://radiopaedia.org/articles/herpes-simplex-encephalitis. Used with permission.)

Chronic Meningitis Syndrome

Signs and symptoms of meningeal inflammation are more subtle in chronic meningitis and evolve over weeks to months. Chronic meningitis may be due to either infectious or noninfectious causes. Delayed presentation with apathy or altered mentation can occur. The CSF profile typically shows long-term inflammatory changes. The causative agents include *Brucella*, *Nocardia*, spirochetes (eg, syphilis, Lyme disease), fungi (eg, *Cryptococcus, Coccidioides, Histoplasma, Blastomyces*), mycobacteria, and parasites.

Other Causes of Central Nervous System Infections

Poliovirus

Although wild-type polio has been eliminated from the Western Hemisphere, it continues to be endemic in parts of Asia and Africa. Disease still can be imported from these areas. Polio is most often an asymptomatic infection. The virus affects the nuclei of cranial nerves and anterior motor neurons of the spinal cord, causing a flaccid paralysis. When paralysis develops, it is usually asymmetrical. A polio like illness in the United States, without personal travel or exposure, should also raise suspicion for West Nile virus.

Rabies

A high index of suspicion is a requisite for antemortem diagnosis of rabies. Cardinal clinical manifestations are hydrophobia and copious salivation. Rabies should be considered in any case of encephalitis or myelitis of unknown cause, especially in persons who have recently traveled outside the United States. The virus spreads along peripheral nerves to the central nervous system. The most common source of exposure in the world is dogs; in the United States, bats, foxes, raccoons, and skunks are often implicated.

Rabies acquisition in the United States is predominantly related to bat bites, which may not be apparent, especially when they occur during sleep. Aerosol spread is possible, and it is most often due to exposure to bats during spelunking or working in a medical laboratory. Annually, 1 or 2 cases of rabies are reported in the United States. From 1995 to 2006, 7 of the 37 cases in the United States were due to exposure to rabid animals outside the country, whereas the majority of the rest (28, including 4 transplant recipients who had a donor with rabies) were from exposure to bats in the United States.

Definitive diagnosis of rabies encephalitis is established by finding Negri bodies on biopsy of the hippocampus. Serum and CSF can be tested for rabies antibodies when trying to diagnose the disease. Direct fluorescent antibody testing of a skin biopsy specimen from the nape of the neck can be used to detect rabies antigen.

Any bite by bats or other animals suspected of carrying rabies should be taken seriously. Postbite management includes observing the animal, if possible; immediate soap and water washing of the wound; administering rabies immunoglobulin (injected into the bite site); and starting the postexposure rabies vaccine schedule. Human rabies

KEY FACTS

✓ Aseptic meningitis syndrome involves acute onset of meningeal symptoms, fever, CSF pleocytosis, and negative CSF bacterial cultures

✓ Empirical therapy for encephalitis should always include intravenous high-dose acyclovir and antibiotics, including doxycycline when risk factors for *Rickettsia* or *Ehrlichia* infection are present

immunoglobulin is widely available; however, rabies immunoglobulin and vaccine are not of benefit after the onset of clinical disease. Preexposure rabies vaccination is advised for patients likely to be in situations that put them at high risk for rabies, such as occupational exposure in veterinary medicine, spelunking, and prolonged stay in rabies-endemic countries. Preexposure vaccination mitigates the need for rabies immunoglobulin and decreases the number of postexposure doses to 2 (days 0 and 3 after the bite).

Slow Viruses and Prion-Associated Central Nervous System Diseases

Progressive Multifocal Leukoencephalopathy

Progressive multifocal leukoencephalopathy is caused by a papovavirus (JC virus) and usually occurs in immunocompromised patients, such as those with acquired immunodeficiency syndrome, leukemia, lymphoma, certain mediations (eg, natalizumab), and immunosuppression for organ transplant. It can cause either diffuse or focal central nervous system abnormalities. Despite its name, progressive multifocal leukoencephalopathy usually causes solitary brain lesions, as seen on computed tomography or magnetic resonance imaging. CSF analysis is normal in most cases, and the diagnosis is based on brain biopsy. Detection of JC virus DNA in CSF with PCR

testing in appropriate clinical context confirms the diagnosis. However, the sensitivity of this test is low. There is no effective therapy directed at the JC virus. However, antiretroviral drugs in patients with AIDS and reduction of immunosuppression in transplant patients usually lead to improvement.

Creutzfeldt-Jakob Disease

This is a rare degenerative and fatal disease of the central nervous system. It occurs equally in both sexes, usually at older ages. The disease has both familial and sporadic forms. It usually presents as rapidly evolving dementia with myoclonic seizures. **Prions** (small proteinaceous infectious particles without nucleic acid) have been proposed as the cause of this disease. Nosocomial transmission of Creutzfeldt-Jakob disease can occur via corneal transplant and exposure to CSF. Creutzfeldt-Jakob disease has no treatment.

Key Definitions

Creutzfeldt-Jakob Disease: *A rare degenerative and fatal disease of the central nervous system with familial and sporadic forms and no treatment.*

Prions: *Small proteinaceous infectious particles without nucleic acid.*

42 HIV Infection[a]

MARY J. KASTEN, MD AND ZELALEM TEMESGEN, MD

Transmission

Human immunodeficiency virus (HIV) is transmitted sexually, perinatally, through parenteral inoculation (eg, intravenous drug injection, occupational exposure), through blood products, and, less commonly, through donated organs or semen (Table 42.1). Sexual transmission is the most common means of infection. Conditions that may increase the risk of sexually acquiring HIV infection include traumatic intercourse (ie, receptive anal), ulcerative genital infections (including syphilis, herpes simplex, and chancroid), and lack of male circumcision. The proper use of latex condoms substantially reduces the risk of HIV transmission. Nonoxynol spermicide increases the risk of HIV transmission; therefore, condoms that do not contain spermicide are preferred for HIV prevention. Condoms with spermicide do offer some protection compared with not using a condom, however. Perinatal transmission can occur in utero, at birth, and through breast milk.

Laboratory Diagnosis

The Centers for Disease Control and Prevention (CDC) updated the testing algorithm for diagnosing HIV in 2014 (Figure 42.1). The recommended testing is a combination immunoassay that detects HIV-1 and HIV-2 antibodies and HIV p24 antigen. Positive specimens undergo secondary testing to differentiate HIV-1 antibodies from HIV-2 antibodies. Specimens that are negative or indeterminate on this secondary testing undergo HIV-1 nucleic acid testing for

Table 42.1 • Risk of HIV Infection by Type of Exposure

Type of Exposure	Risk, %
Transfusion of HIV-positive blood	>90
Percutaneous needlestick	0.3
Receptive anal intercourse	0.5
Receptive penile-vaginal intercourse	0.1
Insertive intercourse	0.05–0.07
Oral intercourse	0.005–0.01
Blood to mucous membranes	0.09
Blood to nonintact skin	<0.1

Abbreviation: HIV, human immunodeficiency virus.

resolution. Specimens that are negative on the nucleic acid testing are considered to be false-positive results. This testing sequence provides a more accurate diagnosis of acute HIV testing than previous screening that involved only antibody testing. The combined immunoassay has an increased likelihood of being positive because of the presence of p24 antigen in the serum, usually by 15 days after infection.

The CDC and the US Preventive Services Task Force both recommend that screening for HIV infection be performed routinely for all patients 13 to 64 years old. An opt-out approach, similar to what has been used successfully for many years with pregnant women, is recommended. With the opt-out approach, testing is performed after the patient is notified, unless the patient declines. Neither separate written consent nor prevention counseling is required.

---

[a] Portions previously published in Warnke D, Barreto J, Temesgen Z. Antiretroviral drugs. J Clin Pharmacol. 2007 Dec;47(12):1570–9. Used with permission; treatment guidelines for opportunistic infections based on Benson CA, Kaplan JE, Masur H, Pau A, Holmes KK; CDC; National Institutes of Health; Infectious Diseases Society of America. Treating opportunistic infections among HIV-infected adults and adolescents: recommendations from CDC, the National Institutes of Health, and the HIV Medicine Association/Infectious Diseases Society of America. MMWR Recomm Rep. 2004 Dec 17;53(RR-15):1–112. Erratum in: MMWR Morb Mortal Wkly Rep. 2005 Apr 1;54(12):311.

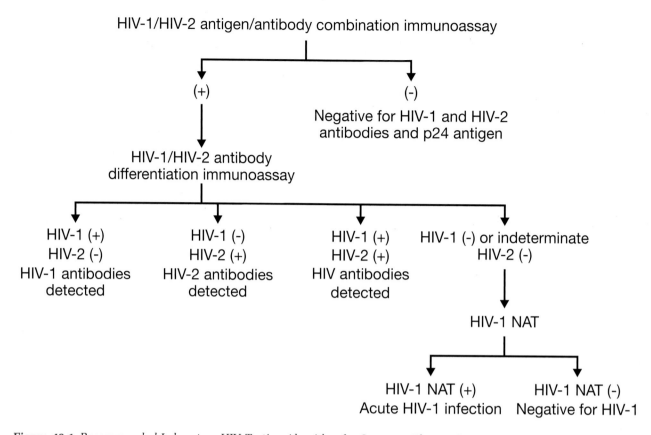

Figure 42.1 *Recommended Laboratory HIV Testing Algorithm for Serum or Plasma Specimens. HIV indicates human immunodeficiency virus; NAT, nucleic acid test; +, reactive test result; -, nonreactive test result.*
(Adapted from Centers for Disease Control and Prevention and National Center for HIV/AIDS, Viral Hepatitis, STD, and TB Prevention. Laboratory testing for the diagnosis of HIV infection: updated recommendations. Published June 27, 2014 [cited 2014 Sep 11] Available from: http://stacks.cdc.gov/view/cdc/23447.)

Patients who engage in behaviors that place them at risk for HIV infection should be screened on a regular basis. All pregnant women should be screened for HIV infection with each pregnancy. Chronic HIV infection should be considered in patients with many different presentations; some of the more common clues are listed in Box 42.1.

KEY FACTS

✓ The CDC updated the testing algorithm for diagnosing HIV infection in 2014. The recommended testing is a combination immunoassay that detects HIV-1 and HIV-2 antibodies and HIV p24 antigen

✓ The current testing sequence provides a more accurate diagnosis of acute HIV testing than previous screening that involved only antibody testing. The combination immunoassay has fewer false negatives because of the presence of p24 antigen in the serum by 15 days after infection

✓ The CDC and the US Preventive Services Task Force both recommend that screening for HIV infection be performed routinely for all patients aged 13 to 64 years

✓ All pregnant women should be screened for HIV infection with each pregnancy

---

Natural History of HIV Disease

Acute HIV Infection

Days to weeks after exposure to HIV, most infected persons present with a brief illness that may last from a few days to a few weeks. This period of illness is associated with an enormous amount of circulating virus, a rapid decline in the CD4 cell count, and a vigorous immune response. Occasionally, CD4 counts decrease to levels at which patients can present with opportunistic illness. Patients often present with a mononucleosis like illness, but the clinical manifestations of acute HIV infection are extremely varied (Table 42.2).

Chronic HIV Infection

After acute HIV infection, CD4 counts rebound, although frequently not to baseline, and the viral load decreases to a set point that often stays stable for years. Over time, most patients have a gradual loss of CD4 cells. Some patients continue to be asymptomatic with relatively preserved CD4 counts for more than a decade; other patients progress to AIDS in 2 to 3 years. The loss of CD4 cells eventually places the person at risk for opportunistic infections and other complications of HIV infection. The CDC defines

Box 42.1 • Common Clinical Clues to Chronic HIV Infection

History of high-risk behavior

History of a sexually transmitted disease

Request for HIV testing

Active tuberculosis

Herpes zoster in a person <50 y old

New severe flare of psoriasis

Unexplained severe skin disorder

Hepatitis B or C virus infection

Cervical cancer or HPV infection

Thrush not related to recent antibiotic use

Unexplained cachexia or weight loss

Diffuse lymphadenopathy

Unexplained thrombocytopenia, leukopenia, or anemia

Unusual neurologic illness

History of unusual infection in an otherwise healthy person

Prolonged unexplained illness

Abbreviations: HIV, human immunodeficiency virus; HPV, human papillomavirus.

Adapted from Kasten MJ. Human immunodeficiency virus: the initial physician-patient encounter. Mayo Clin Proc. 2002 Sep;77(9):957–63. Used with permission of Mayo Foundation for Medical Education and Research.

AIDS as known HIV infection with a CD4 count less than 200 cells/mcL or HIV infection associated with an AIDS-defining illness (Box 42.2).

Key Definition

AIDS: *known HIV infection with a CD4 count less than 200 cells/mcL or HIV infection associated with an AIDS-defining illness.*

The illnesses and conditions associated with HIV infection vary greatly depending on a person's CD4 count and behaviors. Figure 42.2 illustrates the natural history of HIV infection and the stages at which conditions that are commonly associated with HIV infection occur.

KEY FACTS

✓ Patients often present with a mononucleosis like illness, but the clinical manifestations of acute HIV infection are extremely varied

✓ The CDC defines AIDS as known HIV infection with a CD4 count less than 200 cells/mcL or HIV infection associated with an AIDS-defining illness

Table 42.2 • Frequency of Symptoms and Findings Associated With Acute HIV-1 Infection

Symptom or Finding	Patients, %
Fever	>80–90
Fatigue	>70–90
Rash	>40–80
Headache	32–70
Lymphadenopathy	40–70
Pharyngitis	50–70
Myalgia or arthralgia	50–70
Nausea, vomiting, or diarrhea	30–60
Night sweats	50
Aseptic meningitis	24
Oral ulcers	10–20
Genital ulcers	5–15
Thrombocytopenia	45
Leukopenia	40
Elevated hepatic enzyme levels	21

Abbreviation: HIV-1, human immunodeficiency virus type 1.

Adapted from Kahn JO, Walker BD. Acute human immunodeficiency virus type 1 infection. N Engl J Med. 1998 Jul 2;339(1):33–9. Used with permission.

Box 42.2 • AIDS-Defining Conditions in Adults

Candidiasis of bronchi, trachea, or lungs

Candidiasis, esophageal

Cervical cancer, invasive

Coccidioidomycosis, disseminated or extrapulmonary

Cryptococcosis, extrapulmonary

Cryptosporidiosis, chronic intestinal (>1 mo duration)

CMV disease (other than liver, spleen, or nodes)

CMV retinitis (with loss of vision)

Encephalopathy, HIV-related

Herpes simplex: chronic ulcer(s) (>1 mo duration) or bronchitis, pneumonitis, or esophagitis

Histoplasmosis, disseminated or extrapulmonary

Isosporiasis, chronic intestinal (>1 mo duration)

Kaposi sarcoma

Lymphoma, Burkitt (or equivalent term)

Lymphoma, immunoblastic (or equivalent term)

Lymphoma, primary, of brain

Mycobacterium avium complex or *Mycobacterium kansasii*, disseminated or extrapulmonary

Mycobacterium tuberculosis, any site

Mycobacterium, other species or unidentified species, disseminated or extrapulmonary

Pneumocystis jiroveci pneumonia

(continued on next page)

Pneumonia, recurrent

Progressive multifocal leukoencephalopathy

Salmonella septicemia, recurrent

Toxoplasmosis of brain

Wasting syndrome due to HIV infection

Abbreviations: CMV, cytomegalovirus; HIV, human immunodeficiency virus.

Adapted from Schneider E, Whitmore S, Glynn MK, Dominguez K, Mitsch A, McKenna MT. Revised surveillance case definitions for HIV infection among adults, adolescents, and children aged <18 months and for HIV infection and AIDS among children aged 18 months to <13 years—United States, 2008. MMWR Morb Mortal Wkly Rep. 2008 Dec 5;57(RR10):1–8.

Primary Care and HIV Infection

Immunizations

Patients with HIV infection should have routine immunizations, but live virus vaccines should be given cautiously and generally are avoided in patients with CD4 counts less than 200 cells/mcL. Clinicians should consider repeating immunizations for patients immunized when they had low CD4 cell counts after their immune system has improved.

All patients with HIV infection who are not immune to or infected with hepatitis B virus should receive the hepatitis B vaccination series. Antibody response to the hepatitis B vaccine is poorer in HIV-infected patients than noninfected patients, and a "double-dose" vaccine is recommended. Antibody response to the vaccination should be verified after the series is completed. Deferring this vaccination series until the patient's CD4 count is more than 200 cells/mcL is reasonable for improvement of response rates.

Hepatitis A vaccine is recommended for all patients who are at risk, including men who have sex with men, travelers to developing countries, and patients with hepatitis B or C or other liver disease.

All patients with HIV infection should receive the pneumococcal conjugate vaccine (PCV13) unless they have received a dose of pneumococcal polysaccharide vaccine-23 (PPV23) within the past year. These patients should receive the PCV13 a year after their PPV23. If a patient has not had the PPV23 and has a CD4 count of more than 200 cells/mcL, the PCV13 should be given and should be followed with the PPV23 at 8 or more weeks later. A second dose of PPV23 should be given 5 or more years following the first dose. Many providers defer PPV23 in HIV-infected patients until their CD4 count improves, ideally to more than 200 cells/mcL.

The quadrivalent human papillomavirus vaccine is recommended for HIV-infected women and men between ages 11 and 26 years.

All HIV-infected patients should receive an annual inactivated influenza vaccine.

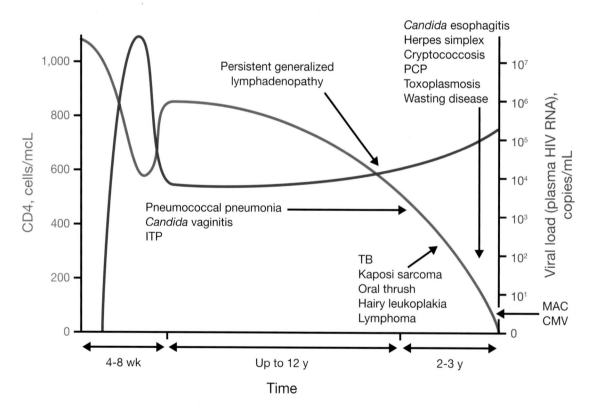

Figure 42.2 *Natural History of HIV Infection: CD4 Counts, Viral Load, and Clinical Manifestations. CMV indicates cytomegalovirus; HIV, human immunodeficiency virus; ITP, idiopathic thrombocytopenic purpura; MAC, Mycobacterium avium complex; PCP, Pneumocystis pneumonia; TB, tuberculosis.*

Prophylaxis Against Opportunistic Infections

HIV-infected persons are susceptible to many unusual infections, depending on their CD4 counts. A few of these infections can be prevented with immunization or appropriate prophylaxis. Recommendations and indications for primary prevention of *Pneumocystis* pneumonia (PCP), *Mycobacterium avium* complex (MAC) infection, and toxoplasmosis are listed in Table 42.3. Primary prophylaxis against other infections is not routinely recommended; primary prophylaxis against PCP and toxoplasmosis can be discontinued when the CD4 count is 200 cells/mcL or more for 3 months or longer. Primary prophylaxis against MAC can be discontinued when the CD4 count is 100 cells/mcL or more for 3 months or longer.

Cancer Screening

Three cancers—Kaposi sarcoma, non-Hodgkin lymphoma, and invasive cervical cancer—have been designated as AIDS-defining cancers. Several other malignancies, although not classified as *AIDS-defining*, seem to be more common among people infected with HIV. HIV-infected patients who are generally well, whether receiving antiretroviral treatment or not, should have routine cancer screening as recommended for uninfected persons, with the exception of the need for more frequent Papanicolaou (Pap) smears. Women with HIV infection should have a cervical Pap smear at the time of diagnosis.

Cotesting—Pap smear and HPV testing—is not recommended for HIV-infected women younger than 30 years. When Pap smears alone are used for cervical cancer screening, the test should be repeated in 12 months if the result is normal. After 3 consecutive normal Pap smears, testing can decrease to every 3 years if Pap smears continue to be normal. Women older than 30 years can be screened with cotesting, and if results are normal, screening every 3 years is recommended. HIV-infected women should have continued screening with either Pap smears or cotesting even after age 65 years unlike for the general population. HIV-infected women with abnormal Pap smears should be monitored by a practitioner with expertise in preventing cervical cancer in HIV infection. An anal Pap smear should be considered for men and women who have a history of receptive anal intercourse, an abnormal Pap smear, or a history of genital warts because of the increased incidence of human papillomavirus–related anal cell cancer.

KEY FACT

✓ HIV-infected women should have a cervical Pap smear at the time of diagnosis. Cotesting—Pap smear and HPV testing—is not recommended for HIV-infected women younger than 30 years. When Pap smears alone are used for cervical screening, the test should be repeated in 12 months if the result is normal

Selected Infections and Conditions Associated With HIV Infection

Pneumocystis Pneumonia

PCP is one of the most common opportunistic infections in patients with AIDS. It typically occurs in patients with CD4 counts less than 200 cells/mcL. The onset of illness is usually insidious, with several days to weeks of fever, exertional dyspnea, chest discomfort, weight loss, malaise, and night sweats. Chest radiography typically shows bilateral interstitial pulmonary infiltrates; a lobar distribution and spontaneous pneumothoraces may also occur. Patients with early disease can have a normal chest radiograph. Thin-section computed tomography usually shows patchy ground-glass infiltrates. Arterial blood gas analysis usually shows hypoxemia and respiratory alkalosis. Levels of $1\text{-}3\text{-}\beta\text{-}D\text{-}glucan$ levels are elevated (>80 pg/mL) and are supportive of a PCP diagnosis.

Definitive diagnosis of PCP is made through visualization of the organism. In HIV-infected persons, staining for *Pneumocystis* organisms in hypertonic saline-induced expectorated sputum is 55% to 90% sensitive, and bronchoalveolar lavage is 90% to 97% sensitive.

The treatment of choice for PCP is trimethoprim-sulfamethoxazole. The usual recommended dosage is 15 mg/kg per day (trimethoprim component) in 3 or 4 equally divided doses for 21 days. If no improvement occurs 4 to 8 days after treatment is begun, a different drug should be

Table 42.3 • Primary Prophylaxis for PCP, Toxoplasmosis, and MAC

Pathogen/Disease	Indication	First-Choice Therapy
Pneumocystis jiroveci/PCP	CD4 <200 cells/mcL or oropharyngeal candidiasis	TMP-SMX
Toxoplasma gondii/encephalitis	*Toxoplasma* IgG-positive with CD4 <100 cells/mcL	TMP-SMX DS
MAC/MAC disease	CD4 <50 cells/mcL after ruling out active MAC infection	Azithromycin *or* clarithromycin

Abbreviations: DS, double strength; IgG, immunoglobulin G; MAC, *Mycobacterium avium* complex; PCP, *Pneumocystis* pneumonia; TMP-SMX, trimethoprim-sulfamethoxazole.

Adapted from Kaplan JE, Benson C, Holmes KK, Brooks JT, Pau A, Masur H. Guidelines for prevention and treatment of opportunistic infections in HIV-infected adults and adolescents: recommendations from CDC, the National Institutes of Health, and the HIV Medicine Association of the Infectious Diseases Society of America. MMWR Morb Mortal Wkly Rep. 2009 Apr 10;58(RR04):1–198.

Box 42.3 • **Preferred Drug Therapy for PCP**

For moderate to severe PCP

TMP-SMX: 15–20 mg TMP and 75–100 mg SMX/kg daily, IV administered every 6 to 8 h, may switch to orally after clinical improvement

Duration: 21 d

For mild to moderate PCP

Same daily dose of TMP-SMX as above, administered orally in 3 divided doses, *or* TMP-SMX (160 mg/800 mg or DS), 2 tablets 3 times daily

Duration: 21 d

Abbreviations: DS, double strength; IV, intravenously; PCP, *Pneumocystis* pneumonia; TMP-SMX, trimethoprim-sulfamethoxazole.

Adapted from Kaplan JE, Benson C, Holmes KK, Brooks JT, Pau A, Masur H. Guidelines for prevention and treatment of opportunistic infections in HIV-infected adults and adolescents: recommendations from CDC, the National Institutes of Health, and the HIV Medicine Association of the Infectious Diseases Society of America. MMWR Morb Mortal Wkly Rep. 2009 Apr 10;58(RR04):1–198.

Box 42.4 • **Regimens for the Treatment of Latent Tuberculosis**

Isoniazid 300 mg orally daily for 9 mo[a]

Isoniazid 900 mg twice weekly for 9 mo[a]

Rifampin 600 mg orally daily for 4 mo

Isoniazid 15 mg/kg orally once weekly and a weight-based rifapentine dose orally once weekly through directly observed therapy for 12 wk

[a] These regimens are preferred for persons infected with human immunodeficiency virus.

---

considered (Box 42.3). Controlled studies have shown that adjunctive corticosteroid therapy increases survival in patients with moderate to severe disease, defined as room air Po_2 less than 70 mm Hg or an alveolar-arterial Po_2 difference (A-a gradient) greater than 35 mm Hg. When indicated, adjunctive corticosteroid therapy should be started immediately; a delay may compromise its effectiveness.

KEY FACTS

✓ PCP is one of the most common opportunistic infections in persons with AIDS. It typically occurs in those with CD4 counts less than 200 cells/mcL

✓ The treatment of choice for PCP is trimethoprim-sulfamethoxazole

---

Tuberculosis

Tuberculosis (TB) is the most common HIV-associated opportunistic infection globally. TB is a preventable disease in patients with HIV infection; all such patients should be screened with either a tuberculin skin test or an interferon-γ release assay. All HIV-infected patients with a positive test result (≥5 mm for the skin test), a past history of a positive test result, or recent exposure to a person with active TB should be treated for latent TB, provided they have no symptoms or signs to suggest active infection and they have not been treated previously. Effective treatment programs for latent TB are reviewed in Box 42.4.

TB occurs among HIV-infected persons at all CD4 counts. However, clinical manifestations generally differ depending on the degree of immunosuppression. When TB occurs late in the course of HIV infection, it tends to have atypical features, such as extrapulmonary disease, disseminated disease, and an unusual chest radiographic appearance (eg, lower lung zone lesions, intrathoracic adenopathy, diffuse infiltrations, lower frequency of cavitation). Patients with low CD4 counts and TB have a high mortality rate (70%) and often have a fulminant course leading to death in 2 to 3 months. When TB occurs early in the course of HIV infection (CD4 count >350 cells/mcL), it tends to manifest with the classic presentation of upper-lobe fibronodular infiltrates with cavitation.

The diagnosis of TB requires evaluation with a chest radiograph, sputum samples for acid-fast bacillus smear and culture, and aspiration or tissue biopsy when extrapulmonary disease is suspected. Mycobacterial blood cultures are useful in cases of disseminated disease. In patients with relatively intact immune function, the yield of sputum smear and culture is similar to that in HIV-negative patients.

The treatment of HIV-infected patients is complex when they are taking antiretroviral agents and undergoing therapy for active TB. Protease inhibitors and nonnucleoside analogue reverse transcriptase inhibitors have clinically significant interactions with the rifamycins—rifampin, rifabutin, and rifapentine—used to treat mycobacterial infections. TB in HIV-infected persons that is susceptible to all first-line antituberculosis drugs may be treated with the standard 6-month drug program.

Clinicians should consider factors that increase a person's risk of a poor clinical outcome (eg, lack of adherence to TB therapy, delayed conversion of *Mycobacterium tuberculosis* sputum cultures from positive to negative, delayed clinical response) when deciding the total duration of TB therapy. Directly observed therapy is recommended. Patients who have successfully completed a treatment regimen for TB do not require secondary prophylaxis or long-term maintenance therapy. Patients with multiple drug–resistant TB illnesses are at high risk for relapse and treatment failure. Treatment regimens for these patients are complex and require expertise in the management of both TB and HIV infection.

MAC Infection

Organisms of MAC are ubiquitous in the environment and include *M avium* and *Mycobacterium intracellulare*. They cause disseminated infection in HIV-infected persons, especially when immunosuppression is severe (CD4 count <50 cells/mcL). Disseminated MAC infection is a common systemic bacterial infection in patients with AIDS and very low CD4 counts. Common presentations include low-grade fever, night sweats, weight loss, fatigue, abdominal pain, and diarrhea. Hepatomegaly, splenomegaly, and lymphadenopathy may be present. Common laboratory abnormalities include anemia and increased alkaline phosphatase levels. Blood cultures are usually positive; however, organisms can be isolated also from stool, respiratory tract secretions, bone marrow, liver, and other biopsy specimens.

The MAC organisms are resistant to conventional antimycobacterial agents. The current recommended treatment regimen includes one of the newer macrolides (eg, clarithromycin, azithromycin), ethambutol, and 1 or 2 additional drugs with activity against MAC.

Cryptococcus neoformans Disease

Cryptococcus neoformans is a yeast acquired through inhalation. It can cause symptomatic pneumonia, particularly in immunocompromised persons or in persons with lung disease. The organism has a strong propensity for dissemination to the central nervous system. The most common manifestation of *C neoformans* disease in HIV-infected patients is cryptococcal meningitis, which usually occurs when the CD4 count is less than 50 cells/mcL. The onset is insidious; symptoms are nonspecific (eg, fever, headache, malaise) and may have a waxing and waning course. Classic meningeal symptoms (eg, neck stiffness, photophobia) are present in only one-fourth to one-third of patients with

HIV and *C neoformans* disease. Brain imaging findings are nonspecific; cerebral atrophy and ventricular enlargement are the most common findings. Cerebrospinal fluid (CSF) findings may be minimal but frequently include increased opening pressure, mild mononuclear pleocytosis, and increased protein value. Glucose levels may be normal or slightly low. The India ink preparation is positive in more than 70% of cases. The serum and CSF cryptococcal antigen test has a sensitivity of 93% to 99% for cryptococcal meningitis. Cultures of CSF are usually positive. Blood cultures are positive for *C neoformans* in up to 75% of HIV-infected persons with cryptococcal meningitis.

Adverse prognostic factors include altered mental status on presentation and high fungal burden (ie, positive result of India ink test, high antigen titers, and extraneural disease). Increased intracranial pressure is common and may be associated with headache, confusion, or cranial nerve palsies. Aggressive management of intracranial pressure with daily lumbar puncture or placement of lumbar drains substantially minimizes morbidity and death from this illness.

Initial therapy should include amphotericin B with flucytosine for 2 weeks, followed by fluconazole 400 mg daily for a total of 10 weeks. This initial therapy is followed by fluconazole 200 mg daily for long-term maintenance therapy. Such long-term maintenance therapy can be discontinued when the patient continues to be asymptomatic and has a sustained increase in CD4 count to more than 200 cells/mcL for 6 months.

Cytomegalovirus

Serious cytomegalovirus (CMV) disease in HIV infection is not seen until advanced HIV disease (CD4 count <50 cells/mcL). Other risk factors include previous opportunistic infections and a high plasma HIV-1 RNA level (>100,000 copies/mL). Chorioretinitis is the most common clinical manifestation of CMV in patients with HIV infection. The usual symptoms are floaters, visual field deficits, and painless loss of vision. Funduscopic examination shows

Table 42.4 • Drugs Used for Treatment of CMV Disease

Drug	Major Adverse Effect
Systemic anti-CMV therapy	
Ganciclovir IV	Bone marrow suppression
Valganciclovir	Bone marrow suppression
Foscarnet IV	Renal toxicity
Cidofovir IV[a]	Renal toxicity
Local anti-CMV therapy for retinitis	
Ganciclovir intraocular-release device[b]	Retinal detachment
Ganciclovir intravitreal injection[b]	Bone marrow suppression
Foscarnet intravitreal injection[b]	Renal toxicity

Abbreviations: CMV, cytomegalovirus; IV, intravenously.

[a] Vigorous hydration and coadministration of probenecid are required to limit renal toxicity.

[b] Local anti-CMV therapy should be accompanied by systemic therapy, such as oral ganciclovir, to avoid the risk of extraocular diseases.

yellowish or white retinal infiltrates with or without intraretinal hemorrhage. In CMV gastrointestinal disease, the esophagus and colon are most commonly involved, and the disease manifests with dysphagia, abdominal pain, and bloody diarrhea. Hepatitis, pneumonitis, sclerosing cholangitis, encephalitis, adrenalitis, polyradiculopathy, and myelopathy can also be caused by CMV.

Agents used for the treatment of CMV disease and their general characteristics are listed in Table 42.4.

All patients with AIDS should undergo annual funduscopic examination to screen for CMV retinitis and other HIV-related eye disease and should have prompt evaluation of reported visual problems. Routine prophylaxis against CMV is not recommended because of concerns regarding treatment-induced toxicities (including neutropenia and anemia), potential resistance, conflicting reports of efficacy, lack of proven survival benefit, and cost.

KEY FACTS

✓ CMV disease is not seen until advanced HIV disease (CD4 count <50 cells/mcL)

✓ Chorioretinitis is the most common clinical manifestation of CMV in patients with HIV infection

---

Toxoplasmosis

Toxoplasma gondii, a protozoan, is the most common cause of focal central nervous system lesions in patients with AIDS. The most common symptoms of *Toxoplasma* encephalitis include headache and confusion; fever may be absent. Focal neurologic deficits occur in 69% of cases. The median CD4 count at diagnosis is 50 cells/mcL. Multiple ring-enhancing lesions with associated edema are usually

noted on brain imaging studies. Magnetic resonance imaging is more sensitive than computed tomography for identifying lesions. The differential diagnosis of central nervous system mass lesions in patients with AIDS includes not only toxoplasmosis but also lymphoma and other infections, such as TB, cryptococcosis, histoplasmosis, bacterial abscess, and progressive multifocal leukoencephalitis.

Empirical antitoxoplasmosis therapy is indicated in patients with AIDS and positive *Toxoplasma* serologic testing who present with multiple intracranial lesions. The absence of anti–toxoplasma immunoglobulin G (IgG) antibody makes a diagnosis of toxoplasmosis unlikely. Effective treatment should result not only in amelioration of symptoms but also in a reduction of the number, size, and contrast medium enhancement of the brain lesions. If the patient has seronegativity for *Toxoplasma*, has a single mass lesion on both computed tomography and magnetic resonance imaging, or did not achieve the desired response after an empirical course of antitoxoplasmosis therapy for 10 to 14 days, the diagnosis of *Toxoplasma* encephalitis should be questioned and a diagnostic brain biopsy considered.

The initial regimen of choice for the treatment of HIV-associated toxoplasmosis is the combination of pyrimethamine plus sulfadiazine plus leucovorin. All HIV-infected persons with a CD4 count of less than 100 cells/mcL who have seropositivity for *Toxoplasma* should receive primary prophylaxis against *Toxoplasma* encephalitis (Table 42.3).

HIV-infected patients should be tested for IgG antibody to *Toxoplasma* as part of their initial work-up. If the result is negative, they should be counseled about the various potential sources of *Toxoplasma* infection, including consumption of raw or undercooked meat or shellfish and handling of cat litter.

KEY FACTS

✓ *Toxoplasma gondii* is the most common cause of focal central nervous system lesions in patients with AIDS

✓ The most common symptoms of *Toxoplasma* encephalitis include headache and confusion; fever may be absent

✓ The median CD4 count at diagnosis of toxoplasmosis is 50 cells/mcL

✓ Multiple ring-enhancing lesions with associated edema are usually noted on brain imaging studies

✓ All HIV-infected persons with a CD4 count of less than 100 cells/mcL who are seropositive for *Toxoplasma* should receive primary prophylaxis against *Toxoplasma* encephalitis

---

Progressive Multifocal Leukoencephalopathy

Progressive multifocal leukoencephalopathy is a demyelinating disease caused by the JC virus, a polyomavirus.

Symptoms and signs are progressive, variable, and usually long term or subacute. Symptoms include cognitive dysfunction, dementia, seizures, ataxia, aphasia, cranial nerve deficits, and focal deficits, such as hemiparesis and visual field deficits. Fever is usually absent. Occasionally, symptoms present rapidly and progress in a few weeks to dementia or coma.

Key Definition

Progressive multifocal leukoencephalopathy: *a demyelinating disease caused by JC virus, a polyomavirus.*

Diagnosis is based on clinical findings and magnetic resonance imaging, which shows characteristic white matter changes (bright areas on T2-weighted images) without contrast agent enhancement or mass effect. Routine CSF studies are generally nondiagnostic, but identification of JC virus DNA in the CSF through polymerase chain reaction may confirm the diagnosis. Absence of JC virus DNA does not rule out progressive multifocal leukoencephalopathy.

No specific therapy is established for progressive multifocal leukoencephalopathy. The prognosis has improved considerably with antiretroviral therapy (ART), and approximately one-half of patients with a good response to ART have long-term remission. Thus, all patients with progressive multifocal leukoencephalopathy should be receiving effective ART.

KEY FACTS

✓ Progressive multifocal leukoencephalopathy is a demyelinating disease caused by the JC virus

✓ Symptoms include cognitive dysfunction, dementia, seizures, ataxia, aphasia, cranial nerve deficits, and focal deficits (eg, hemiparesis, visual field deficits)

Mucocutaneous Candidiasis

Mucocutaneous disease, such as oral thrush, recurrent vaginitis, and candidal esophagitis, is common among HIV-infected persons. Candidal esophagitis is an AIDS-defining condition. Systemic candidal infection, including candidemia, is rare unless additional risk factors for disseminated fungal infection, such as severe neutropenia and indwelling catheters, are present.

Mucocutaneous disease can often be successfully treated with clotrimazole troches or nystatin suspension or pastilles. Fluconazole is used for the treatment of candidal esophagitis and topical treatment failures. Amphotericin B or caspofungin can be used when azole failures occur.

Diagnosis of oropharyngeal candidiasis is usually clinical and is based on the appearance of lesions. Visualization of the organisms in microscopic examination of scrapings provides supportive diagnostic information.

The diagnosis of esophageal candidiasis is usually made presumptively on clinical grounds (retrosternal burning pain or odynophagia in a patient with a low CD4 count or oral candidiasis). A diagnostic trial of antifungal therapy is recommended before endoscopy is used for identifying the cause of the disease. Fluconazole 100 to 400 mg daily by mouth is usually used for 14 to 21 days to treat esophageal candidiasis.

Long-term maintenance therapy for recurrent oropharyngeal or vulvovaginal candidiasis is not recommended unless recurrences are frequent or severe. Fluconazole 100 to 200 mg daily can be used to prevent esophageal candidiasis or other problematic candidiasis.

KEY FACTS

✓ The diagnosis of esophageal candidiasis in HIV-infected patients is usually made presumptively on clinical grounds (retrosternal burning pain or odynophagia in a patient with a low CD4 count or oral candidiasis)

✓ A diagnostic trial of antifungal therapy is recommended before endoscopy is used to identify the cause of the disease

---

Selected AIDS-Associated Malignancies

Kaposi Sarcoma

Kaposi sarcoma, a vascular tumor, is an AIDS-defining illness and is most common in men who have sex with men. Human herpesvirus 8 (HHV-8), also known as *Kaposi sarcoma–associated herpesvirus*, has been established as the etiologic agent of Kaposi sarcoma. HHV-8 appears to be sexually transmitted. With HIV, it synergistically acts to induce the changes of Kaposi sarcoma. Histologically, whorls of spindle-shaped cells and abnormal proliferation of small blood vessels are seen. Skin, lung, and the gastrointestinal tract are the commonly affected organs. Early on, skin lesions are often mistaken for benign vascular lesions.

Key Definition

Kaposi sarcoma: *vascular cancerous tumor that is AIDS-defining.*

Treatment options include local therapy (eg, radiotherapy, intralesional chemotherapy, cryotherapy) and systemic therapy (eg, chemotherapy, interferon-α). Liposome-encapsulated anthracycline chemotherapeutic agents enable delivery of high doses of effective drug with fewer adverse effects than with other agents. ART has resulted in a substantial reduction in the incidence of Kaposi sarcoma and has been associated with a reduction in tumor burden and disease progression. Therefore, ART is recommended for all HIV-infected patients with Kaposi sarcoma.

Non-Hodgkin Lymphoma

Non-Hodgkin lymphoma is much more common (as high as a 200-fold increased risk) among HIV-infected patients than in the general population. It is a heterogeneous group of malignancies with varying biologic behavior and occurs in patients with widely ranging levels of immune function. The vast majority of non-Hodgkin lymphomas in patients with HIV infection are of B-cell origin. Intermediate- or high-grade B-cell non-Hodgkin lymphoma in a patient with HIV infection is a CDC-defined AIDS diagnosis. As patients with AIDS live longer, this complication is likely to become more frequent. Non-Hodgkin lymphomas commonly present with constitutional symptoms (fever, night sweats, and weight loss), lymphadenopathy, and involvement of extranodal sites, such as the central nervous system, bone marrow, gastrointestinal tract, and liver. Involvement of the brain in non-Hodgkin lymphoma can manifest as an isolated disease (primary central nervous system lymphoma) or as leptomeningeal involvement in the context of spread of lymphoma elsewhere.

The optimal treatment of HIV-associated non-Hodgkin lymphoma has not been well defined. Current recommendations suggest that most patients should receive standard-dose chemotherapy, PCP prophylaxis (regardless of CD4 count), and growth factor support. In addition, highly active ART should be a component of therapy.

KEY FACT

✓ Non-Hodgkin lymphoma is much more common (as high as a 200-fold increased risk) among HIV-infected patients than in the general population

---

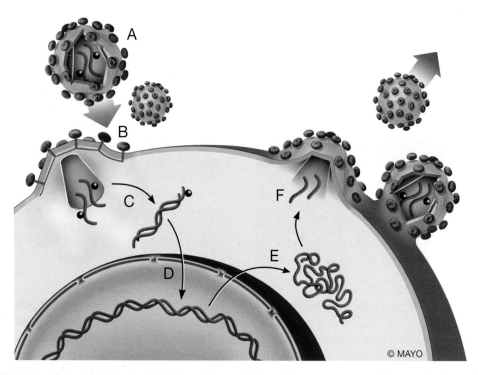

Figure 42.3 *Life Cycle of Human Immunodeficiency Virus. A, The virus is an enveloped virus that contains viral genomic RNA and various Gag and Pol protein products. B, The interaction between the envelope proteins of the virus and CD4 receptor and other receptors of the host cell leads to the binding of the viral envelope and the host cytoplasmic membrane. C, The viral reverse transcriptase enzyme catalyzes the conversion of viral RNA into DNA. D, The viral DNA enters the nucleus and becomes inserted into the chromosomal DNA of the host cell. E, Expression of the viral genes leads to production of viral RNA and proteins. F, These viral proteins, as well as viral RNA, are assembled at the cell surface into new viral particles and leave the host cell in a process called* budding. *During budding, they acquire the outer layer and envelope. At this stage, the protease enzyme cleaves the precursor Gag and Gag-Pol proteins into their mature products.*

Antiretroviral Agents

The Replication Cycle of HIV

A working knowledge of the HIV replication cycle is essential for understanding the mechanism of action of antiretroviral agents. Figure 42.3 reviews the interaction between the virus and the host cell that leads to production of infectious virions.

The 6 classes of antiretroviral drugs are nucleoside and nucleotide analogue reverse transcriptase inhibitors, nonnucleoside analogue reverse transcriptase inhibitors, protease inhibitors, fusion inhibitors, integrase inhibitors, and chemokine coreceptor antagonists. For details about common adverse effects of these medications, see Tables 42.5 through 42.8. A single fusion inhibitor enfuvirtide, also called *T20*, is only available in an injectable form and causes significant local site reactions and hypersensitivity reactions. Maraviroc is the only available chemokine coreceptor antagonist and can only be used for patients who have viruses that use the CCR5 receptor for entry into the CD4 cell. This characteristic can be measured with a tropism assay. Both enfuvirtide and maraviroc are used only in salvage programs and therefore are not further discussed.

Table 42.5 • General Characteristics of Nucleoside Analogue Reverse Transcriptase Inhibitors (NRTIs)*1 Commonly Used in the United States

Drug Name (Alias)	Toxic/Adverse Effects[a]
Abacavir (ABC)	Diarrhea, anorexia, nausea, vomiting, headache, fatigue **Contraindicated if HLA-B*5701 negative because of potential for fatal hypersensitivity reactions**
Emtricitabine (FTC)	Hyperpigmentation of skin, rash, diarrhea, nausea, vomiting, headache, adverse effects rare
Lamivudine (3TC)	Decrease in appetite, nausea, vomiting, headache, fatigue, adverse effects rare
Tenofovir (TDF)	Diarrhea, nausea, vomiting, **osteopenia, renal impairment**
Zidovudine (ZDV)	Headache, nausea, anorexia, vomiting, **anemia, leukopenia,** myopathy, lipoatrophy, hyperlipidemia

[a] *1 Class effect of lactic acidosis that presents with gastrointestinal prodrome and can rapidly progress to organ failure; risk is increased when more NRTIs are in a program.

Adapted from Panel on Antiretroviral Guidelines for Adults and Adolescents: Guidelines for the use of antiretroviral agents in HIV-1–infected adults and adolescents. Department of Health and Human Services. Apr 8, 2015; [cited 2015 Jul 23]. Available from: http://www.aidsinfo.nih.gov/ContentFiles/AdultandAdolescentGL.pdf.

Table 42.6 • General Characteristics of Nonnucleoside Reverse Transcriptase Inhibitors Commonly Used in the United States

Drug Name (Alias)	Toxic/Adverse Effects
Efavirenz (EFV)	Rash, **central nervous system (CNS) symptoms** (dizziness, light-headedness, abnormal dreams, difficulty with concentration), hepatotoxicity
Etravirine (ETR)	Rash, hypersensitivity reaction
Rilpivirine (RPV)	Headache, insomnia, depression (less CNS symptoms than EFV), transient rash, increased transaminase levels, increased total and LDL-C levels, may prolong QT interval **Requires acid for absorption**

Abbreviation: LDL-C, low-density lipoprotein cholesterol.

Adapted from Panel on Antiretroviral Guidelines for Adults and Adolescents: Guidelines for the use of antiretroviral agents in HIV-1–infected adults and adolescents. Department of Health and Human Services. Apr 8, 2015; [cited 2015 Jul 23]. Available from: http://www.aidsinfo.nih.gov/ContentFiles/AdultandAdolescentGL.pdf.

Guidelines for Use of ART for HIV Infection

Guidelines addressing the issue of ART in different populations and situations have been developed and receive regular updates electronically as new information becomes available (http://www.aidsinfo.nih.gov/). The benefits of ART are increasingly evident. Its benefit in reducing HIV-related illness and death has been clearly established.

An independent association between cumulative exposure to replicating virus over time and death has also been observed. Thus, although ART is beneficial even when started later in the course of HIV disease, experts are finding that the damage done by unchecked replication early in the HIV disease course may be irreparable. Furthermore, the public health benefit of ART has been recognized and the concept of "treatment as prevention" has been fully accepted as an important attribute of ART. A recent landmark study, HPTN 052, involving nearly 2,000 HIV-serodiscordant couples with CD4 counts of 350 to 550 cells/mm³ showed the benefit of early ART with a relative reduction of 96% in HIV-1 transmission to uninfected partners compared with delayed ART. Thus, ART is now recommended for all HIV-infected persons to both reduce the risk of disease progression and prevent HIV transmission.

KEY FACT

✓ ART is recommended for all HIV-infected persons to reduce risk of disease progression and to prevent HIV transmission

Table 42.7 • General Characteristics of Protease Inhibitors Commonly Used in the United States

Drug Name (Alias)	Toxic/Adverse Effects
Atazanavir (ATZ)	**Indirect hyperbilirubinemia**; prolonged PR interval, including symptomatic first-degree AV block; **nephrolithiasis**; hyperglycemia; fat maldistribution[a] **Requires acid for absorption**
Darunavir (DRV)	Rash, hepatotoxicity, diarrhea, nausea, headache, hyperlipidemia, transaminase increased, hyperglycemia, fat maldistribution[a]
Lopinavir/ ritonavir (LPV/r)	**GI tract intolerance, nausea, vomiting, diarrhea,** asthenia, **hyperlipidemia** (especially hypertriglyceridemia), **increased serum transaminases,** hyperglycemia, fat maldistribution[a]
Ritonavir (RTV)	**GI tract intolerance,** nausea, vomiting, diarrhea, paresthesias (circumoral and extremities), hyperlipidemia (especially hypertriglyceridemia), hepatitis, asthenia, taste perversion, **hyperglycemia,** fat maldistribution[a] Used to boost levels of other protease inhibitors
Saquinavir (SQV)	GI tract intolerance, nausea, diarrhea, headache, increased transaminase enzymes, hyperlipidemia, hyperglycemia, fat maldistribution[a]
Tipranavir (TPV)	Hepatotoxicity, including clinical hepatitis; rash; intracranial hemorrhages; hyperlipidemia (especially hypertriglyceridemia); hyperglycemia; fat maldistribution[a]

Abbreviations: AV, atrioventricular; GI, gastrointestinal.

[a] Possible increased bleeding episodes in patients with hemophilia.

Adapted from Panel on Antiretroviral Guidelines for Adults and Adolescents: Guidelines for the use of antiretroviral agents in HIV-1–infected adults and adolescents. Department of Health and Human Services. Apr 8, 2015; [cited 2015 Jul 23]. Available from: http://www.aidsinfo.nih.gov/ContentFiles/AdultandAdolescentGL.pdf.

Recommended First-Line Antiretroviral Regimens

Many excellent options are available to patients with a new diagnosis of HIV infection. Selection should be guided by resistance test results, toxicity, pill burden, drug-drug interactions, and comorbid conditions. Regimens classified as *recommended* for antiretroviral-naïve patients are those therapies that have shown optimal and durable virologic efficacy in randomized controlled trials, are easy to use, and have favorable tolerability and toxicity profiles. Currently recommended regimens for initial ART are the following:

- Ritonavir-boosted darunavir + tenofovir/emtricitabine
- Raltegravir + tenofovir/emtricitabine

Table 42.8 • General Characteristics of Integrase Inhibitors

Drug Name (Alias)	Adverse Effects
Raltegravir (RAL)	Nausea, headache, diarrhea, fever, **increased creatine kinase**
Elvitegravir (EVG) (only available coformulated with cobi/TDF/FTC)	Nausea, diarrhea, hyperlipidemia
Dolutegravir (DTG)	Hypersensitivity reactions, including rash, constitutional symptoms, and organ dysfunction (eg, liver injury); insomnia; headache

Abbreviations: cobi, cobicistat; FTC, emtricitabine; TDF, tenofovir.

Adapted from Panel on Antiretroviral Guidelines for Adults and Adolescents: Guidelines for the use of antiretroviral agents in HIV-1–infected adults and adolescents. Department of Health and Human Services. Apr 8, 2015; [cited 2015 Jul 23]. Available from: http://www.aidsinfo.nih.gov/ContentFiles/AdultandAdolescentGL.pdf.

- Elvitegravir/cobicistat/tenofovir/emtricitabine
- Dolutegravir/abacavir/lamivudine[a]
- Dolutegravir + tenofovir/emtricitabine

[a]Abacavir can only be used for patients who are HLA-B*5701 negative.

Recommendations for Postexposure Prophylaxis

The risk of infection after exposure is a function of the type of exposure and the infectivity of the exposure source. Infectivity is related to viral load. An undetectable viral load is associated with a small chance of infectivity, but exposure to a source patient with an undetectable serum viral load does not eliminate the possibility of HIV transmission. Exposure to a hollow needle, a deep puncture wound, or an exposure with visible blood on the device or needle is considered a high-risk exposure in the health care setting. Receptive anal intercourse with a partner known to have HIV infection and a high viral load is a high-risk sexual exposure.

Whenever possible, the HIV status of the exposure source patient should be determined; the use of rapid HIV testing of source patients in such cases facilitates timely decision making. However, administration of PEP should not be delayed while waiting for test results.

In source patients who have tested negative for HIV infection, additional investigation to determine whether a source patient might be in the window period is unnecessary unless the acute retroviral syndrome is clinically suspected. If the source patient is found to be HIV negative, PEP should be discontinued, and no follow-up HIV testing for this exposure is indicated.

PEP medication regimens should be started as soon as possible after occupational and high-risk sexual exposure to HIV, and they should be continued for 4 weeks.

The severity of exposure is no longer a criterion to determine the number of drugs to offer in an HIV PEP regimen; a regimen containing at least 3 antiretroviral drugs is now recommended routinely for all PEP. The preferred HIV PEP regimen is a combination of raltegravir plus tenofovir/emtricitabine at standard doses.

Follow-up of the exposed patient includes counseling; baseline and follow-up HIV testing; and monitoring for drug toxicity. Follow-up HIV testing is typically concluded at 6 months after an HIV exposure. However, if the newer fourth-generation HIV p24 antigen/HIV antibody combination test is used for follow-up HIV testing, the HIV testing may be concluded at 4 months after exposure.

KEY FACTS

✓ PEP medication regimens should be started as soon as possible after occupational or sexual exposure to HIV and should continue for 4 weeks

✓ A regimen of at least 3 antiretroviral drugs is recommended routinely for all PEP treatment

✓ The preferred HIV PEP regimen is a combination of raltegravir plus tenofovir/emtricitabine at standard doses for 28 days

43 Immunocompromised Hosts and Microorganism-Specific Syndromes

PRITISH K. TOSH, MD AND M. RIZWAN SOHAIL, MD

Infections in the Immunocompromised Host

Infections in the immunocompromised person may occur in the clinical setting of neutropenia, B-cell and T-cell deficiencies, immunoglobulin deficiencies, complement deficiencies, and leukocyte dysfunction. Some patients have multiple defects due to both the underlying disease and its treatment.

Febrile Neutropenia

Patients with neutropenia are at higher risk for infections with *Pseudomonas* species, gram-positive cocci, *Enterobacteriaceae*, and *Candida* and *Aspergillus* species. Patients who have neutropenia from the cytotoxic effects of chemotherapy, which breach normal mucosal and cutaneous barriers, are at the highest risk for infection. Fever of a patient with an absolute neutrophil count less than 0.5×10^9/L is usually due to translocation of bacteria from impaired mucosal surfaces in the oral cavity (oral mucosa and gingival crevices are rich sites of aerobic and anaerobic streptococci) and the lower gastrointestinal tract (contains gram-negative organisms and anaerobes). Bacteremia occurs in about 20% of neutropenic fever episodes. With prolonged neutropenia, invasive mold disease may occur. Because of the high risk of morbidity, patients with acute leukemia who are expected to have prolonged neutropenia may be given antimicrobial prophylaxis with levofloxacin and a mold-active azole (posaconazole or voriconazole) during the neutropenia period.

Because of high morbidity and mortality rates of patients presenting with febrile neutropenia, empirical antimicrobial therapy should be started urgently. Empirical antimicrobial therapy should have activity against viridans group streptococci and gram-negative bacilli, including *Pseudomonas aeruginosa*. Recommended empirical regimens include monotherapy with cefepime, piperacillin-tazobactam, or an antipseudomonal carbapenem, such as meropenem. Vancomycin should be added to the empirical regimen when a patient has evidence of pneumonia or severe mucositis; has concern for central line infection or for skin or soft tissue infection; or is known to have colonization with methicillin-resistant *Staphylococcus aureus* (MRSA). Empirical vancomycin therapy can be subsequently discontinued in this clinical setting if cultures are negative for MRSA or another resistant gram-positive organism.

Oral ulcerations and odynophagia are common in herpes simplex virus (HSV) infection. The presence of ulcerating papules of ecthyma gangrenosum should suggest disseminated infections due to *Pseudomonas* or other gram-negative bacteria. Bloodstream infection with gram-positive organisms (eg, *S aureus*, coagulase-negative staphylococci, enterococci, viridans group streptococci, *Corynebacterium jeikeium*) is often due to infected central venous catheters. *Streptococcus mitis* bacteremia may occur in mucositis and can be associated with sepsis and acute respiratory distress syndrome, especially in patients with leukemia.

Bacteremia due to anaerobic organisms is uncommon except in cases of perirectal abscess, gingivitis, or neutropenic enterocolitis (typhlitis). Persistent fever and abdominal symptoms in a person with neutropenia should raise this consideration. Anaerobic coverage should be added in these clinical settings.

Disseminated fungal infections often arise during prolonged neutropenia. The development of fever and an increased alkaline phosphatase level during recovery from neutropenia and the finding of microabscesses in the liver and spleen on computed tomography suggest the presence of hepatosplenic candidiasis. The therapy for hepatosplenic candidiasis requires months of antifungal therapy, usually with fluconazole. However, this particular complication is rare in current day because of widespread use of prophylactic antifungal therapy in high-risk neutropenic patients. Nonresolving nodular or consolidative pulmonary infiltrates in the clinical setting of prolonged antibacterial use and neutropenia suggest invasive aspergillosis. Affected patients may have an air crescent sign on computed tomography of the chest, and the diagnosis can be determined from a respiratory or tissue specimen or a positive result on serum *Aspergillus* galactomannan assay.

Antimicrobial agents active against *Aspergillus* include voriconazole, amphotericin B, posaconazole, and the echinocandins, such as caspofungin. The presence of facial numbness, pain, or sinus disease in a patient with prolonged neutropenia raises suspicion for invasive mucormycosis (due most often to *Rhizopus* or *Mucor* species) and invasive aspergillosis. This clinical situation is a medical emergency and requires rapid diagnosis through imaging and biopsy. Optimal treatment of rhinocerebral mucormycosis includes surgical débridement and intravenous (IV) liposomal amphotericin compounds.

KEY FACTS

✓ Because of high morbidity and mortality rates in febrile neutropenia, empirical antimicrobial therapy should begin urgently. It should be effective against viridans group streptococci and gram-negative bacilli, including *Pseudomonas aeruginosa*

✓ Recommended empirical regimens include monotherapy with cefepime, piperacillin-tazobactam, or an antipseudomonal carbapenem, such as meropenem

✓ Vancomycin should be added to the empirical regimen when evidence of pneumonia or severe mucositis is present; concern exists for central line infection, skin, or soft tissue infection or when colonization with MRSA is found

Infections in Transplant Recipients

Recipients of hematopoietic stem-cell transplants receive "conditioning" chemotherapy that often leads to prolonged neutropenia and mucositis in the early transplant period before engraftment. These patients have complications similar to those with febrile neutropenia. In addition, patients who receive allogeneic transplants are at risk for graft-vs-host disease augmenting the degree of immunosuppression.

In solid organ transplant recipients, the risk of specific infection can be classified according to the posttransplant time course and the serologic status of recipient and donor for certain infections (eg, cytomegalovirus [CMV], toxoplasmosis). Most infections in the first month after transplant receipt are common nosocomial infections, such as wound infections, urinary tract infections, and central venous line infections. CMV, a common infection after transplant operation, can present with fever, viremia, hepatitis, colitis, gastritis, retinitis, myocarditis, and pneumonitis. CMV-seronegative

Table 43.1 • Opportunistic Infections in Solid Organ Transplant

Month	Type of Infection After Transplant
1	Bacterial infections (related to wound, venous lines, urinary tract), herpes simplex virus, hepatitis B virus
1–4	Cytomegalovirus, *Pneumocystis carinii*, *Listeria monocytogenes*, *Mycobacterium tuberculosis*, *Aspergillus*, *Nocardia*, *Toxoplasma*, hepatitis B virus, *Legionella*
2–6	Epstein-Barr virus, varicella-zoster virus, hepatitis C virus, *Legionella*
>6	*Cryptococcus neoformans*, *Legionella*

recipients of organs from a seropositive donor are at highest risk for CMV disease. The time of occurrence of opportunistic infections after solid organ transplant is summarized in Table 43.1. Pathogens associated with various immunodeficiency states are listed in Table 43.2.

KEY FACTS

✓ CMV is a common infection after transplantation that can present with fever, viremia, hepatitis, colitis, gastritis, retinitis, myocarditis, and pneumonitis

✓ CMV-seronegative recipients of organs from a CMV-seropositive donor are at highest risk for disease

Immunosuppressive Medications

Commonly used immunosuppressive agents, such as cyclosporin, tacrolimus, sirolimus, mycophenolate mofetil, and azathioprine, often given in combination with corticosteroids, are associated with several T-cell–mediated opportunistic infections. These include *Pneumocystis jiroveci* pneumonia, nocardiosis (pulmonary, brain, and cutaneous), histoplasmosis, cryptococcosis, coccidioidomycosis, listeriosis, CMV, varicella-zoster virus (VZV), and HSV (Table 43.2).

The tumor necrosis factor-α inhibitors infliximab, adalimumab, and etanercept are associated with impaired granuloma formation and infections due to mycobacteria and such endemic fungi as *Histoplasma*.

Natalizumab, an agent used for treatment of multiple sclerosis and Crohn disease, is associated with the development of progressive multifocal leukoencephalopathy.

Infectious Syndromes Caused by Specific Microorganisms

Bacteria

Actinomycetes

Actinomyces israelii, an anaerobic gram-positive, branching, filamentous organism, is the most common cause of

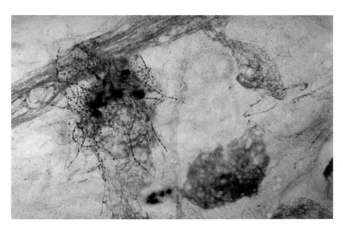

Figure 43.1 Nocardia asteroides *(Modified Acid-Fast Stain, Original Magnification × 450).*

sputum culture is relatively insensitive, specimens obtained by bronchoscopy or open lung biopsy may be needed to confirm the diagnosis. The disease must be differentiated from other causes of chronic pneumonia (such as bacterial, actinomycotic, tubercular, and fungal infections).

Therapy involves drainage of abscesses and high doses of sulfonamide drugs (trimethoprim-sulfamethoxazole is the drug of choice), although some species of *Nocardia* show evidence of sulfonamide resistance. Other antimicrobial agents used for nocardiosis include imipenem, amikacin, minocycline, and cephalosporins. Therapy should be guided by antimicrobial susceptibility testing.

Spirochetes

Leptospirosis

Leptospira interrogans infection is acquired by contact with urine from infected animals (eg, rats, dogs) and should be considered in the differential diagnosis of febrile travelers who were exposed to freshwater. *Leptospira* causes a biphasic illness. The first phase, the leptospiremic phase, is characterized by abrupt-onset headache (98%), fever, chills, conjunctivitis, severe muscle aching, gastrointestinal tract symptoms (50%), changes in sensorium (25%), rash (7%), and hypotension. This phase lasts 3 to 7 days. Improvement in symptoms coincides with disappearance of *Leptospira* organisms from blood and cerebrospinal fluid (CSF).

The second phase, the immune stage, occurs after a relatively asymptomatic period of 1 to 3 days, when fever and generalized symptoms recur. Meningeal symptoms often develop during this period. The second phase is characterized by the appearance of immunoglobulin M antibodies. Most patients recover after 1 to 3 days. However, in serious cases, hepatic dysfunction and renal failure may develop. Death in patients with leptospirosis usually occurs in the second phase as a result of hepatic and renal failure.

The diagnosis of leptospirosis is established on the basis of clinical presentation and of cultures of blood and, rarely, CSF in the first 7 to 10 days of infection. Urine cultures can remain positive in the second week of illness. Serologic testing has high specificity but low sensitivity, especially in the acute phase of disease, although it increases to 89% specificity and 63% sensitivity in the second phase. Treatment with penicillin G is effective only when given within the first 5 days from onset of symptoms. Oral amoxicillin or doxycycline can be used for mild-to-moderate illness.

Lyme Disease

Epidemiologic Factors

Lyme disease is the most common vector-borne (*Ixodes* ticks) disease reported in the United States. The incidence of disease is highest in spring and summer, when exposure to ticks is most common. Ticks must be attached to the skin for more than 36 hours to transmit infection (ticks are engorged with blood on inspection). Although Lyme disease has been reported in most states, it is most common in coastal New England and New York State, the Mid-Atlantic states, Oregon, northern California, and the Upper Midwest. Coinfection with *Babesia* or *Anaplasma* may occur in up to 15% of cases and may increase symptom severity.

Clinical Syndromes

Stage 1 (early stage) occurs from 3 to 32 days after the tick bite. Erythema migrans (solitary or multiple lesions) is the hallmark of Lyme disease and occurs in 80% or more of infected persons. It can be associated with fever, lymphadenopathy, and meningismus. The rash of erythema migrans usually enlarges and resolves over 3 to 4 weeks. *Borrelia burgdorferi* disseminates hematogenously early in the course of the illness.

Stage 2 occurs weeks to months after untreated stage 1 disease. In 10% to 15% of cases, neurologic abnormalities develop (eg, facial nerve palsy, lymphocytic meningitis, encephalitis, chorea, myelitis, radiculitis, peripheral neuropathy). Carditis (reversible atrioventricular block) occurs in 5% to 10%. Conduction abnormalities are mostly reversible, and permanent heart block is rare.

Stage 3, although uncommon, can develop months to years after the initial untreated infection. Monarticular or oligoarticular arthritis occurs in 50% of patients at this stage and becomes chronic in 10% to 20%. Chronic arthritis is more common in those with HLA-DR2 and HLA-DR4. Almost all patients with stage 3 Lyme disease have detectable serum antibodies against *B burgdorferi*. Magnetic resonance imaging may show demyelination.

Diagnosis

Although screening serologic testing may be negative in the acute stage (with the erythema migrans rash) of illness, antibodies to *B burgdorferi* can be detected by enzyme-linked immunosorbent assay (ELISA) after the first 2 to 6 weeks of illness. Western blot test is used to confirm the diagnosis when the screening ELISA test is positive. This 2-step test approach is both sensitive and specific for establishing the diagnosis of Lyme disease. Serologic tests should be ordered only in cases of a clinical syndrome compatible with Lyme disease. False-positive results may occur with infectious mononucleosis, rheumatoid arthritis, systemic lupus erythematosus, echovirus infection, and other spirochetal disease because of antibody cross-reactivity.

Treatment

Patients who reside in or visit endemic areas and have the characteristic skin lesion of erythema migrans should be treated without any serologic testing. For stage 1 (early) Lyme disease in the absence of neurologic involvement or complete heart block, doxycycline (100 mg orally twice daily), amoxicillin (500 mg 3 times daily), and cefuroxime axetil (500 mg twice daily) are effective therapeutic agents. Recommended treatment duration is 14 days (range, 10–21 days).

In Lyme disease carditis, the outcome is usually favorable. In patients with first- or second-degree atrioventricular block, infection should be treated with oral agents, whereas patients with third-degree heart block should be treated with IV ceftriaxone (2 g daily) or IV penicillin G (20 million units daily) for 14 to 21 days. Lyme disease meningitis, radiculopathy, or encephalitis should be treated parenterally.

The outcome in patients with facial palsy in Lyme disease is also usually favorable. If only facial nerve palsy is present (no symptoms of meningitis or radiculoneuritis), oral therapy with doxycycline or amoxicillin is used.

If Lyme disease meningitis is present, treatment with ceftriaxone (2 g daily) or IV penicillin G (20 million units daily) should be administered for 14 to 28 days.

Optimal treatment regimens (oral vs IV) for Lyme disease arthritis are not established yet. Joint rest and repeated joint aspirations are often needed. Response to antibiotics may be delayed. If no neurologic disease is present, doxycycline is given (100 mg orally twice daily) for 28 days. An alternative regimen is amoxicillin and probenecid (500 mg each, 4 times daily) for 28 days or ceftriaxone (2 g IV daily) for 14 to 28 days. Synovectomy may be necessary in the management of persistent monoarticular Lyme disease arthritis that has not responded to antimicrobial therapy.

Rickettsiae

All rickettsial infections are transmitted by an arthropod vector, except *Coxiella burnetii* (Q fever), which spreads by respiratory route. Most are associated with a skin rash, except Q fever and ehrlichiosis.

Rickettsia rickettsii infection (Rocky Mountain spotted fever [RMSF]) is associated with a skin rash that may be indistinguishable from that of meningococcemia. RMSF rash begins on the extremities and moves centrally. RMSF is most common in the Mid-Atlantic states and Oklahoma, not the Rocky Mountain states. Doxycycline is the treatment of choice.

Coxiella burnetii, the cause of Q fever, is acquired by inhalation of contaminated aerosol particles of dust, earth, or feces or by exposure to animal products, especially infected placentas. Cattle and sheep are common sources, but other animals (usually asymptomatic), including cats, can harbor the disease. An isolated febrile illness is the most common disease manifestation, and most such cases present with pneumonitis. Granulomatous hepatitis is seen in 15% of the cases. Endocarditis (1%) and central nervous system (CNS) manifestations are rare. Q fever is one of the causes of culture-negative endocarditis. It usually is diagnosed with serologic testing. Acute Q-fever pneumonitis or hepatitis is treated with 2 weeks of doxycycline or a fluoroquinolone. Endocarditis typically requires prolonged (>18 months) therapy.

Ehrlichia species are gram-negative intracellular bacteria that resemble rickettsial organisms and preferentially infect lymphocytes, monocytes, and neutrophils. *Ehrlichia chaffeensis* infects monocytes (also called *human monocytic ehrlichiosis*), and *Ehrlichia equi* and *Anaplasma phagocytophilum* infect neutrophils (also called *human granulocytic ehrlichiosis* or *anaplasmosis*). Ehrlichiosis is seasonal; peak incidence occurs in summer. The vectors are the common dog tick (*Dermacentor variabilis*) and the lone star tick (*Amblyomma americanum*) for *E chaffeensis*, and *Ixodes scapularis* (deer tick; the same vector as in Lyme disease) for the agent of anaplasmosis. The incubation period is short (average, 7 days), and patients present with acute-onset fever, chills, malaise, headache, and myalgia. Fewer than 50% of patients with anaplasmosis have a rash. Rarely, a rash develops with human monocytic ehrlichiosis. Important laboratory features include leukopenia, thrombocytopenia, and increased levels of hepatic transaminases. Disease severity is variable, but severe complications,

---

KEY FACTS

✓ For Lyme disease, ticks must be attached to the skin for more than 36 hours to transmit infection

✓ Lyme disease is most common in coastal New England states and New York State, the Mid-Atlantic states, Oregon, northern California, and the Upper Midwest

✓ Coinfection with *Babesia* or *Anaplasma* may occur in up to 15% of cases and may increase symptom severity

✓ Stage 1 Lyme disease occurs at 3 to 32 days after the tick bite

✓ Erythema migrans in solitary or multiple lesions is the hallmark of Lyme disease and occurs in 80% or more of cases

including death, can occur. Coinfection with *Babesia* and *B burgdorferi* (Lyme disease) can occur and can be especially severe. Diagnosis is based on serologic testing (indirect immunofluorescent assay) or detection through polymerase chain reaction amplification. Treatment is with doxycycline for 7 to 10 days.

KEY FACTS

✓ RMSF is associated with skin rash that can be indistinguishable from meningococcemia, beginning on the extremities and moving centrally

✓ RMSF is most common in the Mid-Atlantic states and Oklahoma

✓ Doxycycline for 7 to 10 days is the treatment of choice

✓ Q fever is a cause of culture-negative endocarditis and usually is diagnosed through serologic testing

✓ Important laboratory features of RMSF include leukopenia, thrombocytopenia, and increased levels of hepatic transaminases

✓ Diagnosis is based on indirect immunofluorescent assay or detection with PCR amplification

---

Fungi

Coccidioidomycosis

Coccidioides immitis is endemic in the southwestern United States, especially the San Joaquin Valley of California and central Arizona, and in Mexico. Disseminated disease is most likely to occur in men (especially Filipino and black men), pregnant women, and immunocompromised persons, including HIV-infected patients, regardless of sex.

Most primary infections with *C immitis* are subclinical. The most common clinical manifestation is self-limited pneumonitis. Common manifestations are dry cough and fever (called *valley fever*) that may resemble influenza. Associated findings include hilar adenopathy, pleural effusion (12%), thin-walled cavities (5%), and solid "coin" lesions. Disseminated infection predominantly affects the CNS, skin, bones, and joints.

The diagnosis of coccidioidomycosis is primarily based on detecting the organism through culture or biopsy with silver stains. A *C immitis* serologic titer greater than 1:4 is suggestive of infection (≥1:16 indicates likely disseminated infection). The diagnosis of coccidioidomycosis meningitis is usually established by detecting CSF antibodies. A biopsy specimen may show the diagnostic *C immitis* spherule (Figure 43.2). Laboratory abnormalities may include eosinophilia and hypercalcemia.

Fluconazole, itraconazole, and amphotericin B are effective agents for treating coccidioidomycosis. The acute pulmonary form is usually self-limited, and observation may be adequate. However, therapy is indicated when a patient is

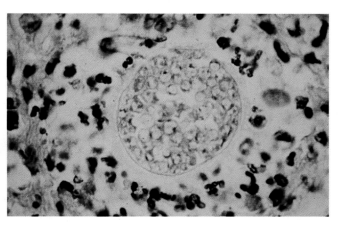

Figure 43.2 Coccidioides immitis *Spherules in a Clinical Specimen (Grocott Methenamine-Silver Stain).*

pregnant, is immunocompromised, or has worsening infection without therapy. Amphotericin B is the drug of choice for severe manifestations and for pregnant women with coccidioidomycosis. An alternative to fluconazole is itraconazole. For meningitis, therapy with high-dose fluconazole is preferred and has largely replaced intrathecal amphotericin B. Because of the high relapse rate of *C immitis* meningitis, long-term suppressive therapy is recommended, usually with fluconazole. Given their risk for teratogenicity, azole antifungals such as fluconazole should be avoided during the first trimester of pregnancy.

Histoplasmosis

Histoplasma capsulatum is also a dimorphic fungus that grows as a small yeast in tissues and as a mold at room temperature. Although present in many areas of the world, histoplasmosis is especially prevalent in the Ohio, Missouri, and Mississippi river valleys and parts of Mexico and Central America. Outbreaks have been associated with large construction projects and exposure to bird or bat droppings. Histoplasmosis is acquired by inhalation of spores, and the risk of acquisition is increased with certain activities, including caving and bridge or other construction. Although healthy individuals may acquire histoplasmosis, patients with AIDS or cell-mediated immune deficiency are particularly susceptible to disseminated disease. *H capsulatum* infection is one of the causes of caseating granulomata.

Primary (acute) histoplasmosis may be clinically indistinguishable from influenza or other upper respiratory tract infections. After resolution, multiple small, calcified granulomas may be seen on subsequent chest radiographs. The progressive (disseminated) form of histoplasmosis is uncommon but serious. The disseminated form and reactivation of prior disease are most likely to occur in infants, elderly men, and immunosuppressed persons, including those with HIV infection or AIDS and those receiving therapy with tumor necrosis factor-α inhibitors, such as etanercept and infliximab. Disseminated histoplasmosis typically involves the reticuloendothelial system—bone marrow, spleen, lymph nodes, and liver. Manifestations may resemble those of lymphoma, with weight loss, fever, anemia, increased erythrocyte sedimentation rate, and splenomegaly. Bone marrow involvement may be associated with pancytopenia. Mucosal ulcers, which can occur throughout the gastrointestinal tract and mouth, are not infrequent. Chronic cavitary pulmonary disease due to *Histoplasma* may resemble tuberculosis and tends to occur in patients with preexistent pulmonary disease, such as chronic obstructive pulmonary disease.

Positive serologic findings are helpful for confirming the diagnosis of histoplasmosis, although the sensitivity may be decreased in immunosuppressed patients. Biopsy, silver stain, and cultures of infected tissues are the best means of establishing the diagnosis. Detection of *Histoplasma* antigen in urine, CSF, or serum is sensitive, especially for the diagnosis of disseminated disease and to follow up on treatment response.

The mild, acute forms of histoplasmosis are usually self-limited and do not require therapy. Amphotericin B is the drug of choice for initial therapy for all severe, life-threatening cases. Itraconazole is effective for most non-meningeal, non–life-threatening cases and to complete the treatment course of severe disease. Patients with AIDS require long-term maintenance therapy.

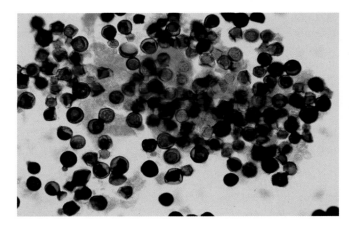

Figure 43.3 Blastomyces dermatitidis *in Bronchoalveolar Lavage (Silver Stain, Original Magnification ×450).*

In culture at room temperature, a mycelial form grows. Blastomycosis is endemic in the southeastern United States and the Upper Midwest. Primary pulmonary blastomycosis may be asymptomatic, but organisms may disseminate hematogenously to skin, bone (especially vertebrae), male genitalia (ie, prostate, epididymis, and testis), and the CNS. Granulomas occur, but calcification is less frequent than with histoplasmosis or tuberculosis.

The pulmonary form has no characteristic findings: Pleural effusion is rare, hilar adenopathy develops occasionally, and cavitation is infrequent. It often mimics carcinoma of the lung. Cutaneous involvement with blastomycosis is common. Lesions, especially on the face, are characteristically painless and nonpruritic and have a sharp, spreading border. Chronic crusty lesions may occur.

The diagnosis of blastomycosis is based on results of biopsy, fungal stains, and cultures. Serologic and skin testings are rarely helpful. Urine antigen is sensitive in disseminated disease. Amphotericin B is reserved primarily for life-threatening infections. Mild-to-moderate nonmeningeal blastomycosis can be treated with itraconazole for 6 months.

Sporotrichosis

Sporothrix schenckii, another dimorphic fungal pathogen, is seen as round, cigar-shaped yeast in tissues, but culture at room temperature yields a mycelial form. *Sporothrix schenckii* is most often found in soil and plants. Sporotrichosis is usually transmitted through cutaneous inoculation (so-called rose gardener disease) and, rarely, through inhalation causing chronic pneumonitis (with cavitation and empyema).

Cutaneous sporotrichosis presents as characteristic crusty lesions with suppuration and granulomatous reaction. New lesions develop along the lymphatic system of the extremities from the initial site of infection. Similar lesions may be produced by infection with *Mycobacterium*

KEY FACTS

✓ Histoplasmosis is especially prevalent in the Ohio, Missouri, and Mississippi river valleys and parts of Mexico and Central America

✓ Primary acute histoplasmosis may be indistinguishable from influenza or other upper respiratory tract infections. After its resolution, multiple small, calcified granulomas may be seen on chest radiographs

✓ Dissemination and reactivation of prior disease are most likely in infants, elderly men, and immunosuppressed persons, including those with HIV infection or AIDS or receiving tumor necrosis factor-α inhibitors

✓ Disseminated histoplasmosis typically involves bone marrow, spleen, lymph nodes, and liver

✓ Manifestations may resemble lymphoma, with weight loss, fever, anemia, increased erythrocyte sedimentation rate, and splenomegaly. Bone marrow involvement may be associated with pancytopenia

Blastomycosis

Blastomyces dermatitidis is another dimorphic fungal pathogen. In tissue, the yeast has thick walls and has broad-based buds (±10 mm in diameter) (Figure 43.3).

marinum and *Nocardia* or by cutaneous leishmaniasis. Septic arthritis can occasionally occur.

The diagnosis of sporotrichosis may be difficult and depends on clinical recognition of the cutaneous lesions in most instances. Biopsy, fungal culture, and serologic testing can help establish the diagnosis.

For the cutaneous or lymphocutaneous form, itraconazole is the therapy of choice. An effective alternative is supersaturated solution of potassium iodide. Amphotericin B is recommended for disseminated disease (pulmonary and joint), although such disseminated disease may respond poorly to therapy.

Aspergillosis

Aspergillus is an opportunistic pathogen that causes infection in immunocompromised persons, particularly those with prolonged neutropenia. Although any *Aspergillus* species can cause disease, *Aspergillus fumigatus* is the most common pathogen. The organisms have large, septated hyphae branching at 45° angles (Figure 43.4). In contrast, Zygomycetes have aseptate, ribbonlike hyphae with wide-angle branching. In neutropenic persons, *Aspergillus* may invade blood vessels, producing a striking thrombotic angiitis. Metastatic foci may cause suppurative abscess formation.

The form of aspergillosis disease primarily is determined by the nature of the immunologic deficit in the infected person. Neutropenia predisposes to rapidly invasive bronchopulmonary disease with early dissemination to the brain and other tissues. The longer the duration of neutropenia is, the higher the risk of invasive aspergillosis. Prompt therapy with voriconazole or large doses of amphotericin B and the resolution of neutropenia are necessary to control the disease. Diagnosis should be suspected when *Aspergillus* is isolated from any source in a susceptible person.

Aspergillus frequently colonizes the respiratory tract. Hence, isolating the organism from the sputum of an immunocompetent person usually does not indicate disease and does not require treatment.

However, *Aspergillus* may cause localized disease in persons with normal immunologic function. It may produce a "fungus ball" in preexisting lung bullae or cavities (eg, previous tuberculosis, emphysema). Hemoptysis is the main symptom. Surgical excision may be necessary to prevent lethal hemorrhage.

The symptoms of allergic bronchopulmonary aspergillosis resemble those of asthma. It is characterized by migratory pulmonary infiltrates; thick, brown, tenacious mucous plugs in the sputum; eosinophilia; and high titers of anti-*Aspergillus* antibodies; it typically occurs in the clinical setting of chronic asthma.

Cryptococcosis

Cryptococcus neoformans is a yeast in both tissue and culture. It is 4 to 7 mcm in diameter and has a characteristic narrow-based budding and a thick capsule (Figure 43.5). *Cryptococcus neoformans* is an opportunistic pathogen infecting persons with T-cell deficiency or dysfunction (eg, patients with Hodgkin lymphoma, hematologic malignancy, organ transplant, exogenous corticosteroid therapy, chronic liver disease, or AIDS).

Cryptococcus neoformans is acquired by inhalation. From the lungs, it disseminates widely and easily crosses into the CNS. Pneumonia and meningitis are the most common forms of cryptococcosis. Meningitis may be insidious, with headache as the only symptom. Cranial nerve involvement may develop (including blindness with optic nerve involvement).

Cryptococcal infection can be diagnosed with fungal culture (eg, CSF, blood, sputum, urine) and silver stain of biopsy tissue. The cryptococcal antigen test is the most helpful of all fungal serologic tests; it detects capsular antigen, whereas most other fungal serologic tests measure antibody response. If *C neoformans* is isolated from any source

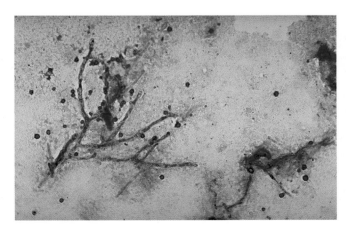

Figure 43.4 Aspergillus fumigatus *in Bronchoalveolar Lavage (Original Magnification × 450).*

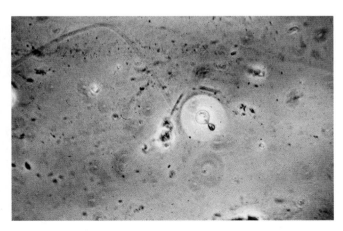

Figure 43.5 Cryptococcus neoformans *in Cerebrospinal Fluid (Original Magnification ×450).*

(eg, sputum, urine, blood) in an immunosuppressed patient, a lumbar puncture should be done to rule out meningitis, even in the absence of symptoms.

Choice of therapy depends on the extent of disease and host immune function. Mild-to-moderate non-CNS cryptococcosis can be treated with fluconazole for 6 to 12 months. However, in cases of severe presentation, immunocompromised hosts, and CNS involvement, treatment with IV amphotericin B in combination with flucytosine should be provided for 2 weeks, followed by fluconazole therapy for 6 to 12 months. Oral fluconazole therapy is continued indefinitely for patients with severe immunosuppression and poor immune reconstitution.

Candidiasis

Candida is a normal part of human microflora. It grows as both yeast and hyphal forms simultaneously. Although *Candida albicans* is the most common species, numerous other species can cause human disease. *Candida* causes mucosal and cutaneous infections in both normal and immunocompromised persons. Invasive disease primarily occurs in neutropenic hosts and as a nosocomial bloodstream infection.

Examples of candidiasis in a healthy person include diaper rash and intertrigo, in which *Candida* growth on moist skin surfaces produces irritation. Vulvovaginal candidiasis is common, especially in women after antibiotic therapy for bacterial infection. Treatment with topical antifungal agents or a single dose of oral fluconazole is usually curative for candida vaginitis. Diabetes mellitus, corticosteroid therapy, oral contraceptives, obesity, and HIV infection predispose to recurrent vulvovaginal candidiasis. Oral thrush may result from these same risk factors.

Candida species cause 5% to 10% of nosocomial bloodstream infections. Candidemia most often occurs in critically ill patients receiving broad-spectrum antibiotics and parenteral nutrition. Neutropenia is another predisposing factor. Current blood culture techniques usually detect *Candida*, but culture results may be delayed. All IV catheters should always be removed or replaced when bloodstream infection with *Candida* is discovered. Metastatic abscesses can occur in any site after an episode of candidemia. *Candida* osteomyelitis or joint infections can occur as complications after an episode of central venous catheter–related candidemia. Endophthalmitis may present as long as 1 month after initial fungemia. For central venous catheter–related candidemias, catheter removal followed by antifungal therapy with fluconazole, an echinocandin (such as caspofungin), or amphotericin B, based on susceptibility testing, should be administered.

Injection drug use is a risk factor for *Candida* endocarditis (and joint space infections, especially of the sternoclavicular joint). It is often caused by species other than *C albicans*.

Candida urinary tract infection is common in patients with urinary catheters and those receiving antibacterial drugs. Removal of the catheter is the primary therapy. If necessary, treatment with fluconazole or bladder irrigation with dilute amphotericin B may be curative, although recurrence is common.

Hepatosplenic candidiasis, also called *chronic disseminated candidiasis*, typically occurs during the recovery phase after prolonged neutropenia. This condition is now rare because of frequent use of azole prophylaxis in neutropenic patients in current practice. When it does occur, fever, abdominal pain, and increased alkaline phosphatase level suggest the diagnosis. Typical "bull's-eye lesions" can be seen with ultrasonography, computed tomography, or magnetic resonance imaging of the infected liver. Fluconazole is the preferred antifungal agent in clinically stable patients; however, amphotericin B or an echinocandin is an option in ill patients or patients with refractory disease.

Candida esophagitis is a common cause of odynophagia in immunosuppressed patients, especially those with AIDS. Endoscopy is necessary to prove the diagnosis. *Candida* esophagitis is clinically indistinguishable from, and may coexist with, CMV and HSV esophagitis. Fluconazole is effective therapy for oral or esophageal candidiasis, although amphotericin B or an echinocandin may be needed for resistant organisms.

KEY FACTS

- ✓ Injection drug use is a risk factor for *Candida* endocarditis (and infections of joint space, especially the sternoclavicular joint). It is often caused by species other than *C albicans*

- ✓ *Candida* esophagitis is a common cause of odynophagia in immunosuppressed patients, especially those with AIDS. Endoscopy is necessary to prove the diagnosis

---

Mucormycosis (*Rhizopus* Species, *Zygomycetes*)

Mucormycosis is a term used to describe infections caused by fungi of the order *Mucorales*, such as *Mucor* and *Rhizopus*. Mucormycosis is a disease of immunocompromised hosts, primarily persons with impaired neutrophil number or function. Pulmonary, nasal, and sinus infections are the most common manifestations. Facial pain, headache, and fever are common symptoms. Rhinocerebral mucormycosis results from direct extension into the brain. Diabetic ketoacidosis, neutropenia, renal failure, and deferoxamine therapy are all risk factors for this life-threatening infection. The diagnosis of mucormycosis depends on finding the typical black necrotic lesions (usually in the nose or on the palate) and is confirmed by biopsy. Treatment involves reversing the predisposing condition as much as possible, surgical débridement of necrotic tissue, and high-dose amphotericin B therapy.

Viruses

Herpesviruses

There are now 8 known human herpesviruses: HSV types 1 and 2, VZV, Epstein-Barr virus (EBV), CMV, human herpesvirus (HHV) 6 (HHV-6), HHV-7 (not yet known to be associated with a clinical disease), and HHV-8. All herpesviruses are DNA viruses that establish latency after primary infection, with or without symptoms.

Serologic evidence of infection is common by adulthood: HSV-1, 87%; HSV-2, 20%; VZV, 90%; EBV, 95%; and CMV, 50%. The rate of infection is greater in populations of lower socioeconomic status than of high socioeconomic status.

Herpes Simplex Virus

Primary infection with HSV results from exposure of skin or mucous membranes to intact viral particles. Latent infection is then established in sensory nerve ganglia. Genital HSV infection is caused by HSV type 2 in 80% of cases and by HSV type 1 in the remaining 20%. The reverse is true for oral HSV infection. Genital HSV infection is more likely to recur when caused by HSV type 2. Recurrence rates of oral and genital HSV infection can be decreased by 80% with long-term use of antiviral drugs. Acyclovir, valacyclovir, and famciclovir are effective antiviral medications for treatment of primary or recurrent HSV infection.

Herpes simplex encephalitis is a nonseasonal, life-threatening illness usually caused by HSV type 1. It causes confusion, fever, and seizures. Simultaneous herpes labialis is present in 10% to 15% of cases. Magnetic resonance imaging of the brain, which shows characteristic temporal lobe involvement, and PCR for HSV from CSF are extremely sensitive. Detecting periodic lateralized epileptiform discharges with electroencephalography is suggestive of HSV encephalitis. Older age, poor neurologic status at presentation, and encephalitis of longer than 4 days before the initiation of therapy with IV acyclovir are associated with a poor outcome.

Neonatal HSV infection is acquired at the time of vaginal delivery. The mortality rate is high (20%) despite antiviral therapy. In neonates who survive, neurologic sequelae and recurrent HSV lesions are common. Cesarean section is recommended when a woman has active herpetic lesions at the time of delivery.

HSV pneumonia is rare and usually occurs in immunosuppressed persons. When HSV is isolated from a respiratory source, it most commonly represents shedding from the oral mucosa rather than the lungs. HSV also is associated with visceral disease (such as esophagitis). Biopsy is required to reliably distinguish HSV from CMV or *Candida* esophagitis. **Herpetic whitlow** is a painful HSV infection of a finger that is most commonly acquired through contact with oral secretions. Health care professionals at risk are respiratory technicians, dentists, and anesthesiologists.

KEY FACT

✓ Genital HSV infection is caused by HSV-2 in 80% of cases and by HSV-1 in the remaining 20%

Key Definition

Herpetic whitlow: *A painful HSV infection of a finger that is most commonly acquired through contact with oral secretions.*

Varicella-Zoster Virus

Before the availability of routine vaccination against VZV, primary infection with the virus commonly occurred in childhood and caused chickenpox, an illness characterized by fever and a generalized vesicular eruption (dew drop on a rose petal). Illness with chickenpox is more likely to be severe in adults and immunocompromised persons. Varicella pneumonia occurs in 5% to 50% of chickenpox cases. Pregnant women are especially vulnerable and should be treated with high-dose IV acyclovir. Pneumonia develops within 1 to 6 days after the onset of illness with primary VZV infection. Encephalomyelitis is another serious complication, occurring predominantly in children. Typical onset is 3 to 14 days after the appearance of rash.

After primary infection, VZV DNA persists in a latent state in sensory nerve ganglia. Reactivated infection causes zoster (shingles), which manifests as a painful vesicular rash in a dermatomal distribution. Involvement of the fifth cranial nerve, especially the ophthalmic branch, may threaten the person's vision. Neurologic complications of VZV include motor paralysis (localized to the dermatomal distribution of rash), encephalitis, and myelitis.

Varicella immune globulin can prevent primary VZV infection and is recommended within 10 days of exposure in the following: 1) all persons without immunity to VZV, 2) immunocompromised patients, and 3) neonates whose mothers have signs and symptoms of varicella around the time of delivery (ie, 5 days before through 2 days after delivery).

Chickenpox (primary VZV infection) is treated with acyclovir, valacyclovir, or famciclovir to reduce the severity and duration of illness, as well as to reduce complications from infection. Zoster should also be treated with acyclovir, valacyclovir, or famciclovir to reduce illness duration, as well as prevent postherpetic neuralgia. Corticosteroid use for the prevention of postherpetic neuralgia is controversial. For disseminated zoster infections (eg, encephalitis, cranial neuritis), high-dose IV acyclovir decreases the duration of hospitalization.

Two effective live-virus vaccines for VZV are available. One VZV vaccine (Varivax; Merck and Co, Inc) is part of the routine childhood vaccine series for primary prevention of varicella infection. A higher-dose vaccine (Zostavax; Merck and Co, Inc) is recommended for shingles prevention (and resultant postherpetic neuralgia) in patients older than 60 years. Both vaccines are contraindicated in pregnancy and in patients with impaired cellular immunity caused by such entities as AIDS, leukemia, lymphoma, chemotherapy, bone marrow or organ transplant, long-term corticosteroid therapy, or other cellular immunodeficiency states.

Epstein-Barr Virus

Most acute EBV infections are asymptomatic. Symptomatic infectious mononucleosis due to EBV infection causes the clinical triad of fever, pharyngitis (in 80% of cases), and adenopathy. Splenomegaly occurs in 50% of cases. A rare, but serious, complication of mononucleosis is splenic rupture (may occur spontaneously, typically at 1–2 weeks after initial symptoms). Other complications include hemolytic anemia, airway obstruction, encephalitis, and transverse myelitis. Associated laboratory abnormalities include atypical lymphocytosis, thrombocytopenia, and mild increases in liver enzyme values.

Corticosteroids are indicated for hemolytic anemia, severe thrombocytopenia, and acute airway obstruction. Ampicillin or amoxicillin given during infectious mononucleosis commonly causes a diffuse macular rash.

Table 43.3 differentiates EBV from other causes of mononucleosis. The diagnosis of infectious mononucleosis depends on detection of heterophile antibodies (monospot test) or specific EBV immunoglobulin M antibodies. False-negative results of the monospot test are more likely with increasing patient age.

Uncomplicated cases of EBV require symptomatic care only. The patient should not participate in contact sports for several months because of the risk of splenic rupture.

KEY FACT

✓ Symptomatic infectious mononucleosis causes the clinical triad of fever, pharyngitis (in 80% of cases), and adenopathy

---

Corticosteroids are not indicated for uncomplicated infection. Acyclovir and other antiviral drug therapy are not effective against EBV.

Cytomegalovirus

Primary CMV infection is usually asymptomatic, but it can cause a heterophile-negative mononucleosis syndrome. It is a substantial cause of neonatal disease. Perinatal infection can occur in utero, intrapartum, or postpartum and can cause congenital malformations. Primary infection of a woman during pregnancy results in a 15% chance of fetal cytomegalic inclusion disease. Young children in day care centers commonly shed CMV in their urine and saliva. Parents are at risk of acquiring primary infection from asymptomatic children. CMV can cause fever of unknown origin in healthy adults, especially in those with children of day care age.

In persons with impaired cellular immunity (such as persons with AIDS or organ and bone marrow transplant recipients), CMV causes serious infections—retinitis, pneumonia, gastrointestinal tract ulcerations, encephalitis, and adrenalitis. The diagnosis is most often established through isolation of CMV from blood or from culture, CMV blood PCR, or histopathologic evidence of CMV infection in involved tissue (eg, liver, lung, gastrointestinal tract) or through clinical findings alone (such as CMV retinitis).

CMV disease in persons with advanced AIDS is almost always caused by reactivation of latent infection. Finding CMV in the blood or urine of patients with AIDS is common and has a low predictive value for symptomatic CMV disease. CMV retinitis occurs in 20% to 30% of patients with advanced AIDS. Its diagnosis is based on ophthalmologic examination (from a finding of "ketchup and mustard retina"). The relapse rate for CMV retinitis in AIDS is high, even with long-term antiviral therapy.

Solid organ and bone marrow transplant recipients are another group of patients at risk for CMV disease.

Symptomatic disease (called *CMV syndrome*) usually develops in the first 4 to 8 weeks after a solid organ transplant and causes fever, leukopenia, increases in liver enzyme values, and end-organ involvement. CMV serum

---

Table 43.3 • Infectious Mononucleosislike Syndromes

Disease	Pharyngitis	Adenopathy	Splenomegaly	Atypical Lymphocytes	Heterophile	Other Test
Infectious mononucleosis	++++	++++	+++	+++	+	Specific EBV antibody + (VCA IgM)
CMV	–	–	+++	++	–	CMV IgM
Toxoplasmosis	–	++++	+++	++		Toxoplasmosis serology
HIV infection	+	+++	–	++	–	HIV serology (will likely be negative in acute infection) HIV viral load

Abbreviations and symbols: CMV, cytomegalovirus; EBV, Epstein-Barr virus; HIV, human immunodeficiency virus; IgM, immunoglobulin M; VCA, viral capsid antigen; –, absent; +, ++, +++, and ++++, present to various degrees.

antigen testing or CMV blood PCR helps confirm the diagnosis. Patients who have had bone marrow transplant are especially at risk for CMV pneumonia. The mortality rate approaches 50% despite therapy.

Immunocompetent patients with CMV typically do not require treatment. Ganciclovir is the treatment of choice for most CMV infections in immunocompromised hosts. Full-dose induction therapy is given for 2 to 3 weeks, followed by maintenance therapy for 2 to 3 months. Oral valganciclovir has excellent bioavailability and can be used for maintenance therapy or suppression.

KEY FACT

✓ Primary CMV infection is usually asymptomatic, but it can cause a heterophile-negative mononucleosis syndrome

---

Human Herpesvirus 6

HHV-6 is a recently discovered lymphotropic virus. It causes the mild childhood infectious exanthem known as *roseola infantum*. Similar to CMV, the reactivation of HHV-6 infection occurs after organ transplant. HHV-6 has been associated with encephalitis and pneumonitis after bone marrow transplant.

Human Herpesvirus 8

HHV-8 is associated with Kaposi sarcoma in patients with HIV infection. HHV-8 has also been linked to other body cavity–based lymphomas in patients with AIDS and Castleman disease.

Measles (Rubeola)

Measles cases have undergone a substantial increase, starting in the late 1990s in unvaccinated children. Prodromal upper respiratory tract symptoms are prominent. Blue-grey oral lesions (Koplik spots) precede the measles rash.

Complications of measles include encephalitis and pneumonia. Encephalitis is often severe and usually occurs after a period of apparent improvement of measles infection. Secondary bacterial infection is more common than primary measles pneumonia. *Staphylococcus aureus* and *Haemophilus influenzae* are the most common bacterial pathogens.

Rubella

The prodromal symptoms of rubella are mild (unlike those of measles). Posterior cervical lymphadenopathy, arthralgia (70% in adult cases), transient erythematous rash, and fever are characteristic. Infection is subclinical in many cases. CNS complications and thrombocytopenia are rare. The greatest danger from rubella is fetal infection in unimmunized pregnant women, which can result in congenital rubella syndrome or fetal demise. The risk varies from 40% to 60% when infection occurs during the first 2 months of gestation to 10% by the fourth month. Intravenous gamma globulin may mask symptoms of rubella in pregnant woman, but it does not protect the fetus.

From 6% to 11% of young adults continue to be susceptible to rubella after receiving the rubella vaccine. A pregnant woman should not be given rubella vaccine because it can cause congenital abnormalities. Women of childbearing age should be warned not to become pregnant within 2 to 3 months from the time of immunization. Transient arthralgias develop in 25% of immunized women. Fever, rash, and lymphadenopathy also may develop. Symptoms may occur as long as 2 months after vaccination.

Mumps

Mumps virus can be transmitted by direct contact with respiratory droplets, saliva, or contaminated fomites. The incubation period is 16 to 18 days (range, 12–25 days) from exposure to onset of symptoms. Mumps virus commonly affects glandular tissue. Parotitis, pancreatitis, and orchitis are characteristic manifestations. Orchitis occurs in 20% of boys and men with mumps. It is unilateral in approximately 75%. Orchitis often is associated with recrudescence of fever, malaise, chills, and testicular pain. Sterility is uncommon, even after bilateral infection. Before mumps vaccination became routine, mumps meningoencephalitis was one of the most common nonseasonal viral meningitides. It can cause low glucose levels in CSF, mimicking bacterial meningitis. Although mumps cases are uncommon in the United States, outbreaks have been identified, largely in unvaccinated children.

Clinical suspicion of mumps can be confirmed by serologic test (immunoglobulin M for mumps) within 5 days of illness onset or sending a parotid duct swab or other samples such as CSF for viral cultures.

KEY FACT

✓ Parotitis, pancreatitis, and orchitis are characteristic manifestations of mumps

---

Parvovirus B19

Parvovirus B19 is a single-stranded DNA virus that infects the erythrocyte precursors in bone marrow, with resulting reticulocytopenia. It is the cause of erythema infectiosum (fifth disease) in children, transient arthritis in adults (which is symmetrical, involves small joints, and can mimic rheumatoid arthritis), and aplastic crisis in persons with hemolytic anemias. Infection during pregnancy results in a 5% chance of hydrops fetalis or fetal death. Serologic testing is the preferred diagnostic method in immunologically competent persons.

Parvovirus B19 infection may persist in immunosuppressed patients, resulting in red blood cell aplasia. Diagnosis is established by demonstration of giant pronormoblasts in bone marrow or the identification of viral DNA in bone marrow or peripheral blood. Most patients respond to administration of immune globulin infusions for 5 to 10 days. No treatment is recommended for parvovirus infections in immunocompetent patients.

KEY FACT

✓ Parvovirus is the cause of transient arthritis in adults (which is symmetrical, involves small joints, and can mimic rheumatoid arthritis) and aplastic crisis in persons with hemolytic anemias

---

Human T-Cell Lymphotropic Viruses

Human T-cell lymphotropic virus (HTLV) types I and II are non-HIV human retroviruses. HTLV-I is endemic in parts of Japan, the Caribbean basin, South America, and Africa. It can be transmitted through sexual contact, infected cellular blood products (not clotting factor concentrates), and injection drug use. Vertical transmission (eg, breast-feeding, transplacental) also occurs. HTLV-I is associated with human T-cell leukemia/lymphoma and tropical spastic paraparesis (also known as *HTLV-I–associated myelopathy*). However, clinical disease never develops in 96% of persons infected with HTLV-I. An HTLV-II infection does not cause clinical disease.

Parasites

Helminths

Neurocysticercosis is an infection of the CNS with a larval stage of the pork tapeworm, *Taenia solium*. It is acquired by ingesting tapeworm eggs from fecally contaminated food (not from eating undercooked pork). It is endemic in Latin America, Asia, and Africa. Cases have been reported among household contacts of foreign-born persons (working as domestic employees). The most common presentation is seizures. Brain imaging reveals cystic or calcified brain lesions. Serum or CSF serologic testing can aid in the diagnosis. Treatment with praziquantel or albendazole may be beneficial. The coadministration of corticosteroids often is used to decrease cerebral inflammation associated with therapy.

Strongyloides stercoralis is unique among the intestinal nematode infections. Unlike with the other helminths, the larvae of this organism can mature in the human host (autoinfection). In immunocompromised hosts (eg, persons with neutropenia, corticosteroid therapy, or AIDS), a superinfection can develop with larval migration throughout the body. Gram-negative bacteremia is a common coinfection, resulting from disruption of the intestinal mucosa by the invasive larvae. Treatment is with ivermectin.

Trichinosis is acquired from eating undercooked meat, particularly bear or cougar. Features include muscle pain (especially diaphragm, chest, and tongue), eosinophilia, and periorbital edema. Treatment is with mebendazole or albendazole.

Hookworm (*Necator americanus*) infection causes anemia. It is found mainly in tropical and subtropical regions. The larval form can penetrate intact skin. Walking barefoot is a risk factor for infection. Treatment is with mebendazole or albendazole.

Ascariasis infection may cause intestinal obstruction or pancreatitis (ie, the worm migrates up the pancreatic duct). Treatment is with mebendazole or albendazole.

Schistosomiasis is a tropical disease that causes hepatic cirrhosis, hematuria, and carcinoma of the bladder. It is acquired by direct penetration of the *Schistosoma cercariae* from contaminated water (eg, lakes, rivers). Praziquantel is the drug of choice for schistosomiasis.

Protozoan Parasites

Acanthamoeba, a free-living ameba, can cause amebic keratitis in persons swimming in freshwater while wearing soft contact lenses. The diagnosis is based on microscopic examination of scrapings of the cornea. Treatment is with topical antifungal agents. Patients often respond poorly to therapy and have progressive corneal destruction.

Symptomatic infection with *Entamoeba histolytica* (amebiasis) may cause diarrhea (often, bloody diarrhea), abdominal pain, and fever. Metronidazole administration, followed by a luminal agent such as iodoquinol or paromomycin, is the preferred therapy (metronidazole does not kill amebae in the intestinal lumen). Asymptomatic carriage of amebic cysts should be treated with one of the luminal agents.

Invasive amebiasis may lead to distant abscesses (primarily of the liver, but other organs can be involved). An amebic liver abscess usually is a sole abscess commonly located in the right lobe of the liver. The anatomical location and the fact that it is usually a single abscess may help to distinguish amebic hepatic abscess from bacterial abscess. Serologic tests are positive in more than 90% of patients with amebic abscess. Hepatic abscess may rupture into the peritoneal cavity or through the diaphragm into the right pleural space.

Giardia lamblia infection characteristically produces sudden onset of watery diarrhea with malabsorption, bloating, and flatulence. Prolonged disease that is refractory to standard therapy may occur in patients with immunoglobulin A deficiency. The organism may be detected in stool specimens through antigen testing, which has high sensitivity. Metronidazole, tinidazole, or nitazoxanide is effective for treating giardiasis.

Toxoplasma gondii is acquired from eating undercooked meat or being exposed to cat feces. Primary toxoplasmosis is usually asymptomatic. In immunocompetent persons, it may cause a heterophile-negative mononucleosislike syndrome. *Toxoplasma* chorioretinitis can occur in immunocompetent persons during primary infection. A person with toxoplasmosis may present with fever and blurry vision. On ophthalmologic examination, an acute retinochoroiditis causes marked vitreous reaction overlying the retinal infection, leading to the characteristic fundus picture of the optic nerve appearing as a "headlight in the fog." Reactivation disease can cause brain and eye lesions and pneumonia in patients with AIDS and other immunocompromising conditions. Toxoplasmosis can be treated effectively with pyrimethamine in combination with either sulfadiazine or clindamycin.

Malaria is caused by *Plasmodium* parasites and is endemic in many parts of the world. It is transmitted by *Anopheles* species mosquitoes that typically bite at night and predawn. After it enters human blood from mosquito bite, the parasite first matures in the liver and then infects erythrocytes. Spiking fevers, rigors, headache, and hemolytic anemia are the hallmarks of malaria. It is diagnosed through examination of Giemsa-stained thick and thin blood smears (Figure 43.6). PCR tests are available to confirm the diagnosis microscopically or in the clinical setting of low-level parasitemia. *Plasmodium falciparum* is the most common cause of fever in a traveler returned from Africa and is more likely to cause malarial complications, such as cerebral malaria, pulmonary edema, and death. With *P falciparum* malaria, fevers may be irregular or continuous. *Plasmodium vivax* and *Plasmodium malariae* infections cause regular episodic fevers (malarial paroxysms). *Plasmodium vivax* and *Plasmodium ovale* have hypnozoite forms that can remain latent in the liver and cause relapsing infection.

Chloroquine is the preferred treatment of infection caused by *P ovale, P vivax, P malariae*, and known chloroquine-susceptible strains of *P falciparum*. Chloroquine-resistant strains of *P falciparum* may respond

to quinine and doxycycline, atovaquone-proguanil hydrochloride, mefloquine, or artemisinin derivatives (available in the United States only through the Centers for Disease Control and Prevention). For severe *P falciparum* infection, IV quinidine gluconate is effective; however, resistant cases of *P falciparum* might require treatment with doxycycline or clindamycin. Exchange transfusion may be beneficial for severely ill patients with parasitemia of more than 10%. Primaquine is used to eradicate the exoerythrocytic phase of *P ovale* and *P vivax* infections, thereby preventing relapses.

Prophylaxis for malaria is increasingly difficult because of drug-resistant *P falciparum*. Personal protection should always be used (such as mosquito nets, insect repellents containing DEET). For travelers to chloroquine-sensitive areas—Central America, Mexico, Haiti, the Dominican Republic, and the Middle East—chloroquine is still effective therapy. In chloroquine-resistant areas, mefloquine, doxycycline, or an atovaquone-proguanil combination tablet is suggested. Travelers to the mefloquine-resistant areas of the Thai-Myanmar and Thai-Cambodian borders should use doxycycline or atovaquone-proguanil. Protection resulting from these medications ranges from 90% to 95%. All patients should be advised to seek medical attention if fever develops within 1 year after return from an endemic area.

Leishmaniasis is a protozoan disease transmitted by the bite of a sand fly. Visceral leishmaniasis (kalaazar, caused by *Leishmania donovani*) causes fever, hepatosplenomegaly, cachexia, and pancytopenia. Bone marrow examination (Giemsa stain) is often diagnostic. Cutaneous leishmaniasis (caused by *Leishmania tropica, Leishmania major, Leishmania braziliensis*, and *Leishmania mexicana*) occurs as a painless papule that progresses to an ulcer and may be self-limited. Cutaneous leishmaniasis has occurred in military personnel returning from Iraq (the so-called Baghdad boil) and Afghanistan. Cutaneous leishmaniasis lesions are often destructive and should be treated. Leishmaniasis treatment is antimony compounds or amphotericin B or its liposomal formulations.

Babesia microti is a tick-borne illness transmitted by the same *Ixodes* tick that is responsible for Lyme disease and

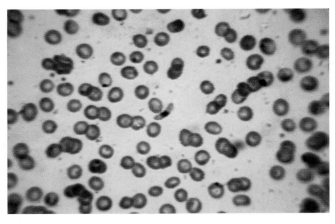

Figure 43.6 *Banana-Shaped Gametocyte of* Plasmodium falciparum *in Thin Blood Smear.*

KEY FACTS

✓ Chloroquine is the preferred treatment of infection by *P ovale, P vivax, P malariae*, and the known chloroquine-susceptible strains of *P falciparum*

✓ Chloroquine-resistant strains of *P falciparum* may respond to quinine and doxycycline, atovaquone-proguanil, mefloquine, or artemisinin derivatives (available in the United States only through the Centers for Disease Control and Prevention)

✓ Leishmaniasis is a protozoan disease transmitted through the bite of a sand fly

> **Key Definition**
>
> Neurocysticercosis: *An infection of the CNS with the larval stage of the pork tapeworm,* Taenia solium.

ehrlichiosis. This parasite infects erythrocytes and causes fever, myalgias, and hemolytic anemia. Often asymptomatic in healthy persons, severe disease may develop in asplenic individuals. Babesiosis is endemic in the northeastern United States, especially around Nantucket, Martha's Vineyard, and Cape Cod, Massachusetts. The diagnosis is established through examination of a peripheral blood smear or PCR amplification of *Babesia* DNA from peripheral blood. Treatment is with clindamycin and quinine or atovaquone plus azithromycin. Exchange transfusion has been needed in severely ill patients with high-level parasitemia. Simultaneous infection with babesiosis and Lyme disease may be especially severe.

44 Infective Endocarditis and Health Care–Associated Infections

M. RIZWAN SOHAIL, MD AND PRITISH K. TOSH, MD

Health Care–Associated Infections

Hospital-Acquired Pneumonia, Ventilator-Associated Pneumonia, and Health Care–Associated Pneumonia

Hospital-acquired pneumonia (HAP), ventilator-associated pneumonia (VAP), and health care–associated pneumonia (HCAP) cause 25% of all infections in the intensive care unit and are the basis for 50% of all antimicrobials prescribed in the hospital. These are primarily bacterial infections and are associated with high morbidity and mortality rates. However, pneumonias occurring before the fifth day of hospitalization are generally caused by organisms that are more susceptible to antimicrobials and have a better prognosis than those occurring on or after the fifth hospital day. The diagnostic and therapeutic approaches to HAP, VAP, and HCAP are similar.

HAP is pneumonia that develops in a nonintubated patient more than 48 hours after hospital admission. VAP develops in a patient more than 48 hours after intubation. By comparison, HCAP develops within 90 days of contact with a health care system (ie, inpatient or outpatient care, care in a hemodialysis center, or residence in a nursing home or long-term care facility) or within 30 days of receipt of antimicrobials, chemotherapy, or wound care.

> ### Key Definition
>
> **Hospital acquired pneumonia (HAP):** *HAP is pneumonia that develops in a nonintubated patient more than 48 hours after hospital admission.*

The common microbiologic causes of HAP, VAP, and HCAP are summarized in Box 44.1. The general principles

> ### Box 44.1 • Common Microbiologic Causes of HAP, VAP, and HCAP
>
> *Pseudomonas aeruginosa*
>
> *Klebsiella* spp
>
> *Serratia* spp
>
> *Escherichia coli*
>
> *Staphylococcus aureus*, including methicillin-resistant *S aureus*
>
> *Proteus mirabilis*
>
> *Citrobacter* spp
>
> *Enterobacter* spp
>
> *Acinetobacter* spp
>
> *Stenotrophomonas maltophilia*
>
> Abbreviations: HAP, hospital-acquired pneumonia; HCAP, health care–associated pneumonia; VAP, ventilator-associated pneumonia.

for treatment and prevention of HAP, VAP, and HCAP are listed in Box 44.2.

HAP, VAP, or HCAP should be suspected when a patient has clinical signs of lower respiratory tract infection, such as fever, purulent sputum, leukocytosis, decline in oxygenation, and a new infiltrate on chest imaging. Blood cultures and culture of lower respiratory tract secretions (eg, obtained with bronchoalveolar lavage in intubated patients) should be performed before starting or changing antimicrobial therapy. However, initiation of antimicrobial therapy should not be delayed while awaiting culture results. If a patient has marked clinical improvement within 48 to 72 hours of starting empirical antimicrobial therapy and sputum tests are negative, use of antimicrobials can safely be discontinued.

Box 44.2 • General Principles for Treatment and Prevention of HAP, VAP, and HCAP

1) Early recognition and start of empirical therapy (because morbidity and mortality rates increase with delays in initiation of antimicrobial treatment)

2) Choice of empirical therapy based on regional bacteriologic findings and susceptibility data

3) Antimicrobials stewardship to reduce unnecessary antimicrobial use and selection pressure for resistant organisms

4) Implement prevention strategies

   General
      Staff education and hand hygiene
      Surveillance of infections in the intensive care unit, including susceptibility testing

   Aspiration precautions
      Semirecumbent position (30°–45°), rather than supine
      Preference of enteral feeding over parenteral nutrition

   Intubation and mechanical ventilation
      Strategies to avoid re-intubation
      Noninvasive ventilation should be used when possible in selected patients
      Orotracheal and orogastric tubes are preferred over nasotracheal and nasogastric tubes
      Continuous aspiration of subglottic secretions should be performed
      Endotracheal tube cuff pressure maintenance at >20 cm H_2O
      Contaminated condensate should be carefully removed from ventilator circuits
      Protocols to reduce sedation and accelerate weaning should be enacted

Abbreviations: HAP, hospital-acquired pneumonia; HCAP, health care–associated pneumonia; VAP, ventilator-associated pneumonia.

Empirical antimicrobial therapy should be based on local microbiologic and susceptibility data. In general, empirical therapy should include an antipseudomonal β-lactam (eg, cefepime, ceftazadime, imipenem, meropenem, doripenem, piperacillin-tazobactam) *plus* an antipseudomonal aminoglycoside or fluoroquinolone (eg, amikacin, gentamicin, tobramycin, ciprofloxacin, levofloxacin) *plus* vancomycin or linezolid for coverage of methicillin-resistant *Staphylococcus aureus* (MRSA). In patients with recent antimicrobial exposure, antimicrobials of a different drug class should be used for empirical therapy. Antimicrobial therapy should be adjusted when the cause and antimicrobial susceptibilities are known. If started early, antimicrobial therapy can be stopped after 8 days, with the exception of pneumonia caused by *Pseudomonas*, for which 14 or more days of therapy is often recommended.

KEY FACTS

✓ HAP, VAP, and HCAP cause 25% of the intensive care unit infections. They are the reason for 50% of all antimicrobials prescribed in US hospitals

✓ HAP, VAP, and HCAP are primarily bacterial infections that are associated with high morbidity and mortality rates.

Catheter-Related Bloodstream Infection

In the United States, approximately 5 million central venous catheters are placed annually. About 1 in 20 of these catheters becomes infected. Indeed, catheter-related bloodstream infection (CR-BSI) is the most common cause of health care–associated bacteremia in the United States. CR-BSI is associated with substantial cost (about $28,000 per survivor), increased length of stay (average, 6.5 days), and a substantial mortality rate (10%–25%).

Catheter infection may present with local manifestations (port, tunnel, or exit site infection) or CR-BSI. Local infections are easy to recognize and always necessitate removal of the infected catheter. However, CR-BSI may present with no inflammatory signs or drainage from the exit site or tunnel. In these situations, blood should be simultaneously drawn from the catheter and a peripheral site. If cultures of blood drawn from the catheter have positive results 2 hours before the cultures from the peripheral site (differential time to positivity), this finding has high correlation (>80%) with catheter infection. If the catheter is urgently removed (eg, because of absence of an alternative source of infection, because of hemodynamic instability of the patient), the catheter tip should be submitted for culture. Growth of more than 15 colony-forming units (per milliliter) of bacteria is highly suggestive of the catheter being the source of bloodstream infection.

Removal of the infected catheter is always the preferred method for treating CR-BSI. Short-term catheters (temporary central venous catheters or peripherally inserted central catheter) should always be removed to treat CR-BSI. However, long-term tunneled catheters (for hemodialysis, chemotherapy, or parenteral nutrition) may be salvaged in patients who are clinically stable, have infection with a low-virulence organism (such as *Staphylococcus epidermidis*), and where bloodstream infection quickly resolves on therapy. Antibiotic lock therapy, in combination with systemic antimicrobial agents, is a key ingredient of catheter salvage attempts. A clinically unstable patient, presence of local or systemic complications, and infection with virulent organisms (such as *S aureus*, *Candida*, or gram-negative bacteria) warrant removal of an infected, long-term, tunneled catheter.

Box 44.3 • Modified Duke Criteria for the Diagnosis of Infective Endocarditis

Definite infective endocarditis

Pathologic criteria

Microorganisms on culture or histologic examination of a vegetation, a vegetation that has embolized, or an intracardiac abscess specimen,

or

Pathologic lesions; vegetation or intracardiac abscess confirmed by histologic examination showing active endocarditis

Clinical criteria[a]

2 major criteria, *or*

1 major criterion and 3 minor criteria, *or*

5 minor criteria

Possible infective endocarditis

1 major criterion and 1 minor criterion, *or*

3 minor criteria

Rejected

Firm alternative diagnosis explaining evidence of infective endocarditis,

or

Resolution of infective endocarditis syndrome with antibiotic therapy for ≤4 d, *or*

No pathologic evidence of infective endocarditis at surgery or autopsy, with antibiotic therapy for ≤4 d, *or*

Does not meet criteria for possible infective endocarditis, as above

---

[a] See Box 44.4 for definitions of major and minor criteria.

Adapted from Li JS, Sexton DJ, Mick N, Nettles R, Fowler VG Jr, Ryan T, et al. Proposed modifications to the Duke criteria for the diagnosis of infective endocarditis. Clin Infect Dis. 2000 Apr;30(4):633–8. Epub 2000 Apr 3. Used with permission.

Box 44.4 • Definitions of Terminology Used in the Modified Duke Criteria for the Diagnosis of Infective Endocarditis

Major criteria

Blood culture positive for infective endocarditis

Typical microorganisms consistent with infective endocarditis from 2 separate blood cultures

Viridans group streptococci, *Streptococcus bovis*, HACEK group, *Staphylococcus aureus,* or

Community-acquired enterococci, in the absence of a primary focus, *or*

Microorganisms consistent with infective endocarditis from persistently positive blood cultures, defined as follows:

At least 2 positive cultures of blood samples drawn >12 h apart, *or*

All of 3 or a majority of ≥4 separate blood cultures, with first and last samples drawn at least 1 h apart

Single blood culture positive for *Coxiella burnetii* or anti–phase I immunoglobulin G antibody titer ≥1:800

Evidence of endocardial involvement

Echocardiogram positive for infective endocarditis (TEE recommended in patients with prosthetic valves, rated at least "possible infective endocarditis" by clinical criteria, or complicated infective endocarditis [paravalvular abscess]; TTE as first test in other patients), defined as follows:

Oscillating intracardiac mass on valve or supporting structures, in the path of regurgitant jets, or on implanted material in the absence of an alternative anatomical explanation, *or*

Abscess, *or*

New partial dehiscence of prosthetic valve

New valvular regurgitation (worsening or changing of preexisting murmur not sufficient)

Minor criteria

Predisposition: predisposing heart condition or injection drug use

Fever: >38.0°C (>100.4°F)

Vascular phenomena: major arterial emboli, septic pulmonary infarcts, mycotic aneurysm, intracranial hemorrhage, conjunctival hemorrhages, Janeway lesions

Immunologic phenomena: glomerulonephritis, Osler nodes, Roth spots, rheumatoid factor

Microbiologic evidence: positive blood culture but not meeting major criteria as noted previously[a] *or* serologic evidence of active infection with organisms consistent with infective endocarditis

Echocardiographic minor criteria eliminated

Abbreviations: HACEK, *Haemophilus* spp, *Actinobacillus actinomycetem comitans, Cardiobacterium hominis, Eikenella* spp, and *Kingella kingae*; TEE, transesophageal echocardiography; TTE, transthoracic echocardiography.

[a] Excluding single positive cultures for coagulase-negative staphylococci and organisms that do not cause endocarditis.

Adapted from Li JS, Sexton DJ, Mick N, Nettles R, Fowler VG Jr, Ryan T, et al. Proposed modifications to the Duke criteria for the diagnosis of infective endocarditis. Clin Infect Dis. 2000 Apr;30(4):633–8. Epub 2000 Apr 3. Used with permission.

valve involvement is common in injection drug users and patients with health care–associated endocarditis due to central venous catheters or implanted cardiac devices.

Starting empirical antibiotic therapy before obtaining blood cultures is the most common cause of culture-negative endocarditis. Other reasons for culture-negative endocarditis include infection with fastidious organisms that are difficult to cultivate in blood cultures (Box 44.5). Several of these can be diagnosed with serologic tests or molecular assays. The HACEK group (*Haemophilus* species, *Actinobacillus actinomycetemcomitans, Cardiobacterium hominis, Eikenella* species, and *Kingella kingae*) has become a less frequent cause of culture-negative endocarditis because the organisms are more easily detected with contemporary blood culturing systems.

Treatment guidelines for native valve infective endocarditis are listed in Table 44.2.

Valvular endocarditis may be complicated by invasion and destruction of the valve or endocardium or by distant embolization. Large vegetations (>15 mm) increase the risk of embolization. The risk of embolization

---

Box 44.5 • Common Causes of Culture-Negative Infective Endocarditis

Administration of antibiotics before obtaining blood cultures

HACEK group organisms:

Haemophilus spp
Actinobacillus actinomycetemcomitans
Cardiobacterium hominis
Eikenella spp
Kingella kingae

Nutritionally variant streptococci (*Abiotrophia*, *Granulicatella*, and *Gemella* spp)

Fungi

Mycobacteria

Coxiella burnetii (causative agent of Q fever)

Chlamydia spp

Mycoplasma spp

Legionella spp

Bartonella spp

Tropheryma whipplei

Brucella spp

---

is greatest before the receipt of appropriate antimicrobials and decreases after the first week of therapy. Large vegetations may be seen in patients with delayed diagnosis or infection due to group B streptococci, HACEK, and fungi. Embolization may lead to strokes, mycotic aneurysms, and splenic, hepatic, and renal abscesses. Distant abscesses should be drained before valve replacement surgery. The indications for surgical treatment of endocarditis are listed in Box 44.6.

There is a well-recognized association between *Streptococcus bovis* bacteremia and carcinoma of the colon or other colonic disease.

KEY FACTS

✓ Mitral valve prolapse, bicuspid aortic valves, and aortic sclerosis are the principal predisposing valvular lesions in the absence of prosthetic materials

✓ *Streptococcus bovis* bacteremia and carcinoma of the colon or other colonic disease have a well-recognized association

---

Prosthetic Valve Endocarditis

Prosthetic valve endocarditis accounts for 1% to 5% of all endocarditis cases. However, the increasing number of patients with prosthetic valves and pacemakers is increasing the population at risk. Prosthetic valve endocarditis can be broadly categorized into early and late onset. Early-onset prosthetic valve endocarditis is an infection occurring within 2 months after valve replacement surgery, whereas late-onset prosthetic valve endocarditis occurs more than 2 months postoperatively.

Staphylococci are the leading cause of prosthetic valve endocarditis. The aortic valve is affected more often than the mitral valve. Most early-onset cases are due to infections introduced in the perioperative setting and are caused by staphylococci. In contrast, late-onset cases are frequently due to hematogenous seeding of prosthetic valves from a distant focus of infection. Therefore, the microbiologic nature of late-onset prosthetic valve endocarditis has certain similarities to that of community-acquired native valve endocarditis. Persistent bacteremia, heart failure, abscess formation, and stroke are predictors of higher death rate in patients with prosthetic valve endocarditis.

Treatment regimens for prosthetic valve endocarditis are summarized in Table 44.3.

Daptomycin therapy at 6 mg/kg daily has an efficacy similar to that of standard therapy in *S aureus* bacteremia and endocarditis and causes less nephrotoxicity than β-lactam–based or vancomycin-based regimens. However, longer use of daptomycin is associated with more frequent increases in the creatine kinase level.

Combination therapy with rifampin should be used only in cases of prosthetic valve endocarditis due to staphylococci. Use of rifampin in uncomplicated cases of *S aureus* bacteremia and native valve endocarditis has been associated with prolonging the duration of bacteremia and increased mortality.

Specific Pathogens Causing Endocarditis

Staphylococcus aureus
See the section Health Care–Associated Infections.

Viridans Group Streptococci
These bacteria are part of normal oral and enteric flora. This group is a common cause of subacute bacterial endocarditis, which should be suspected when viridans group streptococci are found in blood cultures. Similar to the pneumococci, they are increasingly likely to show variable resistance to penicillin.

Enterococci
Enterococci are an increasingly important cause of bacterial endocarditis. Enterococci are resistant to many antimicrobial agents, including all cephalosporins. Even for susceptible strains, penicillin or vancomycin monotherapy only inhibits bacterial growth and is not bactericidal. Moreover, strains that are resistant to both the penicillins and vancomycin (vancomycin-resistant enterococci) are spreading worldwide. Linezolid, dalfopristin/quinupristin,

Table 44.2 • Treatment of Native Valve Infective Endocarditis

Microorganisms	Therapy[a]	Alternative Therapy[a]
Penicillin-sensitive viridans group streptococci and *Streptococcus bovis* (MIC, ≤0.1 mcg/mL)	Aqueous crystalline penicillin G, 12–18 ×10^6 U/24 h IV either continuously or in 6 equally divided doses for 4 wk *Or* Ceftriaxone sodium 2 g IV or IM for 4 wk[c] *Or* Aqueous penicillin G, 12–18 ×10^6 U/24 h IV either continuously or in 6 equally divided doses for 2 wk *Plus* Gentamicin sulfate,[d] 1 mg/kg IV or IM every 8 h for 2 wk	Vancomycin,[b] 30 mg/kg IV in 2 equally divided doses, not to exceed 2 g/24 h unless serum levels are monitored for 4 wk Vancomycin therapy is recommended for patients allergic to β-lactams (immediate-type hypersensitivity); serum concentration of vancomycin should be obtained 1 h after completion of the infusion and should be in the range of 30–45 mcg/mL for twice-daily dosing
Relatively penicillin-resistant viridans group streptococci (MIC, >0.1 mcg/mL and <0.5 mcg/mL)	Aqueous crystalline penicillin G, 24 ×10^6 U/24 h IV either continuously or in 4–6 equally divided doses for 4 wk *Plus* Gentamicin sulfate,[d] 1 mg/kg IV or IM every 8 h for 2 wk	Vancomycin,[b] 30 mg/kg IV in 2 equally divided doses, not to exceed 2 g/24 h unless serum levels are monitored for 4 wk Vancomycin therapy is recommended for patients allergic to β-lactams (immediate-type hypersensitivity); serum concentration of vancomycin should be obtained 1 h after completion of the infusion and should be in the range of 30–45 mcg/mL for twice-daily dosing
Enterococci (gentamicin- or vancomycin-susceptible) or viridans group streptococci with MIC ≥0.5 mcg/mL or nutritionally variant streptococci (all enterococci causing endocarditis must be tested for antimicrobial susceptibility in order to select optimal therapy)	Aqueous crystalline penicillin G, 18–30 ×10^6 U/24 h IV either continuously or in 6 equally divided doses for 4–6 wk *Or* Ampicillin sodium, 12 g/24 h IV either continuously or in 6 equally divided doses *Plus* Gentamicin sulfate,[d] 1 mg/kg IV or IM every 8 h for 4–6 wk (4-wk therapy recommended for patients with symptoms ≤3 mo in duration; 6-wk therapy recommended for patients with symptoms >3 mo in duration)	Vancomycin,[b] 30 mg/kg IV in 2 equally divided doses, not to exceed 2 g/24 h unless serum levels are monitored for 4–6 wk *Plus* Gentamicin,[d] 1 mg/kg IV or IM every 8 h for 4–6 wk Vancomycin therapy is recommended for patients allergic to β-lactams (immediate-type hypersensitivity); serum concentration of vancomycin should be obtained 1 h after completion of the infusion and should be in the range of 30–45 mcg/mL for twice-daily dosing Cephalosporins are not acceptable alternatives for patients allergic to penicillin
High-level aminoglycoside-resistant *Enterococcus faecalis*: ceftriaxone 2 g IV every 12 h *plus* ampicillin 2 g IV every 4 h for 4–6 wk	Linezolid, 1,200 mg/24 h IV or orally in 2 divided doses for ≥8 wk *Or* Dalfopristin/quinupristin, 22.5 mg/kg per 24 h IV in 3 divided doses for ≥8 wk	Patients with endocarditis caused by these strains should be treated in consultation with an infectious diseases specialist Cardiac valve replacement may be necessary for bacteriologic cure. Cure with antimicrobial therapy alone may be <50% Severe, usually reversible thrombocytopenia may occur with use of linezolid, especially after 2 wk of therapy Dalfopristin/quinupristin is effective against *E faecium* only and can cause severe myalgias, which may require discontinuation of therapy Only a small number of patients have reportedly been treated with imipenem/cilastatin-ampicillin or ceftriaxone + ampicillin

(continued)

Table 44.2 • Continued

Microorganisms	Therapy[a]	Alternative Therapy[a]
E faecalis	Imipenem/cilastatin, 2 g/24 h IV in 4 equally divided doses for ≥8 wk *Plus* Ampicillin sodium, 12 g/24 h IV in 6 divided doses for ≥8 wk *Or* Ceftriaxone sodium, 2 g/24 h IV or IM in 1 dose for ≥8 wk *Plus* Ampicillin sodium, 12 g/24 h IV in 6 divided doses for ≥8 wk *Pediatric dose* (should not exceed that of a normal adult): linezolid, 30 mg/kg per 24 h IV or orally in 3 divided doses; dalfopristin/quinupristin, 22.5 mg/kg per 24 h IV in 3 divided doses; imipenem/cilastatin, 60–100 mg/kg per 24 h IV in 4 divided doses; ampicillin, 300 mg/kg per 24 h IV in 4–6 divided doses; ceftriaxone, 100 mg/kg per 24 h IV or IM once daily	
Staphylococcus aureus[e] methicillin-sensitive	Nafcillin sodium or oxacillin sodium, 2.0 g IV every 4 h for 4–6 wk *Plus* Gentamicin sulfate (optional),[d] 1 mg/kg every 8 h IV or IM for first 3–5 d Benefit of additional aminoglycoside has not been established	Cefazolin (or other first-generation cephalosporins in equivalent dosages), 2 g IV every 8 h for 4–6 wk *Plus* Gentamicin (optional),[d] 1 mg/kg every 8 h IV or IM for first 3–5 d Cephalosporins should be avoided in patients with immediate-type hypersensitivity to penicillin Vancomycin,[b] 30 mg/kg IV in 2 equally divided doses, not to exceed 2 g/24 h unless serum levels are monitored for 4–6 wk Vancomycin therapy is recommended for patients allergic to β-lactams (immediate-type hypersensitivity); serum concentration of vancomycin should be obtained 1 h after completion of the infusion and should be in the range of 30–45 mcg/mL for twice-daily dosing Daptomycin, 6 mg/kg once daily, may be used as an alternative in right-sided endocarditis due to MSSA or MRSA
S aureus[e] methicillin-resistant	Vancomycin,[b] 30 mg/kg IV in 2 equally divided doses, not to exceed 2 g/24 h unless serum levels are monitored for 4–6 wk	Consult an infectious diseases specialist Daptomycin, 6 mg/kg once daily, may be used as an alternative in right-sided endocarditis due to MSSA or MRSA
HACEK group	Ceftriaxone sodium, 2 g IV or IM for 4 wk[c] *Or* Ampicillin[f]-sulbactam 12 g/24 h IV in 4 divided doses for 4 wk *Or* Ciprofloxacin 1,000 mg/24 h orally or 800 mg/24 h IV in 2 divided doses if unable to tolerate alternatives Cefotaxime sodium or other third-generation cephalosporins may be substituted	Consult an infectious diseases specialist
Neisseria gonorrhoeae	Ceftriaxone, 1–2 g every 24 h for ≥4 wk	Aqueous crystalline penicillin G, 20 ×10^6 U/24 h IV either continuously or in 6 equally divided doses for 4 wk, for penicillin-susceptible isolates

Table 44.2 • Continued

Microorganisms	Therapy[a]	Alternative Therapy[a]
Gram-negative bacilli	Most effective single drug or combination of drugs IV for 4–6 wk	
Urgent empirical treatment for culture-negative endocarditis	Vancomycin,[b] 30 mg/kg IV in 2 equally divided doses, not to exceed 2 g/24 h unless serum levels are monitored for 6 wk *Plus* Gentamicin sulfate,[d] 1.0 mg/kg IV every 8 h for 6 wk	
Fungal endocarditis	Amphotericin B *Plus* Flucytosine (optional) *Plus* Cardiac valve replacement (flucytosine levels should be monitored)	
Suspected *Bartonella*, culture negative	Ceftriaxone sodium, 2 g/24 h IV or IM in 1 dose for 6 wk *Plus* Gentamicin sulfate, 3 mg/kg per 24 h IV or IM in 3 divided doses for 2 wk *With or without* Doxycycline, 200 mg/kg per 24 h IV or orally in 2 divided doses for 6 wk	Consult an infectious diseases specialist

Abbreviations: HACEK, *Haemophilus* spp, *Actinobacillus actinomycetemcomitans*, *Cardiobacterium hominis*, *Eikenella* spp, and *Kingella kingae*; IM, intramuscularly; IV, intravenously; MIC, minimal inhibitory concentration; MRSA, methicillin-resistant *Staphylococcus aureus*; MSSA, methicillin-sensitive *Staphylococcus aureus*.

[a] Dosages recommended are for patients with normal renal function.

[b] Vancomycin dosage should be reduced in patients with impaired renal function. Vancomycin given on an mg/kg basis produces higher serum concentrations in obese patients than in lean patients. Therefore, in obese patients, dosing should be based on ideal body weight. Each dose of vancomycin should be infused over at least 1 h to reduce the risk of the histamine-release "red man" syndrome.

[c] Patients should be notified that IM injection of ceftriaxone is painful.

[d] Dosing of gentamicin on an mg/kg basis produces higher serum concentrations in obese patients than in lean patients. Therefore, in obese patients, dosing should be based on ideal body weight. (Ideal body weight for men is 50 kg + 2.3 kg per inch taller than 5 feet, and ideal body weight for women is 45.5 kg + 2.3 kg per inch taller than 5 feet.) Relative contraindications to the use of gentamicin are age older than 65 years, renal impairment, or impairment of the eighth nerve. Other potentially nephrotoxic agents (such as nonsteroidal anti-inflammatory drugs) should be used cautiously in patients receiving gentamicin.

[e] For treatment of endocarditis due to penicillin-susceptible staphylococci (MIC, <0.1 mcg/mL), aqueous crystalline penicillin G, 12–18 ×10⁶ U/24 h IV either continuously or in 6 equally divided doses for 4 to 6 weeks, can be used instead of nafcillin or oxacillin. Shorter antibiotic courses have been effective in some injection drug users with right-sided endocarditis due to *S aureus*. The routine use of rifampin is not recommended for treatment of native-valve staphylococcal endocarditis.

[f] Ampicillin should not be used when laboratory tests show β-lactamase production.

Data from Wilson WR, Karchmer AW, Dajani AS, Taubert KA, Bayer A, Kaye D, et al; American Heart Association. Antibiotic treatment of adults with infective endocarditis due to streptococci, enterococci, staphylococci, and HACEK microorganisms. JAMA. 1995 Dec 6;274(21):1706–13; adapted from Steckelberg JM, Guiliani ER, Wilson WR. Infective endocarditis. In: Giuliani ER, Fuster V, Gersh BJ, McGoon MD, McGoon DC, editors. Cardiology: fundamentals and practice. 2nd ed. Vol 2. St. Louis (MO): Mosby Year Book; c1991. p. 1739–72. Used with permission of Mayo Foundation for Medical Education and Research; and adapted from Baddour LM, Wilson WR, Bayer AS, Fowler VG Jr, Bolger AF, Levison ME, et al. Infective endocarditis: diagnosis, antimicrobial therapy, and management of complications: a statement for healthcare professionals from the Committee on Rheumatic Fever, Endocarditis, and Kawasaki Disease, Council on Cardiovascular Disease in the Young, and the Councils on Clinical Cardiology, Stroke, and Cardiovascular Surgery and Anesthesia, American Heart Association: executive summary. Circulation. 2005 Jun 14;111(23):3167–84. Used with permission.

and daptomycin are used in cases of vancomycin-resistant enterococci infection. However, these agents are also bacteriostatic and not bactericidal. Of note, dalfopristin/quinupristin is active against only *Enterococcus faecium* and not against *E faecalis*.

To achieve the bactericidal activity necessary to cure endocarditis due to enterococci, a combination of penicillin (or ampicillin) plus gentamicin (or streptomycin) is required. The choice of aminoglycoside depends on the results of susceptibility testing (Tables 44.3 and 44.4). Four weeks of therapy is adequate for native valve endocarditis that has been present for less than 3 months and is uncomplicated. When a patient is symptomatic for more than 3 months, has a prosthetic heart valve, or is allergic to penicillin—in which case vancomycin needs to be used—6 weeks of therapy is recommended. Vancomycin is considered less effective than penicillin and therefore should be used only in cases of penicillin resistance or if a patient is

> **Box 44.6 • Indications for Valve Replacement Surgery in Infective Endocarditis**
>
> Heart failure refractory to medical management
>
> More than 1 systemic embolic episode while receiving appropriate therapy
>
> Persistent bacteremia despite appropriate antimicrobial therapy
>
> Perivalvular extension of infection or abscess formation
>
> New electrocardiographic changes suggestive of heart block
>
> Persistent unexplained fever
>
> Fungal endocarditis

allergic to penicillin. A valve replacement procedure may increase the chance of successful treatment in these cases.

Haemophilus Species Other Than *Haemophilus influenzae*

Haemophilus parainfluenzae, Haemophilus aphrophilus, and *Haemophilus paraphrophilus* are part of the normal oral flora and are members of the HACEK group of organisms. Blood cultures positive for these organisms should raise suspicion for endocarditis. Large valvular vegetations with systemic emboli are frequent with HACEK endocarditis. Treatment of HACEK endocarditis is summarized in Table 44.2.

Echocardiography in Infective Endocarditis

Transesophageal echocardiography is superior to transthoracic echocardiography (TTE) for the diagnosis and

Table 44.3 • Treatment of Prosthetic Valve Infection

Organism	Therapy[a]	Alternative Therapy/Comments[a]
Staphylococcus aureus or coagulase-negative staphylococci: methicillin-resistant	Vancomycin,[b] 30 mg/kg IV in 2 equally divided doses, not to exceed 2 g/24 h unless serum levels are monitored for ≥6 wk *Plus* Rifampin,[c] 300 mg orally every 8 h for ≥6 wk *Plus* Gentamicin sulfate,[d] 1 mg/kg IV or IM every 8 h for first 2 wk of therapy. (If organism is not susceptible to gentamicin, ciprofloxacin may be substituted when the organism is susceptible in vitro)	Rifampin increases the amount of warfarin sodium required for antithrombotic therapy
Staphylococcus aureus or coagulase-negative staphylococci: methicillin-susceptible	Nafcillin sodium or oxacillin sodium, 2 g IV every 4 h for ≥6 wk *Plus* Rifampin,[c] 300 mg orally every 8 h for ≥6 wk *Plus* Gentamicin sulfate,[d] 1 mg/kg IV or IM every 8 h for first 2 wk of therapy (if organism is not susceptible to gentamicin, ciprofloxacin may be substituted when the organism is susceptible in vitro)	Rifampin increases the amount of warfarin sodium required for antithrombotic therapy First-generation cephalosporins or vancomycin should be used in patients allergic to β-lactams Cephalosporins should be avoided in patients with immediate-type hypersensitivity to penicillin or to methicillin-resistant staphylococci
Enterococci (gentamicin- or vancomycin-susceptible) or viridans group streptococci or nutritionally variant streptococci or *Streptococcus bovis* (all streptococci causing endocarditis must be tested for antimicrobial susceptibility in order to select optimal therapy)	Aqueous crystalline penicillin G, 18–30 ×10⁶ U/24 h IV either continuously or in 6 equally divided doses for 6 wk *Or* Ampicillin sodium, 12 g/24 h IV either continuously or in 6 equally divided doses for 6 wk *Plus* Gentamicin sulfate,[d] 1 mg/kg IV or IM every 8 h for 6 wk	Vancomycin,[b] 30 mg/kg IV in 2 equally divided doses, not to exceed 2 g/24 h unless serum levels are monitored for 4–6 wk *Plus* Gentamicin sulfate,[d] 1 mg/kg IV or IM every 8 h for 4–6 wk Vancomycin therapy is recommended for patients allergic to β-lactams (immediate-type hypersensitivity); serum concentration of vancomycin should be obtained 1 h after completion of the infusion and should be in the range of 30–45 mcg/mL for twice-daily dosing Cephalosporins are not acceptable alternatives for patients allergic to penicillin

Table 44.3 • Continued

Organism	Therapy[a]	Alternative Therapy/Comments[a]
Enterococcus faecium	Linezolid, 1,200 mg/24 h IV or orally in 2 divided doses for ≥8 wk *Or* Dalfopristin/quinupristin, 22.5 mg/kg per 24 h IV in 3 divided doses for ≥8 wk	Patients with endocarditis caused by these strains should be treated in consultation with an infectious diseases specialist Cardiac valve replacement may be necessary for bacteriologic cure Cure with antimicrobial therapy alone may be <50% Severe, usually reversible thrombocytopenia may occur with use of linezolid, especially after 2 wk of therapy Dalfopristin/quinupristin is only effective against *E faecium* and can cause severe myalgias, which may require discontinuation of therapy Only a small number of patients have reportedly been treated with imipenem/cilastatin-ampicillin or ceftriaxone *plus* ampicillin
Enterococcus faecalis	Imipenem/cilastatin, 2 g/24 h IV in 4 equally divided doses for ≥8 wk *Plus* Ampicillin sodium, 12 g/24 h IV in 6 divided doses for ≥8 wk *Or* Ceftriaxone sodium, 2 g/24 h IV or IM in 1 dose for ≥8 wk *Plus* Ampicillin sodium, 12 g/24 h IV in 6 divided doses for ≥8 wk *Pediatric dose* (should not exceed that of a normal adult): linezolid, 30 mg/kg per 24 h IV or orally in 3 divided doses; dalfopristin/quinupristin, 22.5 mg/kg per 24 h IV in 3 divided doses; imipenem/cilastatin, 60–100 mg/kg per 24 h IV in 4 divided doses; ampicillin, 300 mg/kg per 24 h IV in 4–6 divided doses; ceftriaxone, 100 mg/kg per 24 h IV or IM once daily	

Abbreviations: IM, intramuscularly; IV, intravenously.

[a] Dosages recommended are for patients with normal renal function.

[b] Vancomycin dosage should be reduced in patients with impaired renal function. Vancomycin given on an mg/kg basis produces greater serum concentrations in obese patients than in lean patients. Therefore, in obese patients, dosing should be based on ideal body weight. Each dose of vancomycin should be infused over at least 1 h to reduce the risk of the histamine-release "red man" syndrome.

[c] Rifampin has a unique role in the eradication of staphylococcal infection involving prosthetic material; combination therapy is essential to prevent emergence of rifampin resistance.

[d] Dosing of gentamicin on an mg/kg basis produces greater serum concentrations in obese patients than in lean patients. Therefore, in obese patients, dosing should be based on ideal body weight. (Ideal body weight for men is 50 kg + 2.3 kg per inch over 5 feet, and ideal body weight for women is 45.5 kg + 2.3 kg per inch over 5 feet.) Relative contraindications to the use of gentamicin are age older than 65 years, renal impairment, or impairment of the eighth nerve. Other potentially nephrotoxic agents (such as nonsteroidal anti-inflammatory drugs) should be used cautiously in patients receiving gentamicin.

Data from Wilson WR, Karchmer AW, Dajani AS, Taubert KA, Bayer A, Kaye D, et al; American Heart Association. Antibiotic treatment of adults with infective endocarditis due to streptococci, enterococci, staphylococci, and HACEK microorganisms. JAMA. 1995 Dec 6;274(21):1706–13; and adapted from Baddour LM, Wilson WR, Bayer AS, Fowler VG Jr, Bolger AF, Levison ME, et al. Infective endocarditis: diagnosis, antimicrobial therapy, and management of complications: a statement for healthcare professionals from the Committee on Rheumatic Fever, Endocarditis, and Kawasaki Disease, Council on Cardiovascular Disease in the Young, and the Councils on Clinical Cardiology, Stroke, and Cardiovascular Surgery and Anesthesia, American Heart Association: executive summary. Circulation. 2005 Jun 14;111(23):3167–84. Used with permission.

Table 44.4 • Regimens for a Dental Procedure

| Situation | Agent | Single Dose 30–60 Min Before Procedure | |
		Adults	Children
Oral	Amoxicillin	2 g	50 mg/kg
Unable to take oral medication	Ampicillin *Or*	2 g IM or IV	50 mg/kg IM or IV
	Cefazolin or ceftriaxone	1 g IM or IV	50 mg/kg IM or IV
Allergic to penicillins or ampicillin—oral	Cephalexin[a,b] *Or*	2 g	50 mg/kg
	Clindamycin *Or*	600 mg	20 mg/kg
	Azithromycin or clarithromycin	500 mg	15 mg/kg
Allergic to penicillins or ampicillin and unable to take oral medication	Cefazolin or ceftriaxone[b] *Or*	1 g IM or IV	50 mg/kg IM or IV
	Clindamycin	600 mg IM or IV	20 mg/kg IM or IV

Abbreviations: IM, intramuscularly; IV, intravenously.

[a] Or other first- or second-generation oral cephalosporin in equivalent adult or pediatric dosage.

[b] Cephalosporins should not be used in a patient with a history of anaphylaxis, angioedema, or urticaria with penicillins or ampicillin.

Adapted from Wilson W, Taubert KA, Gewitz M, Lockhart PB, Baddour LM, Levison M, et al. Prevention of infective endo-carditis: guidelines from the American Heart Association: a guideline from the American Heart Association Rheumatic Fever, Endocarditis, and Kawasaki Disease Committee, Council on Cardiovascular Disease in the Young, and the Council on Clinical Cardiology, Council on Cardiovascular Surgery and Anesthesia, and the Quality of Care and Outcomes Research Interdisciplinary Working Group. Circulation. 2007 Oct 9;116(15):1736–54. Epub 2007 Apr 19. Used with permission.

assessment of complications of endocarditis. The sensitivity of TTE for diagnosing endocarditis is less than 50% in most series, whereas it is more than 95% with TEE. Moreover, TEE is superior for detection of cardiac abscesses or mycotic aneurysms, visualization of vegetations less than 5 mm in size, pulmonic valve infection, and vegetation attached to prosthetic valves or cardiac device leads.

Infections of Cardiovascular Implantable Electronic Devices

Permanent pacemakers, implantable cardioverter-defibrillators, and other cardiac devices are being increasingly used. Infections associated with these devices may present as localized generator-pocket infection or systemic infection associated with bacteremia or lead endocarditis. Staphylococci (*S aureus* and CoNS) account for two-thirds of the cases. Regardless of the infecting pathogen and clinical presentation, complete removal of the infected device (including

Box 44.7 • Guidelines for the Diagnosis and Management of Cardiac Device Infections

All patients should have at least 2 blood cultures drawn at initial evaluation

Generator tissue should be obtained for Gram stain and culture, and lead tip tissue should be obtained for culture at device removal

Patients who have blood culture positivity should undergo TEE to assess for device-related endocarditis. Sensitivity of TTE is low, thus it is not the preferred evaluation test for evaluating for device-related endocarditis

All patients with device infection should undergo complete device removal, including all leads, regardless of clinical presentation

Most device leads (even with lead vegetations) can be safely removed percutaneously by experienced operator. Surgical consultation is recommended for lead vegetation >3 cm

Blood cultures should be repeated for all patients after device explantation to document cure of infection and plan for reimplantation of new device

Duration of antimicrobial therapy should also be extended to 4–6 wk in patients with complicated infection (eg, endocarditis, septic venous thrombosis, osteomyelitis, metastatic seeding)

Adequate débridement of generator pocket and control of bloodstream infection should be achieved before reimplantation of a new device

Reevaluation of the continued need for the device should be performed before a new device placement. On average, one-third of patients may no longer need a new device

If an infected cardiac device cannot be removed, then long-term suppressive antibiotic therapy should be administered after completing an initial course of parenteral therapy. Opinion of an infectious diseases expert should be sought for appropriate selection of long-term suppressive therapy

Abbreviations: TEE, transesophageal echocardiography; TTE, transthoracic echocardiography.

Adapted from Sohail MR, Uslan DZ, Khan AH, Friedman PA, Hayes DL, Wilson WR, et al. Management and outcome of permanent pacemaker and implantable cardioverter-defibrillator infections. J Am Coll Cardiol. 2007 May 8;49(18):1851–9. Epub 2007 Apr 23. Used with permission.

generator and transvenous leads) is a requisite for curing these infections.

Box 44.7 and Figure 44.1 summarize Mayo Clinic guidelines for the diagnosis and management of infections of cardiac devices. The American Heart Association endorsed these guidelines in its updated Scientific Statement, published in 2010.

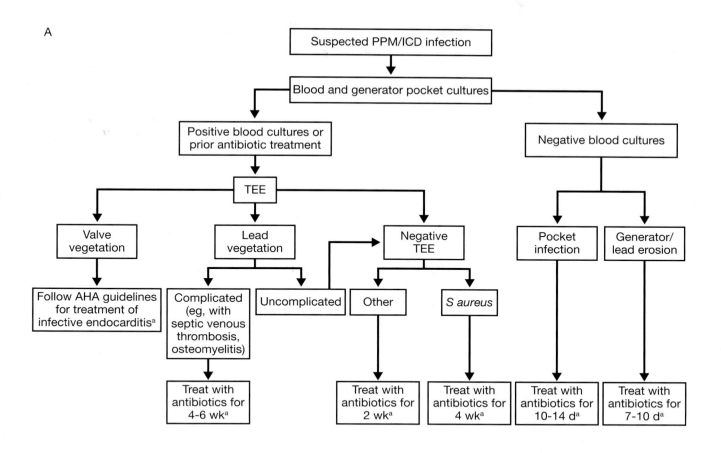

A

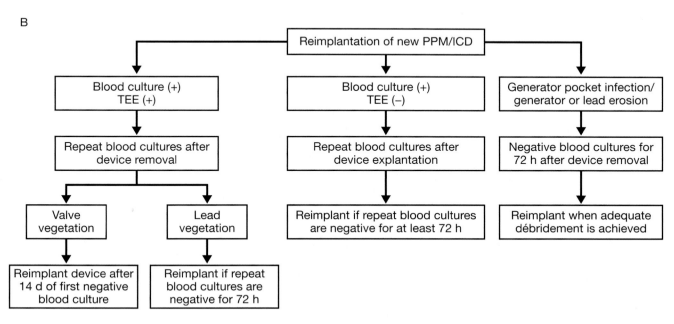

B

Figure 44.1 *Algorithm for Management of Cardiac Device Infection. A, Approach to management of infection in adults (also see Box 44.8). This algorithm applies only to patients with complete device explantation. B, Guidelines for reimplantation of new device (also see Box 44.7).* [a] *Duration of antibiotic treatment should be counted from the day of device explantation. AHA indicates American Heart Association; ICD, implantable cardioverter-defibrillator; PPM, permanent pacemaker; S aureus, Staphylococcus aureus; TEE, transesophageal echocardiography; +, positive; −, negative.*

(Adapted from Sohail MR, Uslan DZ, Khan AH, Friedman PA, Hayes DL, Wilson WR, et al. Management and outcome of permanent pacemaker and implantable cardioverter-defibrillator infections. J Am Coll Cardiol. 2007 May 8;49[18]:1851–9. Epub 2007 Apr 23. Used with permission.)

Box 44.8 • Cardiac Conditions for Which Endocarditis Prophylaxis With Dental Procedures Is Recommended

Prosthetic heart valve

History of infective endocarditis

CHD[a]

1) Unrepaired cyanotic CHD, including palliative shunts and conduits
2) Congenital heart defect completely repaired with prosthetic material or device, whether placed through surgery or catheter intervention, during the first 6 mo after the procedure[b]
3) Repaired CHD with residual defects at or adjacent to the site of a prosthetic patch or prosthetic device (which inhibit endothelialization)
4) Cardiac transplant recipients who have valvulopathy of the transplanted heart

Abbreviation: CHD, congenital heart disease.

[a] Only for these conditions; antibiotic prophylaxis is no longer recommended for any other form of CHD.

[b] Prophylaxis is recommended because endothelialization of prosthetic material occurs within 6 mo after the procedure.

Adapted from Wilson W, Taubert KA, Gewitz M, Lockhart PB, Baddour LM, Levison M, et al. Prevention of infective endocarditis: guidelines from the American Heart Association: a guideline from the American Heart Association Rheumatic Fever, Endocarditis, and Kawasaki Disease Committee, Council on Cardiovascular Disease in the Young, and the Council on Clinical Cardiology, Council on Cardiovascular Surgery and Anesthesia, and the Quality of Care and Outcomes Research Interdisciplinary Working Group. Circulation. 2007 Oct 9;116(15):1736–54. Epub 2007 Apr 19. Used with permission.

Prevention of Bacterial Endocarditis

Recommendations for the prevention of bacterial endocarditis were extensively revised and simplified in 2007. Endocarditis prophylaxis is no longer recommended before genitourinary or gastrointestinal procedures, regardless of the cardiac lesions. Prophylaxis for infective endocarditis is now recommended only in patients with high-risk cardiac lesions (Box 44.8). For these high-risk patients, prophylaxis is indicated before dental procedures that involve manipulation of the gingival tissue or the periapical region of the teeth or involve perforation of the oral mucosa. Current recommendations for antibiotic prophylaxis before a dental procedure are summarized in Table 44.4.

KEY FACTS

✓ Endocarditis prophylaxis is no longer recommended before genitourinary or gastrointestinal procedures regardless of the cardiac lesions

✓ Prophylaxis for infective endocarditis is now recommended only in patients with high-risk cardiac lesions.

Pulmonary and Mycobacterial Infections

PRITISH K. TOSH, MD AND ELIE F. BERBARI, MD

Viral Infections

Influenza

Influenza causes annual, seasonal epidemics that lead to tens of thousands of deaths each year in the United States. Two influenza A strains (H3N2 and H1N1) and 1 or 2 influenza B strains typically circulate during winter months and undergo minor antigenic mutations (**antigenic drift**) resulting in annual seasonal epidemics. Influenza pandemics occur more rarely (every 20–30 years) and are the result of major antigenic changes (**antigenic shift**) leading to large numbers of infections due to low levels of population immunity. In seasonal epidemics, 80% to 90% of deaths due to influenza occur in persons older than 65 years. Complications include 1) primary influenza pneumonia and 2) secondary bacterial infection, which usually is caused by *Streptococcus pneumoniae*, *Haemophilus* sp, or *Staphylococcus aureus*.

Key Definitions

Antigenic drift: *Minor antigenic mutations that occur during a season.*

Antigenic shift: *Major antigenic mutations that occur and result in pandemics.*

Amantadine and rimantadine are effective against only the influenza A viruses, not influenza B. Neuraminidase inhibitors (oseltamivir and zanamivir) are effective against disease caused by influenza A and influenza B. Oseltamivir or zanamivir can reduce the duration of symptoms by 1 day when given within 48 hours after symptom onset. Because of seasonal changes in antiviral resistance of circulating strains, recommendations for treatment from the Centers for Disease Control and Prevention should be consulted each year.

KEY FACT

✓ Amantadine and rimantadine are effective against influenza A viruses only. Neuraminidase inhibitors (oseltamivir and zanamivir) are effective against both influenza A and B viruses. When given within 48 hours after symptom onset, both oseltamivir and zanamivir reduce symptom duration by 1 day

---

Inactivated injectable and live attenuated intranasal influenza vaccines are used for disease prevention. Inactivated influenza vaccine is recommended for everyone older than 6 months, but target groups for vaccination include persons older than 50 years, residents of long-term care facilities, persons with cardiopulmonary disorders, children older than 6 months who are receiving long-term aspirin therapy (to prevent Reye syndrome), health care personnel, employees of long-term care facilities, providers of home health care, and persons sharing the same household as someone at high risk for influenza. The live attenuated vaccine is approved only for healthy immunocompetent persons between the ages of 2 and 49 years. Adverse reactions to both vaccines include fever, myalgias, and hypersensitivity. For persons at high risk for influenza complication who did not receive the vaccine, antiviral prophylaxis can be used for influenza prevention and is effective after exposure to a person with influenza.

Respiratory Syncytial Virus

Respiratory syncytial virus (RSV) is a common cause of winter-time respiratory illness, especially in children. Lower respiratory tract infection with RSV is uncommon in immunocompetent adults. However, it can be life-threatening in adults who are severely immunocompromised, such as a recipient of solid organ transplant or bone marrow transplant. For these highly immunocompromised adults who have evidence of RSV pneumonia, treatment with oral or inhaled ribavirin with or without intravenous immunoglobulin should be considered.

Adenovirus

Adenovirus can cause viral pneumonia in immunocompetent adults and is classically associated with conjunctivitis and diarrhea. Although usually self-limiting, adenovirus-related lower respiratory tract infections can be severe and antivirals such as foscarnet should be considered in severe cases or for immunocompromised patients.

KEY FACT

✓ Adenovirus can cause viral pneumonia in adults who are immunocompetent and is classically associated with conjunctivitis and diarrhea

Varicella

In adults, varicella (chickenpox) pneumonia is a severe illness. In adults with chickenpox, the most important predictors of varicella pneumonia are cough (which occurs in 25% of patients), profuse rash, fever for more than 1 week, and age 35 years or older. Early therapy with intravenous acyclovir is recommended for patients at risk for pneumonia.

Cytomegalovirus

Cytomegalovirus (CMV) pneumonia typically occurs in immunocompromised patients, such as those with AIDS who have CD4 counts less than 50/mcL, transplant recipients, and patients with hematologic malignancies. Diffuse, small nodular or hazy infiltrates are seen on chest radiographs of 15% of patients with pneumonia caused by CMV. Interstitial pneumonia due to CMV occurs in 50% of bone marrow graft recipients. Diagnosis of CMV pneumonia is made by finding characteristic inclusion bodies in affected cells, isolating the virus, or detecting CMV antigens or nucleic acids. Isolation of CMV from respiratory tract secretions does not always establish that infection is present.

KEY FACTS

✓ Cytomegalovirus (CMV) pneumonia typically occurs in immunocompromised patients

✓ Diagnosis of CMV pneumonia is made through finding characteristic inclusion bodies in affected cells, virus isolation, or detection of CMV antigens or nucleic acids

✓ CMV isolation from respiratory tract secretions does not always establish the presence of infection

Bacterial Infections

Community-Acquired Pneumonia

Each year in the United States, more than 900,000 cases of community-acquired pneumonia (CAP) occur in persons older than 65 years. Despite the use of antimicrobials, its mortality rate continues to be high. CAP and influenza combine to be the seventh leading cause of death in the United States. Common microbiologic causes of CAP are *S pneumoniae*, *Mycoplasma pneumoniae*, *Haemophilus influenzae*, *Chlamydophila (Chlamydia) pneumoniae*, *Legionella* sp, *S aureus*, and respiratory viruses (most commonly, influenza and RSV) (Table 45.1).

KEY FACT

✓ Common microbiologic causes of community-acquired pneumonia (CAP) are *Streptococcus pneumoniae*, *Mycoplasma pneumoniae*, *Haemophilus influenzae*, *Chlamydophila (Chlamydia) pneumoniae*, *Legionella* sp, *Staphylococcus aureus*, and various respiratory viruses (most commonly, influenza and respiratory syncytial virus)

The medical unit where a patient receives therapy for CAP is important because unnecessary hospitalizations for this condition increase treatment costs. In addition, patients transferred from a hospital ward to an intensive care unit for CAP care have worse outcomes than those who are admitted directly to the intensive care unit. Although not meant to supplant good clinical judgment, CAP risk stratification indices help clinicians decide the site of care for CAP patients. The most validated index is the Pneumonia Severity Index, which calculates the risk of death through 20 demographic characteristics, comorbidity, physical examination, and laboratory risk factors. CURB-65, an alternative index, is validated and easier to

KEY FACTS

✓ CAP risk stratification indices help clinicians decide the location of care for CAP patients. The Pneumonia Severity Index is the most validated index

✓ CURB-65, an alternative index, is validated and easier to use. For a patient with suspected CAP, 1 point is given for each of the following criteria: *confusion*, *uremia* (serum urea nitrogen >19 mg/dL), *respiratory* rate (>30 breaths per min), *blood* pressure (systolic <90 mm Hg or diastolic ≤60 mm Hg), and *age* 65 years or greater

✓ For patients with suspected CAP who do not have laboratory data available, a modified index (CRB-65) can be used. For its calculation, the uremia risk factor is removed

Table 45.1 • Organisms of Community-Acquired Pneumonia

Organism	Diagnostic Testing	Treatment
Streptococcus pneumoniae	Culture, urine antigen	Penicillins, cephalosporins, respiratory fluoroquinolones
Legionella	Culture on special media, urine antigen	Fluoroquinolones, macrolides
Mycoplasma pneumoniae	Serology	Fluoroquinolones, macrolides, tetracyclines
Chlamydophila pneumoniae	Serology	Fluoroquinolones, macrolides, tetracyclines
Moraxella catarrhalis	Culture	Fluoroquinolones, trimethoprim-sulfamethoxazole, amoxicillin-clavulanate
Bordatella pertussis	Polymerase chain reaction or culture	Macrolides
Klebsiella, Enterobacter, and *Serratia*	Culture	Fluoroquinolones, trimethoprim-sulfamethoxazole, fourth-generation cephalosporins, carbapenems

Table 45.2 • CURB-65 and CRB-65 Severity Scores for Community-Acquired Pneumonia

Clinical Factor	Points
Confusion	1
Serum urea nitrogen >19 mg/dL	1
Respiratory rate ≥30 breaths/min	1
Systolic blood pressure <90 mm Hg or diastolic blood pressure ≤60 mm Hg	1
Age ≥65 y	1
Total points:	

Score	Deaths/Total No. of Patients (%)[a]	Recommendation[b]
CURB-65		
0	7/1,223 (0.6)	Low risk; consider home treatment
1	31/1,142 (2.7)	
2	69/1,019 (6.8)	Short inpatient hospitalization or closely supervised outpatient treatment
3	79/563 (14.0)	Severe pneumonia; hospitalize and consider admitting to intensive care unit
4 or 5	44/158 (27.8)	
CRB-65[c]		
0	2/212 (0.9)	Very low risk of death; usually does not require hospitalization
1	18/344 (5.2)	Increased risk of death; consider hospitalization
2	30/251 (12.0)	
3 or 4	39/125 (31.2)	High risk of death; urgent hospitalization

Abbreviations: CRB-65, confusion, respiratory rate, blood pressure, age ≥65 y; CURB-65, confusion, urea nitrogen, respiratory rate, blood pressure, age ≥65 y.

[a] Data are weighted averages from validation studies.[1,2]

[b] Recommendations are consistent with British Thoracic Society guidelines.[3] Clinical judgment may overrule the guideline recommendation.

[c] A CRB-65 score can be calculated by omitting the serum urea nitrogen value, which gives a point range of 0 to 4. This score is useful when blood tests are not readily available.

Adapted from Fish D. Pneumonia. In: Mueller BA, Bertch KE, Dunsworth TS, et al, editors. Pharmacotherapy Self-Assessment Program (PSAP). 4th ed. Book 4 (Infectious Diseases). Kansas City (MO): American College of Clinical Pharmacy; c2002. p. 202. Used with permission.

1. Aujesky D, Auble TE, Yealy DM, Stone RA, Obrosky DS, Meehan TP, et al. Prospective comparison of three validated prediction rules for prognosis in community-acquired pneumonia. *Am J Med.* 2005;118:384–392.
2. Lim WS, van der Eerden MM, Laing R, Boersma WG, Karalus N, Town GI, et al. Defining community acquired pneumonia severity on presentation to hospital: an international derivation and validation study. *Thorax.* 2003;58:377–382.
3. British Thoracic Society Pneumonia Guidelines Committee. BTS guidelines for the management of community-acquired pneumonia in adults: 2004 update. Available at http://www.brit-thoracic.org.uk/c2/uploads/MACAPrevisedApr04.pdf. Accessed March 20, 2006.

use (Table 45.2). For a patient in whom CAP is suspected, 1 point is given for each of the following criteria: confusion, uremia (serum urea nitrogen >19 mg/dL), respiratory rate (≥30 breaths/min), blood pressure (systolic <90 mm Hg or diastolic ≤60 mm Hg), and age of 65 years or more. Among patients for whom CAP is suspected but laboratory data are not available, a modified index (CRB-65) can be used. In this index, the uremia risk factor is removed from the calculation.

Chest imaging is a requirement for the diagnosis of CAP. Computed tomography is more sensitive than chest radiography, but chest radiography is usually sufficient. The usefulness of other diagnostic tests is controversial because they generally have low yield and infrequently affect clinical care. However, they can be helpful for certain patients and provide data for epidemiologic purposes. Other testing is optional for patients receiving outpatient care for CAP. Pretreatment culture of blood and sputum should be performed for all patients hospitalized with CAP, and urinary antigen testing for *Legionella pneumophila* and *S pneumoniae* should be performed on patients requiring care in an intensive care unit. During influenza season, influenza testing should be performed on all CAP patients who require hospitalization.

KEY FACTS

✓ Chest imaging is required for CAP diagnosis

✓ Pretreatment blood and sputum culturing should be performed for all hospitalized CAP patients. Urinary antigen testing for *Legionella pneumophila* and *S pneumoniae* should be performed on CAP patients who need treatment in an intensive care unit

✓ During influenza season, influenza tests should be performed on all patients with CAP who require hospitalization

Empirical treatment of CAP should be directed toward the suspected pathogens on the basis of a patient's risk factors. For a summary of risk factors, see Box 45.1.

KEY FACT

✓ Empirical CAP treatment should be directed toward the pathogens suspected because of risk factors

If the microbiologic cause of CAP is determined, antimicrobial therapy can be directed toward that pathogen. For hospitalized patients, an intravenously administered antimicrobial can be switched to the oral form when the patient is hemodynamically stable, improving clinically, and able to take medications orally. The oral antimicrobial should be the same agent or of the same drug class as the intravenous antimicrobial. The duration of antimicrobial therapy for CAP differs but generally ranges between 7 and 10 days. Patients should be treated for a minimum of 5 days and until all but 1 of the following criteria occur before antimicrobial treatment is discontinued: temperature, 37.8°C or less; heart rate, 100 beats per minute or less; respiratory rate, 24 breaths per minute or less; systolic blood pressure, 90 mm Hg or less; oxygen saturation, 90% or more while

KEY FACTS

✓ The duration of antimicrobial therapy for CAP differs, but its general range is 7 and 10 days

✓ Patients should be treated for at least 5 days. Before antimicrobial treatment is discontinued, all but 1 of the following criteria need to occur: temperature, 37.8°C or less; heart rate, 100 beats per minute or fewer; respiratory rate, 24 breaths per minute or fewer; systolic blood pressure, 90 mm Hg or less; oxygen saturation, 90% or more while breathing room air; ability to take oral medication; and normal mental status

Box 45.1 • Summary of Risk Factors for Community-Acquired Pneumonia

For previously healthy patients who have not received antimicrobials in the prior 3 mo, reside in locations with <25% macrolide resistance in *Streptococcus pneumoniae*, and will be treated as outpatients, macrolide monotherapy (eg, erythromycin, azithromycin, or clarithromycin) is recommended, and doxycycline is recommended as an alternative

For patients with clinically significant medical comorbidities who have received antimicrobials in the prior 3 mo, have >25% macrolide resistance in *S pneumoniae*, and will be treated as outpatients, treatment options are as follows:

a. A respiratory fluoroquinolone as monotherapy (eg, levofloxacin, moxifloxacin) *or*

b. A β-lactam antibiotic *and* a macrolide *or* doxycycline

For patients with clinically significant medical comorbidities or who have received antimicrobials in the prior 3 mo and will be treated as inpatients, treatment options are as follows:

a. A respiratory fluoroquinolone as monotherapy (eg, levofloxacin, moxifloxacin) *or*

b. A β-lactam antibiotic *and* a macrolide *or* doxycycline

For patients who require disease management in an intensive care unit, recommended treatment is with a β-lactam antibiotic (eg, cefotaxime, ceftriaxone, ampicillin-sulbactam) *and* azithromycin or a respiratory fluoroquinolone (eg, levofloxacin, moxifloxacin)

Empirical treatment of methicillin-resistant *Staphylococcus aureus* with the addition of vancomycin or linezolid should be considered for patients with such clinical risk factors as end-stage renal disease, injection drug use, recent influenza infection, and prior use of antimicrobials, especially fluoroquinolones

breathing room air; ability to take oral medication; and normal mental status.

Streptococcus pneumoniae (pneumococcus) is a leading cause of community-acquired infections that cause such conditions as pneumonia, meningitis, otitis media, and sinusitis. Similar to many organisms, *S pneumoniae* is becoming increasingly resistant to traditional antibiotics. Potential complications of pneumococcal pneumonia include empyema and pericarditis from direct extension of

KEY FACT

✓ Empyema should be suspected when a patient's fever persists despite appropriate antibiotic therapy for pneumococcal pneumonia infection. Empyema should be suspected when fever persists despite appropriate antibiotic therapy for pneumococcal pneumonia.

Asplenia predisposes to severe infections with *S pneumoniae* (and other encapsulated organisms). After splenectomy, fulminant (purpura fulminans) pneumococcal bacteremia with disseminated intravascular coagulation occurs more commonly and is often fatal. Similarly, *S pneumoniae* infections are more frequent and unusually severe in smokers and patients who have asthma, sickle cell disease, multiple myeloma, alcoholism, human immunodeficiency virus (HIV) infection, or hypogammaglobulinemia.

Two pneumococcal vaccines are available: a polysaccharide vaccine containing the 23 serotypes that most commonly cause pneumococcal infection and a conjugated vaccine containing the 13 serotypes responsible for the most invasive pneumococcal infection. Pneumococcal vaccination is recommended for persons with increased risk of invasive pneumococcal disease or complications. These persons include 1) adults older than 65 years; 2) patients of any age with chronic illness, such as chronic cardiovascular disease (eg, congestive heart failure, cardiomyopathies), chronic pulmonary disease (eg, chronic obstructive pulmonary disease, emphysema), diabetes mellitus, alcoholism, asthma, chronic liver disease (cirrhosis), or asplenia; 3) smokers; 4) persons with cochlear implants; or 5) persons with cerebrospinal fluid leaks.

The vaccine can be given simultaneously with influenza virus vaccine. Pneumococcal vaccine booster is recommended at 5 years after the initial dose for high-risk patients or patients who received the first dose before age 65 years. Immunocompromised patients are recommended to have an initial vaccination with conjugate vaccine followed by booster vaccination with the polysaccharide vaccine 8 weeks later.

Legionella

Legionellae organisms are fastidious gram-negative bacilli. *Legionella pneumophila* causes both CAP and nosocomial pneumonia, typically occurring in summer. Nosocomial legionellosis may be due to contaminated water supplies. Immunocompromised patients, especially those receiving long-term corticosteroid therapy, are especially susceptible to *Legionella* infections. Typical clinical features of legionellosis include weakness, malaise, fever, dry cough, diarrhea, pleuritic chest pain, relative bradycardia, diffuse rales bilaterally, and patchy bilateral pulmonary infiltrates.

Characteristic laboratory features of *Legionella* pneumonia may include decreased sodium and phosphorus values, increased leukocyte level, and increased liver enzyme values. Legionellae organisms will not grow on standard media. Diagnosis depends on assessing the results of special culture, finding organisms by direct fluorescent antibody staining, or detecting an increase in anti-*Legionella* antibody titers. Urine antigen detection is a more sensitive (>80%) and simple diagnostic test for *L pneumophila* infections, but only serogroup 1 is detected.

> **KEY FACT**
>
> ✓ Laboratory results characteristic of *Legionella* pneumonia include decreased sodium and phosphorus levels, increased leukocyte count, and increased liver enzyme values

Legionellae organisms are intracellular parasites. As such, they are resistant to all β-lactam drugs and aminoglycosides. Effective agents for treating *Legionella* infection include macrolides, fluoroquinolones, and, to a lesser extent, doxycycline. Fluoroquinolones are considered drugs of choice for therapy. Some authorities recommend adding rifampin for severe infection.

Mycoplasma pneumoniae

Mycoplasma pneumoniae is one of the smallest microorganisms capable of extracellular replication. Because *Mycoplasma* organisms lack a cell wall, the cell-wall–active antibiotics such as penicillins are ineffective in treating *Mycoplasma* infection. Spread by droplet inhalation, *Mycoplasma* infection primarily infects young, previously healthy persons and presents with rapid onset of headache, dry cough, and fever. Results of physical examination are often unremarkable, with the possible exception of bullous myringitis. Chest radiography usually shows bilateral, patchy pneumonitis. The chest radiographic abnormalities are often out of proportion to the physical findings. Pleural effusion is present in 15% to 20% of cases. Neurologic complications include Guillain-Barré syndrome, cerebellar

> **KEY FACTS**
>
> ✓ *Mycoplasma* infection is spread through droplet inhalation and presents with rapid onset of headache, dry cough, and fever. The organism primarily infects young, previously healthy persons
>
> ✓ Neurologic complications of *Mycoplasma* infection include Guillain-Barré syndrome, cerebellar peripheral neuropathy, aseptic meningitis, and mononeuritis multiplex
>
> ✓ Hemolytic anemia may occur late in *Mycoplasma* infection because of circulating cold hemagglutinins, and erythema multiforme may occur
>
> ✓ The diagnosis of *Mycoplasma* infection is established with specific complement fixation test. In contrast, cold agglutinins are nonspecific and are not reliable for its diagnosis

peripheral neuropathy, aseptic meningitis, and mononeuritis multiplex. Hemolytic anemia may occur late in the illness as a result of circulating cold hemagglutinins. Erythema multiforme may also occur. The diagnosis is established through specific complement fixation test. Cold agglutinins are nonspecific and unreliable for diagnosing *Mycoplasma* infections. Fluoroquinolones, macrolides, and tetracyclines are effective therapies. Because immunity to *Mycoplasma* infection is transient, reinfection may occur. Clinical relapse of pneumonia occurs in up to 10% of *Mycoplasma* pneumonia cases.

Chlamydophila (Chlamydia) pneumoniae

Chlamydophila (Chlamydia) pneumoniae may also cause so-called atypical pneumonia. *Chlamydia trachomatis* and *Chlamydophila psittaci* are the other 2 chlamydial species that cause human disease. In young adults, *C pneumoniae* causes 10% of pneumonia cases and 5% of bronchitis cases. It has caused community outbreaks, and nosocomial transmission has occurred. Half of US adults are seropositive for *C pneumoniae*. Birds are the source of infection with *C psittaci* (psittacosis), but no animal reservoir exists for *C pneumoniae*. Clinical manifestations of infection are usually mild and may resemble those caused by *M pneumoniae*. Pharyngitis occurs 1 to 3 weeks before the onset of pulmonary symptoms, and cough may last for weeks. The diagnosis is based on serologic testing. Treatment is with a fluoroquinolone, doxycycline, or a macrolide. Of note, trimethoprim-sulfamethoxazole and β-lactam antibiotics such as penicillins and cephalosporins are not active against chlamydial species.

Moraxella

Moraxella catarrhalis (formerly called *Branhamella catarrhalis*) is a respiratory tract pathogen primarily causing bronchitis and pneumonia in persons with chronic obstructive pulmonary disease. It also can cause otitis media, sinusitis, meningitis, bacteremia, and endocarditis in immunosuppressed patients. Ampicillin resistance through β-lactamase production is common. Trimethoprim-sulfamethoxazole, the fluoroquinolones, and amoxicillin-clavulanate are effective for therapy.

Bordetella pertussis

Bordetella pertussis infection often results in persistent coughing in older children and adults, but it is potentially

---

KEY FACT

✓ *Bordetella pertussis* infection often causes persistent coughing in older children and adults, but it is potentially fatal in infants. Whooping cough can cause severe lymphocytosis

---

fatal in infants. Whooping cough may cause severe lymphocytosis (>100 lymphocytes ×10^9/L).

Diagnosis of *B pertussis* infection may be difficult. Molecular testing (polymerase chain reaction) of a nasopharyngeal aspirate is more sensitive, rapid, and reliable than cultures. Early treatment of pertussis with a macrolide (erythromycin, clarithromycin, or azithromycin) is recommended. The duration of pertussis treatment is 14 days for the patient and 5 days for persons in close contact with affected patients for prevention, irrespective of age or vaccination status. Aerosolized bronchodilators or corticosteroids may alleviate the persistent coughing. A pertussis-containing tetanus-diphtheria (Tdap) vaccine is recommended for use in adults. It is given as a single booster to replace a dose of tetanus-diphtheria booster. This approach is particularly emphasized for adults who have close contact with infants (eg, parents, health care workers, day care providers). Women should receive Tdap vaccination after 20 weeks' gestation for each pregnancy.

KEY FACT

✓ Early treatment of pertussis with the macrolides erythromycin, clarithromycin, or azithromycin is recommended, with a duration of 14 days for the pertussis patient. Treatment with a macrolide for prevention should be 5 days for persons who have been in close contact with pertussis-affected patients, irrespective of age or vaccination status

---

Klebsiella, Enterobacter, and Serratia

Klebsiella pneumoniae is an important cause of both CAP and nosocomial pneumonia and often is associated with alcoholism, diabetes mellitus, and chronic obstructive pulmonary disease. Red sputum, with the color of red currant jelly, is a characteristic sign. Lung abscess and empyema are more frequent with *K pneumoniae* than with other pneumonia-causing organisms, especially in persons with alcoholism. Third-generation cephalosporins are the drugs of choice for treating most types of *Klebsiella*. Strains of *Klebsiella* have emerged that are resistant to

---

KEY FACTS

✓ *Klebsiella pneumoniae* is an important cause of CAP and nosocomial pneumonia and often is associated with alcoholism, diabetes mellitus, and chronic obstructive pulmonary disease

✓ Sputum the color of red currant jelly is a characteristic sign of *K pneumoniae* infection. Lung abscess and empyema are more frequent with *K pneumoniae* than with other pneumonia-causing organisms, especially in persons with alcoholism

ceftazidime. This resistance is caused by an extended-spectrum β-lactamase. Susceptibility testing results for such strains may erroneously report that they are susceptible to cefotaxime. If they are resistant to ceftazidime, the strains should be considered resistant to all cephalosporins. Resistance to carbapenem antibiotics through *K pneumoniae* carbapenemases has also emerged; treatment with such antimicrobials as colistin may be needed for these organisms.

Enterobacter and *Serratia* are primarily associated with nosocomial infections. *Enterobacter* species, such as *Enterobacter cloacae* and *Enterobacter aerogenes*, often are resistant to third-generation cephalosporins, such as cefotaxime. Despite in vitro data suggesting their susceptibility, β-lactamase production is induced when *Enterobacter* and *Serratia* are grown in the presence of cephalosporins. Carbapenems, such as imipenem or meropenem, fluoroquinolones, cefepime, and trimethoprim-sulfamethoxazole, are usually active against these strains.

Nocardia Pneumonia

Nocardia asteroides, *Nocardia brasiliensis*, and *Nocardia otitidiscaviarum* can cause pneumonia in susceptible persons. *Nocardia asteroides* is a weakly acid-fast saprophytic bacterium present in soil, dust, plants, and water. Infection is more common among immunosuppressed patients. Primary infection leads to necrotizing pneumonia with abscess formation. Pulmonary nodules suggestive of cancer metastases and dense alveolar infiltrates are common chest radiographic findings. *Nocardia* infection may produce pleural effusion. Lymphohematogenous spread occurs in 20% of affected patients; in nearly all these patients, a brain abscess develops.

Isolation of the *Nocardia* organism from the sputum of immunocompetent patients might represent colonization because the saprophytic state is well recognized. However, in an immunocompromised patient, this colonization should be considered a true infection. Most *Nocardia* isolates are susceptible to trimethoprim-sulfamethoxazole. Nevertheless, use of an initial combination therapy with the addition of imipenem, ceftriaxone, or amikacin should be considered in severe or complicated cases.

Aspiration Pneumonia

Aspiration pneumonia can be acute or chronic. The acute type usually results from aspiration of a liquid volume larger than 50 mL and with a pH less than 2.4. The aspiration produces classic aspiration pneumonia that is often sterile; the role of antibiotics in the absence of supporting cultures is unclear and controversial. Predisposing factors include use of a nasogastric tube, anesthesia, coma, seizures, central nervous system problems, diaphragmatic hernia with reflux, and tracheoesophageal fistula.

Nosocomial aspiration pneumonia is caused by *Escherichia coli*, *S aureus*, *K pneumoniae*, and *Pseudomonas aeruginosa*. Community-acquired aspiration pneumonias are caused by infections due to anaerobes. Preventive measures are important for patients with the identified predisposing factors.

Chronic aspiration pneumonia results from recurrent aspiration of small volumes. Examples include patients with reflux aspiration who have granuloma caused by mineral oil. Symptoms include chronic cough, patchy lung infiltrates, and nocturnal wheeze.

Lung Abscess

Lung abscess is a circumscribed collection of pus in the lung that leads to cavity formation; the cavity has an air-fluid level on chest radiography. Lung abscess usually is caused by bacteria, particularly anaerobic bacilli (30%–50% of cases); aerobic gram-positive cocci (25%); and aerobic gram-negative bacilli (5%–12%). Polymicrobial infections are the most common causes of lung abscess. Suppuration leading to lung abscess can result from primary, opportunistic, and hematogenous lung infection. Primary lung abscess is caused by oral infection; aspiration accounts for up to 90% of all abscesses. Alcohol abuse and dental caries also contribute. Lung abscesses caused by opportunistic infections occur in elderly patients with a blood dyscrasia and in patients with cancer of the lung or oropharynx. In patients with advanced HIV infection, lung abscess can develop in association with a broad spectrum of pathogens, including opportunistic organisms. These patients have a poor prognosis.

KEY FACT

✓ Primary lung abscess is caused by oral infection. Aspiration accounts for up to 90%, and alcohol abuse and dental caries also contribute

---

Hematogenous lung abscesses occur with septicemia, septic embolism, and sterile infarcts (3% of cases). A history of any of these conditions in association with fever, cough with purulent or bloody sputum, weight loss, and leukocytosis suggests the diagnosis. Chest radiography may show cavitated lesions. The abscess may rupture into the pleural space and cause empyema. Bronchoscopy may be necessary to obtain samples for culture, to drain the abscess, and to exclude obstructing lesions. High morbidity and mortality rates (20%) are associated with lung abscess despite antibiotic therapy. The prognosis is worse for patients with a large abscess and those infected with *S aureus*, *K pneumoniae*, and *P aeruginosa*. Treatment includes drainage (physiotherapy, postural, and broncho-scopic), antibiotic therapy for 4 to 6 weeks, and surgical treatment if medical therapy fails.

KEY FACTS

✓ High morbidity and mortality rates (20%) are associated with lung abscess despite antibiotic treatment. The prognosis is worse for patients with a large abscess and those with *S aureus, K pneumoniae,* and *P aeruginosa* infections

✓ Treatment includes physiotherapy, postural, and bronchoscopic drainage; antibiotic therapy for 4 to 6 weeks; and surgical treatment if medical therapy fails

---

Mycobacterial Infections

Mycobacterium tuberculosis

Worldwide, *Mycobacterium tuberculosis* causes the most common type of human-to-human chronic infection due to mycobacteria. The most common mode of transmission is inhalation of droplet nuclei. Of persons exposed to *M tuberculosis*, 30% become infected. Among infected persons, active primary disease occurs in less than 5%; active disease from reactivation develops in less than 5%. Active infection is diagnosed through documenting *M tuberculosis* in clinical specimens. Sputum and gastric washings have an approximately 30% diagnostic yield. Bronchoscopy with bronchoalveolar lavage has a 40% di-agnostic yield, which increases to almost 95% with biopsy. Culture of pleural fluid alone has a low sensitivity, but culture of pleural biopsy specimens has a 70% diagnostic yield. Faster culture results are available with broth cul-ture systems (results within 1.5–2 weeks) and nucleic acid amplification (results within 8 hours). **Latent tuberculosis infection** is the current term for the condition in a person who is infected with *M tuberculosis* (positive purified pro-tein derivative [PPD] skin test) but does not have active tuberculosis.

Key Definition

Latent tuberculosis infection: *The condition of* Mycobacterium tuberculosis *infection (positive purified protein derivative skin test) without active tuberculosis.*

A PPD tuberculin skin test can be positive within 4 weeks after exposure to *M tuberculosis*. The test is negative in 25% of patients who have active tuberculosis. A false-negative

PPD result can also occur when the following factors are pres-ent: concomitant infections with viruses or bacteria, receipt of live virus vaccinations, chronic renal failure, nutritional deficiency, lymphoid malignancies, leukemias, corticoste-roid and immunosuppressive drug therapies, newborn or elderly patients, recent or overwhelming infection with my-cobacteria, and acute stress. The annual risk of active tuber-culosis for those who have a positive PPD skin test depends on the underlying medical condition: HIV-positive (annual risk, 8%–10%), recent converters (2%–5%), abnormal chest radiograph (2%–4%), intravenous drug abuse (1%), end-stage renal disease (1%), and diabetes mellitus (0.3%). PPD skin testing should use a 5-tuberculin-unit preparation; the widest induration is read at 48 and 72 hours. Prior vaccina-tion with bacille Calmette-Guérin (BCG) is not a contraindi-cation for the test. No method can reliably distinguish posi-tive PPD test results caused by BCG vaccination from those caused by mycobacterial infections, although large reactions (≥20 mm) are not likely caused by BCG. The classification of PPD test results is summarized in Table 45.3.

KEY FACTS

✓ Purified protein derivative (PPD) skin testing should be done with a 5-tuberculin-unit preparation; the widest induration is read at 48 and 72 hours

✓ Prior vaccination with bacille calmette-Guérin (BCG) is not a contraindication for the test. No diagnostic method can reliably distinguish positive PPD skin test results caused by BCG vaccination from those caused by mycobacterial infections, although large reactions (≥20 mm) are not likely caused by BCG

The role of the serum interferon-γ release assay (eg, QuantiFERON-TB Gold [Cellestis], T-SPOT.*TB* [Oxford Immunotec, Inc]) continues to evolve and has the promise of increased specificity of testing to identify latent tuber-culosis. This assay may help distinguish latent tuberculous infection from nontuberculous mycobacterial infection and BCG vaccination. Current Centers for Disease Control and Prevention guidelines suggest that the assay may be used in all circumstances in which the PPD skin test is used. Compared with the PPD skin test, the assay is probably less subject to reader bias and error, requires only a single health care visit, and is less likely to be positive after BCG vaccine. Like the PPD skin test, the assay may be negative in patients who have active tuberculosis.

In the United States, 4% of all tuberculous patients have pleural involvement, and pleural tuberculosis con-stitutes 23% of the extrapulmonary tuberculosis cases. Effusions usually occur 3 to 6 months after the primary infection. Acute presentation (cough, fever, and pleu-ritic chest pain) is more common in younger patients than older ones. Bilateral exudative effusions occur in

Table 45.3 • Targeted Tuberculin Testing for Latent TB Infection

Induration of ≥5 mm is considered positive in the following:	**Induration of ≥10 mm** is considered positive in the following:	**Induration of ≥15 mm** is considered positive in any person, including persons with no known risk factors for TB infection. However, targeted skin testing programs should be conducted only among high-risk groups
HIV-infected persons	Recent (<5 y) immigrants from high-prevalence countries	
Persons in recent contact with persons who have active TB disease	Injection drug users	
Persons with fibrotic changes seen on chest radiograph that are consistent with prior TB infection	Residents of and employees at high-risk congregate settings	
Patients with organ transplants	Mycobacteriology laboratory personnel	
Persons who are immunosuppressed for other reasons (eg, taking the equivalent of >15 mg/d of prednisone for ≥1 mo, taking TNF-α antagonists)	Persons with clinical conditions that place them at high risk	
	Children age <4 y	
	Infants, children, and adolescents exposed to adults in high-risk categories	

Abbreviations: HIV, human immunodeficiency virus; TB, tuberculosis; TNF-α, tumor necrosis factor α.

Adapted from American Thoracic Society. Targeted tuberculin testing and treatment of latent tuberculosis infection. MMWR Recomm Rep. 2000 Jun 9;49(RR-6):1–51.

up to 8% of patients, and the PPD skin test is positive in more than 66%. The effusions typically have high protein levels (>5 g/dL), lymphocytosis (>50%), and low glucose levels (<50 mg/dL). A low pleural fluid pH occurs in 20% of patients who have pleural tuberculosis. Pleural biopsy specimens show caseous granulomas in up to 80% of patients, and cultures of biopsy specimens are positive in more than 75%. Cultures of pleural fluid are positive in only 20% to 40% of patients, and sputum is positive in 40%. Bronchopleural fistula is a complication of biopsy in pleural tuberculosis.

KEY FACTS

✓ The serum interferon-γ release assay may help distinguish latent tuberculous infection from nontuberculous mycobacterial infection and BCG vaccination

✓ Compared with the PPD skin test, the serum interferon-γ release assay is probably less subject to reader bias and error, requires a single health care visit, and is less likely to be positive after BCG vaccination. Similar to the PPD skin test, the assay may be negative for patients with active tuberculosis

---

Miliary tuberculosis constitutes 10% of cases of extrapulmonary tuberculosis. It is clinically characterized by the diffuse presence of small (<2 mm) nodules throughout the body. The spleen, liver, and lung are frequently involved. The disease can be acute and fatal or insidious in onset and slowly progressive. Chest radiography shows typical miliary lesions in more than 65% of patients. Among patients with miliary tuberculosis, sputum findings are negative in up to 80%, and the PPD skin test is negative in approximately 50%. Mortality rate is high (30%) even with therapy.

Tuberculous lymphadenitis (ie, scrofula) is the most common form of extrapulmonary tuberculosis. It is more common in children and young adults than in older persons. Cervical lymph nodes are affected most commonly. *Skeletal tuberculosis* is becoming less common; when identified, it is more often seen in the young than in older adults. Any bone can be involved, but the vertebrae are involved in 50% of skeletal tuberculosis cases. Pott disease is *tuberculous spondylitis* and may produce severe kyphosis. *Tuberculous meningitis* is the most common form of central nervous system involvement and is localized mainly to the base of the brain. It occurs more commonly in immunocompromised patients. Tuberculous meningitis is often insidious in onset.

Therapy is indicated for all patients with culture-positive tuberculosis. Treatment usually should include multidrug therapy (>2 drugs at a minimum; the use of 4 drugs is recommended) for all patients who have active tuberculosis (Tables 45.4 and 45.5; Figures 45.1 and 45.2). With strictly administered 6-month regimens, more than 90% of patients are smear-negative after 2 months of therapy, more than 95% are cured, and less than 5% have relapse. A 9-month regimen provides a cure rate higher than 97% and a relapse rate less than 2%. All treatment programs should be recommended and preferably undertaken by physicians and health care workers experienced in the management of mycobacterial diseases. The most important impediment to lack of adequate therapy worldwide is the lack of adherence to the treatment. Cavitary tuberculosis is often treated for 9 months. Extrapulmonary

---

KEY FACT

✓ Therapy is indicated for patients with culture-positive tuberculosis. It usually should include multidrug therapy (>2 drugs at a minimum; 4-drug treatment is recommended) for patients with active tuberculosis

tuberculosis can be treated effectively with either a 6- or 9-month regimen. However, miliary tuberculosis, bone and joint tuberculosis, and tuberculous meningitis in infants and children may require treatment for 12 months or more.

Drug-resistant tuberculosis is an increasingly recognized problem. Drug resistance can develop against a single first-line drug. *Multidrug-resistant tuberculosis* (MDR-TB) refers to resistance that develops to at least both isoniazid and rifampin. *Extensively drug-resistant tuberculosis* (XDR-TB) is defined as resistance to at least both isoniazid and rifampin and resistance to fluoroquinolones or aminoglycosides.

Treatment of latent tuberculosis infection is indicated for persons with a positive PPD skin test who do not have active infection. When latent tuberculosis infection is likely caused by an isoniazid-sensitive organism, treatment options include isoniazid at a dose of 300 mg daily or

KEY FACT

✓ Treatment of latent tuberculosis infection is indicated for persons with a positive PPD skin test who do not have active infection

---

Table 45.4 • Drug Regimens for Culture-Positive Pulmonary Tuberculosis Caused by Drug-Susceptible Organisms

Initial Phase			Continuation Phase			No. of Total Doses, Range (Minimal Duration)	Rating[a] (Evidence)[b]	
Regimen	Drugs	Interval and Doses[c] (Minimal Duration)	Regimen	Drugs	Interval and Doses[c,d] (Minimal Duration)		HIV Negative	HIV Positive
1	INH RIF PZA EMB	7 d/wk for 56 doses (8 wk) *or* 5 d/wk for 40 doses (8 wk)[e]	1a	INH/RIF	7 d/wk for 126 doses (18 wk) *or* 5 d/wk for 90 doses (18 wk)[e]	182–130 (26 wk)	A (I)	A (II)
			1b	INH/RIF	Twice weekly for 36 doses (18 wk)	92–76 (26 wk)	A (I)	A (II)[f]
			1c[g]	INH/RPT	Once weekly for 18 doses (18 wk)	74–58 (26 wk)	B (I)	E (I)
2	INH RIF PZA EMB	7 d/wk for 14 doses (2 wk), *then* twice weekly for 12 doses (6 wk) *or* 5 d/wk for 10 doses (2 wk)[e], *then* twice weekly for 12 doses (6 wk)	2a	INH/RIF	Twice weekly for 36 doses (18 wk)	62–58 (26 wk)	A (II)	B (II)[f]
			2b[g]	INH/RPT	Once weekly for 18 doses (18 wk)	44–40 (26 wk)	B (I)	E (I)
3	INH RIF PZA EMB	3 times weekly for 24 doses (8 wk)	3a	INH/RIF	3 times weekly for 54 doses (18 wk)	78 (26 wk)	B (I)	B (II)
4	INH RIF EMB	7 d/wk for 56 doses (8 wk) *or* 5 d/wk for 40 doses (8 wk)[e]	4a	INH/RIF	7 d/wk for 217 doses (31 wk) *or* 5 d/wk for 155 doses (31 wk)[e]	273–195 (39 wk)	C (I)	C (II)
			4b	INH/RIF	Twice weekly for 62 doses (31 wk)	118–102 (39 wk)	C (I)	C (II)

Abbreviations: EMB, ethambutol; INH, isoniazid; PZA, pyrazinamide; RIF, rifampin; RPT, rifapentine.

[a] Definitions of ratings: A, preferred; B, acceptable alternative; C, offer when A and B cannot be given; E, should never be given.

[b] Definitions of evidence: I, randomized clinical trial; II, data from clinical trials that were not randomized or were conducted in other populations; III, expert opinion.

[c] When directly observed therapy is used, drugs may be given 5 days weekly and the necessary number of doses adjusted accordingly. Although no studies have compared 5 daily doses with 7 daily doses, extensive experience indicates this regimen would be an effective practice.

[d] Patients with cavitation on initial chest radiograph and positive cultures at completion of 2 months of therapy should receive therapy for a 7-month continuation phase (31 weeks; either 217 doses [daily] or 62 doses [twice weekly]).

[e] Drugs given for 5 days weekly are always given through directly observed therapy. Rating for these regimens is A (III).

[f] Not recommended for human immunodeficiency virus (HIV)-infected patients with CD4+ cell counts <100/mcL.

[g] Options 1c and 2b should be used only in HIV-negative patients who have negative sputum smears at completion of 2 months of therapy and do not have cavitation on initial chest radiograph. For patients receiving this regimen and found to have a positive culture from the 2-month specimen, treatment should be extended an extra 3 months.

Adapted from Blumberg HM, Burman WJ, Chaisson RE, Daley CL, Etkind SC, Friedman LN, et al. American Thoracic Society/Centers for Disease Control and Prevention/Infectious Diseases Society of America: treatment of tuberculosis. Am J Respir Crit Care Med. 2003 Feb 15;167(4):603–62. Used with permission.

Table 45.5 • First-Line Drug Therapies for Tuberculosis[a,b]

Drug	Dose, mg/kg						Adverse Reactions	Monitoring
	Daily		2 Times Weekly[c]		3 Times Weekly[c]			
	Children[d]	Adults	Children[d]	Adults	Children[d]	Adults		
INH[e] (maximal dose in mg)	10–20 (300)	5 (300)	20–40 (900)	15 (900)	20–40 (900)	15 (900)	Elevated liver enzyme level, hepatitis, peripheral neuropathy, mild effects on central nervous system, drug interactions	Baseline measurements of liver enzymes for adults. Repeat measurements when baseline results are abnormal, when patient is at high risk for adverse reactions, or when patient has symptoms of adverse reactions
RIF[f] (maximal dose in mg)	10–20 (600)	10 (600)	10–20 (600)	10 (600)	10–20 (600)	10 (600)	GI upset, drug interactions, hepatitis, bleeding problems, flulike symptoms, rash	Baseline measurements for adults: CBC, platelets, liver enzymes. Repeat measurements when baseline results are abnormal or when patient has symptoms of adverse reactions
PZA[g] (maximal dose in mg)	15–30 (2,000)	15–30 (2,000)	50–70 (4,000)	50–70 (4,000)	50–70 (3,000)	50–70 (3,000)	Hepatitis, rash, GI upset, joint aches, hyperuricemia, gout (rare)	Baseline measurements for adults: uric acid, liver enzymes. Repeat measurements when baseline results are abnormal or when patient has symptoms of adverse reactions
EMB[h]	15–25	15–25	50	50	25–30	25–30	Optic neuritis	Baseline and monthly tests: visual acuity, color vision
SM[i] (maximal dose in mg)	20–40 (1,000)	15 (1,000)	25–30 (1,500)	25–30 (1,500)	25–30 (1,500)	25–30 (1,500)	Ototoxicity (hearing loss or vestibular dysfunction), renal toxicity	Baseline and repeat as needed: hearing, kidney function

Abbreviations: CBC, complete blood cell count; EMB, ethambutol; GI, gastrointestinal tract; INH, isoniazid; PZA, pyrazinamide; RIF, rifampin; SM, streptomycin.

[a] Adjust weight-based dosages as patient's weight changes.
[b] INH, RIF, PZA, and EMB are administered orally; SM is administered intramuscularly.
[c] Directly observed therapy should be used with all regimens administered 2 or 3 times weekly.
[d] Age <12 years.
[e] Hepatitis risk increases with age and alcohol consumption. Pyridoxine can prevent peripheral neuropathy.
[f] Severe interactions with methadone, oral contraceptives, and many other drugs. Drug colors the body fluids orange and may permanently discolor soft contact lenses.
[g] Treat hyperuricemia only when patient has symptoms.
[h] Not recommended for children too young to be monitored for changes in vision, unless tuberculosis is drug-resistant.
[i] Avoid or decrease dose in adults age >60 years.

Adapted from American Thoracic Society; CDC; Infectious Diseases Society of America. Treatment of tuberculosis. MMWR Recomm Rep. 2003 Jun 20;52(RR-11):1–77. Erratum in: MMWR Recomm Rep. 2005 Jan 7;53(51):1203. Dosage error in article text.

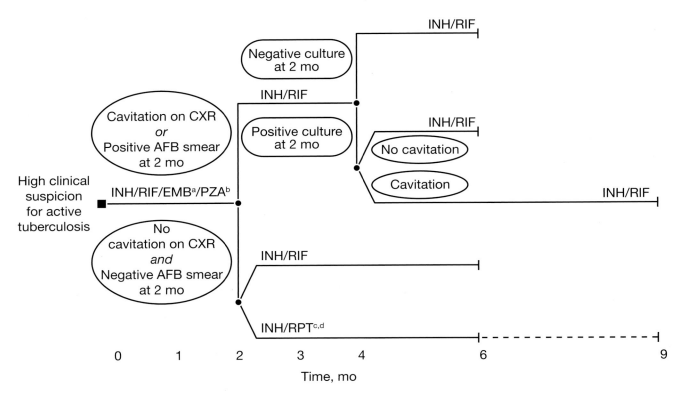

Figure 45.1 *Treatment Algorithm for Tuberculosis. Patients in whom tuberculosis is proved or strongly suspected should have treatment initiated with isoniazid (INH), rifampin (RIF), pyrazinamide (PZA), and ethambutol (EMB) for the first 2 months. Another acid-fast bacilli (AFB) smear and culture should be performed after 2 months of treatment. If cavities were seen on initial chest radiograph (CXR) or the AFB smear is positive at completion of 2 months of treatment, the continuation phase of treatment should consist of INH and RIF daily or twice weekly for 4 months (total, 6 months of treatment). If cavitation was present on initial CXR and if the culture at completion of 2 months of therapy is positive, the continuation phase should be lengthened to 7 months (total, 9 months of treatment). If the patient has human immunodeficiency virus (HIV) infection and a CD4+ cell count <100/mcL, the continuation phase should consist of daily or 3-times-weekly doses of INH and RIF. For patients without HIV infection who have no cavitation on CXR and negative AFB smears at completion of 2 months of treatment, the continuation phase may consist of either once-weekly doses of INH and rifapentine (RPT) or daily or twice-weekly doses of INH and RIF (total of 6 months) (bottom of figure). Patients receiving INH and RPT and whose 2-month cultures are positive should have treatment extended by 3 additional months (total, 9 months of treatment). [a]Use of EMB may be discontinued when results of drug susceptibility testing indicate no drug resistance. [b]Use of PZA may be discontinued after 2 months (56 doses). [c]RPT should not be used for HIV-infected patients with tuberculosis or patients with extrapulmonary tuberculosis. [d]Therapy should be extended to 9 months if the 2-month culture is positive.*
(Adapted from Blumberg HM, Burman WJ, Chiasson RE, Daley CL, Etkind SC, Friedman LN, et al. American Thoracic Society/Centers for Disease Control and Prevention/Infectious Diseases Society of America: treatment of tuberculosis. Am J Respir Crit Care Med. 2003 Feb 15;167[4]:603–62. Used with permission.)

900 mg biweekly. Pyridoxine is usually added to prevent peripheral neuropathy, which is particularly common in patients with diabetes mellitus, alcohol abuse, or kidney disease. Rifampin (600 mg daily) is an alternative option. The recommended duration for therapy of latent tuberculosis infection is 6 to 9 months with isoniazid. Rifampin is typically given for 4 months; isoniazid and rifapentine, 3 months.

Nontuberculous Mycobacteria

Mycobacteria other than *M tuberculosis* and *Mycobacterium leprae* are commonly classified as *nontuberculous mycobacteria* (NTM), even though tubercle formation occurs. Most NTMs have been isolated from natural water and soil. Human-to-human spread has not been documented.

Chronic pulmonary disease is caused most frequently by *M avium* complex and *Mycobacterium kansasii*. Pulmonary

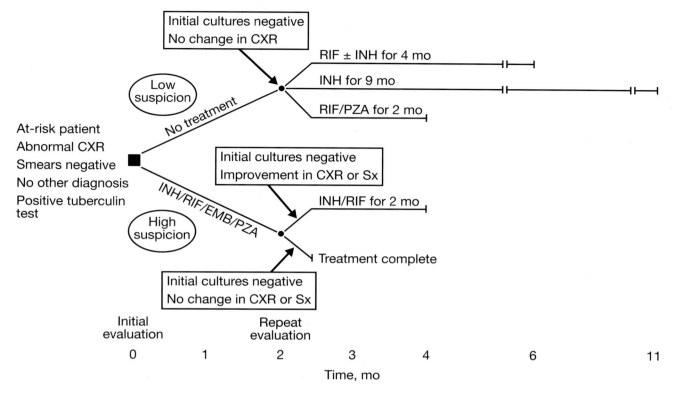

Figure 45.2 *Treatment Algorithm for Active, Culture-Negative Pulmonary Tuberculosis (TB) and Inactive TB. The decision to begin treatment of a patient with sputum smears that are negative depends on the degree of clinical suspicion that the patient has TB. If suspicion is high (bottom of figure), multidrug therapy should be initiated before acid-fast smear and culture results are known. If the diagnosis is confirmed by a positive culture, treatment can be continued to complete a standard course of therapy (see Figure 45.1). If initial cultures continue to be negative and treatment has consisted of multiple drugs for 2 months, 2 options are available depending on reevaluation at 2 months (bottom of figure): 1) If the patient shows symptomatic or radiographic improvement without another apparent diagnosis, a diagnosis of culture-negative TB can be inferred. Treatment should be continued with isoniazid (INH) and rifampin (RIF) alone for an additional 2 months. 2) If the patient shows neither symptomatic nor radiographic improvement, prior TB is unlikely and therapy is complete after treatment including at least 2 months of RIF and pyrazinamide (PZA) has been administered. For patients whose clinical suspicion is low and who are not initially receiving treatment (top of figure), if cultures remain negative, the patient has no symptoms, and the chest radiograph (CXR) is unchanged at 2 to 3 months, the 3 treatment options are as follows: 1) INH for 9 months, 2) RIF with or without INH for 4 months, or 3) RIF and PZA for 2 months. The RIF-PZA 2-month regimen should be used only for patients who are not likely to complete a longer course of treatment and can be monitored closely. EMB indicates ethambutol; Sx, signs and symptoms.*
(Adapted from Blumberg HM, Burman WJ, Chaisson RE, Daley CL, Etkind SC, Friedman LN, et al. American Thoracic Society/Centers for Disease Control and Prevention/Infectious Diseases Society of America: treatment of tuberculosis. Am J Respir Crit Care Med. 2003 Feb 15;167[4]:603–62. Used with permission.)

disease is more common in older adults, those with underlying chronic obstructive pulmonary disease, smokers, persons who abuse alcohol, and some children with cystic fibrosis. Most of these patients (>90%) have bronchiectasis or small nodules without predilection for any lobe. High-resolution computed tomography may show associated multifocal bronchiectasis with small (<5 mm) nodular infiltrates. Bilateral nodular or interstitial lung disease (or both), isolated disease in the right middle lobe, or lingular disease is more predominant in elderly, nonsmoking women. Hypersensitivity pneumonitis caused by exposure to *Mycobacterium avium* complex growing in a hot tub has been reported. *Mycobacterium avium* complex is responsible for 5% of the cases of mycobacterial lymphadenitis in adults and more than 90% of the cases in children. Lymphadenopathy is usually unilateral and nontender. Disseminated disease caused by NTM manifests as a fever of unknown origin in immunocompromised patients without AIDS.

HIV-infected persons are at high risk for NTM infections. More than 95% of NTM disease in HIV-infected persons is caused by the *M avium* complex. In persons with AIDS, disseminated infection occurs in up to 40% and localized infection in 5%; dissemination is more likely in those with a CD4 cell count less than 50/mcL. The risk of disseminated infection is 20% per year when the CD4 cell count is less than 100/mcL. Most patients present with high fever; sweats, anemia, and increased alkaline phosphatase levels are common. Dissemination is usually documented with positive blood cultures (sensitivity, 90%).

Mycobacterium kansasii is the second most common cause of NTM pulmonary disease in the United States. Approximately 90% of patients with *M kansasii* disease have cavitary infiltrates. *Mycobacterium kansasii* infection can be clinically indistinguishable from tuberculosis; however, its symptoms may be less severe and more long term than with tuberculosis. In HIV-negative patients, common symptoms are cough (90%), purulent sputum (85%), weight loss (55%), and dyspnea (50%). In immunocompromised patients, including those with AIDS, the lung is most commonly involved and symptoms include fever, chills, night sweats, cough, weight loss, dyspnea, and chest pain. Disseminated *M kansasii* infection occurs in 20% of HIV-positive patients who have *M kansasii* pulmonary disease.

Specific skin tests are not available for the diagnosis of NTM. Routine cultures of sputum, blood, or stool are not recommended for asymptomatic patients. All specimens positive for acid-fast bacilli must be considered to indicate *M tuberculosis* until final culture results are available. Bronchoscopy or open lung biopsy is required for diagnosis in nearly 50% of cases. *Mycobacterium avium* complex is generally treated with at least 12 months of clarithromycin, rifabutin, and ethambutol. The current recommendation for treatment of pulmonary disease caused by *M kansasii* in adults is isoniazid, rifampin, and ethambutol.

Pneumocystis jiroveci Infection

Pneumocystis jiroveci (formerly *Pneumocystis carinii*) is a fungus with trophic and cyst forms. *Pneumocystis jiroveci* infections occur in immunosuppressed persons, especially those with AIDS (CD4 cell count ≤200/mcL) or malignancy and after organ transplant. Clinical features in patients with AIDS include the gradual onset of dyspnea, fever, tachypnea, and hypoxia. In patients without AIDS, the onset is more abrupt, and progression to respiratory failure occurs quickly. Patients typically have relatively normal findings on lung examination and a patchy or diffuse interstitial or alveolar process on chest radiography. The typical computed tomographic finding is ground-glass attenuation. Although the level of lactate dehydrogenase may be elevated, routine laboratory data are often unhelpful. The diagnosis can be made with microscopic examination or polymerase chain reaction of induced sputum, bronchoalveolar lavage, or lung biopsy.

Parasitic Diseases

Parasitic infections of the lung are less common in the United States than in many other parts of the world. Travelers to endemic regions may be at risk. Dirofilariasis is indigenous to the eastern and southeastern United States. Other parasitic infections, including helminthic infestations, also occur in the United States. The parasites most likely to cause pulmonary infections include *Paragonimus westermani* (paragonimiasis), *Echinococcus granulosus* (echinococcosis or hydatid disease), *Dirofilaria immitis* (dirofilariasis), *Schistosoma japonicum* and *Schistosoma mansoni* (schistosomiasis), and *Entamoeba histolytica* (amebiasis). Protozoal infections are more likely in persons with suppressed cellular immunity.

Dirofilariasis, caused by the heartworm that infects dogs, is transmitted to humans by mosquitoes. The disease is endemic to the Mississippi River Valley, southeastern United States, and the Gulf Coast. Characteristically, the infection manifests as a defined solitary lung nodule or multiple lung nodules that have a diameter of 1.5 to 2.5 cm. Eosinophilia occurs in less than 15% of patients. Serologic tests may aid in the diagnosis.

Echinococcosis has occurred in Alaska, the Upper Peninsula of Michigan, and the US Southwest. When persons have echinococcosis lung disease, chest radiography shows well-defined round or oval cystic or solid lesions up to 15 cm in diameter. Cyst rupture can cause anaphylactic shock, hypersensitivity reactions, and seeding of adjacent anatomical areas. Liver involvement (which develops in 40% of lung disease cases) and positive serologic findings are common.

Paragonimiasis is more likely in immigrants from Southeast Asia, but sporadic cases occur in the United States. It is transmitted typically through consumption of raw or undercooked crabs or crayfish. Respiratory characteristics resemble those of chronic bronchitis, bronchiectasis, or tuberculosis. Profuse, brown-colored sputum and hemoptysis can be seen. Pleural effusion is relatively common; peripheral eosinophilia also is common. Ova can be found in pleural fluid, bronchial wash, or sputum.

Strongyloidiasis involving the lungs may mimic asthma with eosinophilia. Risk factors include corticosteroid use, age greater than 65 years, chronic lung disease, and chronic debilitating illness. Pulmonary signs and symptoms include cough, shortness of breath, wheezing, and hemoptysis in more than 90% of patients, and pulmonary infiltrates in 90%. A series of 20 patients with pulmonary strongyloidiasis showed that acute respiratory distress syndrome developed in 9 patients (45%). Preexisting chronic lung disease and the development of acute respiratory distress syndrome are important predictors of a poor prognosis.

46 Sexually Transmitted, Urinary Tract, and Gastrointestinal Tract Infections[a]

M. RIZWAN SOHAIL, MD

Sexually Transmitted Infections

Sexually transmitted infections (STIs) remain a major public health burden. About 19 million STIs occur annually in the United States. Rates of STIs are higher in young African American women and in men who have sex with men. The most common STIs are human papillomavirus (HPV) infection, chlamydia, herpes simplex virus (HSV) infection, and trichomoniasis. Although selected types of HPV are preventable with vaccination, other STIs require effective barriers to prevent transmission. These infections are characterized by their clinical presentations: 1) genital ulcers and lesions, 2) urethritis, 3) pelvic inflammatory disease (PID), 4) vulvovaginitis and cervicitis, and 5) urinary tract infections.

Genital Ulcers and Lesions

Chancroid

In the United States, patients who present with genital ulcers usually have genital herpes, syphilis, or chancroid. These conditions are associated with an increased risk of human immunodeficiency virus (HIV) infection. The combination of a painful genital ulcer (Figure 46.1) and tender suppurative inguinal adenopathy (Figure 46.2) is highly suggestive of chancroid, which is caused by *Haemophilus ducreyi*. Nevertheless, clinical inspection may not distinguish these 3 conditions, and all patients with genital ulcers should have syphilis serologic testing and HSV cell culture or polymerase chain reaction (PCR) test. In areas where chancroid is prevalent, such as Africa and other tropical and subtropical regions, specialized culture for *H ducreyi* can be performed.

KEY FACT

✓ In the United States, patients who present with genital ulcers usually have genital herpes, syphilis, or chancroid

---

Chancroid is treated with azithromycin (1 g orally once), ceftriaxone (250 mg intramuscularly once), or ciprofloxacin (500 mg orally twice daily for 3 days). Persons who have had sexual contact with an index patient during the 10 days preceding the patient's onset of symptoms should receive prophylactic treatment.

---

[a] Portions previously published in Workowski KA, Berman S; Centers for Disease Control and Prevention (CDC). Sexually transmitted diseases treatment guidelines, 2010. MMWR Recomm Rep. 2010 Dec 17;59(RR-12):1–110. Erratum in: MMWR Recomm Rep. 2011 Jan 14;60(1):18. Dosage error in article text; Workowski KA, Berman SM; Centers for Disease Control and Prevention. Sexually transmitted diseases treatment guidelines, 2006. MMWR Recomm Rep. 2006 Aug 4;55(RR-11):1–94. Erratum in: MMWR Recomm Rep. 2006 Sep 15;55(36):997; Centers for Disease Control and Prevention. Updated recommended treatment regimens for gonococcal infections and associated conditions: United States, April 2007 [Internet]. Atlanta (GA): Centers for Disease Control and Prevention; c2007 [cited 2015 Oct 22]. Available from: http://www.cdc.gov/STD/treatment/2006/updated-regimens.htm; and Workowski KA, Bolan GA; Centers for Disease Control and Prevention. Sexually transmitted diseases treatment guidelines, 2015. MMWR Recomm Rep. 2015 Jun 5;64(RR-03):1–137.

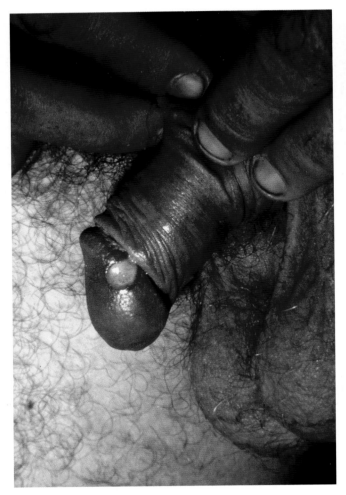

Figure 46.1 *Painful Genital Ulcer Caused by* Haemophilus ducreyi *(Chancroid).*
(Adapted from Centers for Disease Control and Prevention. Penile chancroid lesion [Internet]. Atlanta [GA]: Centers for Disease Control and Prevention; c1974 CDC/Joe Miller. Available from: http://phil.cdc.gov/phil/details.asp?pid=3728.)

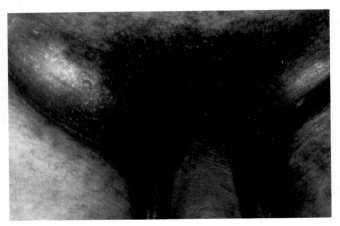

Figure 46.2 *Tender Suppurative Inguinal Adenopathy in a Patient With Chancroid.*
(Adapted from Centers for Disease Control and Prevention. Chancroid infection spread to inguinal lymph nodes [Internet]. Atlanta [GA]: Centers for Disease Control and Prevention; c1971 CDC/Susan Lindsley. Available from: http://phil.cdc.gov/phil/details.asp?pid=5811.)

KEY FACT

✓ Antivirals are beneficial when they treat first and recurrent episodes or when used as daily suppressive therapy

---

Herpes Simplex Virus

At least 50 million persons in the United States are infected with HSV type 1 or type 2. Most of them have not received a diagnosis of genital herpes. Infected persons intermittently shed virus from the genital tract despite a lack of symptoms, thereby leading to transmission. Symptomatic infection typically presents as a few painful, clustered vesicles with an erythematous base (Figure 46.3). Isolation of HSV in cell culture or PCR from genital lesions is the preferred virologic test.

Antivirals are helpful when they are used to treat first and recurrent episodes or when used as daily suppressive therapy. Recommended regimens for a first episode of genital HSV include acyclovir (400 mg orally 3 times a day), famciclovir (250 mg orally 3 times a day), and valacyclovir (1 g orally twice a day). Treatment duration for first episode is 7 to 10 days.

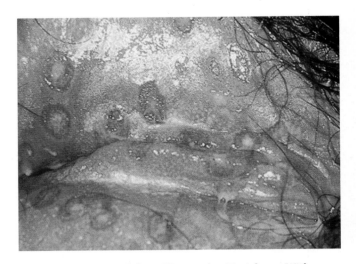

Figure **46.3** *Painful, Clustered Vesicles With an Erythematous Base Due to Herpes Simplex Virus.*
(Adapted from SOA-AIDS Amsterdam. SOA-Herpes-genitalis-female [Internet]. AIDS Fonds: Amsterdam [Netherlands] [cited 2015 Nov 25]. Available from: http://www.aidsfonds.nl/.)

Because recurrences are common, especially with HSV type 2, episodic or continuous suppressive antiviral therapy with acyclovir (400 mg orally twice a day), famciclovir (250 mg orally twice a day), or valacyclovir (500 mg or 1g orally once a day) is equally effective in reducing the frequency of recurrences. Daily treatment with valacyclovir (500 mg a day) decreases the rate of HSV type 2 transmission in discordant, heterosexual couples.

HSV in Pregnancy

In the first trimester of pregnancy, development of primary HSV infection may be associated with chorioretinitis and microcephaly in the fetus. The risk of HSV transmission to the baby from an infected mother is 30% to 50% among women who acquire genital herpes near the time of delivery, 3% for women with a recurrence at delivery, and <1% among women with histories of recurrent herpes but no lesions at delivery. Prevention of neonatal herpes relies on preventing acquisition of genital HSV late in pregnancy and avoiding exposure of the infant to herpetic lesions during delivery. Women without known genital herpes should be counseled to avoid intercourse during the third trimester with partners known to have genital herpes or in whom it is suspected. Pregnant women without known orolabial herpes should be advised to avoid receptive oral sex during the third trimester with partners known to have orolabial herpes or in whom it is suspected.

KEY FACT

✓ In the first trimester of pregnancy, development of a primary HSV infection may be associated with chorioretinitis and microcephaly in the fetus

---

At the onset of labor, all women should be questioned about symptoms of genital herpes, including prodromal symptoms, and be examined carefully for herpetic lesions. Women without symptoms or signs of genital herpes or its prodrome can deliver vaginally. Acyclovir treatment late in pregnancy reduces the frequency of cesarean sections among women who have recurrent genital herpes because it diminishes the frequency of recurrences at term. Women with recurrent genital herpetic lesions at the onset of labor should deliver by cesarean section to prevent neonatal herpes.

Syphilis

Syphilis is caused by the spirochete *Treponema pallidum*. The incidence of syphilis is highest in large, inner-city minority populations and in men who have sex with men. Called the *great masquerader*, syphilis may present with various manifestations, depending on the stage of disease and including a painless genital ulcer or chancre at the infection site; rash; mucocutaneous lesions; lymphadenopathy; cardiac, neurologic, and ophthalmic manifestations; auditory abnormalities; gummatous lesions; or simply a positive serologic test result. Because of the wide variation and transient nature of its manifestations, syphilis is often overlooked.

KEY FACT

✓ Called the *great masquerader*, syphilis may present with various manifestations, depending on disease stage and including a painless genital ulcer or chancre at the infection site; rash; mucocutaneous lesions; lymphadenopathy; cardiac, neurologic, and ophthalmic signs; auditory abnormalities; gummatous lesions; and positive serologic test result

---

Serologic tests for syphilis differ by laboratory. Some centers use the enzyme immunoassay for syphilis immunoglobulin M and immunoglobulin G as a screening test, followed by the nontreponemal test of rapid plasma reagin (RPR). Other centers use the RPR test initially and confirm its result with a more specific test, such as the fluorescent treponemal antibody absorption test (Table 46.1). Results of this test are positive before Venereal Disease Research Laboratory (VDRL) testing (nontreponemal test), and thus they may be positive without a positive VDRL result in primary syphilis cases. VDRL results may be negative in 30% of patients with primary syphilis and can be negative also in late-latent infections (those that occur >1 year after secondary syphilis).

A **chancre** (clean, indurated ulcer) is the main manifestation of primary syphilis (Figure 46.4). It occurs at the site of inoculation and is usually painless. The incubation period is 3 to 90 days. Chancre should be distinguished from HSV (painful) and **chancroid** (painful exudative ulcer). Diagnosis

---

Key Definitions

Chancre: *A clean, indurated ulcer and the main manifestation of primary syphilis, usually painless.*

Chancroid: *A painful exudative ulcer.*

Table 46.1 • Laboratory Diagnosis of Syphilis

Syphilis	Test, % Positive		
	VDRL	**FTA-ABS**	**MHA-TP**
Primary	70	85	50–60
Secondary	99	100	100
Tertiary	70	98	98

Abbreviations: FTA-ABS, fluorescent treponemal antibody absorption; MHA-TP, microhemagglutination assay for *Treponema pallidum*; VDRL, Venereal Disease Research Laboratory.

Adapted from Hook EW III. Syphilis. In: Goldman L, Schafer AI, editors. Goldman-Cecil medicine. 25th ed. Philadelphia (PA): Elsevier Saunders; c2016. p. 2013–20.e2. Used with permission.

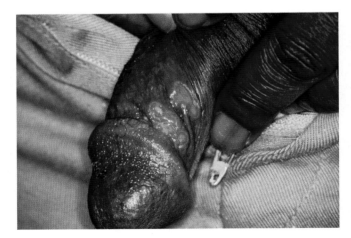

Figure 46.4 *Painless Ulcer (Chancre) Due to Primary Syphilis.*
(Adapted from Centers for Disease Control and Prevention. Chancres on the penile shaft due to a primary syphilitic infection caused by Treponema pallidum bacteria [Internet]. Atlanta [GA]: Centers for Disease Control and Prevention; c1978 CDC/M. Rein. Available from: http://phil.cdc.gov/phil/details.asp?pid=6803.)

of primary syphilis can be made with dark-field examination of a specimen taken from the genital ulcer.

The manifestations of secondary syphilis result from hematogenous dissemination and usually occur 2 to 8 weeks after appearance of the chancre. Constitutional symptoms occur, in addition to a rash, mucocutaneous lesions (Figure 46.5), alopecia, **condylomata lata** (ie, broad and flat verrucous syphilitic lesions located in warm, moist

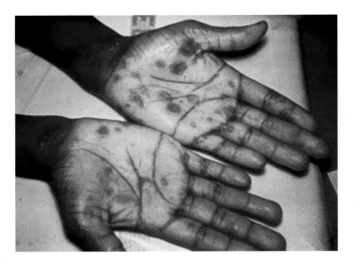

Figure 46.5 *Cutaneous Lesions in Secondary Syphilis.*
(Adapted from Centers for Disease Control and Prevention. Papulosquamous syphilids, or cutaneous eruptions of syphilis [Internet]. Atlanta [GA]: Centers for Disease Control and Prevention; c1971 CDC/Susan Lindsley. Available from: http://phil.cdc.gov/phil/details.asp?pid=2369.)

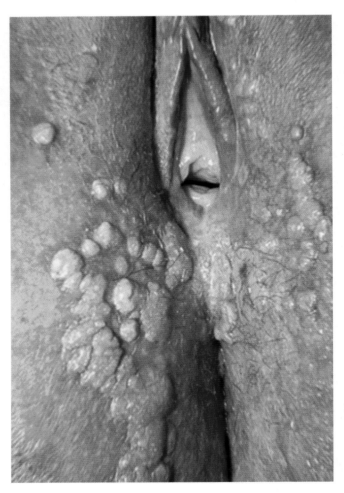

Figure 46.6 *Condylomata Lata in Secondary Syphilis.*
(Adapted from Science Source. Secondary syphilitic lesions: image number BT4983 [Internet]. Science Source Images: New York [NY] [cited 2015 Nov 25]. Available from: http://images.sciencesource.com/preview/BT4983.html. Used with permission.)

intertriginous areas, especially about the anus and genitals [Figure 46.6]), lymphadenopathy, and various other symptoms and signs. The diagnosis is based on clinical findings and the results of serologic testing. The condition resolves spontaneously without treatment.

Key Definition

Condylomata lata: *Broad, flat verrucous syphilitic lesions occurring in warm, moist intertriginous areas, especially in the anal and genital areas.*

Latent syphilis is the asymptomatic stage after symptoms of secondary syphilis subside. Cases of secondary syphilis that occur after 1 year are classified as *late latent*.

The diagnosis is based on the results of serologic testing. For latent syphilis, examination of cerebrospinal fluid (CSF) is indicated before treatment of patients with neurologic or ophthalmic abnormalities (Argyll Robertson pupils [accommodation reflex present and light reflex absent]), treatment of patients with other evidence of active tertiary syphilis (eg, aortitis, gummas), before re-treatment of relapses, and treatment of patients with HIV infection, especially those with a CD4 count <350 cells/mcL and a serum RPR titer >1:32.

Tertiary syphilis can involve any body system (eg, cardiovascular aortitis involving the ascending aorta, which can cause aneurysms and aortic regurgitation; gummatous osteomyelitis; hepatitis). However, neurosyphilis is the most common manifestation of tertiary syphilis in the United States. Neurosyphilis is often asymptomatic. Symptomatic disease is divided into several clinical syndromes that may overlap and occur at any time after primary infection. CSF abnormalities in neurosyphilis may include mononuclear pleocytosis and an increased protein value. CSF VDRL testing is only 30% to 70% sensitive. By comparison, CSF fluorescent treponemal antibody absorption test is highly sensitive (>90% sensitivity). Any CSF abnormality in a patient who is seropositive for syphilis must be investigated. The spectrum of neurosyphilis includes meningovascular syphilis (occurs 4–7 years after infection and presents with stroke or cranial nerve abnormalities) and parenchymatous syphilis (occurs decades after infection and may present as general paresis or chronic progressive dementia or as tabes dorsalis resulting in sensory ataxia, lightning pains, autonomic dysfunction, and optic atrophy).

KEY FACT

✓ Neurosyphilis is the most common manifestation of tertiary syphilis in the United States

---

Treatment of syphilis is summarized in Table 46.2. After treatment (especially in early syphilis), 10% to 25% of patients may experience a Jarisch-Herxheimer reaction, manifested by varying degrees of fever, chills, myalgias, headache, tachycardia, and hypotension. This reaction lasts 12 to 24 hours and can be managed symptomatically.

Pregnant patients should receive a penicillin-based regimen for treatment of all stages of syphilis. If a pregnant patient has a penicillin allergy, she should receive therapy for desensitization to penicillin.

For early and secondary syphilis, follow-up clinical and serologic testing (ie, RPR) should be performed at 6 and 12 months. Re-treatment with 3 weekly injections of 2.4 million U of benzathine penicillin G should be given to patients with signs or symptoms that persist or whose RPR result shows a sustained 4-fold increase in titer. HIV testing should be performed if not done previously. If the RPR titer

Table 46.2 • Treatment of Syphilis

Condition	Recommended Regimen	Alternative Regimen
Early syphilis (primary, secondary, or early latent [<1 y])[a]	Benzathine penicillin G (2.4 million U given IM once)	Doxycycline (100 mg twice daily for 14 d) *Or* Tetracycline (500 mg orally 4 times daily for 14 d) *Or* Erythromycin (500 mg orally 4 times daily) (least-effective treatment)
Late syphilis (cardiovascular disease, gumma, or late latent [≥1 y])	Benzathine penicillin (2.4 million U given IM weekly for 3 wk)	Doxycycline (100 mg orally twice daily for 4 wk) *Or* Tetracycline (500 mg orally 4 times daily)
Neurosyphilis	Aqueous penicillin G (12 million-24 million U given IV daily for 10 to 14 d)	Procaine penicillin (2.4 million U given IM daily) *plus* probenecid (500 mg 4 times daily) for 10 to 14 d

Abbreviations: IM, intramuscularly; IV, intravenously.

does not decrease 4-fold within 6 months, consideration also should be given to re-treatment.

Patients with latent syphilis should have follow-up testing at 6, 12, and 24 months. If the RPR result increases 4-fold, if a high titer (>1:32) fails to decrease 4-fold within 12 to 24 months, or if signs or symptoms attributable to syphilis occur, a CSF examination should be repeated to rule out neurosyphilis, and re-treatment should be done accordingly.

Follow-up in patients who receive therapy for neurosyphilis should include testing of CSF every 6 months if CSF pleocytosis was present initially; this testing is done until the results are normal. If the cell count is not decreased at 6 months or the CSF is not entirely normal at 2 years, re-treatment should be considered.

Urethritis Syndromes

The clinical syndrome of urethral pain and discharge is often associated with gonorrhea, chlamydia, and other causes of nongonococcal urethritis. A diagnosis of urethritis is made on the basis of the following findings: mucopurulent or purulent discharge, a Gram stain of urethral secretions with ≥5 leukocytes per oil immersion field, or a positive result of leukocyte esterase test on first-void urine. The presence of gram-negative intracellular diplococci on

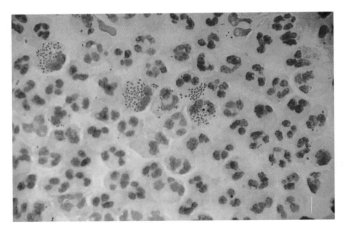

Figure 46.7 Gram-Negative Intracellular Diplococci in Gonococcal Urethritis (Gram stain).
(Adapted from Centers for Disease Control and Prevention. Histopathology in an acute case of gonococcal urethritis using Gram-stain technique [Internet]. Atlanta [GA]: Centers for Disease Control and Prevention. Available from: http://phil.cdc.gov/phil/details.asp?pid=4085.)

a urethral smear (Figure 46.7) is indicative of gonorrhea infection and is often accompanied by chlamydial infection. Nongonococcal urethritis is diagnosed when microscopy indicates inflammation without gram-negative intracellular diplococci. Urine or urethral exudates should be tested for gonorrhea and *Chlamydia trachomatis*. A frequent cause of nongonococcal urethritis (15%–55% of cases), *C trachomatis* nevertheless varies in prevalence by age-group, with lower prevalence among older men. The etiologic agent of most cases of nonchlamydial nongonococcal urethritis is unknown; however, *Mycoplasma genitalium* is emerging as an increasingly recognized cause. Complications of nongonococcal urethritis among men infected with *C trachomatis* include epididymitis, prostatitis, and Reiter syndrome.

> ### KEY FACT
>
> ✓ Urethritis diagnosis is based on finding mucopurulent or purulent discharge, Gram stain of urethral secretions with 5 leukocytes or more per oil-immersion field, or positive result of leukocyte esterase test on first-void urine

Gonorrhea

Neisseria gonorrhoeae is a gram-negative intracellular diplococcus. Although rates of gonorrhea have remained stable in the United States, resistance to antimicrobials has increased. The infection often causes symptomatic urethritis and discharge in men, but it has few symptoms in women and may lead to cervicitis, infertility, ectopic pregnancy, and chronic pelvic pain. In women, concomitant proctitis is common, and all women with proctitis should have rectal cultures. Gonococcal pharyngitis is often asymptomatic. The diagnosis of gonorrhea may be made with Gram stain of urethral exudate of men showing intracellular gram-negative diplococci (Figure 46.7) or by nucleic acid amplification tests (NAAT) of a urine or urethral-cervix base.

> ### KEY FACT
>
> ✓ Although gonorrhea rates have stayed stable in the United States, antimicrobial resistance in gonorrhea has increased

Resistance to penicillin, tetracycline, and, most recently, fluoroquinolones has limited the gonorrhea treatment options to the cephalosporins solely. Because chlamydial infection often is concomitant, a second agent is frequently included in the treatment regimen. Primary treatment is ceftriaxone (125 mg intramuscularly) plus doxycycline (100 mg orally twice daily for 7 days) or azithromycin (a sole 1-g dose) to treat chlamydial infection in addition. Cefixime (400 mg once daily) is available as a first-line oral option; a test of cure is required 1 week after treatment using culture or using NAAT when culture is not available. Alternative therapies are limited for patients who are allergic to β-lactam. Spectinomycin is not available in the United States. Limited data suggest that high-dose azithromycin (2 g in 1 dose) therapy might be an option, although this regimen should generally be avoided as solitary treatment of gonorrhea because of concern about drug resistance. Pharyngeal infection is best treated with ceftriaxone. Therapy recommended for pregnant women includes ceftriaxone (125 mg intramuscularly) or cefixime (400 mg orally) plus azithromycin (1 g orally). Follow-up NAAT at 3 weeks after treatment is recommended for all pregnant women. All patients with a sexually transmitted disease should be tested for HIV infection. Sexual partners should be offered evaluation and treatment. Table 46.3 outlines the treatment of gonococcal infections.

In 1% to 3% of patients with *N gonorrhoeae*, the infection may lead to disseminated gonococcal infection. Risk factors include complement deficiency, pharyngeal infection, pregnancy, and menstruation. The disseminated infection occurs most often in women during menstruation, when sloughing of endometrium allows access to a blood supply, enhanced growth of gonococci due to necrotic tissue, and change in pH. Two distinct phases occur in *N gonorrhoeae* infection. The bacteremic phase may manifest as tenosynovitis (around the wrists or ankles [also called *lover's heels*]); painful, distally distributed skin lesions (macular or pustular with a hemorrhagic component); and polyarthralgias involving knees and elbows (the classic

Table 46.3 • Treatment Regimens for Gonococcal Infections and Associated Conditions

Infection	Recommended Regimen	Alternative Regimen
Cervix, urethra, rectum[a]	Ceftriaxone (125 mg IM in single dose) *Or* Cefixime[c] (400 mg orally in single dose or 400 mg in suspension [200 mg/5 mL]) *Plus* Treatment of *Chlamydia* infection if not ruled out	Spectinomycin[b] (2 g IM in a single dose) *Or* Single-dose cephalosporin regimen
Pharynx[a]	Ceftriaxone (125 mg IM in single dose) *Plus* Treatment of *Chlamydia* infection if not ruled out	

Disseminated gonococcal infection[d]	Ceftriaxone (1 g IM or IV every 24 h)	Cefotaxime (1 g IV every 8 h)
		Or
		Ceftizoxime (1 g IV every 8 h)
		Or
		Spectinomycin[b] (2 g IM every 12 h)
		After 24 to 48 h of clinical improvement, switch therapy[e]
		   Cefixime (400 mg orally twice daily)
		Or
		   Cefixime[c] (400 mg in suspension [200 mg/5 mL])
		Or
		   Cefpodoxime (400 mg orally twice daily)

Pelvic inflammatory disease[f]	Parenteral A
	   Cefotetan (2 g IV every 12 h)
	Or
	   Cefoxitin (2 g IV every 6 h)
	Plus
	   Doxycycline (100 mg orally or IV every 12 h)
	Parenteral B
	   Clindamycin (900 mg IV every 8 h)
	Plus
	   Gentamicin[g]
	
	Oral[h]
	   Ceftriaxone (250 mg IM in single dose)
	Plus
	   Doxycycline (100 mg orally twice daily for 14 d) *with or without* metronidazole (500 mg orally twice daily for 14 d)
	Or
	   Cefoxitin (2 g IM in single dose) and probenecid (1 g orally concurrently in single dose)
	Plus
	   Doxycycline (100 mg orally twice daily for 14 d) *with or without* metronidazole (500 mg orally twice daily for 14 d)
	
	Or
	   Other parenteral third-generation cephalosporin[j]
	Plus
	   Doxycycline 100 mg orally twice daily for 14 d *with or without* metronidazole 500 mg orally twice daily for 14 d
		Parenteral
		   Ampicillin-sulbactam (3 g IV every 6 h)
		Plus
		   Doxycycline (100 mg orally or IV every 12 h)
		
		Fluoroquinolones[i]
		Levofloxacin (500 mg orally once daily) or oxacin (400 mg twice daily for 14 d) *with or without* metronidazole (500 mg orally twice daily for 14 d)

(continued)

Table 46.3 • (Continued)

Infection	Recommended Regimen	Alternative Regimen

Epididymitis	Ceftriaxone 250 mg IM in a single dose
	Plus
	    Doxycycline 100 mg orally twice daily for 10 d
	    Ofloxacin[k] 300 mg orally twice daily for 10 d
	Or
	    Levofloxacin 500 mg orally once daily for 10 d	

Abbreviations: IM, intramuscularly; IV, intravenously.

[a] These regimens are recommended for all adult and adolescent patients, regardless of travel history or sexual behavior.

[b] Spectinomycin is currently not available in the United States.

[c] The tablet formulation of cefixime is currently not available in the United States.

[d] A cephalosporin-based IV regimen is recommended for the initial treatment of disseminated gonococcal infection. This use is particularly important when gonorrhea is detected at mucosal sites through nonculture tests.

[e] Switch to 1 of the following regimens for at least 1 wk of antimicrobial therapy: cefixime[c] 400 mg orally twice daily *or* cefixime 400 mg by suspension (200 mg/5 mL) twice daily *or* cefpodoxime 400 mg orally twice daily.

[f] Parenteral and oral therapies seem to have similar clinical efficacy for women with pelvic inflammatory disease of mild or moderate severity. Clinical experience should guide decisions regarding transition to oral therapy, which usually can be initiated within 24 hours of clinical improvement.

[g] Loading dose (2 mg/kg) IV or IM, followed by maintenance dose (1.5 mg/kg) every 8 hours. Single daily dosing may be substituted.

[h] Oral therapy can be considered for women with mild to moderately severe acute pelvic inflammatory disease because the clinical outcomes with oral therapy are similar to those with parenteral therapy. Women whose disease does not respond to oral therapy within 72 hours should be reevaluated to confirm the diagnosis and should be administered parenteral therapy on either an outpatient or an inpatient basis.

[i] If parenteral cephalosporin therapy is not feasible, use of fluoroquinolones with or without metronidazole may be considered when the community prevalence and individual risk of gonorrhea are low. Tests for gonorrhea must be performed before initiating therapy.

[j] Ceftizoxime or cefotaxime.

[k] For acute epididymitis most likely caused by enteric organisms or with negative gonococcal culture or nucleic acid amplification test.

Adapted from Workowski KA, Bolan GA; Centers for Disease Control and Prevention. Sexually transmitted diseases treatment guidelines, 2015. MMWR Recomm Rep. 2015 Jun 5;64(RR-03):1–137.

dermatitis arthritis syndrome). Synovial fluid testing is frequently negative. The nonbacteremic phase follows 1 week later and may present as monoarticular infectious arthritis of the knee, wrist, and ankle; results of joint culture are positive in about 50% of cases. Culture specimens should be obtained from the urethra, cervix, rectum, and pharynx.

> **KEY FACT**
>
> ✓ Risk factors for disseminated *N gonorrhoeae* infection include complement deficiency, pharyngeal infection, pregnancy, and menstruation

Treatment of disseminated gonococcal infection is with ceftriaxone (1 g intravenously each day for 7 to 10 days). An alternative option is ceftriaxone for 3 or 4 days or until clinical improvement, followed by oral cefixime (400 mg daily for 7 to 10 days). If the gonorrhea strain is tested and found to be penicillin-susceptible, treatment is intravenous and includes penicillin G (10 million U daily) for 3 or 4 days and then oral amoxicillin to finish a 7- to 10-day course.

Nongonococcal Urethritis and Cervicitis

Chlamydia trachomatis genital infection is the most common reportable STI. This organism causes urethritis in men and mucopurulent cervicitis, endometritis, and PID in women. Its sequelae include tubal infertility, chronic pelvic pain, and ectopic pregnancy. Because this infection may be asymptomatic in one-half of affected men and three-fourths of affected women, screening for *C trachomatis* is recommended for all sexually active women age 24 years or younger.

> **KEY FACT**
>
> ✓ *Chlamydia trachomatis* genital infection is the most common reportable sexually transmitted infection

The diagnosis is most often made from NAATs or from urine or urethrocervical specimens. Treatment of infected persons, whether the infection is symptomatic or not, reduces *C trachomatis* transmission. Two regimens are highly effective, and the treatment choice depends on patient compliance. Doxycycline (100 mg twice daily for 7 days) or azithromycin (a single 1-g oral dose) is standard treatment. Infected persons should abstain from sexual activity until 1 week after treatment is completed. Women with *C trachomatis* cervicitis should be rescreened with NAAT at 3 to 4 months posttreatment. *Ureaplasma urealyticum, Trichomonas vaginalis, M genitalium*, and HSV are less common causes of nongonococcal urethritis. If urethritis fails to resolve and reinfection or relapse of a chlamydial infection has been excluded, *Trichomonas* or tetracycline-resistant *Ureaplasma* infection should be considered. In this situation, empirical treatment consists of metronidazole (2 g orally in a single dose) plus an erythromycin-base treatment (500 mg orally 4 times daily for 7 days).

Epididymitis

This condition usually presents as a unilateral, painful scrotal swelling. In men who are sexually active and young (age <35 years), *C trachomatis* and *N gonorrhoeae* are the common pathogens of epididymitis. Sexually transmitted acute epididymitis is usually accompanied by asymptomatic urethritis and absence of bacteruria. In contrast, aerobic gram-negative rods and enterococci predominate in older men with epididymitis, which is frequently associated with urinary tract abnormalities or instrumentation. Although epididymitis is primarily a clinical diagnosis, ultrasonography has a sensitivity of 70% and a specificity of 88% for diagnosing acute epididymitis. The diagnostic evaluation of men in whom epididymitis is suspected should include a Gram stain of urethral secretions, a leukocyte esterase test of first-void urine, and microscopic examination of first-void urine sediment (positive result, ≥10 leukocytes per high-power field).

Empirical treatment includes ceftriaxone (250 mg intramuscularly) plus doxycycline (100 mg orally twice daily for 10 days). In older men with test results that are negative for gonorrhea and *Chlamydia*, the treatment advised is empirical therapy with oral levofloxacin (500 mg daily for 10 days) or treatment based on culture results (if positive).

Pelvic Inflammatory Disease

In reproductive-age women, PID is associated with considerable long-term sequelae, such as infertility, ectopic pregnancy, tubo-ovarian abscess, and chronic pelvic pain. The organisms responsible include *N gonorrhoeae, C trachomatis, Mycoplasma hominis*, and various aerobic gram-negative rods and anaerobes. Fitz-Hugh-Curtis syndrome is an acute perihepatitis caused by direct extension of *N gonorrhoeae* or *C trachomatis* infection to the liver capsule. *Actinomyces* species can be a pathogen in patients with an intrauterine device. Diagnosis of PID is based on clinical findings, including lower abdominal or adnexal tenderness, cervical motion tenderness, fever, abnormal cervical discharge, and evidence of *N gonorrhoeae* or *C trachomatis* infection. Early empirical therapy is recommended for women at risk. Sonography and laparoscopy are reserved for complicated cases.

KEY FACT

✓ Pelvic inflammatory disease in reproductive-age women is associated with such long-term sequelae as infertility, ectopic pregnancy, tubo-ovarian abscess, and chronic pelvic pain

The goal of treatment is to prevent complications. Most women can receive treatment as outpatients and be reassessed within 1 to 3 days. Hospitalization is indicated when the outpatient therapy is precluded by severe nausea and vomiting; the diagnosis is uncertain; pelvic abscess or peritonitis is present; the patient is pregnant or an adolescent; or noncompliance is suspected. Table 46.3 outlines the treatment of PID.

Tubo-ovarian abscess may be characterized by an adnexal mass on physical examination or radiographic examination or by failure of antimicrobial therapy. Most abscesses less than 5 cm in diameter respond to medical therapy alone with the preferred regimen of ampicillin, gentamicin, and clindamycin. Large abscesses (>10 cm) often necessitate operation.

Vaginitis

Vaginitis is characterized by vaginal discharge or vulvar itching, odor, or irritation. The 3 entities most frequently associated with vaginal discharge are bacterial vaginosis, trichomoniasis, and vulvovaginal candidiasis.

Bacterial Vaginosis

Bacterial vaginosis is the most common vaginal infection affecting women of child-bearing age. It occurs because of a change in local vaginal ecologic characteristics from a flora of predominant lactobacilli to one of various anaerobic bacteria. Organisms associated with the syndrome include *Atopobium vaginae, Gardnerella* species, *Prevotella* species, *Mobiluncus* species, and *M hominis*. Risk factors for bacterial vaginosis include new or multiple sex partners, excessive douching, and a lack of vaginal lactobacilli. Bacterial vaginosis has been associated with increased risk for STIs and low-birth-weight infants.

KEY FACT

✓ Risk factors for bacterial vaginosis include new or multiple sex partners, douching, and a lack of vaginal lactobacilli

Bacterial vaginosis can be diagnosed with clinical or microbiologic criteria. Clinical criteria require 3 of the following: grayish white discharge that is homogeneous and coats the vaginal walls; bacteria obscuring the borders of vaginal epithelial cells, giving them a stippled appearance (so-called clue cells) on wet-mount examination (Figure 46.8); a vaginal fluid pH >4.5; and a fishy smell when secretion is mixed with 10% potassium hydroxide (a positive "whiff" test). Microbiologic criteria require microscopic examination with Gram stain that shows predominantly *Gardnerella* or *Mobiluncus* morphotype, or both, with few or absent lactobacilli. Rapid nucleic acid test using DNA probe–based

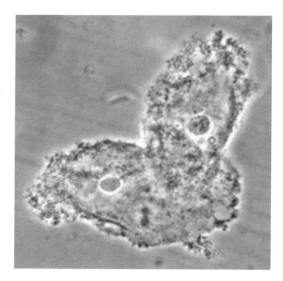

Figure 46.8 *Clue Cells With Bacteria Obscuring the Borders of Vaginal Epithelial Cells in a Patient With Bacterial Vaginosis.*

(Adapted from Centers for Disease Control and Prevention. Bacteria adhering to vaginal epithelial cells [Internet]. Atlanta [GA]: Centers for Disease Control and Prevention; c1978 CDC/M. Rein. Available from: http://phil.cdc.gov/phil/details.asp?pid=3720.)

assessment for high concentrations of *Gardnerella vaginalis* may also be used. Culture for *G vaginalis* is not recommended because it is frequently present in women without bacterial vaginosis.

KEY FACT

✓ Clinical criteria for bacterial vaginosis require 3 of the following: grayish white, homogeneous discharge that coats the vaginal walls, clue cells (bacteria obscuring the borders of vaginal epithelial cells, giving a stippled appearance) on wet-mount examination, vaginal fluid pH greater than 4.5, and a fishy smell when secretion is mixed with 10% potassium hydroxide

---

Recommended treatment regimens include metronidazole (500 mg orally twice daily for 7 days), clindamycin (300 mg orally twice daily for 7 days), topical clindamycin cream (2% for 7 days), or metronidazole gel (0.75% intravaginal applicator nightly for 5 days). Topical clindamycin cream appears less efficacious than metronidazole. Single-dose metronidazole therapy should not be used. Recurrence of bacterial vaginosis is common. Treatment of recurrent disease should include re-treatment followed by a prolonged course of twice-weekly metronidazole gel.

Bacterial vaginosis has been associated with adverse pregnancy outcomes. All symptomatic pregnant women should receive treatment. In pregnant patients, systemic therapy with metronidazole (500 mg twice daily for 7 days) or clindamycin (300 mg orally twice daily for 7 days) is recommended, rather than topical therapy. Some experts also recommend treatment of asymptomatic pregnant women at high risk for preterm delivery.

Trichomoniasis

Trichomonas vaginitis (trichomoniasis) presents as malodorous yellow-green vaginal discharge with vulvar irritation, dysuria, or dyspareunia. Petechial lesions may be noted on the cervix (called *strawberry cervix*) with colposcopy. The diagnosis is established from wet-mount examination of vaginal secretions showing the motile organisms. The vaginal pH is usually greater than 4.5. New rapid tests for *Trichomonas* in women include the 10-minute dipstick assay (OSOM *Trichomonas* Rapid Test; Sekisui Diagnostics, LLC) and the 45-minute nucleic acid probe test (Affirm VPIII; Becton, Dickinson and Co). Both these tests are performed on vaginal secretions and have a sensitivity greater than 83% and a specificity greater than 97%. These rapid tests are much more sensitive than the direct wet-mount examination.

KEY FACT

✓ *Trichomonas* vaginitis presents as malodorous yellow-green vaginal discharge with vulvar irritation, dysuria, or dyspareunia. Petechial lesions may be seen on the cervix at colposcopy

---

Treatment is with a single 2-g dose of metronidazole or tinidazole. A 7-day course of metronidazole (500 mg twice daily) is an alternative regimen. Gastrointestinal tolerance may be better with tinidazole. All partners should be examined and treated. Symptomatic pregnant women should receive a single 2-g dose of metronidazole.

Vulvovaginal Candidiasis

Vulvovaginal candidiasis is the second most common cause of vaginitis. The majority of cases are due to *C albicans*; a smaller number are due to *Candida glabrata*. The predominant symptoms of this condition are itching, soreness, burning, and dyspareunia although not discharge. Usually there is no odor, and the discharge is scant, watery, and white. A so-called cottage cheese curd material may adhere to the vaginal wall. Microscopy with 10% potassium hydroxide added to the discharge may show characteristic pseudohyphae; however, it is insensitive for diagnosis, and culture may be needed. Complicated cases include recurrent episodes (>4 per year), have severe symptoms, involve non-*albicans Candida*, or occur in the clinical setting of immunosuppression, diabetes mellitus, or pregnancy. In severe or recurrent cases, patients should be tested for HIV infection. For uncomplicated vulvovaginal candidiasis, any of a number of topical antifungal azole agents may be used for 1 to 7 days, or a single 150-mg oral dose of fluconazole may be used. Multiple-dose oral azole therapy is reserved for severe, refractory cases. In recurrent vulvovaginal candidiasis due to *C albicans*, treatment with fluconazole (150 mg every 3 days for 3 doses, followed by 150 mg once weekly) may be effective.

> **KEY FACT**
>
> ✓ The predominant symptoms of vulvovaginal candidiasis are itching, soreness, burning, and dyspareunia but not discharge. Usually, no odor is present, and discharge is scant, watery, and white. Whitish material that resembles cottage cheese curds may adhere to the vaginal wall

Urinary Tract Infections

In Women

Urinary tract infections (UTIs) are common in young women. Because urethritis or cystitis can occur with low colony counts of bacteria (ie, 10^3 colony-forming units/mL), routine urine cultures in young women with dysuria are not recommended. Urinalysis should be done with or without evaluation with a Gram stain. If pyuria and uncomplicated UTI are present, short-course treatment (3 days) should be initiated with no further testing. Appropriate culture and sensitivity test should be performed only when upper urinary tract disease, a complicated UTI, or sexually transmitted disease is suspected. Risk factors for complications include emergency department presentation, low socioeconomic status, hospital-acquired infection, pregnancy, urinary catheter placement, recent instrumentation, known urologic abnormality, UTI at age less than 12 years, acute pyelonephritis or 3 UTIs or more in 1 year, symptoms for more than 7 days, recent antibiotic use, diabetes, and immunosuppression. Common causative organisms include *Escherichia coli*, *Staphylococcus saprophyticus*, *Proteus mirabilis*, and *Klebsiella pneumoniae*.

> **KEY FACT**
>
> ✓ When pyuria and uncomplicated UTI are present, short-course treatment (3 days) should be initiated with no further testing

Staphylococcus saprophyticus is a distinct species of coagulase-negative staphylococcus that is a common cause of UTIs in young, sexually active women. Coagulase-negative staphylococci are usually resistant to the β-lactam antibiotics. However, *S saprophyticus* and *Staphylococcus*

lugdunensis (another cause of UTI) are exceptions because they usually are susceptible to the penicillins, trimethoprim-sulfamethoxazole, and many other antibiotics.

> **KEY FACT**
>
> ✓ *Staphylococcus saprophyticus* is a distinct coagulase-negative staphylococcus species that commonly causes UTIs in young, sexually active women

For the first episode of cystitis or urethritis, treatment is given but no investigation is needed. Short-course (3 days) treatment has fewer adverse effects than standard (7 to 10 days) therapy, and risk of infection relapse is the same. Trimethoprim-sulfamethoxazole, nitrofurantoin, and fosfomycin are considered first-line antimicrobial options for uncomplicated UTIs. In patients whose condition does not improve in 48 hours of treatment with first-line therapy, drug resistance should be suspected and an oral fluoroquinolone should be considered. Rates of trimethoprim-sulfamethoxazole resistance among *E coli* approach 20% in some populations. If recurrence develops after 3-day therapy, subclinical pyelonephritis or drug resistance should be considered. Urologic evaluation is usually not necessary. It should be performed, however, for patients with multiple relapses, painless hematuria, a history of childhood UTI, renal lithiasis, and recurrent pyelonephritis.

Asymptomatic bacteriuria ($>10^5$ colony-forming units/mL) in a midstream urine specimen should be treated only in pregnant women and in patients undergoing urinary tract instrumentation. For acute uncomplicated pyelonephritis, levofloxacin (750 mg once daily for 5 days) is equal in efficacy to 10 days of twice-daily therapy with ciprofloxacin. In patients who are sufficiently ill to require hospitalization, a third-generation cephalosporin or a fluoroquinolone can be used as empirical therapy over 10 to 14 days. If enterococci are suspected on the basis of the gram-stain evaluation, ampicillin or piperacillin should be used. Cephalosporins and trimethoprim-sulfamethoxazole should not be used to treat enterococcal UTI. Oral regimens can be substituted quickly as the patient improves. A repeat urine culture (test of cure) is recommended 1 to 2 weeks after completion of therapy only in pregnant women, children, and patients with recurrent pyelonephritis for whom suppressive therapy is being considered.

> **KEY FACT**
>
> ✓ Asymptomatic bacteriuria ($>10^5$ colony-forming units/mL) in a midstream urine specimen should be treated only in pregnant women and patients having urinary tract instrumentation

Recurrent UTIs may occur in women even without an anatomic abnormality. Prophylaxis may be offered to women who have 2 or more symptomatic UTIs within 6 months or 3 or more over 12 months. For these patients, 3 options have been shown to be effective: continuous prophylaxis, postcoital prophylaxis, and intermittent self-treatment, depending on clinical circumstances. For postmenopausal women, vaginal estrogen supplementation is beneficial.

In Men

UTI is less common in men, but its frequency increases with age. Urologic abnormalities (such as benign prostatic enlargement) are common in older men with UTIs. Men with symptomatic dysuria should be evaluated for sexually transmitted diseases and prostatism. When a UTI is suspected, urine culture and sensitivity testing should be done. Causative organisms include *E coli* in 50% of cases, other gram-negative organisms in 25%, enterococci in 20%, and other organisms in 5%. If signs and symptoms of epididymitis, acute prostatitis, and pyelonephritis are present, these conditions should be treated accordingly. All UTIs in men are treated as complicated conditions (10 to 14 days of antimicrobial therapy even for cystitis). If symptoms persist or relapse, urine culture should be repeated. If results are positive again and no abnormalities are noted on imaging, a 6-week treatment may be considered for presumed prostatitis. If culture results are negative, consider further evaluation for one of the chronic prostatitis–chronic pelvic pain syndromes.

KEY FACT

✓ Men with symptomatic dysuria should receive evaluation for sexually transmitted diseases and prostatism

---

Gastrointestinal Infections

Bacterial and Toxigenic Diarrhea

The principal causes of toxigenic diarrhea are listed in Table 46.4, and those of invasive diarrhea are listed in Table 46.5. Fecal leukocytes are usually absent in toxigenic diarrhea. In invasive diarrhea, fecal leukocytes may be present. The travel and exposure history is critical for appropriate work-up.

Campylobacter jejuni

Campylobacter jejuni is the most common cause of sporadic acute bacterial diarrhea. Outbreaks, although infrequent, are associated with consumption of unpasteurized dairy products and undercooked poultry. The incidence of disease peaks in summer and early fall. Diarrhea may be bloody, and fever is usually present. The diagnosis is established by isolation of the organism from stool culture or PCR. Treatment is usually symptomatic because the disease tends to be self-limited. Fluoroquinolone resistance is common, especially in Asia. Erythromycin (500 mg twice daily for 5 days) or azithromycin can be used when symptoms are prolonged and severe or the host is immunocompromised.

KEY FACT

✓ *Campylobacter jejuni* is the most common cause of sporadic acute bacterial diarrhea. Outbreaks, although less common, are associated with consumption of unpasteurized dairy products and undercooked poultry

---

Staphylococcal Enterotoxin

Preformed enterotoxins produced by *S aureus* are a common cause of food poisoning in the United States. The toxins are heat stable and therefore are not destroyed by cooking the contaminated foods. Preformed toxin of *S aureus* is ingested in contaminated food. It has a short incubation period of 4 to 6 hours. Onset is abrupt, with severe vomiting (often predominates), diarrhea, and abdominal cramps. The duration of infection is 8 to 24 hours. Diagnosis is based on rapid onset, absence of fever, and history. Treatment is supportive.

Clostridium perfringens

Bacterial diarrhea caused by *Clostridium perfringens* is associated with ingestion of bacteria that produce toxin in vivo, often in improperly prepared or stored precooked

---

Table 46.4 • Causes of Toxigenic Bacterial Diarrhea

Organism	Onset After Ingestion, h	Preformed Toxin	Fever Present	Vomiting Predominates
Staphylococcus aureus	2–6	Yes	No	Yes
Clostridium perfringens	8–16	No	No	No
Escherichia coli	12	No	No	No
Vibrio cholerae	12	No	Yes, due to dehydration	No
Bacillus cereus				
a	1–6	Yes	No	Yes
B	8–16	No	No	No

Table 46.5 • Causes of Invasive Bacterial Diarrhea

Organism[a]	Bloody Diarrhea Present	Antibiotics Effective
Shigella species	Yes	Yes
Salmonella non-*typhi*	No	No
Vibrio parahaemolyticus	Yes (occasionally)	No
Escherichia coli O157:H7	Yes	No
Campylobacter	Yes	Yes
Yersinia	Yes (occasionally)	Sometimes

[a] For all organisms listed, fever is present.

foods (meat and poultry products). Food is precooked and toxin is destroyed, but spores survive; when food is re-warmed, spores germinate. When the contaminated food is ingested, toxin is produced. Diarrhea is more severe than vomiting, and abdominal cramping is prominent. Onset of symptoms is later than with *S aureus* infection. Duration of illness is 24 hours. The diagnosis is based on the later onset of symptoms, a typical history. Treatment is supportive.

Bacillus cereus Toxin

Two types of food poisoning are associated with *Bacillus cereus* infection. Profuse vomiting follows a short incubation period (1 to 6 hours); this is associated with the ingestion of a preformed toxin (usually in fried rice). A disease with a longer incubation occurs 8 to 16 hours after consumption; profound diarrhea develops and usually is associated with eating meat or vegetables. The diagnosis is confirmed by isolation of the organism from contaminated food. The illness is self-limited and treatment is supportive.

> **KEY FACT**
>
> ✓ Frequently, food poisoning due to *Bacillus cereus* has a short incubation period and is associated with ingestion of a preformed toxin (usually in fried rice)

Escherichia coli

Diarrhea caused by *E coli* can be either enterotoxigenic or enterohemorrhagic. Enterotoxigenic *E coli* is the most common etiologic agent of traveler's diarrhea. Treatment consists of fluid and electrolyte replacement along with loperamide plus a fluoroquinolone or rifaximin. Medical evaluation should be sought if fever and bloody diarrhea occur. For prophylaxis, travelers should use food and water precautions. Routine prophylactic use of antibiotics such as trimethoprim-sulfamethoxazole, ciprofloxacin, and doxycycline is not recommended. Use of bismuth

subsalicylate as primary prophylaxis for travelers reduces the incidence of enterotoxigenic *E coli*–associated diarrhea by up to 60%.

> **KEY FACT**
>
> ✓ Diarrhea caused by *E coli* can be enterotoxigenic or enterohemorrhagic. Enterotoxigenic *E coli* is the most common etiologic agent of traveler's diarrhea

Escherichia coli O157:H7 causes an uncommon form of bloody diarrhea. This agent has been identified as the cause of waterborne illness, outbreaks in nursing homes and child care centers, and sporadic cases. It also has been transmitted by eating undercooked beef and other contaminated food products. Bloody diarrhea, severe abdominal cramps, fever, and profound toxicity characterize this enterohemorrhagic illness. It may mimic ischemic colitis. In persons at extremes of age (old and young), the infection may produce hemolytic uremic syndrome (HUS) and death. This organism should be considered in all patients with HUS. Antibiotics are not known to be effective and may increase the likelihood of HUS.

Shigella

Diarrhea caused by *Shigella* species is often acquired outside the United States. It frequently is spread from person to person or through consumption of contaminated food or water. Bloody diarrhea is characteristic, bacteremia may occur, and fever is present. The diagnosis is confirmed by stool culture and blood culture (occasionally positive). Treatment is with ampicillin, trimethoprim-sulfamethoxazole, ciprofloxacin, or azithromycin. However, resistance to these antimicrobials has been reported. The illness may precede the onset of spondyloarthropathy (reactive arthritis) in persons with HLA-B27 and group B *Shigella flexneri*.

Salmonella

In the United States, *Salmonella* (non-*typhi*)–associated illness most commonly is caused by *Salmonella enteritidis* and *Salmonella typhimurium*. It is associated with consumption of contaminated foods or exposure to reptiles and snakes, pet turtles, ducklings, and iguanas. Large outbreaks have been associated with produce and even contaminated peanut butter—food sources previously not connected with this infection.

Salmonella infection is a common cause of severe diarrhea and may cause septicemia in patients with sickle cell anemia or AIDS. *Salmonella* bacteremia can lead to hematogenous seeding of abdominal aortic plaques, resulting in mycotic aneurysms. In *Salmonella* enteritis, fever is usually present and bloody diarrhea often absent (a characteristic distinguishing it from *Shigella* infection). The diagnosis is based on stool culture or PCR. Treatment is supportive, and most cases of *Salmonella* gastroenteritis resolve without therapy. Antibiotics may prolong the carrier state and do not affect the course of the disease. Antibiotics are used if blood cultures are positive or if the host is older (age >50 years), has valvular heart disease or severe atherosclerosis, has intravascular prosthesis, or is immunocompromised. Reactive arthritis may be a complication of this illness. Nontyphoidal *Salmonella* species may also cause UTIs. The UTIs caused by *Salmonella* occur particularly in patients who are coinfected with *Schistosoma haematobium*.

Salmonella serotype *typhi* is rare in the United States; often, it is found in travelers who have returned from endemic regions and who present with fever. Patients with typhoid fever have relative bradycardia and skin rash (macular, rose-colored spots occur in 50% of cases). Leukocyte counts may be decreased. Blood cultures usually are positive within approximately 10 days of symptom onset, whereas stool cultures become positive later. Antimicrobial resistance is increasingly common with *S typhi*.

Serious or invasive *Salmonella* infections should be treated with a third-generation cephalosporin or fluoroquinolone pending susceptibility data.

Listeria monocytogenes

Listeria monocytogenes is a gram-positive rod often mistaken for a diphtheroid in clinical cultures. Most often recognized as a cause of meningitis, it can be associated with food-borne diarrhea, typically acquired from processed deli meats or hot dogs consumed in the summer. The incubation ranges from 6 hours to 90 days. In most persons, febrile gastroenteritis is self-limited over 2 or 3 days. Infection can be severe and disseminate to involve multiple organs and to cause meningitis in patients with cellular immune defects (eg, those with a transplant or HIV infection, those taking corticosteroids or other immunosuppressive medications). Curiously, in pregnant women, *Listeria* can cause placental infection that may lead to fetal death or premature birth. Neonatal infection, also called **granulomatosis infantiseptica**, may result from transplacental transmission of *Listeria*. Diagnosis is made through stool or blood culture. Severe listerial infections are usually treated with ampicillin plus gentamicin.

KEY FACT

✓ *Listeria monocytogenes* can be associated with food-borne diarrhea, typically acquired from processed deli meats or hot dogs consumed in summer

---

Key Definition

Granulomatosis infantiseptica: *Neonatal infection resulting from transplacental transmission of Listeria.*

Vibrio Species

In the United States, consumption of raw or undercooked shellfish such as oysters is the most common source of infection with pathogenic vibrios (eg, *Vibrio parahaemolyticus, Vibrio vulnificus*). *Vibrio parahaemolyticus* is appearing with increasing frequency in the United States along the Atlantic Gulf Coast and on cruise ships. Acute onset of explosive, watery diarrhea and fever are characteristic. The diagnosis is determined with stool culture. Disease usually manifests as self-limited enteritis, and antibiotic therapy is not required.

Cholera, a toxigenic bacterial diarrhea caused by *Vibrio cholerae*, continues to cause periodic pandemics, the most recent affecting South America and Central America, with the latest occurrence in Haiti. Cholera is rare in the United States and Canada, even among travelers. Fluid replacement therapy is the mainstay of its management. Antibiotics (eg, macrolides, tetracyclines, quinolones) administered for 1 to 3 days can shorten the duration of illness. Azithromycin (1g oral once) is probably the drug of choice.

Yersinia enterocolitica

Yersinia enterocolitica is the etiologic agent of several major clinical syndromes: enterocolitis, mesenteric adenitis, erythema nodosum, polyarthritis, Reiter syndrome, and bacteremia associated with contaminated blood products. Approximately 20% of infected patients have sore throat. Infection with *Y enterocolitica* causing mesenteric adenitis can mimic acute appendicitis. Acquisition of infection is thought to be associated with eating contaminated food products. *Y enterocolitica* has been cultured from chocolate milk, meat, mussels, poultry, oysters, and cheese. Enterocolitis and lymphadenitis are usually self-limited, and antibiotic therapy is not necessary. For severe or complicated infection requiring hospitalization, a 5-day course of ciprofloxacin, trimethoprim-sulfamethoxazole, or doxycycline is effective.

KEY FACT

✓ *Yersinia enterocolitica* is the causative agent in the major clinical syndromes of enterocolitis, mesenteric adenitis, erythema nodosum, polyarthritis, Reiter syndrome, and bacteremia associated with contaminated blood products

Clostridium difficile

Clostridium difficile infection should be distinguished from other forms of antibiotic-associated diarrhea (ie, it causes watery stools and no systemic symptoms, with negative tests for *C difficile* toxin). Symptoms often occur after exposure to antibiotics and health care settings. Antibiotics with high biliary concentrations and broad aerobic and anaerobic activity are associated with higher risk of *C difficile* infection. This infection is more common in elderly persons and is associated with an increased morbidity rate. The disease spectrum ranges from mild diarrhea to severe, life-threatening colitis. Typical features are profuse, watery stools; crampy abdominal pain; constitutional illness; unexplained leukocytosis; presence of fecal leukocytes; and positive result of *C difficile* toxin assay. If enzyme-linked immunosorbent assay for toxin A and B detection is used alone, the sensitivity may be suboptimal. When clinical suspicion is high and the assay result is negative, PCR should be requested or empirical therapy provided. In selected cases, proctoscopy or flexible sigmoidoscopy can be used to look for pseudomembranes.

Disease can be localized to the cecum (for example, postoperatively with clinical ileus) and can present as fever of unknown origin. A new toxigenic strain (North America pulsed-field type 1) associated with a binary toxin has become epidemic and is associated with fluoroquinolone resistance and more severe disease. Indications for hospitalization for *C difficile* infection are listed in Box 46.1.

KEY FACT

✓ Symptoms of *C difficile* infection often develop after exposure to antibiotics and health care facilities

---

Treatment of *C difficile* infection differs depending on the severity of illness and whether it is the first infection episode or recurrent disease (Table 46.6). Besides promptly initiating appropriate antimicrobial therapy directed at *C difficile*, use of unnecessary other antibiotics and acid-suppression medications (eg, proton pump inhibitors, histamine blockers) should be discontinued, and antiperistaltic agents should be avoided. Test of cure following treatment is not recommended.

KEY FACT

✓ Therapy for *C difficile* infection depends on illness severity and whether the infection is the first episode or recurrent disease

---

Box 46.1 • Indications for Hospitalization in *Clostridium difficile* Infection[a]

Patient has an unstable condition and presents with the following:

> Intractable vomiting
> Dehydration
> Hypotension
> Sepsis
> Severe abdominal pain
> Bowel perforation or megacolon[b]

[a] Use clinical judgment when determining whether a patient's condition is unstable and whether the patient needs hospitalization. Patient should be kept in contact isolation during the hospital stay.

[b] Megacolon or bowel perforation can complicate *C difficile* infection. If a patient has abdominal distention with continued abdominal pain despite resolution of or decrease in diarrhea, a diagnosis of toxic megacolon with or without perforation should be suspected. Plain abdominal radiographs should be obtained.

Relapse is frequent (>15% of cases) and necessitates re-treatment. Recurrent *C difficile* infection is defined as symptom recurrence **and** a positive stool test for *C difficile* present within 56 days of prior infection after symptom resolution. Reinfection is defined as symptom recurrence with a positive stool test for *C difficile* beyond 56 days of prior infection after symptom resolution. Patients with recurrent infection should be treated in accordance with guidelines outlined for recurrent infection; patients with reinfection may be treated as de novo infection (Table 46.6).

Currently, the use of probiotics in patients with *C difficile* infection is not recommended because of insufficient evidence of efficacy and the possibility of potential harm in immunocompromised patients. In addition, no evidence shows that adding cholestyramine to the treatment regimen decreases the risk of recurrence. Moreover, cholestyramine binds to vancomycin and is contraindicated.

Total colectomy may be lifesaving in severe cases. Indications for surgical consultation include hypotension requiring vasopressor therapy, clinical signs of sepsis and organ dysfunction (renal and pulmonary), mental status changes, certain laboratory results (WBC count ≥50,000 cells/mcL and lactate ≥5 mmol/L), and failure to improve from medical therapy after 5 days.

Fecal microbiota transplant may be helpful for patients who have refractory or symptomatically recurrent *C difficile* infection despite treatment with conventional antibiotic therapies. The transplantation involves infusion of processed fecal material from a screened, approved donor to replenish the normal bacterial flora of a patient's colon. Although not approved by the US Food and Drug Administration, this procedure has been highly effective in patients with refractory and recurrent *C difficile* infection. Indications for a fecal microbiota transplant are listed in Box 46.2.

Table 46.6 • Treatment of *Clostridium difficile* Infection

Severity	First Episode or First Recurrence	Second (or Subsequent) Recurrence
Mild or moderate Diarrhea with no additional signs or symptoms of severe or severe-complicated infection	**Metronidazole** 500 mg orally every 8 h for 10 d (consider change to vancomycin if no response after 5–7 d; for patients who do not tolerate or are allergic to metronidazole and for pregnant or breastfeeding women, vancomycin should be used at standard dosing)	**Vancomycin** 125 mg 4 times daily for 14 d; then 125 mg 2 times daily for 7 d; then 125 mg once daily for 7 d; then 125 mg once every other d for 8 d; then 125 mg once every 3 d for 15 d
Severe (WBC count ≥15,000/mm³, creatinine ≥1.5 × baseline, or albumin <3 g/dL)	**Vancomycin** 125 mg oral or NG tube every 6 h for 10 d	**Vancomycin** 125 mg 4 times daily for 14 d; then 125 mg 2 times daily for 7 d; then 125 mg daily for 7 d; then 125 mg once every other d for 8 d; then 125 mg once every 3 d for 15 d
Severe-Complicated[a] Any of the following attributable to *Clostridium difficile* infection: admission to ICU, hypotension, ileus or significant abdominal distention, WBC count ≥35,000/mm³ or <2,000/mm³, serum lactate levels >2.2 mmol/L, end-organ failure (eg, mechanical ventilation, renal failure; includes shock and megacolon)	**Vancomycin**[b] 500 mg oral or via NG tube every 6 h for 14 d *And* **Metronidazole** 500 mg IV every 8 h for 14 d	**Vancomycin** 500 mg oral or via NG tube every 6 h for 14 d *And* **Metronidazole** 500 mg IV every 8 h for 14 d *Then* **Vancomycin** 125 mg 4 times daily for 14 d; then 125 mg 2 times daily for 7 d; then 125 mg daily for 7 d; then 125 mg once every other d for 8 d; then 125 mg once every 3 d for 15 d

Abbreviations: ICU, intensive care unit; IV, intravenously; NG, nasogastric; WBC, white blood cells.

[a] On significant clinical improvement (eg, decrease in diarrhea, improvement of vital signs, resolution of sepsis or megacolon), IV metronidazole therapy can be discontinued and treatment should be continued with oral vancomycin and a decrease in dose from 500 mg to 125 mg.

[b] If patient has ileus, vancomycin retention enemas can be considered, but they come with a risk of rectum or colon perforation. Clinician should obtain gastroenterology consult.

KEY FACT

✓ Fecal microbiota transplant may be helpful for refractory or symptomatically recurrent *C difficile* infection, despite treatment with conventional antibiotic therapies

---

Box 46.2 • Indications for Fecal Microbiota Transplant

≥3 episodes of *Clostridium difficile* infection

Previous treatment with first-line therapies for *C difficile* infection (vancomycin, metronidazole, or fidaxomicin)

Previous treatment of ≥1 courses of a 6- to 8-week vancomycin treatment taper or vancomycin treatment followed by rifaximin for 2 weeks

Refractory moderate to severe *C difficile* diarrhea that fails vancomycin therapy after >1 week

---

Viral Diarrhea

Many types of viral diarrhea can be defined by their seasonal epidemiologic factors. Rotavirus infection is the most common cause of sporadic mild diarrhea in children. It may be spread from children to adults. It usually occurs during the winter. Vomiting is a more common early manifestation than watery diarrhea. Hospitalization for dehydration is often needed for young children. Diagnosis is made with detection of antigen in stool. Treatment is symptomatic.

Noroviruses are a common cause of epidemic diarrhea and so-called winter vomiting disease in older children and adults. These viruses have high secondary attack rates. Outbreaks have been reported from day-care facilities, nursing homes, hospitals, family gatherings, and cruise ships. Various contaminated foods and liquids, such as shellfish, undercooked fish, cake frosting, salads, and water, have been implicated. The condition is explosive and self-limited (36 hours) with severe nausea, vomiting, watery diarrhea, and dehydration. Treatment is symptomatic.

Parasitic Diarrhea

The histories of travel and exposure are critical to identifying causative pathogens in parasitic diarrhea. The parasitic conditions most common in the United States are giardiasis, amebiasis, and cryptosporidiosis.

Giardiasis may present with abdominal bloating, weight loss, and flatulence. Hosts at risk are men who have sex with men, hikers with exposures to fresh water streams, day-care contacts, and persons with immunoglobulin A deficiency or HIV infection. A wet-preparation examination of stool or a *Giardia* antigen test can establish the diagnosis. Treatment is with metronidazole or tinidazole.

KEY FACT

✓ Giardiasis may present with abdominal bloating, weight loss, and flatulence. Hosts at risk for giardiasis are men who have sex with men, hikers with exposures to fresh water streams, day-care contacts, and persons with immunoglobulin A deficiency or HIV infection

---

Entamoeba histolytica infection is acquired through ingestion of *E histolytica* cysts in contaminated water or food. Amebiasis is more common in immigrants from regions with high endemic rates of the disease, such as Central America and South America. Infected patients may present with a subacute onset of colitis or liver abscess. Diagnosis is made by stool testing for ova or by serum antibody tests. Treatment is with metronidazole (750 mg 3 times daily for 7 to 10 days). After treatment, the intestinal carrier state is eradicated with paromomycin or iodoquinol.

Cryptosporidium parvum is an important cause of diarrhea, especially in persons with AIDS, who may have a chronic, debilitating illness. Cryptosporidiosis is also a cause of self-limited diarrhea in otherwise healthy persons. Waterborne outbreaks have been reported in Georgia and Wisconsin. They occur most often in late summer and fall. The organism is resistant to chlorination and can best be eliminated from water sources by microfiltration. Among patients, 35% have a coinfection, most commonly with *Giardia*. The stool *Cryptosporidium* antigen test, based on enzyme-linked immunosorbent assay, has a sensitivity of 87%, a specificity of 99%, and a positive predictive value of 98%. No effective therapy is available for treating *Cryptosporidium*. Nitazoxanide is the drug of choice for therapy.

Cyclospora cayetanensis is a protozoan that can cause persistent diarrhea, fever, and profound fatigue. It has been linked to consumption of contaminated food shipped to the United States (eg, raspberries from Guatemala). Like *Cryptosporidium*, the organism may not be detected on routine stool examinations; therefore, tests specific to the organism should be ordered. Trimethoprim-sulfamethoxazole is the preferred drug for treatment. Ciprofloxacin is an alternative treatment for patients with sulfa allergy.

Intra-abdominal Abscesses

Hepatic abscesses can be bacterial (more frequently) or nonbacterial in origin. Common nonbacterial causes include *Candida* and *E histolytica* (amebic abscess). Bacterial hepatic abscesses can be a result of portal vein bacteremia from an enteric source (such as appendicitis or diverticulitis), a biliary source, or a nonabdominal source. Fever, malaise, and abdominal pain are the usual symptoms. Computed tomography is the preferred imaging method. Causative pathogens include enteric gram-negative rods (such as Enterobacteriaceae) and anaerobes (such as *Bacteroides*). Blood cultures and amebic serologic tests are recommended for the patient's work-up. If the amebic serologic results are negative, aspiration (diagnostic and therapeutic) and culture are recommended. Therapy should be guided by culture results.

Splenic abscesses are frequently due to hematogenous seeding (eg, from endocarditis). Unexplained thrombocytosis in the clinical setting of fever should raise the concern for splenic abscess. Small abscesses (<3 cm) can be managed with percutaneous drainage and directed antimicrobial therapy. Large abscesses usually require splenectomy.

Psoas abscesses arise with the contiguous spread from perivertebral, genitourinary, or gastrointestinal foci. Hematogenous seeding occurs with *S aureus* bacteremia. The psoas muscle is also a site of tuberculous abscesses.

Pancreatic abscesses usually occur in cases of infected pancreatic necrosis. The abscesses are often polymicrobial and reflect the biliary and intestinal flora. Treatment is endoscopic or percutaneous drainage and culture-directed antimicrobial therapy.

47 Skin, Soft Tissue, Bone, and Joint Infections

ELIE F. BERBARI, MD

Skin and Soft Tissue Infections

Specific skin and soft tissue infections can be characterized by their visual appearance, including vesicles, bullae, folliculitis, crusted lesions, papular lesions, ulcerations, and cellulitis.

Nonpurulent cellulitis is an acute, spreading infection of the dermis and subcutaneous tissue. Cellulitis (Figure 47.1) is most common in tissue damaged by trauma and in extremities with impaired venous or lymphatic drainage (eg, the arm after mastectomy, the leg after saphenous vein harvest for coronary artery bypass grafting). Minor inflammation or disruption of skin integrity from tinea pedis may serve as a portal of entry for β-hemolytic streptococci (Figure 47.2). The involved area—usually on the lower extremity—is tender, warm, erythematous, and swollen. It lacks sharp demarcation from uninvolved skin. Cellulitis may recur in patients with a history of dermatitis or malignancy or a prior history of ipsilateral limb cellulitis. Severe infection with

Key Definition

Nonpurulent cellulitis: *Acute, spreading infection of the dermis and subcutaneous tissue.*

KEY FACTS

✓ Cellulitis is most common in tissue damaged by trauma and in extremities with diminished venous or lymphatic drainage

✓ In cellulitis, minor inflammation or disruption in skin integrity from tinea pedis may serve as an entry portal for β-hemolytic streptococci

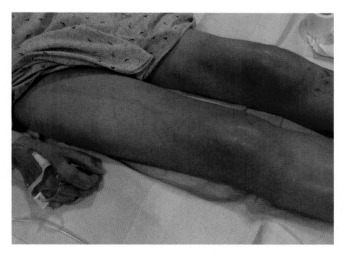

Figure 47.1 *Cellulitis With Lymphangitic Streaking due to* Yokenella regensburgei.

(Adapted from Bhowmick T, Weinstein MP. A deceptive case of cellulitis caused by a Gram-negative pathogen. J Clin Microbiol. 2013 Apr;51[4]:1320–3. Epub 2013 Jan 30. Used with permission.)

group A streptococci can complicate dermatomal varicella zoster virus infection.

Acute purulent cellulitis is often due to community-acquired methicillin-resistant *Staphylococcus aureus* (CA-MRSA) infection. Other organisms, such as methicillin-sensitive *S aureus* (MSSA) or β-hemolytic streptococci, may also have a role. CA-MRSA cellulitis should be suspected in patients 1) with recurrent furunculosis, 2) with cellulitis who have a prior personal history of or a family member or close contact with CA-MRSA, and 3) who do not respond to antimicrobial coverage for MSSA and streptococci. Options for treatment in these cases include trimethoprim-sulfamethoxazole, clindamycin, or doxycycline with or

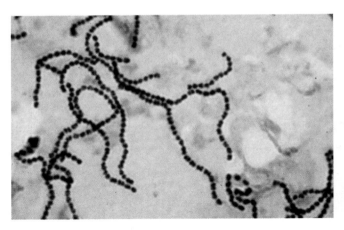

Figure 47.2 Chaining of β-Hemolytic Streptococcus in a Blood Culture (Gram Stain).

without rifampin. Use of vancomycin, daptomycin, or linezolid should be strongly considered for patients who do not respond to initial therapy with a β-lactam, who have serious illness at initial presentation, and in whom multidrug-resistant *S aureus* is suspected.

KEY FACT

✓ Acute purulent cellulitis is often the result of community-acquired methicillin-resistant *Staphylococcus aureus*. Other organisms, such as methicillin-sensitive *S aureus* or β-hemolytic streptococci, may also be causes

The approach to treatment of cellulitis is guided by the type of skin and soft tissue infection and the severity of clinical presentation. Empirical antibiotic therapy should include MRSA coverage when MRSA is suspected on the basis of local epidemiologic factors. When a patient presents with a purulent lesion, it should be drained and sent for Gram stain and bacterial culture, to exclude CA-MRSA.

Importantly, clinicians should exclude animal or human bites, hot-tub folliculitis, necrotizing fasciitis, fish tank or water exposures, and mixed infections in patients with diabetes mellitus. In most cases, cellulitis is due to β-hemolytic streptococci. A first-generation oral or parenteral cephalosporin (ie, cephalexin or cefazolin) is the usual initial choice when MRSA is not suspected.

KEY FACT

✓ Exclusion of animal or human bites, hot-tub folliculitis, necrotizing fasciitis, fish tank or water exposures, and mixed infections is important

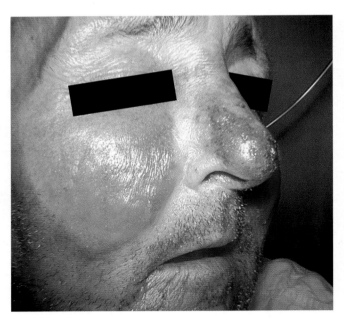

Figure 47.3 Erysipelas.
(Adapted from Centers for Disease Control and Prevention. Facial erysipelas manifested as severe malar and nasal erythema and swelling [Internet]. Atlanta [GA]: Centers for Disease Control and Prevention; c1963 CDC/Thomas F. Sellers. Available from: http://phil.cdc.gov/phil/details.asp?pid=2874.)

Erysipelas (Figure 47.3) is a superficial cellulitis with prominent lymphatic involvement, presenting with an indurated peau d'orange appearance that has a raised border well demarcated from normal skin. This infection is painful and most often occurs in elderly persons. Recent reports have associated erysipelas with "toxic strep syndrome."

Key Definition

Erysipelas: *Superficial cellulitis with lymphatic involvement, with peau d'orange appearance and a raised border.*

KEY FACT

✓ A superficial cellulitis, erysipelas has prominent lymphatic involvement and presents with an indurated peau d'orange and a raised border well demarcated from healthy skin

The term *impetigo* describes a superficial skin infection. Historically, *Streptococcus pyogenes* was the most common cause of impetigo. Since the 1980s, however, most cases of impetigo have been caused by *S aureus* or mixed infections with *S aureus* and β-hemolytic streptococci.

Unusual causes of soft tissue infection are *Eikenella corrodens* and oral anaerobes after human bites (eg, knuckles cellulitis after a fist fight), *Pasteurella multocida* after cat or dog bites, *Capnocytophaga canimorsus* after dog bites, *Aeromonas hydrophila* after freshwater exposure or exposure to leeches, *Vibrio vulnificus* after salt water exposure, *Erysipelothrix rhusiopathiae* and *Streptococcus iniae* after fish exposure, and *Pseudomonas aeruginosa* after hot-tub exposure.

Several severe complications can occur with soft tissue infections. They include necrotizing fasciitis (usually due to a polymicrobial infection or a toxin-producing group A *Streptococcus*) and pyomyositis (usually due to *S aureus*). Necrotizing infections are best managed with surgery and directed antimicrobial therapy, including a protein synthesis inhibitor such as clindamycin and a β-lactam antibiotic for invasive group A streptococcal syndromes (Figure 47.2).

KEY FACT

✓ A complication of soft tissue infections is necrotizing fasciitis, usually caused by a polymicrobial infection or toxin-producing group A *Streptococcus*

The mortality rate associated with streptococcal necrotizing fasciitis is 30%, even in previously healthy patients and with appropriate treatment. Most patients require débridement or amputation of affected tissues. Effective treatment requires early recognition of the illness, with prompt initiation of antibiotic treatment and early and aggressive surgical débridement of devitalized tissue when indicated.

KEY FACTS

✓ Streptococcal necrotizing fasciitis has a mortality rate of 30%, even in previously healthy patients and with appropriate treatment

✓ Most patients with streptococcal necrotizing fasciitis require débridement or amputation of affected tissues

Unlike many other pathogens, group A streptococci continue to be susceptible to the penicillins. First-generation cephalosporins and vancomycin are effective alternative drugs. Erythromycin-resistant strains have been reported,

KEY FACT

✓ Growing evidence indicates that clindamycin and penicillin in combination are the most effective antibiotic treatment of streptococcal necrotizing fasciitis

but so far they are uncommon in the United States. Mounting evidence indicates that clindamycin in combination with penicillin is the most effective antibiotic for treating streptococcal necrotizing fasciitis.

Toxic Shock Syndrome

Group A streptococci produce many disease-causing exotoxins. Scarlet fever may develop in persons with no previous immunity to erythrogenic toxin. Production of hyaluronidase causes the rapidly advancing margins characteristic of cellulitis due to β-hemolytic streptococci. Streptococcal exotoxin A has similarities with the toxin produced by *S aureus*, which causes toxic shock syndrome.

Streptococcal toxic shock syndrome is similar to staphylococcal toxic shock syndrome (see below). Patients with invasive group A streptococcal infection have associated hypotension and 2 of the following: renal impairment, coagulopathy, liver impairment, adult respiratory distress syndrome, rash (which may desquamate), or soft tissue necrosis. Symptoms are caused by production of streptococcal toxin (pyrogenic exotoxin A). Most patients have skin or soft tissue infection, are younger than 50 years, and are otherwise healthy. These characteristics compare with those of patients who have invasive group A streptococcal infections without the streptococcal toxic shock syndrome. This latter patient group may present with only severe limb pain and no skin lesions. Most patients have bacteremia (in contrast to toxic shock syndrome due to *S aureus*).

Treatment of streptococcal toxic shock syndrome includes early administration of antibiotics, supportive care, and surgical débridement as needed. The case fatality rate is 30%. Although no reported resistance to penicillin has been reported, clindamycin plus high-dose penicillin G is the preferred regimen because clindamycin may suppress exotoxin and M-protein production, in addition to its activity against group A streptococci. In severe cases, consideration should be given to the use of early intravenous immunoglobulin therapy.

Staphylococcal toxic shock syndrome is caused by the establishment or growth of a toxin-producing strain of *S aureus* in a nonimmune person. Clinical scenarios associated with this syndrome include prolonged, continuous use of tampons in young menstruating women, postoperative and nonoperative wound infections, localized abscesses, and *S aureus* pneumonia developing after influenza. Staphylococcal toxic shock syndrome is a multisystem disease. Clinical criteria include fever, hypotension, erythroderma (often leads to desquamation, particularly on palms and soles), and involvement of 3 or more organ systems. Onset is acute; blood culture results are usually negative. The condition is caused by production of staphylococcal toxin (toxic shock syndrome toxin 1). Treatment is supportive; subsequent episodes are treated with a β-lactam antibiotic, which decreases the frequency and severity of subsequent attacks. The relapse rate may be as high as 40% (in menstruation-related disease). The mortality rate is 5% to 10%.

Infections due to Other, Unusual Organisms

Pasteurella multocida

Pasteurella multocida is a common cause of acute cutaneous infection after a cat or dog bite. Soft tissue infection after a dog or cat bite should be treated with amoxicillin-clavulanate or a combination of fluoroquinolone and clindamycin, to cover the pathogens in the oral flora of the biting animal and the skin flora of the infected person.

Capnocytophaga canimorsus (Formerly Called DF-2)

This organism may cause rapidly progressive soft tissue infection, bacteremia, and fulminant sepsis in asplenic persons who are bitten by domestic animals, such as dogs. Treatment of *Capnocytophaga canimorsus* infection is with penicillins or cephalosporins.

Vibrio vulnificus

Vibrio vulnificus can cause a severe bullous soft tissue infection in persons with underlying cirrhosis or hemochromatosis. Disease is usually acquired by the ingestion of raw oysters or through injury sustained in warm salt water. Chronic liver disease predisposes to the infection. After the abrupt onset of fever and hypotension, multiple hemorrhagic bullae develop. Clinical syndromes associated with *V vulnificus* include bloodstream infection, gastroenteritis, and cellulitis. Even with prompt therapy, the mortality rate exceeds 30%. Blood stream infection or cellulitis is treated with tetracycline, cefotaxime, or ciprofloxacin. *Vibrio vulnificus* is not uniformly susceptible to aminoglycosides.

KEY FACTS

✓ *Vibrio vulnificus* can cause a severe, bullous soft tissue infection in persons with underlying cirrhosis or hemochromatosis

✓ *Vibrio vulnificus* disease is acquired usually through ingestion of raw oysters or through injury obtained in warm salt water

---

Bone and Joint Infections

Acute Bacterial Arthritis (Nongonococcal)

Acute bacterial arthritis is most commonly due to hematogenous seeding of the joint and most commonly occurs in persons with underlying crystalline or rheumatoid arthritis, injection drug users, and patients undergoing hemodialysis. The hip and knee joints are the 2 most commonly involved joints. These infections are often caused by *S aureus* (most frequent cause) and β-hemolytic streptococci. *Salmonella* septic arthritis is proportionally more common in persons with sickle cell disease. Septic arthritis due to gram-negative aerobic bacilli causes 20% of septic arthritis cases and is more common in elderly persons. By comparison, *P aeruginosa* infection is associated with injection drug use.

KEY FACTS

✓ Acute bacterial arthritis most commonly results from hematogenous seeding of the joint (ie, through injection drug use and hemodialysis) and most commonly occurs in persons with underlying crystalline or rheumatoid arthritis

✓ Hip and knee joints are the joints most commonly involved in acute bacterial arthritis

✓ These infections are commonly caused by *S aureus* (most often) and β-hemolytic streptococci

✓ Persons with sickle cell disease may have *Salmonella* septic arthritis

✓ Septic arthritis due to gram-negative aerobic bacilli causes 20% of cases and is more common in elderly persons

---

Clinical features of acute bacterial arthritis include fever, joint pain, and swelling. All suspected septic joints should undergo a diagnostic aspiration. Infected synovial fluid is usually turbid, and the leukocyte count generally exceeds 40×10^9/L (>75% polymorphonuclear neutrophils). This condition may overlap and be confused with other inflammatory arthropathies. Gram stain shows positivity in 50% of cases; joint culture results are typically positive. Radiographs are not helpful in early cases because destructive changes may take up to 2 weeks to occur. The duration of antimicrobial therapy is 2 to 4 weeks. Empirical therapy should include agents directed against *S aureus* and aerobic gram-negative bacilli. Percutaneous, arthroscopic, or open surgical débridement is an essential part of therapy. Hip,

---

KEY FACTS

✓ A diagnostic aspiration should be performed of all septic joints in which acute bacterial arthritis is suspected

✓ The duration of antimicrobial therapy is 2 to 4 weeks for acute bacterial arthritis

✓ Empirical therapy for acute bacterial arthritis should include agents directed against *S aureus* and aerobic gram-negative bacilli

✓ Percutaneous, arthroscopic, or open surgical débridement are an essential part of therapy for acute bacterial arthritis

shoulder, and sternoclavicular joint involvement, development of loculations, and persistently positive blood or joint culture are indications for arthroscopy or open surgical débridement.

Viral Arthritis

Viral arthritis often presents as transient, self-limited polyarthritis. It may be caused by rubella, hepatitis B, mumps, coxsackievirus, adenovirus, parvovirus B19, human immunodeficiency virus, Ross River virus, and chikungunya virus infections in travelers. Parvovirus can cause a chronic symmetrical, small-joint arthritis that mimics rheumatoid arthritis, especially in women.

> **KEY FACT**
>
> ✓ Parvovirus can cause a chronic symmetrical, small-joint arthritis that mimics rheumatoid arthritis, especially in women

Chronic Monoarticular Arthritis

Tuberculosis, nontuberculous mycobacteria, and fungi should be considered in patients presenting with insidious-onset arthritis and chronic arthritis. Exposure to fish tank or brackish water should raise the possibility of *Mycobacterium marinum* septic arthritis, which typically involves the small hand joints. A history of travel to the southwestern United States or being a gardener should raise the possibility of *Coccidioides immitis* and *Sporothrix schenckii*, respectively. In patients with chronic monoarticular arthritis of the knee and a history of tick exposure, positive Lyme serology, or erythema migrans, clinicians should consider a diagnosis of chronic Lyme arthritis.

Osteomyelitis

Osteomyelitis can be a result of hematogenous seeding, contiguous spread of infection to bone from adjacent soft tissues and joints, or direct inoculation of infection into the bone due to trauma or a surgical procedure. Hematogenous osteomyelitis is usually monomicrobial, whereas osteomyelitis due to contiguous spread or direct inoculation is usually polymicrobial. Acute hematogenous osteomyelitis is more common in children, but it can occur in adults who have prolonged bloodstream infection, intravenous drug use, dialysis, and sickle cell disease. *Staphylococcus aureus*, coagulase-negative staphylococci, and aerobic gram-negative bacilli are the most common organisms in osteomyelitis. In long bone involvement, the acute onset of pain and fever is typical. In vertebral infection, pain may be the sole characteristic. To establish the diagnosis, clinicians may use compatible imaging changes and image-guided bone biopsy for culture and pathologic examination. Results of blood culture may be positive for a microbial cause. Specific parenteral antibiotic therapy is used for 4 to 6 weeks on the basis of culture and sensitivity test results. Surgical débridement in acute hematogenous osteomyelitis is often not necessary unless a sequestrum is present or in cases of neurologic compromise.

Chronic, contiguous osteomyelitis more commonly occurs in adults, particularly when wounds, vascular insufficiency, and diabetic foot ulcers are present. The infections are usually mixed, but *S aureus* is the single most commonly isolated organism. In the presence of foreign bodies (such as plate, screws, or prosthetic joint), coagulase-negative staphylococci is often the culprit. Local pain, tenderness, erythema, and draining sinuses are common. Fever is atypical unless concurrent cellulitis is present. Compatible radiographic changes (often vague) and bone biopsy for culture and pathologic examination are used to establish the diagnosis. Blood culture results are rarely positive. Adequate débridement, removal of dead space and foreign bodies, soft tissue coverage, and fixation of infected fractures are essential. Specific parenteral antibiotic therapy is given for 4 to 6 weeks. If a foreign body is retained in patients with staphylococcal osteomyelitis, a rifampin-based therapy such as the combination of fluoroquinolones and rifampin is warranted.

> **KEY FACTS**
>
> ✓ Chronic, contiguous osteomyelitis occurs more commonly in adults than children, particularly when adults have traumatic wounds, vascular insufficiency, and diabetic foot ulcers
>
> ✓ Osteomyelitis infections are usually mixed, but *S aureus* is the single most commonly isolated organism
>
> ✓ When a patient with osteomyelitis has an imbedded foreign body (eg, bone plate, screws, prosthetic joint), coagulase-negative staphylococci are often the culprit bacteria

Diskitis and Vertebral Infections

Infection of the intervertebral disk and the adjacent vertebrae may occur with or without associated epidural or psoas abscesses. These infections most often arise from hematogenous dissemination of infection from the skin and soft tissues, genitourinary tract, infective endocarditis, infected intravenous sites, injection drug use, or respiratory tract infection. The incidence is greatest among male patients, peaks in the fifth decade of life, and is increasing, particularly among the elderly population. Additional risk factors for spine infections include immunocompromise, diabetes mellitus, intravenous drug use, renal failure, bacteremia, malignancy, long-term corticosteroid use, intravascular devices, and recent instrumentation or spine surgery.

The clinical presentation of vertebral osteomyelitis includes localized insidious pain and tenderness in the spine area in 90% of cases. Most commonly affected is the lumbar or lumbosacral region; cervical disease may occur in patients with head and neck infections or in injection drug users. Fever is present in less than one-half of cases. Because of the clinical uncertainty, a delay in diagnosis of weeks to months often occurs, which can lead to motor and sensory deficits in 15% of patients. The erythrocyte sedimentation rate is increased in more than 90% of cases, and the leukocyte count is increased in less than 50%.

KEY FACT

✓ Clinical presentation of vertebral osteomyelitis includes localized insidious pain and tenderness in the spine area

---

Plain radiography may show vertebral end-plate irregularity at 2 to 8 weeks after the onset of symptoms, but it is neither sensitive nor specific. Gadolinium-enhanced magnetic resonance imaging is the most useful test for diagnosis because of its high sensitivity (96%) and high specificity (94%) (Figure 47.4). In patients who cannot undergo magnetic resonance imaging, computed tomography or nuclear scanning may help establish the diagnosis. The best nuclear study for imaging disk space infections is scanning with technetium combined with gallium citrate. Computed tomography–guided percutaneous aspiration or biopsy is often used to identify the causative organism. If the initial result is negative, the test should be repeated before proceeding to an open biopsy procedure.

KEY FACT

✓ Gadolinium-enhanced magnetic resonance imaging is the most useful test for diagnosis because it provides high sensitivity (96%) and high specificity (94%)

Staphylococcus aureus and coagulase-negative staphylococci are the most common microorganisms cultured in vertebral osteomyelitis. *Mycobacterium tuberculosis* and *Brucella* are common in endemic regions. Most patients can be treated conservatively with antimicrobials. Antibiotics

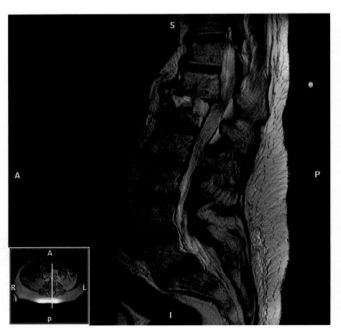

Figure 47.4 *Magnetic Resonance Imaging of the Spine Showing T2 Images of a T12-L1 Disk Space Infection and Associated Contiguous Vertebral Body Involvement. Of note, image shows complete destruction of vertebral end plates. A indicates anterior; I, inferior; L, left; P, posterior; R, right; S, superior.*

should be given parenterally for a minimum of 4 to 6 weeks or given longer when the patient has extensive vertebral destruction or undrained infected collections. Surgical interventions are limited to cases with progressive neurologic deterioration, spinal instability, progressive epidural abscess, or failed medical therapy.

KEY FACTS

✓ *Staphylococcus aureus* and coagulase-negative staphylococci are the microorganisms most commonly cultured in vertebral osteomyelitis

✓ The treatment of most patients with vertebral osteomyelitis can be managed conservatively with antimicrobials given parenterally for a minimum of 4 weeks

✓ Surgical interventions are limited to cases with progressive neurologic deterioration, spinal instability, progressive epidural abscess, or unsuccessful medical treatment

Questions and Answers

Questions

Multiple Choice (choose the best answer)

VII.1. An 87-year-old man presents with pelvic pain and dysuria. He has had 3 urinary tract infections in the past 6 months. A urologic evaluation last month showed an enlarged prostate but normal urodynamics. Urinalysis results are the following: 10 to 20 leukocytes per high-power field, a positive leukocyte esterase test, a negative nitrite test, and numerous gram-negative rods. Which of the following is the best choice for treatment of his symptoms?
a. Nitrofurantoin 100 mg daily for 7 days
b. Amoxicillin 500 mg 3 times daily for 7 days
c. Ciprofloxacin 500 mg twice daily for 28 days
d. Trimethoprim-sulfamethoxazole 1 tablet twice daily for 14 days
e. Levofloxacin 500 mg once daily for 14 days

VII.2. A 51-year-old diabetic woman from India has had unrelenting fever and night sweats for 2 weeks. Blood cultures have been negative, and an abdominal computed tomographic scan shows a 3×6-cm hypodense lesion in the left lobe of her liver. Which of the following should be done next for this patient?
a. Ultrasound-guided needle aspiration
b. Serology test on blood
c. Stool test for ova and parasites
d. Piperacillin-tazobactam 3.375 g intravenously every 6 hours
e. Purified protein derivative (PPD) skin test

VII.3. A 43-year-old morbidly obese diabetic woman, recently treated for abdominal wall cellulitis, now presents with a 3-day history of fever, right flank pain, and dysuria. A urinalysis is esterase positive and a Gram stain shows gram-negative bacilli too numerous to count. Which of the following treatments should you recommend for management of her urinary tract infection?
a. Ceftriaxone 1 g intravenously (IV) daily for 10 days
b. Ampicillin 2 g IV every 6 hours for 10 days
c. Ciprofloxacin 500 mg orally twice daily for 7 days
d. Trimethoprim-sulfamethoxazole (TMP-SMX) 160–480 mg orally twice daily for 7 days
e. Nitrofurantoin 100 mg orally twice daily for 10 days

VII.4. A 67-year-old man with uncomplicated type 2 diabetes mellitus and hypertension presents to his primary care physician with a 3-day history of fever, productive cough, and shortness of breath. He has been in good health otherwise, has never been hospitalized, and has good social support at home. Examination findings include the following: temperature 39.1°C, blood pressure 110/75 mm Hg, heart rate 78 beats per minute with regular rate and rhythm, and respiratory rate 26 breaths per minute. Oxygen saturation is 94% with room air. He is awake and alert and oriented to person, place, and time; he responds to questions appropriately. Inspiratory crackles are audible in the right lower lung field, his abdomen has active bowel sounds and is not tender, and his extremities have no clubbing or cyanosis. Which of the following should be done next?
a. Outpatient observation only with follow-up in 2 days
b. Outpatient consultation with an infectious disease specialist
c. Hospital admission and treatment with levofloxacin
d. Intensive care unit admission and treatment with levofloxacin
e. Outpatient treatment with levofloxacin

VII.5. A 57-year-old woman is admitted to an internal medicine hospital ward with a 3-day history of fever, cough, progressively purulent sputum, and shortness of breath. She has been well otherwise, has never been hospitalized, and has a past medical history of well-controlled type 2 diabetes mellitus and hypertension. She has not had any recent antimicrobial exposure, foreign travel, or animal exposure. She has no known drug allergies. Examination findings include the following: temperature 38.7°C, blood pressure 125/75 mm Hg, heart rate 78 beats per minute with regular rate and rhythm, and respiratory rate 26 breaths per minute. Oxygen saturation is 95% with 2 L of oxygen per minute by nasal cannula. She is awake and alert and oriented to person, place, and time. Inspiratory crackles are audible in the left upper lung field, her abdomen has active bowel sounds and is not tender, and her extremities have no clubbing or cyanosis. The total leukocyte count is 14.4×10⁹/L. Results of serum chemistry tests are normal. The chest radiograph shows a new dense consolidation in the left upper lung field. Which of the following antimicrobial regimens would you initiate?
a. Azithromycin orally
b. Ceftriaxone intravenously (IV) and azithromycin orally
c. Ciprofloxacin IV
d. Ampicillin IV and clindamycin orally
e. Meropenem IV

VII.6. A previously healthy 32-year-old man presents to his primary care physician after his cat bit his arm earlier in the morning. The cat's vaccinations are current, and the cat has not been attacked by other animals. The patient says that the bite was deep enough to draw blood, although the bleeding has stopped. You cleanse the wound, apply a bandage, and update his tetanus-diphtheria vaccination. Examination findings include the following: temperature 37.2°C, blood pressure 125/80 mm Hg, heart rate 72 beats per minute, and respiratory rate 16 breaths per minute. A 1.5-cm laceration is evident on the dorsal aspect of the left forearm without any erythema or purulence. Which of the following antimicrobial regimens should be prescribed?
a. Amoxicillin-clavulanic acid
b. Dicloxacillin

c. Cephalexin
   d. Clindamycin
   e. No antimicrobials

VII.7. A 45-year-old woman presents for evaluation of fever, arthralgias, and a truncal rash. She has a history of steroid-dependent asthma and nasal polyps diagnosed 5 years previously. One month ago, she began using a steroid inhaler and was weaned from oral corticosteroids. On physical examination, her blood pressure is 138/84 mm Hg, her pulse rate is 92 beats per minute, and her respirations are 20 per minute. Physical examination of the nose shows nasal mucosal crusting and bilateral nasal polyps. Scattered wheezes are heard on auscultation of the chest. The leukocyte count is 11×10^9/L (70% neutrophils, 8% lymphocytes, 18% eosinophils, and 5% monocytes), and the serum creatinine level is 1.1 mg/dL. Chest radiography shows bilateral upper lobe infiltrates. Which of the following diagnoses is most likely?
   a. Behçet disease
   b. Granulomatosis with polyangiitis (Wegener)
   c. Churg-Strauss syndrome
   d. Giant cell arteritis
   e. Allergic bronchopulmonary aspergillosis

VII.8. Influenza B is diagnosed in a 67-year-old man who has underlying asthma. Which is the most appropriate treatment for this patient?
   a. Oseltamivir
   b. Amantadine
   c. Zanamivir
   d. Rimantadine
   e. Ribavirin

VII.9. A 31-year-old man underwent septoplasty for a deviated nasal septum and recurrent sinusitis. He presents to the emergency department 48 hours later with headache, fever, chills, myalgia, nausea, vomiting, and abdominal cramping. His temperature is 39.9°C, his pulse is 142 beats per minute, his respiratory rate is 28 breaths per minute, and his blood pressure is 74/30 mm Hg. He has generalized erythroderma. On head and neck examination, the nasal passages are hyperemic but not purulent. Laboratory test results included the following: leukocyte count 14.7×10^9/L, hemoglobin 15.0 g/dL, and platelet count 84×10^9/L. The results of liver function tests, serum creatinine, and amylase were within the reference ranges. Which pathogen is most likely to cause this syndrome?
   a. *Pseudomonas aeruginosa*
   b. *Haemophilus influenzae*
   c. *Moraxella catarrhalis*
   d. *Streptococcus pneumoniae*
   e. *Staphylococcus aureus*

VII.10. A 45-year-old man with diabetes mellitus and severe peripheral vascular disease presents with a 6-week history of erythema and induration surrounding a 3-cm plantar ulcer. Today he is nauseated, febrile, and tachycardic. You can insert a metallic probe through the open wound to the bone surface. There is surrounding redness and drainage of foul-smelling pus. Which of the following would be the next appropriate step in management?
   a. Swab the patient's nose for methicillin-resistant *Staphylococcus aureus* (MRSA).
   b. Perform magnetic resonance imaging (MRI) of the foot.
   c. Treat with parenteral vancomycin and piperacillin-tazobactam.
   d. Perform bone scintigraphy.
   e. Perform plain radiography of the foot.

Answers

VII.1. Answer c.

This elderly man has had recurrent episodes of urinary tract infection. In the absence of a neurogenic bladder or other secondary cause, this almost always reflects an infected prostate. The diagnosis of chronic prostatitis is a clinical one, based on symptoms and signs of recurrent urinary tract infection as seen in this patient. Antibiotics that penetrate well into the prostate include fluoroquinolones, trimethoprim-sulfamethoxazole, and doxycycline. Amoxicillin and nitrofurantoin penetrate poorly into the prostate. The duration of therapy should be prolonged to reduce the rates of recurrence. Thus, a 28-day course of ciprofloxacin would be the best choice for management of this patient's chronic prostatitis due to *Escherichia coli*.

VII.2. Answer b.

This diabetic woman from India has a large abscess in the left lobe of her liver. Since blood cultures have been negative in the absence of antimicrobial therapy, a bacteremic seeding of the liver is less likely. Common bacterial causes of liver abscess include enteric organisms from the biliary tree, viridans group streptococci from the digestive tract, and *Staphylococcus aureus* secondary to bacteremia. In India, *Entamoeba histolytica* infection is common and may manifest as a febrile illness with a focal liver mass. The best test is blood serology for *E histolytica*. Ultrasound-guided needle aspiration is useful for many liver lesions but should be delayed pending the serology results. A stool test for ova and parasites is not specific, and ameba may not be seen at the stage of liver abscess. Empirical antibiotic therapy should be avoided until the diagnosis is established. A PPD skin test is likely to be positive and not helpful in establishing the cause of the liver lesion.

VII.3. Answer c.

This woman has acute uncomplicated pyelonephritis. She has been recently exposed to antimicrobials, so she is at increased risk for resistance to TMP-SMX and ampicillin. Thus, an oral fluoroquinolone is the drug of choice. Intravenous therapy is not necessary. Nitrofurantoin, although effective for cystitis, is not appropriate for pyelonephritis.

VII.4. Answer e.

Initial assessment of the severity of community-acquired pneumonia is important for internal medicine physicians to reduce unnecessary hospitalization and to identify patients who are at higher risk of death or who need more immediate intervention. Illness severity scores, such as the pneumonia severity index (PSI) and CURB-65 (confusion, urea nitrogen, respiratory rate, blood pressure, and 65 years or older), have been developed to help in the decision for site of care for patients with community-acquired pneumonia. In the outpatient setting, the modified CRB-65 (confusion, respiratory rate, blood pressure, and 65 years or older) score is useful since it does not require laboratory or radiographic evidence to determine the severity score. In this question, the patient is not confused, does not have a respiratory rate of 30 breaths per minute or more, does not have a systolic blood pressure less than 90 mm Hg or a diastolic blood pressure of 60 mm Hg or less, but is 65 years or older. His CRB-65 score is 1. Patients with scores of 0 or 1 can generally be treated as outpatients if they can reliably take oral antimicrobials and have outpatient support resources.

VII.5. Answer b.

This question is related to appropriate initial antimicrobial treatment of community-acquired pneumonia in a patient with medical comorbidities who requires hospitalization but not admission to an intensive care unit. Recommended treatment is either a respiratory fluoroquinolone or a β-lactam antibiotic in combination with a macrolide antibiotic. Azithromycin alone is not a recommended regimen in patients with medical comorbidities, including diabetes mellitus. Ciprofloxacin does not have sufficient coverage for *Streptococcus pneumoniae* and is thus not considered a respiratory fluoroquinolone. Although IV ampicillin would be an acceptable β-lactam antibiotic antimicrobial choice, clindamycin is not a macrolide antibiotic and the patient does not have risk factors to warrant empirical coverage of methicillin-resistant *Staphylococcus aureus*. Meropenem is a very broad-spectrum antimicrobial and is not recommended for routine use in hospitalized patients with community-acquired pneumonia who do not have risk factors for infection with *Pseudomonas aeruginosa*.

VII.6. Answer a.

This question is based on an understanding of the microbiology and subsequent antimicrobial prophylaxis ramifications of cat bites. Major pathogens isolated from cat bites include numerous anaerobes, streptococci, and staphylococci but most commonly *Pasteurella multocida*. Prophylactic antimicrobials are recommended unless the bite wound is very superficial, and *P multocida* is generally resistant to dicloxacillin, cephalexin, clindamycin, and erythromycin but is generally susceptible to amoxicillin-clavulanic acid.

VII.7. Answer c.

This patient has features of Churg-Strauss syndrome, which had previously been controlled with oral corticosteroids. Her presenting symptoms indicate a flare of vasculitis as the oral corticosteroid dosage was tapered. The difficult-to-control asthma, nasal polyps, infiltrates on chest radiography, and peripheral blood eosinophilia all point to Churg-Strauss syndrome as the correct diagnosis. A dramatic response can be expected with high doses of systemic corticosteroids.

VII.8. Answer a.

Amantadine and rimantadine can be used to treat and prevent influenza A but are not active against influenza B. Zanamivir and oseltamivir can be used to treat both influenza A and influenza B, and oseltamivir can also be used for prevention of influenza A and influenza B. Inhaled zanamivir is not recommended for use in patients with underlying lung disease such as chronic obstructive pulmonary disease or asthma because bronchospasm and decreased respiratory function have been reported with its use. Treatment with any of these drugs can shorten the duration of illness by approximately 1 day if treatment is started within the first 2 days of illness.

VII.9. Answer e.

This patient has staphylococcal toxic shock syndrome, which may be associated with retained packing after the nasal procedure. Often patients receive clindamycin until the packing is removed. The features of staphylococcal toxic shock syndrome are due to toxin-mediated cytokine activation and can occur 1) after surgical and postpartum procedures; 2) with mastitis, sinusitis, burns, and skin and soft tissue infections (especially of the extremities, perianal area, and axillae); and 3) with respiratory infections after influenza.

VII.10. Answer c.

This diabetic man has peripheral vascular disease and a fetid foot ulcer with surrounding cellulitis, which can be probed to the bone. He is manifesting systemic toxicity. The first step in management would be to begin antimicrobial therapy to cover MRSA and a mixed infection.

The infection will be polymicrobial, and a culture would have limited value. A nasal swab for MRSA does not establish the presence of MRSA in the wound. An MRI offers no additional immediate value at this stage, especially since the wound can be probed to the bone and is likely osteomyelitic.

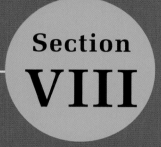

Section
VIII

Nephrology

Acid-Base Disorders

48

QI QIAN, MD

Determination of Acid-Base Status

Simple acid-base disorders are defined by changes in pH and the initial change in 1 of the 2 variables, serum bicarbonate (HCO_3^-) and Pco_2. Low pH indicates acidosis, and high pH indicates alkalosis. If 1 of the 2 components (HCO_3^- or Pco_2) decreases, the other component also decreases (a compensatory change that minimizes the change in the ratio and the pH) and vice versa, as shown in the Henderson-Hasselbalch equation. Emphasis has been placed on the Henderson-Hasselbalch equation because the equation describes the 4 acid-base disorders and their compensatory changes (Figure 48.1).

The adequacy of the compensation can be evaluated by the Winter formula for patients who have metabolic acidosis and by the +15 rule for patients with serum HCO_3^- 10 to 40 mmol/L. An example is shown in Box 48.1.

Metabolic Acid-Base Disorders

Metabolic acidosis is characterized by a decrease in pH, a decrease in serum HCO_3^-, and a compensatory decrease in Pco_2. Metabolic alkalosis is characterized by an increase in pH, an increase in HCO_3^-, and a compensatory increase in Pco_2.

	Initial Change	With Compensation
Metabolic acidosis	$\downarrow pH = pK_a + \dfrac{\downarrow HCO_3^-}{Pco_2}$	$\downarrow pH = pK_a + \dfrac{\downarrow HCO_3^-}{\downarrow Pco_2}$
Metabolic alkalosis	$\uparrow pH = pK_a + \dfrac{\uparrow HCO_3^-}{Pco_2}$	$\uparrow pH = pK_a + \dfrac{\uparrow HCO_3^-}{\uparrow Pco_2}$
Respiratory acidosis	$\downarrow pH = pK_a + \dfrac{HCO_3^-}{\uparrow Pco_2}$	$\downarrow pH = pK_a + \dfrac{\uparrow HCO_3^-}{\uparrow Pco_2}$
Respiratory alkalosis	$\uparrow pH = pK_a + \dfrac{HCO_3^-}{\downarrow Pco_2}$	$\uparrow pH = pK_a + \dfrac{\downarrow HCO_3^-}{\downarrow Pco_2}$

Figure 48.1 Four Types of Simple Acid-Base Disorders. The initial insult of acid or base influx causes large changes in pH and in 1 of the 2 components of the Henderson-Hasselbalch equation (bicarbonate [HCO_3^-] or Pco_2). With compensation, the other component changes accordingly to minimize the net change in the ratio and blood pH. The arrow size indicates the relative amount of increase ($\uparrow$) or decrease ($\downarrow$). pK_a indicates the negative logarithm of the acid dissociation constant.

Box 48.1 • Example of Acid–Base Determination

Patient: A 37-year-old woman with a history of Sjögren syndrome and hypothyroidism was admitted for shortness of breath. Evaluation showed significant electrolyte and acid-base imbalance. Physical examination findings were unremarkable except for mild tachypnea. Laboratory test results included the following: sodium 134 mmol/L, potassium 2.6 mmol/L, chloride 115 mmol/L, bicarbonate (HCO_3^-) 10 mmol/L, and creatinine 0.6 mg/dL. Arterial blood gas results were pH 7.25 and P_{CO_2} 25 mm Hg.

Question: What is the patient's acid-base status?

Answer: With the Henderson-Hasselbalch equation, first look at the blood pH. The patient's blood pH is decreased, indicating acidemia. Next identify which of the 2 variables (P_{CO_2} or HCO_3^-) decreases like the blood pH. Her serum HCO_3^- is decreased, like the blood pH (low HCO_3^- and low blood pH), indicating metabolic acidosis. Then look at whether the patient has an appropriate degree of compensation, which indicates a singular metabolic acidosis without any other primary abnormality. If the compensation is much more or much less than expected, there is likely a second, primary respiratory abnormality. For example, if the P_{CO_2} is lower than the expected compensation, there is a primary respiratory alkalosis in addition to a primary metabolic acidosis; a P_{CO_2} higher than expected indicates the existence of an additional primary respiratory acidosis.

One of 2 methods is used to determine the expected respiratory compensation (P_{CO_2}):

1. Winter formula: Expected $P_{CO_2} = (1.5 \times HCO_3^-) + 8 \pm 2$. For this patient, expected $P_{CO_2} = 23 \pm 2$ mm Hg. This formula is used when the patient's serum HCO_3^- is in the acidemic range (<24 mmol/L).

2. +15 Rule: Expected $P_{CO_2} = HCO_3^- + 15$. The value (25 for this patient) should equal the last 2 digits of the pH if the patient has a single acidosis with adequate respiratory compensation. The +15 rule is relatively simple and applicable when the HCO_3^- ranges between 10 and 40 mmol/L.

On the basis of the calculation, this patient has a pure non–anion gap acidosis with appropriate compensation.

Metabolic acidosis can be categorized as normal gap acidosis or anion gap (AG) acidosis. The **AG** is the difference between the serum sodium concentration and the sum of the chloride and HCO_3^- concentrations.

Key Definition

AG: *sodium – (chloride + HCO_3^-).*

Box 48.2 • Common Causes of Metabolic Acidosis and Metabolic Alkalosis

Metabolic acidosis
  Normal gap acidosis
    Renal tubular acidosis
    Diarrhea
    Stage 2 or 3 chronic kidney disease
    Ureterosigmoid fistula
    Drugs such as carbonic anhydrase inhibitors
      (eg, acetazolamide)
  Anion gap acidosis[a]
    Glycols (ethylene and propylene)
    Oxoproline
    L-lactate
    D-lactate
    Methanol
    Aspirin
    Renal failure
    Ketones
Metabolic alkalosis
  Chloride-responsive alkalosis
    Volume contraction
    Diuretics
    Vomiting
    Gastric suction
  Chloride-resistant alkalosis
    Hyperaldosteronism
    Corticosteroids
    Renal artery stenosis
    Bartter syndrome
    Gitelman syndrome
    Severe hypokalemia
    Milk-alkali syndrome

[a] *GOLDMARK* is the mnemonic for the major causes of anion gap acidosis.

Common causes of non-AG and AG acidosis are listed in Box 48.2.

Renal Tubular Acidoses

There are 3 main types of renal tubular acidosis (Table 48.1):

1. Type 1—distal tubular acidosis due to defects in hydrogen ion excretion in the collecting duct
2. Type 2—proximal tubular acidosis due to defects in proximal tubular HCO_3^- reclamation
3. Type 4—hyporeninemic hypoaldosteronism

AG Acidosis

AG acidosis is characterized by a decrease in blood pH, a decrease in serum HCO_3^-, and an AG greater than 12 mmol/L (AG reference range, 8–12 mmol/L). Regardless of the

Table 48.1 • Features of 3 Types of Renal Tubular Acidosis

Feature	Type 1: Distal Tubular	Type 2: Proximal Tubular	Type 4: Hyporeninemic Hypoaldosteronism
Defect	H⁺ excretion in distal tubule	HCO_3^- reabsorption in proximal tubule	Low renin, low aldosterone
Etiology and clinical setting	Acquired: connective tissue diseases, interstitial renal diseases Drugs: amphotericin B Hereditary: rare	Acquired: dysproteinemia (MM), interstitial renal diseases (less frequently), lead or mercury toxicity Drugs: ifosfamide Hereditary: glycogen storage disease, hereditary fructose intolerance, mitochondrial diseases, cystinosis, Wilson disease	DM, mild-moderate CKD, heparin, NSAIDs, ACEI/ARB
Serum potassium	Low	Low	High
Urine pH	Always high (>5.3)	Low (when HCO_3^- <Tm)	Variable
Urinary loss of glucose, amino acids, and phosphate (Fanconi syndrome)	No	Yes	No
Nephrocalcinosis or nephrolithiasis	Yes	No	No
Acidemia	Severe if no treatment	Self-limited	Mild
Alkali treatment	Small requirement	Large requirement; treat the cause	Small requirement
FE-HCO_3^-	<5%	Can be high with alkali treatment	Variable

Abbreviations: ACEI/ARB, angiotensin-converting enzyme inhibitor/angiotensin receptor blocker; CKD, chronic kidney disease; DM, diabetes mellitus; FE, fractional excretion; H+, hydrogen ion; HCO_3^-, bicarbonate; MM, multiple myeloma; NSAID, nonsteroidal anti-inflammatory drug; Tm, tubular transport maximum.

blood pH, the AG should always be calculated, because with concurrent acid-base alterations, an AG acidosis may not be apparent. The AG should be corrected for low serum albumin: For each decrease of 1 g/dL in serum albumin, the AG decreases by 2.5 mmol/L. Paraproteinemia can decrease the AG to less than 8 mmol/L.

KEY FACTS

✓ Use the Winter formula to determine the expected respiratory compensation in metabolic acidosis (serum HCO_3^- <24 mmol/L)

✓ Use the +15 rule to determine the expected respiratory compensation when HCO_3^- is 10–40 mmol/L

✓ Acid-base problems—calculate the AG regardless of the blood pH

✓ Correct the AG for low serum albumin

In recent years, several new anion-generating acids have been recognized as causes of AG metabolic acidosis. The new mnemonic for the major causes of AG metabolic acidosis is **GOLDMARK** (Box 48.2).

Key Definition

GOLDMARK: *mnemonic for major causes of AG metabolic acidosis (glycols [ethylene and propylene], oxoproline, L-lactate, D-lactate, methanol, aspirin, renal failure, and ketones).*

Diagnosis and Therapy

In most cases, the clinical scenario indicates the cause of acidosis. Among the causes of AG acidosis, L-lactic acidosis is common, especially in critically ill patients. L-lactic acidosis can be subdivided into 2 types: Type A lactic acidosis develops with tissue hypoxia, as in shock, severe anemia, and hypoxia from pulmonary diseases. Type B lactic acidosis develops in conditions of mitochondrial oxidative impairment, including MELAS syndrome (mitochondrial encephalomyopathy, lactic acidosis, and strokelike episodes), cyanide intoxication, and use of certain medications (metformin, linezolid, and reverse transcriptase inhibitors).

D-lactic acidosis occurs mainly in patients with short gut syndrome and overgrowth of gut bacteria. The bacteria generate D-lactate, which causes AG acidosis. Notably, most clinical laboratories test for L-lactate but not D-lactate unless requested. Therefore, when D-lactic acidosis is suspected, measurement of D-lactate must be requested specifically.

When toxic alcohol ingestion is suspected, the osmolal gap should be calculated in addition to the AG. The toxic alcohols (especially methanol and ethylene glycol) are osmotically active molecules. Methanol is metabolized to formic acid, causing blindness. Ethylene glycol is metabolized to glycolic acid and oxalic acid; the lines in calcium oxalate crystals resemble the lines on the back of an envelope.

Before their conversion to toxic acids, the alcohols generate an osmolal gap (ie, the measured serum osmolality exceeds the calculated serum osmolality by >10 mOsm/kg).

$$\text{Calculated Serum Osmolality} = [2(\text{Sodium} + \text{Potassium})] + (\text{Serum Urea Nitrogen}/2.8) + (\text{Glucose}/18)$$

When the osmolal gap is elevated, treatment should be instituted immediately to block the toxic alcohols (parent

Table 48.2 • Metabolic Alkalosis

Cause	Pathophysiology (Major)	Diagnostic Features in Addition to Metabolic Alkalosis	Therapy
Vomiting and gastric suction	Gastric acid loss Renal HCO_3^- absorption	↓ BP or normal BP Low urine Cl^- (<20 mmol/L)	Normal saline
Hyperaldosteronism	↑ Renal H^+ excretion ↑ Proximal renal tubular HCO_3^- absorption	. . .	. . .
Primary hyperaldosteronism	. . .	↑ BP, high urine Cl^- (≥20 mmol/L)	Correct the causes
Secondary hyperaldosteronism	. . .	. . .	Treat underlying cause
Renal artery stenosis		↑ BP, stenosis apparent with renal ultrasonography	
Volume depletion Diuretic use		↓ BP, low Cl^- (<20 mmol/L) ↓ BP, high Cl^- (≥20 mmol/L), hypokalemia	
Severe hypokalemia	↑ Renal H^+ excretion	Normal BP, polyuria	Potassium repletion
Exogenous alkali intake ($CaHCO_3$ and $NaHCO_3$)	Analogous to milk-alkali syndrome	Hypercalcemia, usually in patients with CKD	Discontinue alkaline intake
Posthypercapnic state	Net loss of $CO_2(H_2CO_3)$	Mechanical ventilation in patients with severe COPD	↓ Ventilation
Liddle syndrome	Autosomal dominant inheritance Epithelial sodium channel mutation in collecting duct results in increased activity	↑ BP, hypokalemia, metabolic alkalosis	Potassium repletion and diuretics (amiloride preferred)
Glucocorticoid-remediable aldosteronism	Autosomal dominant inheritance Aldosterone synthesis is stimulated by corticotropin	↑ BP, hypokalemia ↑ Aldosterone ↓ Renin activity	Glucocorticoids
Apparent glucocorticoid excess	Defects in 11β-hydroxysteroid dehydrogenase Genetic defect (autosomal recessive inheritance), acquired (excessive licorice intake), or Cushing syndrome	↑ BP, hypokalemia ↓ Renin activity ↓ Aldosterone level ↑ Urine cortisol to cortisone ratio	Mineralocorticoid receptor blockade Symptomatic treatment
Bartter syndrome	Autosomal recessive inheritance with 5 types of genetic defects	Neonatal or childhood onset ↓ BP Hypokalemia Hypercalciuria High urine Cl^- (≥20 mmol/L)	Sodium and potassium repletion
Gitelman syndrome	Autosomal recessive inheritance Mutations in distal sodium-Cl^- cotransporters	Adolescence or adulthood onset ↓ BP or normal BP Hypokalemia Hypocalciuria High urine Cl^- (≥20 mmol/L)	Sodium and potassium repletion

Abbreviations: ↓, decreased; ↑, increased; BP, blood pressure; $CaHCO_3$, calcium bicarbonate; Cl^-, chloride; $CO_2(H_2CO_3)$, carbonic acid; CKD, chronic kidney disease; COPD, chronic obstructive pulmonary disease; H^+, hydrogen ion; HCO_3^-, bicarbonate; $NaHCO_3$, sodium bicarbonate.

Box 48.3 • Respiratory Acid-Base Alterations

Causes of respiratory acidosis

CNS respiratory depression

Injury: trauma, infarct, hemorrhage, tumor
Drugs: opiates, sedatives, anesthetics
Hypoventilation of obesity (eg, pickwickian syndrome)
Cerebral hypoxia

Nerve or muscle

Guillain-Barré syndrome, myasthenia gravis, various myopathies
Diaphragmatic factors: paralysis or splinting, muscle relaxants
Toxins (eg, organophosphates, snake venom)

Chest wall, airway, lung

Airway: upper and lower airway obstruction
Chest wall trauma: flail chest, contusion, hemothorax, pneumothorax
Lung: pulmonary edema, ARDS, aspiration

Carbon dioxide excess

Hypercatabolic states: malignant hyperthermia
Addition of CO_2 to inspired gas
Insufflation of CO_2 into body cavity (eg, for laparoscopic surgery)

Causes of respiratory alkalosis

CNS respiratory stimulation

Pain, hyperventilation syndrome, anxiety, psychosis, infection, trauma, cerebrovascular accident

Hypoxia

High altitude, severe anemia, right-to-left shunts

Drugs

Progesterone, methylxanthines, salicylates, catecholamines, nicotine

Endocrine conditions

Progesterone (pregnancy)

Pulmonary conditions

Pneumonia, edema, embolism, asthma

Miscellaneous

Sepsis, hepatic failure, recovery phase of metabolic acidosis

Abbreviations: ARDS, acute respiratory distress syndrome; CNS, central nervous system; CO_2, carbon dioxide.

---

compounds) from being metabolized. Inhibitors of alcohol dehydrogenase, such as fomepizole (4-methylpyrazole), effectively block toxic alcohol metabolism. In severe cases, hemodialysis is necessary.

Salicylate intoxication in adults typically causes AG acidosis and respiratory alkalosis, but it does not cause an osmolal gap.

Metabolic Alkalosis

Metabolic alkalosis can result from a net loss of acid or a net gain of HCO_3^-. Clinical manifestations include weakness, muscle cramps, hyperreflexia, alveolar hypoventilation, and arrhythmias. The major causes, pathophysiology, diagnostic features, and therapy are summarized in Table 48.2.

Diagnosis and Therapy

Metabolic alkalosis associated with hypovolemia is characterized by a low urine chloride concentration (<20 mmol/L) and is responsive to volume expansion with isotonic saline infusion or oral salt tablets (Box 48.2). Metabolic alkalosis associated with primary mineralocorticoid excess is usually characterized by hypervolemia, a high urine chloride concentration (≥20 mmol/L), and resistance to therapy with saline but responsiveness to acetazolamide diuresis and mineralocorticoid antagonizers. These treatments should be given only after serum potassium is repleted, since both alkalosis and treatment with acetazolamide are associated with kaliuresis.

Respiratory Acid-Base Alterations

Respiratory acidosis is characterized by a decreased pH, an increased P_{CO_2}, and a compensatory increase in serum HCO_3^-. *Respiratory alkalosis* is characterized by an increased pH, a decreased P_{CO_2}, and a compensatory decrease in serum HCO_3^-.

Respiratory acidosis and respiratory alkalosis can be caused by defects in the central nervous system respiratory center, the chest wall (ribs, nerves, and muscles), and the lung parenchyma. Causes of respiratory acid-base alterations and expected metabolic compensations for acute and chronic respiratory acid-base alterations are summarized in Box 48.3.

KEY FACTS

✓ Lactic acidosis—rule out medications as the cause

✓ For patients with acid-base disorder and decreased mental status (eg, toxic alcohol ingestion), calculate both the osmolal gap and the AG

✓ Salicylate intoxication in adults—AG acidosis and respiratory alkalosis

---

Therapy for respiratory acid-base alterations is directed to the specific causes.

49 Acute Kidney Injury

SUZANNE M. NORBY, MD AND KIANOUSH B. KASHANI, MD

Definition

The term *acute kidney injury* (AKI) has replaced *acute renal failure* in contemporary medical literature. AKI denotes a rapid deterioration of kidney function (glomerular filtration rate [GFR]) within hours to weeks, resulting in the accumulation of nitrogenous metabolites in addition to fluid, electrolyte, and acid-base imbalances.

The definition of *AKI* was refined by the Kidney Disease: Improving Global Outcomes group (KDIGO) to a 3-stage definition (Table 49.1), with criteria for stage 1 as follows: 1) an absolute increase in serum creatinine (SCr) by at least 0.3 mg/dL from baseline within 48 hours; *or* 2) a relative increase in SCr to at least 1.5 times baseline within the past 7 days; *or* 3) urine output decreased to less than 0.5 mL/kg/h for 6 hours. Use of SCr as a marker of AKI, however, has disadvantages. For example, many

conditions interfere with SCr measurement and, therefore, can overestimate or underestimate the actual GFR (Table 49.2). Changes in serum urea nitrogen are less reliable for diagnosing AKI than changes in SCr. Novel biomarkers of AKI have been validated, and these biomarkers are now used for early recognition of AKI, estimation of the intensity of injury, and prognosis for recovery from AKI. A relatively common biomarker used for GFR estimation is cystatin C, which is synthesized by all nucleated cells and released into the blood at a relatively constant rate. As with SCr, factors other than GFR influence the cystatin C level (Table 49.2).

Epidemiology

The incidence of AKI over the past few decades has increased significantly for multiple reasons, including longer survival and aging of the general population, medical comorbidities, and increased incidence of chronic kidney disease. In addition, from 2000 to 2009 the number of patients with AKI who required dialysis increased from 250 per million patients to 630 per million patients.

The traditional classification subdivides AKI into prerenal, intrinsic renal, and postrenal categories (Figure 49.1). Although AKI has a dominant cause in some patients, multiple factors usually contribute to its development.

Prerenal AKI

Prerenal AKI or *functional AKI* is defined as decreased GFR due to decreased renal perfusion *without* ischemic injury to tubules, resulting from volume depletion, low cardiac output, drugs, or peripheral vasodilatation (eg, sepsis) (Box 49.1).

Table 49.1 • Classification and Staging System for Acute Kidney Injury		
Stage	**Serum Creatinine Concentration**	**Urine Output**
1	Increase of ≥0.3 mg/dL *or* Increase to 1.5–1.9 times baseline	<0.5 mL/kg/h for 6–12 h
2	Increase to 2.0–2.9 times baseline	<0.5 mL/h for ≥12 h
3	Increase to 3.0 times baseline *or* Increase to ≥4.0 mg/dL *or* Initiation of renal replacement therapy	<0.3 mL/kg/h for ≥24 h *or* anuria for ≥12 h

Adapted from Kidney Disease: Improving Global Outcomes (KDIGO) Acute Kidney Injury Work Group. KDIGO clinical practice guideline for acute kidney injury. Kidney Int Suppl. 2012 Mar;2(1):1–138. Used with permission.

Table 49.2 • Conditions That Change Serum Creatinine Level Independently of Glomerular Filtration Rate (GFR)

Analyte	GFR-Independent Increase	GFR-Independent Decrease
Serum creatinine	Decreased tubular secretion	Low muscle mass
	Trimethoprim	Small body habitus
	Cimetidine	Female sex
	Amiloride	Amputation
	Probenecid	Advanced age
	Spironolactone	Advanced liver disease
	Triamterene	
	Male sex	Muscle wasting disorders
	Rhabdomyolysis	
	Vigorous exercise	Neuromuscular diseases
	Large muscle mass	
	Ingestion of cooked meat	Malnutrition
	Increased muscle mass	Dietary protein restriction
	Jaffe reaction	Renal disease
	Ketotic states	Liver disease
	Hyperglycemia	Vegetarian diet
		Amputation
		Jaffe reaction
		Hyperbilirubinemia
Serum urea nitrogen	Hypercatabolism	Aggressive volume expansion
	High-protein diet	Pregnancy
	Decreased intravascular volume	SIADH
	Diuretics	Dietary protein restriction
	Glucocorticoids	Liver disease
	Tetracyclines	
	Gastrointestinal tract bleeding	
Cystatin C	Advanced age	Female sex
	Male sex	Lower body mass
	Greater body mass	Corticosteroids
	Smoking	Hypothyroidism
	Inflammatory states	
	Hyperthyroidism	

Abbreviation: SIADH, syndrome of inappropriate secretion of antidiuretic hormone.

Adapted from Bagshaw SM, Gibney RTN. Conventional markers of kidney function. Crit Care Med. 2008;36(Suppl 4):S152–8. Used with permission.

Intravascular volume depletion could be due to external loss of fluids and electrolytes (vomiting, diarrhea, and dehydration), loss of plasma volume (burns), internal fluid losses (third spacing, as occurs in severe pancreatitis), and hemorrhage. Physical findings of volume depletion include orthostatic hypotension, dry mucous membranes, and decreased skin turgor. Management involves administration of oral or intravenous fluids.

Kidney hypoperfusion results from various factors. Decreased cardiac output, as occurs in congestive heart failure (cardiorenal syndrome), can cause prerenal AKI. Physical findings include elevated jugular venous pressure, bibasilar crackles in the lungs, peripheral edema, and a third heart sound gallop. Management includes optimization of cardiac function, which often includes use of diuretics. Kidney hypoperfusion also occurs in sepsis because of peripheral vasodilatation and abnormal vascular tone, along with the effects of inflammatory mediators and other pathways that are beginning to be further understood. Another cause of impaired perfusion to the kidneys is intra-abdominal hypertension, sometimes referred to as abdominal compartment syndrome. Conditions that increase intra-abdominal pressure include ascites, ileus, interstitial fluid accumulation (as occurs with administration of large volumes of blood products or fluids and with pancreatitis), trauma, and abdominal surgery.

Renal artery occlusion due to thrombosis, stenosis, emboli, or vasculitis of the main renal arteries or several intrarenal arteries can result in a rapid decline in renal function. If not promptly addressed, renal artery occlusion causes ischemic acute tubular necrosis (ATN).

Nonsteroidal anti-inflammatory drugs (NSAIDs) inhibit cyclooxygenase and decrease vasodilatory prostaglandin production. Patients who take NSAIDs and have underlying renal insufficiency, volume depletion, advanced liver disease, or congestive heart failure are at risk for AKI. Angiotensin-converting enzyme inhibitors (ACEIs) and angiotensin receptor blockers (ARBs) increase the risk of AKI when renal blood flow is decreased. These medications interfere with the action of angiotensin II, which serves to maintain GFR when renal blood flow is decreased. If AKI develops while a patient is taking an ACEI or ARB, the medication should be withheld until renal function improves. Also, drugs in the calcineurin inhibitor class of immunosuppressants (eg, cyclosporine and tacrolimus) cause renal vasoconstriction and kidney hypoperfusion.

Hepatorenal syndrome (HRS) is a rapid decline in kidney function in the presence of severe liver disease. HRS is a functional renal failure induced by intrarenal vasoconstriction in the presence of circulatory dysfunction with splanchnic vasodilatation and relatively insufficient cardiac output, leading to effective hypovolemia. Precipitating events may be worsening liver function, bleeding, infection (such as spontaneous bacterial peritonitis), and large-volume paracentesis without albumin replacement. Diagnostic criteria for HRS in a patient with hepatic failure and portal hypertension are listed in Box 49.2.

Key Definition

Hepatorenal syndrome: *functional renal failure associated with severe liver disease and induced by intrarenal vasoconstriction with circulatory dysfunction, splanchnic vasodilatation, insufficient cardiac output, and hypovolemia.*

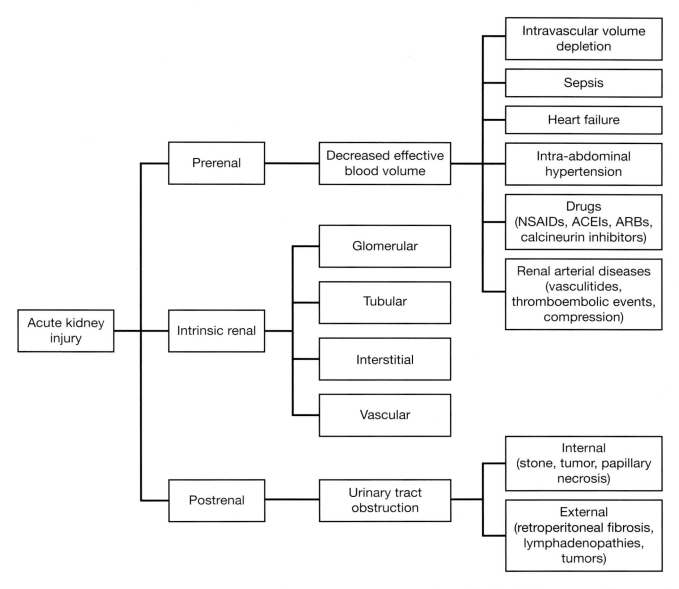

Figure 49.1 *Classification of Acute Kidney Injury. Acute kidney injury is traditionally classified as prerenal (functional), intrinsic renal, and postrenal. ACEI indicates angiotensin-converting enzyme inhibitor; ARB, angiotensin receptor blocker; NSAID, nonsteroidal anti-inflammatory drug.*

In type 1 HRS, the decline in kidney function is rapid. Type 2 HRS manifests with a more gradual decline in kidney function and, often, refractory ascites. Administration of albumin and vasoconstrictors (such as vasopressin analogues) or midodrine plus octreotide may improve the historically poor short-term prognosis. Transjugular intrahepatic portosystemic shunt may also improve HRS. Liver transplant is the preferred therapy for appropriate candidates.

Box 49.1 · Characteristics of Prerenal Acute Kidney Injury

Increased reabsorption of sodium and water leading to concentrated urine

Increased reabsorption of urea resulting in elevation of serum urea nitrogen (SUN) out of proportion to creatinine (SUN: creatinine ratio >20:1)

Rapid reversibility if the underlying cause is treated

KEY FACTS

✓ AKI—common (incidence is increasing) and associated with significant morbidity and mortality

✓ Cystatin C—relatively common biomarker for estimating GFR

✓ Type 1 HRS—rapid decline in kidney function

✓ Type 2 HRS—gradual decline in kidney function, often with refractory ascites

Box 49.2 • Diagnostic Criteria for Hepatorenal Syndrome in a Patient With Hepatic Failure and Portal Hypertension

SCr >1.5 mg/dL

No improvement in SCr after 2 d of diuretic withdrawal and volume expansion with albumin

No other apparent reason for acute kidney injury, such as recent administration of nephrotoxic drugs or shock

Normal findings on renal ultrasonography

Typically, proteinuria <500 mg daily and microhematuria <50 RBCs per high-power field; however, another coexisting kidney disease would not preclude the development of superimposed hepatorenal syndrome

Abbreviations: RBC, red blood cell; SCr, serum creatinine.

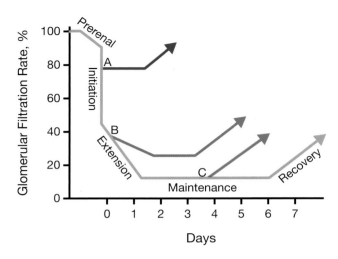

Figure 49.2 *Time Course of Acute Tubular Necrosis. A, B, and C indicate therapy for preventing (A) or limiting (B) the extension phase and therapy for established acute tubular necrosis (C).*

(Adapted from Molitoris BA. Transitioning to therapy in ischemic acute renal failure. J Am Soc Nephrol. 2003 Jan;14[1]:265–7. Used with permission.)

Intrinsic Renal AKI

Glomerular Disease and Vasculitis

Glomerular disease occurring in combination with AKI, called rapidly progressive glomerulonephritis, and vasculitis are discussed in Chapter 52, "Renal Parenchymal Diseases."

Acute Tubular Necrosis

The natural history of ATN depends on its cause, which can be ischemia (from a decrease in oxygen delivery), inflammation, or nephrotoxic injury. Many toxins, both endogenous and exogenous, can cause tubular damage. The timeline of ATN development and recovery is based on the clinical picture. If prerenal ischemia lasts long enough, overt tubular damage ensues. Extension of the injury after reperfusion is usually from the infiltration of inflammatory cells. The typical course of ischemic ATN begins with a rapid decrease in urine output, accompanied by an increase in the SCr level (Figure 49.2). During the maintenance phase, oliguria is usually followed by polyuria before tubules regain their concentrating capacity. The longer the duration of the oliguric phase before recovery, the smaller the chance of complete recovery of kidney function. In the recovery phase, the SCr level begins to decrease, and urine output normalizes.

Contrast-induced nephropathy is typically defined as an increase in SCr of 0.5 mg/dL or 25% within 3 days after administration of a contrast agent if no other cause is identified. In most patients, urine output decreases and SCr increases 24 to 48 hours after administration of the dye and returns to normal within 7 to 10 days. If a patient's risk factors for contrast-induced nephropathy are identified, steps can be taken to reduce the risk (Box 49.3).

Key Definition

Contrast-induced nephropathy: *SCr increase of 0.5 mg/dL or 25% within 3 days after contrast agent administration if no other cause is identified.*

Tubular cells can be directly damaged by many medications and agents, including aminoglycosides, amphotericin B, vancomycin, calcineurin inhibitors, cisplatin, methotrexate, ifosfamide, pentamidine, contrast agents, foscarnet, and cidofovir.

Pigment Nephropathy

Pigment nephropathy can occur with rhabdomyolysis or intravascular hemolysis, in which abnormal amounts of myoglobin or free hemoglobin in the serum are filtered by the kidney. These pigments are directly toxic to renal tubular cells and can also form intratubular casts. The key to diagnosis of pigment nephropathy is urine dipstick positivity for blood without finding red blood cells (RBCs) with urine microscopy. During rhabdomyolysis or hemolysis, management includes aggressive intravenous fluid administration to achieve a high rate of urine flow (200–300 mL/h). Urine alkalization has been advocated but is controversial.

Atheroembolic Disease

Atheroembolic disease usually occurs after vascular manipulations during arterial catheterization or vascular

Box 49.3 • CIN Risk Factors and Risk Reduction

Risk factors for CIN

Advanced age
Diabetes mellitus
CKD (especially with estimated GFR <30 mL/min/
  1.73 m^2)
Congestive heart failure
Acute myocardial infarction within 24 h
Peripheral vascular disease
Intravascular volume depletion
Concomitant use of other nephrotoxins

Steps to reduce the incidence or severity of CIN in
  high-risk patients

Use low or iso-osmolar contrast agents
Limit the dose of contrast agent
Increase the time between repeated dye loads
Withhold medications that alter renal blood flow
  or intrarenal hemodynamics (ACEIs, ARBs, and
  NSAIDs)
Optimize intravascular effective blood volume with
  intravenous isotonic crystalloid solution

Abbreviations: ACEI, angiotensin-converting enzyme
  inhibitor; ARB, angiotensin receptor blocker; CIN, contrast-
  induced nephropathy; CKD, chronic kidney disease;
  GFR, glomerular filtration rate; NSAID, nonsteroidal
  anti-inflammatory drug.

operations in patients who have severe atherosclerosis. The timeline for development of atheroembolic disease after a procedure is variable, ranging from hours to weeks. About 20% of patients with atheroembolic disease do not report a history of vascular procedures. Livedo reticularis may be seen on the back, flank, abdomen, or extremities. On ophthalmoscopic examination, atheroemboli manifest as Hollenhorst plaques. Other clinical manifestations are bowel ischemia and AKI. Although the diagnosis is mostly clinical, the definitive diagnosis of atheroembolic disease is made by kidney or skin biopsy showing cholesterol crystals in small arterioles with distal necrosis. A high erythrocyte sedimentation rate or C-reactive protein level and decreased complement levels are suggestive of athero-embolic disease. The prognosis for kidney recovery after atheroembolic disease is poor, and recovery is usually incomplete. Treatment is supportive, including cholesterol-lowering agents and renal replacement therapy as needed. Anticoagulation is relatively contraindicated because it can destabilize the atheromatous plaques and, therefore, cause additional cholesterol emboli.

Acute Interstitial Nephritis

Acute interstitial nephritis (AIN) is an inflammatory process characterized by a mononuclear cell infiltrate within the renal interstitium. Relatively common, AIN accounts for approximately 10% to 15% of cases of AKI. AIN is idiopathic in 10% to 20% of cases, but it is most frequently associated with drugs, infections, autoimmune systemic diseases, and malignancies (Box 49.4).

Diagnosis of AIN may require renal biopsy. Clinically, AIN has a sudden onset, usually after the patient has had several days of exposure if the cause is related to a medication. Systemic manifestations of a hypersensitivity reaction in patients with drug-induced AIN include fever, maculopapular rash, and arthralgias (25% of patients). Flank pain caused by distention of the renal capsule occurs in about 50% of patients. Abnormal renal function, occurring in about 60% of patients, varies from a mild increase in the SCr level to severe AKI requiring dialysis. Tubular damage can impair the urinary concentration mechanism and result in polyuria. Other urinary abnormalities are listed in Box 49.5. Peripheral eosinophilia is common (about 50% of patients).

Therapy for AIN includes identification and elimination of inciting factors. For patients with drug-induced

Box 49.4 • Common Causes of Acute Interstitial Nephritis

Drugs

Antibiotics—penicillin, methicillin (anti–tubular
  basement membrane antibodies), ampicillin,
  rifampin, sulfa drugs, ciprofloxacin, pentamidine
NSAIDs—not dose-dependent; recurs; possibly
  T-cell–mediated; allergic signs and symptoms
  are absent; interstitial nephritis with nephrotic
  syndrome and renal insufficiency may have a
  latent period
Diuretics—thiazides, furosemide, bumetanide (sulfa
  derivatives)
Cimetidine
Proton pump inhibitors
Allopurinol, phenytoin, phenindione
Cyclosporine

Infections

Bacteria— *Legionella, Brucella, Streptococcus,*
  Staphylococcus, pneumococci
Viruses—Epstein-Barr virus, CMV, *Hantavirus,* HIV,
  hepatitis B virus, *Polyomavirus*
Fungi—*Candida, Histoplasma*
Parasites—*Plasmodium, Toxoplasma, Schistosoma,*
  Leishmania

Systemic diseases

Systemic lupus erythematosus
Sjögren syndrome
Sarcoidosis
Lymphoma, leukemic infiltration
Renal transplant rejection

Idiopathic

Abbreviations: CMV, cytomegalovirus; HIV, human
  immunodeficiency virus; NSAID, nonsteroidal
  anti-inflammatory drug.

Box 49.5 • Urinary Abnormalities in Acute Interstitial Nephritis (AIN)

Pyuria (in almost all patients)

Microscopic hematuria

Low-grade proteinuria (<1 g/1.73 m²/24 h)

Eosinophiluria (>1% eosinophils)—may be suggestive of AIN but is also seen in other unrelated renal diseases; relatively low sensitivity and specificity limit the utility of this test

AIN, administration of corticosteroids for 2 to 4 weeks may be beneficial. Corticosteroids are not indicated in infection-related AIN. Although AIN has traditionally been considered to be reversible, recent studies have shown that impaired renal function can persist long-term in up to 40% of patients.

Acute Phosphate Nephropathy

Acute phosphate nephropathy occurs in patients who receive oral sodium phosphate–based laxatives, commonly when preparing for colonoscopy (Box 49.6). AKI results from interstitial inflammation due to precipitation of calcium phosphate in the renal tubules and interstitium.

The treatment is intravascular volume expansion, and in the majority of cases, removal of phosphorus is recommended. Seizures and tetany may result from severe hypocalcemia, and calcium must be replaced cautiously because it may increase the chance of calcium phosphate crystal precipitation. In the majority of patients, recovery of kidney function is only partial.

Acute Uric Acid Nephropathy

Acute uric acid nephropathy is associated with the tumor lysis syndrome that develops after chemotherapy, myelo-proliferative disorders, heat stroke, status epilepticus, and Lesch-Nyhan syndrome. AKI is caused by uric acid crystal formation in the renal tubular lumens, causing intrarenal

tubular obstruction. This condition is generally reversible. Prevention includes forced diuresis, allopurinol, and ras-buricase. In some cases, hemodialysis is needed.

Crystal Deposition Due to Medications or Toxins

Medications that may cause crystal deposition include acyclovir, indinavir, sulfonamide, methotrexate (doses >50 mg/kg), and triamterene. Crystal deposition is mainly a pH-dependent process. Treatment includes optimizing the intravascular volume, alkalizing the urine, and withdrawing the offending medication. Excessive oxalate production occurs after ethylene glycol ingestion. Precipitation of calcium oxalate crystals contributes to AKI, which is also mediated by direct tubular toxicity of glycolate, another metabolite of ethylene glycol. Treatment consists of urine alkalization, administration of the alcohol dehydrogenase inhibitor fomepizole, and hemodialysis.

Hypercalcemia

Hypercalcemia induces nephrogenic diabetes insipidus. Dehydration and interstitial nephritis can result in manifestations of AKI. Treatment is directed at decreasing the serum calcium concentration and addressing the underlying cause of hypercalcemia.

Postrenal AKI

Postrenal AKI is defined as obstructed urinary flow at any level of the urinary tract. Obstruction can result from any of several causes (Box 49.7).

Postrenal AKI is often accompanied by pain, hypertension, and normal anion gap acidosis. Postrenal causes should be excluded in all patients with anuria. For this purpose, ultrasonography is recommended because it is noninvasive, widely available, and very sensitive for established hydronephrosis. Postrenal AKI is usually reversible with prompt relief of the obstruction. Additionally, partial or unilateral obstruction may occur without an increase in SCr.

Box 49.6 • Risk Factors for Acute Phosphate Nephropathy

Advanced age

Hypertension

Preexisting chronic kidney disease

Volume depletion

Use of angiotensin-converting enzyme inhibitors or angiotensin receptor blockers

Box 49.7 • Causes of Urinary Flow Obstruction

Bladder outlet obstruction (eg, prostate cancer or benign prostatic hypertrophy in men and genitourinary cancer in women)

Neurogenic bladder

Ureteral obstruction (eg, urolithiasis, tumor, necrosed renal papillae, and blood clots)

Extrinsic compression of the genitourinary tract (eg, malignancies and retroperitoneal fibrosis)

Inadvertent surgical ligation of a ureter

Diagnostic Approach to AKI

Obtaining a medical history and performing a physical examination are the first steps in differentiating the causes of AKI. Past medical history is important for identifying risk factors such as diabetes mellitus, hypertension, allergies, and medications along with any family history of kidney disease. Physical signs and symptoms of AKI are nonspecific and can include polyuria, oliguria, anuria, hematuria, dysuria, decreased appetite, nausea and vomiting, altered mental status, increased respiratory rate due to respiratory compensation, hypervolemia, and hypertension.

The physical examination should assess fluid balance to distinguish between prerenal causes and intrinsic or postrenal causes.

Laboratory Studies

Findings on urinalysis and urine chemistry testing can help to distinguish between causes of AKI (Table 49.3). In prerenal AKI, urine osmolality is increased and the urinary sediment is usually benign, with only hyaline casts. Urinary sodium and fractional excretion of sodium are low because sodium is retained by the kidney in states of low renal perfusion. In ATN, urine is usually isosmotic with the serum. Fractional excretion of sodium is of low utility in patients who are not oliguric.

Although examination of urinary sediment has low sensitivity, specificity is high for renal disorders. Specific findings in ATN are renal tubular epithelial cells, granular casts, and epithelial cell casts. In AIN, leukocytes, leukocyte casts, and urinary eosinophils are present. Dysmorphic RBCs and RBC casts indicate glomerular bleeding, consistent with glomerulonephritis or other damage to the glomerular basement membrane. With severe glomerular inflammation, leukocytes and leukocyte casts may also be seen. Nondysmorphic RBCs may suggest obstruction due to genitourinary cancer or urolithiasis.

Imaging

Ultrasonography can be helpful in differentiating among the causes of AKI (Table 49.4). For postrenal AKI, ultrasonography is the test of choice to determine whether hydronephrosis is present. If the use of contrast media is avoided, other imaging techniques can be useful on a case-by-case basis.

Biopsy

Kidney biopsy is often indicated when renal parenchymal involvement is suspected, such as when a patient has a rapid decline in kidney function in the presence of progressive or massive proteinuria or abnormal urinary sediment that includes glomerular hematuria (RBC casts or dysmorphic RBCs), granular casts, sterile pyuria, and leukocyte casts. In addition, clinicians may choose kidney biopsy when progressive kidney dysfunction is unexplained by noninvasive tools.

Table 49.3 • Comparison of Test Results in Prerenal Failure and Acute Tubular Necrosis

Laboratory Test or Urinary Index	Prerenal Failure	Acute Tubular Necrosis
Urine osmolality, mOsm/kg	>500	<400
Urine specific gravity	>1.018	Approximately 1.010
Urinary sodium level, mmol/L	<20	>40
Fractional excretion of sodium, %[a]	<1	>2
Fractional excretion of urea, %	<35	>35
Urinary sediment	Normal; occasional hyaline or fine granular casts	Renal tubular epithelial cells; granular and muddy brown casts

[a]Fractional Excertion of sodium

$$= \frac{[\text{Urinary sodium}] \times [\text{Plasma Creatinine}]}{[\text{Plasma sodium}] \times [\text{Urinary Creatinine}]} \times 100$$

Adapted from Schrier RW, Wang W, Poole B, Mitra A. Acute renal failure: definitions, diagnosis, pathogenesis, and therapy. J Clin Invest. 2004 Jul;114(1):5–14. Erratum in: J Clin Invest. 2004 Aug;114(4):598. Used with permission.

Table 49.4 • Use of Ultrasonography in Differential Diagnosis of Acute Kidney Injury

Ultrasonographic Finding	Diagnosis
Shrunken kidneys	Chronic kidney disease
Normal-sized kidneys	
Echogenic	Acute glomerulonephritis Acute tubular necrosis
Normal echo pattern	Prerenal acute renal failure Acute renal artery occlusion
Enlarged kidneys	Malignancy Renal vein thrombosis Diabetic nephropathy HIV-associated nephropathy
Hydronephrosis	Obstructive nephropathy

Abbreviation: HIV, human immunodeficiency virus.

Adapted from Lameire N, Van Biesen W, Vanholder R. Epidemiology, clinical evaluation, and prevention of acute renal failure. In: Feehally J, Floege J, Johnson RJ, editors. Comprehensive clinical nephrology. 3rd ed. Philadelphia (PA): Mosby Elsevier; c2007. p. 771–85. Used with permission.

Biomarkers

Since the early 2000s, many tubular cell injury biomarkers have been discovered. Proteins such as neutrophil gelatinase-associated lipocalin (NGAL) and kidney injury molecule-1 (KIM-1) could potentially be used for the differential diagnosis of AKI and for the early diagnosis of AKI along with prognostication of outcomes.

Management of AKI

The management of patients with AKI is mostly supportive. Determining and managing the risk factors associated with AKI are essential steps to decrease the extent of the injury (Box 49.8).

KEY FACTS

✓ Urinary sediment examination for renal disorders—very specific but not sensitive

✓ Oliguric patients—measurement of fractional excretion of sodium helps distinguish prerenal azotemia from ATN

✓ Kidney biopsy—indicated when renal parenchymal diseases are suspected from history, physical examination, and urinary sediment

✓ Management of AKI—early diagnosis and risk factor mitigation with mainly supportive therapy

Renal Replacement Therapy

The goals for renal replacement therapy in AKI are to maintain fluid, electrolyte, acid-base, and solute balance and to prevent further insult and promote healing. Renal

---

Box 49.8 • Management Recommendations According to the Stage of Acute Kidney Injury

High risk

Discontinue all nephrotoxic agents when possible
Ensure volume status and perfusion pressure
Consider functional hemodynamic monitoring
Monitor serum creatinine and urine output
Avoid hyperglycemia
Consider alternatives to radiocontrast procedures

Stage 1

All the above *and*
Perform noninvasive diagnostic workup
Consider invasive diagnostic workup

Stage 2

All the above *and*
Check for changes in drug dosing
Consider renal replacement therapy
Consider admission to intensive care unit

Stage 3

All the above *and*
Avoid use of subclavian catheter if possible

Adapted from Kidney Disease: Improving Global Outcomes (KDIGO) Acute Kidney Injury Work Group. KDIGO clinical practice guideline for acute kidney injury. Kidney Int Suppl. 2012 Mar;2(1):1–138. Used with permission.

---

replacement therapy should be considered for patients who have diuretic-resistant volume overload, severe electrolyte disorders (typically hyperkalemia with electrocardiographic changes), acid-base disorders, and uremic symptoms (metabolic encephalopathy or other evidence of nervous system toxicity, pericarditis, and bleeding believed to be due to uremic platelet dysfunction).

50 Chronic Kidney Disease

CARRIE A. SCHINSTOCK, MD

Epidemiology

Chronic kidney disease (CKD) is a worldwide public health problem. In the United States, the prevalence of end-stage renal disease (ESRD) is increasing, especially among patients older than 65 years. More than 20 million people in the United States are thought to have CKD, and this population consumes a disproportionate amount of health care resources. CKD is also associated with increased mortality, particularly from cardiovascular causes.

Certain ethnic groups have an increased incidence of CKD. In the United States, African Americans have the highest incidence of CKD, followed by American Indians and Alaskan natives; Asian Americans, native Hawaiians, and other Pacific Islanders; Hispanics; and whites. The main risk factors for the development of CKD include diabetes mellitus and hypertension. Other major causes include glomerulonephritis, inherited disorders such as polycystic kidney disease, congenital urologic abnormalities, renal obstruction, and autoimmune disease.

Definition and Staging

Chronic kidney disease is defined by the presence of kidney damage or decreased kidney function (as indicated by decreased glomerular filtration rate [GFR]) for 3 or more months. **Kidney damage** refers to abnormal renal histology, abnormal urine sediment (ie, white or red blood cell casts), or albuminuria (>30 mg/dL).

Key Definition

Chronic kidney disease: *kidney damage or decreased kidney function (as indicated by decreased GFR) for ≥3 months.*

Key Definition

Kidney damage: *abnormal renal histology, abnormal urine sediment (ie, white or red blood cell casts), or albuminuria (>30 mg/dL).*

GFR is most often estimated with various equations that are based on the serum creatinine level in some combination with age, sex, race, and body size (Box 50.1). The use of serum creatinine alone is not optimal for assessing

---

Box 50.1 • Equations for Estimating Glomerular Filtration Rate

MDRD Study equation

$$\text{eGFR (mL/min/1.73 m}^2) = 175 \times (\text{SCr})^{-1.154} \times \text{Age}^{-0.203} \times 0.742 \text{ (if Female)} \times 1.212 \text{ (if African American)}$$

CKD-EPI equation

$$\text{eGFR} = 141 \times \min (\text{SCr}/\kappa, 1)^{\alpha} \times \max(\text{SCr}/\kappa, 1)^{-1.209} \times 0.993^{\text{Age}} \times 1.018 \text{ (if Female)} \times 1.159 \text{ (if African American)}$$

κ is 0.7 for females and 0.9 for males
α is −0.329 for females and −0.411 for males
min indicates the minimum of SCr/κ or 1
max indicates the maximum of SCr/κ or 1

Cockroft-Gault formula

$$\text{eGFR} = 0.85 \text{ (if Female)} \times [(140 - \text{Age})/(\text{SCr})] \times (\text{Weight}/72)$$

Abbreviations: CKD-EPI, Chronic Kidney Disease Epidemiology Collaboration; eGFR, estimated glomerular filtration rate; MDRD, Modification of Diet in Renal Disease; SCr, serum creatinine.

Data from United States Renal Data System, 2014 Annual Data Report: Epidemiology of Kidney Disease in the United States. Bethesda, MD: National Institutes of Health, National Institute of Diabetes and Digestive and Kidney Diseases; 2014.

Table 50.1 • Stages of Chronic Kidney Disease

Stage	GFR, mL/min/1.73 m²
1	>90[a]
2	60–89
3a	45–59
3b	30–44
4	15–29
5	<15

Abbreviation: GFR, glomerular filtration rate.
[a] With signs of renal damage (eg, proteinuria).

Table 50.2 • Stages of Albuminuria

Stage	Albumin Excretion Rate, mg/24 h
1	<30
2	30–300
3	>300

the level of kidney function. Currently, the most commonly used equation is the Modification of Diet in Renal Disease (MDRD) Study equation, but the Chronic Kidney Disease Epidemiology Collaboration (CKD-EPI) equation is more reliable for patients with GFR greater than 60 mL/min/1.73 m² and is increasingly being used. However, the CKD-EPI equation is still being validated, and this equation has not been implemented for widespread use. The Cockcroft-Gault formula was historically used most often, but it is considered less accurate than the MDRD equation in many cases.

Although the gold standard for measuring GFR is based on measuring the clearance of exogenous substances, such as inulin, iothalamate, and other radiolabeled markers, methods of determining an estimated GFR (eGFR) are considered the best overall indexes of the level of kidney function because they are readily available and have been most fully evaluated. The serum concentration of cystatin C is another marker of kidney function that is not completely validated for regular use in clinical practice. Calculating a 24-hour creatinine clearance with serum creatinine level and 24-hour urine collection is also suboptimal because of the tubular secretion of creatinine, especially with renal dysfunction and the difficulty with obtaining a reliable, timed urine collection. All these equations are unreliable in pediatric patients, in patients with unstable creatinine concentrations, and in patients with extremes in muscle mass or diet.

CKD and albuminuria are classified in stages to help guide management. CKD is staged from 1 to 5 (Table 50.1), and albuminuria is staged from 1 to 3 (Table 50.2). A patient is considered to have ESRD when dialysis is required.

Screening for CKD in High-Risk Patients

There is insufficient evidence to support screening for CKD in asymptomatic adults. However, screening can be considered for patients who are at high risk for CKD. Clinical factors that increase the risk of CKD include having diabetes mellitus, hypertension, autoimmune disease, systemic

infection, urinary tract infection, nephrolithiasis, urinary tract obstruction, malignancy, family history of CKD, history of acute kidney injury (AKI), small kidney mass (ie, low birth weight), or exposure to certain drugs (ie, amphotericin). Other factors include being elderly, being in an ethnic minority, or having a low socioeconomic status. Monitoring blood pressure, serum creatinine, and urine albumin are reasonable screening tests for patients at higher risk.

Management of CKD

The general management approach for CKD includes the following: 1) recognize and treat the reversible causes of renal failure; 2) prevent the progressive decline in renal function; 3) manage the complications of renal failure; 4) ensure that medications are dosed appropriately according to GFR; 5) educate the patient about the increased risk of AKI; and 6) refer the patient to a nephrologist for AKI, complex CKD care, and preparation for renal replacement therapy (Box 50.2).

Recognize and Treat Reversible Causes of Renal Failure

Recognition of recent (<3 months) renal dysfunction is important because it is more likely to be reversible than CKD. Major causes of AKI are summarized in Box 50.3. The diagnosis and management of AKI are reviewed in Chapter 49, "Acute Kidney Injury."

Box 50.2 • Approach for Managing Chronic Kidney Disease

1. Treat reversible causes of renal failure
2. Prevent further worsening of renal function
3. Manage complications of renal failure
4. Dose medications according to glomerular filtration rate
5. Educate the patient about the increased risk of acute kidney injury
6. Refer the patient to a nephrologist for acute kidney injury, complex chronic kidney disease, or preparation for renal replacement therapy

---

> ### Box 50.3 • Major Causes of Acute Kidney Injury
>
> Prerenal
>
> > Renovascular disease
> > Hypovolemia
> > Angiotensin-converting enzyme inhibitors
> > Angiotensin receptor blockers
> > Nonsteroidal anti-inflammatory drugs
>
> Intrinsic renal
>
> > Glomerulonephritis
> > Interstitial nephritis
> > Nephrotoxic medications
> > Cystic renal disease
>
> Postrenal
>
> > Renal obstruction (prostate enlargement, renal or
> > bladder stones, mass lesions)
> > Congenital ureteral abnormalities

Prevent Progressive Decline in Renal Function

Most importantly, identify the cause of renal dysfunction and treat appropriately if possible. Several factors are associated with the progression of renal dysfunction, including proteinuria, hypertension, African American race, *APOL1* risk alleles, nephrolithiasis, low socioeconomic status, male sex, obesity, diabetes mellitus, hyperlipidemia, smoking, high-protein diet, phosphate retention, and metabolic acidosis. Often these risk factors are irreversible, and the treatment of other risk factors has not been proved to effectively reduce the progression of renal dysfunction.

Blood pressure control, reduction in proteinuria, glycemic control (target hemoglobin A_{1c} <7%), smoking cessation, and treatment of chronic metabolic acidosis have all been independently shown to prevent the progression of renal disease. Several organizations have developed guidelines to aid in managing hypertension. Controversy exists regarding the optimal blood pressure target for patients with CKD, but most organizations support a blood pressure of less than 140/90 mm Hg because there is insufficient evidence that a blood pressure goal of less than 130/80 mm Hg delays the progression of CKD.

Angiotensin-converting enzyme (ACE) inhibitors and angiotensin receptor blockers (ARBs) are recommended for patients with proteinuria. These agents can be used in patients at any stage of CKD but should be initiated when the renal function is stable. Serum creatinine and potassium levels should be checked 2 to 3 weeks after initiation.

Manage Complications of CKD

Volume Overload and Sodium Disorders

In advanced stages of CKD, the kidney loses its ability to appropriately dilute or concentrate urine, leading to disorders in sodium balance (hyponatremia or hypernatremia).

Additionally, sodium retention occurs with CKD; particularly when the GFR is less than 10 mL/min/1.73 m². Sodium retention contributes to hypertension, edema, and congestive heart failure. Sodium restriction (<2 g daily) and diuretics are often necessary.

Hyperkalemia

Potassium excretion is impaired in advanced CKD, particularly when oliguria leads to hyperkalemia. Concomitant metabolic acidosis, which causes a shift of potassium from the intracellular space to the extracellular space, can exacerbate this electrolyte disturbance. Moreover, hyporeninemic hypoaldosteronism, which often occurs in tubulointerstitial disease and diabetes mellitus, is also associated with hyperkalemia. The mainstay of treatment is dietary restriction, but loop diuretics and potassium-binding resins are occasionally needed. Complete review of prescription and nonprescription medications is also necessary. Drugs that are commonly associated with hyperkalemia include ACE inhibitors, ARBs, potassium-sparing diuretics, β-blockers, aldosterone antagonists, nonsteroidal anti-inflammatory drugs, and calcineurin inhibitors. Hyperkalemia associated with electrocardiographic change is a nephrologic emergency and an indication for dialysis if not rapidly treated medically.

> ### KEY FACTS
>
> ✓ Stages of CKD and albuminuria—useful for guiding management
> ✓ Prevent progression of renal disease with blood pressure control, reduction in proteinuria, glycemic control (hemoglobin A_{1c} <7%), smoking cessation, and treatment of chronic metabolic acidosis
> ✓ Potassium excretion—impaired in advanced CKD

Anemia of Chronic Disease

Anemia is a common complication of CKD and contributes to fatigue and reduced quality of life in patients with CKD. CKD is associated with inappropriate erythropoietin production, but reduced bone marrow erythropoiesis and decreased iron absorption also contribute to this condition. The reduced bone marrow erythropoiesis is associated with chronic inflammation. Decreased iron absorption is also related to inflammation, which induces the liver to produce hepcidin. This protein interferes with the iron export protein ferroportin, thereby inhibiting iron absorption.

Initial diagnostic studies for patients with suspected anemia of chronic disease include the following: 1) complete blood cell count with a differential leukocyte count, reticulocyte index, and peripheral smear and 2) serum iron studies, including serum iron level, total iron-binding capacity, and transferrin saturation. Anemia of chronic disease in the absence of other causes of anemia is normocytic and normochromic. The serum iron concentration and transferrin level (also measured as total iron-binding capacity) are both low, and the transferrin saturation is usually normal or low-normal. In contrast, with iron deficiency the transferrin level is increased and transferrin saturation is low. Ferritin is an unreliable marker of iron stores in CKD because it can be elevated in the presence of inflammation. A coexisting iron deficiency is often present.

Treatment of anemia in CKD patients who are not receiving dialysis should be limited mainly to patients with symptoms. Treatment includes erythropoietin-stimulating agents, red blood cell transfusion, or supplemental iron if needed (parenteral iron is most effective because gastrointestinal absorption of iron is abnormal in CKD). Erythropoietin-stimulating agents are associated with thromboembolism; therefore, these agents should be held if hemoglobin approaches 12 g/dL.

Metabolic Acidosis

Metabolic acidosis is a common complication of CKD and occurs as a result of reduced ammonium excretion, retention of hydrogen ions, and reduced excretion of titratable acid. The prevalence of metabolic acidosis increases as the stage of CKD increases: A bicarbonate concentration less than 22 mmol/L is present in less than 5% of patients with stage 1 CKD, but it is present in approximately 25% of patients with stage 5 CKD who are not yet receiving dialysis. Lower serum bicarbonate has been associated with a higher risk of progressive renal dysfunction in several observational and randomized studies. Other potential benefits of bicarbonate therapy include the prevention of osteopenia and bone disease associated with renal hyperparathyroidism, improved nutritional status, and improved lean body mass.

Mineral and Bone Disorder

CKD results in disordered calcium and phosphorus metabolism, leading to a broad spectrum of disorders, including hyperparathyroidism (Figure 50.1), abnormal bone turnover, and vascular and soft tissue calcification (Table 50.3). Calcium and phosphorus homeostasis can be restored as the parathyroid increases the release of parathyroid hormone (PTH) in response to hypocalcemia from reduced production of calcitriol (also called 1,25-dihydroxycholecalciferol or dihydroxyvitamin D$_3$) and in response to hyperphosphatemia from decreased renal excretion of phosphate.

PTH is a calcemic hormone that targets the kidney, bone, and gastrointestinal tract and promotes calcium conservation by increasing reabsorption of calcium, promoting calcitriol synthesis, increasing calcium efflux from bone, and increasing calcium absorption from the gastrointestinal tract. In addition, PTH leads to a reduction in phosphorus absorption by the kidney but also to increased phosphorus absorption by the gastrointestinal tract and increased

phosphorus efflux by the bone. The main phosphaturic hormone is fibroblast growth factor 23 (FGF23). Over time, hyperparathyroidism leads to disruptions in bone turnover, including high bone turnover, osteitis fibrosis, defective mineralization (osteomalacia), and low bone turnover–adynamic bone disease. The result of these bone defects is fracture. Besides having detrimental effects on bone, hyperparathyroidism leads to calcification of soft tissues, blood vessels, heart valves, and skin. Increased cardiovascular calcification is thought to be involved in the increased cardiovascular mortality of patients with CKD, particularly ESRD. One of the most devastating forms of calcification is calcemic uremic arteriopathy or calciphylaxis. This is a form of vascular calcification in which the patient presents with extensive calcifications of the skin, muscles, and subcutaneous tissues leading to ulcerations and necrosis.

Phosphate retention in CKD leads to an increase in serum FGF23, which increases urinary phosphorus excretion and thereby maintains serum phosphorus levels. This biomarker is elevated in the early stages of CKD before alterations in PTH or serum phosphorus are detected. FGF23 also leads to decreased levels of calcitriol.

Monitoring for hyperparathyroidism involves regular monitoring of calcium, phosphorus, PTH, and calcitriol. Treatment is aimed at normalizing the levels of serum calcium, phosphate, and PTH while minimizing the risks of therapy. In addition to dietary phosphorus restriction, other commonly used therapies are phosphorus binders, vitamin D metabolites, calcimimetic agents, and parathyroidectomy.

Cardiovascular Disease

A large body of evidence indicates that patients with CKD have a substantially higher cardiovascular risk that can be explained in part by an increase in traditional risk factors such as hypertension, diabetes mellitus, and the metabolic syndrome. However, CKD alone is also an independent risk factor for cardiovascular disease. Among patients with CKD, the risk of death, particularly death due to cardiovascular disease, is much higher than the risk of eventually requiring dialysis. CKD is considered an equivalent to coronary artery disease in terms of risk for future cardiovascular events; thus, cardiovascular risk factors (diabetes mellitus, hyperlipidemia, and hypertension) should be aggressively managed. Lipid-lowering therapy has been an intense area of interest for patients with CKD. The effect of lipid-lowering therapy varies according to the stage of CKD. Lipid-lowering therapy, particularly with statins, is most helpful in patients with CKD who are not undergoing hemodialysis.

Hypoalbuminemia

Hypoalbuminemia is common in patients with CKD, particularly patients with nephrotic syndrome or ESRD who are undergoing hemodialysis. In nephrotic syndrome,

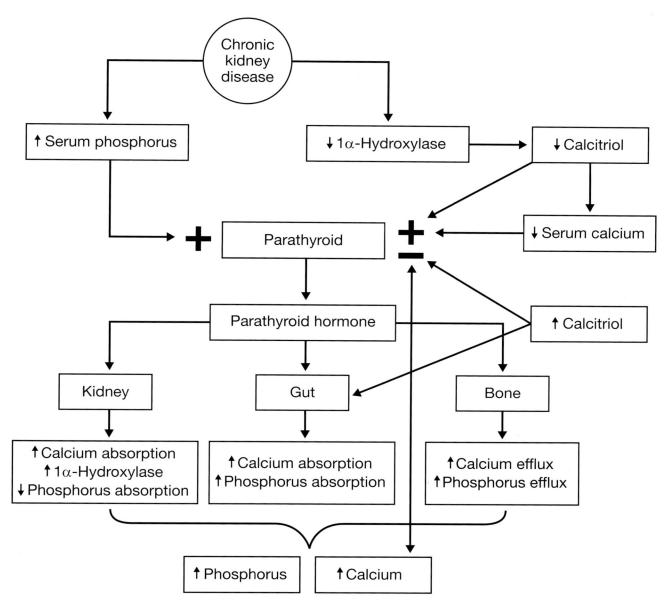

Figure 50.1 *Mechanisms of Hyperparathyroidism in Chronic Kidney Disease. Calcitriol is the active form of vitamin D. Plus signs indicate positive feedback; negative sign, negative feedback.*

hypoalbuminemia results from ongoing renal protein losses. In ESRD, reduced protein synthesis and increased protein breakdown in the presence of chronic systemic inflammation is the most common cause of hypoalbuminemia. Hypoalbuminemia is a poor prognostic factor. Albumin supplementation is not beneficial in CKD.

Cutaneous Manifestations

Pruritus, pallor, ecchymosis, and hyperpigmentation are usually signs of advanced CKD and often indicate the need for initiating dialysis. Pruritus often improves (but not always) with the initiation of dialysis. The mechanism leading to pruritus is not clear, but secondary hyperparathyroidism, dry skin, peripheral neuropathy, high aluminum levels, hyperphosphatemia, and hypervitaminosis A are potential contributors.

Neurologic Manifestations

Advanced stages of CKD are associated with several neurologic manifestations, including cognitive impairment, depression, fatigue, confusion, irritability, anxiety, and peripheral neuropathy. Indications for the initiation of dialysis include severe neurologic manifestations such as lethargy, stupor, and coma.

Table 50.3 • Chronic Kidney Disease Complications Stratified by Glomerular Filtration Rate (GFR)[a]

Complication	GFR, mL/min/1.73 m²				
	≥90	60–89	45–59	30–44	<30
Anemia	4.0	4.7	12.3	22.7	51.5
Hypertension	18.3	41.0	71.8	78.3	82.1
Calcitriol deficiency	14.1	9.1	10.7	10.7	27.2
Acidosis	11.2	8.4	9.4	18.1	31.5
Hyperphosphatemia	7.2	7.4	9.2	9.3	23.0
Hypoalbuminemia	1.0	1.3	2.8	9.0	7.5
Hyperparathyroidism	5.5	9.4	23.0	44.0	72.5

[a] Values are percentages of affected patients.

Adapted from Inker LA, Coresh J, Levey AS, Tonelli M, Muntner P. Estimated GFR, albuminuria, and complications of chronic kidney disease. J Am Soc Nephrol. 2011 Dec;22(12):2322–31. Epub 2011 Sep 30. Used with permission.

Uremic Syndrome

The gradual decline in function in patients with CKD is initially asymptomatic. As patients progress to ESRD, uremia is manifested by loss of appetite and weight loss, nausea, vomiting, pericarditis, peripheral neuropathy, and confusion. Severe uremia can result in seizures, coma, and death in the absence of dialysis. No direct correlation exists between signs and symptoms of ESRD and creatinine or serum urea nitrogen level.

Ensure Appropriate Dosing of Medications According to GFR

When medications excreted by the kidney are prescribed, the GFR must be estimated, usually with the various estimating equations. However, assessing kidney function with alternative methods, such as measured creatinine clearance or measured GFR with the use of exogenous filtration markers, may be useful in the following situations: when prescribing drugs with a therapeutic window, when eGFR and creatinine clearance provide discrepant results, or when eGFR is likely inaccurate or unreliable (eg, from extremes of diet, body mass, or fluctuations in GFR).

Educate About Increased Risk of AKI

AKI is not only a risk factor for the development of CKD, but it is also a risk factor for progression in CKD. Progression occurs even when renal function appears to have recovered. The risk of progressive CKD is most pronounced in patients requiring temporary dialysis; all those patients should be followed by a nephrologist. Patients must be educated about the importance of avoiding known causes of preventable AKI, including nephrotoxic medications, nonsteroidal anti-inflammatory drugs, iodinated contrast agents, volume depletion, and hypotension.

KEY FACTS

✓ Anemia in CKD—from inappropriate erythropoietin production, reduced bone marrow erythropoiesis, and decreased iron absorption

✓ Disordered calcium and phosphorus metabolism in CKD causes hyperparathyroidism, abnormal bone turnover, and vascular and soft tissue calcification

✓ AKI—risk factor for development and progression of CKD

Consider Referral to a Nephrologist

Referral to a nephrologist should be considered when patients have AKI, stage 4 CKD (GFR <30 mL/min/1.73 m²), significant proteinuria (albumin to creatinine ratio ≥300 mg/g or protein to creatinine ratio >500 mg/g), unexplained hematuria or red blood cell casts, resistant hypertension, hereditary kidney disease, electrolyte abnormalities, or recurrent nephrolithiasis. Nephrologists can identify and treat causes of renal insufficiency, manage complications of CKD, and plan for renal replacement therapy with renal transplant, dialysis (in-center hemodialysis, peritoneal dialysis, or home hemodialysis), or both transplant and dialysis.

51 Electrolyte Disorders

QI QIAN, MD

Disorders of Sodium Balance and Volume Regulation

Volume expansion can be general (as in patients with congestive heart failure, cirrhosis, or nephrotic syndrome) or regional (as in patients with regional capillary leak, venous insufficiency, or lymphatic obstruction). Volume depletion is associated primarily with gastrointestinal tract (GI) fluid loss, excessive sweating, and renal sodium loss related to diuretic use or, rarely, renal salt wasting.

Diagnosis

The cause of a volume disorder can be determined by physical examination. Elevated systemic blood pressure with or without edema signifies total body sodium excess. In congestive heart failure and cirrhosis, the kidneys are stimulated to retain sodium because the systemic blood pressure is low from low arterial effective volume (arterial underfill) due to pump failure and circulation derangements. Sodium retention leads to a net positive sodium balance and edema. Regional volume expansion is typically obvious on physical examination: Vital signs are normal, and the areas of fluid retention are confined. Volume depletion is manifested by hypotension and tachycardia.

Therapy

Management of volume disorders is 2-fold: 1) volume repletion for hypovolemia and volume removal for hypervolemia with diuretics or dialysis (or both) when appropriate and 2) correction of the underlying causes. For patients with volume depletion, infusion of isotonic fluids and oral sodium restores volume status. In patients with congestive heart failure, measures that optimize cardiac function may improve renal perfusion and, therefore, facilitate diuresis. In cirrhosis, reduction of portal hypertension (ie,

transjugular intrahepatic portosystemic shunt) and liver transplant can improve hemodynamics. In nephrotic syndrome, correcting proteinuria restores sodium homeostasis and volume balance. Diuresis, in general, is unnecessary in patients with regional fluid retention (except for regional edema involving the airway).

Disorders of Water Balance

Hyponatremia (Water Excess)

Hyponatremia can be categorized as hypovolemic, euvolemic, or hypervolemic. Hypovolemia is a potent stimulus for secretion of antidiuretic hormone (ADH), also known as arginine vasopressin, leading to renal water retention and hyponatremia. Increased plasma osmolality is the other major stimulus for ADH secretion. Euvolemic hyponatremia includes 1) psychogenic polydipsia and beer potomania, in which water or hypotonic beer ingestion exceeds the capacity of renal water excretion; 2) **syndrome of inappropriate secretion of ADH** (SIADH), in which ADH-mediated water retention is independent of serum osmolality and volume status; and, rarely, 3) hypothyroidism and adrenal insufficiency. Hypervolemic hyponatremia mainly occurs in patients with congestive heart failure or cirrhosis. Arterial underfill in both conditions signals volume depletion and activates ADH-mediated water retention, resulting in hyponatremia. In patients with moderate to advanced renal failure, dilutional hyponatremia may develop because of the diminished capacity of renal water excretion.

Key Definition

Syndrome of inappropriate secretion of ADH: *ADH-mediated water retention that is independent of serum osmolality and volume status.*

Diagnosis

The initial step in evaluating patients with hyponatremia is to determine the serum osmolality. Hyperlipidemia and elevated total serum protein (ie, multiple myeloma) can cause pseudohyponatremia, when serum osmolality is normal. Hyperglycemia can cause hyperosmolar hyponatremia. As shown in Figure 51.1, if serum osmolality is reduced (true hyponatremia), the differential diagnosis is narrowed to 3 categories—hypovolemic, euvolemic, or hypervolemic hyponatremia—on the basis of the patient's volume status determined by physical examination. Urine osmolality and urinary sodium concentration can then further help with delineating the underlying cause of hyponatremia.

In patients with euvolemic hyponatremia, if the urine is not maximally diluted (>150 mOsm/kg) and the urinary sodium concentration is greater than 20 mmol/L (with a regular diet), thyroid disease and adrenal insufficiency must be ruled out before considering the diagnosis of SIADH. Patients with thiazide diuretic–induced hyponatremia may present with euvolemic hyponatremia that is indistinguishable from SIADH. Clinical history is critical in establishing causation. Postoperative pain can be associated with transient SIADH. Drugs associated with euvolemic hyponatremia include selective serotonin reuptake inhibitors, carbamazepine, chlorpromazine, vasopressin analogues, 3,4-methylenedioxymethamphetamine (also called MDMA or Ecstasy), and, rarely, theophylline and amiodarone.

Therapy

For isosmotic and hyperosmotic hyponatremia, management should be directed toward correcting the underlying cause.

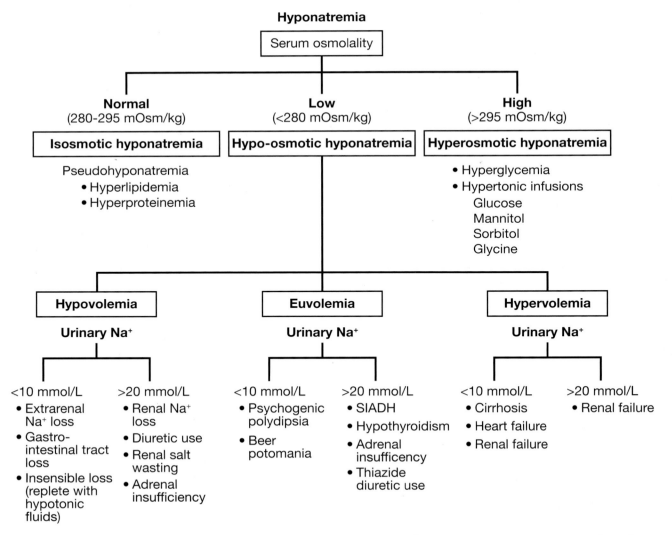

Figure 51.1 *Diagnosis of Hyponatremia. Na⁺ indicates sodium; SIADH, syndrome of inappropriate secretion of antidiuretic hormone.*

For hypovolemic hyponatremia, restoring intravascular volume eliminates the stimulatory signal for ADH. For patients with normal renal clearance, renal water unloading normalizes serum sodium concentration and osmolality.

For hypervolemic hyponatremia, symptomatic treatment directed toward reducing both total body water and sodium (aquaresis more than natriuresis) is necessary. Loop diuretics are usually effective. Correcting the underlying cardiac and hepatic abnormalities, if possible, will ultimately correct the water dysregulation.

For euvolemic hyponatremia, including SIADH, treatment options include restricting free water, discontinuing use of all potential contributors of hyponatremia, initiating low-dose loop diuretics in combination with oral sodium chloride, and, when symptomatic, administering high-concentration (3%) saline. Currently, lithium, demeclocycline, and long-term use of vasopressin receptor antagonists are not recommended. Specific attention should be paid to the rate of serum sodium correction. When hyponatremia develops over more than 2 days, correction should be gradual (≤10 mmol/L in the first 24 hours and <18 mmol/L in the first 48 hours). Rapid correction could lead to osmotic demyelination syndrome (also known as central pontine myelinolysis), a devastating neurologic complication including quadriplegia, coma, and the "locked-in" state. Underlying causes of SIADH should always be sought and, when possible, corrected.

KEY FACTS

✓ Management of volume disorder—volume repletion for hypovolemia, volume removal for hypervolemia, and correction of underlying cause

✓ ADH secretion—stimulated by hypovolemia and by increased plasma osmolality

✓ Evaluation of hyponatremia—first determine serum osmolality

✓ Euvolemic hyponatremia—with urine osmolality >150 mOsm/kg and urinary sodium >20 mmol/L, rule out thyroid disease and adrenal insufficiency before considering SIADH

✓ Drugs that can cause euvolemic hyponatremia—selective serotonin reuptake inhibitors, carbamazepine, chlorpromazine, vasopressin analogues, MDMA (Ecstasy), theophylline, and amiodarone

✓ Serum sodium correction for hyponatremia—gradual (≤10 mmol/L in first 24 hours and <18 mmol/L in first 48 hours) to avoid osmotic demyelination syndrome

Hypernatremia (Water Deficiency)

Hypernatremia (Figure 51.2) occurs with 1) decreased oral water intake (insufficient water provision or impairment of central nervous system thirst response); 2) increased renal water loss (diabetes insipidus [DI] or diuretic or aquaretic medications), osmotic diuresis from hyperalimentation, GI water loss (osmotic diarrhea), or insensible water loss (sweat and respiration); and 3) hypertonic sodium-containing fluid administration (intravenous administration of concentrated sodium bicarbonate solution). There is almost always a degree of overlap in excessive water loss and insufficient water intake. Hypernatremia occurs mostly in the elderly and infants and increases mortality among hospitalized patients.

Diagnosis

Unlike hyponatremia, for which confirmation of hypo-osmolality is necessary, hypernatremia is always associated with hyperosmolality; hence, there is no need to measure serum osmolality.

Urine osmolality and volume help differentiate renal from extrarenal water loss. Renal water wasting is typically associated with dilute urine and high urine volume (>3 L/d), whereas extrarenal water loss is associated with maximally concentrated urine (>900 mOsm/kg) and urine output is usually low-normal (<1.0–1.5 L/d).

Renal water wasting can be confirmed by determining random urinary sodium and potassium concentrations. Renal water wasting is signified if the sum of the urinary sodium and potassium concentrations is less than the serum sodium concentration. Investigations for osmotic diuresis and DI are indicated.

Osmotic Diuresis

Patients with osmotic diuresis may present with polyuria and hypernatremia. The osmolality of their urine is typically similar to the plasma osmolality. Osmotic diuresis can be confirmed by calculating the total daily solute excretion. Normal solute excretion for an adult is approximately 700 to 1,000 mOsm/d (about 10 mOsm/kg/d). If solute excretion in a 24-hour urine sample is greater than normal, the presence of osmotic diuresis is confirmed.

Diabetes Insipidus

DI can be classified into 2 major types: central DI and nephrogenic DI. **Central DI** is due to insufficiency or absence of endogenous ADH. **Nephrogenic DI** is due to a partial or complete unresponsiveness of the renal tubular cells to ADH. Nephrogenic DI can be caused by genetic disorders, but more commonly it is caused by various acquired conditions. Lithium, demeclocycline, and amphotericin B are well-known drugs that can cause renal concentration defect and nephrogenic DI.

Key Definitions

Central diabetes insipidus: *insufficient or absent endogenous ADH.*

Nephrogenic diabetes insipidus: *renal tubular cells partially or completely unresponsive to ADH.*

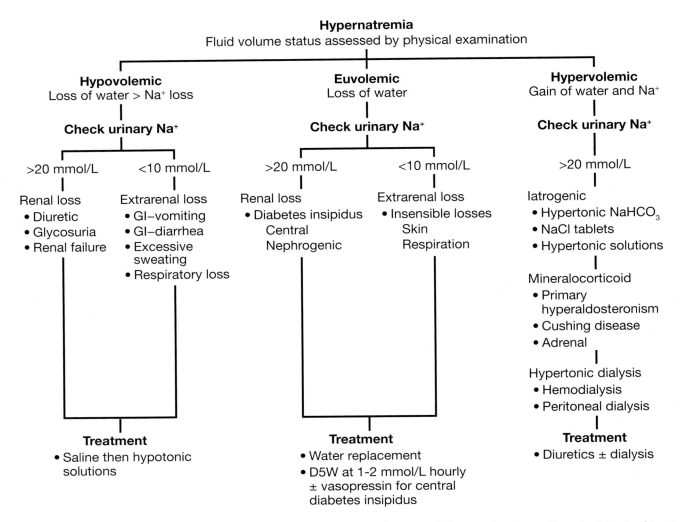

Figure 51.2 *Diagnosis and Management of Hypernatremia. D5W indicates 5% dextrose in water; GI, gastrointestinal tract; Na⁺, sodium; NaCl, sodium chloride; NaHCO₃, sodium bicarbonate.*

Diagnosis

DI is diagnosed with a water deprivation study, during which the combination of high serum sodium concentration (>145 mmol/L) and low urine osmolality (<150 mOsm/kg) constitutes a positive result and is diagnostic for DI.

If a patient presents with both hypernatremia (>145 mmol/L) and dilute urine (<150 mOsm/kg) without receiving any aquaretic medications, those findings are sufficient to establish a diagnosis of DI. A water deprivation study is not necessary.

After a diagnosis of DI is made, intranasal or intravenous desmopressin may be administered to differentiate central DI from nephrogenic DI. Desmopressin should be administered only when the serum sodium concentration is greater than 145 mmol/L. Central DI is diagnosed if the urine osmolality increases in response to desmopressin.

Nephrogenic DI is diagnosed if there is no change in urine osmolality with desmopressin.

DI-associated polyuria should be differentiated from psychogenic polydipsia. Determination of the serum sodium concentration helps with the differentiation. In patients with psychogenic polydipsia, polyuria is driven by excessive water intake; thus, serum sodium concentration is typically in the lower end of the reference range (<140 mmol/ L). Patients with DI, however, typically have serum sodium concentrations that are in the upper end of the reference range (>140 mmol/ L) or greater.

Therapy

The same principles for correcting hyponatremia apply to correcting hypernatremia. When hypernatremia develops over the course of more than 2 days, correction of sodium concentration should be gradual (≤10 mmol/L/d).

Disorders of Potassium Balance

Hypokalemia

Hypokalemia can be associated with pseudohypokalemia, transcellular shift, inadequate intake, GI loss, or renal loss. Hypokalemia (excluding pseudohypokalemia) can cause cellular hyperpolarization. Manifestations of hypokalemia include electrocardiographic (ECG) changes (blunted T wave and appearance of U wave as in Figure 51.3), muscle weakness, ileus, polyuria (functional nephrogenic DI), and, in severe cases, rhabdomyolysis and asystole.

Diagnosis

Pseudohypokalemia due to active cellular potassium uptake in the test tube (leukocytosis or leukemia) should be

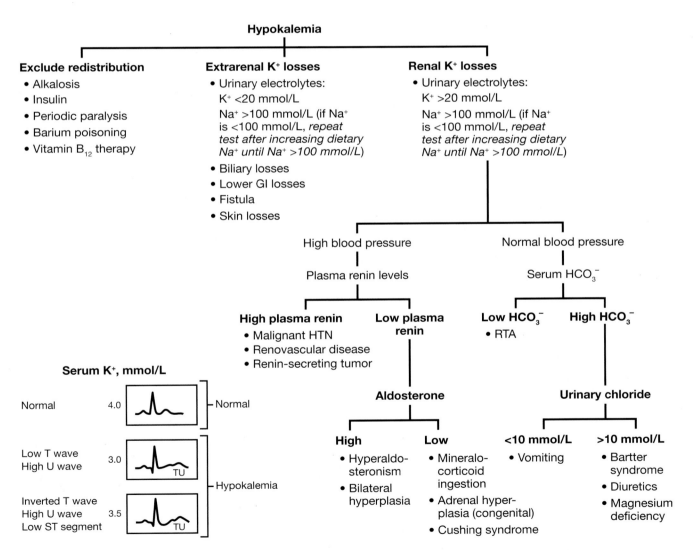

Figure 51.3 *Diagnosis of Hypokalemia. GI indicates gastrointestinal tract; HCO$_3$⁻, bicarbonate; HTN, hypertension; K⁺, potassium; Na⁺, sodium; RTA, renal tubular acidosis.*

ruled out when appropriate. If the plasma is immediately separated from the blood sample, this error can be avoided.

Hypokalemia caused by transcellular shift is typically transient. Pertinent clinical history provides key diagnostic clues, especially for rare hereditary types of hypokalemic paralysis.

As shown in Figure 51.3, quantifying urinary potassium is a key step in delineating the underlying (GI or renal) causes of hypokalemia.

Therapy

Potassium repletion can be achieved with oral or intravenous supplementation. Intravenous potassium infusion is indicated for patients who have severe symptomatic hypokalemia or who lack GI access. Intravenous potassium should be given in a saline-based solution rather than a dextrose-containing solution because sugar stimulates insulin secretion, shifting potassium intracellularly and exacerbating hypokalemia. A central line is preferred for the infusion since potassium can be corrosive to peripheral vessels. The rate of potassium infusion should not exceed 10 mmol/h.

Hyperkalemia

Hyperkalemia (Figure 51.4) can be associated with pseudohyperkalemia, excessive potassium intake, transcellular shift,

and impaired secretion of renal potassium. Hyperkalemia (excluding pseudohyperkalemia) can cause cellular depolarization. Clinical manifestations include ECG changes (peaked T wave, shortened QT interval, and prolonged PR interval with widened QRS complex, as in Figure 51.4) and muscle weakness or frank paralysis. These manifestations may occur when the serum potassium concentration exceeds 6.5 to 7.0 mmol/L. Severe hyperkalemia can cause lethal cardiac arrhythmia (sine wave or complete absence of electrical activity—cardiac standstill), although a precise numerical correlation between the ECG changes and serum potassium concentrations has not been established.

Diagnosis

Rule out pseudohyperkalemia due to cell lysis during or after blood sampling from use of a small needle and inadequate technique. Use of a needle of an appropriate size and optimal technique can eliminate the problem.

Hyperkalemia caused by increased potassium intake occurs typically in patients with some degree of kidney dysfunction, and impaired kidney function is a major cause of persistent hyperkalemia. Urinary tract outlet obstruction (eg, benign prostatic hypertrophy) can cause hyperkalemia due to impaired collecting duct potassium excretion.

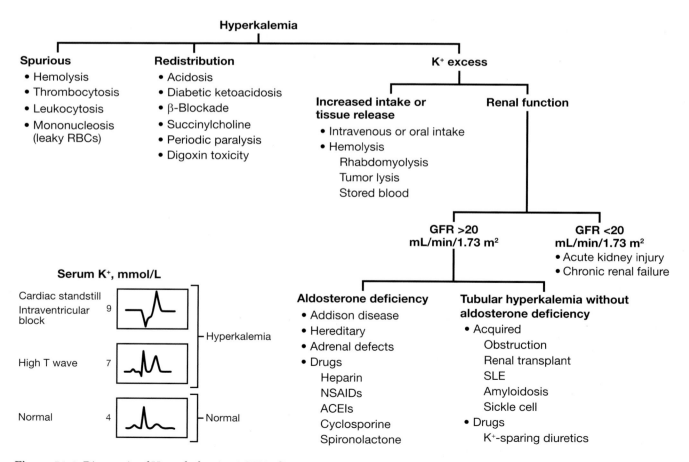

Figure 51.4 *Diagnosis of Hyperkalemia. ACEI indicates angiotensin-converting enzyme inhibitor; GFR, glomerular filtration rate; K+, potassium; NSAID, nonsteroidal anti-inflammatory drug; RBC, red blood cell; SLE, systemic lupus erythematosus.*

Cellular breakdown (rhabdomyolysis and tumor lysis syndrome) can acutely release cellular potassium into the circulation. Nonorganic metabolic acidosis and hyperosmolality (hyperglycemia or administration of osmotically active solutions) can shift intracellular potassium out to the extracellular space. Other conditions that can cause hyperkalemia include hyporeninemic hypoaldosteronism and medications such as potassium-sparing diuretics, nonsteroidal anti-inflammatory drugs, calcineurin inhibitors, angiotensin-converting enzyme inhibitors, angiotensin receptor blockers, and heparin.

Therapy

Therapy is dictated by the severity and underlying causes of hyperkalemia. For patients with ECG changes, urgent intravenous administration of calcium is indicated to stabilize the myocardium. Simultaneously, intravenous insulin, dextrose solution (5% or 10%), and inhaled β-agonist should be administered to promote an intracellular potassium shift. If acidosis is present, sodium bicarbonate may be given to correct it. When appropriate, non–potassium-sparing diuretics and potassium-exchange resin (sodium polystyrene) may be used to promote renal and GI potassium excretion. For asymptomatic patients with mild to moderate hyperkalemia (<6 mmol/L), dietary potassium restriction, non–potassium-sparing diuretics, and potassium-exchange resin may suffice. For patients with advanced renal failure or hyperkalemia that is refractory to conservative measures, dialysis is necessary.

While the above measures mitigate hyperkalemia, steps should be taken to correct the underlying causes. Correcting a urinary tract obstruction can increase urinary potassium excretion. Medication-induced hyperkalemia should be corrected by adjusting the medication regimen.

KEY FACTS

✓ Hypokalemia—ECG shows blunted T wave and appearance of U wave

✓ Therapy for hypokalemia—replete potassium before correcting acidemia

✓ Hyperkalemia—ECG shows peaked T wave, shortened QT interval, and prolonged PR interval with widened QRS complex

✓ Diagnosis of hyperkalemia—rule out pseudohyperkalemia due to cell lysis; consider kidney dysfunction, cellular breakdown, urinary tract outlet obstruction, and medications

✓ Drugs that can cause hyperkalemia—potassium-sparing diuretics, nonsteroidal anti-inflammatory drugs, calcineurin inhibitors, angiotensin-converting enzyme inhibitors, angiotensin receptor blockers, and heparin

✓ Therapy for severe hyperkalemia with ECG changes—urgent intravenous calcium; also, intravenous insulin and dextrose and inhaled β-agonist

✓ Therapy for mild to moderate hyperkalemia—dietary potassium restriction, non–potassium-sparing diuretics, and potassium-exchange resin

52 Renal Parenchymal Diseases

SUZANNE M. NORBY, MD AND FERNANDO C. FERVENZA, MD, PHD

Tubulointerstitial Disease

Acute and chronic interstitial inflammation can result in injury to renal tubules, leading to tubular dysfunction and, chronically, tubular atrophy. Acute interstitial nephritis is discussed in Chapter 49, "Acute Kidney Injury." Causes of chronic tubulointerstitial damage include autoimmune and hereditary causes, analgesic nephropathy, uric acid, lithium, heavy metals, mercury, lead, and oxalate. Proteinuria (usually <1.5 g/1.73 m²/24 h) and sterile pyuria may be present.

Analgesic Nephropathy

Analgesic nephropathy is a slowly progressive chronic interstitial nephritis caused by long-term consumption of mixed analgesic preparations, frequently complicated by papillary necrosis and resulting in bilateral renal atrophy. Renal damage can develop from the use of acetaminophen in combination with aspirin and from long-term use of nonsteroidal anti-inflammatory drugs (NSAIDs). Noncontrast computed tomographic imaging of the kidneys has become the standard method for diagnosing analgesic nephropathy. No specific treatment is available. Patients with analgesic nephropathy are at an increased risk for uroepithelial tumors, particularly transitional cell carcinomas (in the renal pelvis, ureter, bladder, and proximal urethra). Tumors frequently occur simultaneously at different sites in the urinary tract, and close urologic follow-up with regular urinary cytologic examination is recommended.

Other Causes

Other causes of chronic tubulointerstitial damage include the following: *Interstitial uric acid crystal formation* in the renal parenchyma causes chronic uric acid nephropathy. It is associated with tophaceous gout and has limited reversibility. *Lithium* induces nephrogenic diabetes insipidus and microcystic changes in the renal tubules along with interstitial fibrosis. *Heavy metals* (eg, cadmium, certain pigments, and substances involved in manufacturing glass, plastic, metal alloys, electrical equipment, and some cigarettes) induce proximal renal tubular acidosis and tubulointerstitial nephritis. *Mercury* in its organic salt form can induce chronic tubulointerstitial nephritis and membranous nephropathy (MN) or acute tubular necrosis. *Chronic lead intoxication* can cause lead nephropathy, a form of chronic interstitial nephritis. Patients typically present with hypertension, elevated serum creatinine level, little or no proteinuria, bland urinary sediment, and hyperuricemia. A history of nontophaceous gout is common. *Oxalate deposition* from primary or secondary hyperoxaluria causes renal and extrarenal oxalate deposition. Secondary causes of oxalate deposition include enteric hyperoxaluria, ethylene glycol ingestion, methoxyflurane, high doses of ascorbic acid, and vitamin B₆ deficiency.

Clinical Manifestations

Clinical manifestations in patients with tubulointerstitial disease include tubular proteinuria (mainly retinol binding protein, α_1-microglobulin, or light chains), proximal tubule dysfunction, distal tubule dysfunction, medullary concentration defects, abnormal urinary sediment, azotemia, and renal insufficiency (Box 52.1).

Cystic Renal Disease

Autosomal dominant polycystic kidney disease (ADPKD) is the most common hereditary renal disease. It occurs in both males and females and is characterized by multiple bilateral renal cysts and cysts in other organs (eg, liver, spleen, and pancreas). ADPKD is most often associated with mutations in 2 genes that code for interacting proteins found in renal tubular cells and in primary cilia: The *PKD1* gene, localized on chromosome 16p, encodes polycystin 1 (85%–90% of cases), and the *PKD2* gene, localized on chromosome 4, encodes polycystin 2.

Box 52.1 • Clinical Manifestations of Tubulointerstitial Disease

Tubular proteinuria ($<$1.5–2 g/1.73 m^2/24 h; mainly retinol binding protein, α_1-microglobulin, or light chains)

Proximal tubule dysfunction

Distal tubule dysfunction

Medullary concentration defects

Abnormal urinary sediment

Azotemia and renal insufficiency

The diagnosis of ADPKD relies on the clinical and family history and imaging of the kidneys. In a patient with a family history of ADPKD, ultrasonographic criteria for diagnosis vary by age (Table 52.1):

- Age 15–39 years: 3 cysts in 1 or both kidneys
- Age 40–59 years: ≥2 cysts in each kidney
- Age ≥60 years: ≥4 cysts in each kidney

In certain settings, genetic testing is required for a definitive diagnosis.

Manifestations of renal involvement can include hypertension, flank or back pain, macroscopic or microscopic hematuria, chronic kidney disease, urinary tract infection, and inferior vena cava obstruction.

Extrarenal manifestations of ADPKD include polycystic liver disease (most common) and intracranial aneurysm (ICA). The incidence of ICA is 5% to 22%, depending on whether the patient has a positive family history of ICA. Risk of rupture depends on ICA diameter (if $<$5 mm, risk is minimal; if $>$10 mm, risk is high). Screening for ICA in all patients who have ADPKD is not recommended. Instead, screening should be reserved for the following:

- Patients with prior known ICA, family history of ICA, or intracerebral bleeding
- Patients undergoing surgical procedures that may cause hemodynamic instability
- Patients with occupations that may place others at risk (eg, aircraft pilots, bus drivers)

Table 52.1 • Ultrasonographic Criteria for Diagnosis of ADPKD in a Patient With a Family History of ADPKD

Age, y	Criterion
15–39	3 cysts in 1 or 2 kidneys
40–59	≥2 cysts in each kidney
≥60	≥4 cysts in each kidney

Abbreviation: ADPKD, autosomal dominant polycystic kidney disease.

Glomerular Disease

Clinical Manifestations

Clinical manifestations of glomerular injury vary. They include painless hematuria and proteinuria. *Painless hematuria* is defined as 3 or more red blood cells (RBCs) per high-power field in a freshly centrifuged urinary sediment sample. Dysmorphic RBCs or RBC casts (or both) may be present. Urine is often brown (tea- or cola-colored), rather than bright red, as a result of methemoglobin formation in acidic urine. *Proteinuria* may be nonnephrotic (0.3–3.5 g/1.73 m^2/24 h) or nephrotic ($>$3.5 g/1.73 m^2/24 h). Patients may report foamy urine. Proteinuria may be detected with a urine dipstick test for protein, which detects albumin. Therefore, the urine dipstick test is negative for protein when proteinuria is due to immunoglobulin light chains or tubular proteinuria.

In general, glomerular disorders are considered to be predominantly *nephritic* (characterized by hematuria and modest proteinuria) or *nephrotic* (characterized by a higher level of proteinuria), but in practice, overlap may exist (Table 52.2).

Renal biopsy provides a definitive diagnosis and is usually indicated in the presence of any of the following:

- Active urinary sediment (dysmorphic RBCs, RBC casts, or white blood cell casts)
- Proteinuria (usually $>$1 g/1.73 m^2/24 h)
- Reduced glomerular filtration rate
- Acute kidney injury (AKI) lasting $>$3–4 weeks
- Atypical course of diabetic nephropathy
- Suspicion of systemic diseases associated with renal manifestations (eg, systemic lupus erythematosus [SLE], paraproteinemias and amyloidosis, systemic vasculitis, Alport syndrome, or Fabry disease)

Table 52.2 • Presentation of Glomerular Diseases in Relation to Degree of Proteinuria and Nephritic Features

Disease	Proteinuria	Nephritic Features
Minimal change nephropathy	+++++	–
Diabetic nephropathy	++++	–
Focal segmental glomerulosclerosis	++++	±
Membranous nephropathy	++++	±
IgA nephropathy	++	+++
Membranoproliferative GN	++	+++
Acute infection–related GN	+	++++
Crescentic glomerulonephritis	+	++++
Thrombotic microangiopathy	±	±

Abbreviations: GN, glomerulonephritis; Ig, immunoglobulin; –, absent; +, present (number of symbols indicates relative degree of presence); ±, present or absent.

Renal biopsy is rarely indicated for patients with small, shrunken kidneys because of an increased risk of bleeding and the low probability of providing a diagnosis. Typical characteristics of select glomerular diseases are summarized in Table 52.3.

Nephrotic Syndrome

Nephrotic syndrome is defined as the presence of urinary protein greater than 3.5 g/1.73 m²/24 h, hypoalbuminemia (<3.5 g/dL), peripheral edema, hypercholesterolemia, and lipiduria (Box 52.2). Edema can be prominent. Urinalysis shows waxy casts, free fat, oval fat bodies, and lipiduria ("Maltese crosses").

Complications of nephrotic syndrome include the following:

- Hypogammaglobulinemia—increases the risk of infection, especially cellulitis and spontaneous peritonitis
- Vitamin D deficiency—due to loss of vitamin D–binding protein
- Iron deficiency anemia—due to hypotransferrinemia
- Thrombotic complications—due to increased levels of prothrombotic factors and decreased antithrombin III and antiplasmin
- Renal vein thrombosis

> ### Key Definition
>
> Nephrotic syndrome: *urinary protein >3.5 g/1.73 m²/24 h, hypoalbuminemia (<3.5 g/dL), peripheral edema, hypercholesterolemia, and lipiduria.*

Table 52.3 • Characteristics of Select Glomerular Diseases

Disease	Clinical Features	Characteristic Renal Biopsy Findings	Initial Disease-Specific Treatment
Minimal change nephropathy	Abrupt onset of nephrotic syndrome with edema GFR usually preserved	LM, IF: no structural abnormalities EM: diffuse podocyte foot process effacement	ACEI or ARB Responds well to corticosteroids, although relapses are common
Focal segmental glomerulosclerosis (FSGS)	May present with full-blown nephrotic syndrome (usually primary) or asymptomatic proteinuria (secondary—see text)	LM: segmental areas of sclerosis within glomeruli EM: diffuse podocyte foot process effacement in primary FSGS; segmental in secondary FSGS	ACEI or ARB Primary: corticosteroids; may require cyclophosphamide or cyclosporine Secondary: treat underlying cause
Membranous nephropathy	Nephrotic syndrome Thrombotic complications are more common than in other disorders with nephrotic syndrome GFR usually preserved Most patients (70%–80%) are positive for antiphospholipase A₂ receptor (anti-PLA₂R)	LM: diffuse glomerular capillary thickening; spikes on silver stain IF: granular capillary IgG, C3 EM: subepithelial deposits	Conservative management with ACEI or ARB alone in patients at low risk for progression; corticosteroids and either a cytotoxic agent or a calcineurin inhibitor
IgA nephropathy	Various degrees of proteinuria with intermittent gross or microscopic hematuria and reduced GFR	LM: mesangial matrix expansion and mesangial cell proliferation IgA: granular mesangial IgA	ACEI or ARB High-dose corticosteroids Benefit of fish oil is controversial but likely not harmful
Membranoproliferative glomerulonephritis (MPGN)	Various degrees of proteinuria and hematuria with reduced GFR May have low C3 level and presence of C3 nephritic factor Associated with monoclonal proteins, infections, autoimmune disorders, and abnormalities of alternate complement pathway	LM: endocapillary proliferation IF: immunoglobulins and complement *or* complement alone EM: subendothelial deposits; electron-dense osmophilic deposits replacing lamina densa	Control underlying disease ACEI or ARB
Anti-GBM disease	Rapidly progressive GN; pulmonary hemorrhage may occur	LM: crescentic GN IF: linear deposition of IgG in glomerular capillary loops	High-dose corticosteroids, cyclophosphamide, plasma exchange

Abbreviations: ACEI, angiotensin-converting enzyme inhibitor; ARB, angiotensin II receptor blocker; EM, electron microscopy; GBM, glomerular basement membrane; GFR, glomerular filtration rate; GN, glomerulonephritis; IF, immunofluorescence microscopy; Ig, immunoglobulin; LM, light microscopy.

Box 52.2 • Clinical Manifestations of Nephrotic Syndrome

Urinary protein >3.5 g/1.73 m²/24 h

Hypoalbuminemia (<3.5 g/dL)

Peripheral edema

Hypercholesterolemia

Lipiduria

General management of nephrotic syndrome regardless of the cause includes managing edema with diuretics, controlling blood pressure, limiting dietary protein and sodium, treating hyperlipidemia, and using angiotensin-converting enzyme inhibitors (ACEIs) or angiotensin II receptor blockers (ARBs). The use of an ACEI in combination with an ARB is no longer routinely recommended because the incidence of AKI and hyperkalemia is increased when both are used together in some patient populations.

KEY FACTS

✓ Analgesic nephropathy—slowly progressive chronic interstitial nephritis, often with papillary necrosis and resulting in bilateral renal atrophy

✓ ADPKD—the most common hereditary renal disease

✓ Clinical manifestations of glomerular disease—painless hematuria and proteinuria (nonnephrotic or nephrotic), which may be accompanied by other features, including dysmorphic RBCs, RBC casts, brown urine, and foamy urine

✓ Management of proteinuric renal diseases—ACEI or ARB to control blood pressure and reduce proteinuria

Glomerular Diseases Usually Manifesting as Nephrotic Syndrome

Minimal Change Nephropathy

Minimal change nephropathy (MCN) is defined by the absence of structural glomerular abnormalities, except for the widespread fusion of epithelial cell foot processes seen on electron microscopy, in patients with nephrotic syndrome. It is the most common cause of nephrotic syndrome in children. The presence of nephrotic syndrome in a child with normal urinalysis results indicates MCN until proved otherwise. Among patients with nephrotic syndrome, MCN is the cause in 70% to 90% of children younger than 10 years, in 50% of adolescents and young adults, and in less than 20% of adults.

The typical presentation is abrupt onset of nephrotic syndrome. Hematuria is unusual. In adults, hypertension and acute kidney injury may be present. The pathogenesis of MCN is unknown and may be a consequence of T-lymphocyte abnormalities, with T cells producing a lymphokine that is toxic to glomerular epithelial cells. In some patients, MCN may have a secondary cause, such as viral infections, drugs, malignancy (eg, lymphoma), or allergies.

Treatment includes high-dose corticosteroid therapy continued for 4 to 8 weeks after remission is achieved. In adolescents and adults, response to therapy is high (>80%), but the response is slow and may require up to 16 weeks. Approximately 75% of patients who initially respond to corticosteroids have at least 1 relapse. Other immunosuppressive agents (eg, cyclophosphamide or cyclosporine) are used in patients with frequent relapses or corticosteroid dependence or resistance. The overall prognosis is excellent, with patients maintaining long-term renal function. If there is no response to therapy or if progressive renal failure develops, an alternative diagnosis (such as focal segmental glomerulosclerosis [FSGS]) must be considered.

Focal Segmental Glomerulosclerosis

FSGS accounts for about 25% of cases of adult nephrotic syndrome. FSGS is considered the most common cause of idiopathic nephrotic syndrome in African Americans, in whom FSGS is associated with variations in the apolipoprotein A1 gene. Patients with FSGS may present with either asymptomatic proteinuria or full-blown nephrotic syndrome. Nephrotic-range proteinuria may occur in patients with secondary FSGS, but full-blown nephrotic syndrome is unusual in adults with secondary FSGS.

Secondary causes of FSGS include drugs (eg, heroin, pamidronate, anabolic steroids, and interferon), infections (eg, human immunodeficiency virus and parvovirus), sickle cell disease, obesity, vesicoureteral reflux, decreased renal mass (eg, unilateral renal agenesis and decreased renal mass), healed lesions of prior inflammatory disorders in glomeruli, and aging.

Treatment of primary FSGS includes prolonged (>4 months) high-dose corticosteroid therapy, with a remission rate up to 40% to 60%. For patients who do not respond to corticosteroids, alternative therapy includes other immunosuppressants (eg, cyclophosphamide, cyclosporine, or tacrolimus) either alone or in combination with corticosteroids. For patients with secondary forms of FSGS, treatment should target the underlying cause whenever possible. In all patients, treatment with an ACEI or an ARB may substantially reduce proteinuria and prolong renal survival. The prognosis is better for patients with a smaller degree of proteinuria and for those who respond to corticosteroids.

Membranous Nephropathy

MN occurs in persons of all ages and races. It is the most common cause of nephrotic syndrome in white adults and is most often diagnosed in middle age, with the incidence peaking during the fourth and fifth decades of life. The

---

Box 52.3 • Clinical Manifestations of Membranous Nephropathy

High-grade proteinuria (>2.0 g/1.73 m^2/24 h in >80% of patients and >10 g/1.73 m^2/24 h in as many as 30%)

Preserved renal function initially in the majority of patients

Absence of hypertension at diagnosis (>80% of patients)

Microscopic hematuria (approximately 30% of patients)

Thrombotic complications (eg, renal vein thrombosis, deep vein thrombosis, pulmonary embolism)

Most patients (70%–80%) are positive for antiphospholipase A_2 receptor (anti-PLA$_2$R)

Box 52.4 • Clinical Manifestations of Nephritic Syndrome

Oliguria

Edema

Hypertension

Proteinuria (usually <3.5 g/1.73 m^2/24 h)

Active urinary sediment

KEY FACTS

✓ MCN—no structural glomerular abnormalities except for widespread fusion of epithelial cell foot processes on EM if patient has nephrotic syndrome

✓ FSGS—present in about 25% of adults with nephrotic syndrome; the most common form of idiopathic nephrotic syndrome in African Americans

✓ MN—the most common cause of nephrotic syndrome in white adults (usually occurs in middle age)

Key Definition

Nephritic syndrome: *oliguria, edema, hypertension, proteinuria (usually <3.5 g/1.73 m^2/24 h), and active urinary sediment.*

---

male to female ratio is 2:1. Approximately 70% of the patients are positive for a circulating antiphospholipase A_2 receptor (anti-PLA$_2$R) autoantibody.

Patients present with the following: high-grade proteinuria (>2.0 g/1.73 m^2/24 h in >80% of patients and >10 g/1.73 m^2/24 h in as many as 30%), preserved renal function initially in the majority of patients, absence of hypertension at diagnosis (>80% of patients), microscopic hematuria (approximately 30% of patients), and thrombotic complications (eg, renal vein thrombosis, deep vein thrombosis, and pulmonary embolism) (Box 52.3).

Secondary causes of MN include autoimmune diseases (eg, SLE), infections (eg, hepatitis B, hepatitis C, and syphilis), drugs (eg, NSAIDs, penicillamine, and gold), and malignancies (solid tumors such as colon, breast, and lung cancer), with the association increasing with age, reaching up to 20% among patients over age 60.

Initial therapy consists of general measures for management of nephrotic syndrome as discussed above. The probability of renal survival is more than 80% at 5 years and 60% at 15 years. With initiation of ACEI or ARB therapy, nearly 25% of patients have spontaneous complete remission, and 50% have partial remission. Immunosuppressive therapies should be considered for patients who remain nephrotic after a 6-month trial of a maximal dose of ARB and should include use of corticosteroids in combination with a cytotoxic agent (eg, cyclophosphamide or chlorambucil), cyclosporine, tacrolimus, or rituximab. Patients with persistent nephrotic syndrome unresponsive to immunosuppressive therapy are likely to progress to end-stage renal disease (ESRD).

Nephritic Syndrome

Nephritic syndrome is defined as the presence of oliguria, edema, hypertension, proteinuria (usually <3.5 g/1.73 m^2/24 h), and active urinary sediment (Box 52.4). General management includes sodium restriction and use of loop diuretics to reduce the risk of fluid overload and to help control hypertension.

Glomerular Disease Manifesting With Nephritic Syndrome

Infection-Related Glomerulonephritis

Classic poststreptococcal glomerulonephritis (GN) develops after pharyngitis (1–3 weeks) or skin infection (2–4 weeks) due to specific (nephritogenic) strains of group A β-hemolytic streptococci. Cultures are usually negative since the infection is no longer active. Titers for antistreptolysin O (ASO) and antideoxyribonuclease B (anti-DNase B) may provide evidence of recent streptococcal infection. Infection-related GN may be rapidly progressive and can occur after or concomitant with other infections, such as staphylococcal, meningococcal, and pneumococcal infections; bacterial endocarditis; and infections of ventriculoatrial shunts.

A typical manifestation is the abrupt onset of nephritic syndrome. Treatment is supportive, with appropriate antibiotic therapy for persistent infections and, if applicable, for persons who are contacts (to prevent new cases). In some patients, microscopic hematuria, proteinuria, hypertension, and renal dysfunction may persist for years. These cases of atypical postinfectious GN are associated with abnormalities in the alternate pathway of complement.

Immunoglobulin A Nephropathy

Immunoglobulin (Ig) A nephropathy (IgAN) is the most common glomerulopathy worldwide, with an incidence approaching 1:100 in some countries (eg, Japan). IgAN is a mesangial proliferative GN characterized by diffuse deposition of IgA in the mesangium of glomeruli.

The majority of patients with IgAN are asymptomatic. This disorder may be identified when microscopic hematuria with or without proteinuria is found on routine urinalysis. Some patients, typically young adults in the second or third decade of life, may present with episodic macroscopic hematuria, often accompanying an upper respiratory tract infection ("synpharyngitic hematuria"). Proteinuria is common, but nephrotic syndrome occurs in less than 10% of all patients. Patients with nephrotic syndrome may have MCN superimposed on IgAN.

Patients who are normotensive with proteinuria less than 500 mg/1.73 m²/24 h and normal renal function at presentation usually have a good long-term prognosis. However, in 20% to 40% of patients, the disease progresses to ESRD within 10 to 25 years. Progression may be slowed by use of an ACEI or an ARB and administration of high doses of corticosteroids. The use of fish oil to prevent progression of IgAN is controversial. Persistent proteinuria, uncontrolled hypertension, impaired renal function at diagnosis, and fibrosis identified in renal biopsy specimens predict a poor outcome. For patients with rapidly progressive renal failure due to crescentic IgAN, a regimen of corticosteroids and cyclophosphamide, with the addition of plasma exchange or pulse methylprednisolone, has been tried with variable results.

Henoch-Schönlein Purpura

Henoch-Schönlein purpura is a systemic form of IgAN. Patients usually present with microscopic or gross hematuria (or both), RBC casts, purpura, and abdominal pain. Generally, the prognosis is good for children and variable for adults. In patients with normal kidney function, treatment is supportive only. Patients with progressive renal failure should be considered for treatment with high-dose corticosteroids with or without cytotoxic medication.

Membranoproliferative Glomerulonephritis

Membranoproliferative glomerulonephritis (MPGN) is a pattern of glomerular injury resulting from predominantly subendothelial and mesangial deposition of immune complexes or complement factors (or both) and their products along with proliferative changes in glomeruli. MPGN can be classified according to patterns found with immunofluorescence microscopy (IF): 1) deposits of immunoglobulins and complement factors or 2) deposits of predominantly complement factors.

Immune complex–mediated MPGN shows deposition of both immunoglobulin and complement factor on IF. Immune complex–mediated MPGN usually results from chronic infection (eg, hepatitis C), cryoglobulinemia, autoimmune diseases (eg, SLE), or monoclonal gammopathies.

Complement-mediated MPGN results from dysregulation of the alternate pathway of complement and shows predominantly complement factors without significant immunoglobulin deposition on IF. Complement-mediated MPGN can be further classified with electron microscopy into C3 glomerulonephritis (C3 GN) and dense deposit disease (DDD) (formerly known as type II MPGN). DDD can be differentiated from C3 GN by the presence of electrondense, osmophilic deposits replacing the lamina densa and producing a smooth, ribbonlike thickening found on electron microscopy.

Clinical presentation is variable and can include both nephrotic and nephritic features. In patients with cryoglobulinemic MPGN, the levels of C3, C4, and total complement (with the CH50 assay) are persistently low, reflecting activation of both complement pathways. In contrast, patients with C3 GN and DDD may have a persistently low level of C3 but a normal level of C4. Many patients have a C3 nephritic factor (an autoantibody to alternative pathway C3 convertase, resulting in persistent breakdown of C3).

Treatment is aimed at resolving or controlling the underlying disease (ie, infection, SLE, or monoclonal gammopathy). Optimal treatment of patients with idiopathic MPGN is unclear: Available data come from studies performed when the use of ACEIs and ARBs was inconsistent and currently accepted pathophysiologic processes had not yet been elucidated. Patients with normal kidney function, no active urinary sediment, and proteinuria less than the nephrotic range have favorable long-term outcomes and may be treated conservatively with ACEIs or ARBs. Follow-up is required to detect early deterioration in kidney function, which may prompt use of immunosuppressive therapy. Patients who present with advanced renal insufficiency and severe tubulointerstitial fibrosis on renal biopsy are unlikely to benefit from immunosuppressive therapy.

Rapidly Progressive (Crescentic) GN

Rapidly progressive GN is defined as an acute, rapidly progressive (days to weeks or months) deterioration of renal function associated with an active urinary sediment and a focal necrotizing crescentic GN seen on light microscopic examination of renal biopsy specimens. Oliguria is common. The following immunofluorescence patterns are seen in renal biopsy specimens (Figure 52.1 and Box 52.5): *Type I* has linear IgG deposition along glomerular basement membranes (GBM), as seen in Goodpasture disease and anti-GBM nephritis. *Type II* has granular immune complexes, as seen in SLE, infection-related GN, IgA nephropathy, cryoglobulinemic GN, and MPGN. *Type III* is pauci-immune, with negative or weak immunoglobulin deposition seen on IF, as seen in antineutrophil

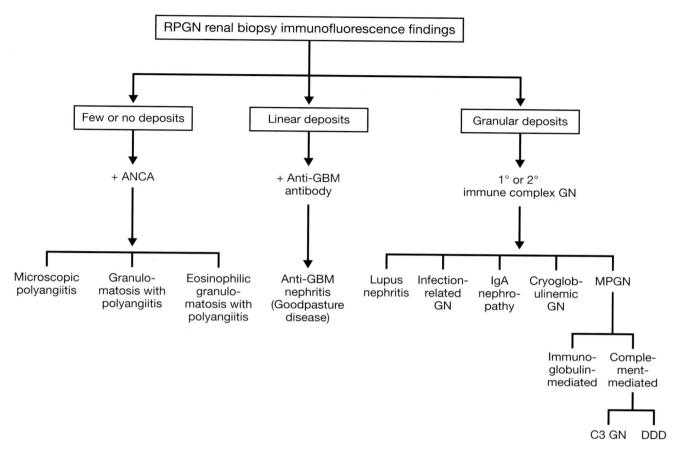

Figure 52.1 *Rapidly Progressive Glomerulonephritis (RPGN). Diagnostic algorithm for glomerular disorders that may present with RPGN. Classification is based on immunofluorescence microscopy findings in renal biopsy specimens. ANCA indicates antineutrophil cytoplasmic autoantibody; DDD, dense deposit disease; GBM, glomerular basement membrane; GN, glomerulonephritis; Ig, immunoglobulin; MPGN, membranoproliferative glomerulonephritis; +, presence of; 1°, primary; 2°, secondary.*

cytoplasmic autoantibody (ANCA) vasculitis. Pulmonary-renal syndrome occurs frequently and can be due to anti-GBM disease, SLE, cryoglobulinemia, and ANCA-associated vasculitis (AAV) (microscopic polyangiitis,

granulomatosis with polyangiitis [formerly known as Wegener granulomatosis], and eosinophilic granulomatosis with polyangiitis [formerly known as Churg-Strauss syndrome]).

Box 52.5 • Immunofluorescence Patterns in Rapidly Progressive Glomerulonephritis (GN)

Type I—linear IgG deposition along glomerular basement membranes (GBM): Goodpasture disease, anti-GBM nephritis

Type II—granular immune complexes: SLE, infection-related GN, IgA nephropathy, cryoglobulinemic GN, MPGN

Type III—pauci-immune, with negative or weak immunoglobulin deposition seen on IF: antineutrophil cytoplasmic autoantibody (ANCA)-associated vasculitis

Abbreviations: IF, immunofluorescence microscopy; Ig, immunoglobulin; MPGN, membranoproliferative glomerulonephritis; SLE, systemic lupus erythematosus.

Key Definition

Rapidly progressive glomerulonephritis: *acute, rapidly progressive deterioration of renal function with active urinary sediment and focal necrotizing crescentic glomerulonephritis.*

ANCA-Associated Vasculitis

AAV is characterized by inflammation and necrosis of small blood vessels of the kidney and other organs in association with autoantibodies against antigens present in lysosomal granules in the cytoplasm of neutrophils: myeloperoxidase (MPO) and proteinase 3 (PR3). AAV is the most common cause of rapidly progressive GN in patients older than 60 years and

Box 52.6 • Signs and Symptoms of ANCA-Associated Vasculitis

Cutaneous purpura, nodules, and ulcerations

Peripheral neuropathy (mononeuritis multiplex)

Abdominal pain and blood in stools

Hematuria, proteinuria, and renal failure

Hemoptysis and pulmonary infiltrates or nodules

Necrotizing (hemorrhagic) sinusitis

Myalgias and arthralgias

Muscle and pancreatic enzymes in blood

Abbreviation: ANCA, antineutrophil cytoplasmic autoantibody.

may present with a wide range of signs and symptoms (Box 52.6). The classification of AAV is outlined in Table 52.4.

Microscopic polyangiitis is a necrotizing vasculitis of small vessels (ie, capillaries, venules, and arterioles) with few or no immune deposits (pauci-immune) on immunofluorescence. Necrotizing GN with crescents is common, and pulmonary capillaritis often occurs. A necrotizing arteritis involving small and medium-sized arteries can be present. Fifty percent of patients are MPO-ANCA–positive, 40% are PR3-ANCA–positive, and a few are ANCA-negative.

Granulomatosis with polyangiitis is characterized by granulomatous inflammation involving the respiratory tract and necrotizing vasculitis affecting small and medium-sized vessels (ie, capillaries, venules, arterioles, and arteries). Necrotizing GN is common. Seventy-five percent of patients are PR3-ANCA–positive, and 20% are MPO-ANCA–positive.

Eosinophilic granulomatosis with polyangiitis is characterized by peripheral blood eosinophilia, asthma or other form of atopy, an eosinophil-rich granulomatous inflammation involving the respiratory tract, and a necrotizing vasculitis affecting small and medium-sized vessels. Sixty percent of patients are MPO-ANCA–positive.

Treatment of AAV includes high-dose corticosteroids in combination with either cyclophosphamide or rituximab (anti-CD20 monoclonal antibody) until remission is achieved (3–6 months). Rituximab is equivalent to cyclophosphamide for induction therapy. For patients with pulmonary hemorrhage who require ventilatory support treatment, plasma exchange should be added. Patients with severe renal failure (serum creatinine >5.5 mg/dL or receiving dialysis) can also be considered for plasma exchange. Patients who have granulomatosis with polyangiitis and are nasal carriers of *Staphylococcus aureus* benefit from long-term treatment with trimethoprim-sulfamethoxazole.

A drug-induced AAV syndrome has been reported with the use of propylthiouracil, methimazole, carbimazole, hydralazine, minocycline, levamisole-contaminated cocaine, and penicillamine. Although uncommon, drug-induced AAV should be considered in patients with vasculitis. The clinical presentation is similar to that in cases that are not

KEY FACTS

✓ Poststreptococcal GN—after pharyngitis (1–3 weeks) or skin infection (2–4 weeks) from nephritogenic group A β-hemolytic streptococci

✓ IgAN—most common glomerulopathy worldwide (incidence in Japan, 1:100), but most are asymptomatic

✓ Immune-complex–mediated MPGN—deposition of immunoglobulin and complement factor

✓ Complement-mediated MPGN—predominantly complement factors with relatively little immunoglobulin deposition

✓ Pulmonary-renal syndrome occurs with rapidly progressive GN and may be due to anti-GBM disease, AAV vasculitis, SLE, or cryoglobulinemia

✓ AAV—inflammation and necrosis of small blood vessels in kidneys and other organs; associated with autoantibodies against MPO and PR3

Table 52.4 • Classification of ANCA-Associated Vasculitis

ANCA-Associated Vasculitis	Pulmonary and Renal Features	Size of Affected Blood Vessels	Types of Antibodies, Percentage of Patients
Microscopic polyangiitis (MPA)	Pauci-immune necrotizing GN, with or without pulmonary capillaritis	Small	MPO-ANCA, 50% PR3-ANCA, 40% ANCA-negative, few patients
Granulomatosis with polyangiitis (GPA)	Granulomatous inflammation of respiratory tract with pauci-immune necrotizing vasculitis	Small and medium	PR3-ANCA, 75% MPO-ANCA, 20%
Eosinophilic granulomatosis with polyangiitis	Peripheral blood eosinophilia, asthma or atopy, eosinophil-rich granulomatous inflammation of respiratory tract with pauci-immune necrotizing vasculitis	Small and medium	MPO-ANCA, 60%

Abbreviations: ANCA, antineutrophil cytoplasmic antibody; GN, glomerulonephritis; MPO, myeloperoxidase; PR3, proteinase 3.

drug related (Box 52.6). Most patients have MPO-ANCA, frequently in very high titers, as well as antibodies to elastase or to lactoferrin.

Polyarteritis Nodosa

Polyarteritis nodosa (PAN) is a rare disease characterized by necrotizing inflammation of small or medium-sized arteries without GN or vasculitis in arterioles, capillaries, or venules. It affects males and females equally, with onset most frequently between the ages of 40 and 60 years. PAN is ANCA-negative. In some patients, it is associated with hepatitis B virus infection. Diagnosis is made by finding aneurysms on angiography or nerve biopsy. Treatment of patients who do not have evidence of hepatitis B virus infection includes high-dose corticosteroids and cyclophosphamide. Patients with hepatitis B–associated PAN should be treated with a short course of corticosteroids in combination with antiviral therapy and plasma exchange.

Anti-GBM Antibody–Mediated GN (Goodpasture Disease)

Anti-GBM disease is a pulmonary-renal syndrome caused by circulating anti-GBM antibodies directed against the α3 chain of type IV collagen. Approximately 25% to 30% of patients with anti-GBM antibodies are also ANCA-positive. Pulmonary hemorrhage may be absent or not clinically apparent.

Treatment consists of high-dose corticosteroids (pulse intravenous methylprednisolone followed by oral prednisone) in combination with oral cyclophosphamide and plasma exchange. Patients who have 100% circumferential crescents on renal biopsy and are receiving dialysis do not recover renal function and should not be treated with the immunosuppressive regimen outlined above unless pulmonary hemorrhage is present. The prognosis depends on the percentage of circumferential crescents of the renal biopsy specimen, the presence of oliguria, and the need for dialysis. Anti-GBM disease rarely recurs.

Systemic Diseases Associated With Glomerular Disorders

Diabetic Nephropathy

Diabetic nephropathy (DN) is the most common cause of ESRD in the United States. It occurs in 30% to 40% of patients with type 1 diabetes mellitus (DM) and in 20% to 30% of patients with type 2 DM. In type 1 DM, the peak onset of nephropathy is between 10 and 15 years after the initial presentation with diabetes. DN is unlikely to develop in patients who do not have proteinuria after 25 years of diabetes. The main risk factors for the development of DN are a positive family history of DN, hypertension, and poor glycemic control. The risk is greater in some ethnic groups (eg, Pima Indians and African Americans).

The initial manifestation of DN is the onset of microalbuminuria (defined as urinary albumin excretion of 20–200 mcg/min or 30–300 mg/1.73 m^2/24 h), which can evolve into overt proteinuria (>300 mg/1.73 m^2/24 h) and subsequent nephrotic-range proteinuria, although full-blown nephrotic syndrome is uncommon. After overt proteinuria develops, the progression toward ESRD is relentless, although rates of decline vary among patients (over a period of 5–15 years). The degree of proteinuria correlates approximately with the renal prognosis. Among patients with type 1 DM, there is a strong correlation between the development of nephropathy and other signs of diabetic microvascular compromise, such as diabetic retinopathy. This correlation is weaker for patients with type 2 DM; however, nephropathy develops in up to one-third of patients with type 2 DM *without* evidence of diabetic retinopathy.

The pathogenesis of DN involves increased glycosylation of proteins, with accumulation of advanced glycosylation end products that cross-link with collagen, in combination with glomerular hyperfiltration and hypertension. Renal biopsy may not be necessary for patients with long-term DM, especially if retinopathy is present and other causes of proteinuria are excluded. Renal biopsy is indicated for patients if the disease has an atypical course or if progressive loss of renal function occurs rapidly.

Progression of DN can be slowed by tight glycemic control (glycated hemoglobin <7.0%) and the use of ACEIs or ARBs. Patients with ESRD due to DN are candidates for a solitary kidney or combined kidney-pancreas transplant, which afford better long-term survival and quality of life than the alternatives of hemodialysis and peritoneal dialysis.

Lupus Nephritis

Lupus nephritis (LN), one of the most serious manifestations of SLE, is observed in up to 50% of patients with SLE. Renal involvement usually occurs early in the course of the disease and is rarely the sole manifestation of SLE.

Renal biopsy findings are used in the classification of LN, which includes focal proliferative LN (class III); diffuse proliferative LN (class IV); and membranous LN (class V). For patients with severe LN (class III or IV), the use of a high-dose corticosteroid (depending on severity, either prednisone orally or pulsed doses of intravenous methylprednisolone) in combination with intravenous cyclophosphamide was the most effective form of therapy until more recent studies showed that mycophenolate mofetil in combination with prednisone is as effective as cyclophosphamide in combination with prednisone. The subtype of class V LN is characterized by proteinuria, weakly positive or negative antinuclear antibody results, and no erythrocyte casts. Initial therapy is supportive, using an ACEI or an ARB to reduce proteinuria. Immunosuppressive treatment should be considered for patients with class V LN who are nephrotic.

Table 52.5 • Cryoglobulins and Associated Diseases

Cryoglobulin Type	Immunoglobulin Class	Associated Diseases
I. Monoclonal immunoglobulins	M>G>A>BJP	Myeloma, Waldenström macroglobulinemia
II. Mixed cryoglobulins with monoclonal immunoglobulins	M/G>>G/G	Sjögren syndrome, Waldenström macroglobulinemia, lymphoma, essential cryoglobulinemia
III. Mixed polyclonal immunoglobulins	M/G	Infection, SLE, vasculitis, neoplasia, essential cryoglobulinemia

Abbreviations: BJP, Bence Jones protein; SLE, systemic lupus erythematosus.

Cryoglobulinemic GN Associated With Hepatitis Infection

Type II or mixed essential cryoglobulins (Table 52.5) are commonly found in patients with hepatitis C virus (HCV) infection. Cryoglobulins contain HCV RNA and anti-HCV IgG, which precipitate in the glomeruli, bind complement, activate a cytokine cascade, and trigger an inflammatory response. Patients may present with proteinuria, microscopic hematuria, nephrotic syndrome, or renal impairment. Hypertension is common and may be severe, particularly with acute nephritic syndrome. Cryoglobulinemic GN is usually associated with low levels of C3 and C4. Cryoglobulin levels correlate poorly with disease activity, and 30% to 40% of patients do not have detectable cryoglobulins. Modern antiviral treatments are effective in clearing HCV from the circulation and result in improvement of proteinuria and renal function. Relapses after discontinuation of antiviral therapy are common. For patients with acute nephritis, treatment with prednisone and cytotoxic agents is indicated, with the addition of plasmapheresis, depending on the severity. The renal prognosis is usually favorable.

KEY FACTS

✓ PAN—rare; necrotizing inflammation of small or medium-sized arteries without GN or vasculitis in arterioles, capillaries, or venules.

✓ Anti-GBM disease—a pulmonary-renal syndrome caused by circulating anti-GBM antibodies directed against the α3 chain of type IV collagen

✓ DN—the most common cause of ESRD in the United States

✓ Initial manifestation of DN—microalbuminuria (urinary albumin excretion, 20–200 mcg/min or 30–300 mg/1.73 m²/24 h)

Human Immunodeficiency Virus—Associated Nephropathy

Human immunodeficiency virus (HIV)-associated nephropathy characterized by progressive renal insufficiency in patients with nephrotic-range proteinuria (frequently massive) but often little edema. Ultrasonography shows large, echogenic kidneys. Renal biopsy specimens show a collapsing form of FSGS. HIV-associated nephropathy is typically seen in African Americans. Treatment includes the use of highly active antiretroviral therapy, treatment of underlying infections, and an ACEI to reduce proteinuria.

Other types of renal disease can be encountered in HIV-infected patients. These include IgAN, MPGN, MCN, MN, infection-related GN, thrombotic microangiopathy, and a lupus-like immune complex–mediated GN. Intratubular obstruction can result from crystal precipitation after the administration of sulfadiazine or intravenous acyclovir. Renal calculi or nephropathy (or both) can occur after administration of indinavir.

Paraproteinemia-Associated Renal Diseases

Multiple Myeloma

Multiple myeloma has renal manifestations that may manifest as AKI or as chronic progressive disease occurring at any time during the course of the disease. Other renal manifestations include pseudohyponatremia, low anion gap, and type 2 (proximal) renal tubular acidosis with Fanconi syndrome. Virtually all patients with multiple myeloma have monoclonal immunoglobulins or light chains in the serum or urine (or in both). AKI occurs as a result of intraluminal precipitation of proteinaceous casts (cast nephropathy) and the resulting interstitial inflammatory reaction (myeloma kidney). Intratubular cast formation is facilitated by increased urinary concentrations of calcium, sodium, and chloride (eg, after the use of a loop diuretic); conditions that reduce flow rates (eg, intravascular depletion and the use of NSAIDs); and use of radiocontrast agents.

Treatment of cast nephropathy includes vigorous hydration with normal saline, correction of hypercalcemia, avoidance of nephrotoxic or precipitating agents, alkalization of the urine to maintain a pH greater than 7 (possibly beneficial in some patients), and consideration of plasmapheresis (which quickly removes light chains from the circulation) for patients with AKI and high serum levels of free light chains or hyperviscosity syndrome.

Amyloidosis

Amyloidosis may be primary (AL amyloidosis), secondary (AA amyloidosis), or familial. AL amyloidosis is characterized by systemic extracellular deposition of antiparallel, β-pleated sheet, nonbranching, 8- to 12-nm fibrils that stain positive with Congo red (showing green birefringence with polarized light) or thioflavin T.

Patients with primary (AL) amyloidosis are typically older than 50 years, and the kidneys are affected in 50% of patients. New advances in treatment of amyloidosis, including stem cell transplant, have greatly improved the previously dismal prognosis.

Secondary (AA) amyloidosis is most common in patients who have rheumatoid arthritis, inflammatory bowel disease, chronic infection, or familial Mediterranean fever and in persons who subcutaneously inject illicit drugs such as heroin. The treatment of AA amyloidosis is directed at the underlying inflammatory process.

Light Chain Deposition Disease

Light chain deposition disease is characterized by immunoglobulin light chain deposition along the GBM. It is strongly associated with the development of myeloma, lymphoma, and Waldenström macroglobulinemia. Renal involvement is manifested by proteinuria, nephrotic syndrome, and renal insufficiency. As in amyloidosis and multiple myeloma, treatment can lead to stabilization or improved renal function in some patients.

Thrombotic Microangiopathies

Different types of thrombotic microangiopathy (TMA) are characterized by renal failure along with microangiopathic hemolytic anemia and thrombocytopenia. Recently, much has been learned to clarify the pathogenesis of various disorders that present as TMA, and the terminology is evolving. Diagnostic features include anemia with schistocytes on peripheral blood smear, high reticulocyte count, elevated levels of indirect bilirubin and lactate dehydrogenase, decreased haptoglobin level, and presence of urinary hemoglobin without RBCs on microscopy. Making a diagnostic distinction between hemolytic uremic syndrome (HUS) and thrombotic thrombocytopenic purpura (TTP) can be difficult. Traditionally, HUS is more commonly associated with AKI, and patients with TTP typically present with fever, neurologic signs, and purpura.

Hemolytic Uremic Syndrome

The sporadic or diarrhea-associated form of HUS (D+HUS) is strongly linked to ingestion of meat or other foods contaminated with *Escherichia coli* O157:H7, which produces a Shiga-like toxin that binds to a glycolipid receptor on renal endothelial cells and triggers endothelial damage. The treatment is supportive; antibiotics should not be used because they can cause additional release of toxins. Children with D+HUS have a good prognosis (90% recover renal function), but older patients have an increased mortality rate and unfavorable long-term renal survival.

Thrombotic Thrombocytopenic Purpura

Typically, fluctuating neurologic signs and symptoms along with purpura are more commonly associated with TTP. TTP may result from autoantibody to the von Willebrand factor–cleaving protease ADAMTS13 (acute form) or from deficiency of ADAMTS13 (chronic-relapsing form). An ADAMTS13 activity measurement greater than 5% excludes severe ADAMTS13 deficiency (congenital or acquired TTP). In addition, TTP can occur in association with drugs (eg, cocaine, quinidine, ticlopidine, oral contraceptives, cyclosporine, tacrolimus, mitomycin C, bleomycin, and vascular endothelial growth factor inhibitors), HIV infection, malignancies, radiotherapy, SLE, antiphospholipid antibody syndrome, and scleroderma renal crisis. In general, treatment of TTP consists of plasma exchange, although scleroderma renal crisis is treated with ACEIs.

Complement-Mediated TMA

Atypical HUS is now recognized to be a complement-mediated form of TMA, resulting from various inherited and acquired abnormalities of the proteins involved in the alternate pathway of complement activation. It may be acquired (formation of antibody to Factor H) or genetic (mutations in the genes coding for C3, CD46, and complement factors H, I, and B).

Eculizumab, an inhibitor of the C5 complement component that blocks formation of the C5b-9 membrane attack complex, has been approved for the treatment of patients with atypical HUS. Eculizumab or plasma exchange (or both) may also be considered in the treatment of children with D+HUS and severe central nervous system involvement (eg, seizures or coma).

Diseases With Intrinsic GBM Abnormalities

Alport Syndrome

Alport syndrome is characterized by a progressive nephritis manifested by persistent or intermittent hematuria and proteinuria that increases with age. It is frequently associated with sensorineural hearing loss and ocular abnormalities. In virtually all male patients, the syndrome progresses to ESRD, often by age 16 to 35 years. This disorder is usually mild in heterozygous females, although ESRD develops in some women, usually after age 50 years. The rate of progression to ESRD is fairly constant among affected males within individual families but varies markedly from family to family.

The diagnostic abnormality is the absence of α3, α4, and α5 chains of type IV collagen from the GBM and distal tubular basement membrane. This abnormality occurs only in patients with Alport syndrome. More than 50% of patients have a mutation in the gene (*COL4A5*) that codes for the α5 chain of type IV collagen, α5(IV). It is X-linked in at least 80% of the patients. Additionally, autosomal recessive and autosomal dominant patterns of inheritance have been described. In families with a previously defined mutation, molecular diagnosis of affected males or gene-carrying females is possible. For families in which mutations have not been defined, genetic linkage analysis can determine whether an at-risk person carries the mutant gene, provided that at least 2 other affected members are available for testing.

No specific treatment is available. Tight control of blood pressure and moderate dietary protein restriction are recommended, and ACEI use may retard the progression of renal disease. Renal replacement therapy is eventually required. If the defect is in the α5(IV) chain, these patients are a phenotypic knockout for the α3(IV) chain, Thus, patients with Alport syndrome who receive a kidney transplant have a 5% to 10% risk of Goodpasture disease developing because of the presence of the α3(IV) chain (the location of the "Goodpasture antigen") in the transplanted kidney.

KEY FACTS

✓ HIV-associated nephropathy—progressive renal insufficiency and proteinuria (frequently massive) but often little edema

✓ Thrombotic microangiopathies (eg, HUS and TTP)—microangiopathic hemolytic anemia, thrombocytopenia, and renal failure

✓ Alport syndrome—progressive nephritis with persistent or intermittent hematuria and proteinuria (increases with age); frequently associated with sensorineural hearing loss and ocular abnormalities

---

Thin Basement Membrane Nephropathy

Thin basement membrane nephropathy (TBMN), sometimes referred to as benign familial hematuria, is a relatively common condition characterized by *isolated* glomerular hematuria (proteinuria is usually absent) associated with the renal biopsy finding of an excessively thin GBM (typically <250 nm in adults). Although TBMN is transmitted in a dominant fashion, patients with TBMN can be considered carriers of the autosomal recessive Alport syndrome since mutations (homozygous or compound heterozygous) in both alleles of *COL4A3* or *COL4A4* cause autosomal recessive Alport syndrome.

The clinical presentation includes persistent or intermittent hematuria that is first detected in childhood or during a routine urinalysis and is sometimes not manifested until adulthood. Macroscopic hematuria is not uncommon and may occur in association with an upper respiratory tract infection. Blood pressure is typically normal. When TBMN is first detected in young adults, 60% have proteinuria less than 500 mg/1.73 m²/24 h. In contrast to patients with Alport syndrome, patients with TBMN do not have hearing loss, ocular abnormalities, or a strong family history of ESRD. The diagnosis of TBMN requires a renal biopsy and electron microscopy with measurement of GBM thickness. For the majority of patients who have isolated hematuria and a negative family history of ESRD, the condition is benign, requires no specific treatment, and carries an excellent long-term prognosis. In some patients, progressive proteinuria and renal failure may develop and can eventually result in ESRD. TBMN has been reported to occur in association with other glomerular diseases.

Questions and Answers

Questions

Multiple Choice (choose the best answer)

VIII.1. A 38-year-old woman who has had Sjögren syndrome for 2 years presents with diffuse muscle weakness. The only medication she uses is artificial tears. Physical examination findings and laboratory test results are shown in Table VIII.Q1. A computed tomographic scan of the abdomen is shown in Figure VIII.Q1.

Table VIII.Q1

Component	Finding
Body mass index	19
Blood pressure, mm Hg	98/60
Pulse, beats per minute	98
Respiratory rate, breaths per minute	20
Edema	Absent
Sodium, mmol/L	134
Potassium, mmol/L	2.3
Chloride, mmol/L	114
Bicarbonate, mmol/L	12
Serum creatinine, mg/dL	0.8
Anion gap, mEq/L	8
Arterial blood gas	
pH	7.27
Pco_2, mm Hg	27
Urinalysis	
pH	6.7
Protein	Trace
Glucose	Negative
Red blood cells per high-power field	3–10

What is the diagnosis?
a. Proximal renal tubular acidosis (RTA)
b. Distal RTA
c. Idiopathic nephrolithiasis
d. Hyporeninemic hypoaldosteronism
e. Gout

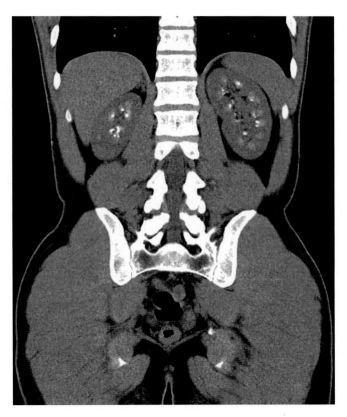

Figure VIII.Q1

VIII.2. A 68-year-old woman presents with new-onset back pain, weakness, episodic light-headedness, and a recent spontaneous left rib fracture. Physical examination findings and laboratory test results are shown in Table VIII.Q2.
What is the diagnosis?
a. Proximal renal tubular acidosis (RTA)
b. Distal RTA
c. Drug-induced diarrhea
d. Hypoaldosteronism
e. Multiple myeloma

VIII.3. A 47-year-old man who has a history of polysubstance abuse presents with delirium. Reportedly, he ingested an unknown

Table VIII.Q2

Component	Finding
Blood pressure, mm Hg	98/50
Pulse, beats per minute	106
Respiratory rate, breaths per minute	20
Heart examination	Unremarkable
Lung examination	Unremarkable
Edema	Extremities: pitting edema (trace)
Hemoglobin, g/dL	10.5
Sodium, mmol/L	134
Potassium, mmol/L	3.4
Chloride, mmol/L	116
Bicarbonate, mmol/L	17
Serum creatinine, mg/dL	1.6
Phosphorus, mg/dL	2.0
Uric acid, mg/dL	1.9
Glucose, mg/dL	99
Arterial blood gas	
pH	7.32
Pco_2, mm Hg	32
Urinalysis	
pH	5.1
Protein	1+
Glucose	2+
Red blood cells per high-power field	1–3

Table VIII.Q3

Component	Finding
Mental status	Disoriented
Blood pressure, mm Hg	110/70
Pulse, beats per minute	110 (normal heart rhythm)
Respiratory rate, breaths per minute	34
Lung fields	Clear
Edema	Absent
Sodium, mmol/L	138
Potassium, mmol/L	3.8
Bicarbonate, mmol/L	14
Chloride, mmol/L	100
Serum urea nitrogen, mg/dL	20
Serum creatinine, mg/dL	1.5
Arterial blood gas	
pH	7.43
Pco_2, mm Hg	20
Po_2, mm Hg	85

Table VIII.Q4

Component	Finding
Hemoglobin, g/dL	11.1
Leukocyte count, $\times 10^9$/L	7.5
Platelet count, $\times 10^9$/L	187
Sodium, mmol/L	142
Potassium, mmol/L	5.2
Bicarbonate, mmol/L	22
Chloride, mmol/L	105
Serum creatinine, mg/dL	3.2
Serum urea nitrogen, mg/dL	50
Calcium, mg/dL	13.1
Albumin, g/dL	3.9
Phosphorus, mg/dL	3.3
Urinalysis	
Protein	1+
Microscopic examination	Occasional granular casts
Sodium, mmol/L	68
Creatinine, mg/dL	31

substance. Physical examination findings and laboratory test results are shown in Table VIII.Q3.

What is the patient's acid-base status?

a. Metabolic acidosis with respiratory compensation
b. Metabolic acidosis and respiratory acidosis
c. Metabolic acidosis and respiratory alkalosis
d. Acute respiratory alkalosis with appropriate metabolic compensation
e. Chronic respiratory alkalosis and metabolic compensation

VIII.4. A 73-year-old man who has a history of hypertension and metastatic prostate cancer presents with dizziness and weakness. He has no known history of kidney disease; his creatinine was 1.2 mg/dL 2 months ago. His medications include lisinopril-hydrochlorothiazide (20 mg–12.5 mg daily), multivitamin daily, tramadol (50 mg 2–3 times daily as needed for pain), and leuprolide (30 mg intramuscularly every 4 months). His blood pressure is 130/86 mm Hg, his pulse is 90 beats per minute, and his temperature is 36.9°C. On examination, he appears fatigued, his heart sounds are normal, his lungs are clear, and he has pretibial edema (trace). Laboratory test results are shown in Table VIII.Q4. Renal ultrasonography shows no evidence of hydronephrosis.

What is the most likely cause of this patient's acute renal failure?

a. Membranous nephropathy
b. Acute tubular necrosis
c. Dehydration
d. Obstruction
e. Tumor lysis syndrome

VIII.5. A 54-year-old woman who had been previously healthy is evaluated for a rash on her lower extremities that has been present for 1 week. She has noticed tea-colored urine for several weeks. She takes no medications. Her temperature is 37.3°C, her pulse is 88 beats per minute, and her blood pressure is 154/90 mm Hg. Palpable purpura is present on both legs and feet. The remainder of the examination findings are unremarkable. Results of laboratory studies are notable for creatinine

1.8 mg/dL. The erythrocyte sedimentation rate is 80 mm/h. Antinuclear antibody, antibodies to double-stranded DNA, myeloperoxidase, and proteinase 3 assays are negative. The C4 complement level is low, and the results of cryoglobulin testing are positive. Urinalysis shows proteinuria (2+) and hematuria (3+). Urine microscopy shows 31 to 40 erythrocytes per high-power field (HPF) and 3 to 10 leukocytes per HPF. Which of the following viruses is most likely to be associated with this disorder?

a. Epstein-Barr virus
b. Cytomegalovirus
c. Human immunodeficiency virus
d. Parvovirus B19
e. Hepatitis C virus

VIII.6. A 51-year-old truck driver is referred for evaluation of persistent asymptomatic microhematuria. He has not seen a physician since he was first told about blood in his urine during a Department of Transportation physical examination 9 years ago. At that time, he had a computed tomographic scan of the abdomen and pelvis, cystoscopy with retrograde pyelograms, and urine cytology. He was told last year that his blood glucose level was elevated. He has never smoked and takes no medications other than ibuprofen 400 mg approximately twice monthly for headaches. Physical examination findings and laboratory test results are shown in Table VIII.Q6. Results of erythrocyte sedimentation rate, antinuclear antibody testing, testing for antibodies to myeloperoxidase and proteinase 3, serum protein electrophoresis, and hepatitis B and C and human immunodeficiency serologies all are negative or normal. Renal biopsy is performed.

Table VIII.Q6

Component	Finding
Blood pressure, mm Hg	164/94
Pulse, beats per minute	76
Weight, kg	92
Height, cm	185
Heart, lungs, and abdomen	Normal
Jugular venous distention	Absent
Pitting edema	Both lower extremities (trace)
Rashes	Absent
Serum creatinine, mg/dL	2.1
Fasting blood glucose, mg/dL	130
Spot urine microalbumin, mg/g	1,586
Urinalysis	
Blood	3+
Protein	3+
24-h total protein, g	2.1

What is the most likely diagnosis?

a. Minimal change nephropathy
b. Membranous nephropathy
c. Chronic interstitial nephritis
d. Diabetic nephropathy
e. Immunoglobulin (Ig)A nephropathy

VIII.7. A 34-year-old woman presents to the emergency department with diffuse myalgias. Her past medical history is significant for arthroscopic knee surgery 3 years ago. She has no history of recent trauma. She admits to using cocaine regularly. She takes an oral contraceptive tablet daily and ibuprofen 400 mg 2 to 3 times daily as needed for pain, most recently this morning. On auscultation, the heart rhythm is regular with no murmur, rub, or gallop, and the lungs are clear. Findings on abdominal examination are normal. There is diffuse tenderness in both upper and lower extremities without any ecchymoses or rashes. Ankle edema (trace) is present bilaterally. Additional physical examination findings and laboratory test results are shown in Table VIII.Q7.

Table VIII.Q7

Component	Finding
Blood pressure, mm Hg	158/90
Pulse, beats per minute	100
Temperature, °C	37.5
Hemoglobin, g/dL	12.1
Leukocyte count, ×10^9/L	8.3
Platelet count, ×10^9/L	189
Sodium, mmol/L	137
Potassium, mmol/L	5.8
Bicarbonate, mmol/L	17
Chloride, mmol/L	108
Serum creatinine, mg/dL	2.8
Serum urea nitrogen, mg/dL	39
Creatine kinase, U/L	12,870
Urinalysis	
Color	Brown
Blood	3+
Protein	2+
Leukocytes	1–3
Microscopic examination	Granular casts, epithelial casts, renal epithelial cells (11–20)

What is the most likely cause of her renal failure?

a. Rhabdomyolysis
b. Acute interstitial nephritis
c. Thrombotic thrombocytopenic purpura (TTP)
d. Membranoproliferative glomerulonephritis (MPGN)
e. Anti–glomerular basement membrane nephritis

VIII.8. A 56-year-old woman who is doing well is seeing you for her annual checkup. Her medical history is significant for type 2 diabetes mellitus for 20 years, hypertension, and diabetic neuropathy. On physical examination, she is obese and has decreased sensation in her feet. Other physical examination findings and laboratory test results are shown in Table VIII.Q8. Her current medications are metformin 1,000 mg twice daily, simvastatin 40 mg daily, gabapentin 300 mg 3 times daily, and atenolol 50 mg twice daily.

What additional tests should you order for this patient?

a. Renal ultrasonography
b. A 24-hour urine protein collection

Table VIII.Q8

Component	Finding
Heart rate, beats per minute	65
Blood pressure, mm Hg	125/65
Height, cm	165
Weight, kg	91
Hemoglobin A_{1c}, %	6.5
Serum creatinine, mg/dL	1.2
Total cholesterol, mg/dL	190
Triglycerides, mg/dL	123
High-density lipoprotein cholesterol, mg/dL	34
Low-density lipoprotein cholesterol, mg/dL	89

    c. A 24-hour urine albumin collection
    d. Random urine albumin to creatinine ratio
    e. Creatinine clearance

VIII.9. A 72-year-old woman presents with fatigue, decreased stamina, and loss of appetite. She has a 25-year history of type 2 diabetes mellitus; she has coronary artery disease and has had coronary artery bypass graft surgery; she received a diagnosis of breast cancer 10 years ago and had a mastectomy and radiotherapy; she has hypertension, hyperlipidemia, and a history of gout. Her heart rate is 48 beats per minute, her blood pressure is 132/78 mm Hg, her height is 174 cm, and her weight is 88 kg. On physical examination, she is pale, she is in no acute distress, and she has lower extremity edema; otherwise, examination findings are normal. Laboratory test results are shown in Table VIII.Q9. Results of liver function studies are normal. The patient takes atenolol 50 mg daily, lisinopril 40 mg daily, NPH insulin 30 units twice daily, simvastatin 20 mg daily, and allopurinol 150 mg daily.

Table VIII.Q9

Component	Finding
Hemoglobin, g/dL	9.8
Serum creatinine, mg/dL	2.2
Sodium, mmol/L	140
Bicarbonate, mmol/L	17
Chloride, mmol/L	113
Potassium, mmol/L	5.4
Uric acid, mg/dL	11
Hemoglobin A_{1c}, %	7.6
Urine albumin to creatinine ratio, mg/g	1,800

What should you recommend?
    a. Exchange atenolol for metoprolol.
    b. Increase the dosage of lisinopril to 80 mg daily.
    c. Add losartan 100 mg daily.
    d. Increase the dosage of allopurinol to 600 mg daily.
    e. Add metformin 1,000 mg twice daily.

Answers

VIII.1. Answer b.

This is a classic scenario for distal RTA, which is associated with calcium phosphate nephrolithiasis and nephrocalcinosis. Without treatment, the hypokalemia and non–anion gap metabolic acidosis can become severe. Patients with RTA tend to have slightly low intravascular volume. Therefore, hyporeninemic hypoaldosteronism would not be a possibility. Proximal RTA would not be associated with a severe reduction in serum bicarbonate or with nephrolithiasis.

VIII.2. Answer a.

This patient likely has plasma cell dyscrasia (multiple myeloma or AL amyloidosis, or both). The unusually low anion gap indicates the presence of positively charged paraproteins. The presence of glucosuria with euglycemia indicates a proximal tubular dysfunction. Typically, renin and aldosterone levels are high because the blood pressure is low.

VIII.3. Answer c.

This patient has anion gap acidosis and respiratory alkalosis, which is typical for salicylate intoxication.

VIII.4. Answer b.

Granular casts on urine microscopy and a fractional excretion of sodium that is greater than 3% (4.9% in this patient) are consistent with a diagnosis of acute tubular necrosis. Proteinuria would be higher in membranous nephropathy, which is associated with malignancies. Tumor lysis syndrome is associated with hyperphosphatemia and, typically, hypocalcemia. Absence of hydronephrosis on ultrasonography is not consistent with obstruction.

VIII.5. Answer e.

Cryoglobulinemia can develop in patients with asymptomatic hepatitis C infection, and this can cause a vasculitis involving small vessels (skin) and membranoproliferative glomerulonephritis.

VIII.6. Answer e.

A common manifestation of IgA nephropathy is persistent asymptomatic microhematuria with various degrees of proteinuria. Membranous nephropathy and minimal change nephropathy typically manifest with nephrotic range proteinuria without significant hematuria. Patients who have chronic interstitial nephritis and diabetic nephropathy do not present with persistent microhematuria.

VIII.7. Answer a.

Rhabdomyolysis precipitated by cocaine use can cause acute renal failure from acute tubular necrosis that results from injury to renal tubular epithelial cells after myoglobin is released by myocytes. The urine sediment findings are characteristic of acute tubular necrosis. Urinalysis typically is positive for blood by dipstick since the assay detects myoglobin in addition to hemoglobin, but red blood cells are not seen on urine microscopy. Acute interstitial nephritis would manifest with pyuria; patients with TTP have anemia and thrombocytopenia; and MPGN and anti–glomerular basement membrane nephritis would manifest with hematuria with or without red blood cell casts.

VIII.8. Answer d.

In the United States, only 20% to 30% of patients with type 2 diabetes mellitus are evaluated for diabetic kidney disease (DKD) with testing for proteinuria. Patients with DKD and proteinuria have a higher risk of end-stage renal disease and have a high associated cardiovascular mortality. Initiation of timely screening and appropriate therapy can decrease the rate of progression of DKD.

VIII.9. Answer a.

Exchange atenolol for metoprolol because atenolol is cleared by the kidneys and may accumulate to adverse plasma levels in patients with stage 3 or 4 chronic kidney disease (CKD). The patient has a Modification of Diet in Renal Disease (MDRD) glomerular filtration rate (GFR) of 22 mL/min/1.73 m². Metoprolol is metabolized by the liver and therefore has fewer side effects. Patients with progressive CKD (stages 3 and 4) have decreased elimination of medications that are excreted by the kidneys. These medications can accumulate and lead to adverse effects, such as bradycardia from renally excreted β-blockers (eg, atenolol). Switching to medications metabolized in the liver is more advantageous in these patients. Furthermore, although inhibitors of the renin-angiotensin system decrease progression of CKD and diabetic kidney disease, their benefit is limited in patients with progressive CKD. The adverse effects of these agents from decreasing the GFR and causing hyperkalemia might be harmful.

Neurology

53 Cerebrovascular Diseases

JAMES P. KLAAS, MD AND ROBERT D. BROWN JR, MD

Ischemic Cerebrovascular Disease

Pathophysiologic Mechanisms

The causes of ischemic cerebrovascular disorders, including transient ischemic attack (TIA) and cerebral infarction, can be classified according to the site of the source for the arterial blockage within the vascular system, from most proximal to distal (Figure 53.1):

1. *Cardiac source*: arrhythmias (eg, atrial fibrillation) and structural disease (eg, valve disease, dilated cardiomyopathy, recent myocardial infarction); paradoxical emboli with a right-to-left shunt through a patent foramen ovale, although most patients with patent foramen ovale are asymptomatic
2. *Large-vessel disorders*: most commonly atherosclerosis or dissection in the carotid or vertebrobasilar system; the aorta is uncommonly a source of embolus
3. *Small-vessel occlusive disease*: inflammatory or noninflammatory arteriopathies (eg, hypertension-induced disease is most common; isolated central nervous system angiitis, systemic lupus erythematosus, and others are rare)
4. *Hematologic disorders*: disorders of hemoglobin, white blood cells and platelets (polycythemia, sickle cell anemia, severe leukocytosis caused by blast crisis in the setting of acute leukemia thrombocytosis); hypercoagulable states including antithrombin III deficiency, protein C deficiency, protein S deficiency, hereditary resistance to activated protein C, anticardiolipin antibody syndrome, lupus anticoagulant positivity, and hypercoagulable states caused by carcinoma. Factor V Leiden mutation is a risk factor for venous thrombosis, but in general not for arterial thrombosis

Notably, illicit drug use is a common cause of stroke in young persons; it may cause arrhythmia, inflammatory arteriopathies, and a relative hypercoagulable state.

Risk Factors

Risk factors for atherosclerotic occlusive disease are similar to those for coronary artery disease: hypertension, cigarette smoking, diabetes mellitus, hypercholesterolemia, male sex, and advanced age. Emboli from intracardiac mural thrombi also cause TIA and cerebral infarction. Proven cardiac risk factors are atrial fibrillation (including paroxysmal and persistent atrial fibrillation), atrial flutter, dilated cardiomyopathy, mechanical valve, rheumatic valve disease, recent myocardial infarction, and others (Box 53.1).

Hypertension is the most important modifiable risk factor for stroke, but other modifiable risk factors include cigarette smoking, diabetes mellitus, hypercholesterolemia, metabolic syndrome, sedentary lifestyle, obesity, obstructive sleep apnea, and, possibly, increased homocysteine level. Although low levels of alcohol consumption seem to have a protective effect for ischemic stroke, heavy alcohol consumption increases a person's risk for all types of stroke, particularly intracerebral and subarachnoid hemorrhage.

Transient Ischemic Attacks

A **TIA** is any transient neurologic dysfunction as a result of cerebral ischemia that does not result in cerebral infarction. Patients who experience a TIA are at high risk for subsequent cerebral infarctions: 4% to 10% within 1 year to 33% within a patient's lifetime. Most TIAs last less than 15 minutes; about 90% resolve within 1 hour. Patients with cerebral infarcts, hemorrhages, and mass lesions can present with transient symptoms like those of TIAs.

> **Key Definition**
>
> Transient ischemic attack: *any transient neurologic dysfunction as a result of cerebral ischemia that does not result in cerebral infarction.*

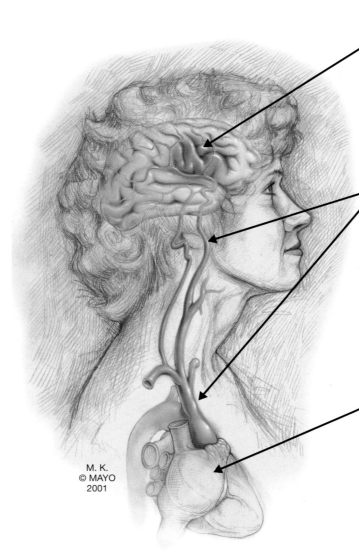

Small artery ~35%
- Noninflammatory
  Atherosclerosis
  Lipohyalinosis
- Inflammatory
  Vasculitis (eg, primary central
  nervous system vasculitis)

Large artery ~25%
Intracranial: cerebral arteries
Extracranial: aorta, vertebral and carotid
arteries
- Noninflammatory
  Atherosclerosis
  Dissection
- Inflammatory
  Vasculitis (eg, giant cell arteritis)

Cardioembolic ~35%
- Arrhythmias
  Atrial fibrillation
- Structural
  Valvular disease
  Recent myocardial infarction
  Patent foramen ovale with
  paradoxical embolus

Coagulopathies ~5%
- Disorders of main blood products
  Sickle cell disease, acute leukemia,
  thrombocytosis
- Other hematologic disorders leading
  to procoagulant state

M. K.
© MAYO
2001

Figure 53.1 *Causes of Ischemic Cerebrovascular Disease. Sites of source for arterial blockage within the vascular system are listed with corresponding frequencies.*

The long-term prognosis for patients who have a TIA generally follows the rule of 3s: one-third will have cerebral infarction, one-third will have at least 1 more TIA, and one-third will have no more TIAs. The following features increase the risk of stroke after TIA: age older than 60 years, hypertension, weakness or speech disturbance with TIA, TIA duration more than 60 minutes, and diabetes mellitus.

TIAs, like stroke, can cause various neurologic symptoms, but classically they produce speech, language, motor, or sensory dysfunction. A classic example is **amaurosis fugax**, which is defined as temporary, partial, or complete

Box 53.1 • Cardiac Risk Factors for Cerebral Infarction or Transient Ischemic Attack

Proven cardiac risk factors

    Atrial fibrillation
    Paroxysmal atrial fibrillation
    Atrial flutter
    Dilated cardiomyopathy
    Mechanical valve
    Rheumatic valve disease
    Recent (within 1 month) myocardial infarction
    Intracardiac thrombus
    Intracardiac mass (ie, atrial myxoma or papillary fibroelastoma)
    Infectious endocarditis
    Nonbacterial thrombotic endocarditis

Putative or uncertain cardiac risk factors

    Sick sinus syndrome
    Patent foramen ovale with or without atrial septal aneurysm
    Atherosclerotic debris in the thoracic aorta
    Spontaneous echocardiographic contrast
    Myocardial infarction 2–6 months earlier
    Hypokinetic or akinetic left ventricular segment
    Calcification of mitral annulus

monocular blindness and is a symptom of carotid artery disease. Glaucoma, vitreous hemorrhage, retinal detachment, papilledema, migrainous aura, temporal arteritis, and even ectopic floaters can mimic amaurosis fugax.

Key Definition

Amaurosis fugax: *temporary, partial, or complete monocular blindness (a symptom of carotid artery disease).*

Carotid Endarterectomy and Carotid Angioplasty With Stent Placement

Carotid endarterectomy markedly decreases the risk of stroke and death of *symptomatic* patients who have a 70% to 99% stenosis of the carotid artery. For a 50% to 69% stenosis, carotid endarterectomy is moderately efficacious in select symptomatic patients. Medical treatment alone is better than carotid endarterectomy for patients with a stenosis of 49% or less. Symptoms must be those of a carotid territory TIA or minor stroke and must be of recent onset (<4 months). To have a favorable risk-benefit ratio, the perioperative complication rate must be low.

Carotid angioplasty with stent placement may be used as an alternative to carotid endarterectomy, particularly for high-risk patients, such as those who previously had carotid endarterectomy, radiotherapy to the neck, or neck dissection; those with a stenosis high in the internal carotid artery; or those otherwise deemed at high risk for the operation. The safety and durability of the endovascular approach compared with endarterectomy are not clear, and the available data are somewhat conflicting.

Select patients with an *asymptomatic* carotid stenosis of at least 60% may also benefit from carotid endarterectomy (ie, they have a decreased risk of future ipsilateral stroke or related death). Clinical trials comparing treatment with aspirin and risk-factor reduction with carotid endarterectomy have found that the risk of stroke is low for patients treated surgically and for those treated medically. In the Asymptomatic Carotid Atherosclerosis Study (ACAS) and the Asymptomatic Carotid Surgery Trial, the 5-year risk of ipsilateral stroke or death was about 2% per year for patients treated medically and 1% per year for those treated surgically. As in symptomatic patients, in order for treatment to be of benefit, the perioperative complication rate must be low (surgeons and hospitals in ACAS had to have perioperative complication rates <3%). As is the case for symptomatic patients, carotid angioplasty with stent placement may be used as an alternative to carotid endarterectomy in select asymptomatic patients.

Patients with asymptomatic carotid occlusive disease who require an operation for another reason (eg, coronary artery bypass graft or abdominal aortic aneurysm repair) usually can have that procedure performed without prophylactic carotid endarterectomy, because in this context the risk of stroke in asymptomatic persons is quite low. For patients with symptoms in the distribution of a stenotic carotid artery, the decision is more complicated. Generally, if a patient with an asymptomatic carotid stenosis has cardiac symptoms (eg, angina), coronary artery bypass grafting or angioplasty is performed first and carotid endarterectomy or carotid angioplasty with stent placement is then performed if the patient is otherwise a good candidate for a carotid procedure.

KEY FACTS

✓ Modifiable risk factors for stroke: hypertension is the most important; others include cigarette smoking, diabetes mellitus, hypercholesterolemia, metabolic syndrome, sedentary lifestyle, obesity, obstructive sleep apnea

✓ Risk for subsequent cerebral infarctions is high for patients who experience a TIA—4%–10% within 1 year to 33% within a patient's lifetime

✓ Carotid endarterectomy—markedly decreases the risk of stroke and death of *symptomatic* patients who have a 70%–99% stenosis of the carotid artery

Antiplatelet Agents

Aspirin, aspirin in combination with extended-release dipyridamole, and clopidogrel are all effective for secondary prevention of non-cardioembolic ischemic stroke or TIA. The optimal dose of aspirin is uncertain, in that trials have examined doses ranging from 20 to 1,300 mg per day. However, most studies have shown 50 to 325 mg per day to be as efficacious as higher doses. The guideline from the American College of Chest Physicians recommends aspirin at a dose of 75 to 100 mg per day. Clopidogrel is given as a single dose, 75 mg daily. A combination of low-dose aspirin and extended-release dipyridamole provides another useful alternative to aspirin alone for prevention of stroke. The combination may be slightly more effective than aspirin alone in secondary stroke prevention.

Ticlopidine is also an effective antiplatelet agent, but it is rarely used because of associated neutropenia (thus, a complete blood cell count must be monitored every 2 weeks for the first 3 months of treatment) and thrombotic thrombocytopenic purpura, which has rarely been reported with clopidogrel.

The use of clopidogrel in combination with aspirin may be beneficial in select circumstances, such as use for 90 days in patients with symptomatic intracranial stenosis. It is also being evaluated for short-term (90 day) use after a minor stroke or TIA, a strategy that was noted to be effective in stroke reduction in a clinical trial performed in China. The use of aspirin plus clopidogrel for longer periods does not provide additional benefit, but it does increase the risk of significant bleeding; therefore, the combination is not commonly used as long-term stroke prevention.

Warfarin

Warfarin is used for secondary prevention in select patients who have TIA or cerebral infarction and 1) specific cardiac sources of embolus (eg, atrial fibrillation, left atrial or ventricular clot, mechanical heart valves, recent myocardial infarction with left ventricular thrombus, valvular thrombus) or 2) hypercoagulable states. Warfarin may also be recommended for patients with TIA or cerebral infarction and aortic arch thrombus and for those with extracranial dissection; no clinical trial data support this treatment approach, though, and aspirin is sometimes recommended for these conditions instead of warfarin. In a clinical trial with patients who had symptomatic intracranial stenosis, warfarin was not more effective than aspirin for reducing ischemic stroke risk and was associated with a higher risk of hemorrhage.

Management of Acute Cerebral Infarction

If a patient has a severe neurologic deficit caused by an acute cerebral infarction, the immediate decision in the emergency department is whether the patient is a candidate for thrombolytic therapy (tissue plasminogen activator [tPA]). The initial therapeutic approach to ischemic infarction depends greatly on the time from the onset of symptoms to the presentation for emergency medical care. If the onset of symptoms was less than 3 hours before the evaluation, emergency thrombolytic therapy should be considered. If a patient awakens from sleep with the deficit, thrombolytic therapy should not be considered unless the duration of the deficit is clearly less than 3 hours. Some data do suggest that select patients may benefit from the use of tPA up to 4.5 hours after symptom onset.

Computed tomographic findings are important in selecting patients for tPA. A noncontrast computed tomogram should not show any evidence of intracranial hemorrhage, mass effect, early evidence of significant cerebral infarction (greater than one-third distribution of the cerebral hemisphere), or midline shift. Patients may be excluded by the following clinical criteria: rapidly improving deficit, obtunded or comatose status or presentation with seizure, history of intracranial hemorrhage or bleeding diathesis, blood pressure elevation persistently greater than 185/110 mm Hg, gastrointestinal tract hemorrhage or urinary tract hemorrhage within the previous 21 days, traumatic brain injury or cerebral infarction within 3 months, or mild deficit. Eligible patients should have marked weakness in at least 1 limb or severe aphasia. Laboratory abnormalities that may preclude treatment are heparin use within the previous 48 hours with an increased activated partial thromboplastin time, international normalized ratio (INR) greater than 1.7, or blood glucose concentration less than 50 mg/dL.

Intravenous tPA improves neurologic status at 3 months after stroke compared with placebo. In one clinical trial, a greater proportion (about 12% greater) of subjects who received tPA had minimal or no deficit at 3 months after the event, and there was no increase in the proportion of persons who died. This finding is particularly important because there was an increased occurrence of symptomatic hemorrhage in the tPA group (6.4% compared with 0.6%).

Stroke Risks With Nonvalvular Atrial Fibrillation

Atrial fibrillation is associated with up to 24% of ischemic strokes. The stroke rate for the entire cohort of patients with chronic atrial fibrillation is generally about 5% per year. However, patients younger than 60 years with lone atrial fibrillation have a lower risk for stroke than other patients with atrial fibrillation and often receive treatment with only aspirin, depending on their CHADS2 score (congestive heart failure, hypertension, age ≥75 years, diabetes mellitus, and previous stroke) (see Table 3.4) or CHADS-VASc score (congestive heart failure, hypertension, age, diabetes, history of stroke or TIA or thromboembolism, vascular disease, female sex). Patients with atrial fibrillation whose predictive scores suggest an intermediate or high risk for a thromboembolic event generally should receive anticoagulation with warfarin (INR, 2.0–3.0), and those at low risk should receive aspirin. Some patients with atrial fibrillation requiring anticoagulation are treated with newer oral anticoagulants including direct factor Xa inhibitors (apixaban or rivaroxaban) or direct thrombin inhibitors (dabigatran).

For patients receiving anticoagulant therapy with warfarin, the dominant risk factor for intracranial hemorrhage is the INR, but age is another risk factor for subdural hemorrhage. An INR of 2.0 to 3.0 is probably an adequate level of anticoagulation for nearly all warfarin indications except for preventing embolization from mechanical heart valves. Generally, the lowest effective intensity of anticoagulant therapy should be given.

KEY FACTS

- ✓ Aspirin, aspirin in combination with extended-release dipyridamole, and clopidogrel—all are effective for secondary prevention of non-cardioembolic ischemic stroke or TIA

- ✓ Use of aspirin plus clopidogrel for long periods (>90 days)—does not provide additional benefit but does increase the risk of significant bleeding; thus, the combination is not commonly used as long-term stroke prevention

- ✓ Warfarin—used for secondary prevention in select patients who have TIA or cerebral infarction and 1) specific cardiac sources of embolus or 2) hypercoagulable states

- ✓ Management of acute cerebral infarction—

  - emergency thrombolytic therapy should be considered if symptom onset was <3 hours before evaluation

  - if patient awakens from sleep with the deficit, thrombolytic therapy should not be considered unless the duration of the deficit is clearly <3 hours

  - for selecting use of tPA, noncontrast computed tomogram should not show any evidence of intracranial hemorrhage, mass effect, early evidence of significant cerebral infarction (more than one-third distribution of cerebral hemisphere), or midline shift

- ✓ Treatment of patients with atrial fibrillation—those whose predictive scores suggest an intermediate or high risk for a thromboembolic event generally should receive anticoagulation with warfarin (INR, 2.0–3.0); those at low risk should receive aspirin

---

Hemorrhagic Cerebrovascular Disease

Intracerebral Hemorrhage

Intracerebral hemorrhage (ICH) is the second most common cause of stroke, accounting for 10% to 30% of all nonischemic strokes. Hypertension and cerebral amyloid angiopathy account for most primary hemorrhages, but trauma and structural lesions (eg, primary and metastatic tumors, arteriovenous malformation, cavernous malformation) can also cause ICH. Hypertension commonly affects deep penetrating cerebral vessels, especially those supplying the basal ganglia, cerebral white matter, thalamus, pons, and cerebellum. Therefore, most hemorrhages due to hypertension occur in these regions of the brain. The opposite pattern is seen with cerebral amyloid angiopathy, which usually causes lobar hemorrhages.

Patients with ICH can present with symptoms identical to those of an ischemic stroke. Patients with ICH often complain of a headache, although not always. Imaging is therefore necessary to differentiate between ischemia and hemorrhage.

Surgical evacuation of intracerebral hematomas may be necessary for patients who have signs of increased intracranial pressure or for those whose condition is worsening. However, apart from data for select patients with lobar hemorrhages, there are no data that clearly show that surgery is beneficial for intracerebral hemorrhage.

Prognosis depends on the size and location of the hemorrhage. Factors that increase mortality are age older than 80 years, hemorrhage volume more than 30 mL, initial Glasgow Coma Scale score less than 13, extension of the hemorrhage into the ventricular system, and infratentorial hemorrhage location.

Cerebellar Hemorrhage

It is important to recognize cerebellar hemorrhage because surgical drainage may be lifesaving. The important clinical findings are vomiting and inability to walk (ataxia). Long-tract signs, such as hemiparesis, usually are not present. Cerebellar hemorrhage can cause obstructive hydrocephalus, and patients may have ipsilateral gaze palsy (cranial nerve VI palsy) or ipsilateral facial weakness (cranial nerve VII palsy). They may or may not have headache, vertigo, or lethargy.

Subarachnoid Hemorrhage

Subarachnoid hemorrhage (SAH) accounts for about 5% of strokes, including about half of those in patients younger than 45 years; the peak age ranges from 35 to 65 years. The most common cause of nontraumatic SAH is intracranial saccular aneurysm. In up to 50% of cases of SAH, a patient with an aneurysm may have a small sentinel bleed with a warning headache, or the expansion of an aneurysm may cause focal neurologic signs or symptoms (eg, an incomplete cranial nerve III palsy). The prognosis is related directly to the state of consciousness at the time of intervention. Onset of the headache is characteristically sudden (thunderclap), and although one-third of SAHs occur during exertion, one-third occur during rest or minimal activity, and one-third occur during sleep. Complications of SAH include intracranial arterial vasospasm, which peaks in incidence between days 4 and 12 after the initial hemorrhage. Other potential SAH complications include hyponatremia associated with a cerebral salt-wasting syndrome or the syndrome of inappropriate secretion of antidiuretic hormone, communicating hydrocephalus, seizures, and aneurysm rebleeding. In addition to the initial hemorrhage, vasospasm and subsequent hemorrhage are the leading causes of morbidity and death among patients who have SAH. The outpouring of catecholamines may cause myocardial damage and accompanying electrocardiographic abnormalities, pulmonary edema, and arrhythmias. Arrhythmias can be both supraventricular and ventricular and are most likely to occur during the initial hours or days after a moderate-to-severe SAH.

Initial treatment is supportive, often in an intensive care unit. Prevention of vasospasm is best achieved by maintaining normal or increased blood pressure and intravascular volume as well as using the calcium channel blocker nimodipine. If the SAH is from a ruptured aneurysm, an experienced team often does early intervention (surgical clipping or endovascular coiling).

The differential diagnosis of subtypes of hemorrhagic cerebrovascular disease is outlined in Box 53.2.

KEY FACTS

✓ Most common cause of nontraumatic SAH—intracranial saccular aneurysm

✓ Onset of headache in SAH—characteristically is sudden (thunderclap)

✓ Complications of SAH—intracranial arterial vasospasm, hyponatremia associated with a cerebral salt-wasting syndrome or the syndrome of inappropriate secretion of antidiuretic hormone, communicating hydrocephalus, seizures, and aneurysm rebleeding

✓ Outpouring of catecholamines in SAH—may cause myocardial damage and accompanying electrocardiographic abnormalities, pulmonary edema, and arrhythmias

✓ Arrhythmias in SAH—can be both supraventricular and ventricular and are most likely to occur during the initial hours or days after a moderate-to-severe SAH

Box 53.2 • Differential Diagnosis of Subtypes of Hemorrhagic Cerebrovascular Disease

Hemorrhage into parenchyma
  Hypertension
  Amyloid angiopathy
  Aneurysm
  Vascular malformation

   Arteriovenous malformation
   Cavernous malformation
   Venous malformation (rare cause of hemorrhage)

  Trauma—primarily frontal and temporal
  Hemorrhagic infarction
  Secondary to brain tumors (primary and secondary neoplasms)
  Inflammatory diseases of vasculature
  Disorders of blood-forming organs (blood dyscrasia, especially leukemia and thrombocytopenic purpura)
  Anticoagulant or thrombolytic therapy
  Increased intracranial pressure (brainstem) (Duret hemorrhages)
  Illicit drug use (cocaine or amphetamines)
  Postsurgical
  Fat embolism (petechial)
  Hemorrhagic encephalitis (petechial)
  Undetermined cause (normal blood pressure and no other recognizable disorder)

Hemorrhage into subarachnoid space (subarachnoid hemorrhage)
  Trauma
  Aneurysm

   Saccular (berry, congenital)
   Fusiform (arteriosclerotic)—rarely causes hemorrhage
   Mycotic

  Arteriovenous malformation
  Many of the same causes listed under "Hemorrhage into parenchyma" above

Subdural and epidural hemorrhage (hematoma)

  Mainly traumatic (especially during anticoagulation)
  Many of the same causes listed under "Hemorrhage into parenchyma" above

Hemorrhage into pituitary (pituitary apoplexy)

54 Headache, Facial Pain, and "Dizziness"

BERT B. VARGAS, MD

Headache and Facial Pain

Headache is considered to be a nearly universal experience. Approximately 98% of the population will experience some form of headache in a lifetime. The number of migraineurs worldwide is approximately 1 billion, and nearly 1 in every 4 households in the United States has at least one family member who experiences migraine. Persons with headache disorders also present frequently to outpatient clinics; they are the reason for approximately 1 in every 10 consultations with a primary care physician. Migraine, in particular, poses a considerable economic burden because it typically affects persons during ages associated with peak productivity.

Distinguishing Primary From Secondary Headache

The primary goal in the evaluation of any patient with headache should be to identify concerning features or red flags that may suggest the presence of an underlying and potentially sinister secondary cause of headache. A useful pneumonic to help identify concerning headache features that warrant additional evaluation is "to SNOOP4 red flags" (Box 54.1).

Box 54.1 • SNOOP4 Red Flags: Indications of a Headache That May Have a Secondary Cause

*S*ystemic disease or symptoms

*N*eurologic signs or symptoms

*O*nset that is sudden

*O*lder than age 40 years

*P*rogressive worsening

*P*ostural

*P*recipitated by Valsalva maneuver or exertion

*P*revious headache history with new features

Thunderclap, or sudden-onset, **headache** is defined as a headache that is severe (typically described as the worst headache of one's life) and reaches maximal severity in less than 1 minute. Thunderclap headache is a medical emergency and warrants special attention and proper evaluation for underlying causes such as subarachnoid hemorrhage. Emergency computed tomography of the head is needed; if the result is negative, lumbar puncture should be done. Additional investigations, including magnetic resonance imaging of the brain and cerebrovascular imaging (either magnetic resonance imaging or computed tomography), should strongly be considered because several possible underlying causes of thunderclap headache (many of which are vascular) may evade detection on routine noncontrast computed tomography of the head (Box 54.2).

Key Definition

Thunderclap headache: *a headache that is severe (worst headache of one's life) and reaches maximal severity in less than 1 minute.*

KEY FACTS

✓ Thunderclap headache—

- a medical emergency and warrants evaluation for subarachnoid hemorrhage
- emergency computed tomography of the head is needed; if results are negative, lumbar puncture is done
- other imaging (magnetic resonance imaging of brain and cerebrovascular imaging) should strongly be considered because underlying causes of thunderclap headache (many vascular) may evade detection on routine noncontrast computed tomography

---

Box 54.2 • Serious Causes of Headache in Which Routine Computed Tomography of the Head May Have Normal Results

Reversible cerebral vasoconstriction syndrome

Giant cell or temporal arteritis

Glaucoma

Trigeminal or glossopharyngeal neuralgia

Lesions around sella turcica

Warning leak of aneurysm (sentinel bleed)

Cerebral venous sinus thrombosis

Third ventricle colloid cyst

Pseudotumor cerebri

Low intracranial pressure syndromes (cerebrospinal fluid leaks)

Cervical artery dissection

In persons older than 50 years with new-onset headache, evaluation should include laboratory investigations to help rule out giant cell arteritis, including complete blood count, sedimentation rate, and C-reactive protein. These tests should be done even in the absence of classic features such as vision change, jaw claudication, palpable temporal artery abnormalities, and scalp allodynia.

Differentiation and Treatment of Common Headache Disorders

Although tension-type headache is the most common primary headache in the general population, migraine is overwhelmingly the most common primary headache disorder evaluated in outpatient primary care clinics. Despite its relatively high prevalence (17% of women and 6% of men), migraine is underdiagnosed and therefore undertreated. Because a large number of migraineurs have been misidentified at some point as having tension-type headache, sinus headache, or cluster headache, both patients and providers should be aware of the key differentiating features among primary headache subtypes (Table 54.1). The complete diagnostic criteria for migraine, tension-type headache, and cluster headache, as published in the International Classification of Headache Disorders, 3rd edition (beta), are listed in Box 54.3.

Migraine is defined by multiple attacks of moderate to severe headache, often unilateral, which last several hours if untreated and accompanied by photophobia, phonophobia, and osmophobia; nausea; a pounding quality to the headache; and an increase in intensity with light activity. Approximately one-third of migraineurs experience an aura before the headache onset, most commonly described as visual, with flashing lights, jagged lines, or scintillating scotomas. Tension-type headaches can be severe but are often bilateral, squeezing or tight in quality, and lack other associated features that occur in migraine. Although tension-type headache is the most common primary headache subtype in the general population, it makes up only 3% of the headache disorders evaluated in outpatient primary care clinics.

Several medications with evidence-based efficacy are available for the abortive treatment of migraine both at home and in the acute-care setting. These include nonsteroidal anti-inflammatory drugs, acetaminophen, triptans, and dihydroergotamine (Table 54.2). When considering an abortive medication, several factors should be considered, including time to peak severity of headache (suggesting a need for medications with a rapid onset) and the presence of nausea or vomiting (suggesting a need for routes of administration other than oral).

To avoid medication overuse headache, measures should be taken to prevent the misuse or overuse of abortive medications. Strategies to prevent overuse of abortive medications include establishing limits to the frequency of use and providing preventive medications to reduce headache frequency. Triptans and ergotamines are vasoconstrictive and contraindicated in patients with coronary artery disease, uncontrolled hypertension, history of stroke or heart attack,

Table 54.1 • Distinguishing Characteristics of Migraine, Cluster, and Tension-Type Headache

Characteristic	Migraine	Cluster	Tension-Type
Duration	4–72 h	15–180 min	30 min-7 days
Location	Unilateral (but may be bilateral)	Unilateral, orbital, or temporal (typically side-locked)	Typically bilateral
Pain quality	Moderate to severe intensity Typically pulsating or throbbing	Excruciating	Mild to moderate intensity Typically pressing or tightening
Associated features	Must be associated with nausea or vomiting or photophobia and phonophobia	Must be associated with ipsilateral autonomic features (ie, conjunctival injection, lacrimation, nasal congestion, eyelid edema) or a sense of restlessness or agitation	Must not be associated with nausea or vomiting and no more than one of either photophobia or phonophobia

Box 54.3 • Diagnostic Criteria for Migraine Without Aura, Cluster Headache, and Tension-Type Headache

Migraine without aura

A. At least 5 attacks fulfilling criteria B-D
B. Attacks lasting 4–72 hours (untreated or unsuccessfully treated)
C. At least 2 of the following 4 characteristics:
   1. Unilateral
   2. Pulsating
   3. Moderate or severe
   4. Aggravation by or causing avoidance of routine physical activity
D. During headache, at least 1 of the following:
   1. Nausea or vomiting
   2. Photophobia and phonophobia

Cluster headache

A. At least 5 attacks fulfilling criteria B-D
B. Severe unilateral orbital, supraorbital, or temporal pain lasting 15–180 minutes (if untreated)
C. Either or both of the following:
   1. At least 1 of the following signs or symptoms ipsilateral to the headache:
      a. Conjunctival injection or lacrimation
      b. Nasal congestion or rhinorrhea
      c. Eyelid edema
      d. Forehead and facial sweating
      e. Forehead and facial flushing
      f. Sensation of fullness in the ear
      g. Miosis or ptosis
   2. A sense of restlessness or agitation
D. Frequency between 1 every other day and 8 per day for more than half the time when the disorder is active

Tension-type headache

A. At least 10 episodes occurring <1 day per month on average and fulfilling criteria B-D
B. Lasting from 30 minutes to 7 days
C. At least 2 of the following 4 characteristics:
   1. Bilateral
   2. Pressing or tightening (nonpulsating) quality
   3. Mild or moderate
   4. Not aggravated by routine physical activity
D. Both of the following:
   1. No nausea or vomiting
   2. No more than 1 of phonophobia or photophobia

Adapted from Headache Classification Committee of the International Headache Society (IHS). The International Classification of Headache Disorders, 3rd edition (beta version). Cephalalgia. 2013 Jul;33(9):629–808. Used with permission.

13% actually receive it. Guidelines for the initiation of prophylactic treatment have been published by the American Academy of Family Physicians, American College of Physicians, and the American Society of Internal Medicine with assistance from the American Headache Society and include the following scenarios:

1. More than 1 attack per week
2. Use of an abortive medication more than 2 days per week
3. Patients in whom abortive medications are contraindicated, not tolerated, or ineffective
4. Uncommon migraine conditions in which some abortive medications are contraindicated (ie, hemiplegic migraine)
5. Patient preference

Drugs frequently used for migraine prophylaxis include antihypertensives, tricyclic antidepressants, and anticonvulsants. Current American Academy of Neurology guidelines for the prophylaxis of migraine are listed in Table 54.3. Currently, the only medications approved by the US Food and Drug Administration for the prophylaxis of migraine include propranolol, timolol, divalproex sodium, and topiramate. Despite the common understanding that valproic acid has substantial teratogenic potential, current research indicates that the use of topiramate also has the potential for serious and deleterious effects on embryologic and fetal development. The use of divalproex sodium or topiramate in women of childbearing potential should be accompanied with documented counseling about potential risks and the use of birth control while taking these medications. Amitriptyline is a useful medication in patients with either migraine or chronic-type tension headache because the commonly occurring sedative adverse effects can be effectively utilized at bedtime when patients have a coexisting complaint of disrupted sleep or insomnia. Although the level of evidence is strongest

KEY FACTS

✓ Strategies to prevent overuse of abortive medications in migraine—establish limits to the frequency of use and provide preventive medications to reduce headache frequency

✓ Triptans and ergotamines in migraine—they are contraindicated in coronary artery disease, uncontrolled hypertension, history of stroke or heart attack, and basilar or hemiplegic migraine

✓ Valproic acid and topiramate—have the potential for serious and deleterious effects on embryologic and fetal development

✓ Amitriptyline—a useful medication for either migraine or chronic-type tension headache with a coexisting complaint of disrupted sleep or insomnia because it has sedative adverse effects

and certain migraine subtypes such as basilar migraine and hemiplegic migraine.

Despite the fact that 40% of all migraineurs may be eligible for treatment with prophylactic medications, only

Table 54.2 • Evidence-Based Recommendations for Abortive Treatment of Migraine

Level A: Established Efficacy (≥2 Class I Trials)	Level B: Probably Effective (1 Class I or 2 Class II Studies)	Level C: Possibly Effective (1 Class II Study)	Level U: Inadequate or Conflicting Data
Acetaminophen (PO)	Chlorpromazine (IV)	Valproate (IV)	Celecoxib (PO)
Dihydroergotamine (IN/INH)	Droperidol (IV)	Ergotamine (PO)	Lidocaine (IV)
Aspirin (PO)	Metoclopramide (IV)	Phenazone (PO)	Hydrocortisone (IV)
Diclofenac (PO)	Prochlorperazine (IV/IM/PR)	Butorphanol (IM)	
Ibuprofen (PO)	Dihydroergotamine (IV/IM/SC)	Codeine (PO)	
Naproxen (PO)	Flurbiprofen (PO)	Meperidine (IM)	
Butorphanol (IN)	Ketoprofen (PO)	Methadone (IM)	
Almotriptan (PO)	Ketorolac (IV/IM)	Tramadol (IV)	
Eletriptan (PO)	Magnesium sulfate (IV/IM)	Dexamethasone (IV)	
Frovatriptan (PO)	Isometheptene (PO)	Butalbital (PO)	
Naratriptan (PO)	Codeine/acetaminophen (PO)	Lidocaine (IN)	
Rizatriptan (PO)	Tramadol/acetaminophen (PO)	Butalbital/acetaminophen/ caffeine/codeine (PO)	
Sumatriptan (PO/SC/IN/ patch)		Butalbital/acetaminophen/ caffeine (PO)	
Zolmitriptan (IN/PO)			
Acetaminophen/aspirin/ caffeine (PO)			
Sumatriptan/naproxen (PO)			

Abbreviations: IM, intramuscularly; IN/INH, intranasally/intranasal inhalation; IV, intravenously; PO, orally; PR, rectally; SC, subcutaneously.

Table 54.3 • Evidence-Based Recommendations for the Prophylactic Treatment of Migraine

Level A: Established Efficacy (≥2 Class I Trials)	Level B: Probably Effective (1 Class I or 2 Class II Studies)	Level C: Possibly Effective (1 Class II Study)	Level U: Inadequate or Conflicting Data
Divalproex sodium	Amitriptyline	Lisinopril	Acetazolamide
Sodium valproate	Venlafaxine	Candesartan	Acenocoumarol
Topiramate	Atenolol	Clonidine	Coumadin
Metoprolol	Nadolol	Guanfacine	Picotamide
Propranolol		Carbamazepine	Fluvoxamine
Timolol		Nebivolol	Fluoxetine
		Pindolol	Gabapentin
		Cyproheptadine	Protriptyline
			Bisoprolol
			Nicardipine
			Nifedipine
			Nimodipine
			Verapamil
			Cyclandelate

for β-blockers among the antihypertensive medications, other blood pressure medications with weaker levels of evidence are commonly used and can be effective in select populations.

Cluster Headache

Cluster headache is one subtype of a general class of headache disorders known as the trigeminal autonomic cephalgias (TACs). Unlike migraine, which predominantly affects women, the male to female ratio for cluster headache is 3 to 1. TACs are characterized by their side-locked unilateral distribution, are typically periorbital or retroorbital in location, have a rapid time to peak severity of minutes, and occur with at least one of several prominent autonomic features, including conjunctival injection, lacrimation, rhinorrhea, ptosis, miosis, facial flushing or sweating, eyelid or periorbital edema, or a sense of restlessness or agitation.

The TACs are further subdivided by attack frequency and duration; cluster headache typically lasts 15 to 180 minutes and occurs anywhere from 1 attack every other day to 8 in a day. The episodic form of cluster often respects a circadian rhythmicity and seasonal periodicity in that it may occur at or near a specific time in the day or night during certain seasons of the year. Chronic cluster headache is defined by attacks that occur for more than 1 year without remission or with periods of remission of less than 1 month.

The American Academy of Neurology guidelines for the abortive and prophylactic treatment of cluster headache are summarized in Table 54.4. Abortive treatments with the highest level of evidence for cluster attacks include subcutaneous sumatriptan, intranasal zolmitriptan, and high-flow (6–12 L/min) oxygen via non-rebreather facemask.

Although strong evidence is lacking to support any one prophylactic agent for the treatment of cluster headache, first-line treatments typically include verapamil, melatonin, occipital nerve blockade, lithium, and brief courses of corticosteroid. Other treatments that seem to be promising but currently lack strong supportive evidence include sphenopalatine ganglion blockade, pregabalin, short courses of corticosteroid, and both occipital and sphenopalatine ganglion stimulation.

Other TACs include paroxysmal hemicrania and short-lasting unilateral neuralgiform headache with conjunctival injection and tearing, which have features identical to those of cluster headache but last 2 to 30 minutes in the case of paroxysmal hemicrania or 1 to 600 seconds in short-lasting unilateral neuralgiform headache with conjunctival injection and tearing.

"Chronic Daily" Headache

Primary headache disorders should never be diagnosed as "chronic daily" headache because numerous primary and secondary headaches can present as chronic and daily. This point is especially important because correct diagnosis of the underlying headache disorder is key to the identification of appropriate treatment options and portends a better outcome for patients. The most commonly presenting primary "chronic daily" headache is chronic migraine, which is defined by the International Classification of Headache Disorders, 3rd edition (beta), as headache for more than 15 days per month for more than 3 months with at least 8 headache days meeting the criteria for migraine with or without aura (Box 54.4).

A key differentiation between many chronic headache disorders is the duration of acute attacks (if untreated). A 4-hour time frame differentiates disorders such as chronic migraine and chronic tension-type headache from short-lasting headache disorders such as chronic cluster

---

Table 54.4 • Evidence-Based Recommendations for the Abortive and Prophylactic Treatment of Cluster Headache

Type of Treatment	Level A: Established Efficacy (≥2 Class I Trials)	Level B: Probably Effective (1 Class I or 2 Class II Studies)	Level C: Possibly Effective (1 Class II Study)	Level U: Inadequate or Conflicting Data
Abortive	Sumatriptan (subcutaneous)	Sumatriptan (intranasal)	Octreotide	Dihydroergotamine (intranasal)
	Zolmitriptan (intranasal)	Zolmitriptan (oral)		Somatostatin
	Oxygen			Prednisone
Prophylactic		Civamide	Melatonin	Capsaicin
		Occipital nerve block	Verapamil	Nitrate tolerance
		Sodium valproate	Cimetidine/ chlorpheniramine	Prednisone
		Sumatriptan	Lithium	
			Misoprostol	
			Oxygen	

Box 54.4 • **Diagnostic Criteria for Chronic Migraine**

A. Headache (tension-type–like or migraine-like) on ≥15 days per month for >3 months and fulfilling criteria B and C

B. Occurring in a patient who has at least 5 attacks fulfilling criteria for migraine with or without aura

C. On ≥8 days per month for >3 months, fulfilling any of the following:

1. Criteria for migraine without aura

2. Criteria for migraine with aura

3. Believed by the patient to be migraine and relieved by a triptan or ergot

Adapted from Headache Classification Committee of the International Headache Society (IHS). The International Classification of Headache Disorders, 3rd edition (beta version). Cephalalgia. 2013 Jul;33(9):629–808. Used with permission.

headache and chronic paroxysmal hemicrania (Box 54.5). Hemicrania continua is characterized by a continuous unilateral side-locked pain with superimposed attacks of no specific duration that are accompanied by any number of autonomic features of other TACs. New daily persistent headache may have features of either migraine or tension-type headache but is characterized by persistent daily headache of rather abrupt onset with no prior headache history. Affected patients frequently present with a history of their daily unremitting headache beginning on a specific day.

Some medications effective for the prophylaxis of episodic migraine are also used for the prophylaxis of chronic migraine; however, no formalized prophylactic treatment guidelines exist. The only treatment approved by the US Food and Drug Administration for the prophylaxis of chronic migraine is botulinum toxin injections.

Potentially modifiable risk factors for the progression of episodic to chronic migraine include frequency of attacks, obesity, caffeine and medication overuse, depression, and sleep disorders. In general, patients should be encouraged to limit their use of abortive medications to no more than 2 or 3 days per week, especially when using opioids or barbiturates, which have a higher likelihood of dependence or abuse. Definitions for medication overuse are summarized in Box 54.6.

The management of daily or refractory headache should include transitional, abortive, and prophylactic treatments. Transitional treatments are designed to temporarily treat refractory pain and serve as a bridge to the long-term care plan. Transitional treatments may include hospitalization, outpatient infusion of abortive medications, brief courses of oral corticosteroid or nonsteroidal anti-inflammatory drugs simultaneous with lifestyle modifications, trigger avoidance, and withdrawal of overused medications. Although many overused medications can be withdrawn abruptly, caution should be exercised with opioids and barbiturates, both of which may need to be withdrawn gradually.

Of note, TACs such as chronic paroxysmal hemicrania and hemicrania continua often have rapid and full remission with therapeutic doses of indomethacin.

Trigeminal Neuralgia

Trigeminal neuralgia is characterized by sharp, electric-shock–like paroxysmal facial pain lasting seconds and occurring numerous times in a day, typically in association with tactile triggers including touching the affected area, brushing one's teeth, drinking hot or cold liquids, chewing or swallowing, talking, or exposure to wind against the face. The pain can occur in any 1 of the 3 distributions of the trigeminal nerve, but it most commonly affects the second or third division with pain often radiating into the teeth. Although many cases of trigeminal neuralgia are idiopathic, vascular contact with or compression of the trigeminal nerve is a frequent underlying cause and can sometimes be corrected with microvascular decompression surgery in

Box 54.5 • **Differentiation of Common "Chronic Daily" Headaches by Duration of Attack**

Short-lasting (<4 h)

Cluster headache
Paroxysmal hemicranias
SUNCT

Long-lasting (>4 h)

Chronic migraine
Chronic tension-type headache
New daily persistent headache
Hemicrania continua

Abbreviation: SUNCT, short-lasting unilateral neuralgiform headache with conjunctival injection and tearing.

Box 54.6 • **Diagnostic Criteria for Medication Overuse Headache**

A. Headache present on ≥15 days per month

B. Regular overuse for >3 months of acute medications defined by the following:

1. Ergot, triptan, opioid, or butalbital analgesics ≥10 days per month

2. Nonopioid analgesics ≥15 days per month

3. All acute drugs ≥15 days/month

Data from Headache Classification Committee of the International Headache Society (IHS). The International Classification of Headache Disorders, 3rd edition (beta version). Cephalalgia. 2013 Jul;33(9):629–808.

medically refractory cases. Trigeminal neuralgia is typically a unilateral phenomenon and most often occurs in the elderly; thus, if it occurs in younger patients or if it occurs bilaterally, underlying secondary causes should be strongly considered.

Treatment options for trigeminal neuralgia include carbamazepine, oxcarbazepine, phenytoin, baclofen, gabapentin, clonazepam, and lamotrigine. Surgical treatments include alcohol blocks, radiofrequency ablation of the gasserian ganglion (cranial nerve V), gamma knife radiosurgery, and section of the trigeminal nerve.

KEY FACTS

✓ Abortive treatments for cluster headache—subcutaneous sumatriptan, intranasal zolmitriptan, and high-flow oxygen via a non-rebreather facemask have the highest level of evidence

✓ Prophylaxis of chronic migraine—botulinum toxin injections are the only treatment approved by the US Food and Drug Administration

✓ Trigeminal neuralgia—characterized by sharp, electric-shock–like paroxysmal facial pain lasting seconds and occurring numerous times a day

✓ Typical triggers of trigeminal neuralgia—touching the affected area, brushing one's teeth, drinking hot or cold liquids, chewing or swallowing, talking, or exposure to wind against the face

---

"Dizziness"

"Dizziness" is a nonspecific term that can describe any one of several subjective experiences, including light-headedness, vertigo, imbalance and unsteadiness, or ataxia. Because each of these complaints suggests different possible diagnoses and treatment options, it is always important to obtain a detailed history with specific attention to the patient's definition of "dizzy" and to specific details about timing, onset, duration, triggers, and the presence of neurologic signs or symptoms.

Accurate visual, vestibular, proprioceptive, tactile, and auditory perceptions are necessary for normal spatial orientation. These inputs are integrated in the brainstem and cerebral hemispheres. The outputs are the cortical, brainstem, and cerebellar motor systems. Impairment of any of these functions or their input, integration, or output causes a complaint of "dizziness" (a sensation of altered orientation or space). Dizziness, vertigo, and dysequilibrium are common complaints. The results of diagnostic tests are often normal. Diagnosis depends mainly on the medical history, and physical examination findings are required in some cases. Vestibular tests rarely provide an exact diagnosis. The types of dizziness are listed in Box 54.7.

Box 54.7 • Types of Dizziness

Vertigo
    Peripheral
    Central

Presyncopal light-headedness
    Orthostatic hypotension
    Vasovagal attacks
    Impaired cardiac output
    Hyperventilation

Psychophysiologic dizziness
    Acute anxiety
    Agoraphobia (fear and avoidance of being in public places)
    Chronic anxiety

Dysequilibrium
    Lesions of basal ganglia, frontal lobes, and white matter
    Hydrocephalus
    Cerebellar dysfunction

Ocular dizziness
    High magnification and lens implant
    Imbalance in extraocular muscles
    Oscillopsia

Multisensory dizziness
    Physiologic dizziness
        Motion sickness
        Space sickness
        Height vertigo

Presyncope and Light-headedness

Presyncope is frequently reported as feeling faint or light-headed and is rarely neurologic in origin. It commonly results from pancerebral hypoperfusion and may indicate orthostatic hypotension, usually due to decreased blood volume, chronic use of antihypertensive drugs, or autonomic dysfunction. Other causes include vasovagal attacks, which are induced when emotions such as fear and anxiety activate medullary vasodepressor centers. Vasodepressor episodes can also be precipitated by acute visceral pain or sudden severe attacks of vertigo. Impaired cardiac output causes presyncopal light-headedness, as does hyperventilation. Chronic anxiety with associated hyperventilation is the most common cause of persistent presyncopal light-headedness in young patients, although postural orthostatic tachycardia syndrome is also common in this population. In most persons, a moderate increase in respiratory rate can decrease the $Paco_2$ level to 25 mm Hg or less in a few minutes.

The 5 types of syncopal attacks that are especially common in elderly patients are listed in Box 54.8.

Vertigo

Vertigo is an illusion of movement (usually that of rotation) and the feeling of vertical or horizontal rotation of

Box 54.8 • Syncopal Attacks Common in Elderly Patients

Orthostatic—from multiple causes

Autonomic dysfunction—from peripheral (ie, postganglionic) or central (ie, preganglionic) involvement

Reflex—such as carotid sinus syncope or cough or micturition syncope

Vasovagal syncope—occurs less frequently in elderly patients than in young patients; however, the prognosis is worse for the elderly, with about 16% of them having major morbidity or mortality in the following 6 months compared with less than 1% of patients younger than 30 years (common precipitating events in the elderly include emotional stress, prolonged bed rest, prolonged standing, and painful stimuli)

Cardiogenic—from conditions such as arrhythmias or valvular disease

either the person or the environment around the person. Most patients report this as a "spinning" or "rotational" sensation. In contrast to vertigo, **dysequilibrium** is a feeling of unsteadiness or insecurity about the environment, without a rotatory sensation. Vertigo occurs when there is imbalance, especially acute, between the left and right vestibular systems. The sudden unilateral loss of vestibular function is dramatic; the patient complains of severe vertigo and nausea and vomiting and is pale and diaphoretic. With acute vertigo, the patient also has problems with equilibrium and vision, often described as "blurred vision" or diplopia. Autonomic symptoms are common—sweating, pallor, nausea, and vomiting—and occasionally can cause vasovagal syncope.

Key Definitions

Vertigo: *illusion of movement (usually that of rotation) and feeling of vertical or horizontal rotation or either the person or the environment around the person.*

Dysequilibrium: *feeling of unsteadiness or insecurity about the environment, without a rotatory sensation.*

Meniere Disease

Fluctuating hearing loss, aural fullness, and tinnitus are characteristic of Meniere disease. Abrupt complete unilateral deafness and vertigo occur with viral involvement of the labyrinth or cranial nerve VIII (or both) and with ischemia of the inner ear. Patients who slowly lose vestibular function bilaterally, as may happen with the use of ototoxic drugs, often do not complain of vertigo but have

oscillopsia with head movements and instability with walking. Even if unilateral vestibular loss occurs slowly (eg, acoustic neuroma), patients usually do not complain of vertigo; they typically present with unilateral hearing loss and tinnitus. Vertigo frequently occurs in episodes. Common vestibular disorders with a genetic predisposition include migraine, Meniere disease, otosclerosis, neurofibromatosis, and spinocerebellar degeneration.

Benign Positional Vertigo

Benign positional vertigo is the most common cause of vertigo. Symptoms include brief episodes of vertigo that usually last 30 seconds up to 1 to 2 minutes and are specifically associated with positional change (eg, turning over in bed, getting in or out of bed, bending over and straightening up, and extending the neck to look up). Typically, the underlying cause is due to displaced otoliths in one of the semicircular canals disrupting the normal flow of endolymphatic fluid and creating a false sense of motion. In about half the patients who do not have benign positional vertigo, no cause is found. For the other half, the most common causes are posttraumatic and postviral neurolabyrinthitis.

Typically, bouts of benign positional vertigo are intermixed with variable periods of remission. Although episodes of vertigo are typically short-lasting, patients may complain of more prolonged nonspecific dizziness that lasts hours to days after a flurry of episodes (eg, light-headedness or a swimming sensation associated with nausea). Management includes reassurance, positional exercises (ie, vestibular exercises), and canalith repositioning maneuvers such as the Epley maneuver. Although pharmacologic treatment is typically of little utility, meclizine and promethazine are frequently used and may provide some modest benefit. Rarely, in intractable cases, surgical treatment (section of the ampullary nerve) may be needed.

Cerebellar Lesions

Vertigo of central nervous system origin can be caused by acute cerebellar lesions (hemorrhages or infarcts) or acute brainstem lesions (especially the lateral medullary syndrome [also called Wallenberg syndrome]). Vertebrobasilar arterial disease can also cause brief transient episodes of vertigo, but it rarely occurs without other focal or localizing neurologic signs and symptoms such as dysarthria, dysphagia, diplopia, facial numbness, crossed syndromes, hemiparesis or alternating hemiparesis, ataxia, and visual field defects.

Psychophysiologic Dizziness

Patients usually describe psychophysiologic dizziness as "floating," "swimming," or "fogginess," but they can also be completely unable to describe their symptoms. The symptoms are not associated with an illusion of movement or movement of the environment or with nystagmus.

Commonly associated symptoms include tension headache, heart palpitations, gastric distress, urinary frequency, backache, and a generalized feeling of weakness and fatigue. Psychophysiologic dizziness can also be associated with panic attacks.

Dysequilibrium

Patients who slowly lose vestibular function on one side, as with an acoustic neuroma, usually do not have vertigo but often describe a vague feeling of imbalance and unsteadiness on their feet. Dysequilibrium may be a presenting symptom of lesions involving motor centers of the basal ganglia and frontal lobe (eg, Parkinson disease, hydrocephalus, and multiple lacunar infarctions). The broad-based ataxic gait of persons with cerebellar disorders is readily distinguished from milder gait disorders that occur with vestibular or sensory loss or with senile gait.

Multifactorial Dizziness and Imbalance

Multifactorial dizziness and imbalance is common in elderly patients and in patients with systemic disorders such as diabetes mellitus. A typical combination includes, for example, mild peripheral neuropathy that causes diminished touch and proprioceptive input, decreased visual acuity, impaired hearing, and decreased baroreceptor function. In affected patients, an added vestibular impairment, as from an ototoxic drug, can be devastating.

The resulting sensation of dizziness and imbalance is usually present only when the patient walks or moves and not when the patient is supine or seated. There is a feeling of insecurity of gait and motion. The patient is usually helped by walking close to a wall, using a cane, or by holding on to another person. Drugs should not be prescribed for this disorder. Instead, the use of a cane or walker is important to improve support and to increase somatosensory signals. A thorough review of the patient's medications should be conducted, and laboratory investigations should be considered when peripheral neuropathy is thought to be contributory. Common laboratory investigations include electromyography; determination of levels of vitamin B_{12} and folate, thyroid-stimulating hormone, and hemoglobin A_{1c} or 2-hour glucose tolerance test; and serum protein electrophoresis.

KEY FACTS

✓ Meniere disease—fluctuating hearing loss, aural fullness, and tinnitus are characteristics

✓ Multifactorial dizziness and imbalance—common in elderly patients and patients with systemic disorders such as diabetes mellitus

✓ Sensation of dizziness and imbalance—usually present only when a patient walks or moves and not when supine or seated

✓ In patients with dizziness and imbalance—use of a cane or walker improves support and increases somatosensory signals

55 Inflammatory and Autoimmune Central Nervous System Diseases and the Neurology of Sepsis

ANDREW MCKEON, MB, BCH, MD

Inflammatory Central Nervous System Diseases

Multiple Sclerosis

The most common inflammatory demyelinating disease of the central nervous system is multiple sclerosis, a disabling disorder that affects predominantly young adults between 20 and 50 years old. It affects women twice as often as men. Multiple sclerosis has a complex immunopathogenesis, variable prognosis, and an unpredictable course. Polygenic and environmental (possibly viral) factors probably have a substantial effect on susceptibility to multiple sclerosis. The disease attacks white matter and (in both early and late stages) axons of the cerebral hemispheres, brainstem, cerebellum, spinal cord, and optic nerve. Most patients (80%–85%) present with relapsing-remitting symptoms. In about 15% of patients, the disease is progressive from onset (primary progressive). Over time, in 70% of patients with the relapsing-remitting form, secondary progressive multiple sclerosis develops. A minority have a primary progressive course without a preceding relapsing course.

Symptoms reflect multiple white matter lesions disseminated in space and time. Typical syndromes include optic neuritis, myelitis, brainstem syndromes, and paroxysmal attacks. Optic neuritis manifests with unilateral visual loss frequently associated with eye pain on movement. Myelitis manifests with sensory symptoms, including a bandlike sensation in the abdomen and chest, spastic weakness of the limbs, and bladder and bowel dysfunction. Other typical symptoms include diplopia (due to internuclear ophthalmoplegia) and ataxia. Paroxysmal symptoms, including trigeminal neuralgia and hemifacial spasm, in a young patient should increase awareness of multiple sclerosis. Other important symptoms are memory and cognitive dysfunction and depression. Associated features that suggest multiple sclerosis include excessive unexplained fatigue and exacerbation of symptoms on exposure to heat.

The diagnosis is primarily based on clinical and magnetic resonance imaging (MRI) data that show lesions disseminated in space and time. Abnormalities on MRI are most helpful and include multifocal lesions of various ages in the periventricular white matter, corpus callosum, brainstem, cerebellum, and spinal cord. Gadolinium-enhanced lesions are presumed to be active lesions of inflammatory demyelination. In patients with clinically isolated syndromes, such as optic neuritis, myelopathy, or brainstem syndrome, abnormal MRI findings are a strong predictor of the eventual clinical diagnosis of multiple sclerosis in the next 5 years. Cerebrospinal fluid findings include oligoclonal bands, increased immunoglobulin (Ig)G synthesis or synthesis rate, and moderate lymphocytic pleocytosis (<50 mononuclear cells/mcL). Visual and somatosensory evoked potential studies are less helpful.

Many other disorders mimic multiple sclerosis and should be considered when patients have atypical findings. Important examples include vasculitis, infections (eg, human immunodeficiency virus infection or Lyme disease), paraneoplastic disorders, neurosarcoidosis, systemic lupus erythematosus, Behçet syndrome, and lymphoma.

Predictors associated with a more favorable long-term course of multiple sclerosis include age younger than 40 years at onset, female sex, optic neuritis or isolated sensory symptoms as the first clinical manifestation, and relatively infrequent attacks. Prognostic factors associated with a poor outcome include age older than 40 years at onset, male sex, cerebellar or pyramidal tract findings at initial presentation, relatively frequent attacks during the first 2 years, incomplete remissions, and a chronically progressive course. However, no single clinical variable is sufficient to predict the course or outcome of this disease. There is evidence that a subset of patients with multiple sclerosis has very benign disease; hence, not every patient with multiple sclerosis must receive long-term treatment.

The recommended therapy for acute exacerbations of multiple sclerosis is a 3- to 5-day course of a high dose of intravenous methylprednisolone (1.0 g daily). Severe or steroid-unresponsive exacerbations are treated with plasma exchange.

Several parenterally administered immunomodulatory agents may reduce the rate of disease relapse in patients with relapsing-remitting disease. Evidence that these drugs have utility in the progressive phases of multiple sclerosis is limited. In clinical trials, reduction in the relapse rate has varied from 33% for interferon beta-1a, interferon beta-1b, and glatiramer acetate to 70% for natalizumab. Newer oral agents include fingolimod, dimethyl fumarate, and teriflunomide. Important adverse effects include depression (interferon therapies), injection site reactions (interferons and glatiramer acetate), and life-threatening opportunistic infection (natalizumab and fingolimod). For patients receiving interferon beta, periodic monitoring includes liver function tests and complete blood cell counts. In 5% to 30% of patients receiving interferon beta, neutralizing antibodies develop and block its effects.

Several drugs are used to treat specific symptoms of multiple sclerosis. Trigeminal neuralgia, flexor spasms, and other paroxysmal symptoms respond to carbamazepine, and spasticity responds to baclofen and tizanidine. Fatigue, a disabling symptom of multiple sclerosis, occasionally responds to amantadine, modafinil, or stimulants.

KEY FACTS

✓ Multiple sclerosis—most common inflammatory demyelinating disease of the central nervous system

✓ Most patients with multiple sclerosis (80%-85%) present with relapsing-remitting symptoms

✓ Typical syndromes in multiple sclerosis—optic neuritis, myelitis, brainstem syndromes, and paroxysmal attacks

✓ The diagnosis of multiple sclerosis—primarily based on clinical and MRI data that show lesions disseminated in space and time

✓ Cerebrospinal fluid findings in multiple sclerosis—oligoclonal bands, increased IgG synthesis or synthesis rate, and moderate lymphocytic pleocytosis (<50 mononuclear cells/mcL)

✓ Recommended therapy for acute exacerbations of multiple sclerosis—3- to 5-day course of a high dose of intravenous methylprednisolone (1.0 g daily); severe or steroid-unresponsive exacerbations are treated with plasma exchange

---

Monophasic Inflammatory Disorders

Some patients have single-episode acute demyelinating events not evolving into multiple sclerosis. Some of these events are hypothesized to occur as parainfectious inflammatory disorders. They can be single episodes of optic neuritis or transverse myelitis. These disorders are usually mild and self-limiting. However, acute disseminated encephalomyelitis usually presents in children or young adults with widespread neurologic dysfunction and diffuse inflammatory-appearing lesions on brain and spinal cord imaging. The treatment of all of these disorders described is the same as that of acute attacks of multiple sclerosis: corticosteroids, in the first instance, and plasma exchange, if necessary.

Other Inflammatory Central Nervous System Disorders

Neurosarcoidosis is likely the most common chronic central nervous system inflammatory disorder after multiple sclerosis. Neurologic manifestations are protean, and it is often referred to as the "great mimicker" of other common central nervous system disorders, including multiple sclerosis and tumors. MRI shows unifocal or multifocal inflammatory lesions of both parenchyma and pial meninges. Clinical examination and imaging of nonneurologic organs can raise suspicion for a multisystem disorder and provide a site for biopsy more accessible than brain from which to obtain a tissue diagnosis. Other, rare inflammatory central nervous system disorders include Langerhans cell histiocytosis, Erdheim-Chester disease, and Susac syndrome.

Autoimmune Central Nervous System Diseases

Paraneoplastic and Other Autoimmune Disorders

Broadly speaking, a paraneoplastic disorder occurs because of the remote effects of malignancy, rather than because of direct tumor invasion. Paraneoplastic neurologic disorders come about because of vigorous immune responses directed against antigens expressed in tumors. The vigor of the immune response usually ensures that neoplasm is confined to the primary organ and regional lymph nodes. The neurologic presentation is often the first clue to the existence, or recurrence, of cancer. Autoimmune neurologic disorders may also arise in nonparaneoplastic contexts (eg, stiff-man syndrome, Lambert-Eaton syndrome, and neuropsychiatric lupus).

The most common neural antibodies, common neurologic findings, and oncologic associations of autoimmune neurologic disorders are listed in Table 55.1. Neurologic presentations are protean and may affect any level of the

Table 55.1 • Autoimmune Neurologic Disorders

Antibody	Oncologic Association	Neurologic Presentation
Amphiphysin IgG	Small cell carcinoma, breast adenocarcinoma	Encephalitis, stiff-man syndrome, myelopathy, neuropathy
ANNA-1 (anti-Hu)	Small cell carcinoma	Encephalitis, brainstem encephalitis, autonomic neuropathies, peripheral neuropathies
ANNA-2 (anti-Ri)	Small cell carcinoma, breast adenocarcinoma	Encephalitis, brainstem encephalitis, myelopathy, neuropathy
Calcium channels (P/Q- and N-types)	Small cell carcinoma, or nonparaneoplastic	Lambert-Eaton myasthenic syndrome, encephalitis, myelopathy
GAD65	Usually no cancer found	Stiff-man syndrome, ataxia, encephalitis, parkinsonism, myelopathy
Ma1, Ma2	Testicular (Ma2 only); breast, colon, testicular (Ma1 and Ma2 together)	Encephalitis, brainstem encephalitis
Muscle AChR	Thymoma or nonparaneoplastic	Myasthenia gravis
Neuronal AChR	Adenocarcinomas, thymoma in 30%. Nonparaneoplastic in 70%	Autoimmune dysautonomia
NMDA receptor	Ovarian teratoma (50% of patients)	Anxiety, psychosis, seizures, encephalitis, dyskinesias
PCA-1 (anti-Yo)	Ovarian or other gynecologic tract adenocarcinoma, breast adenocarcinoma	Cerebellar ataxia, brainstem encephalitis, myelopathy, neuropathies
PCA-Tr	Hodgkin lymphoma	Cerebellar ataxia
VGKC complex	Various in about 20%, or nonparaneoplastic	Limbic encephalitis, amnestic syndrome, executive dysfunction, personality change, disinhibition, hypothalamic disorder, brainstem encephalitis, ataxia, extrapyramidal disorders, myoclonus, peripheral and autonomic neuropathy

Abbreviations: AChR, acetylcholine receptor; ANNA, antineuronal nuclear antibody; CRMP5, collapsin-response mediator-protein 5; GAD65, 65 kDa isoform of glutamic acid decarboxylase; Ig, immunoglobulin; NMDA, *N*-methyl-ᴅ-aspartate; PCA, Purkinje cytoplasmic antibody; Tr, Trotter (named after John Trotter who first described this antibody); VGKC, voltage-gated potassium channel.

neuraxis. Symptoms are usually subacute in onset and rapidly progress. In any individual patient, the neurologic presentation may be a classic unifocal disorder (eg, pure limbic encephalitis in a patient with voltage-gated potassium channel complex antibody) or multifocal disorder (eg, stiff-man syndrome and ataxia in a patient with gadolinium acid decarboxylase [GAD]65 antibody positivity). Nonneural antibodies such as markers of lupus and thyroid antibodies may be clues to an autoimmune diagnosis. In addition to IgG antibody markers, testing that aids confirmation of an autoimmune diagnosis includes imaging, neurophysiologic, and cerebrospinal fluid evaluations. One or more of an increased cerebrospinal fluid protein, white cell count, IgG index, IgG synthesis rate, and oligoclonal bands are supportive of an autoimmune neurologic diagnosis. The search for cancer may be aided by detection of a specific antibody. Cerebrospinal fluid testing for paraneoplastic antibodies may complement serologic testing for cases in which the latter has been negative.

The primary therapy for autoimmune neurologic disorders is treatment of the cancer in the standard way (one or more of surgery, chemotherapy, and radiation). One or more immunotherapies (corticosteroids, intravenous Ig, plasma exchange, cyclophosphamide) may provide additional

neurologic improvements when cancer remission has been achieved, although responses are variable.

Neuromyelitis Optica

Neuromyelitis optica, an example of an autoimmune central nervous system disorder, is a recurrent severe demyelinating disease that may mimic multiple sclerosis. In contrast to multiple sclerosis, the pathophysiology of this disorder is relatively well understood. Antibody targets the central nervous system-predominant water channel, aquaporin 4, resulting in a cascade of inflammatory events leading to attacks of neurologic symptoms. The diagnosis is based on the following: 1) presence of severe optic neuritis or transverse myelitis, or both; 2) MRI evidence of contiguous spinal cord lesions spanning more than 3 vertebral segments; and 3) presence of neuromyelitis optica–IgG (aquaporin 4–IgG) in serum. Encephalitis occasionally occurs, most often in children. Twelve percent of patients present with intractable vomiting due to brainstem encephalitis. Unlike in multiple sclerosis, the cerebrospinal fluid in neuromyelitis optica often shows polynuclear pleocytosis (>50 cells/mcL) and usually an absence of oligoclonal bands. Exacerbations may respond to intravenous methylprednisolone or plasma exchange. The presence of neuromyelitis optica–IgG antibodies indicates risk of recurrence and warrants long-term immunosuppression with azathioprine, mycophenolate, or rituximab.

Key Definition

Neuromyelitis optica: *an autoimmune central nervous system disorder; a recurrent severe demyelinating disease that may mimic multiple sclerosis.*

Neurology of Sepsis

The nervous system is commonly affected in sepsis syndrome. The neurologic conditions encountered are septic encephalopathy, critical illness polyneuropathy or myopathy (or both), cachexia, and panfascicular muscle necrosis. Neurologic complications also occur in intensive care units for critical medical illness. These complications include metabolic encephalopathy, seizures, hypoxic-ischemic encephalopathy, and stroke.

Septic Encephalopathy

Septic encephalopathy is brain dysfunction in association with systemic infection without overt infection of the brain or meninges. Early encephalopathy often begins before failure of other organs and is not due to single or multiple organ failure. Endotoxin does not cross the blood-brain barrier and so probably does not directly affect adult brains. Cytokines, important components of sepsis syndrome, may contribute to encephalopathy. Gegenhalten, or paratonic, rigidity occurs in more than 50% of patients, and tremor, asterixis, and multifocal myoclonus occur in about 25%. Seizures and focal neurologic signs are rare.

Electroencephalography is a sensitive indicator of encephalopathy. The mildest abnormality is diffuse excessive low-voltage theta activity (4–7 Hz). The next level of severity is intermittent rhythmic delta activity (<4 Hz). As the condition worsens, delta activity becomes arrhythmic and continuous. Typical triphasic waves occur in severe cases, especially in hepatic failure. In these cases, MRI and computed tomography of the brain may be normal.

Critical Illness Polyneuropathy and Myopathy

Critical illness polyneuropathy occurs in 70% of patients with sepsis and multiple-organ failure. There is often an unexplained difficulty in weaning from mechanical ventilation. Nerve biopsy specimens show primary axonal degeneration of motor and sensory fibers without inflammation. Critical illness myopathy is also recognized in patients with sepsis. Similarly, biopsy shows degenerative changes without inflammation. Most patients have findings of both myopathy and neuropathy. Recovery is satisfactory if the patient survives sepsis and multiple-organ failure. Treatment is supportive care and rehabilitation.

KEY FACTS

✓ Primary therapy for autoimmune neurologic disorders—treatment of the cancer in the standard way

✓ Diagnosis of neuromyelitis optica—based on 1) presence of severe optic neuritis or transverse myelitis, or both; 2) MRI evidence of contiguous spinal cord lesions spanning more than 3 vertebral segments; and 3) presence of neuromyelitis optica–IgG (aquaporin 4–IgG) in serum

✓ Critical illness polyneuropathy—occurs in 70% of patients with sepsis and multiple-organ failure

✓ Recovery from critical illness polyneuropathy and myopathy is satisfactory if the patient survives sepsis and multiple-organ failure; treatment is supportive care and rehabilitation

56 Movement Disorders

ANHAR HASSAN, MB, BCh AND EDUARDO E. BENARROCH, MD

Movement disorders are common in adult clinical practice. An important first step in evaluation and management of these disorders is identification of a potentially reversible cause, most commonly medication effect. All patients younger than 50 years presenting with any type of movement disorder should be evaluated for Wilson disease.

Tremor

Tremor is an oscillatory rhythmic movement that may occur in isolation, as in the case of essential tremor, or as part of another condition such as Parkinson disease or cerebellar disorders. *Rest tremor* is observed with the limb fully relaxed and supported, with the arms lying in the lap or hanging at the side (for example while walking) or the legs hanging over the examining table. The most common cause of rest tremor is Parkinson disease. Several types of action tremor are triggered by muscle contraction. *Postural tremor* occurs when the body part is held in a sustained posture (eg, arms held outstretched or head held erect). Postural tremor includes exaggerated physiologic tremor, essential tremor, tremor induced by drugs (eg, methylxanthines, β-adrenergic agonists, lithium, and amiodarone) or toxic-metabolic conditions (such as stimulant overuse or alcohol withdrawal), and neuropathic tremor. *Intention tremor* is worsened with action, as in finger-to-nose testing, especially the terminal part of the movement. This type of tremor occurs with diseases of the cerebellum or its connections. *Task-related tremor* occurs during specific tasks and includes primary writing tremor (which may occur in association with writer's cramp) and orthostatic tremor, which occurs only when a patient is in the standing position.

Essential Tremor

Essential tremor is the most common movement disorder and can be differentiated from Parkinson disease tremor (Table 56.1). It is most common in middle and older age. There is often a positive family history. The hands are most frequently affected, with both postural and intention tremor, followed by the head and voice. Head tremor can be either horizontal ("no-no") or vertical ("yes-yes"). Head tremor almost never occurs in Parkinson disease, although patients with Parkinson disease may have tremor of the mouth, lips, tongue, and jaw. The legs and trunk (affected in orthostatic tremor) are affected less frequently in essential tremor. Essential tremor is slowly progressive, and its pathophysiologic mechanism is not known.

The most effective agent to decrease essential tremor is alcohol. First-line medications are propranolol (40 mg/day, up to 320 mg/day) (or other β-blockers) and primidone (25–250 mg at bedtime). Second-line drugs are clonazepam, gabapentin, and topiramate. Deep brain stimulation of the thalamus is effective for all types of medication-refractory tremor with functional disability.

Parkinson Disease

Patients with Parkinson disease present with tremor (the initial symptom in 50%–70%, but 15% never have tremor), rigidity, or bradykinesia. The gait is unsteady, slow, and shuffling. Decreased blink rate, lack of facial expression, small handwriting, and asymptomatic orthostatic hypotension are also common. Parkinson disease includes motor manifestations (Box 56.1) and nonmotor manifestations (Box 56.2). The classic motor manifestations of Parkinson disease are rest tremor, muscle stiffness (rigidity), and slowness of movement (bradykinesia), which typically start asymmetrically and respond to levodopa therapy. Late motor manifestations, including difficulty swallowing, postural instability, and freezing of gait, are much less responsive to treatment. At late stages of the disease after prolonged dopamine replacement therapy, motor fluctuations or dyskinesia (chorea-like movements of the limbs,

Table 56.1 • Differential Diagnosis of Tremor

Feature	Parkinson Disease	Essential Tremor
Tremor type and frequency	Rest >> postural; 3–5 Hz	Postural, kinetic; 8–12 Hz
Affected by tremor	Hands, legs, chin, jaw	Hands, head, voice
Rigidity and bradykinesia	Yes	No
Family history	15%	60%
Alcohol response	Inconsistent	Consistent
Therapy	Levodopa, dopamine agonists, anticholinergics	Propranolol, primidone, gabapentin (botulinum toxin for head tremor)
Surgical treatment	Subthalamic, globus pallidus interna stimulation	Thalamic (Vim) stimulation

Abbreviations: Vim, subnucleus ventralis intermedius; >>, much greater than.

Box 56.2 • Nonmotor Manifestations of Parkinson Disease

Autonomic
  Constipation[a]
  Orthostatic hypotension
  Bladder dysfunction
Sleep disorders
  Excessive diurnal somnolence
  Insomnia
  RBD[a]
  Periodic leg movement disorder
Cognitive symptoms
  Depression[a]
  Anxiety
  Apathy
  Hallucinations
  Mild cognitive impairment, dementia
Sensory symptoms
  Impaired olfaction[a]

Abbreviation: RBD, rapid eye movement (REM)–sleep behavior disorder.
[a] May precede the diagnosis of disease.

trunk, or head) develop. Some nonmotor manifestations may precede the diagnosis of Parkinson disease (Box 56.2).

The differential diagnosis of Parkinson disease includes disorders caused by drugs (Box 56.3), toxins (eg, carbon monoxide, manganese), neurometabolic disorders (particularly Wilson disease in patients younger than 50 years), and other neurodegenerative disorders in which parkinsonism is a prominent feature (atypical parkinsonian syndromes) (Table 56.2). Manifestations that suggest a disorder other than Parkinson disease ("red flags") include a lack of response to levodopa, early postural instability with falls, orthostatic hypotension or urinary incontinence, cerebellar findings (ataxia), corticospinal signs (increased deep tendon reflexes, spasticity, or extensor plantar response), and early dementia.

Treatment of the motor manifestations of Parkinson disease is summarized in Table 56.3. The initial treatment options include levodopa combined with carbidopa or

dopamine agonists. Anticholinergic agents can suppress tremor but are rarely used now and should be avoided in patients older than 65 years because of frequent adverse effects, such as memory loss, delirium, urinary hesitancy, and blurred vision. Patients with disabling symptoms

Box 56.1 • Motor Manifestations of Parkinson Disease

Early manifestations (typically asymmetric in onset and responsive to levodopa)
  Rest tremor
  Rigidity
  Bradykinesia
Late manifestations (less responsive to levodopa)
  Gait and postural instability
  Dysphagia
  Motor fluctuations (wearing-off and on-off phenomena)
  Levodopa-induced dyskinesia

Box 56.3 • Drugs That Induce Parkinsonism or Tremor

Antagonist of dopamine D_2 receptors
  Neuroleptics (eg, haloperidol, risperidone, reserpine)
  Antiemetics (metoclopramide, prochlorperazine)
Other psychiatric drugs
  Selective serotonin reuptake inhibitors
  Tricyclics
  Lithium
Cardiovascular drugs
  Amiodarone
  Calcium channel blockers (flunarizine)
  Atorvastatin
Anticonvulsants
  Valproate
Others
  Cyclosporine
  Metronidazole
  Caffeine and other methylxanthines
  α-Adrenergic agonist
  Thyroxine
  Prednisone

Table 56.2 • Differential Diagnosis of Atypical Parkinsonian Syndromes

Manifestation	Suspect
Poor response to levodopa	Any atypical parkinsonian syndrome (MSA and PSP may respond)
Early falls	PSP or MSA
Severe OH, urologic symptoms, anosmia, or RBD	MSA
Cerebellar signs	MSA or spinocerebellar degeneration
Vertical gaze palsy	PSP
Asymmetric apraxia	Corticobasal degeneration
Early dementia	Lewy body dementia Creutzfeldt-Jakob disease

Abbreviations: MSA, multiple system atrophy; OH, orthostatic hypotension; PSP, progressive supranuclear palsy; RBD, rapid eye movement, (REM)–sleep behavior disorder.

should receive carbidopa-levodopa. The initial dosage is a 25/100 tablet (25 mg carbidopa/100 mg levodopa) by mouth 3 times daily on an empty stomach. Starting with dopamine agonists reduces the risk of motor complications compared with long-term levodopa therapy, but these agents are less efficacious than levodopa. Dopamine agonists include pramipexole and ropinirole. The main adverse effects of levodopa and dopamine agonists are nausea, orthostatic hypotension, and hallucinations. All can cause unpredictable daytime sleepiness. An important adverse effect of dopamine agonists is impulse control disorders, manifested as compulsive gambling, compulsive shopping, or pathologic hypersexuality. Patients and their families should be counseled about these problems before initiation of dopaminergic agonist therapy.

Selegiline or rasagiline (monoamine oxidase inhibitors type B) may give mild symptomatic relief in early Parkinson disease and delay levodopa therapy. Adverse effects include nausea, hallucinations, confusion, dyskinesias, and orthostatic hypotension.

Long-term levodopa therapy leads to dyskinesias and motor fluctuations. Management strategies for motor fluctuations include the use of smaller and more frequent doses of levodopa, long-acting levodopa preparations, dopamine agonists, and inhibitors of catechol *O*-methyltransferase. Apomorphine can be administered subcutaneously for severe akinesia at end-of-dose wearing-off times. Restricting protein to mealtimes may decrease unpredictable off times. Reducing the dose of levodopa can improve dyskinesia. Amantadine, a glutamate receptor antagonist, is used as adjuvant treatment in patients with levodopa-induced dyskinesias.

Deep brain stimulation of the subthalamic nucleus or globus pallidus can relieve motor symptoms in eligible patients with levodopa-responsive Parkinson disease and medication-resistant tremor, severe motor fluctuations, or dyskinesia. Patient selection is critical to ensure maximal benefit of this therapy. Patients who have cognitive or

Table 56.3 • Management of Motor Manifestations of Parkinson Disease

Drug[a]	Indications	Complications/Adverse Effects
Carbidopa-levodopa (25/100,[b] 50/200[c])	Most efficacious treatment Give early in patients with marked impairment	Nausea, vomiting, OH Motor fluctuations with long-term treatment
Dopaminergic agonists Pramipexole Ropinirole Rotigotine	Early use in young patients, either alone or associated with small dose of levodopa Motor fluctuations in patients taking levodopa	Nausea, vomiting, OH More likely than levodopa to produce excessive diurnal somnolence, impulse control disorder (eg, gambling), hallucinations, or peripheral edema
COMT inhibitors Entacapone	Prolong the duration of action of levodopa in patients with wearing-off effect	Diarrhea
MAO-B inhibitors Selegiline Rasagiline	Delay the need to start levodopa therapy May be neuroprotective	Insomnia (with selegiline); nausea, hallucinations, confusion, dyskinesias, OH
Amantadine	Adjuvant treatment in patients with levodopa-induced dyskinesia	Dizziness, livedo reticularis, edema
Surgical treatment GPi or STN DBS	Levodopa responsive, motor fluctuations, disabling dyskinesia, medication-refractory tremor	Does not help gait instability; contraindicated in moderate-severe cognitive impairment Cognitive and psychiatric symptoms may follow STN DBS

Abbreviations: COMT, catechol *O*-methyltransferase; DBS, deep brain stimulation; GPi, globus pallidus, pars interna; MAO, monoamine oxidase; OH, orthostatic hypotension; STN, subthalamic nucleus.

[a] Anticholinergics (eg, trihexyphenidyl) are used only rarely and are contraindicated in patients older than 65 years because of prominent autonomic and cognitive adverse effects.

[b] Carbidopa 25 mg, levodopa 100 mg.

[c] Controlled release formulation: carbidopa 50 mg, levodopa 200 mg.

Table 56.4 • Management of Nonmotor Manifestations of Parkinson Disease

Manifestation	Mechanism	Management
Orthostatic hypotension	Loss of sympathetic ganglion neurons and effects of dopaminergic agonists	Increase sodium and water intake Fludrocortisone, midodrine, pyridostigmine
Constipation	Loss of enteric neurons	Bulk agents, enema
Insomnia	Wearing off; PLMS	Nightly dose of levodopa
REM sleep behavior disorder	Early manifestation	Clonazepam, melatonin
Hallucinations	Medication effect (exclude DLB)	Discontinue use of anticholinergics, MAO-B inhibitors, and amantadine Reduce or discontinue use of dopamine agonists Quetiapine or olanzapine
Depression	Loss of serotonergic neurons?	SSRIs Optimize dopaminergic therapy
Anxiety	Akathisia, stressors	Optimize dopaminergic therapy
Cognitive impairment	Frontal lobe dysfunction Development of DLB	Cholinesterase inhibitors Optimize dopaminergic therapy
Impulse dyscontrol (compulsive gambling, compulsive shopping, pathologic hypersexuality)	Activation of dopamine D_3 receptors in limbic striatum	Warn the patients Reduce or discontinue use of dopaminergic agonist Quetiapine or SSRI may help
Fatigue	Multifactorial	Optimize dopaminergic therapy
Pain	Early morning dystonia Immobility	Increase levodopa Mobilization, physical therapy
Arm paresthesia	May reflect insufficient levodopa treatment	Increase levodopa Exclude other causes
Diplopia	Medication effect Poor convergence	Reading glasses or prisms instead of bifocals

Abbreviations: DLB, dementia with Lewy bodies; MAO, monoamine oxidase; PLMS, periodic leg movement disorder; REM, rapid eye movement; SSRI, selective serotonin reuptake inhibitor.

psychiatric disorders or who do not respond to levodopa are not eligible. Manifestations such as dysphagia, postural instability, and gait freezing do not respond to the procedure. Deep brain stimulation of the subthalamic nucleus may result in transient cognitive or psychiatric manifestations. Suicide has been reported in some patients.

The management of nonmotor manifestations of Parkinson disease is summarized in Table 56.4. Orthostatic hypotension, constipation, bladder dysfunction, and other autonomic manifestations develop in many patients with parkinsonism. In these patients, Parkinson disease should be distinguished from multiple system atrophy. Findings suggestive of multiple system atrophy include lack of a predictable response to levodopa, cerebellar or pyramidal signs, severe orthostatic hypotension and urinary incontinence, and laryngeal stridor. The management of orthostatic hypotension includes eliminating potentially offending drugs (eg, vasodilators, diuretics, dopamine agonists), increasing sodium and water intake, elevating the head of the bed, and wearing compression garments. Drug treatment includes fludrocortisone, midodrine, pyridostigmine, or the recently introduced norepinephrine precursor dihydroxyphenylserine (droxidopa).

New-generation antipsychotic drugs, such as quetiapine or clozapine, are preferably used to manage drug-induced psychosis or hallucinations because they have a lower risk of exacerbating parkinsonism. Typical neuroleptics (eg,

KEY FACTS

✓ The first principle to consider in every patient with any type of movement disorder—potential adverse effect of medication

✓ Wilson disease—should be considered in young patients (<50 years old) with any type of movement disorder

✓ First-line treatment for essential tremor—β-blockers or primidone

✓ Manifestations that suggest an atypical parkinsonian syndrome—poor response to levodopa, early postural instability with falls, severe orthostatic hypotension, and early dementia

✓ Neuroleptics and other dopaminergic-blocking medications should be avoided in patients with parkinsonism or suspected Lewy body dementia

haloperidol) and other dopaminergic-blocking medications (eg, metoclopramide) should be avoided in patients with parkinsonism or suspected Lewy body dementia.

Dystonia

Dystonia is a movement disorder defined as sustained muscle contractions that produce involuntary twisting and repetitive movements and abnormal postures (choreoathetosis). There is inappropriate co-contraction of agonist and antagonist muscles. Dystonia is classified by etiology, distribution, or age at onset. Etiology can be primary (hereditary or idiopathic) or secondary. Distribution can be focal (1 limb or body part), segmental, multifocal, hemidystonia, or generalized. In children, it typically starts in a limb and becomes generalized and is often hereditary. In adults, it is typically focal at onset (eg, cervical dystonia, writer's cramp, orofacial dystonia), with limited spread. Dystonia is usually induced by action and absent at rest; it may be task-specific (eg, writer's cramp, musician's dystonia). There is often a sensory trick (eg, touching the affected body part) to suppress dystonia.

Young patients with focal, segmental, and generalized dystonia should undergo a trial with carbidopa-levodopa because some forms may be very sensitive to dopaminergic medication. Other medications for focal or generalized dystonia include anticholinergics, baclofen, or clonazepam. Deep brain stimulation of bilateral globus pallidus pars interna, is used for severe medication-refractory dystonia, and benefit can take weeks to months.

The first-line treatment for focal dystonia is botulinum toxin. Botulinum toxin, which blocks the neuromuscular junction, is effective therapy for cervical dystonia, blepharospasm, hemifacial spasm, spasmodic dysphonia, oromandibular dystonia, and limb dystonia, including occupational dystonias.

Acute dystonic reactions, including oculogyric crises, may be triggered, particularly in young patients, by drugs that block dopamine receptors, including antiemetics such as metoclopramide and antipsychotic agents (particularly first-generation drugs such as haloperidol). In older patients, these drugs may typically trigger parkinsonism. Chronic use of dopaminergic agonists may result in *tardive dyskinesia*, characterized by stereotyped movements affecting the face, mouth, or other body parts.

> **Key Definition**
>
> Dystonia: *a movement disorder with sustained muscle contractions that produce involuntary twisting and repetitive movements and abnormal postures (choreoathetosis).*

Chorea, Athetosis, and Ballismus

Chorea is characterized by rapid, random, flowing movements that may affect the face, neck, or limbs. Patients may appear restless and can maintain postures only briefly (motor impersistence), such as inability to keep the tongue protruded or sustain a handgrip. There are many causes, including vascular, postinfectious, autoimmune (including antiphospholipid antibody syndrome), pregnancy, drugs (such as psychostimulants), toxic-metabolic (thyrotoxicosis), or paraneoplastic. Chorea is the typical motor manifestation of Huntington disease, in which it is associated with dementia and behavioral abnormalities. Antichorea medications include dopamine-depleting agents (eg, tetrabenazine), amantadine, and dopaminergic-blocking agents (typical and atypical antipsychotics, such as haloperidol and quetiapine).

Athetosis is a slow, writhing involuntary movement of the distal aspect of a limb caused by chorea superimposed on dystonia. If chorea is more prominent, the term *choreoathetosis* is used, and this is most commonly found in cerebral palsy.

Ballismus is a severe form of chorea, with large-amplitude flailing movements, especially seen in the proximal aspects of limbs. It typically affects only 1 side of the body, hence "hemiballismus." It is commonly due to a lesion of the contralateral subthalamic nucleus.

Myoclonus

Myoclonus is defined as sudden, lightning-like jerks of an entire muscle that moves a joint. In comparison, fasciculations or myokymia occurs in a segment of muscle and does not cause movement across the joint. These are simple movements and can be observed at rest or accentuated with posture or action. They can be low or high amplitude. They are not rhythmic like tremor and are briefer than tics. Asterixis is the opposite of myoclonus (negative myoclonus) and is due to loss of muscle tone. Myoclonus occurs in many toxic-metabolic and some neurodegenerative disorders. Important examples are hypoxic-ischemic encephalopathy, medication effect (eg, opiates, tramadol, antidepressants), renal or hepatic failure, and Creutzfeldt-Jakob disease.

> **Key Definition**
>
> Myoclonus: *sudden, lightning-like jerks of an entire muscle that moves a joint.*

Tics

These are sudden, rapid, involuntary movements (motor tics) or vocalizations (vocal tics) of varying intensity, frequency, and duration. They can be simple (eg, eye blink, head turn, cough, sniff) or complex (eg, kicking, jumping, vocalizing words). They wax and wane and are exacerbated with stress, anxiety, fatigue, and excitement. They can reduce with concentration and are absent during sleep. A premonitory sensation (urge, tension) often occurs before the tics. They can be briefly suppressed, which leads to increased tension followed by relief after the tics occur. Tics begin in childhood or adolescence and improve in late teenage years and early adulthood. Causes include genetic risk such as family history of tics or Tourette syndrome, autoimmune disorders, medications, or brain lesion.

Tourette syndrome is a disorder in which tics occur before age 21 years, with multiple motor tics and at least one vocal tic for at least 12 months. Associated psychiatric comorbidities are obsessive-compulsive disorder, attention-deficit/hyperactivity disorder, anxiety, or depression.

Treatment includes education, behavioral therapy for tic suppression, and medications. The medications are α_2-adrenergic agonists (eg, clonidine, guanfacine), dopamine blockers (eg, fluphenazine, risperidone, aripiprazole, quetiapine, haloperidol, pimozide), dopamine-depleting agents (eg, tetrabenazine), dopamine agonists (eg, pramipexole), baclofen, topiramate, levetiracetam, clonazepam, and botulinum toxin (for simple motor tics). Deep brain stimulation can be used for severe tics refractory to medication.

Ataxia

This is a disorder of the cerebellum or its connections. Symptoms include unsteady gait, slurred speech, clumsy limbs, and diplopia. The signs include ataxic gait, dysarthria, finger-nose and heel-shin ataxia and dysmetria, intention tremor, nystagmus, impaired saccades, and rebound. Ataxia is hereditary, acquired, or sporadic, and the cause depends on the age at onset, speed of progression (sudden, acute, subacute, or chronic), and presence of family history. There are many causes of ataxia, including vascular (eg, cerebellar stroke), infectious (eg, varicella, Lyme disease, Whipple disease), demyelinating (eg, multiple sclerosis), immune-mediated (eg, celiac disease), paraneoplastic (eg, ovarian cancer), neoplastic (eg, cerebellar metastasis), toxic (eg, alcohol, antiepileptic drugs, toluene, heavy metals, chemotherapy), metabolic (eg, thiamine deficiency, hypothyroidism, vitamin E deficiency), prion disorders (eg, Creutzfeldt-Jakob disease), and genetic. The presence of comorbidities or other neurologic signs can help with the diagnosis. For patients with a positive family history of ataxia, genetic testing can be performed for autosomal dominant (spinocerebellar ataxia), and autosomal

recessive genes (eg, Friedreich ataxia). In the absence of a reversible cause, treatment is mainly supportive with physical, occupational, and speech therapy.

Restless Legs Syndrome and Periodic Limb Movements of Sleep

Restless legs syndrome is a common movement disorder, characterized by an unpleasant sensation (crawling, paresthesia) in the lower limbs (occasionally upper limbs) that typically emerges when sitting or lying down in the evening. It is relieved by limb movement or ambulation and is worsened by holding the limbs still. It occurs during wakefulness. Risk factors are family history, anemia, pregnancy, drugs, and alcohol. It is improved by correcting anemia (ferritin value >50), hydration, exercise, and avoiding alcohol. First-line treatment is gabapentin (or pregabalin) or a dopamine agonist (ropinirole, pramipexole; patient should be counselled about risk for impulse control disorders). Second-line agents are opioids or benzodiazepines.

Periodic leg movements of sleep are repetitive rhythmic leg flexion movements that only arise during sleep, and they sometimes lead to arousals from sleep. They differ from restless legs syndrome in that they are painless and the patient is asleep at onset and has no awareness of them. They frequently occur with restless legs syndrome, however. Typically, a spouse reports these movements, which wake him or her from sleep. They are confirmed by history and polysomnography. Treatments include dopamine agonists and gabapentin.

KEY FACTS

- ✓ Acute onset of unilateral dystonia, chorea, or ballismus—suggests a vascular lesion in the contralateral cerebral hemisphere
- ✓ Subacute onset of generalized chorea or other movement disorder—suggests an immune cause, including paraneoplastic syndrome
- ✓ Treatment of focal dystonia—botulinum toxin
- ✓ Primary treatment of restless legs syndrome and periodic limb movements of sleep—dopaminergic agonist or gabapentin (or pregabalin)
- ✓ Patients receiving dopamine agonist therapy for Parkinson disease, restless legs syndrome, or periodic limb movements of sleep should be made aware of the risk for development of impulse control disorders, including compulsive gambling, pathologic hypersexuality, or compulsive shopping

Neoplastic Diseases

57

ALYX B. PORTER, MD

Primary Neoplasms of the Central Nervous System

Brain tumors may manifest with focal progressive neurologic deficits, increased intracranial pressure (causing headache, vomiting, and papilledema), new-onset seizures, or progressive cognitive and behavioral changes. The most common primary brain tumors in adults are meningioma, astrocytoma, oligodendroglioma, and lymphoma.

The main risk factors associated with meningioma are syndromes associated with genetic predisposition and ionizing radiation (Figure 57.1). Treatment options vary according to patient age, comorbid conditions, tumor size, location, progression, and histologic characteristics. Small asymptomatic tumors should be observed with follow-up computed tomography or magnetic resonance imaging every 6 to 12 months. If symptoms develop or there is clear tumor growth, surgical resection is indicated. Postoperative radiotherapy is indicated after incomplete resection, for tumors with aggressive histologic features (anaplastic or malignant meningiomas), or for disease recurrence. Stereotactic radiosurgery is a treatment option in some cases.

Of all primary central nervous system neoplasms, 40% are gliomas, which occur in all areas of the brain and spinal cord. They are classified as grades 1 through 4 according to their histologic features. Patients with gliomas, which are infiltrative tumors, may present with various presenting symptoms based on tumor location. Prognosis depends on the patient's age at diagnosis, performance status, resectability, and tumor type. Among patients with low-grade astrocytomas, median survival is 6 to 8 years; among patients with oligodendrogliomas, about 10 years. Clinical and radiologic observation is a reasonable approach for patients with stable lesions in a nonresectable area of the brain. Patients with large lesions and mass effect are candidates for surgical resection. The role of postoperative radiotherapy and chemotherapy is still controversial.

High-grade astrocytomas, including anaplastic (grade 3) astrocytoma and glioblastoma multiforme (grade 4), are associated with low survival (about 17.7% at 1 year) (Figure 57.2). Surgical therapy is important for

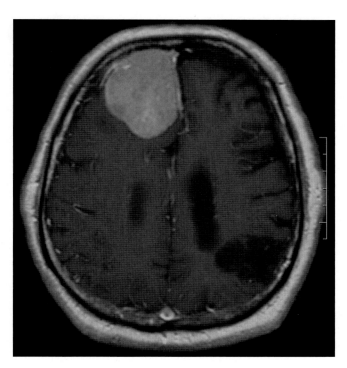

Figure 57.1 *Magnetic Resonance Imaging of a Large Right Frontal Meningioma. Characteristic dural tail and near homogeneous enhancement (gadolinium-enhanced axial T1-weighted sequence) are seen.*

(Adapted from Mowzoon N, Vernino S. Neoplasms of the nervous system and related topics. In: Mowzoon N, Flemming KD, editors. Neurology board review: an illustrated study guide. Rochester [MN]: Mayo Clinic Scientific Press and Florence [KY]: Informa Healthcare USA; c2007. p. 627–78. Used with permission of Mayo Foundation for Medical Education and Research.)

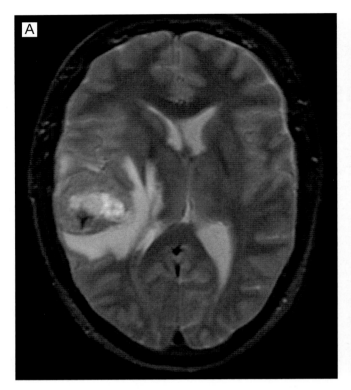

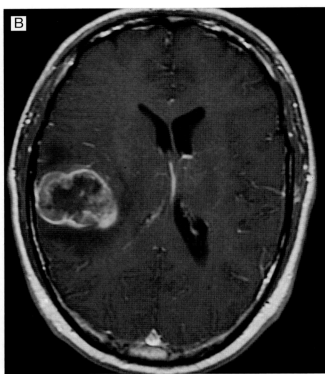

Figure 57.2 Magnetic Resonance Imaging for a 33-Year-Old Patient With Glioblastoma Multiforme. A, T2-weighted and, B, contrast-enhanced T1-weighted images show peripherally enhancing mass with a heterogeneous signal within the lesion, situated in the junction of right posterior frontotemporal operculum and insula. Note vasogenic edema in the white matter surrounding lesion, associated with mass effect and right-to-left midline shift.

(Adapted from Mowzoon N, Vernino S. Neoplasms of the nervous system and related topics. In: Mowzoon N, Flemming KD, editors. Neurology board review: an illustrated study guide. Rochester [MN]: Mayo Clinic Scientific Press and Florence [KY]: Informa Healthcare USA; c2007. p. 627–78. Used with permission of Mayo Foundation for Medical Education and Research.)

obtaining a tissue diagnosis, reducing the mass effect, and removing the majority of the lesion. Surgical therapy is followed by radiotherapy at the site of the lesion. Patients who receive concurrent temozolomide and radiotherapy have longer survival than those who receive radiotherapy alone.

Primary central nervous system lymphoma is a lymphoma that is confined to the brain and the spinal cord and is becoming more common in both immunosuppressed and immunocompetent patients. Imaging features are typically consistent with homogeneously enhancing lesions that may be multifocal (Figure 57.3). These lesions may also be necrotic or ring-enhancing in their appearance, particularly in patients who are immunosuppressed. Diagnosis is made by cytologic analysis of cerebrospinal fluid or brain biopsy. Surgical resection is indicated only for reduction of considerable mass effect. Treatment has been geared toward chemotherapy and stem-cell transplant; radiation therapy is used mainly for disease recurrence and palliation. With improved treatment techniques, median survival has increased to approximately 2 years.

Key Definition

Primary central nervous system lymphoma: *a lymphoma that is confined to the brain and the spinal cord.*

Neurologic Manifestations in Patients With Systemic Cancer

The most common neurologic symptoms of patients with systemic cancer are back pain, altered mental status, and headache. However, the most common neurologic complication of systemic cancer is metastatic disease, of which cerebral metastasis is most frequent. In patients with cancer and back pain, epidural metastasis and direct vertebral metastasis are common, but 15% to 20% of patients have no malignant diagnosis. Nonstructural causes are the most common reasons for headache. Identified causes include fever, adverse effects

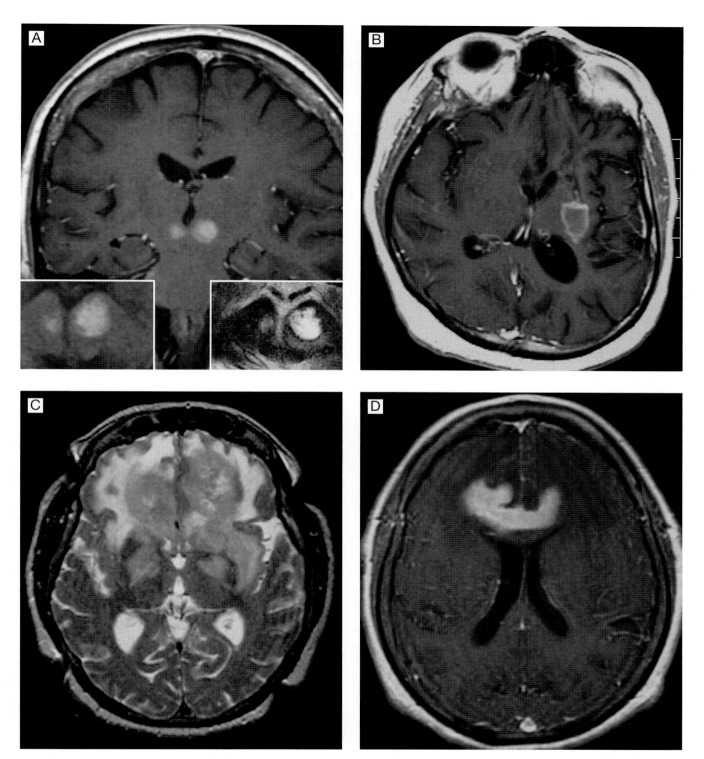

Figure 57.3 *Magnetic Resonance Imaging of Primary Central Nervous System Lymphoma. A, A 64-year-old woman with diffuse large B-cell lymphoma presented with worsening mental status. Gadolinium-enhanced T1-weighted image shows lesions in deep gray matter appearing as mirror images. Both pregadolinium T1- (left inset) and T2- (right inset) weighted images showed increased signal, suggestive of subacute hemorrhage into the mass. B, Gadolinium-enhanced T1-weighted image of an 18-year-old girl with diffuse large B-cell lymphoma shows ring-enhancement outlining the lesion in deep gray matter (common location for lymphoma). C, T2-weighted image and, D, gadolinium-enhanced T1-weighted image of a different patient with diffuse large B-cell lymphoma shows large intraparenchymal mass in frontal lobes bilaterally, extending through genu of corpus callosum and involving deep gray matter. There appears to be extensive perilesional vasogenic edema and mass effect on the frontal horns of the lateral ventricles.*

(Adapted from Mowzoon N, Vernino S. Neoplasms of the nervous system and related topics. In: Mowzoon N, Flemming KD, editors. Neurology board review: an illustrated study guide. Rochester [MN]: Mayo Clinic Scientific Press and Florence [KY]: Informa Healthcare USA; c2007. p. 627–78. Used with permission of Mayo Foundation for Medical Education and Research.)

of therapy, lumbar puncture, metastasis (cerebral, lepto-meningeal, or base of skull), and intracranial hemorrhage (thrombocytopenia or hemorrhage due to intracranial metastasis). The most common cause of altered mental status is toxic-metabolic encephalopathy, which is also the most common nonmetastatic manifestation of systemic cancer. Less common causes include intracranial metastatic disease (parenchymal and meningeal), paraneoplastic limbic encephalitis, intracranial hemorrhage, primary dementia, cerebral infarction, psychiatric disorder, known primary brain tumor, bacterial meningitis, and transient global amnesia.

Many neurologic problems in patients with cancer can be diagnosed from the medical history and findings on neurologic examination and require knowledge of both nonmetastatic- and noncancer-related neurologic illness.

The neurologic complications of systemic cancer are listed in Box 57.1.

KEY FACTS

✓ Brain tumors—may manifest with focal progressive neurologic deficits, increased intracranial pressure (causing headache, vomiting, and papilledema), new-onset seizures, or progressive cognitive and behavioral changes

✓ Most common primary brain tumors in adults—meningioma, astrocytoma, oligodendroglioma, and lymphoma

✓ Treatment of primary central nervous system lymphoma—geared toward chemotherapy and stem-cell transplant; radiation therapy is used mainly for disease recurrence and palliation

---

Metastasis to the Brain

Brain metastases are the most common brain tumors (Figure 57.4). Approximately 30% of cancer patients have brain metastasis at presentation or later. Metastatic lung cancer is the most common (40%–50% of cases), followed by breast cancer, colon cancer, melanoma, and unknown primary cancer. Melanoma produces a disproportionate number of metastases in the central nervous system. Evaluation includes detailed history and examination, assessment of medical and neurologic performance status, and imaging studies (magnetic resonance imaging of the brain with gadolinium; computed tomography of the chest, abdomen, and pelvis; positron emission tomography). Brain metastases are frequently associated with surrounding edema. Dexamethasone (4 mg 2–4 times daily) is indicated in these cases, but additional treatment is required to prolong survival. Among untreated patients, median survival is 1 to 2 months; among treated patients, 2 to 10 months.

Box 57.1 • Neurologic Complications of Systemic Cancer

Metastatic: parenchymal, leptomeningeal, epidural, subdural, brachial plexus, lumbosacral plexus, and nerve infiltration; these complications are common

Infectious: unusual central nervous system infections because of immunosuppression

Complications of systemic metastases: hepatic encephalopathy

Vascular complications: cerebral infarction from hypercoagulable states, nonbacterial thrombotic endocarditis, and radiation damage to carotid arteries; cerebral hemorrhage (eg, from thrombocytopenia and hemorrhagic metastases)

Toxic-metabolic encephalopathies: usually from multiple causes, hypercalcemia, syndrome of inappropriate secretion of antidiuretic hormone, medications, and systemic infections

Complications of treatment (radiotherapy, chemotherapy, or surgery): radiation necrosis of the brain, radiation myelopathy, radiation plexopathy, fibrosis of the carotid arteries, neuropathies, encephalopathies, and cerebellar ataxia

Paraneoplastic (ie, nonmetastatic or "remote" effect of cancer): rare syndromes have been described from the cerebral cortex through the central and peripheral neuraxes to muscle

Miscellaneous: various systemic and neurologic illnesses unrelated to cancer

---

Survival depends on patient age, performance status, presence or absence of extracranial metastasis, and control of the primary tumor. Surgical resection of single accessible lesions increases survival among patients with good prognostic factors. Most patients receive postoperative whole-brain radiotherapy. Stereotactic radiosurgery can be used to treat multiple lesions in a single session and is associated with decreased risk of cognitive impairment.

Metastasis to the Spinal Cord, Leptomeninges, or Peripheral Nerves

Epidural spinal cord compression is the most common cause of spinal cord dysfunction in patients with cancer and is frequently preceded by vertebral metastasis. The most common causes are lung, breast, and prostate cancer, followed by non-Hodgkin lymphoma, multiple myeloma, and colorectal or renal carcinoma. About 60% of all cases involve the thoracic spine, and multiple sites are involved in one-third of the patients. The cardinal symptom is back pain, followed by weakness, sensory loss, and bladder or bowel dysfunction. Epidural spinal cord compression should be considered in all patients with any type of cancer and back or radicular pain.

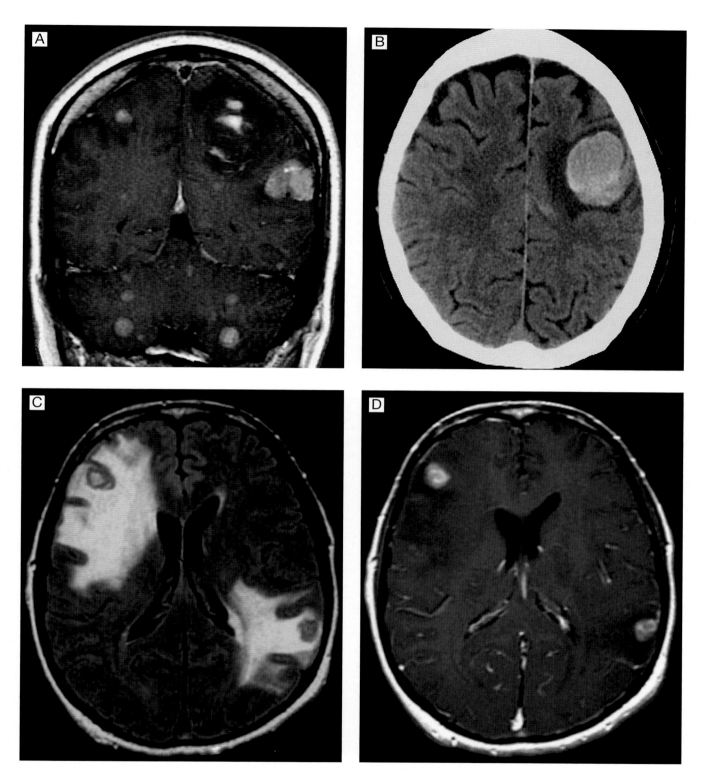

Figure 57.4 *Neuroimaging of Metastatic Cancer. Single or multiple enhancing lesions are seen at junction of gray and white matter with various degrees of surrounding vasogenic edema, hemorrhage, or necrosis. A, Gadolinium-enhanced coronal T1-weighted image of metastatic melanoma shows numerous enhancing masses throughout brain. B, Unenhanced computed tomogram of a different patient with metastatic melanoma shows subacute hemorrhage into the metastatic focus at parasagittal posterior left frontal cortex. C, Axial fluid-attenuated inversion recovery and, D, enhanced axial T1-weighted images show 2 enhancing foci of metastasis at junction of gray and white matter, with surrounding vasogenic edema. The primary tumor was metastatic lung adenocarcinoma.*

(Adapted from Mowzoon N, Vernino S. Neoplasms of the nervous system and related topics. In: Mowzoon N, Flemming KD, editors. Neurology board review: an illustrated study guide. Rochester [MN]: Mayo Clinic Scientific Press and Florence [KY]: Informa Healthcare USA; c2007. p. 627–78. Used with permission of Mayo Foundation for Medical Education and Research.)

Dexamethasone is highly effective at ameliorating symptoms. In many patients, radiotherapy is efficacious for preventing further tumor growth and neural damage. The therapeutic response is better with radiosensitive tumors (eg, multiple myeloma, lymphoma, and prostate, breast, and small cell lung carcinoma) than with relatively radioresistant tumors (eg, melanoma, renal cell carcinoma). Surgery is indicated for patients with spinal instability, bone impingement on the spinal cord, worsening deficits during or despite radiotherapy, radioresistant epidural tumors with limited tumor elsewhere, or a diagnosis that is in doubt.

Meningeal metastases occur in lung and breast cancer, melanoma, leukemia, and lymphoma. Patients typically present with symptoms and signs reflecting involvement at many levels of the nervous system: headache, encephalopathy, seizures, cranial nerve involvement (most commonly diplopia or facial weakness), back pain, or spinal root involvement. Diagnosis is suggested by the presence of meningeal enhancement on gadolinium magnetic resonance imaging and is confirmed by cerebrospinal fluid cytologic findings. Subsequent cerebrospinal fluid samples may be necessary; the yield is 90% after the third lumbar puncture.

Intramedullary spinal cord metastases are much less frequent than epidural metastases and most commonly result from small cell lung carcinoma. Brachial plexus involvement is most frequent with lung and breast cancer as a result of direct tumor invasion. Colorectal cancer causes local pelvic metastasis and is the most frequent cause of neoplastic plexopathy. Head and neck cancers are the most frequent sources of metastasis to the base of the skull.

Paraneoplastic Disorders

Paraneoplastic disorders are associated with increased levels of circulating antibodies (onconeural antibodies) directed against neoplastic cells and attacking membrane ion channels or intracellular (nuclear or cytoplasmic) proteins in neurons. The most common underlying malignancies are small cell lung carcinoma and breast cancer. Others include ovarian or testicular carcinoma, thymoma, Hodgkin disease, and parotid tumors. Paraneoplastic syndromes can affect any level of the central nervous system or peripheral nervous system (Box 57.2). Important examples include limbic encephalitis (characterized by behavioral and memory abnormalities and seizures), brainstem encephalitis, opsoclonus-myoclonus, cerebellar ataxia, myelopathy,

---

Box 57.2 • Classification of Paraneoplastic Neurologic Disorders

Central nervous system
    Encephalomyelitis
    Limbic encephalitis
    Cerebellar degeneration
    Brainstem encephalitis
    Opsoclonus-myoclonus
    Stiff person syndrome
    Chorea
    Necrotizing myelopathy
    Motor neuronopathy

Dorsal root ganglion and peripheral nerves
    Subacute sensory neuronopathy
    Gastroparesis or intestinal pseudo-obstruction
    Acute autonomic ganglionopathy
    Acquired neuromyotonia
    Neuropathy associated with plasma cell dyscrasia or lymphoma
    Vasculitis of nerve or muscle

Neuromuscular junction
    Lambert-Eaton myasthenic syndrome
    Myasthenia gravis

Muscle
    Dermatomyositis
    Polymyositis
    Acute necrotizing myopathy

Eye and retina
    Cancer-associated retinopathy
    Optic neuropathy

---

peripheral neuropathy, stiff person syndrome (with axial and limb rigidity), sensory ganglionopathies, Lambert-Eaton myasthenic syndrome, dermatomyositis, and retinopathy. These syndromes are characterized by an acute or subacute onset and increased levels of 1 or more antibodies (Table 57.1). A paraneoplastic neurologic syndrome precedes the diagnosis of cancer in 60% of cases and develops after tumor diagnosis or at tumor recurrence in 40%.

Treatment of the underlying neoplasm is the main factor associated with neurologic stabilization. Immunotherapy with corticosteroids, intravenous immunoglobulin, plasma exchange, cyclophosphamide, or rituximab may be helpful in paraneoplastic disorders related to antibodies against membrane antigens such as P/Q type voltage-gated calcium channels (Lambert-Eaton myasthenic syndrome) or voltage-gated potassium channels (limbic encephalitis) (Figure 57.5).

Table 57.1 • Paraneoplastic Antibodies Associated With Cancer and Syndromes

Antibody	Associated Cancer	Associated Syndromes
Anti-Hu (ANNA-1)	SCLC	Encephalomyelitis Limbic encephalitis Cerebellar degeneration SSN Autonomic ganglionopathy
Anti-Ri (ANNA-2)	Breast, gynecologic, SCLC	Ataxia Opsoclonus-myoclonus Brainstem encephalitis
Anti-Yo (PCA-1)	Breast, ovary	Cerebellar degeneration
CRMP-5	SCLC, thymoma	Chorea, myelopathy, optic neuritis, retinopathy, and others
Amphiphysin	Breast, SCLC	Stiff person syndrome Encephalomyelitis
Anti-Ma2	Testicular germinoma	Limbic encephalitis Brainstem encephalitis
P/Q type VGCC	SCLC	LEMS
Muscle nAChR	Thymoma	Myasthenia gravis
Ganglionic nAChR	SCLC	Autonomic ganglionopathy
Voltage-gated potassium channel	Thymoma, SCLC	Neuromyotonia Limbic encephalitis
NMDA receptor	Ovarian teratoma	Limbic encephalitis Rigidity Hypoventilation Dysautonomia

Abbreviations: ANNA, antineuronal nuclear antibody; CRMP, collapsin response mediator protein; LEMS, Lambert-Eaton myasthenic syndrome; nAChR, nicotinic acetylcholine receptor; NMDA, N-methyl-D-aspartate; PCA, Purkinje cell antibody; SCLC, small cell lung carcinoma; SSN, subacute sensory neuronopathy; VGCC, voltage-gated calcium channels.

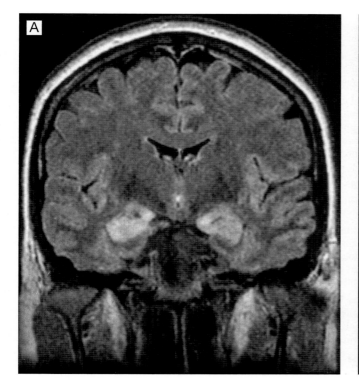
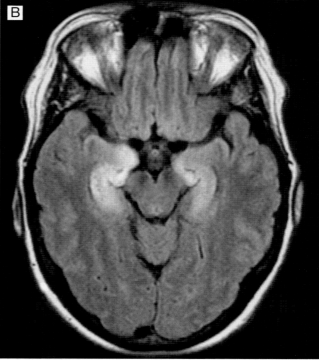

Figure 57.5 *Magnetic Resonance Imaging Characteristics of Paraneoplastic Limbic Encephalopathy in a Patient With Small Cell Lung Carcionoma. Coronal (A) and axial (B) fluid-attenuated inversion recovery sequences show increased signal within mesial temporal lobes bilaterally. The lesions were nonenhancing (not shown).*
(Adapted from Mowzoon N, Vernino S. Neoplasms of the nervous system and related topics. In: Mowzoon N, Flemming KD, editors. Neurology board review: an illustrated study guide. Rochester [MN]: Mayo Clinic Scientific Press and Florence [KY]: Informa Healthcare USA; c2007. p. 627–78. Used with permission of Mayo Foundation for Medical Education and Research.)

Neurologic Complications of Cancer Treatment

Treatment of cancer with chemotherapeutic and biologic agents is frequently complicated by the development of neurotoxicity. Typical examples are listed in Table 57.2.

Table 57.2 • Examples of Neurotoxicity of Chemotherapeutic Agents

Agent	Typical Manifestations of Neurotoxicity
Platinum compounds (cisplatin, oxaliplatin)	Sensory (large fiber) neuropathy (sensory ataxia) Autonomic neuropathy Ototoxicity Encephalopathy, cortical blindness, seizures Retrobulbar neuritis Retinal injury
Vinca alkaloids	Sensorimotor peripheral neuropathy Autonomic neuropathy
Taxanes (eg, paclitaxel)	Predominantly sensory peripheral neuropathy Occasional motor neuropathies Transient scotomata
Methotrexate	Acute chemical arachnoiditis (intrathecal administration) Acute, reversible, strokelike syndrome Subacute encephalopathy Transverse myelopathy Chronic demyelinating encephalopathy
5-Fluorouracil	Cerebellar dysfunction Acute encephalopathy Subacute extrapyramidal syndrome Leukoencephalopathy (when combined with levamisole)
Cytarabine (ara-C)	Cerebellar dysfunction Cognitive impairment Necrotizing leukoencephalopathy Peripheral neuropathy Seizures, parkinsonism, myelopathy
Ifosfamide	Encephalopathy with agitation, visual and auditory hallucinations, behavioral and memory changes Hemiparesis, seizures, coma Cerebellar, extrapyramidal, or cranial nerve dysfunction
Nitrosoureas	Encephalopathy
Busulfan	Seizures
L-Asparaginase	Encephalopathy Cerebral venous thrombosis

58

Seizure Disorders

LILY C. WONG-KISIEL, MD

Seizures are electroclinical events, and *epilepsy* indicates a tendency for recurrent unprovoked seizures. The updated classification for seizures is given in Table 58.1.

The proper treatment of epilepsy depends on accurate diagnosis of the seizure type, identification of the cause (if possible), and management of psychosocial problems. Electroencephalography (EEG) (preferably after the patient is sleep deprived) can be important in the classification of seizure type. Magnetic resonance imaging is also used to evaluate for focal or structural lesions. Much of the diagnosis rests on a supportive history. An aura and a period of altered mental status after the spell (*postictal confusion*) are highly suggestive of an epileptic seizure.

Causes

Seizures occur at any age, but approximately 70% of all patients with epilepsy have their first seizure before age 20 years. Age distribution for the onset of epilepsy is bimodal, with the second most common group being the elderly population. Both the cause and the type of epilepsy are related to age at onset. However, the cause may not be found in many patients.

Neonatal seizures are often due to congenital defects or prenatal injury, and head trauma is often the cause of focal seizures in young adults. Brain tumors and vascular disease are major known causes of seizures in later life. Seizures often occur during withdrawal from alcohol, barbiturates, or benzodiazepines in young and old adults. Seizures also occur with the use of drugs such as cocaine, usually in young adults. Metabolic derangements (eg, hypoglycemia, hypocalcemia, hyponatremia, and hypernatremia) can occur at any age, as can infections (eg, meningitis and encephalitis). Metabolic abnormalities usually cause primary generalized tonic-clonic seizures and rarely focal or multifocal seizures. Central nervous system infections usually cause partial and secondary generalized tonic-clonic seizures.

In contrast to epileptic seizures, **psychogenic nonepileptic events or episodes** (ie, pseudoseizures or psychogenic nonepileptic seizures) are sudden changes in behavior or mentation not associated with any physiologic cause or abnormal paroxysmal discharge of electrical activity from the brain. Events are frequent and resistant to antiepileptic treatment, affecting about 30% of patients referred for medically refractory epilepsy. A favorable outcome may be associated with an independent lifestyle, the absence of coexisting epilepsy, and a formal psychologic approach to therapy. There is growing evidence for the efficacy of cognitive behavior therapy.

> ### Key Definition
>
> Psychogenic nonepileptic events or episodes (ie, pseudoseizures or psychogenic nonepileptic seizures): *sudden changes in behavior or mentation not associated with any physiologic cause or abnormal paroxysmal discharge of electrical activity from the brain.*

Clinical and Laboratory Diagnostic Evaluations

Magnetic resonance imaging investigates the underlying structural abnormality, and EEG is important for deciding whether to treat a first unprovoked seizure. The risk of recurrent seizures is high if the initial EEG shows epileptiform activity and low if the EEG findings are normal. Laboratory tests for inherited neurometabolic, developmental, and degenerative disorders can be considered in children and patients with a progressive course. Lumbar puncture for cerebral spinal fluid should be considered in those with febrile illness to assess for central nervous system infections.

Table 58.1 • Seizure Types and Terminology Used in 1981 Classification of Seizures and Recommended in 2010 Report

Mode of Onset	1981 Seizure Types	2010 Seizure Descriptions

Focal	Simple partial seizures
	  Simple partial sensory
	  Simple partial motor
	  Simple partial special sensory (unusual smells
	    or tastes)
	  Speech arrest or unusual vocalization
		Without impairment of consciousness or awareness:
		  With observable motor or autonomic components
		  Involving subjective sensory or psychic phenomena
		    only (aura)

	Complex partial seizures
	  Consciousness impaired at onset
	  Simple partial onset followed by impaired
	    consciousness
		With impairment of consciousness or awareness
		  (dyscognitive)

	Evolving to generalized tonic-clonic convulsions
	  (secondary generalized tonic-clonic seizures)
	  Simple evolving to generalized tonic-clonic
	  Complex evolving to generalized tonic-clonic
	    (including those with simple partial onset)
		Evolving to a bilateral, convulsive seizure

Generalized	Tonic-clonic
	Myoclonic
	Absence and atypical absence
		Tonic-clonic
		Myoclonic
		Absence
		  Typical
		  Atypical
		  With special features

	Clonic Tonic Atonic	Clonic Tonic Atonic
Not clear	Unclassified	Unknown (including epileptic spasms)

Data from Berg AT, Millichap JJ. The 2010 revised classification of seizures and epilepsy. Continuum (Minneap Minn). 2013 Jun;19(3):571–97.

KEY FACTS

✓ EEG (preferably after the patient is sleep deprived)—important for the classification of seizure type

✓ Magnetic resonance imaging—used to evaluate for focal or structural lesions

✓ Diagnosis of epilepsy—much of the diagnosis rests on a supportive history

✓ Features highly suggestive of an epileptic seizure—an aura and a period of altered mental status after the spell (postictal confusion)

Anticonvulsant Therapy

Drugs used to treat seizures are listed in Table 58.2. Monotherapy is the treatment of choice. The dosage of the drug may be increased as high as necessary and to as much as can be tolerated. The coadministration of antiepileptic drugs has not been shown to have more antiseizure efficacy than the administration of only 1 drug without concurrently increasing toxicity. In studies of a large population, a particular drug may be shown to be more efficacious and less toxic, but for a given patient, another drug may be more effective or have fewer adverse effects. Older antiepileptic drugs include phenytoin, carbamazepine, valproic acid, benzodiazepines, and ethosuximide. The newer antiepileptic drugs include gabapentin, tiagabine, lamotrigine, topiramate, felbamate, zonisamide, oxcarbazepine, levetiracetam, pregabalin, lacosamide, rufinamide, vigabatrin, clobazam, perampanel, and ezogabine. These agents generally have less potential for drug interactions and fewer adverse effects than the older drugs.

Choice of antiepileptic drug depends on seizure type or epilepsy syndrome. Some antiepileptic drugs have a narrow spectrum and are effective for selected seizure type or epilepsy syndrome (ethosuximide for childhood absence epilepsy). Other antiepileptic drugs may in fact exacerbate certain seizure types: carbamazepine, gabapentin, oxcarbazepine, pregabalin, and tiagabine may aggravate myoclonic and absence seizures. When classification of focal or generalized seizures cannot be made, a broad-spectrum antiepileptic drug able to treat both focal and generalized epilepsy is preferred. Because the efficacy, cost, and dosing schedule (twice daily) are similar for many of these new anticonvulsants, tolerability is frequently the major determinant in choosing a particular drug.

Anticonvulsants have both neurologic and systemic adverse effects. Dose-initiation adverse effects such as fatigue, dizziness, incoordination, and mental slowing are common in most patients and can be prevented with slow introduction of the drug. Dose-related effects may limit the use of a particular drug in a given patient. A dose-related adverse effect common to most drugs is cognitive impairment. Other neurologic adverse effects include cerebellar ataxia (phenytoin), diplopia (carbamazepine), tremor (valproic acid and lamotrigine), and chorea or myoclonus (phenytoin

Table 58.2 • Guidance for Use of Antiepileptic Drugs

Criteria	Possibilities	Drug
Type of seizures	Focal seizures with or without secondary GTCSs	PHT, CBZ, oxcarbazepine, pregabalin, tiagabine, lacosamide, ezogabine, perampanel
	Focal and generalized seizures	VPA, PB, benzodiazepines, lamotrigine, levetiracetam, topiramate, zonisamide, felbamate
	Absence seizures	Ethosuximide, VPA, lamotrigine
	Myoclonic seizures	VPA, clonazepam, lamotrigine, zonisamide
	Atonic, akinetic, or mixed seizures	VPA, felbamate, topiramate, lamotrigine, rufinamide
Use of other drugs metabolized in the liver	Drugs that do not affect metabolism of other drugs	Gabapentin, pregabalin, tiagabine, lamotrigine, zonisamide, levetiracetam, rufinamide, lacosamide
Avoidance of oral contraceptive pill failure	Drugs with no or minimal effect on contraceptive metabolism	VPA, clonazepam, gabapentin, pregabalin, tiagabine, lamotrigine, zonisamide, levetiracetam, lacosamide, ezogabine

Abbreviations: CBZ, carbamazepine; GTCS, generalized tonic-clonic seizure; PB, phenobarbital; PHT, phenytoin; VPA, valproic acid.

and carbamazepine). Idiosyncratic adverse effects are rare, unpredictable, severe, and sometimes life-threatening. Idiosyncratic and systemic adverse effects are listed in Table 58.3.

Many antiepileptic drugs are metabolized in the liver and are responsible for important drug interactions. Liver enzyme inducers (eg, carbamazepine, phenobarbital, phenytoin, primidone, oxcarbazepine, felbamate, and topiramate) increase metabolism and decrease the efficacy of oral contraceptives in preventing pregnancy. Valproic acid and

felbamate are enzyme inhibitors and increase the levels of other anticonvulsants.

Special issues must be considered when managing epilepsy in pregnancy. Seizure control is attempted first with monotherapy, with the lowest possible dose of anticonvulsant and monitoring of drug levels. Essentially all anticonvulsant drugs have the potential to cause developmental abnormalities. Valproic acid and, to a lesser extent, carbamazepine are selectively associated with an increased risk of neural tube defects.

Table 58.3 • Systemic Adverse Effects of Antiepileptic Drugs

Adverse Effect	Drug Most Commonly Involved
Rash and Stevens-Johnson syndrome	10% risk with lamotrigine, CBZ, or PHT; 5% risk with other AEDs; least risk with VPA *Note*: Topiramate and zonisamide are contraindicated for patients with allergy to sulfa drugs
Liver failure	Highest risk with VPA and felbamate Risk increased in infants with mental retardation and receiving polytherapy or with underlying metabolic disease or poor nutritional status
Bone marrow suppression	Highest risk with felbamate and CBZ
Gum hypertrophy, hirsutism, acne, osteoporosis	Phenytoin
Weight gain, hair loss, tremor	VPA
Weight loss	Felbamate, topiramate
Headache, insomnia	Felbamate
Behavioral and cognitive disturbances	Barbiturates, benzodiazepines, topiramate, levetiracetam
Kidney stones	Topiramate, zonisamide
Hyponatremia	CBZ, oxcarbazepine
Atrioventricular conduction defect	CBZ, PHT
Neural tube defect	VPA > CBZ, but all AEDs are potentially teratogenic

Abbreviations: AED, antiepileptic drug; CBZ, carbamazepine; PHT, phenytoin; VPA, valproic acid.

KEY FACTS

✓ Management of seizure disorders—treatment of choice is monotherapy

✓ Dosage of drug used for treatment of seizure disorders—may be increased as high as necessary and to as much as can be tolerated

✓ Coadministration of antiepileptic drugs—has not been shown to have more antiseizure efficacy than the administration of only 1 drug without concurrently increasing toxicity

✓ Metabolism of antiepileptic drugs—many are metabolized in the liver and are responsible for important drug interactions; liver enzyme inducers increase metabolism and decrease the efficacy of oral contraceptives in preventing pregnancy

✓ Valproic acid and felbamate are enzyme inhibitors and increase the levels of other anticonvulsants

When to Start and Stop Anticonvulsant Therapy

Decisions about when to start and stop anticonvulsant therapy are difficult, and there is simply no easy algorithm on which to rely. The decision to begin anticonvulsant therapy after a first seizure should be individualized for each patient. The decision depends on the risk of additional seizures, the risk of seizure-related injury, the loss of employment or driving privileges, and other psychosocial factors. An important decision is whether a single generalized tonic seizure is provoked, for example, by sleep deprivation, alcohol, or concurrent illness. After the first seizure, the risk of recurrence ranges from 30% to 60%, and risks are higher for patients with an abnormal EEG and an identifiable cause (Box 58.1). After

Box 58.1 • Risk Factors for Recurrence After the First Seizure

Age >60 y

No precipitating factor identified (eg, no sleep deprivation or alcohol use)

Focal seizure

Abnormal neurologic examination

Abnormal electroencephalogram (spikes or focal slowing)

Abnormal imaging study

Other factors

    Family history of seizures (in first-degree relative)
    History of febrile seizures
    Onset during sleep
    Postictal Todd paralysis

Occupational risk

a second seizure, the risk of recurrence increases to 80% to 90%.

For many patients who have been seizure free for 1 to 2 years, anticonvulsant therapy can be discontinued. The benefit of discontinuing therapy should be weighed against the possibility of seizure recurrence and its potential adverse consequences. In adults, relapse occurs in 26% to 63% of patients within 1 to 2 years after therapy is discontinued. Predictors of relapse are an abnormal EEG before or during medication withdrawal, abnormal findings on neurologic examination, frequent seizures before entering remission, or mental retardation. To lessen the chance of seizures after discontinuing therapy, withdrawal should not proceed faster than a 20% reduction in dose every 5 half-lives.

Anticonvulsant Blood Levels

Measurement of anticonvulsant blood levels is readily available and helps attain the best control of seizures. It is important to remember that therapeutic levels are represented by a bell-shaped curve and that patients with well-controlled seizures are included under the bell-shaped curve. Seizures are well controlled in many patients who have anticonvulsant blood levels below or above the therapeutic range. The anticonvulsant dose should *never* be changed on the basis of blood levels alone. Remember that toxicity is a clinical phenomenon, *not* a laboratory phenomenon. Measurement of anticonvulsant blood levels ensures that patients are taking their medication and helps determine whether new symptoms might be related to toxicity from the medication.

If a patient is receiving therapy for epilepsy and has breakthrough seizures, several factors should be considered, including the following:

1. Compliance issues
2. Excessive use of alcohol or other recreational drugs
3. Psychologic and physiologic stress (eg, anxiety or lack of sleep)
4. Systemic disease of any type, organ failure of any type, or systemic infection
5. A new cause of seizures (eg, neoplasm)
6. Newly prescribed medication, including other anticonvulsants (ie, polypharmacy) and over-the-counter drugs
7. Toxic levels of anticonvulsants (with definite clinical toxicity)
8. Nonepileptic spells (eg, psychogenic spells)
9. Progressive central nervous system lesion not identified previously with neuroimaging or lumbar puncture

If no cause is found, the anticonvulsant dosage must be readjusted or the drug replaced with another.

Confirm diagnosis by observing seizure activity

↓

Administer oxygen; control airway; evaluate for intubation
Obtain and record vital signs; establish ECG recording
Obtain IV access; keep open with 0.9% saline
Draw venous blood for glucose, chemistry panel, hematology, toxicology, and antiepileptic drug levels
Determine arterial blood gases

↓

Administer 100 mg of thiamine IV and then 50 mL of 50% dextrose IV

↓

Administer IV lorazepam (2 mg/min, up to 4 mg) or diazepam (5 mg/min, up to 20 mg)

↓

Load with IV fosphenytoin (20 mg/kg, up to a phenytoin equivalent of 150 mg/min)

↓

If status persists after 20 mg/kg of fosphenytoin, give additional drug up to a maximum of 30 mg/kg

↓

If status persists, transfer patient to ICU because intubation, ventilation, or vasopressor may be needed
Phenobarbital 20 mg/kg IV, up to 60 mg/min
If status persists, give general anesthesia with pentobarbital, midazolam, or propofol

Figure 58.1 *Algorithm for the Management of Status Epilepticus. ECG indicates electrocardiographic; ICU, intensive care unit; IV, intravenous.*

Status Epilepticus

Status epilepticus is a medical emergency and a life-threatening condition. It can be defined by the duration of the seizure (eg, >5 minutes) or by whether repetitive seizures occur without recovery between seizures. The most common causes of status epilepticus include stopping the use of an anticonvulsant agent, alcohol toxicity or withdrawal, recreational drug toxicity, and central nervous system trauma or infection. Rarely, status epilepticus is the initial presenting sign of epilepsy. The management of status epilepticus is summarized in Figure 58.1.

Nonconvulsive status epilepticus may cause an acute confusional state or stupor and coma, especially in the elderly. In these cases, there is often very subtle rhythmic motor activity in the limbs or face. Electroencephalography is a critical diagnostic tool because nonconvulsive status epilepticus must be treated as quickly and vigorously as convulsive status epilepticus.

KEY FACTS

✓ Risk of recurrence of seizure—30%–60% after the first seizure; risks are higher for patients with an abnormal EEG and an identifiable cause; risk increases to 80%–90% after a second seizure

✓ Blood levels of anticonvulsants—the anticonvulsant dose should *never* be changed on the basis of blood levels alone

✓ Status epilepticus—a medical emergency and a life-threatening condition; can be defined by the duration of the seizure (eg, >5 minutes) or by whether repetitive seizures occur without recovery between seizures

✓ Nonconvulsive status epilepticus—may cause an acute confusional state or stupor and coma, especially in the elderly; there is often very subtle rhythmic motor activity in the limbs or face; EEG is a critical diagnostic tool because the condition must be treated as quickly and vigorously as convulsive status epilepticus

59 Spinal, Peripheral Nerve, and Muscle Disorders

LYELL K. JONES JR, MD AND BRIAN A. CRUM, MD

Diseases affecting the spinal cord, peripheral nerves, and skeletal muscles are common in clinical practice. These conditions may present in isolation or as an associated feature (or complication) of non-neurologic disease. The clinical history and examination provide the greatest usefulness for establishing the diagnosis, which can be firmly established with diagnostic testing. Electrodiagnostic tests (nerve conduction studies and electromyography [EMG]) are among the most useful in patients with nerve or muscle disease. Treatments are targeted to the underlying mechanism of disease.

Myelopathy

Spinal cord dysfunction, or myelopathy, may cause motor, sensory, and sphincter disturbances at or below the level of the lesion. Myelopathy frequently results in muscle weakness, which typically occurs in the arms and legs if the lesion is at the cervical level or only in the legs if the lesion is below the lower cervical level. An upper motor neuron pattern weakness (elbow and wrist extensors and interosseous muscles in the upper limbs; hip flexors, knee flexors, and foot dorsiflexors in the lower limbs) is present and often bilateral. Sensory symptoms in the affected extremities and bowel and bladder difficulties are frequent. Other findings on examination include spasticity and increased muscle stretch reflexes below the level of the lesion. Extensor plantar reflexes (Babinski signs) may also be elicited. Sensory findings are often noted, and a sensory level can be a very powerful localizing finding on clinical examination. Extramedullary cord lesions are usually heralded by radicular pain. Intramedullary cord lesions are usually painless but may have an ill-described nonlocalizable pain, sensory dissociation, and sacral sparing. Conus

medullaris lesions are often indicated by "saddle anesthesia" and early involvement of the urinary bladder. Selected causes of myelopathy are listed in Box 59.1.

Patients suspected of having myelopathy require thorough evaluation. Magnetic resonance imaging of the relevant portion of the spinal cord should be done, and contrast medium should be administered if possible. Patients who are not candidates for magnetic resonance imaging (because of body habitus, claustrophobia, or implanted devices) may undergo computed tomography myelography, understanding that structural or compressive lesions may be recognized but intrinsic abnormalities in the spinal cord will not be apparent. In patients who do not have an apparent structural cause of myelopathy, a complete review for predisposing conditions needs to be performed. Cerebrospinal fluid examination is particularly useful for identifying inflammatory, infectious, and neoplastic spinal cord disorders. Treatment is targeted to the identified cause. Inflammatory disorders of the spinal cord (as may occur in the setting of multiple sclerosis, neuromyelitis optica, sarcoid, or others) may respond to high-dose parenteral corticosteroids or other immunomodulatory therapies. All patients with myelopathy should have careful physiatric monitoring for mobility safety, bowel and bladder regimens, and spasticity management as indicated.

Cervical Spondylosis

Magnetic resonance imaging in combination with plain radiography is the preferred approach for evaluating patients who have cervical spondylosis, or degenerative joint disease of the spine. Results of surgery for the relief of symptoms of cervical radiculopathy are better when the cause is a soft disk herniation rather than when spondylitic radiculopathy and myelopathy are present. **Cervical spondylitic**

Box 59.1 • Causes of Myelopathy

Spinal cord infarction (eg, from vasculitis)

Spinal cord vascular malformation (cavernous malformation, arteriovenous malformation, dural arteriovenous fistula)

Spinal epidural abscess or osteomyelitis with compression

Tuberculoma

Infectious myelitis

Viral: Enterovirus (polio), Flavivirus (West Nile), herpes virus, CMV, varicella zoster, EBV, HIV, HTLV-1, hepatitis A

Bacterial: *Treponema pallidum, Mycoplasma* pneumonia, *Mycobacterium* tuberculosis, neuroborreliosis, dengue, *Bartonella henselae,* Whipple disease

Fungal

Parasitic: schistosomiasis, cysticercosis, hydatid disease

Idiopathic transverse myelitis

Multiple sclerosis

Neuromyelitis optica

Neurosarcoidosis

Sjögren syndrome

Systemic lupus erythematosus

Behçet disease

Scleroderma

Postvaccinal or postinfectious

Tumors (metastasis, ependymoma, neurofibroma, meningioma, astrocytoma)

Paraneoplastic (antibodies to CRMP-5, amphiphysin IgG)

Vitamin B_{12} or folate deficiency

Vitamin E deficiency

Copper deficiency or zinc toxicity (medications or supplements with zinc; denture cream)

Superficial siderosis

Nitrous oxide toxicity

Syringomyelia or hematomyelia

Cervical spondylosis

Hereditary spastic paraplegia

Adrenomyeloneuropathy

Trauma

Radiation injury

Abbreviations: CMV, cytomegalovirus; CRMP, collapsin response-mediated protein 5; EBV, Epstein-Barr virus; HIV, human immunodeficiency virus; HTLV-1, human T-lymphotropic virus 1; IgG, immunoglobulin G.

---

myelopathy is a condition in which the spinal cord is damaged either directly by compression or indirectly by arterial deprivation or venous stasis as a consequence of proliferative bony changes in the cervical spine.

Key Definition

Cervical spondylitic myelopathy: *condition in which the spinal cord is damaged either directly by compression or indirectly by arterial deprivation or venous stasis as a consequence of proliferative bony changes in the cervical spine.*

Lumbar Spine Disease

Asymptomatic bulging disks after the age of 30 years are common and are generally unlikely to cause nerve root compression. Bulging disks appear round and symmetric compared with herniated disks, which appear angular and asymmetric and extend outside the disk space. The criteria for surgical treatment of lumbar disk herniations include the presence of disk herniation on anatomical imaging; dermatome-specific reflex, sensory, or motor deficits; and failure of 6 to 8 weeks of conservative treatment.

The lateral recess syndrome is usually caused by an osteophyte on the superior articular facet; its features are summarized in Box 59.2. Lumbar spinal stenosis is most frequently caused by degenerative changes in the lumbar spine resulting in encroachment on multiple lumbosacral nerve roots. Its features are summarized in Box 59.3. Decompressive operations for lumbar stenosis can be performed with low morbidity despite the advanced age of most patients. A very high initial success rate can be expected, although about 25% of patients become symptomatic again within 5 years. On reoperation, three-fourths of patients ultimately have a successful outcome; failures result from progression of stenosis at levels not previously decompressed or restenosis at levels previously decompressed.

Musculoskeletal low back pain (without leg pain) is treated best with a formal program of physical therapy and exercise, weight reduction, and education on postural principles.

Radiculopathy

Nerve root lesions (radiculopathies) usually are indicated by pain that is sharp and lancinating, follows a dermatomal or myotomal pattern, and is worsened by increasing

---

Box 59.2 • Clinical Features of the Lateral Recess Syndrome

Radicular pain is unilateral or bilateral with paresthesias in the distribution of L5 or S1

Pain is provoked by standing and walking and is relieved by sitting

Results of the straight leg–raising test are usually negative

Little or no back pain

Box 59.3 • Clinical Features of Lumbar Spinal Stenosis

Most patients are older than 50 years

Neurogenic intermittent claudication (pseudoclaudication)

Symptoms are usually bilateral but can be asymmetric or unilateral

Pain usually has a dull, aching quality

Whole lower extremity is generally involved

Pain is provoked while walking or standing

Sitting or leaning forward provides relief

intraspinal pressure (eg, sneezing and coughing) or by stretching of the nerve root. Paresthesias and pain occur in a dermatomal pattern. Findings are in the root distribution and include weakness, sensory impairment, and decreased muscle stretch reflexes. Radiculopathies have many causes, including compressive lesions (eg, osteophytes, ruptured disks, and neoplasms) and noncompressive lesions (eg, postinfectious and inflammatory radiculopathies and metabolic radiculopathies, as in diabetes). Indications for emergency neurologic and neurosurgical consultation are increasing weakness, bowel or bladder dysfunction, or intractable pain with an appropriate lesion seen on magnetic resonance imaging. Large disk protrusions can cause minimal symptoms and are not by themselves grounds for urgent surgical intervention.

Motor Neuron Disease

Amyotrophic Lateral Sclerosis

Degenerative disorders that affect the motor neurons in the cerebral cortex and the anterior horn cells are called motor neuron diseases. The most common is amyotrophic lateral sclerosis (ALS). This disorder should be considered in any patient who has progressive, painless weakness. Typically, patients present with asymmetric weakness that begins distally and is associated with cramps and fasciculations. Footdrop and hand weakness are the most common first complaints. Often the initial (but incorrect) diagnosis is stroke, radiculopathy, carpal tunnel syndrome, or ulnar neuropathy. The diagnosis is often delayed. Bulbar weakness (eg, dysarthria more so than dysphagia) can be the presenting problem and is always eventually present. Bowel and bladder difficulties are very uncommon, and sensory abnormalities are rare. Findings on examination include weakness, atrophy, fasciculations, spasticity, and abnormal muscle stretch reflexes and extensor plantar responses. The hallmark is the mixture of both upper and lower motor neuron signs. Because of the progressive weakness affecting the limbs, bulbar muscles, and diaphragm, the disease

is devastating, and patients have an average life span of about 3 years after the onset of symptoms.

ALS is sporadic in 80% to 90% of cases. A number of genes have been implicated in familial ALS, including *SOD1* and *C9orf72*. No drug has been found to be effective in reversing the progressive course of this disease, although treatment with riluzole had a 3-month survival benefit in a randomized controlled clinical trial. Currently, riluzole is the only medication approved by the US Food and Drug Administration for the treatment of ALS. Treatment of ALS focuses on rehabilitation issues, nutrition, mobility, and communication; a multidisciplinary approach is useful. Many agents hold promise and are being studied, including stem cells, although no clear indication exists for their use outside of a clinical trial.

Multifocal Motor Neuropathy

Multifocal motor neuropathy is a rare syndrome of purely lower motor neuron weakness that can mimic ALS. Treatment of multifocal motor neuropathy with intravenous immunoglobulin (IVIG) can be very effective in slowing the progression of weakness. It is often distal and asymmetric, accompanied by motor conduction block on nerve conduction studies and EMG, and may be associated with high titers of serum antibodies to GM1 gangliosides.

Kennedy Disease

Kennedy disease (or spinobulbar muscular atrophy) is a pure lower motor neuron degenerative process that is X-linked and caused by an excess of CAG repeats in the

KEY FACTS

✓ Myelopathy—frequently results in muscle weakness, typically in the arms and legs if the lesion is at the cervical level or only in the legs if the lesion is below the lower cervical level

✓ Criteria for surgery of lumbar disk herniations—presence of disk herniation on anatomical imaging; dermatome-specific reflex, sensory, or motor deficits; and failure of 6–8 weeks of conservative treatment

✓ Best treatment of musculoskeletal low back pain (without leg pain)—physical therapy and exercise, weight reduction, and education on postural principles

✓ Indications of nerve root lesions (radiculopathies)—pain that is sharp and lancinating, follows a dermatomal or myotomal pattern, and is worsened by increasing intraspinal pressure (eg, sneezing, coughing) or by stretching the nerve root

✓ Examination findings in ALS—weakness, atrophy, fasciculations, spasticity, and abnormal muscle stretch reflexes and extensor plantar responses; hallmark finding is the mixture of both upper and lower motor neuron signs

androgen receptor gene. This most commonly affects elderly men and also leads to gynecomastia, diabetes mellitus, and a sensory peripheral neuropathy. Genetic testing is widely available. There is no effective treatment, although the disease is much more slowly progressive than ALS.

Peripheral Nerve Disorders

Peripheral nerve disorders may occur in patterns ranging from diffuse to focal and can be unimodal or multimodal in affected functions (eg, motor, sensory, or autonomic). Patterns of peripheral nerve disease and common causes are summarized in Table 59.1.

Length-Dependent Sensorimotor Peripheral Neuropathy

The most common pattern of peripheral nerve dysfunction is the length-dependent sensorimotor peripheral

Table 59.1 • Patterns of Neuropathy and Their Causes

Pattern of Neuropathy	Common or Important Causes
Length-dependent distal (stocking-and-glove) sensorimotor neuropathy	Diabetes mellitus Alcohol abuse Uremia Toxins (hexacarbons) Hereditary neuropathy Vitamin B_{12} deficiency Hypothyroidism Copper deficiency
Acute motor polyradiculo-neuropathy	AIDP (Guillain-Barré syndrome) Lyme disease HIV neuropathy Porphyria Toxins (arsenic, thallium) Carcinomatous or lymphomatous meningitis
Chronic motor or sensorimotor polyradiculopathy	CIDP Paraproteinemia (eg, osteosclerotic myeloma) Hereditary neuropathy (eg, Charcot-Marie-Tooth disease) Lead toxicity Diabetes mellitus Amyloidosis
Sensory ataxic neuropathy	Sjögren syndrome Paraneoplastic disorder Diabetes mellitus Paraproteinemia Vitamin B_{12} deficiency HIV infection Cisplatin Vitamin B_6 excess Hereditary neuropathy

Table 59.1 • Continued

Pattern of Neuropathy	Common or Important Causes
Painful peripheral neuropathy	Diabetes mellitus Vasculitis Hereditary amyloidosis Toxins (arsenic, thallium) Hepatitis C Cryoglobulinemia HIV neuropathy CMV polyradiculoneuropathy in HIV-positive patients Alcoholism Fabry disease

Neuropathy with prominent autonomic involvement	Acute or subacute
	  Guillain-Barré syndrome
	  Subacute pandysautonomia
	  Paraneoplastic pandysautonomia
	  Porphyria
	  Vincristine neuropathy
	  Botulism
	Chronic
	  Diabetes mellitus
	  Amyloidosis
	  Sjögren syndrome

Mononeuropathy	Compressive neuropathy
	  Idiopathic
	  Tumor
	  Trauma
	  Diabetes mellitus
	  HNPP

Mononeuropathy multiplex	Diabetes mellitus Vasculitis Lyme disease HIV neuropathy Sarcoidosis Leprosy Multifocal motor neuropathy HNPP

Abbreviations: AIDP, acute inflammatory demyelinating polyradiculoneuropathy; CIDP, chronic inflammatory demyelinating polyradiculoneuropathy; CMV, cytomegalovirus; HIV, human immunodeficiency virus; HNPP, hereditary neuropathy with liability to pressure palsies.

neuropathy and will be used interchangeably with *peripheral neuropathy* for the purpose of this discussion. Peripheral neuropathies are usually characterized by distal weakness and distal sensory changes, and usually axonal loss predominates over demyelination. They are typically symmetric and more severe in the legs than in the arms. Clumsy gait is often associated with distal numbness and paresthesias or footdrop. Examination findings include distal weakness, sensory loss, atrophy, and, sometimes, fasciculations. Muscle stretch reflexes usually are decreased. The evaluation of peripheral neuropathy is summarized in Box 59.4. An extensive search usually uncovers the cause in 70% to 80% of cases. A high percentage of cases of "idiopathic neuropathy" referred to

---

Box 59.4 • Evaluation of Peripheral Neuropathy

Basic laboratory investigations

    CBC with platelets
    Erythrocyte sedimentation rate
    Fasting blood glucose
    Serum electrolytes
    Serum creatinine
    Liver function tests
    Serum and urine electrophoresis and
       immunoelectrophoresis
    Urinalysis
    Chest radiography
    Electromyography
    Thyroid function test
    Vitamin B_{12}

Special investigations in selected patients

    Vitamin E
    Cholesterol and triglycerides
    HIV serology
    Lyme serology
    Hepatitis serology
    Cryoglobulins
    Angiotensin-converting enzyme
    Antineutrophil cytoplasmic antibodies
    Antinuclear antibodies
    Antibodies against extractable nuclear antigens
    Gliadin antibodies, endomysial and tissue
       transglutaminase antibodies
    Paraneoplastic antibodies
    GM1 antibodies
    Porphyrins
    Heavy metal screen
    Serum copper and ceruloplasmin
    Autonomic function tests
    Cerebrospinal fluid analysis (when inflammatory,
       infectious, or neoplastic disorders are suspected)
    Sural nerve biopsy (when amyloidosis, vasculitis, or
       lymphoma is suspected)
    Investigation for inborn errors of metabolism
    Genetic studies
    MRI of nerve roots or plexus

Abbreviations: CBC, complete blood cell count; HIV, human immunodeficiency virus; MRI, magnetic resonance imaging.

---

specialty centers are in fact hereditary neuropathies. On examination, the finding of high arches (ie, pes cavus) or fallen arches (ie, pes planus) with hammertoe deformities is a clue to a long-standing or hereditary neuropathy. Also, examination or close questioning of family members may secure a diagnosis.

Acute Inflammatory Demyelinating Polyradiculoneuropathy

A progressive neuropathy of rapid onset that affects both distal and proximal nerves suggests acute inflammatory demyelinating polyradiculoneuropathy (AIDP), or Guillain-Barré syndrome. The weakness and paresthesias ascend over several days, often accompanied by severe back pain. On examination, the reflexes are absent. There may also be respiratory muscle weakness, cranial neuropathy (particularly facial palsy, which can be bilateral), and autonomic instability. Typically, it is associated with an increased cerebrospinal fluid protein concentration but no pleocytosis. There are characteristic nerve conduction study and EMG findings with conduction block and temporal dispersion. About 50% of patients have a mild respiratory or gastrointestinal tract infection 1 to 3 weeks before the neurologic symptoms appear. In the other patients, the syndrome may be preceded by surgery, viral exanthems, or vaccinations. Also, the syndrome may develop in patients who have autoimmune disease or a lymphoreticular malignancy. This syndrome has no particular seasonal, age, or sex predilection. Either plasma exchange or IVIG is effective in AIDP. Corticosteroids are not effective. Attention must be paid to other complications of the disease: deep vein thrombosis, pain, constipation, back pain, tachyarrhythmias and hypertension, peptic ulcers, decubital ulcers, and accumulation of secretions in the respiratory tract and aspiration.

Chronic Demyelinating Neuropathies

Chronic, predominantly motor or sensorimotor neuropathies include chronic inflammatory demyelinating polyradiculoneuropathy (CIDP), paraproteinemic neuropathies (eg, associated with polyneuropathy, organomegaly, endocrinopathy, monoclonal protein, and skin changes [POEMS] syndrome, amyloidosis, or osteosclerotic myeloma), hereditary neuropathies, lead toxicity, and diabetes mellitus (which often has axonal features as well). Most of these neuropathies are length-dependent, but occasionally there is predominant proximal weakness, which suggests AIDP, CIDP, or porphyria. In sharp contrast to its lack of success in AIDP, corticosteroid therapy works well in CIDP. Plasma exchange and IVIG are also effective. Other potential causes are connective tissue diseases, vasculitis, vitamin B_{12} deficiency, copper deficiency, sarcoidosis, paraneoplastic syndromes, gluten sensitivity, and medications.

Most neuropathies associated with monoclonal gammopathies are not associated with underlying lymphoproliferative disorders, but some are associated with multiple myeloma, POEMS syndrome, amyloidosis, lymphoma, or leukemia. Affected patients usually are older than 50 years and present early with symmetric sensorimotor polyradiculoneuropathy. The cerebrospinal fluid protein concentration is usually increased. Immunoglobulin (Ig) M is more common than IgG or IgA and is generally more resistant to treatment. Plasma exchange can be effective therapy. Other immunosuppressive therapy, such as IVIG and perhaps rituximab, may also be effective.

Sensory Ataxic Neuropathy

Sensory ataxic neuropathies are characterized by severe proprioceptive sensory loss, ataxia, and areflexia. Some neuropathies are due to peripheral nerve demyelination and others to selective loss of large dorsal root ganglion neurons. A predominantly sensory polyneuropathy suggests paraneoplastic disorder, Sjögren syndrome, diabetes mellitus, paraproteinemias, human immunodeficiency virus infection, vitamin B_{12} deficiency, cisplatin toxicity, vitamin B_6 excess, or hereditary neuropathy.

Painful (Small Fiber) Neuropathy

Some peripheral neuropathies affect predominantly the small-diameter nociceptive fibers or their dorsal root ganglion neurons and are characterized by severe burning pain distally in the extremities. The examination findings are normal except for the distal loss of pain and temperature sensation. Typical causes are diabetes mellitus, vasculitis, amyloidosis, toxins, hepatitis C, cryoglobulinemia, some human immunodeficiency virus–associated neuropathies, and alcoholism. Randomized, double-blind, placebo-controlled studies in diabetic neuropathy have shown that the following medications are helpful to manage neuropathic pain: amitriptyline, tramadol, gabapentin, pregabalin, and duloxetine. Others that are useful when these agents are not useful or when they lead to adverse effects include carbamazepine, lidocaine patch (5%), narcotics, lamotrigine, mexiletine, and venlafaxine.

Autonomic Neuropathy

Neuropathy with autonomic dysfunction (eg, orthostatic hypotension, urinary bladder and bowel dysfunction, and impotence) suggests Guillain-Barré syndrome, acute pandysautonomia, paraneoplastic dysautonomia, porphyria, diabetes mellitus, amyloidosis, or familial neuropathy.

Acute pandysautonomia is a heterogeneous, monophasic, usually self-limiting disease that involves the sympathetic and parasympathetic nervous systems. It may produce orthostatic hypotension, anhidrosis, diarrhea, constipation, urinary bladder atony, and impotence. The syndrome usually evolves over a few days to a few months, and recovery is generally prolonged and partial. This may be an immunologic disorder, but it is indistinguishable from paraneoplastic autonomic neuropathy. Some patients may have antibodies against the ganglion-type nicotinic acetylcholine receptor. IVIG treatment limits the duration and reduces the long-term disability of patients with acute pandysautonomia.

Key Definition

Acute pandysautonomia: *a heterogeneous, monophasic, usually self-limiting disease that involves the sympathetic and parasympathetic nervous systems.*

Diabetic Neuropathy

Diabetes mellitus may result in many different patterns of peripheral nerve dysfunction, ranging from focal to diffuse. It may cause cranial nerve III neuropathy; affected patients usually present with sudden diplopia, eye pain, impairment of the muscles supplied by cranial nerve III, and relative sparing of the pupil. With compressive cranial nerve III lesions, the pupil usually is involved early. Painful diabetic neuropathies include cranial nerve III neuropathy, acute thoracoabdominal (ie, truncal) radiculopathies, acute distal sensory neuropathy, acute lumbar radiculoplexopathy, and chronic distal small-fiber neuropathy.

Acute or subacute muscle weakness can occur in various forms of diabetic neuropathy. Weakness, atrophy, and pain affect the pelvic girdle and thigh muscles (asymmetrical or unilateral). This condition has been termed *diabetic lumbosacral radiculoplexus neuropathy* (previously described with various terms such as diabetic amyotrophy) and is due to a microvasculitis of the nerve. A course of intravenous corticosteroids may speed the recovery and reduce pain.

Mononeuropathy

Mononeuropathy is characterized by impairment of a single nerve. The usual cause is compression, as in compressive ulnar neuropathy at the elbow, compressive median neuropathy in the carpal tunnel, and compression of the peroneal nerve as it winds around the fibular head. Diabetes mellitus is a common predisposing factor in patients with multiple compression mononeuropathies.

Mononeuropathy Multiplex

Mononeuropathy multiplex consists of asymmetric involvement of several nerves either simultaneously or sequentially. It suggests such causes as trauma or compression, diabetes mellitus, vasculitis, Lyme disease, human immunodeficiency virus neuropathy, sarcoidosis, leprosy, tumor infiltration, multifocal motor neuropathies, or hereditary neuropathy with predisposition to pressure palsies.

KEY FACTS

✓ Characteristics of peripheral neuropathies—distal weakness and distal sensory changes, usually axonal loss predominates over demyelination, symmetric, and more severe in the legs than in the arms

✓ "Idiopathic neuropathy"—a high percentage of cases are hereditary neuropathies; finding of high arches or fallen arches with hammertoe deformities is a clue to long-standing or hereditary neuropathy

✓ AIDP—progressive neuropathy of rapid onset that affects both distal and proximal nerves; can be preceded by mild respiratory or gastrointestinal tract infection in about 50% of patients and by surgery, viral exanthems, or vaccinations in other patients

✓ Treatment of AIDP—plasma exchange or IVIG; corticosteroids are not effective

✓ Characteristics of small fiber neuropathy—severe burning pain distally in the extremities; examination findings are normal except for the distal loss of pain and temperature sensation

Neuromuscular Junction Disorders

Patients with neuromuscular transmission disorders present with fluctuating weakness manifested as fatigable weakness in the limbs, eyelids (causing ptosis), tongue and palate (causing dysarthria and dysphagia), and extraocular muscles (causing diplopia). Sensation, muscle tone, and reflexes usually are normal except in Lambert-Eaton myasthenic syndrome, in which the weakness is more constant and the reflexes are diminished. Certain drugs may exacerbate neuromuscular junction kinetics; for example, penicillamine can cause a syndrome that appears similar to myasthenia gravis. Three major clinical syndromes of the neuromuscular junction are myasthenia gravis, Lambert-Eaton myasthenic syndrome, and botulism. Several drugs adversely affect neuromuscular transmission and may exacerbate weakness in these disorders. They include aminoglycoside antibiotics, quinine, quinidine, procainamide, propranolol, calcium channel blockers, and iodinated radiocontrast agents.

Myasthenia Gravis

Myasthenia gravis (MG) usually occurs in young women and older men and is often heralded by such cranial nerve findings as diplopia, dysarthria, dysphagia, and dyspnea. The deficits are usually fatigable, worsening with repetition or late in the day. However, muscle stretch reflexes, sensation, mentation, and sphincter function are normal. The diagnosis of MG is classically characterized by the detection of serum nicotinic acetylcholine receptor antibodies and the presence of decremental responses to repetitive electrical stimulation of motor nerves detected on EMG. Administration of a short-acting acetylcholine esterase inhibitor (eg, edrophonium) can immediately reverse weakness due to MG; this can be used as a diagnostic test (although it is prone to false-positive results). Acetylcholine receptor antibodies are rare in conditions other than MG (ie, they do not occur in patients with congenital MG and they occur in only about 50% of those with purely ocular MG). Some patients who have MG without acetylcholine receptor antibodies have muscle-specific kinase antibodies that are also diagnostic for MG. These patients may have more severe weakness, often bulbar, and may be more resistant to treatments. Of the 30% of patients who have MG without acetylcholine receptor antibodies, half have antibodies to muscle-specific kinase.

Treatment strategies for MG include the use of acetylcholinesterase inhibitors and immunomodulatory agents. Acetylcholinesterase inhibitors, such as pyridostigmine bromide, are often given as initial therapy for MG. This therapy provides symptomatic improvement for most patients. Thymectomy is recommended for selected patients younger than 60 years with generalized weakness and for all patients with thymoma. Computed tomography should be performed in all patients with MG to evaluate for thymoma. Prednisone is the most commonly used immunomodulatory agent, but initial administration of high doses may exacerbate the weakness in about 10% of patients. Plasma exchange and IVIG are effective short-term therapies for patients with severe weakness and are particularly useful for a recent exacerbation, for preoperative preparation, or for initiating corticosteroid therapy. Long-term immunomodulatory treatments include azathioprine, mycophenolate, cyclosporine, and methotrexate. Rituximab has also been used for refractory cases.

Lambert-Eaton Myasthenic Syndrome

Patients with Lambert-Eaton myasthenic syndrome often have proximal weakness in the legs and absent or decreased muscle stretch reflexes (sometimes reflexes are elicited after brief exercise). This syndrome usually is diagnosed in middle-aged men who often have vague complaints such as diplopia, impotence, urinary dysfunction, paresthesias, mouth dryness, and other autonomic dysfunctions (eg, orthostatic hypotension). The syndrome is due to the presence of antibodies directed against presynaptic voltage-gated P/Q-type calcium channels. It often is associated with small cell lung carcinoma. Treatment is focused on the underlying malignancy, if present. Pyridostigmine can be helpful, as in MG. Patients may also respond to the potassium channel blocker 3,4-diaminopyridine, as well as to immunomodulatory treatments, as used in MG.

Botulism

Botulism should be suspected when more than 1 person has a syndrome that resembles MG or when a patient has abdominal and gastrointestinal tract symptoms that precede a syndrome that resembles MG. Bulbar and respiratory weakness is common, and pupillary abnormalities are distinctive compared with findings in MG. Botulism occurs after the ingestion of improperly canned vegetables, fruit, meat, or fish contaminated with the exotoxin of *Clostridium botulinum*. Paralysis is caused by toxin-mediated inhibition of acetylcholine release from axon terminals at the neuromuscular junction. Although an antitoxin is available, treatment is mainly supportive, especially respiratory, because the signs and symptoms are reversible.

Muscle Disorders

Patients with muscle disease typically present with symmetric proximal weakness (legs more than arms) and with weakness of neck flexors and, occasionally, of cardiac muscle. Muscle stretch reflexes and sensory examination findings are usually normal. Common patient complaints are difficulty arising from a chair or raising the arms over the head. Dysphagia is uncommon. Some myopathies have more prominent distal involvement or result in peculiar patterns of weakness (eg, myotonic dystrophy, inclusion body myosisis, and distal muscular dystrophies). In myotonic dystrophy, atrophy and weakness begin distally and in the face and especially in the sternocleidomastoid muscles. An interesting feature of this dystrophy is *contraction myotonia* (ie, normal contraction of muscle with slow relaxation). Tests for myotonia include striking the thenar eminence with a reflex hammer (looking for percussion myotonia) and shaking the patient's hand, noting that the patient cannot let go quickly.

Muscle disease may be an acquired or progressive hereditary disease. *Myopathy* is a general term for muscle disease. Progressive, genetically mediated myopathy resulting in muscle tissue destruction is called *dystrophy*. However, patients with a muscular dystrophy may not have a family history positive for muscle disease. A classification of myopathies is given in Box 59.5. The diagnosis of myopathy is based on the history and physical examination, increased levels of creatine kinase, EMG, muscle biopsy results, and selected genetic testing.

Inflammatory Myopathy

Inflammatory myopathies include polymyositis, dermatomyositis, necrotizing myopathy, and inclusion body myositis. With inflammatory myopathies, especially dermatomyositis, an underlying cancer may also be present. Necrotizing myopathy can also be associated with an underlying cancer or autoimmune disease or exposure to toxic

---

Box 59.5 • Classification of Myopathies

Dystrophic myopathies (childhood or adult onset, progressive)

Congenital myopathies (congenital onset; slowly progressive or nonprogressive)

Inflammatory myopathies

    Infectious and viral—toxoplasmosis, trichinosis
    Granulomatous—sarcoidosis
    Idiopathic—polymyositis, dermatomyositis, necrotizing myopathy, IBM
    Inflammatory myopathy with collagen vascular disease

Metabolic myopathies

    Glycogenoses
    Mitochondrial disorders
    Defects of fatty acid oxidation
    Endocrinopathy
    Steroid myopathy

Periodic paralyses

Toxic—statin drugs, emetine, chloroquine, vincristine

Miscellaneous

    Amyloidosis
    Critical illness myopathy

Abbreviation: IBM, inclusion body myositis.

---

medications, such as statins (see below). Muscle biopsy should be used to confirm the diagnosis of an inflammatory myopathy, although it may be suggested by the history and examination findings, increased serum levels of creatine kinase, and EMG results. Inclusion body myositis occurs mainly in men older than 60 years; they have asymmetric weakness of proximal and distal muscles, with a predilection for quadriceps, biceps, and finger flexors (this pattern is highly suggestive of inclusion body myositis). Inclusion body myositis is not associated with collagen vascular diseases or neoplasms, and the creatine kinase level may be normal or slightly increased. Inclusion body myositis does not respond to immunosuppression.

Prednisone is the cornerstone for treatment of other inflammatory myopathies such as polymyositis, dermatomyositis, and necrotizing myopathy. The most common pitfall in treating these conditions is treating with doses of prednisone that are too low and are given for an insufficient time. Dermatomyositis, unlike inclusion body myositis or polymyositis, responds to IVIG. In polymyositis, dermatomyositis, and necrotizing myopathy, other immunomodulatory agents (including azathioprine, methotrexate, mycophenolate mofetil, cyclosporine, or cyclophosphamide) are indicated if relapse occurs while the prednisone dose is being tapered, if unacceptable adverse effects develop from prednisone, or if there is no response to prednisone or the response is slow. Plasma exchange is ineffective for polymyositis, dermatomyositis, and inclusion body myositis. A regular exercise program is important, and it has been shown that physical therapy and exercise are not detrimental to patients with myopathies.

Statin-Induced Myopathy

Statin drugs (3-hydroxy-3-methylglutaryl coenzyme A [HMG-CoA] reductase inhibitors) may produce an acute necrotizing myopathy characterized by myalgia, weakness, myoglobinuria, and a marked increase in the level of creatine kinase. This toxic effect is potentiated by fibric acid–derivative drugs and cyclosporine. A more subacute to chronic myopathy can also occur with statins. Symptoms of cramps and myalgias can occur, occasionally with little or no muscle weakness or creatine kinase elevation. How

---

soon symptoms abate after discontinuing use of the drug is unknown, although 3 to 6 months may be needed. Also, in some patients, statins likely unmask a presymptomatic acquired or genetic myopathy. The myopathic symptoms persist in some patients even after they discontinue the use of the statin medication, in some cases attributable to anti-HMG-CoA reductase antibodies.

Steroid Myopathy

Occasionally, myopathic proximal muscle weakness develops in patients receiving long-term therapy with glucocorticoid medications. The serum creatine kinase level is often not increased in these patients, and electrodiagnostic abnormalities may be subtle or absent. Muscle biopsy is often unremarkable, and the diagnosis is often confirmed with observation of improvement after discontinuing steroid use.

Electrolyte Imbalance

Severe hypokalemia (potassium level <2.5 mEq/L) and hyperkalemia (potassium level >7 mEq/L) produce muscle weakness, as do hypercalcemia, hypocalcemia, and hypophosphatemia. Familial periodic paralysis of the hypokalemic, hyperkalemic, or normokalemic type consists of episodes of acute paralysis that last 2 to 24 hours and can be precipitated by a carbohydrate-rich meal or strenuous exercise; cranial or respiratory muscle paralysis does not occur. The diagnosis is difficult to establish and is based on the potassium levels during an attack, family history, EMG, and genetic testing for causative sodium and calcium channel mutations.

Endocrine Diseases

Hyperthyroidism and hypothyroidism, hyperadrenalism and hypoadrenalism, acromegaly, and primary and secondary hyperparathyroidism cause muscle weakness.

KEY FACTS

- ✓ Presentations of neuromuscular transmission disorders—fluctuating weakness manifested as fatigable weakness in the limbs, eyelids (ptosis), tongue and palate (dysarthria and dysphagia), and extraocular muscles (diplopia)

- ✓ Characteristics of MG—usually occurs in young women and older men, heralded by cranial nerve findings such as diplopia, dysarthria, dysphagia, and dyspnea

- ✓ Lambert-Eaton myasthenic syndrome—often associated with small cell lung carcinoma; treatment is focused on the underlying malignancy, if present

- ✓ Inflammatory myopathies—polymyositis, dermatomyositis, necrotizing myopathy, and inclusion body myositis; an underlying cancer may be present

- ✓ Statin-induced myopathy—an acute necrotizing myopathy caused by statin drugs and characterized by myalgia, weakness, myoglobinuria, and a marked increase in creatine kinase

Questions and Answers

Questions

Multiple Choice (choose the best answer)

IX.1. A 52-year-old woman is evaluated for dizziness. She has a history of well-controlled diabetes mellitus and treated hypertension. On neurologic examination, she has a moderate loss of all sensory modalities distally and to the knees and wrists symmetrically. Her blood pressure is 146/84 mm Hg in the supine position (with a heart rate of 85 beats per minute). Upon standing, her blood pressure is 100/70 mm Hg (with a heart rate of 88 beats per minute), and she reports having a "dizzy sensation." Which of the following interventions should be instituted first?
  a. Administer fludrocortisone.
  b. Perform magnetic resonance angiography.
  c. Discontinue use of antihypertensive drugs.
  d. Perform a vestibular evaluation.
  e. Perform magnetic resonance imaging of the cervical spine.

IX.2. A 37-year-old man has a 1-month history of fluctuating difficulties with his speech and swallowing. He notes that with long conversations he has increasing difficulty speaking; this is apparent during the history when his speech becomes nearly unintelligible. He describes several choking episodes and nasal regurgitation of liquids when swallowing. On examination, he has normal eye movements at baseline, but after 2 minutes of sustained upgaze, asymmetrical ptosis (worse on the left) and right hypertropia occur. Strength is initially normal, but with sequential strong contractions of the deltoid and iliopsoas muscles, mild weakness develops. Sensation, muscle stretch reflexes, coordination, and alternating motion rates are normal. Which of the following would be the most appropriate next step in his evaluation?
  a. Autonomic testing, including tilt table testing
  b. Urgent magnetic resonance imaging of the cervical spine
  c. Cerebrospinal fluid examination
  d. Muscle biopsy
  e. Serum acetylcholine receptor antibody testing

IX.3. A 42-year-old woman presents with a 3-day history of difficulty walking. She has also noted a tingling sensation in her fingers and toes. On neurologic examination, she has a normal mental status and normal neurovascular examination findings. She cannot rise from the couch without assistance, and she cannot ambulate without assistance. She appears somewhat short of breath. Cranial nerve examination findings are normal except for mild symmetrical facial weakness. On motor testing, distal muscle weakness is greater than proximal muscle weakness. Vibratory sensation is decreased distally. Reflexes are absent. The Babinski test is negative. Coordination is difficult to test because of weakness. Which of the following would be expected on further evaluation?
  a. Magnetic resonance imaging (MRI) of the head showing multiple areas of increased T2 signal in the subcortical white matter
  b. Cerebrospinal fluid (CSF) examination showing an increased protein level and a normal cell count
  c. Ophthalmoscopic examination showing optic disc pallor bilaterally
  d. Elevated blood glucose concentration
  e. Electroencephalography showing left temporal sharp waves

IX.4. An 83-year-old man has an abrupt, painless onset of right upper limb weakness and "garbled" speech. On examination in the emergency department 2.5 hours after the onset of symptoms, he has moderate weakness of the right deltoid, triceps, and intrinsic hand muscles and a mild right foot drop. His speech is halting, and he appears frustrated when trying to speak, but he follows commands without difficulty. His blood pressure is 163/87 mm Hg, with a heart rate of 85 beats per minute. His electrocardiogram indicates atrial fibrillation. What is the most appropriate next step in the evaluation and management of this patient?
  a. Infusion of intravenous (IV) tissue plasminogen activator (tPA)
  b. Initiation of warfarin therapy
  c. Computed tomography (CT) of the head
  d. Infusion of IV labetalol
  e. Electroencephalography (EEG)

IX.5. A 53-year-old woman has a 6-week history of increasing clumsiness with both hands and imbalance that has led to several falls. Her family has also noted that her speech "sounds drunk." On neurologic examination, she has a wide-based, cautious, unstable gait. Alternating motion rates of the limbs are of normal frequency and amplitude, but they are irregular and imprecise. Finger-to-nose testing is inaccurate, and the patient becomes tearful during the examination. Her strength, sensation, and muscle stretch reflexes are normal, and magnetic resonance imaging (MRI) of her brain is normal. Which of the following is the most appropriate next step in her evaluation?
  a. Serum paraneoplastic antibodies, including Purkinje cell cytoplasmic autoantibody type 1 (PCA-1) (also known as anti-Yo)
  b. Consultation with a psychiatrist
  c. Cervical spine MRI with contrast medium
  d. Nerve conduction studies, including needle electromyography
  e. Sural nerve biopsy

IX.6. A 20-year-old man is evaluated for spells during which he appears alert but stares ahead, is unresponsive to the environment, and exhibits automatic lip-smacking movements. Results of his neurologic examination are normal. Magnetic resonance imaging of the head shows atrophy of the left hippocampus.

649

Results of awake electroencephalography (EEG) are normal. The spells, which occur up to 3 times weekly despite treatment with maximally tolerated doses of carbamazepine and valproate over the past 10 months, have prevented him from driving and working. Which of the following is the most appropriate approach?

a. Substitute topiramate for valproate.
b. Add gabapentin or levetiracetam.
c. Substitute phenytoin for carbamazepine.
d. Perform prolonged video-EEG monitoring for possible anterior temporal lobectomy.
e. Discontinue use of valproate and consider vagus nerve stimulation.

IX.7. A 38-year-old obese woman has a history of depression, chronic obstructive pulmonary disease, constipation, and recurrent migraine headaches. Up to 3 years ago, the headaches averaged 1 attack every 2 to 4 months and responded to sumatriptan. Over the past 3 months, they have increased in frequency to 1 to 3 attacks weekly. Results of neurologic and ophthalmoscopic examinations are normal. Which of the following is the most appropriate prophylactic therapy for these headaches?

a. Daily long-acting triptan
b. Valproate
c. Topiramate
d. Propranolol
e. Amitriptyline

Answers

IX.1. Answer c.

Orthostatic hypotension is an important cause of "dizziness," particularly in patients at risk of autonomic failure, such as those with diabetic neuropathy or synucleinopathies (eg, parkinsonism). The hallmark of orthostatic hypotension due to autonomic failure is an inability to increase the heart rate when the blood pressure decreases profoundly upon standing. The first step in managing orthostatic hypotension is to correct potentially reversible causes, particularly the use of vasodilators, diuretics, and anticholinergics. Simple maneuvers, such as increasing salt and water intake, elevating the head of the bed, and performing postural maneuvers, should be tried before pharmacologic management.

IX.2. Answer e.

Myasthenia gravis is an autoimmune disorder of the neuromuscular junction. It causes fatigable weakness of the axial musculature or bulbar muscles (or both). Diplopia, ptosis, speech slurring, and difficulty with chewing or swallowing are typical symptoms of the fatigable weakness of the bulbar muscles.

Additional diagnostic studies include electromyography, which shows a decrement in amplitude of compound muscle action potentials with repetitive stimulation. Computed tomography of the chest should be performed because thymoma is occasionally associated with myasthenia gravis. Thymectomy has a role in the treatment of myasthenia gravis, particularly in a person with generalized myasthenia gravis and in younger patients who are not at significant surgical risk. Acetylcholine receptor antibody testing is also useful for diagnosis. The Tensilon (edrophonium chloride) test involves the administration of edrophonium, a short-acting acetylcholinesterase inhibitor, which temporarily increases the concentration of acetylcholine in the synaptic cleft, so that the signs of myasthenia gravis are temporarily improved. Atropine should be available because of the potential for bradycardia or other cholinergic symptoms. Autoimmune thyroid disease can also occur in myasthenia gravis, and appropriate blood tests should be performed. Fatigable weakness argues against muscle disease, and muscle biopsy is not useful in myasthenia gravis. Another neuromuscular junction disease, botulism, occurs typically several hours after ingesting food containing *Clostridium botulinum*. Patients who have botulism present with diplopia, dysphagia, dysarthria, ptosis, and weakness of the jaw muscles. Autonomic symptoms can also occur (eg, constipation, dilation of the pupils, and urinary dysfunction), and systemic symptoms, such as nausea and vomiting and diarrhea, may precede these symptoms.

IX.3. Answer b.

Weakness may be caused by abnormalities in many areas of the central nervous system and peripheral nervous system. Central nervous system abnormalities causing weakness include supratentorial, infratentorial, and spinal cord lesions, each of which would cause an upper motor neuron pattern of weakness with increased reflexes and extensor plantar responses. The weakness is usually associated with other findings that localize the lesion somewhere along the corticospinal tract. Disorders of the nerve roots (ie, radiculopathies) causing weakness are often associated with pain, they may be associated with decreased reflexes, and they are commonly associated with sensory complaints. Disorders of the muscle are associated with normal reflexes early in the disease but may be diminished later. Weakness is typically greater proximally than distally. Plantar responses are flexor, and there is no sensation loss. Neuromuscular diseases such as myasthenia gravis may cause fatigable weakness of both the axial and the bulbar muscles. Reflexes are typically normal, and sensation is intact.

Peripheral nerve disorders typically cause more diffuse weakness that is greater distally than proximally. They are often associated with some degree of sensory loss (there are more pure motor neuropathies that are associated with minimal sensory symptoms). Reflexes are often decreased early in the course and the plantar responses are flexor.

Guillain-Barré syndrome (GBS) is an acute inflammatory demyelinating disorder of the peripheral nerves and nerve roots. Patients present with subacute onset of weakness and sensory symptoms (eg, paresthesias) that slowly progress proximally from the hands and feet. The weakness usually begins in the legs but may occur simultaneously in the upper and lower extremities. Facial weakness occurs later in 50% of patients. The reflexes are diminished early with "large fiber" joint position and vibratory sensation loss. Antecedent infections with viral or bacterial infections occur from 1 to several weeks before symptom onset. Further findings include abnormal CSF with an elevated protein level and a normal cell count (ie, albuminocytologic dissociation). In most GBS patients, these abnormalities can be found within 1 week after onset. MRI is not needed because the lesion is localized to the peripheral nerve. Electromyographic findings may be normal early but later show conduction block and nerve conduction velocity slowing, with findings more apparent on motor testing than on sensory testing; fibrillation potentials indicating denervation also occur within 2 weeks of symptom onset.

Patients with GBS are usually hospitalized and closely monitored for respiratory compromise. Treatment is usually initiated with plasmapheresis or intravenous immunoglobulin and is effective particularly if it is started early. Close attention is also paid to deep vein thrombosis prophylaxis, risk of aspiration pneumonia, constipation, back pain, and autonomic instability (variable heart rate and blood pressure).

IX.4. Answer c.

The patient's presentation suggests an acute ischemic cerebral infarction in the distribution of the anterior division of the left middle cerebral artery, but to exclude the management-changing possibility of cerebral hemorrhage, CT of the head is required. The commonly accepted window for IV thrombolysis is 3 hours, but imaging, laboratory tests, and a careful history cannot be sacrificed to beat the deadline. Selected patients may be considered for IV tPA after 3 hours, and intra-arterial intervention can be considered up to 6 or more hours after the onset of symptoms. Anticoagulation does not typically have a role in the management of acute ischemic cerebral infarction, particularly before imaging has excluded hemorrhage, although it will likely be considered for secondary prevention of stroke in this patient who has atrial fibrillation. The treatment of mild, asymptomatic hypertension in this patient could lead to neurologic deterioration. An EEG might be helpful if a postictal paresis were suspected (Todd paralysis), but the patient has no history of seizure.

IX.5. Answer a.

Gait ataxia, limb dysmetria, and ataxic dysarthria all suggest a cerebellar disorder, and the subacute onset of the symptoms increases the likelihood of an autoimmune or paraneoplastic mechanism. In this patient, the most appropriate next step among the choices listed is assessment for paraneoplastic antibodies, such as PCA-1, that may mediate a cerebellar syndrome. These antibodies and this syndrome are predictive of gynecologic malignancies such as ovarian carcinoma or breast carcinoma. Other diagnostic considerations for this patient might include structural cerebellar lesions such as a tumor (effectively excluded by the normal imaging), intoxication with anticonvulsant medications or alcohol, or infectious cerebellitis.

IX.6. Answer d.

This young man has temporal lobe epilepsy with complex partial seizures. The condition is intractable since it is not responding to 2 medications. Typically, if a patient does not achieve seizure control with 2 medications, additional medical therapy will not help. The next consideration for this patient is a surgical procedure to remove the epileptogenic portion of his brain. Continuous EEG monitoring is done in a hospitalized setting, often with withdrawal of the seizure medications, to map the seizure onset. If it localizes to the temporal lobe, the patient has about a 90% chance of being free of seizures after temporal lobectomy. Vagus nerve stimulation is done in patients who are not surgical candidates.

IX.7. Answer c.

Preventive medication is appropriate for this patient because of the frequency of the migraine headaches. Answer choices *b* through *e* would be reasonable for prevention of migraine, but triptans are abortive agents and would not be used daily. A patient's comorbidities must be reviewed before an appropriate preventive agent is chosen. Since this patient has lung disease, depression, and obesity, topiramate would be the best choice. Potential adverse effects of topiramate include paresthesias, cognitive clouding, taste perturbation (particularly with carbonated beverages), anorexia, and nephrolithiasis.

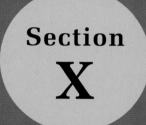

Oncology

60 Breast Cancer

TUFIA C. HADDAD, MD AND TIMOTHY J. MOYNIHAN, MD

Magnitude of the Problem

In the United States, approximately 235,000 new cases of breast cancer are diagnosed annually. Breast cancer will develop in approximately 1 in 8 women who achieve a normal life expectancy and is the second most common cause of cancer death among women in the United States (lung cancer is the most common). The incidence decreased in the early 2000s and has leveled off since then.

Risk Factors

The risk factors for breast cancer are outlined in Table 60.1. Breast cancer–associated genes (*BRCA1* and *BRCA2*) occur in less than 5% to 10% of cases of breast cancer, but the women who carry these genes have a 50% to 80% chance for breast cancer developing in their lifetime. Less than 25% of women with breast cancer have known high-risk factors.

Pathology

Breast cancer by definition is invasive, with malignant cells penetrating from their site of origin within the breast into the surrounding stroma. In situ carcinomas of the breast are noninvasive, and they can be characterized as precancerous lesions (ductal carcinoma in situ [DCIS]) or as markers for increased risk of breast cancer (lobular carcinoma in situ [LCIS]). Of the invasive breast cancers, approximately 90% are classified as ductal or lobular carcinomas, originating within the ducts and lobules of the normal breast (Figure 60.1). Infiltrating ductal carcinoma is the most common histologic type (75% of breast cancers). Invasive lobular carcinoma accounts for 5% to 15% of breast cancers, is more frequently multifocal and bilateral, and is less likely to be seen with mammography. Invasive (sometimes called infiltrating)

breast cancer has the potential for systemic spread, as opposed to carcinoma in situ, which does not have metastatic potential, because by definition, the malignant cells have not invaded through the basement membrane.

DCIS is noninvasive; however, if left untreated it can progress to invasive disease. Whether DCIS should be considered a cancer or a precancerous lesion is controversial. LCIS is not a precursor for invasive disease, but rather it is a marker for increased risk of future development of invasive carcinoma in the ipsilateral or contralateral breast.

Staging

The staging system of the American Joint Committee on Cancer is shown in Box 60.1. Prognosis, which is associated with stage, is improving for patients with breast cancer at any stage. The current 5-year overall survival for patients with breast cancer is 89.2% (98.6% for local disease confined to the breast, 84.4% for regional disease confined to the breast and regional lymph nodes, and 24.3% for stage IV disease that has metastasized to other organs).

Natural History and Prognostic Factors

General Principles

The clinical outcomes for invasive breast cancer depend primarily on whether cancer cells have spread to other organs hematogenously. No established tests can detect the presence of microscopic metastatic disease. The most important predictor for the presence of micrometastatic disease is lymphatic spread from the primary tumor to the ipsilateral axillary lymph nodes. Tumor grade and size, the presence or absence of lymph node involvement, hormone receptor status, and HER2/neu overexpression are the key prognostic characteristics for breast cancer.

Table 60.1 • Risk Factors for Breast Cancer

Risk Factor	High Risk (RR, >4.0)	Low to Moderate Risk (RR, 1–4)
Age	Advanced	
Race		White
Endogenous hormones		Menarche before age 12 y Menopause after age 55 y Nulliparous Age >30 y at first full-term pregnancy
Exogenous hormones		Long duration (≥15 y) of estrogen replacement therapy
Personal medical history	BRCA1 or BRCA2 mutation History of breast cancer History of breast biopsy with benign proliferative changes with atypia Heterogeneously or extremely dense breast tissue on mammography Prior history of chest radiotherapy	Obesity in postmenopausal women History of ovarian or endometrial cancer
Family medical history	First-degree family member with BRCA1 or BRCA2 mutation 2 first-degree family members with breast cancer Other rare familial syndromes associated with breast cancer	1 first-degree family member with premenopausal (RR, 3.3) or postmenopausal (RR, 1.8) breast cancer
Lifestyle		Moderate alcohol intake

Abbreviation: RR, relative risk.

Hormone Receptor Status

Breast cancer cells may or may not express the hormone receptors, estrogen receptor (ER) and progesterone receptor (PR). In general, when the stage of disease is equal,

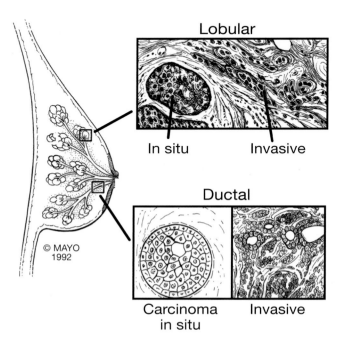

Figure 60.1 *Breast Carcinomas: Lobular and Ductal, In Situ and Invasive.*

patients with ER-positive tumors have a better prognosis than patients with ER-negative tumors. For patients with ER-positive breast cancer, the risk of relapse in the first 5 years after treatment is less than that for patients with ER-negative disease (probably because of the benefit from adjuvant hormonal therapy), and the risk slowly decreases but persists for several decades thereafter. For patients with ER-negative breast cancer, the recurrence risk is higher within the first 5 years after treatment and becomes negligible after 10 years.

Extent of ER-positivity may be important in treatment outcome; the greater the expression of tumor cells staining positive for ER, the more likely they will be sensitive to adjuvant hormonal therapies.

Status of Human Epidermal Growth Factor Receptor 2

Human epidermal growth factor receptor 2 (HER2) is a transmembrane protein that is overexpressed in approximately 20% of breast cancers. Tumors that are HER2-positive are associated with a higher risk of recurrence and an overall worse prognosis. Adjuvant therapies targeting the HER2 pathway, such as trastuzumab and pertuzumab, greatly improve the prognosis. HER2-positive breast cancer is associated with a significantly increased risk of recurrence within the central nervous system.

Triple-Negative Breast Cancer

Cancer cells that are ER negative, PR negative, and negative for overexpression of HER2 are frequently referred to

Box 60.1 • Staging of Breast Cancer

Primary tumor (T)

TIS	Carcinoma in situ
T1	Primary tumor ≤2 cm
T2	Primary tumor 2.1–5 cm
T3	Primary tumor >5 cm
T4	Primary tumor of any size with direct extension to chest wall or skin

Regional lymph node (N)

N0	No involved lymph nodes
N1	Movable ipsilateral axillary lymph nodes
N2	Matted or fixed lymph nodes, or in clinically apparent ipsilateral internal mammary lymph nodes in the absence of clinically evident axillary lymph node metastasis
N3	Metastasis in ipsilateral infraclavicular lymph nodes

Distant metastasis (M)

M0	None detected
M1	Distant metastasis present (includes ipsilateral supraclavicular lymph nodes)

Stage grouping

Stage I[a]	T1 N0
Stage IIA[a]	T0 N1
	T1 N1
	T2 N0
Stage IIB[a]	T2 N1
	T3 N0
Stage IIIA[b]	T0 N2
	T1 N2
	T2 N2
	T3 N1,N2
Stage IIIB[b]	T4, any N
Stage IIIC[c]	any T, N3
Stage IV[d]	any T, any N, M1

[a] Operable disease.

[b] Locally advanced disease.

[c] Advanced disease.

[d] Advanced or metastatic disease.

Data from Singletary SE, Allred C, Ashley P, Bassett LW, Berry D, Bland KI, et al. Revision of the American Joint Committee on Cancer staging system for breast cancer. J Clin Oncol. 2002 Sep 1;20(17):3628–36.

as **triple-negative breast cancer**. These cancers tend to be the most responsive to chemotherapy, yet they are associated with a poorer overall prognosis. Patients with triple-negative disease who show no evidence of recurrence after 5 years are at lower risk for late, distant recurrence.

Key Definition

Triple-negative breast cancer: *cancer cells that are ER-negative, PR-negative, and negative for overexpression of HER2.*

Grade

Tumor grade reflects the aggressiveness of the cancer. Grade can be useful in making adjuvant treatment decisions.

Molecular Profiling

Analysis of the tumor genome is another way that the prognosis can be established. The Oncotype DX Breast Cancer Assay (Genomic Health, Inc), a 21-gene, polymerase chain reaction–based assay, has been validated as a prognostic molecular tool in ER-positive, HER2-negative, lymph node–negative breast cancer. This gene expression analysis can stratify a patient's risk of recurrence as low, intermediate, or high. Furthermore, it is predictive of benefit from adjuvant chemotherapy.

Therapy

Treatment decisions for all breast cancers must take into account not only the breast cancer stage, grade, and hormone and HER2 receptor status, but they must also carefully integrate each patient's comorbidities, life expectancy, and preferences. Risks and benefits of treatment must be individualized to each patient.

Ductal Carcinoma in Situ

DCIS is primarily treated with local therapy only—either lumpectomy (also known as breast conservation surgery) with or without breast radiotherapy or mastectomy. For ER-positive DCIS, the selective ER modulator, tamoxifen, is frequently considered as adjuvant therapy. In the next 10 years, tamoxifen decreases the risk of a subsequent breast event (defined as either recurrent DCIS or the development of an invasive breast cancer in the ipsilateral or contralateral breast) from 13% to 8%. It is not associated with an increase in survival, however, and it may convey risk for adverse effects.

Early-Stage (Stages I-III) Invasive Breast Cancer

Local-Regional Therapy

Surgical resection of invasive breast cancer is achieved by either lumpectomy (also known as a wide local excision or breast conservation surgery) or mastectomy. Several randomized controlled clinical trials that compared mastectomy to lumpectomy plus radiotherapy have demonstrated equivalent survival. Patients who elect to receive breast radiotherapy after lumpectomy have lower rates of recurrence of ipsilateral breast cancer compared with women who are treated by lumpectomy without radiotherapy. Those who undergo mastectomy have rates of ipsilateral breast cancer recurrence similar to those who receive breast conservation therapy plus radiotherapy.

All women with invasive breast cancer should have a sentinel lymph node biopsy performed in conjunction with their definitive breast surgery. If a sentinel node is positive for malignancy, an axillary lymph node dissection should be completed. If the sentinel lymph node does not have metastatic tumor cells, the probability of other lymph nodes being affected is less than 5%. When compared with axillary lymph node dissection, sentinel lymph node biopsy decreases late complications such as lymphedema.

Adjuvant Therapy

After surgical resection of breast cancer, systemic treatment (ie, adjuvant therapy) has been shown to decrease the risk of systemic recurrence and improve overall survival. The goal of adjuvant therapy is to eliminate microscopic metastatic disease present at the time of diagnosis. Adjuvant treatment may include chemotherapy, hormonal therapy, HER2-directed therapy, or various combinations for specific patients. The benefit of chemotherapy may be conferred to patients regardless of the tumor's ER or HER2 status. Hormonal therapy, however, benefits only patients with ER-positive disease, and HER2-directed therapy benefits only patients with HER2-positive disease.

Adjuvant systemic treatment should generally be offered to patients with breast cancer with an intermediate or high risk of relapse, including the majority of patients with lymph node–positive disease. Adjuvant therapy has been shown to decrease the risk of recurrence and improve overall survival among patients with lymph node–negative or lymph node–positive cancer. For those with lymph node–negative disease, chemotherapy is typically advised for more biologically aggressive or proliferative tumors (more commonly triple-negative or HER2-positive disease). Chemotherapy is associated with more acute and long-term toxic effects than hormonal or HER2-directed therapy.

Neoadjuvant Therapy

Systemic therapy given before surgical resection is becoming more common practice. Relapse rates and breast cancer survival are not affected by whether adjuvant therapy is administered before or after definitive breast surgery. Neoadjuvant (ie, preoperative) systemic therapy is used for large primary tumors in women desiring a chance at breast conservation therapy, for inflammatory breast cancer, and for clinical trials that study the effects of therapy on breast cancer. Advantages of neoadjuvant therapy include being able to determine the responsiveness of cancer to systemic treatment and allowing a change in therapy for patients without a response, increasing the chance for a breast conserving operation, and providing a unique opportunity to study the biology of the tumor in vivo. Patients who have a pathologic complete response to neoadjuvant therapy at the time of operation (ie, no residual cancer is identified in the surgical specimen) are known to have a more favorable overall prognosis compared to those with residual disease. Neoadjuvant therapy can be chemotherapy, HER2-directed therapy, or hormonal therapy.

Metastatic (Stage IV) Disease

Approximately 5% to 10% of patients have stage IV disease at the time of initial diagnosis. The majority of patients with stage IV disease, however, experience systemic relapse after prior therapy for early-stage disease. In particular, patients with ER-positive breast cancer are at risk for "late" recurrences occurring beyond the initial 5 years after treatment.

We currently lack curative therapy for metastatic breast cancer. The median duration of survival with recurrent disease is 2.5 years, but the spectrum of survival is wide. In 2013, 5-year survival for stage IV disease was 24%. Survival is generally longer for patients with bone-only or soft tissue disease than it is for patients with visceral metastases. It is also generally longer for patients with ER-positive or HER2-positive metastatic disease than it is for patients with triple-negative breast cancer.

Because treatment is not curative, the goals of treatment are to optimize quality of life and prolong life for as long as possible. The initial systemic treatment of patients with hormone receptor–positive advanced disease is usually hormonal. Chemotherapy is used when resistance to hormonal therapy has occurred in patients with hormone receptor–positive disease. An increasing number of HER2-directed therapy agents are available for patients with HER2-positive metastatic disease. These agents can be administered alone or in combination with another. Frequently, however, HER2-directed therapy is used in combination with hormonal therapy for patients with ER-positive disease or with chemotherapy regardless of tumor ER status. Chemotherapy is the only standard option for treatment of patients with triple-negative breast cancer. Combination chemotherapy has not been shown to improve survival when compared with sequential administration of single-agent chemotherapeutics. It does, however, enhance the odds of tumor cytoreduction, but this approach should be reserved for patients who have symptomatic disease, rapid tumor progression, or imminent end-organ failure.

KEY FACTS

✓ Lobular carcinoma in situ—
  - a marker for increased risk of invasive carcinoma in either breast
  - not a precursor for invasive disease

✓ Ductal carcinoma in situ—a precancerous lesion that can develop into invasive cancer

✓ ER-positive breast cancer—generally portends a better prognosis than ER-negative breast cancer (if stage of disease is equal)

✓ HER2-positive tumors—associated with a higher risk of recurrence and a worse prognosis

✓ DCIS therapy—
  - local therapy only (mastectomy or lumpectomy with or without radiotherapy)
  - if ER-positive, consider adjuvant tamoxifen after lumpectomy

✓ Surgical resection of invasive breast cancer—lumpectomy or mastectomy

✓ Metastatic (stage IV) breast cancer
  - most patients have had a relapse after treatment of early-stage disease, which may have occurred years or decades earlier (especially with ER-positive disease)
  - treatment is palliative

Therapeutic Agents

Chemotherapy

Many chemotherapeutic drugs are active against breast cancer. The anthracyclines (eg, doxorubicin and epirubicin) and the taxanes (eg, paclitaxel and docetaxel) are the most effective agents for breast cancer. Notably, a very small, but real, increased risk for secondary leukemias exists for women receiving adjuvant chemotherapy, especially anthracycline-based chemotherapy. The anthracyclines are also associated with a dose-dependent increase in the risk of irreversible cardiomyopathy. The taxanes may induce peripheral neuropathy.

Hormonal Therapy

Tamoxifen is a selective ER modulator that is commonly used to treat both premenopausal and postmenopausal breast cancer. On some tissue (eg, breast), tamoxifen acts like an ER antagonist; whereas on other tissue (eg, bones, lipids, and uterus), it acts like an ER agonist. Its benefits include 1) antitumor effects on breast cancer cells, 2) decreased risk (by 40%) of contralateral breast cancer, 3) improved bone density, and 4) favorable effects on lipid profiles. Tamoxifen therapy also has adverse effects, including 1) hot flashes, 2) a 2- to 3-fold increase in risk of thromboembolism, 3) an increased risk of endometrial cancer in postmenopausal women, and 4) a slight increase in risk

of cataracts. Tamoxifen is metabolized into its active metabolites by the cytochrome P450 2D6 isozyme (CYP2D6); accordingly, patients who take medications that are strong CYP2D6 inhibitors (eg, paroxetine, cimetidine, and bupropion) should avoid these medications to eliminate drug-drug interactions.

A newer class of hormonal agents, the **aromatase inhibitors**, is being used for the treatment of breast cancer in postmenopausal women. These agents block the peripheral conversion of androgens into estrogen. These drugs show a slight superiority to tamoxifen in reducing the risk of recurrence of breast cancer. They are not associated with an increased risk of thrombotic or endometrial events; however, they do increase the risk of osteoporosis and fractures, arthralgias, and vaginal dryness. These drugs are ineffective for premenopausal women who retain ovarian production of estrogen, and they are not advised for women who experience chemotherapy-induced amenorrhea.

Key Definition

Aromatase inhibitors: *hormonal agents that block peripheral conversion of androgens into estrogen and are used to treat breast cancer in postmenopausal women.*

HER2-Directed Therapy

Trastuzumab is a monoclonal antibody directed against HER2, and it has been shown to have activity against HER2-positive breast cancers. As an adjuvant, the use of trastuzumab therapy for 1 year is associated with an approximately 50% decrease in the risk of breast cancer recurrence in women with HER2-positive breast cancer. Lapatinib is an oral agent that also interferes with the HER2 signaling pathway. It may be effective in women with trastuzumab-refractory HER2-positive breast cancer. Other newer HER2-directed therapies include the antibody drug conjugate, ado-trastuzumab emtansine, and pertuzumab.

Osteoclast Inhibitor Therapy

The use of the bisphosphonates zoledronic acid and pamidronate can reduce the need for palliative radiotherapy, bone fixation, and pain medicine in patients with lytic bone metastases. A recent meta-analysis also suggests that the use of adjuvant zoledronic acid in postmenopausal patients is associated with a decrease in the risk of bony metastatic relapse and improvement in both breast cancer–specific survival and overall survival.

Denosumab is a monoclonal antibody directed against the receptor activator of nuclear factor κB ligand (RANKL), which stimulates osteoclasts. This drug has also been shown to decrease future skeletal events. A major advantage of denosumab is its subcutaneous (as opposed to intravenous) administration; however, compared to the bisphosphonates, it is considerably more expensive and it presents a higher risk (although still rare) of osteonecrosis of the jaw.

Follow-up After Curative Therapy

After definitive therapy for breast cancer, patients are at risk for locoregional or systemic recurrence of the disease or for development of a new primary lesion. Current recommendations for follow-up include history, review of systems, and physical examination every 3 to 6 months for the first 3 years after therapy, every 6 to 12 months for the fourth and fifth years, and annually thereafter. The only diagnostic testing indicated is annual mammography.

In women with a prior history of breast cancer, use of magnetic resonance imaging (MRI) of the breast for surveillance is associated with high sensitivity, good specificity, and high rates of false-positive results. There is no evidence that MRI leads to improved survival, and as such, routine breast MRI surveillance is not justified for the majority of breast cancer survivors. The current American Cancer Society guidelines (2007) state that data are insufficient to support routine use of surveillance MRI of the breast for patients with a prior history of breast cancer or heterogeneously or extremely dense breasts on mammography. Exceptions include breast cancer survivors who 1) retain breast tissue after treatment and are known to have a *BRCA1* or *BRCA2* mutation, 2) are known to have a first-degree family member with an established *BRCA1* or *BRCA2* mutation (but the patient has not been tested), or 3) have a prior history of chest radiotherapy.

Intensive laboratory surveillance (eg, tumor marker tests, liver function tests, and complete blood cell counts) or radiologic surveillance (eg, chest radiography, bone scan, computed tomography [CT], and positron emission tomography [PET]) (or both) has not been shown to improve survival or outcomes, and it is not recommended for asymptomatic patients. Testing should be offered according to the development of new symptoms or suspicious physical examination findings.

Patients who have had breast cancer treatment should be followed for late adverse effects of therapy. These include altered sexual function, mood disturbances, weight gain, and insomnia. Medical complications may include osteoporosis, peripheral neuropathy, myelodysplastic syndrome, and cardiac toxicity. Exercise and maintenance of ideal body weight should be recommended even though they have not been definitively proved to decrease cancer recurrence.

Patterns of Recurrence

Long-term follow-up of women with ER-positive breast cancer is essential because the number of recurrences 5 to 15 years after diagnosis is the same as in the first 5 years after diagnosis. Patients with HER2-positive or triple-negative disease tend to have recurrences within the first 5 years after diagnosis. Relapse after 5 years for women with ER-negative breast cancer is uncommon.

Breast cancer tends to recur in bones, liver, lungs, or brain or locally in the chest wall or residual breast. Patients may have recurrences decades after the initial diagnosis, and this possibility must always be kept in mind when a patient has a history of ER-positive breast cancer. Recent data suggest that HER2-positive tumors have a higher chance of recurrence in the central nervous system.

KEY FACTS

✓ Benefits of adjuvant therapy—
- antitumor effects on breast cancer cells
- decreases risk of ipsilateral and contralateral breast cancer
- decreases risk of systemic relapse
- improves breast cancer–specific and overall survival

✓ Adverse effects of aromatase inhibitors—
- arthralgias
- vaginal dryness
- loss of bone mineral density
- increases risk of bone fractures

✓ Adverse effects of tamoxifen—
- hot flashes
- increases risk of thromboembolism (2- to 3-fold)
- increases risk of endometrial cancer in postmenopausal women
- slightly increases risk of cataracts

✓ Metabolism of tamoxifen—
- metabolized into its active metabolites by CYP2D6
- patients should not use tamoxifen with strong CYP2D6 inhibitors (eg, paroxetine, cimetidine, and bupropion)

✓ Benefits of bisphosphonates (eg, zoledronic acid and pamidronate) for lytic bone metastases—less need for palliative radiotherapy, bone fixation, and pain medicine

✓ Recommended surveillance after curative intent therapy—history, physical examination, and, for those with residual breast tissue, annual mammography

✓ Follow-up that does *not* improve survival or outcomes and is *not* recommended after curative therapy—
- surveillance blood tests (tumor marker tests, liver function tests, and complete blood cell tests)
- other imaging studies (eg, chest radiography, bone scan, CT, and PET)

✓ Patients with history of ER-positive breast cancer may have recurrence decades after the initial diagnosis

61 Cancer of Unknown Primary Origin and Paraneoplastic Syndromes

MICHELLE A. NEBEN WITTICH, MD

Carcinoma of Unknown Primary Origin

Carcinoma of unknown primary origin (CUP) describes a metastatic disease for which the primary cancer cannot be identified. Of all invasive malignancies, 2% to 6% are CUP. The most common tumor associated with CUP is adenocarcinoma. Squamous cell carcinoma and undifferentiated neoplasms make up a smaller portion of CUP. When a pathologic diagnosis is established, additional evaluation should be tailored according to the patient's risk factors (eg, smoking and breast cancer risk), symptoms and signs, sites of metastasis, and the histologic diagnosis. Special consideration should be given to rule out possible curable malignancies (eg, germ cell tumors or lymphoma) or treatable malignancies (eg, breast, ovarian, or prostate cancer).

> ### Key Definition
>
> Carcinoma of unknown primary origin: *a metastatic disease for which the primary cancer cannot be identified.*

Patients with favorable subsets of CUP can have long-term survival with treatment tailored to their most likely disease. Women presenting with axillary adenocarcinomas, with no clear breast primary lesion, should receive therapy for breast cancer. Women with peritoneal carcinomatosis generally undergo exploratory laparotomy with surgical cytoreduction, as they would for ovarian carcinoma. Men presenting with bone metastases, particularly osteoblastic metastases, should have a prostate-specific antigen (PSA) test, and their tumor material should be stained for PSA expression.

Squamous cell carcinoma in isolated cervical lymph nodes should be treated as a locally advanced head and neck cancer, and squamous cell cancer in inguinal lymph nodes should be treated with surgery or radiotherapy (or both). Patients with poorly differentiated neuroendocrine carcinomas can respond well to systemic chemotherapy. Patients with a single small metastatic lesion can be treated with surgery or radiotherapy.

If a potentially treatable neoplasm is ruled out, most patients with CUP have a very poor prognosis, with an expected survival of 4 to 10 months. Some may benefit from palliative treatment (radiotherapy or chemotherapy); many are managed best with supportive care and hospice care.

Paraneoplastic Syndromes

Paraneoplastic syndromes are caused by factors other than direct tumor invasion or compression. They do not necessarily indicate metastatic disease. Paraneoplastic syndromes can be classified as endocrine (Table 61.1), neurologic (Table 61.2), dermatologic (Table 61.3), rheumatologic (Table 61.3), and hematologic (Table 61.4).

> ### Key Definition
>
> Paraneoplastic syndrome: *the presence of symptoms due to factors other than direct tumor invasion or compression.*

> ### Key Definition
>
> Dermatomyositis: *a polymyositis with heliotrope rash (on the upper eyelids), Gottron papules (on bony surfaces), erythematous rash (on the face, neck, chest, back, or shoulders), proximal muscle weakness, swallowing difficulty, respiratory difficulty, and muscle pain.*

Table 61.1 • Paraneoplastic Endocrine Syndromes

Syndrome	Clinical Presentation	Laboratory Findings	Associated Cancers
SIADH	Gait disturbances, falls, headache, nausea, fatigue, muscle cramps, anorexia, confusion, lethargy, seizures, respiratory depression, coma	Hyponatremia: mild, sodium 130–134 mmol/L; moderate, sodium 125–129 mmol/L; severe, sodium <125 mmol/L Increased urine osmolality (>100 mOsm/kg in the context of euvolemic hyponatremia)	SCLC, mesothelioma, bladder, ureteral, endometrial, prostate, oropharyngeal, thymoma, lymphoma, Ewing sarcoma, brain, GI, breast, adrenal
Hypercalcemia	Altered mental status, weakness, ataxia, lethargy, hypertonia, renal failure, nausea and vomiting, hypertension, bradycardia	Hypercalcemia: mild, calcium 10.5–11.9 mg/dL; moderate, calcium 12.0–13.9 mg/dL; severe, calcium ≥14.0 mg/dL Low to normal (<20 pg/mL) PTH level Elevated PTHrP level	Breast, multiple myeloma, renal cell, squamous cell (especially lung), lymphoma (including HTLV-associated lymphoma), ovarian, endometrial
Cushing syndrome	Muscle weakness, peripheral edema, hypertension, weight gain, centripetal fat distribution	Hypokalemia (usually potassium <3.0 mmol/L), elevated baseline serum cortisol (>29.0 mcg/dL), normal to elevated midnight serum ACTH (>100 pg/mL) not suppressed with dexamethasone	SCLC, bronchial carcinoid (neuroendocrine lung tumors account for about 50%-60% of cases of paraneoplastic Cushing syndrome), thymoma, medullary thyroid cancer, GI, pancreatic, adrenal, ovarian
Hypoglycemia	Sweating, anxiety, tremors, palpitations, hunger, weakness, seizures, confusion, coma	For non–islet cell tumor hypoglycemia: low glucose, low insulin (often <1.44–3.60 mcIU/mL), low C-peptide (often <0.3 ng/mL), elevated IGF-2:IGF-1 ratio (often >10:1) For insulinomas: low glucose, elevated insulin, elevated C-peptide, normal IGF-2:IGF-1 ratio	Mesothelioma, sarcomas, lung, GI

Abbreviations: ACTH, corticotropin; GI, gastrointestinal tract; HTLV, human T-lymphotropic virus; IGF, insulinlike growth factor; PTH, parathyroid hormone; PTHrP, parathyroid hormone–related protein; SCLC, small cell lung cancer; SIADH, syndrome of inappropriate secretion of antidiuretic hormone.

Adapted from Pelosof LC, Gerber DE. Paraneoplastic syndromes: an approach to diagnosis and treatment. Mayo Clin Proc. 2010 Sep;85(9):838–54. Erratum in: Mayo Clin Proc. 2011 Apr;86(4):364. Dosage error in article text. Used with permission of Mayo Foundation for Medical Education and Research.

Table 61.2 • Paraneoplastic Neurologic Syndromes

Syndrome	Clinical Presentation	Associated Antibodies	Diagnostic Studies	Associated Cancers
Limbic encephalitis (LE)	Mood changes, hallucinations, memory loss, seizures, and less commonly hypothalamic symptoms (hyperthermia, somnolence, endocrine dysfunction); onset over days to months	Anti-Hu (typically with SCLC) Anti-Ma2 (typically testicular cancer) Anti-CRMP5 (anti-CV2) Antiamphiphysin	EEG: epileptic foci in temporal lobe(s); focal or generalized slow activity FDG-PET: increased metabolism in temporal lobe(s) MRI: hyperintensity in medial temporal lobe(s) CSF analysis: pleocytosis, elevated protein, elevated IgG, oligoclonal bands	SCLC (about 40%-50% of LE patients), testicular germ cell (about 20% of LE patients), breast (about 8% of LE patients), thymoma, teratoma, Hodgkin lymphoma
Lambert-Eaton myasthenic syndrome (LEMS)	Lower-extremity proximal muscle weakness, fatigue, diaphragmatic weakness, bulbar symptoms (usually milder than in MG); later in course, autonomic symptoms (ptosis, impotence, dry mouth) in most patients	Anti-voltage-gated calcium channel (P/Q type)	EMG: low compound muscle action potential amplitude; decremental response with low-rate stimulation but incremental response with high-rate stimulation	SCLC (about 3% of patients have LEMS), prostate, cervical, lymphomas, adenocarcinomas
Myasthenia gravis (MG)	Fatigable weakness of voluntary muscles (ocular-bulbar and limb muscles), diaphragmatic weakness	Anti-acetylcholine receptor	EMG: decremental response to repetitive nerve stimulation	Thymoma (in about 15% of MG patients)

Abbreviations: CSF, cerebrospinal fluid; EEG, electroencephalography; EMG, electromyography; FDG, ^{18}F-fludeoxyglucose; Ig, immunoglobulin; MRI, magnetic resonance imaging; PET, positron emission tomography; SCLC, small cell lung cancer.

Adapted from Pelosof LC, Gerber DE. Paraneoplastic syndromes: an approach to diagnosis and treatment. Mayo Clin Proc. 2010 Sep;85(9):838–54. Erratum in: Mayo Clin Proc. 2011 Apr;86(4):364. Dosage error in article text. Used with permission of Mayo Foundation for Medical Education and Research.

Table 61.3 • Paraneoplastic Dermatologic and Rheumatologic Syndromes

Syndrome	Clinical Presentation	Diagnostic Studies and Laboratory Findings	Associated Cancers
Acanthosis nigricans	Velvety, hyperpigmented skin (usually on flexural regions); papillomatous changes involving mucous membranes and mucocutaneous junctions; rugose changes on palms and dorsal surface of large joints (eg, tripe palms)	Skin biopsy: histologic examination shows hyperkeratosis and papillomatosis	Adenocarcinoma of abdominal organs, especially gastric adenocarcinoma (about 90% of malignancies in patients with acanthosis nigricans are abdominal); gynecologic
Dermatomyositis (DM)	Heliotrope rash (violaceous, edematous rash on upper eyelids); Gottron papules (scaly papules on bony surfaces); erythematous rash (which may be photosensitive) on face, neck, chest, back, or shoulders (on shoulders, is known as *shawl sign*); proximal muscle weakness; swallowing difficulty; respiratory difficulty; muscle pain	Laboratory findings: elevated serum CK, AST, ALT, LDH, and aldolase EMG: increased spontaneous activity with fibrillations, complex repetitive discharges, and positive sharp waves Muscle biopsy: perivascular or interfascicular septal inflammation and perifascicular atrophy	Ovarian, breast, prostate, lung, colorectal, non-Hodgkin lymphoma, nasopharyngeal
Erythroderma	Erythematous, exfoliating, diffuse rash (often pruritic)	Skin biopsy: histologic examination shows dense perivascular lymphocytic infiltrate	Chronic lymphocytic leukemia, cutaneous T-cell lymphoma (including mycosis fungoides), GI (colorectal, gastric, esophageal, gallbladder), adult T-cell leukemia or lymphoma, myeloproliferative disorders
Hypertrophic osteoarthropathy	Subperiosteal new bone formation on phalangeal shafts ("clubbing"), synovial effusions (mainly large joints), pain, swelling along affected bones and joints	Plain radiography: periosteal reaction along long bones Nuclear bone scan: intense and symmetric uptake in long bones	Intrathoracic tumors, metastases to lung, metastases to bone, nasopharyngeal carcinoma, rhabdomyosarcoma
Leukocytoclastic vasculitis	Ulceration, cyanosis, and pain over affected regions (especially digits); palpable purpura, often over lower extremities; renal impairment; peripheral neuropathy	Skin biopsy: histologic examination shows fibrinoid necrosis, endothelial swelling, leukocytoclasis, and RBC extravasation	Leukemia or lymphoma, myelodysplastic syndromes, colon, lung, urologic, multiple myeloma, rhabdomyosarcoma
Paraneoplastic pemphigus (PNP)	Severe cutaneous blisters and erosions (predominantly on trunk, soles, and palms); severe mucosal erosions, including stomatitis	Serum antibodies to epithelia (against plakins and desmogleins) Skin biopsy: histologic examination shows keratinocyte necrosis, epidermal acantholysis, and IgG and complement deposition in epidermal and basement membrane zones	Non-Hodgkin lymphoma, chronic lymphocytic leukemia, thymoma, Castleman disease, follicular dendritic cell sarcoma
Polymyalgia rheumatica (PMR)	Limb girdle pain and stiffness	Laboratory findings: elevated serum ESR (often not as high as in nonparaneoplastic PMR) and CRP	Leukemia or lymphoma, myelodysplastic syndromes, colon, lung, renal, prostate, breast
Sweet syndrome (acute febrile neutrophilic dermatosis)	Acute onset of tender, erythematous nodules, papules, plaques, or pustules on extremities, face, or upper trunk; neutrophilia; fever; malaise	Skin biopsy: histologic examination shows a polymorphonuclear cell dermal infiltrate	Leukemia (especially AML), non-Hodgkin lymphoma, myelodysplastic syndromes, GU, breast, GI, multiple myeloma, gynecologic, testicular, melanoma

Abbreviations: ALT, alanine aminotransferase; AML, acute myeloid leukemia; AST, aspartate aminotransferase; CK, creatine kinase; CRP, C-reactive protein; EMG, electromyography; ESR, erythrocyte sedimentation rate; GI, gastrointestinal tract; GU, genitourinary tract; Ig, immunoglobulin; LDH, lactate dehydrogenase; RBC, red blood cell.

Adapted from Pelosof LC, Gerber DE. Paraneoplastic syndromes: an approach to diagnosis and treatment. Mayo Clin Proc. 2010 Sep;85(9):838–54. Erratum in: Mayo Clin Proc. 2011 Apr;86(4):364. Dosage error in article text. Used with permission of Mayo Foundation for Medical Education and Research.

Table 61.4 • Paraneoplastic Hematologic Syndromes

Syndrome	Clinical Presentation	Laboratory Findings	Associated Cancers
Eosinophilia	Dyspnea, wheezing	Hypereosinophilia (>0.5×10^9/L); elevated serum IL-2, IL-3, IL-5, and GM-CSF	Hodgkin lymphoma, non-Hodgkin lymphoma (B- and T-cell), chronic myeloid leukemia, acute lymphocytic leukemia, lung, thyroid, GI (pancreatic, colon, gastric, liver) renal, breast, gynecologic
Granulocytosis	Asymptomatic (no symptoms or signs of leukostasis, such as neurologic deficits or dyspnea)	Granulocyte (neutrophil) count >8×10^9/L, typically without a shift to immature neutrophil forms; elevated LAP; elevated serum G-CSF	GI, lung, breast, gynecologic, GU, brain, Hodgkin lymphoma, sarcomas
Pure red cell aplasia	Dyspnea, pallor, fatigue, syncope	Anemia (hematocrit <20% not uncommon), low or absent reticulocytes, bone marrow with nearly absent erythroid precursors, platelet and white blood cell counts in reference ranges	Thymoma, leukemia or lymphoma, myelodysplastic syndrome
Thrombocytosis	Asymptomatic (no bleeding or clotting abnormalities)	Elevated platelet count (about 400×10^9/L or more); elevated serum IL-6	GI, lung, breast, gynecologic, lymphoma, renal cell, prostate, mesothelioma, glioblastoma, head and neck

Abbreviations: G-CSF, granulocyte colon-stimulating factor; GI, gastrointestinal tract; GM-CSF, granulocyte-macrophage colony-stimulating factor; GU, genitourinary tract; IL, interleukin; LAP, leukocyte alkaline phosphatase.

Adapted from Pelosof LC, Gerber DE. Paraneoplastic syndromes: an approach to diagnosis and treatment. Mayo Clin Proc. 2010 Sep;85(9):838–54. Erratum in: Mayo Clin Proc. 2011 Apr;86(4):364. Dosage error in article text. Used with permission of Mayo Foundation for Medical Education and Research.

Key Definition

Sweet syndrome (acute febrile neutrophilic dermatosis): *a neutrophilic skin disease with an acute onset that is characterized by tender, erythematous nodules, papules, plaques, or pustules on the extremities, face, or upper trunk; neutrophilia; fever; and malaise.*

KEY FACTS

✓ CUP—2%-6% of all invasive malignancies
✓ Syndrome of inappropriate secretion of antidiuretic hormone (SIADH)—
  • gait disturbances, muscle cramps, falls
  • headache, nausea, anorexia
  • lethargy, fatigue
  • confusion, seizures, respiratory depression, coma
  • hyponatremia
  • increased urine osmolality
✓ SIADH-associated cancers—
  • small cell lung cancer, mesothelioma
  • bladder, ureteral, endometrial, prostate
  • oropharyngeal, gastrointestinal tract
  • thymoma, adrenal
  • Ewing sarcoma
  • brain, breast
✓ Lambert-Eaton myasthenic syndrome (LEMS)—
  • proximal muscle weakness of lower extremities
  • fatigue
  • diaphragmatic weakness
  • bulbar symptoms (milder than in myasthenia gravis)
  • later, autonomic symptoms (ptosis, impotence, dry mouth)
✓ LEMS-associated cancers—
  • small cell lung cancer
  • prostate, cervical
  • lymphomas, adenocarcinomas
✓ Myasthenia gravis—
  • fatigable weakness of voluntary muscles (especially ocular-bulbar and limb muscles), diaphragmatic weakness
  • associated with thymoma in 15% of patients with myasthenia gravis

KEY FACTS

✓ Dermatomyositis-associated cancers—
  • ovarian, breast, prostate
  • lung
  • colorectal
  • non-Hodgkin lymphoma
  • nasopharyngeal
✓ Polymyalgia rheumatica (PMR)—limb girdle pain and stiffness
✓ PMR-associated cancers—
  • leukemia or lymphoma, myelodysplastic syndromes
  • colon, lung, renal
  • prostate, breast
✓ Sweet syndrome–associated cancers—
  • leukemia, non-Hodgkin lymphoma, myelodysplastic syndromes, multiple myeloma
  • genitourinary tract, gynecologic, testicular
  • breast
  • gastrointestinal tract
  • melanoma

62 Gynecologic Cancers: Cervical, Uterine, and Ovarian Cancers

ANDREA E. WAHNER HENDRICKSON, MD

Cervical Cancer

Background

Globally, **cervical cancer** is the second most common type of cancer and the second leading cause of cancer death among women. The incidence varies geographically because of differences in the availability of screening programs and access to them. For example, in Africa, cervical cancer is the leading cause of cancer deaths among women, but in the United States, where screening is more prevalent, cervical cancer is not among the top 10 causes of cancer deaths. In recent decades, the incidence of cervical cancer, as well as the mortality associated with the disease, has markedly decreased. These changes have been attributed to widespread use of cytologic smear screening with the Papanicolaou test (ie, Pap smear).

Risk Factors

Nearly all cervical cancer cases (99%) are associated with persistent human papillomavirus (HPV) infection. Persistent infection with the oncogenic HPV types 16, 18, 33, 35, and 39 (Table 62.1) is the etiologic factor for development of the 2 most common types of cervical cancer (squamous cell carcinoma, which accounts for 75%, and adenocarcinoma, which accounts for 20%–24% of cases). Accordingly, risk factors for cervical cancer include factors related to HPV exposure: first intercourse at an early age, a greater number of sexual partners, and a history of sexually transmitted disease. Smoking and chronic immunosuppression (such as in patients infected with human immunodeficiency virus) increase the risk of persistent HPV infection and are therefore linked to cervical cancer pathogenesis.

Three vaccines against HPV infection have been approved by the US Food and Drug Administration (FDA) for female patients aged 9 through 26 years (Table 62.2). The quadrivalent vaccine protects against the 2 most common oncogenic strains (HPV types 16 and 18) as well as 2 strains that are common causes of genital warts. The quadrivalent vaccine has also been FDA approved for the prevention of genital warts and anal cancer in young men and women. The 9-valent vaccine protects against HPV types 16 and 18 as well, but it also protects against HPV types 31, 33, 45, 52, and 58, which account for approximately 20% of cervical cancer cases. It is important to remember that even after a patient has been vaccinated, cervical cancer screening is still required because the vaccine does not include all oncogenic strains of the virus. (See Chapter 34, "Preventive Medicine," for specific screening recommendations.)

Table 62.1 • Steps in Cervical Cancer Development

Step	Comments
1. Infection of the cervical epithelium with an oncogenic strain of HPV	HPV types 16, 18, 33, 35, and 39 confer the greatest risk HPV types 16 and 18 are found in >70% of cervical cancers
2. Persistence of HPV infection	75%–80% of sexually active adults contract HPV Most infections are transient
3. Progression from persistent viral infection to precancerous lesion	Persistent infection can lead to development of high-grade cervical intraepithelial neoplasia
4. Development of a carcinoma	Cervical cancer develops in <1% of women infected with HPV

Abbreviation: HPV, human papillomavirus.

Table 62.2 • HPV Vaccines

Feature	Gardasil 9[a]	Gardasil[a]	Cervarix[b]
HPV strains	9-valent (HPV 16, 18, 31, 33, 45, 52, 58)	Quadrivalent (HPV 6, 11, 16, and 18)	Bivalent (HPV 16 and 18)
Year of initial FDA approval	2015	2006[c]	2009
Administration schedule	3 injections over 6 mo (at 0, 2, and 6 mo)	3 injections over 6 mo (at 0, 2, and 6 mo)	3 injections over 6 mo (at 0, 1, and 6 mo)

Abbreviations: FDA, US Food and Drug Administration; HPV, human papillomavirus.

[a] Merck and Co, Inc.

[b] GlaxoSmithKline Biologicals SA.

[c] Subsequently, the FDA approved the vaccine for prevention of vulvar and vaginal cancer in females as well as genital warts and anal cancer in males and females.

Clinical Presentation

With most precursor lesions to cervical cancer, patients are asymptomatic. Patients with early cervical cancer can also be asymptomatic, or they may present with abnormal vaginal bleeding, vaginal discharge, or dyspareunia. Patients with late-stage disease may present with pelvic pain, leg pain, back pain, rectal bleeding, and symptoms associated with local spread of the disease. Physical examination findings may include abnormal cervical epithelium that has a white discoloration after application of acetic acid (Figure 62.1); friable tissue, induration, or an exophytic mass on the cervix; or condylomata acuminata (Figure 62.2).

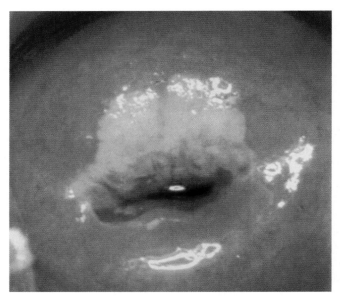

***Figure* 62.1** *Acetowhite Epithelium of the Anterior Lip of the Cervix. Cervical intraepithelial neoplasia, grade 2, was identified on biopsy.*

(Adapted from Massad LS. High-grade squamous intraepithelial lesions. In: Apgar BS, Brotzman GL, Spitzer M, editors. Colposcopy: principles and practice: an integrated textbook and atlas [ebook]. 2nd ed. Philadelphia [PA]: Saunders/Elsevier; c2008. Used with permission.)

Prognosis

Patients with early-stage cervical cancer (stage IA—microscopic tumor) have a good prognosis, with a 5-year overall survival of approximately 93%, whereas patients with stage IV disease have a poor prognosis, with a 5-year overall survival of approximately 15%.

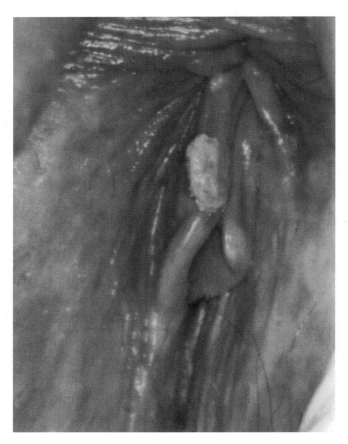

***Figure* 62.2** *Condyloma of the Labia Minora.*

(Adapted from Atlas of external genital condyloma. In: Apgar BS, Brotzman GL, Spitzer M, editors. Colposcopy: principles and practice: an integrated textbook and atlas. Philadelphia [PA]: W. B. Saunders Company; c2002. p. 380–82. Used with permission.)

Treatment

Treatment of a high-grade squamous intraepithelial lesion consists of removal of the affected area with a loop electro-surgical excision procedure (LEEP), cone biopsy, or cryo-surgery. If other symptoms are present (eg, menorrhagia), hysterectomy can be performed. Treatment of invasive cervical cancer depends on the stage, which is determined clinically because of the limited availability of imaging worldwide. In early-stage disease, when the tumor is small (≤4 cm) and confined to the cervix, treatment includes a hysterectomy and possible radiotherapy. For very small (<2 cm) early-stage tumors in women who desire fertility preservation, trachelectomy (removal of the cervix with preservation of the uterus, including the lower uterine segment) with lymphadenectomy can be considered. If the tumor is larger (>4 cm) or involves the surrounding tissues, treatment consists of concurrent chemoradiotherapy and brachytherapy. For distant metastases, the mainstay of therapy is chemotherapy with localized radiotherapy as needed for symptom control.

KEY FACTS

- ✓ Most common types of cervical cancer—squamous cell carcinoma (75% of cases) and adenocarcinoma (20%–24% of cases)
- ✓ Cause of most cervical cancer—persistent infection with HPV types 16 and 18
- ✓ Treatment of cervical cancer—
  - surgery for small tumors
  - chemotherapy and radiotherapy for large tumors
  - removal of affected area with LEEP, cone biopsy, or cryosurgery for high-grade squamous intraepithelial lesion
  - varies for invasive cancer (according to the clinically determined stage)
- ✓ Prevention of cervical cancer—
  - bivalent, quadrivalent, and 9-valent vaccines
  - cervical cancer screening is still required for women who have received the vaccine

---

Uterine Cancer

Background

Uterine cancers are the most common type of gynecologic malignancy in developed countries. Most of these tumors arise from the endometrium, with endometrioid adeno-carcinoma accounting for 90% of uterine cancers, and are referred to as endometrial cancer. Overall, endometrial cancer carries a more favorable prognosis than other types of cancer, and so despite it being the most prevalent type of gynecologic malignancy in the United States, it is not among the top 5 causes of cancer death among US women.

Box 62.1 • Risk Factors Related to Endometrial Cancer

Unopposed estrogen
Tamoxifen therapy
Obesity
Diabetes mellitus
Advanced age
Polycystic ovarian syndrome
Nulliparity
Late menopause

Risk Factors

The majority of endometrial cancers (ie, the type I or endometrioid subtype) are thought to be due, in part, to estrogen excess (long-term, unopposed estrogen exposure). Risk factors for endometrial cancer are listed in Box 62.1. Approximately 10% of patients with endometrial cancer have a genetic predisposition to endometrial cancer. Women with Lynch syndrome have a 40% to 60% lifetime risk of endometrial cancer (Table 62.3). In these women, risk-reducing total hysterectomy is considered after completion of childbearing. Before hysterectomy, or if a woman decides not to have a hysterectomy, the recommended screening is an annual endometrial biopsy starting at age 30 to 35 years or at 5 to 10 years before the earliest age at diagnosis of a Lynch syndrome–related malignancy in the woman's family. The less common histologic subtypes of endometrial cancer, termed type II endometrial cancers, carry a less favorable prognosis and do not seem to depend on estrogen exposure (Table 62.4).

Clinical Presentation

The most common presenting symptom in women with endometrial cancer is abnormal uterine bleeding. The average age of women who have endometrial cancer is 61 years,

---

Table 62.3 • Main Genetic Syndromes and Endometrial Cancer Risk

Syndrome	Associated Malignancies	Lifetime Risk of Endometrial Cancer, %
Lynch syndrome (hereditary nonpolyposis colorectal cancer)	Colorectal and endometrial (also ovarian, gastrointestinal tract, pancreas, hepatobiliary, urologic, and sebaceous)	40–60
Cowden syndrome	Most commonly breast, thyroid, and endometrial	13–19

Table 62.4 • Classification of Endometrial Cancer

Type	Histology	Comment
I	Grades 1 and 2 endometrioid	80% of all endometrial cancers Preceded by an intraepithelial precursor lesion (atypical or complex endometrial hyperplasia) Better prognosis than with type II
II	Grade 3 endometrioid *or* Clear cell, mucinous, squamous, transitional, or undifferentiated	Not clearly associated with estrogen stimulation Often no precursor lesion Higher grade and worse prognosis than with type I

so the uterine bleeding most associated with endometrial cancer is post menopausal. However, abnormal uterine bleeding in women older than 35 years who have atypical glandular cells on a Pap smear should be investigated with an endometrial biopsy to rule out endometrial cancer. Pelvic ultrasonography most often shows a thickened endometrial stripe. Although most cases of postmenopausal bleeding are not endometrial cancer, this must be ruled out. As noted in Box 62.1, tamoxifen therapy has been associated with an increased risk of endometrial cancer. Therefore, postmenopausal women receiving tamoxifen therapy should have an annual gynecologic examination, and they should be monitored and counseled about symptoms of endometrial hyperplasia or cancer. Any abnormal vaginal or uterine symptoms in these patients should be addressed quickly.

Prognosis

Patients who have type I endometrial cancers usually present with abnormal uterine bleeding early in the course of the disease, so those tumors are most often detected early, and the 5-year survival rate for stage I disease is 80% to 90%. Stage IV disease portends a poor prognosis, with 5-year survival rates between 20% and 30%.

Treatment

Surgery is the mainstay of treatment of early-stage disease. With early detection, a total hysterectomy is the treatment of choice, and no adjuvant therapy is required. In more advanced cases, the addition of radiotherapy or chemotherapy (or both) is considered, depending on factors such as tumor grade, size, depth of invasion, and involvement of the lower uterine segment. In recurrent cases, type I tumors can often be treated with endocrine therapy (eg, megestrol acetate).

KEY FACTS

- ✓ Uterine cancer—most (90%) are endometrioid adenocarcinoma (ie, type I endometrial cancer)
- ✓ Endometrial cancer—
  - most are linked to estrogen excess
  - most common presenting symptom is postmenopausal bleeding (but most cases of postmenopausal bleeding are not from endometrial cancer)
  - pelvic ultrasonography shows thickened endometrial stripe
- ✓ Uterine bleeding in a patient receiving tamoxifen must be evaluated

Epithelial Ovarian Cancer

Background

Epithelial ovarian cancer (EOC) is the most lethal of the gynecologic malignancies and is the fifth leading cause of cancer deaths among US women. EOC does not include germ cell tumors or stromal tumors, which are rare. Primary peritoneal and fallopian tube cancers are pathologically similar to EOC and have the same risk factors, interventions, and prognosis. This group of cancers develops primarily in older women (average age at onset, 61 years). It can occur in younger women, but those cases are most likely hereditary.

Risk Factors

Several risk factors are associated with the development of EOC (Box 62.2). In general, conditions that lead to an increased number of ovulatory cycles are thought to increase the risk of EOC; conversely, factors that decrease the number of ovulatory cycles are thought to decrease the risk of EOC. Use of oral contraceptives for more than 5 years

Box 62.2 • Risk Factors Associated With Ovarian Cancer

Increased risk

    Early menarche
    Infertility
    Late menarche
    Family history

Decreased risk

    Oral contraceptive use
    Pregnancy
    Early pregnancy
    Breastfeeding >1 y

Table 62.5 • Main Genetic Syndromes Related to Epithelial Ovarian Cancer

Syndrome	Genetic Changes	Lifetime Risk of Epithelial Ovarian Cancer[a], %
Hereditary breast and ovarian syndrome	*BRCA1* *BRCA2*	14–45 10–20
Lynch syndrome (hereditary nonpolyposis colorectal cancer)	DNA mismatch repair (MMR) genes *MSH2, MLH1, MSH6, PMS1,* and *PMS2*	3–14

[a] Lifetime risk of epithelial ovarian cancer for women in the general population is 1.5%.

can reduce the risk by approximately 50% (30%–60% depending on duration of use). Currently, no screening tests are recommended because no available test (including cancer antigen 125 [CA 125]) has sufficient specificity, sensitivity, or cost-effectiveness to be recommended for the general population. Approximately 85% of EOCs express CA 125, which is released into the circulation. However, it is detectable in only 50% of patients with stage I disease. The highest serum levels of CA 125 are found in patients with EOC, but the serum CA 125 level may be increased in other malignancies and in pregnancy, endometriosis, and menstruation.

The risk of EOC increases if EOC develops in even 1 first-degree relative at any age. Additionally, several genetic syndromes increase the risk of EOC, accounting for approximately 10% of cases of EOC (Table 62.5).

In women who are at high risk for EOC due to genetic predisposition (*BRCA1* or *BRCA2*), the National Institutes of Health Consensus Conference panel of experts recommends pelvic examinations, CA 125 measurements, and pelvic ultrasonography every 6 to 12 months, beginning at age 35 years or at the age that is 5 to 10 years before the first diagnosis in the family. There is no conclusive evidence that this screening affects survival.

In women with *BRCA1* or *BRCA2* mutations, prophylactic bilateral salpingo-oophorectomy is recommended at age 35 years or after completion of childbearing. Although the risk reduction (approximately 90%), is large, these women are still at risk for primary peritoneal carcinoma. The procedure also decreases the risk of breast cancer by approximately 50% in this high-risk population. (See Chapter 60, "Breast Cancer," for details about risk factors for breast cancer.)

Clinical Presentation

Although women may have symptoms secondary to EOC, these symptoms are often overlooked and nonspecific, and

they often are not present until the cancer is quite large or has spread beyond the ovary or fallopian tube. Most women present with gastrointestinal tract complaints, such as bloating, nausea, changes in bowel or bladder habits, and abdominopelvic pain, and approximately 75% of them receive a diagnosis of advanced disease (ie, the disease has spread beyond the pelvis). Occasionally, a patient presents with a pleural effusion (stage IV disease), and further workup will identify ovarian or primary peritoneal cancer.

Prognosis

The prognosis for patients with EOC depends heavily on the stage at diagnosis (Table 62.6). If the disease can be detected at an early stage when the tumor has not spread beyond the inside of the ovary, overall survival is very good. Conversely, if disease is diagnosed when it is advanced, overall 5-year survival is poor. Because of the lack of screening tests, about 75% of cases are detected in an advanced stage (stage III or IV), accounting for an overall 5-year survival for all stages of only 44%.

Treatment

The initial management of patients with EOC includes thorough surgical staging and debulking, if possible. Outcome depends in part on the amount of tumor tissue remaining after the initial staging and debulking. Patients with only microscopic residual disease at the end of the surgical procedure fare better than those with visible disease remaining. The goal is to achieve optimal surgical cytoreduction, which is defined as the patient having no remaining tumor nodule 1 cm or larger after completion of surgery. This cytoreductive surgery should be performed by a gynecologic oncologist to

Table 62.6 • Epithelial Ovarian Cancer Prognosis by Stage

Stage	General Description	5-Year Survival, %
I	Tumor confined to the ovaries	>90 (grade 1; tumor not on surface of ovary) 75–80 (grade 3; clear cell histology; tumor on surface of ovary)
II	Tumor extends into the pelvis	60–70
III	Disease outside the pelvis (peritoneal metastases)	25–40
IV	Distant metastases, including intraparenchymal liver metastases or disease above the diaphragm	10–20

achieve optimal debulking rates. Subsequently, patients receive chemotherapy based on platinum (cisplatin or carboplatin) and taxane (usually paclitaxel). If the disease is not amenable to surgical resection at the time of diagnosis, a few cycles of chemotherapy are given as neoadjuvant chemotherapy before the surgery in an attempt to decrease the tumor burden, decrease the surgical complexity, and increase the chances for an optimal cytoreductive procedure. After an interval debulking surgery, additional chemotherapy is given (as adjuvant chemotherapy).

When EOC is confined to the abdomen, intraperitoneal chemotherapy has been shown to be effective. However, it is more difficult to tolerate and has a higher complication rate. Therefore, it is considered only in a subset of women who are otherwise healthy, have a good performance status, and have minimal to no residual disease after the initial surgical procedure.

In most patients, the tumors respond to the initial therapy, but in the majority of those patients, the tumor recurs. If it recurs within 6 months after the initial chemotherapy, the cancer is termed **platinum resistant** and, in general, single-agent chemotherapy is used, with a response rate of 15% to 25%. If the tumor does not recur within 6 months, the tumor is deemed **platinum sensitive**, and at the time of recurrence, a platinum doublet is again used. If the tumor has recurred, the treatment is palliative.

KEY FACTS

✓ Ovarian cancer—
- no screening tests are available for the general population
- mortality is high because most cases are detected at an advanced stage

✓ Treatment of EOC—
- thorough surgical staging and debulking
- most patients also need chemotherapy (unless EOC is confined to the inside of the ovary) with platinum-taxane doublet

✓ Recommendation for women with *BRCA1* or *BRCA2* mutations—prophylactic bilateral salpingo-oophorectomy at age 35 years or after completion of childbearing

---

Key Definitions

Platinum resistant: *descriptor for ovarian cancer that recurs within 6 months after completion of initial chemotherapy.*

Platinum sensitive: *descriptor for ovarian cancer that does not recur within 6 months after completion of initial chemotherapy.*

63 Colorectal Cancer

JOLEEN M. HUBBARD, MD

Background

Colorectal cancer is diagnosed in approximately 137,000 Americans annually and causes 50,000 deaths each year. It is the third most common cause of cancer death in North America and Europe. The incidence of colorectal cancer has decreased since the early 2000s, after it peaked in the late 1990s. The decrease in colon cancer incidence and mortality is attributed to improved screening methods, consisting mainly of endoscopic surveillance. Screening colonoscopies should be initiated by age 50 years for persons with average risk. Screening may be initiated at a younger age for high-risk patients, such as those with a family history of colorectal cancer, an inherited familial colon cancer syndrome, or inflammatory bowel disease.

Risk Factors

Approximately 10% of colorectal cancer is related to familial syndromes that have been defined or are still undefined. High-risk groups include the following: 1) persons with familial polyposis syndromes (ie, familial adenomatous polyposis [for which a gene has been identified on chromosome 5] and **Gardner syndrome** [gut polyps in combination with desmoid tumors, lipomas, sebaceous cysts, and other abnormalities]), accounting for 1% of colorectal cancer; 2) persons with familial cancer syndromes without polyps (ie, **hereditary nonpolyposis colorectal cancer** [also called **Lynch syndrome**], which is marked by colon cancer with or without endometrial, breast, and other cancers), accounting for 3% to 4% of colorectal cancer; and 3) persons with inflammatory bowel disease (incidence of colorectal cancer, 12% after 25 years).

> **Key Definition**
>
> Gardner syndrome: *a familial polyposis syndrome with gut polyps in combination with desmoid tumors, lipomas, sebaceous cysts, and other abnormalities.*

> **Key Definition**
>
> Hereditary nonpolyposis colorectal cancer (Lynch syndrome): *a familial cancer syndrome without polyps that is marked by colon cancer with or without endometrial, breast, and other cancers.*

The majority of colorectal cancer cases are sporadic, lacking the aforementioned risk factors. Diet and lifestyle are becoming increasingly recognized as risk factors for colorectal cancer. High-fat and low-fiber diets, decreased levels of physical activity, and obesity are all associated with an increased risk of colorectal cancer.

Treatment

Surgery

Surgical resection is the preferred curative treatment of carcinomas of the colon or rectum. Surgical exploration and resection allow for pathologic determination of tumor depth of penetration through the bowel wall and assessment of regional lymph nodes. Prognosis is directly related to the stage of disease (Table 63.1). Five-year survival rates for locoregional disease have improved in recent decades as a result of many factors, including improvements in preoperative staging, surgical technique, adequate lymph

Table 63.1 • Staging of Colorectal Cancer and Survival

AJCC Stage	Depth of Penetration	Lymph Node Status	5-Year Survival, %
I	Submucosa or muscularis	Negative	97
II	Through muscularis or to other organs	Negative	
IIA			86
IIB			80
IIC			58
III	Any	Positive	
IIIA			79–90
IIIB			53–74
IIIC			15–40

Abbreviation: AJCC, American Joint Committee on Cancer.

Data from Edge SB, Byrd DR, Compton CC, Fritz AG, Greene FL, Trotti A 3rd, editors. AJCC cancer staging manual. 7th ed. New York (NY): Springer; c2010. p. 148.

node retrieval, and the use of neoadjuvant (preoperative) and adjuvant (postoperative) therapy.

Adjuvant Therapy

The recommendation for node-positive (stage III) colon cancer is to administer adjuvant chemotherapy with a multidrug regimen that includes oxaliplatin and a fluoropyrimidine (5-fluorouracil or capecitabine) for 6 months. Controversy exists about standard recommendations for deeply invasive but lymph-node negative (stage II) colon carcinomas. Adjuvant chemotherapy is recommended for patients who have high-risk stage II disease and any of the following characteristics: perforation or obstruction, tumor penetrating the visceral peritoneum or adherent to other structures, or less than 10 lymph nodes identified in the surgical specimen. For rectal cancer, a combination of fluoropyrimidine-based chemotherapy and pelvic radiotherapy, preferably administered preoperatively (as neoadjuvant therapy), is standard for stage II and III disease. Postoperative chemotherapy is the same as that recommended for colon cancer.

Metastatic Disease

Certain patients with oligometastatic colorectal cancer in the lung or liver (or both) may be candidates for an attempt at curative resection of the metastatic disease. Of carefully selected patients with minimal metastatic disease, 30% to 40% survive beyond 5 years (many without further evidence of disease recurrence) after resection of metastatic lesions and systemic chemotherapy.

Palliative chemotherapy is the only option for most patients with advanced metastatic colorectal cancer. The median duration of survival is 29 months when patients are given medical therapy and are exposed to all active treatments of this disease.

Doublet cytotoxic chemotherapy regimens (a fluoropyrimidine in combination with oxaliplatin or irinotecan) administered with a biologic agent (bevacizumab, cetuximab, or panitumumab) are the standard of care for first- and second-line treatment of metastatic colorectal cancer. Like other platinum agents, oxaliplatin can cause peripheral neuropathy, and it causes the unique adverse effect of acute sensory neuropathy for cold, which resolves several days after completion of treatment. Irinotecan (a topoisomerase inhibitor) and the fluoropyrimidines are associated with adverse effects that include diarrhea, nausea, vomiting, and cytopenias.

Bevacizumab is a monoclonal antibody targeting the vascular endothelial growth factor (VEGF) ligand that improves survival when combined with cytotoxic chemotherapy. Common adverse effects of bevacizumab include hypertension, epistaxis, proteinuria, and a rare incidence of thrombosis. Bevacizumab should not be administered within 8 weeks before a surgical procedure because of the risk of delayed wound healing and gastrointestinal tract perforation.

Cetuximab and panitumumab are monoclonal antibodies that target the endothelial growth factor receptor (EGFR) and improve survival outcomes when used alone or in combination with cytotoxic chemotherapy. These EGFR inhibitors cause the characteristic adverse effect of an acneiform rash that may be ameliorated with tetracycline and corticosteroid creams. Patients who have tumors with a mutation involving RAS, a protein in the signaling transduction cascade downstream from the EGFR, are not eligible for treatment with either of the EGFR inhibitors.

Regorafenib is an oral multikinase inhibitor recently approved for third-line therapy for metastatic colorectal cancer. Common adverse effects of regorafenib include diarrhea, palmar-plantar erythrodysesthesia, hypertension, and fatigue.

Surveillance After Curative Resection

Current American Society of Clinical Oncology guidelines recommend that the carcinoembryonic antigen (CEA) level be checked preoperatively. After curative treatment of colon cancer in patients with stage II or III disease, the guidelines recommend that the CEA level be checked every 3 to 6 months for 2 years and then every 6 months for a total of 5 years if the patient's general medical condition would allow the patient to be a candidate for surgical intervention or chemotherapy. Monitoring of CEA may also be useful for determining the response of metastatic disease to therapy.

Computed tomography of the abdomen and pelvis, as well as chest imaging, should be performed every 6 to

12 months for the first 3 years after diagnosis and then yearly through the fifth year. Patients must receive adequate endoscopic surveillance for colon cancer recurrence. This surveillance should be performed at 1 and 4 years after surgery and every 5 years thereafter. If a patient's entire colon could not be endoscopically visualized before surgery, a colonoscopy should be performed within 6 months after surgery to assess for a synchronous colon cancer.

KEY FACTS

✓ Screening colonoscopy—begin at age 50 years for persons with average risk for colorectal cancer

✓ Surgical resection—curative treatment of carcinomas of the colon or rectum

✓ Adjuvant chemotherapy—
- recommended for node-positive (stage III) colon cancer
- multidrug regimen (oxaliplatin and either 5-fluorouracil or capecitabine) for 6 months

✓ Oligometastatic colorectal cancer in the lung or liver (or both)—certain patients may be candidates for an attempt at curative resection

✓ CEA levels for surveillance—
- Check CEA preoperatively
- Check CEA every 3–6 months for the first 2 years after curative treatment of colon cancer
- Then check CEA every 6 months for a total of 5 years (if patient is still a candidate for surgical intervention or chemotherapy)

✓ Imaging for surveillance for colon cancer recurrence—
- computed tomography of the abdomen and pelvis *and* chest imaging every 6–12 months for 3 years after diagnosis and then yearly through the fifth year
- endoscopy at 1 and 4 years after surgery and then every 5 years

64

Genitourinary Cancer

BRIAN A. COSTELLO, MD, MS

Prostate Cancer

Background

Approximately 233,000 new cases of prostate cancer occur annually in the United States. It is the most common cancer in US men and is the second leading cause of death from cancer in US men (29,000 deaths annually). Risk factors for prostate cancer include older age, race (African American), family history (first-degree relative), and possibly dietary fat. The lifetime probability of prostate cancer developing in a man is 1 in 6.

Prostate-Specific Antigen

The use of prostate-specific antigen (PSA) for prostate cancer screening is controversial. PSA is produced by normal and neoplastic prostatic ductal epithelium. Its concentration is proportional to the total prostatic mass. The inability to differentiate benign prostatic hyperplasia from carcinoma on the basis of the PSA level renders it inadequate as the sole screening method for prostate cancer. However, PSA is useful for monitoring response to therapy in cases of known prostate cancer, particularly after radical prostatectomy, when PSA should be undetectable.

Prognostic factors for prostate cancer include stage of disease, grade of tumor, and pretreatment PSA level. Box 64.1 shows the TNM classification for the staging of prostate cancer. The Gleason scoring system is used for pathologic grading of tumors. The surgical specimen is graded by adding the grade (1–5) of the predominant pattern of differentiation to the grade (1–5) of the secondary architectural pattern (eg, 3+5=8). Gleason grades 2 through 6 are associated with a better prognosis than Gleason grades of 8 or more. Retrospective results indicate that the pretreatment PSA value is a strong predictor of disease outcome after operation or radiotherapy.

Management

Management of Specific Stages

Prostate cancer is a disease of older men, so comorbid conditions, patient age, and performance status need to be considered when selecting a therapy because more men will die *with* prostate cancer than *of* prostate cancer. In general, patients with T1A prostate tumors are observed without treatment. For organ-confined prostate cancer (T1B, T1C, and T2 tumors), radiotherapy and radical prostatectomy are equally viable options. For T3 or T4 disease (locally advanced), radiotherapy is generally used. For N1 disease (positive pelvic nodes), the management is varied. Divergent approaches include androgen deprivation alone, radiotherapy with or without androgen deprivation, close observation with androgen deprivation at progression, or, infrequently, prostatectomy with androgen deprivation.

Prostatectomy

Prostatectomy is reserved for patients with localized disease. The 15-year disease-specific survival rate after

---

Box 64.1 • TNM Staging System for Prostate Cancer

T1A: incidental focus of tumor in ≤5% of resected tissue

T1B: incidental tumor in >5% of resected tissue

T1C: tumor identified by needle biopsy (performed on basis of increased PSA value)

T2A: tumor ≤50% of 1 lobe

T2B: tumor >50% of 1 lobe but not both lobes

T2C: tumor involvement of both lobes

T3, T4: extracapsular local disease or local invasion

N1: pelvic node involvement

M1: distant disease

Abbreviation: PSA, prostate-specific antigen.

---

prostatectomy is 85% to 90% among these patients. Nerve-sparing prostatectomy preserves sexual potency in 68% to 86% of patients. Risk of impotence increases with increasing age, size of tumor, extent of spread, and preoperative sexual function. Total urinary incontinence is rare (<2% of patients), although many men have some degree of incontinence after prostatectomy.

Radiotherapy

External beam radiotherapy is considered the equivalent of prostatectomy for overall survival. It is preferred for T3 or T4 disease at most centers. Impotence occurs less often than with prostatectomy. Chronic radiation proctitis is not uncommon.

Patients with organ-confined prostate cancer may also be candidates for **brachytherapy**. In this procedure, hundreds of radioactive seeds are placed in the prostate gland through a transrectal approach. This treatment works as well as external beam radiotherapy in appropriately selected patients and is less likely to cause radiation proctitis or impotence, but brachytherapy is less likely to adequately treat patients with extraprostatic spread of disease. Brachytherapy also requires fewer treatments and thus is often attractive to patients who live a long distance from the radiotherapy center.

> ### Key Definition
>
> Brachytherapy: *radiotherapy with the radiation source located near the target; for prostate cancer, many radioactive seeds are placed in the prostate gland through a transrectal approach.*

Androgen Deprivation Therapy

In patients with metastatic (M1) disease, bone is the most frequent site of metastatic disease. Although androgen deprivation therapy (ADT), also known as hormonal therapy, is effective and produces a response in most patients, it is noncurative. The average duration of response to initial hormonal therapy is 18 to 24 months. The average duration of survival is approximately 5 years after diagnosis of metastatic disease.

The sources of androgens in men are the testes (testosterone, 95%) and the adrenal glands (5%). ADT can be accomplished surgically (with orchiectomy) or medically. Potential agents include luteinizing hormone–releasing hormone agonists such as leuprolide, buserelin, and goserelin. They decrease androgen levels through continuous binding of the luteinizing hormone–releasing hormone receptor and subsequent decrease of luteinizing hormone and thus testosterone. They are administered as a depot injection every 1 to 6 months, depending on dosing. ADT can be associated with adverse effects, including decreased libido,

impotence, gynecomastia, osteoporosis, irritability, weight gain (and metabolic syndrome), and an increased risk of myocardial infarction.

Chemotherapy

Previously, prostate cancer was considered refractory to most chemotherapy regimens. Approved by the US Food and Drug Administration (FDA) in 2004, docetaxel in combination with prednisone has resulted in not only considerable responses but also improved survival among men with metastatic, hormone-refractory prostate cancer. More recently, docetaxel has been shown to improve survival for some men when given earlier during metastasis, in the so-called hormone-sensitive phase. Cabazitaxel, which is a novel chemotherapeutic agent, has been approved for use after docetaxel.

Prevention of Skeletal-Related Events

Development of painful and debilitating fractures is a common morbidity in men with bone metastases from prostate cancer. Bisphosphonates and the more recently approved receptor activator of nuclear factor κB (RANK) ligand inhibitors, such as denosumab, reduce the risk of skeletal-related events. Thus far, these agents have been shown to be beneficial only in metastatic castrate-resistant adenocarcinoma of the prostate and not in the metastatic hormone-sensitive state. Although they reduce the morbidity of skeletal-related events, these agents do not improve overall survival.

Novel Therapies for Metastatic Castrate-Resistant Prostate Cancer

In recent years, several new-generation, FDA-approved medications have become available for use in men with metastatic castrate-resistant prostate cancer. Abiraterone is an androgen biosynthesis inhibitor that is given along with prednisone and administered orally once daily. Enzalutamide, an androgen receptor signaling inhibitor, similarly is given orally once daily, but use of prednisone with this agent is not required. Both drugs are approved for use before or after docetaxel chemotherapy. An autologous cellular immunotherapy, sipuleucel-T, is available for use in advanced prostate cancer and works by stimulating the patient's own immune system against the prostate cancer. The newest therapy is radium 223 dichloride, a nuclear medicine therapy (specifically, an alpha emitter) that targets bone metastases with alpha particles. This agent has been shown to benefit patients by increasing the time to first symptomatic skeletal event, improving the quality of life, and increasing overall survival. This treatment, which is generally well tolerated, is given intravenously every 4 weeks for a total of 6 treatments.

Follow-up Recommendations

After curative therapy for prostate cancer (ie, prostatectomy or radiotherapy), the PSA level can be used as a marker for recurrence. PSA should be undetectable after successful primary surgical therapy, but some PSA will persist after radiotherapy. Generally, a biochemical recurrence is indicated by an increasing PSA level compared with either a nondetectable level or the nadir after definitive local therapy. This increase indicates recurrent disease in a patient with no identifiable metastases on radiographic imaging such as bone scan or computed tomographic (CT) scan. When prostate cancer recurs after definitive local therapy and the patient is not receiving ongoing therapy, the median time between identification of an increased PSA level (biochemical recurrence) and development of symptoms from metastatic prostate cancer is 8 years, and the median time to death from recurrent prostate cancer is 13 years. Thus, how closely any individual patient is monitored depends on his overall health, comorbid conditions, and overall life expectancy.

KEY FACTS

✓ PSA level—
- does not distinguish benign prostatic hyperplasia from carcinoma
- inadequate as sole screening method for prostate cancer
- useful after radical prostatectomy (PSA level should be undetectable)

✓ Considerations for prostate cancer therapy—
- comorbid conditions, patient age, and performance status
- more men die *with* prostate cancer than *of* prostate cancer

✓ Therapy for prostate cancer—
- prostatectomy for localized disease
- external beam radiotherapy (similar overall survival as with prostatectomy)
- brachytherapy for some organ-confined cases
- androgen deprivation therapy (hormonal therapy) is effective for metastatic disease but noncurative
- chemotherapy produces responses and may improve survival

Testicular Cancer

Background

Testicular cancer is diagnosed in approximately 8,000 men annually. It is the most common solid malignancy in males 15 to 35 years old, and it is typically curable, even when metastatic. At high risk are males with cryptorchid testes (40-fold relative risk) and Klinefelter syndrome (these patients also have an increased risk of breast cancer). The 2 broad categories of testicular cancer are seminomas and

nonseminomas. Types of nonseminomas include embryonal carcinoma, mature and immature teratoma, choriocarcinoma, yolk sac tumor, and endodermal sinus tumor. Often an admixture of several cell types occurs within nonseminomas. Any nonseminomatous component that is present with a seminoma is treated like a nonseminoma.

Evaluation includes 1) determination of β-human chorionic gonadotropin, alpha fetoprotein, and lactate dehydrogenase (LDH) levels and 2) CT of the abdomen (retroperitoneal lymph nodes) and chest (mediastinal lymph nodes or pulmonary nodules).

Staging

Unlike other malignancies that have 4 stages, testicular cancer has only 3 stages. Stage I disease is confined to the testis, stage II includes infradiaphragmatic nodal metastases, and stage III is spread beyond retroperitoneal nodes. About 85% of nonseminomas are associated with an increased value for β-human chorionic gonadotropin or alpha fetoprotein. Approximately 15% to 20% of advanced seminomas are associated with an increased β-human chorionic gonadotropin level. The alpha fetoprotein value is never increased in pure seminoma; if it is increased, the tumor is nonseminoma and should be treated as such.

Management

Radical inguinal orchiectomy is the definitive procedure for both pathologic diagnosis and local control. Scrotal orchiectomy and biopsy should not be done, because they are associated with a high incidence of local recurrence or spread to inguinal nodes. Thus, a patient with a testicular mass should undergo an ultrasonographic evaluation and be referred to a urologist.

Bladder Cancer

Approximately 72,000 new cases of bladder cancer are diagnosed in the United States each year, and approximately 26,000 people die each year of bladder cancer. The principal risk factor for bladder cancer is smoking, and 50% of cases of bladder cancer in the United States are directly attributable to tobacco use. Active smokers have 4 times the risk of the general population for bladder cancer, and former smokers have 2 times the risk.

Other risk factors include occupational exposures to substances such as dyes, arsenic, and aromatic amines. Previous cyclophosphamide chemotherapy is also a risk factor. In certain developing countries, infection with *Schistosoma haematobium* is a risk factor that accounts for up to 50% of cases.

Histologically, more than 90% of bladder cancers are urothelial carcinomas (also known as transitional cell carcinoma), and a small percentage can be either squamous cell carcinoma or adenocarcinoma. Localized bladder cancers are generally categorized as either non-muscle invasive (superficial) or muscle invasive, in which the bladder tumor invades into or beyond the muscularis propria of the bladder wall. Bladder cancers may spread to the regional lymph nodes and also to more distant sites.

Non-muscle invasive bladder cancer is typically managed by urologists with periodic cystoscopy and resection of recurrent tumors as warranted. Further, BCG or chemotherapy can be instilled into the bladder to help prevent recurrence and progression into muscle invasive disease. If muscle invasive bladder cancer develops, more aggressive treatment is necessary. Typically, the 2 options are 1) neoadjuvant cisplatin-based chemotherapy with subsequent cystectomy and 2) so-called trimodality therapy (cystoscopic resection of the bladder tumor with a subsequent combination of radiotherapy and chemotherapy). Even with aggressive therapy for muscle invasive bladder cancer, patients have a high risk for recurrent metastatic disease. For patients with metastatic disease, the treatment is chemotherapy. (Generally, surgery and radiotherapy are not useful.) Chemotherapy is not curative, and the average survival of patients with metastatic bladder cancer is 12 to 14 months with treatment.

Kidney Cancer

Each year in the United States, 65,000 new cases of kidney cancer are diagnosed, and most of these are localized to the kidney. Approximately 25% to 33% of kidney cancers are metastatic at presentation, and more than 22,000 people die of kidney cancer annually. Half of all kidney cancers are discovered incidentally when patients are asymptomatic and having testing for other reasons. Historically, renal cell carcinoma (RCC) was known as the internist's tumor, with the classic triad of flank pain, hematuria, and palpable abdominal mass, although now only 9% of patients present with this triad.

About 75% of RCCs are clear cell malignancies. Others include papillary RCC, chromophobe RCC, and oncocytomas. Any of these subtypes can be associated with sarcomatoid features, which universally portend a very poor prognosis. About 2% of RCCs are associated with inherited syndromes, most commonly von Hippel-Lindau syndrome.

Localized kidney cancers (and some with regional lymph node involvement) are treated surgically. Radiotherapy is not used for the primary tumor. Some small renal masses found incidentally are observed and treated only if clinically warranted either with surgery or with ablation by an interventional radiologist. In distinction to other metastatic cancers, removal of the primary tumor in the kidney (so-called **cytoreductive nephrectomy**) is considered even if a patient has stage IV disease, because some patients who undergo cytoreductive nephrectomy in combination with

systemic therapy will live longer. If a kidney cancer is localized and treated with surgical removal, there is currently no evidence that adjuvant treatment will help to reduce the risk of recurrence, although this question is under active investigation.

Key Definition

Cytoreductive nephrectomy: *removal of the primary tumor in the kidney.*

For patients who have metastatic disease, the main treatment is systemic therapy. Traditional chemotherapy generally is not used in the treatment of advanced kidney cancer. Since December 2005, the FDA has approved 7 drugs for the treatment of advanced kidney cancer. None is curative, but all of them do slow the progression of the disease, and the average survival with medical therapy for metastatic RCC is 2 to 3 years. Most of these drugs are administered orally.

One category, the tyrosine kinase inhibitors, includes sorafenib, sunitinib, pazopanib, and axitinib. All of these are administered orally. Each has its own adverse effect profile, but some important adverse effects of this class include hypertension, hypothyroidism, fatigue, elevated liver function test results, diarrhea, and congestive heart failure (especially with sunitinib). Another class is the mammalian target of rapamycin (mTOR) inhibitors (oral everolimus and intravenous temsirolimus). Notable adverse

---

KEY FACTS

✓ Testicular cancer—seminoma or nonseminoma

✓ Nonseminomatous component with a seminoma—treat like a nonseminoma

✓ Testicular cancer evaluation—
- determine β-human chorionic gonadotropin, alpha fetoprotein, and LDH levels
- perform CT of the abdomen (retroperitoneal lymph nodes) and chest (mediastinal lymph nodes or pulmonary nodules)

✓ Increased alpha fetoprotein value—rules out pure seminoma; treat tumor like a nonseminoma

✓ Management of non-muscle invasive bladder cancer—periodic cystoscopy and resection of recurrent tumors

✓ Kidney cancer—if localized (including some with regional lymph node involvement), treat surgically

✓ Cytoreductive nephrectomy—
- considered even with stage IV disease (unlike with other metastatic cancers)
- if performed in combination with systemic therapy, it may help some patients live longer

effects with the mTOR inhibitors include hyperlipidemia (especially hypertriglyceridemia), hyperglycemia, diarrhea, and noninfectious pneumonitis. Another agent approved for use in RCC and in other malignancies is bevacizumab, which is an inhibitor that exclusively targets vascular endothelial growth factor and is administered intravenously. Important adverse effects include gastrointestinal tract perforation, which can occur in up to 2.4% of patients, and surgical wound healing complications. Bevacizumab should be discontinued at least 28 days before elective surgery and held at least 28 days after elective surgery and until the surgical wound is fully healed. Bevacizumab carries an increased risk of causing hemorrhage.

65 Lung Cancer and Head and Neck Cancer

MICHELLE A. NEBEN WITTICH, MD AND KATHARINE A. PRICE, MD

Lung Cancer

Each year in the United States, approximately 220,000 new cases of lung cancer are diagnosed and approximately 158,000 people die of lung cancer. Lung cancer accounts for approximately 27% of all cancer deaths. Most patients with a new diagnosis of lung cancer are older than 65 years.

About 95% of lung cancers in men and about 80% of lung cancers in women result from cigarette smoking. Men who smoke 1 to 2 packs per day have up to a 25-fold increased risk for lung cancer compared with men who have never smoked. The risk of lung cancer for a former smoker decreases with time. Passive smoking is associated with an increased risk of lung cancer. Certain occupations (eg, smelter and iron work), chemicals (eg, arsenic and methylethyl ether), and exposure to radioactive agents (radon) and asbestos are associated with increased risks for lung cancer. Electronic cigarettes (e-cigarettes) have increased greatly in popularity, yet clear evidence on their safety is lacking.

Histologic Types and Characteristics

Lung cancer is classified histologically into small cell and non–small cell types (Table 65.1). Manifestations of lung cancer are listed in Box 65.1.

Non–small cell lung cancer (NSCLC) can be classified into squamous, adenocarcinoma, and large cell types. Squamous cell carcinoma may be associated with hypercalcemia due to the secretion of a parathyroid hormone–like peptide. Squamous cell carcinoma tends to occur centrally, whereas large cell and adenocarcinoma types tend to be peripheral. Adenocarcinoma is the most common type of NSCLC and the most frequent histologic subtype in nonsmokers. Patients with **bronchoalveolar carcinoma**, a low-grade NSCLC, frequently present with a patchy infiltrate and recurrent pneumonia.

Small cell lung cancer occurs almost exclusively in smokers and carries the poorest prognosis. The primary tumors are often small but are often associated with bulky mediastinal adenopathy and a high rate of distant metastases. They may be associated with paraneoplastic syndromes, such as syndrome of inappropriate secretion of antidiuretic hormone (SIADH).

KEY FACTS

✓ Lung cancer in the United States—
- 220,000 new cases are diagnosed annually
- 158,000 people die annually
- most patients with a new diagnosis are older than 65 years
- cigarette smoking causes 95% of cases in men and 80% of cases in women

✓ Histologic classification of lung cancer—
- small cell lung cancer
- NSCLC: squamous cell, adenocarcinoma, and large cell

✓ Squamous cell carcinoma—hypercalcemia may be present (from secretion of a parathyroid hormone–like peptide)

✓ Occurrence of NSCLC—
- squamous cell carcinoma: central
- large cell and adenocarcinoma types: peripheral

✓ Adenocarcinoma—
- most common type of NSCLC
- most frequent histologic subtype in nonsmokers

✓ Small cell lung cancer—may be associated with paraneoplastic syndromes (eg, SIADH)

Table 65.1 • Histologic Classification of Lung Cancer

Class	Prevalence, %	Subtypes
Adenocarcinoma	40	Acinar, bronchioalveolar, papillary, solid carcinoma with mucus formation, mixed
Squamous cell carcinoma	25	…
Small cell carcinoma	20	Pure small cell carcinoma, combined small cell carcinoma
Large cell carcinoma	10	Large cell neuroendocrine, basaloid, lymphoepithelial-like, large cell with rhabdoid phenotype
Adenosquamous carcinoma	<5	…
Carcinoid	<5	…
Bronchial gland carcinoma	<5	…

Adapted from Collins LG, Haines C, Perkel R, Enck RE. Lung cancer: diagnosis and management. Am Fam Physician. 2007 Jan 1;75(1):56–63. Used with permission.

Box 65.1 • Common Lung Cancer Manifestations

Primary tumor
  Chest discomfort
  Cough
  Dyspnea
  Hemoptysis
Intrathoracic spread
  Chest wall invasion
  Esophageal symptoms
  Horner syndrome
  Pancoast tumor
  Phrenic nerve paralysis
  Pleural effusion
  Recurrent laryngeal nerve paralysis
  Superior vena cava obstruction
Extrathoracic spread
  Bone pain, fracture
  Confusion, personality change
  Elevated alkaline phosphatase level
  Focal neurologic deficits
  Headache
  Nausea, vomiting
  Palpable lymphadenopathy
  Seizures
  Weakness
  Weight loss

Adapted from Collins LG, Haines C, Perkel R, Enck RE. Lung cancer: diagnosis and management. Am Fam Physician. 2007 Jan 1;75(1):56–63. Used with permission.

Key Definition

Bronchoalveolar carcinoma: *a low-grade NSCLC that often occurs with a patchy infiltrate and recurrent pneumonia.*

Screening

In December 2013, the US Preventive Services Task Force (USPSTF) issued the following lung cancer screening guideline based on the results of recent clinical trials (Ann Intern Med. 2014 Mar;160[4]:330–8):

The USPSTF recommends annual screening for lung cancer with low-dose computed tomography (LDCT) in adults aged 55 to 80 years who have a 30 pack-year smoking history and currently smoke or have quit within the past 15 years. Screening should be discontinued once a person has not smoked for 15 years or develops a health problem that substantially limits life expectancy or the ability or willingness to have curative lung surgery.

Treatment

Non–Small Cell Lung Cancer

General treatment approaches for patients with NSCLC depend on the stage and tumor type. Resection is the treatment of choice for clinical stage I or II disease. Stereotactic radio-surgery can be used for patients with stage I lung cancer who, because of comorbidities and poor pulmonary function, are not healthy enough for standard surgical resection. Patients with stage III NSCLC are treated with chemoradiotherapy, which may be followed by surgery if the cancer is resect-able. The use of adjuvant chemotherapy has been shown to improve survival by 10% to 12% compared with surgery alone in larger tumors or in node-positive disease. The use of adjuvant radiotherapy for selected patients with resected stage II or III disease decreases the likelihood of local recurrence. Patients with locally advanced unresectable NSCLC are treated with concurrent chemotherapy and radiotherapy. Although patients with metastatic disease are not cured, studies have shown that the use of chemotherapy improves overall survival and quality of life compared with the best supportive care.

Advances in the understanding of the genetics of lung cancer cells allow some patients to be treated with drugs that target specific mutations (Table 65.2). Mutations in ana-plastic lymphoma kinase (*ALK*) and the epidermal growth factor receptor (*EGFR*) occur almost exclusively in adeno-carcinoma of the lung and are more frequent in nonsmokers and patients with a minimal smoking history. The US Food

Table 65.2 • Genetic Abnormalities Specific for Non–Small Cell Lung Cancer and Small Cell Lung Cancer

Abnormality	Non–Small Cell Lung Cancer[a]		Small Cell Lung Cancer
	Squamous Cell Carcinoma	Adenocarcinoma	
Precursor			
Lesion	Known (dysplasia)	Probable (atypical adenomatous hyperplasia)	Possible (neuroendocrine field)[b]
Genetic change	*p53* mutation	*KRAS* mutation (atypical adenomatous hyperplasia in smokers); *EGFR* kinase domain mutation (in nonsmokers)	Overexpression of c-MET
Cancer			
KRAS mutation	Very rare	10%–30%[c]	Very rare
BRAF mutation	3%	2%	Very rare
EGFR			
Kinase domain mutation	Very rare	10%–40%[c]	Very rare
Amplification[d]	30%	15%	Very rare
Variant III mutation	5%[e]	Very rare	Very rare
HER2			
Kinase domain mutation	Very rare	4%	Very rare
Amplification	2%	6%	Not known
ALK fusion[f]	Very rare	7%	Not known
MET			
Mutation	12%	14%	13%
Amplification	21%	20%	Not known
TITF-1 amplification	15%	15%	Very rare
p53 mutation	60%–70%	50%–70%[c]	75%
LKB1 mutation	19%	34%	Very rare
PIK3CA			
Mutation	2%	2%	Very rare
Amplification	33%	6%	4%

Abbreviation: c-MET, hepatocyte growth factor receptor.

[a] Non–small cell lung cancer includes squamous cell carcinoma and adenocarcinoma.

[b] Neuroendocrine fields have been detected only in tissue surrounding tumors and have been characterized by extremely high rates of allelic loss and by c-MET overexpression.

[c] Variations are based in part on smoking profiles.

[d] The percentages include increased gene copy numbers from amplification or polysomy and represent percentages from resected cancers. The percentages are higher in primary tumors from patients with metastatic disease. Increased copy numbers have been reported in squamous dysplastic lesions but not in adenocarcinoma precursors.

[e] Genomic *EGFR* variant III mutations have been detected only in lung squamous cell carcinoma, and these tumors are sensitive preclinically to irreversible *EGFR* tyrosine kinase inhibitors. The incidence of 5% is substantially lower than that of 30% to 40% for the detection in squamous cell carcinoma or adenocarcinoma by immunohistochemical analysis or other techniques.

[f] The anaplastic lymphoma kinase (*ALK*) fusion gene (involving chromosome 2p), consisting of parts of *EML4* and *ALK*, is transforming in fibroblasts and occurs in adenocarcinoma but not in other types of non–small cell lung cancer or other nonlung cancers.

Adapted from Herbst RS, Heymach JV, Lippman SM. Lung cancer. N Engl J Med. 2008 Sep 25;359(13):1367–80. Used with permission.

and Drug Administration (FDA)-approved oral drugs erlotinib and gefitinib are treatments of choice for stage IV *EGFR*-mutated lung cancers. The FDA-approved drugs crizotinib and ceritinib are targeted oral drugs used to treat metastatic lung cancers that have *ALK* mutations. The addition of the anti–vascular endothelial growth factor (VEGF) agent bevacizumab to first-line chemotherapy for NSCLC improves response rate, progression-free survival, and overall survival.

Small Cell Lung Cancer

Treatment of limited-stage small cell lung cancer consists of both chemotherapy and chest radiotherapy. Surgical resection has not been shown to improve survival. For patients who have a complete response to chemotherapy and chest radiotherapy, prophylactic cranial radiotherapy is used to decrease the frequency of recurrence in the central nervous system and possibly improve survival. Prophylactic cranial radiotherapy is associated with the risk of delayed leukoencephalopathy, but this risk can be decreased with the administration of radiotherapy in small-dose fractions without concomitant chemotherapy. For limited-stage small cell disease, the median duration of survival is approximately 20 months; 30% to 40% of patients survive 2 years, and 20% survive 5 years.

Chemotherapy is used for extensive-stage (stage IV) small cell lung cancer. Combination chemotherapy is favored over single-agent therapy. Active drugs include etoposide, cisplatin or carboplatin, cyclophosphamide, doxorubicin, and vincristine; the combination of platinum chemotherapy and etoposide is the most frequently used regimen in the United States. Prophylactic cranial radiotherapy improves survival among patients with extensive disease who respond to chemotherapy. The median duration of survival is approximately 12 months, and 10% or fewer survive 5 years.

KEY FACTS

✓ Treatment of NSCLC—knowledge of cancer cell genetics allows use of drugs that target specific mutations

✓ Mutations in *ALK* and *EGFR*—

- occur almost exclusively in adenocarcinoma of the lung

- occur more frequently in nonsmokers and patients with minimal smoking history

✓ Treatment of limited-stage small cell lung cancer—chemotherapy in combination with chest radiotherapy

---

Head and Neck Cancer

Diagnosis

The most common head and neck cancer is squamous cell carcinoma of the upper aerodigestive tract. Head and neck squamous cell carcinoma can occur in the nasopharynx, oropharynx, larynx or hypopharynx, oral cavity, and paranasal sinuses. Uncommon cancers of the head and neck include salivary gland cancers, esthesioneuroblastoma, melanoma, lymphoma, sarcoma, and paraganglioma. Common symptoms at presentation are related to the head and neck and can include throat pain, ear pain, hoarseness, difficulty swallowing, citrus intolerance, and enlarged cervical lymph nodes (Table 65.3).

Risk Factors

Traditional risk factors for the development of head and neck squamous cell carcinoma include tobacco abuse, alcohol use, and chewing betel nuts (Box 65.2). People who consume low amounts of vegetables and fruits also have a higher risk of head and neck cancer. Nasopharyngeal cancer is often associated with Epstein-Barr virus. Human papillomavirus is a common cause of oropharynx squamous cell carcinoma and is now the

Table 65.3 • Clinical Presentations of Patients With Head and Neck Squamous Cell Carcinoma

Subsite	Clinical Presentation
Oral cavity	Sores, ulcers, pain
Oropharynx	Sore throat, chronic dysphagia, odynophagia, otalgia
Hypopharynx	Soreness, dysphagia, otalgia, and hoarseness
Larynx	Persistent hoarseness, shortness of breath
Supraglottis	Neck mass
Nasopharynx	Otitis media unresponsive to antibiotics, unilateral nasal airway obstruction, epistaxis, and cranial nerve palsies

Adapted from Marur S, Forastiere AA. Head and neck cancer: changing epidemiology, diagnosis, and treatment. Mayo Clin Proc. 2008 Apr;83(4):489–501. Erratum in: Mayo Clin Proc. 2008 May;83(5):604. Used with permission of Mayo Foundation for Medical Education and Research.

eighth most common cancer in men in the United States. Patients with tumors related to human papillomavirus have a much better prognosis than patients with tumors related to smoking and alcohol, particularly if the patients have never smoked.

Box 65.2 • Risk Factors for Head and Neck Cancer

Substance use
  Tobacco (primary risk factor)
    Smoking
    Chewing
    Secondhand smoke
  Ethanol
  Ethanol and tobacco together (additive effect)
  Betel nuts
Dietary
  Vitamin A deficiency
  Iron deficiency associated with Plummer-Vinson syndrome
Viruses
  Human papillomavirus types 16, 18, and 31
  Epstein-Barr virus
Occupational exposure
  Asbestos
  Nickel
  Chromium
  Radium
  Mustard gas
  Byproducts of leather tanning and woodworking

Adapted from Marur S, Forastiere AA. Head and neck cancer: changing epidemiology, diagnosis, and treatment. Mayo Clin Proc. 2008 Apr;83(4):489–501. Erratum in: Mayo Clin Proc. 2008 May;83(5):604. Used with permission of Mayo Foundation for Medical Education and Research.

Treatment and Follow-Up

Treatment options for locally advanced head and neck cancer include 1) surgical resection with possible adjuvant radiotherapy with or without chemotherapy and 2) organ preservation with chemotherapy and radiotherapy. Recurrence can be local or distant and generally happens within 5 years. However, follow-up by the patient's oncologist or otorhinolaryngologist should be lifelong. Patients with 1 head and neck cancer have a 25% risk of a second head and neck cancer as a result of the field cancerization effect. Common late adverse effects of treatment include skin fibrosis, decreased neck range of motion, lymphedema, xerostomia, dental problems, hypothyroidism, and swallowing difficulties.

KEY FACTS

- ✓ Most common head and neck cancer—squamous cell carcinoma of the upper aerodigestive tract
- ✓ Common risk factors for head and neck squamous cell carcinoma—using tobacco or alcohol and chewing betel nuts
- ✓ Nasopharyngeal cancer—often associated with Epstein-Barr virus
- ✓ Prognosis with head and neck tumors caused by human papillomavirus—much better than with tumors caused by smoking or alcohol

66 Oncologic Emergencies and Chemotherapy Complications[a]

TIMOTHY J. MOYNIHAN, MD

Hypercalcemia

The most common causes of hypercalcemia are malignancies and primary hyperparathyroidism. Patients with primary hyperparathyroidism have increased serum parathyroid hormone (PTH) values, but PTH is usually suppressed in cancer-associated hypercalcemia. Cancer-related hypercalcemia is often mediated by a PTH-related protein (PTHrP), which is secreted by the tumor and can be measured with current assays. In general, however, measuring PTHrP levels is of academic interest only and should not be done on a routine basis. Local osteolytic effects from tumors within bone can cause hypercalcemia in patients with widespread metastatic breast cancer and multiple myeloma but only rarely in patients with prostate cancer. Tumors can also cause hypercalcemia by secreting other bone-resorbing substances or by enhancing conversion of 25-hydroxyvitamin D to 1,25-dihydroxyvitamin D, a mechanism closely associated with lymphomas.

Accelerated bone resorption is due to activation of osteoclasts by various mediators, primarily PTHrP. The same factors that induce osteoclast-mediated bone resorption also stimulate renal tubular resorption of calcium. The hypercalcemic state interferes with renal resorption of sodium and water, leading to polyuria and eventual depletion of extracellular fluid volume. This reduces the glomerular filtration rate, further increasing the serum calcium level. Immobilization tips the balance toward bone resorption, worsening the hypercalcemia.

Symptoms and signs of hypercalcemia involve the gastrointestinal tract (anorexia, nausea, vomiting, and constipation), kidneys (polyuria, polydipsia, and dehydration), central nervous system (cognitive difficulties, apathy, somnolence, or even coma), and cardiovascular system (hypertension, shortened QT interval, arrhythmias, and enhanced sensitivity to digitalis).

Cancers associated with hypercalcemia include squamous cell carcinomas of the lung and the head and neck, breast cancer, renal cell carcinoma, multiple myeloma, and lymphoma. Patients who have breast cancer or myeloma are the most likely to have bony involvement with their disease.

The magnitude of the hypercalcemia and the degree of symptoms are key considerations for the treatment of hypercalcemia. Generally, patients with a corrected serum calcium value of more than 14 mg/dL, mental status changes, or an inability to maintain adequate hydration should be hospitalized for immediate treatment. However, there is no absolute value of serum calcium at which all patients become symptomatic, and relatively high levels may be well tolerated if the rate of increase has been gradual. The serum calcium value should be adjusted for hypoalbuminemia. The conversion formula is to add 0.8 mg/dL to the measured serum total calcium level for every 1 g of serum albumin less than 4 g/dL.

Patients with clinically symptomatic hypercalcemia almost always have intravascular volume depletion. Initial therapy therefore includes vigorous hydration with intravenously administered normal saline (up to 500 mL/h if heart function is normal). Loop diuretics are not used until after intravascular volume expansion has been completed. Furosemide facilitates urinary excretion of calcium by inhibiting calcium resorption

[a] Portions previously published in Lewis MA, Hendrickson AW, Moynihan TJ. Oncologic emergencies: pathophysiology, presentation, diagnosis, and treatment. CA Cancer J Clin. 2011 Sep-Oct;61(5):287–314. Epub 2011 Aug 19. Used with permission.

in the thick ascending loop of Henle. Use of thiazide diuretics should be avoided because they can worsen hypercalcemia.

The use of intravenous bisphosphonates (zoledronic acid or pamidronate, which is favored for patients with compromised renal function) is standard therapy for hypercalcemia of malignancy. Use of oral agents should be avoided because absorption from the gastrointestinal tract is poor. Bisphosphonates bind to hydroxyapatite and inhibit osteoclasts. In addition to fluids, bisphosphonates have become the mainstay for treatment of hypercalcemia, but they must be used cautiously and infused over longer periods in patients with renal failure.

Denosumab is a monoclonal antibody directed against the receptor activator of nuclear factor κB (RANK) ligand, which stimulates osteoclast activity in metastatic malignancies that cause hypercalcemia. Use of this agent in hypercalcemia is being investigated but has not yet been approved by the US Food and Drug Administration. Studies have reported that denosumab is effective in cases of malignancy-associated hypercalcemia that have become refractory to bisphosphonates.

Calcitonin may be given subcutaneously or intramuscularly; the intranasal form does not effectively decrease calcium levels. Calcitonin has a rapid onset of action and often lowers the calcium level within 12 to 24 hours; thus, it is useful in immediate life-threatening situations, such as cardiac arrhythmias or seizures. However, calcitonin is a relatively weak agent with a short-lived effect, and it should not be used as a single agent because of the potential for rebound hypercalcemia. Salmon-derived calcitonin is associated with a risk of hypersensitivity reaction, and epinephrine should be given for any allergic sequelae beyond flushing, but anaphylaxis is so rare that a test dose is no longer recommended.

Glucocorticoids are useful in hypercalcemia associated with calcitriol production by hematologic malignancies and can have a direct antitumor effect on neoplastic lymphoid tissue.

Calcium-free hemodialysis may be the fastest and least hazardous method of correcting hypercalcemia in patients with diminished kidney function. Dialysis also allows calcium levels to be decreased in patients who have congestive heart failure or other conditions that prevent high-volume fluid infusion.

Tumor Lysis Syndrome

Tumor lysis syndrome results from the release of tumor cell contents into the bloodstream such that overwhelming concentrations of certain substances become life-threatening. It most commonly occurs with cancers that have large tumor burdens and high proliferation rates that are exquisitely sensitive to chemotherapy. Tumor lysis syndrome rarely occurs spontaneously before antitumor therapy begins. Examples include high-grade lymphomas, leukemia, and, much less commonly, solid tumors (small cell lung cancer, anaplastic thyroid cancer, and germ cell tumors). The syndrome is characterized by hyperuricemia, acidosis, hyperkalemia, hyperphosphatemia, and hypocalcemia. These disturbances can lead to renal failure, arrhythmias, tetany, coagulation abnormalities, and death. The syndrome can be diminished with adequate hydration, alkalinization, and administration of allopurinol before chemotherapy. Allopurinol does not decrease uric acid levels that are already increased, and severe hyperuricemia can be treated with rasburicase, which, because of its cost, should be reserved for severe cases.

KEY FACTS

✓ Oncologic emergencies—
- occur at any time during the course of a cancer, from initial manifestation to end-stage disease
- prompt recognition and diagnosis improve patient's survival and quality of life
- patient's overall condition and prognosis should always be considered throughout evaluation and management
- patient should always be offered relief for pain and other symptoms

✓ Hypercalcemia—symptoms and signs involve the gastrointestinal tract, kidneys, central nervous system, and cardiovascular system

✓ Treatment of hypercalcemia—
- hospitalize patients who have a corrected serum calcium >14 mg/dL, who have mental status changes, or who cannot maintain adequate hydration
- initially hydrate with normal saline intravenously (up to 500 mL/h if heart function is normal)
- also administer bisphosphonates intravenously
- calcitonin may be given subcutaneously or intramuscularly (intranasal calcitonin does not decrease calcium levels)

✓ Tumor lysis syndrome—
- caused by release of tumor cell contents into bloodstream, resulting in overwhelming, life-threatening levels of certain substances
- characterized by hyperuricemia, acidosis, hyperkalemia, hyperphosphatemia, and hypocalcemia
- can result in renal failure, arrhythmias, tetany, coagulation abnormalities, and death

Febrile Neutropenia

Febrile neutropenia is defined as a temperature of 38.0°C or more on 1 occasion, or 2 episodes of 38.0°C at least 1 hour apart, *and* an absolute neutrophil count of 500×10^9/L or less (or $<1,000\times10^9$/L with a predicted decrease to $<500\times10^9$/L within 48 hours). Febrile neutropenia most commonly occurs after chemotherapy administration; the risk is dependent on the regimen administered. Febrile neutropenia can also result from any other cause of neutropenia, such as autoimmune conditions, administration of nonchemotherapeutic drugs, or a bone marrow dyscrasia. Although a source of infection is identified in only a minority of patients, any patient with neutropenic fever should have at least 2 sets of peripheral blood samples drawn for cultures, preferably before antibiotics are given. In addition, at least 1 blood sample for culturing should be drawn through each lumen of a multiple-port vascular catheter to determine whether the infection is device-related.

Although management of febrile neutropenia generally involves hospitalization and institution of parenteral broad-spectrum antibiotics, recent extensive clinical experience and multiple randomized clinical trials have shown that outpatient therapy is safe and efficacious for select patients. All patients need to be evaluated by a physician for both medical and social contraindications to outpatient treatment (Box 66.1). Patients who have no contraindication to outpatient treatment should receive oral amoxicillin-clavulanate 875 mg twice daily and oral ciprofloxacin 500 mg every 8 hours. All patients should be reevaluated within 24 hours either by telephone contact or in person.

For inpatients with febrile neutropenia, monotherapy is acceptable only with a sufficiently broad-spectrum agent, such as a fourth-generation cephalosporin (eg,

Box 66.1 • Medical and Social Contraindications to Outpatient Treatment of Febrile Neutropenia

Medical contraindications

Anticipated duration of neutropenia of >7 d (typically patients with leukemia or lymphoma)

Absolute neutrophil count 0.10×10^9/L

Comorbid medical conditions

Hypotension (systolic blood pressure <90 mm Hg)

Hypoxia or tachypnea (respirations >30/min)

Altered mental status

Renal insufficiency (creatinine >2.5 mg/dL)

Hyponatremia (sodium <124 mmol/L)

Bleeding

Dehydration

Poor oral intake

Social contraindications

History of nonadherence to medical therapy or being unreliable with prior medical therapy follow-up

Geographically remote (>50 km from 24-h emergency medical care)

Unable to care for self and lack of reliable caregiver

No telephone

No transportation

cefepime), a carbapenem, or piperacillin-tazobactam, all of which have activity against *Pseudomonas*. Vancomycin can be added for skin and soft tissue infections, pneumonia, or suspicion of an infected device, but it should not be used as monotherapy. Antifungal agents should be added to the regimen if patients have a persistent fever for more than 72 hours while receiving standard broad-spectrum antibiotics or if patients have a prior history of fungal sepsis.

Multiple randomized, placebo-controlled clinical trials have shown that the use of colony-stimulating factors administered at the time of febrile neutropenia does not improve outcomes. Patients who have had prior episodes of febrile neutropenia should receive prophylactic growth factors after subsequent doses of chemotherapy; this has been shown to decrease the risk of febrile neutropenia.

Spinal Cord Compression

Acute spinal cord compression is a neurologic emergency. It usually results from epidural extension of vertebral body metastases from lung, breast, prostate, myeloma, or kidney tumors. Occasionally, compression occurs from tumor invasion through the intervertebral foramen, as seen with lymphoma, sarcomas, and lung cancers in the paraspinous spaces. Occurrence varies by location: 10% of cases occur in the cervical spine, 70% in the thoracic

Table 66.1 • Reflexes and Their Corresponding Roots and Muscles		
Reflex	**Root(s)**	**Muscle**
Biceps	C5–6	Biceps
Triceps	C7–8	Triceps
Knee jerk	L2–4	Quadriceps
Ankle jerk	S1	Gastrocnemius

spine, and 20% in the lumbar spine. Multiple noncontiguous levels are involved in 10% to 40% of cases. The most important prognostic factor in preserving neurologic function is early diagnosis, before neurologic deficits have developed.

More than 90% of patients present with pain. Cervical pain may radiate down the arm. Thoracic pain radiates around the rib cage or abdominal wall; it may be described as a compressing band bilaterally around the chest or abdomen. Lumbar pain may radiate into the groin or down the leg. Pain may be aggravated by coughing, sneezing, or straight-leg raising. Focal neurologic signs depend on the level affected. Paresthesias (tingling and numbness), weakness, and altered reflexes also can be present (Table 66.1). Tenderness over the spine may help localize the level, but absence does not exclude the possibility of spinal cord involvement. Autonomic changes in urinary or fecal retention or incontinence are very concerning and may predict development of motor function loss in the near future.

Imaging studies include bone scanning or plain radiography, which show vertebral metastases in approximately 85% of patients with epidural compression. Magnetic resonance imaging (MRI) of the entire spine is generally recommended. Computed tomographic (CT) myelography can be used if patients cannot undergo MRI.

Treatment usually includes an initial bolus of dexamethasone intravenously. The exact dose is controversial, ranging anywhere from 10 to 100 mg. Higher initial doses are associated with more adverse effects and are not clearly associated with improved outcomes. Thereafter, dexamethasone is given (4 mg 4 times daily), although some physicians favor higher doses for a few days before a rapid taper. Radiotherapy to the involved areas is considered standard, but chemotherapy can also be effective for sensitive tumors (germ cell tumors and lymphomas). The Patchell criteria are used to identify patients who are likely to benefit from emergent surgical resection and stabilization (Box 66.2). Patients with extensive organ involvement, progressive malignancies, a life expectancy of less than 3 months, or poor performance status are unlikely to be able to tolerate an

Box 66.2 • Patchell Criteria for Decompressive Surgery in Patients With Malignant Spinal Cord Compression (MSCC)

Inclusion criteria

Age ≥18 y
Tissue-proven diagnosis of cancer (not of CNS or spinal column origin)
MRI evidence of MSCC (displacement of the spinal cord by an epidural mass)
Any neurologic sign or symptom (including pain)
Not paraplegic for >48 h
MSCC restricted to 1 area (can include several contiguous spinal or vertebral segments)
Expected survival of ≥3 mo
General medical status acceptable for surgery

Exclusion criteria

Multiple discrete lesions
Radiosensitive tumors (lymphomas, leukemia, multiple myeloma, and germ cell tumors)
Mass with compression of only the cauda equina or the spinal roots
Preexisting neurologic problems not directly related to MSCC
Prior radiotherapy that would exclude administration of the study dose

Abbreviations: CNS, central nervous system; MRI, magnetic resonance imaging.

extensive operative procedure and should be treated more conservatively.

Cardiac Tamponade

Pericardial effusions are commonly seen with malignancies, particularly those involving the chest (lymphoma, breast cancer, lung cancer, or metastatic tumors), but cardiac tamponade is rare. Patients present with chest pain, dyspnea, pulsus paradoxus, and electrical alternans on electrocardiography. The hallmark of true tamponade physiology is end-diastolic collapse of the right ventricle on echocardiography. Treatment is pericardiocentesis, which often rapidly relieves symptoms. Pericardial sclerosis or leaving the pigtail drain in place can prevent reaccumulation of the fluid during treatment of the underlying malignancy.

Malignant Airway Obstruction

Malignant airway obstruction can occur with any cancer, but it occurs most commonly with lung or mediastinal

Table 66.2 • Toxic Effects of Common Chemotherapy Drugs

Drug	Toxic Effect	Comment
Anthracyclines		
Doxorubicin	Cardiac	Dose-related over lifetime; may be irreversible
Daunorubicin	Myelosuppression	
Epirubicin	Vesicant	Late secondary MDS or leukemia
Idarubicin		
Mitoxantrone		
Platinum agents		
Cisplatin	Renal insufficiency	
Carboplatin	Peripheral neuropathy	Neuropathy can be irreversible
Oxaliplatin	Myelosuppression	Cold-sensitive neuropathy
	Anaphylaxis	
Taxanes		
Paclitaxel	Peripheral neuropathy	Neuropathy can be irreversible
Docetaxel	Myelosuppression	
	Anaphylaxis	
Antimetabolites		
5-Fluorouracil	Mucositis	Side effects can be severe in patients with DPD deficiency
Capecitabine	Diarrhea	
	Hand-foot syndrome	
	Myelotoxicity	
Methotrexate	Myelosuppression	Caution in patients with pleural effusions or ascites
	Pulmonary toxicity	
	Mucositis	
Cytosine arabinoside (ara-C)	Myelosuppression	
Gemcitabine	Myelosuppression	
Pemetrexed	Myelosuppression	
Alkylating agents		
Cyclophosphamide	Myelosuppression	
Ifosfamide	Hemorrhagic cystitis	
Chlorambucil		
Melphalan		
Temozolomide	Pneumocystis pneumonia	
Dacarbazine	Lymphopenia	
Carmustine (BCNU)	Myelosuppression	
Lomustine		
Topoisomerase inhibitors		
Etoposide (VP-16)	Myelosuppression	Secondary MDS or leukemia; occurs sooner than with anthracyclines
	Secondary MDS or leukemia	
	Anaphylaxis	
Vinca alkaloids		
Vincristine	Peripheral neuropathy	Neuropathy can be irreversible
Vinblastine	Vesicant	
Monoclonal antibodies		
Trastuzumab	Cardiac dysfunction	Usually reversible
Pertuzumab	Cardiac dysfunction	Usually reversible
Cetuximab	Skin rash	
	Diarrhea	

(continued)

Table 66.2 • (Continued)

Drug	Toxic Effect	Comment
Gemtuzumab ozogamicin	Myelosuppression	
Ibritumomab tiuxetan	Lymphopenia	
Ipilimumab	Autoimmune syndromes	
	Panhypophysitis	Severe adrenal insufficiency at presentation
Panitumumab	Rash	
	Diarrhea	
Rituximab	Lymphopenia	

Abbreviations: DPD, dihydropyrimidine dehydrogenase; MDS, myelodysplastic syndrome.

tumors, such as lymphoma or germ cell tumor. Patients present with dyspnea, stridor, and wheezing. A CT scan often shows the location of the obstruction. Bronchoscopy can be both diagnostic and therapeutic with use of either laser or stents to open the bronchus. Tissue can also be obtained for diagnosis.

Intracranial Mass Lesions

Brain involvement from primary or metastatic lesions can lead to increased intracranial pressure and mass effect. This can be exacerbated by acute hemorrhage into a tumor (most commonly in metastatic melanoma, renal cell carcinoma, or primary glioblastoma multiforme). Patients present with headache, severe nausea, vomiting, focal strokelike deficits, or seizures. Imaging with noncontrast CT can show areas of hemorrhage and mass effect, and MRI may further define the extent of the lesion. Immediate therapy involves the use of corticosteroids, specifically dexamethasone (the exact dose is controversial, but an initial bolus of 10–100 mg may be given). The most rapid way to alleviate a severe mass effect is surgical intervention, but consideration must be given to the patient's general condition and overall prognosis. Radiotherapy is commonly used for metastatic or primary tumors.

Chemotherapy Complications

Toxic effects of common chemotherapy drugs are summarized in Table 66.2.

KEY FACTS

✓ Treatment of febrile neutropenia in outpatients (not all patients need to be hospitalized)—oral amoxicillin-clavulanate 875 mg twice daily and oral ciprofloxacin 500 mg every 8 hours

✓ Treatment of febrile neutropenia in inpatients—
- if monotherapy, must use a broad-spectrum agent with activity against *Pseudomonas* (eg, a fourth-generation cephalosporin, a carbapenem, or piperacillin-tazobactam)
- vancomycin is not used for monotherapy but may be added for skin and soft tissue infections, pneumonia, or suspicion of an infected device
- add antifungal agents if patient has persistent fever (>72 hours) while receiving broad-spectrum antibiotics or a history of fungal sepsis
- use of colony-stimulating factors does not improve outcomes

✓ Spinal cord compression—
- MRI of the entire spine
- treat with an initial bolus of dexamethasone intravenously
- radiotherapy to the involved area is standard
- chemotherapy can be effective for germ cell tumors and lymphomas
- Patchell criteria are used to identify patients for emergent surgical resection and stabilization

✓ Intracranial mass lesions—dexamethasone is used for immediate therapy

Questions and Answers

Questions

Multiple Choice (choose the best answer)

X.1. An otherwise healthy 32-year-old man asks you about screening tests for colon cancer. He reports that colon cancer occurred in a sister at age 40, in another sister at age 42, and in his mother at age 40. In addition, his mother had endometrial cancer at age 45, and a maternal aunt had breast cancer at a young age. He notes that no family member had a history of colon polyps. What should you recommend for this patient?
a. Annual fecal occult blood testing
b. Colonoscopy now and every 1 to 2 years thereafter
c. Colonoscopy with random biopsies to look for inflammatory bowel disease (IBD)—if IBD is absent, follow routine screening recommendations for average-risk Americans
d. Prophylactic colectomy
e. Reassurance only, because no polyps were found in family members

X.2. A 72-year-old male smoker with a 42-pack-year history presents with anorexia, cough, and altered mental status. A chest radiograph shows a right-sided mass that, on bronchoscopy, is identified as squamous cell carcinoma. On physical examination, the patient is thin, cachectic, dehydrated, and disoriented with no focal neurologic deficits. The calcium level is elevated (15 mg/dL), creatinine is 2.5 mg/dL, and albumin is 2.2 g/dL. A bone scan shows only some degenerative changes. What is the most appropriate next step in the management of this patient?
a. Cisplatin-based chemotherapy
b. Radiotherapy to the brain
c. Intravenous fluids and bisphosphonates
d. Dexamethasone 100 mg given as an intravenous push
e. Emergent magnetic resonance imaging of the head

X.3. A 55-year-old woman with a history of hypertension, a 30-pack-year history of smoking, mild chronic obstructive pulmonary disease, and moderate obesity presents with a right axillary mass. She has a family history of coronary artery disease and strokes. Current medications include a statin, a diuretic, and a β-blocker. On examination, she is moderately obese and in no distress. Her lungs have increased sound in the expiratory phase diffusely but no frank wheezing or other sounds. Findings from examination of the heart, abdomen, and breasts are unremarkable. On lymph node examination, a palpable right axillary mass is firm, mobile, and not tender. Findings from mammography, breast ultrasonography, and computed tomography of the chest are negative except for the presence of right axillary adenopathy. Biopsy of a lymph node shows a moderately differentiated adenocarcinoma of unknown primary origin. What should be the next step in evaluation of this patient?
a. Perform a mediastinoscopy.
b. Assume that non–small cell carcinoma is present, and treat with cisplatin-based chemotherapy.
c. Clarify the histogenetic origin of the tumor by testing for tumor markers: carcinoembryonic antigen, cancer antigen 15–3, and neuron-specific enolase.
d. Perform breast magnetic resonance imaging (MRI).
e. Recommend bilateral mastectomies.

X.4. A 38-year-old woman presents for intermittent abdominal pain and bloating that has been getting worse for the past several months. She has been reading medical information on the Internet and is very concerned about ovarian cancer. She has no family history of malignancy and has been otherwise healthy. She is not taking any medications. Physical examination findings are remarkable only for some tenderness to movement of the uterus. No pelvic masses are detected. She requests a serum cancer antigen (CA) 125 test; the result is 86 U/mL (reference range <35 U/mL). How should you advise her at this time?
a. Recommend combination chemotherapy with cisplatin and paclitaxel.
b. Tell her that this degree of CA 125 elevation occurs only in ovarian cancer.
c. Tell her that although the CA 125 elevation is concerning, multiple conditions can cause such an elevation, and further investigation is warranted.
d. Recommend exploratory laparotomy with total abdominal hysterectomy, bilateral salpingo-oophorectomy, pelvic lymphadenectomy, omentectomy, and aggressive surgical debulking of all disease.
e. Recommend only observation now, and recheck the CA 125 level in 3 months.

X.5. A 38-year-old woman with recently diagnosed node-positive breast cancer presents to the emergency department with a temperature of 38.3°C. She reports having mild chills and fever but no nausea, vomiting, diarrhea, cough, or dysuria. Seven days ago, she received her third cycle of doxorubicin and cyclophosphamide chemotherapy; thus far, she has tolerated the cycles well. On physical examination, she is pleasant and appears fatigued but in no distress, with the following findings: blood pressure 122/78 mm Hg, pulse 82 beats per minute and regular, respiratory rate 14 breaths per minute, and temperature 38.2°C. The remainder of the examination is remarkable for only alopecia. A chest radiograph is clear of abnormalities. Urinalysis shows no leukocytes. Laboratory data include the following: hemoglobin 11.4 g/dL, leukocyte count 0.8×10^9/L, absolute neutrophil count 0.25×10^9/L, and platelet count 90×10^9/L. She lives in town with her husband and 2 children (aged 10 and 14 years). No one else is ill at home. At this time, what should you do?

a. Admit her to the hospital to receive broad-spectrum antibiotics.

b. Administer granulocyte colony-stimulating factor now.

c. Send her home, and ask her to follow up with her oncologist in the morning.

d. Collect blood and urine samples for cultures, begin therapy with amoxicillin–clavulanate potassium and ciprofloxacin orally, discharge to home, and ask her to follow up with her oncologist by telephone within 24 hours.

e. Obtain a throat swab specimen to test for influenza virus.

X.6. A 67-year-old man with a history of stage II rectal cancer was treated with resection and combined chemotherapy and radiotherapy 6 years ago. He has recovered well from the operations and treatments; he still has some rectal and bladder urgency but no incontinence. He recently retired from his job as an office manager and is physically active. His hypertension is well controlled with a β-blocker, and his cholesterol levels are controlled with diet. He has no relevant family history. His most recent follow-up colonoscopy was done 10 months ago and showed no evidence of recurrence or other disease. He is a lifetime nonsmoker. On physical examination, he is thin and pleasant, and he appears fit. General examination findings are unremarkable. On rectal examination, his prostate feels normal and smooth without palpable masses. A stool sample is negative for heme. Liver function test results are normal, the level of carcinoembryonic antigen (CEA) is within the reference range, and the level of prostate-specific antigen is 1.4 ng/mL. He is concerned about late side effects of his prior therapy, specifically about the development of new cancers. What should you tell him?

a. He is at increased risk for secondary cancers of the bladder, prostate, and rectum, but the risk is only about 1 in 70 at 10 years.

b. He has no need to worry because he has no increased risk for secondary malignancies.

c. He is at high risk for lung cancer, so he should have routine screening chest radiographs.

d. He is right to worry because secondary cancers are very common, and screening should be done at regular intervals.

e. Screening for prostate cancer is no longer necessary because he has had radiotherapy to this area.

X.7. An 82-year-old man comes to your office for routine follow-up care. He has a prior history of chronic obstructive pulmonary disease with a forced expiratory volume in 1 second of 25% of the predicted value, coronary artery disease with mild congestive heart failure, hypertension, and type 2 diabetes mellitus. He reports having no urinary symptoms. He takes the following medications: enalapril 5 mg twice daily, hydrochlorothiazide 25 mg twice daily, lovastatin 20 mg once daily, albuterol inhaler as needed, fluticasone propionate 250 mcg and salmeterol 50 mcg inhalation powder daily, aspirin 325 mg daily, glipizide 10 mg twice daily, and a multivitamin daily. On examination, he has poor breath sounds in all areas, distant heart tones, a normal abdomen, and edema (2+) of the lower extremities bilaterally. On rectal examination, he has an enlarged prostate with a firm nodule. The prostate-specific antigen level is 8.5 ng/mL, and transrectal needle biopsy shows adenocarcinoma (Gleason grade 6). A bone scan shows only some changes consistent with degenerative disease. What can you tell him at this time?

a. Radical prostatectomy is likely to improve his overall survival and decrease his chance of death from prostate cancer.

b. Given his lack of symptoms from prostate cancer, combined with his age and comorbid conditions, a watchful waiting approach is reasonable.

c. External beam radiotherapy is not effective against prostate cancer.

d. Chemotherapy can be used to decrease his risk of recurrence of prostate cancer.

e. Orchiectomy is the standard of care.

Answers

X.1. Answer b.

With his family history, this patient is at very high risk for colon cancer. It is unlikely that he would have a hereditary polyposis syndrome since no family member had polyps. His family history is highly concerning for hereditary non-polyposis colorectal cancer (Lynch syndrome) because multiple first-degree relatives were affected at an early age and because there is a family history of breast and endometrial cancer. This syndrome is associated with a defect in mismatch repair enzymes and leads to microsatellite instability. Screening with fecal occult blood testing is not adequately sensitive for patients at high risk—or even for patients with normal risk. IBD does significantly increase the risk of colon cancer, but nothing in the patient's history suggests that it is present. Prophylactic colectomy would be a consideration only if testing is positive for the defective gene.

X.2. Answer c.

The patient needs intravenous fluids and restoration of intravascular volume along with bisphosphonates to correct the hypercalcemia. In the absence of any focal neurologic deficits, it is unlikely that his disorientation is due to metastatic disease; altered mental status is very common with hypercalcemia. If correction of the hypercalcemia reverses the altered mental status, central nervous system imaging is not required. Cranial radiotherapy should be given only after metastatic disease is identified in a patient with non–small cell carcinoma. Dexamethasone is used to decrease peritumoral edema from intracranial metastases and is not indicated for this patient. Dexamethasone can help to significantly correct hypercalcemia due to multiple myeloma or lymphoma, but it is unlikely to correct hypercalcemia due to squamous cell carcinoma.

X.3. Answer d.

Women presenting with axillary lymph node metastases of adenocarcinoma of unknown primary origin should undergo thorough evaluation for breast cancer. Breast MRI has greater sensitivity than mammography or ultrasonography, and among women who have occult adenocarcinoma in the axillary lymph nodes, MRI can detect a primary lesion in up to 75% of patients. Although breast MRI is helpful for evaluation of women with adenocarcinoma metastatic to axillary lymph nodes, use of breast MRI for routine screening should be limited to high-risk women since it has not been shown to be beneficial for average-risk patients. The detection of hormone receptors in the pathologic specimen has diagnostic and therapeutic implications. Serum tumor markers are rarely useful diagnostic tools (with few exceptions).

X.4. Answer c.

Further investigation is warranted to determine the cause of her discomfort and the reason for her elevated CA 125 level. This nonspecific serum marker can be elevated in many benign conditions, such as endometriosis, pregnancy, menstruation, and peritonitis. The positive predictive value of CA 125 for screening is only about 2% to 3%. Although very high levels (several hundred to several thousand units per milliliter) typically occur only in patients with ovarian cancer, patients with endometriosis can have levels around 200 U/mL with stage IV disease. Chemotherapy is never indicated without tissue confirmation of disease. Extensive resection would be indicated if ovarian carcinoma were diagnosed, and this would typically be followed by systemic chemotherapy. Since the patient's symptoms are worsening, observation only is not warranted.

X.5. Answer d.

Febrile neutropenia is common with many forms of chemotherapy. Most patients have negative culture results. Patients who are medically stable, are able to maintain oral intake, are reliable for close follow up, and live near a medical facility can be safely treated with an outpatient regimen. After neutropenia develops, administration of growth factors is not useful. Observation alone is insufficient since the low absolute neutrophil count puts her at significant risk for sepsis.

X.6. Answer a.

Patients treated with pelvic radiotherapy for rectal or prostate cancer are at increased risk for secondary malignancies in the area, but this risk is low (estimated to be 1 in 125 at 5 years and 1 in 70 at 10 years). Patients should still undergo screening for cancers that they are at risk for, as long as their general health and other medical conditions warrant screening. This patient does not have an increased risk for lung cancer per se, but lung metastases are a common site for recurrence of rectal cancer. The pattern of recurrence is different from that of colon cancer, which much more commonly metastasizes to the liver before traveling to the lung. The venous drainage of the rectum is into the inferior vena cava, while most of the colon's venous drainage is to the portal system. Routine follow-up for otherwise healthy patients who have colorectal cancer includes the following: 1) Evaluate with a history and physical examination every 3 months for 2 years and then every 6 months for a total of 5 years. 2) Perform a colonoscopy in 1 year. If results are abnormal, perform another colonoscopy in 1 year; if results are normal, perform a colonoscopy as clinically indicated. 3) Determine CEA levels every 3 months for 2 years and then every 6 months for years 3 to 5. 4) Consider computed tomography of the chest, abdomen, and pelvis annually for 3 years if the patient is at high risk.

X.7. Answer b.

For patients older than 65, especially those with significant comorbid conditions, it is unclear whether radical prostatectomy improves the patient's overall survival and it certainly has adverse effects on quality of life. Patients in good condition who are younger than 65 do seem to have a survival advantage if treated with radical prostatectomy instead of watchful waiting; however, this elderly patient with other illnesses is unlikely to benefit from aggressive treatment. External beam radiotherapy or brachytherapy would be a reasonable treatment option, but each carries a risk of impotence, rectal injury, and incontinence. Chemotherapy has no role except for patients with metastatic disease. Orchiectomy or hormonal therapies are typically reserved for patients with metastatic or symptomatic disease.

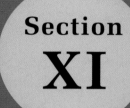

Section
XI

Psychiatry

Mood and Anxiety Disorders

BRIAN A. PALMER, MD

Since 30% to 40% of ambulatory primary care visits have a psychiatric component, successful patient management often hinges on successful treatment of comorbid psychiatric illness.

The key concept when assessing psychiatric symptoms is *whether the symptom interferes with a patient's functioning or causes distress*. For example, a patient may have a fear of heights. If this acrophobia never causes an alteration in activity, intervention is unnecessary. If, however, this acrophobia causes distress and interferes with the patient's functioning, intervention may be warranted.

Mood Disorders

Mood disorders are common, with a prevalence of 8% in the general US population. The essential feature is disturbance of mood in a constellation of other symptoms (mood change alone, such as sadness, is not an illness). Mood disorders are accompanied by related cognitive, psychomotor, neurovegetative, and interpersonal difficulties. Mood disorders may be related to a general medical condition or be substance induced.

Depressive Disorders

Major Depression

Major depression is a serious psychiatric disorder with primary symptoms that include 5 of the 9 criteria in Box 67.1 for at least 2 weeks. Acute mood changes (lasting <2 weeks) from medical causes, such as acute blood loss, are not major depression. The lifetime prevalence of depression is 20% for women and 12% for men. For women, the peak age at onset of depression is 33 to 45 years, and for men, more than 55 years.

If delusions or hallucinations are also present, they are usually less prominent than in schizophrenia, and the disorder is referred to as *major depression with psychotic*

Box 67.1 • Criteria for a Major Depressive Episode[a]

Depressed mood (feeling sad or empty; tearful)[b]

Diminished interest or pleasure in many activities[b]

Notable weight loss or weight gain (>5% of body weight in 1 mo) or decreased or increased appetite

Insomnia or hypersomnia nearly every day

Psychomotor agitation or retardation

Fatigue or loss of energy

Feelings of worthlessness or inappropriate guilt (which may be delusional)

Diminished ability to think or concentrate, or indecisiveness

Recurrent thoughts of death, including suicidal ideation or planning

[a] Symptoms must be present every day or nearly every day for at least 2 weeks. A diagnosis of major depression requires 5 of the 9 criteria.

[b] A diagnosis of major depression requires either a depressed mood or a loss of interest or pleasure in activities.

---

features. These features increase the likelihood of treatment resistance (although they predict a better response to electroconvulsive therapy [ECT]).

Seasonal Affective Disorder

Seasonal affective disorder is a subtype of major depression characterized by the onset of symptoms in autumn or winter. It is twice as common in women as in men and is associated with psychomotor retardation, hypersomnia, overeating (carbohydrate craving), and weight gain (resembling hibernation). Diagnosis requires 3 consecutive years of autumn or winter episodes that resolve by spring or summer. Treatment has relied primarily on phototherapy with a full-spectrum light source of 10,000 lux, which must be used for a minimum of 30 minutes daily. Antidepressant agents are also of benefit in treating this disorder.

Postpartum Depression

Postpartum depression affects 10% of mothers. Although it occurs in all socioeconomic groups, single or poor mothers are at greatest risk. Untreated postpartum depression can adversely affect parent-child bonding. Treatment with antidepressants, although effective, must be balanced with the possible effect on a developing fetus or breast-fed infant, but it is generally accepted that in moderate to severe depression, the risks of not treating depression outweigh the risk of treatment with most antidepressants. Prescribing clinicians should be cognizant of the pregnancy category of the agent they prescribe in this patient group. Bipolar disorder is overrepresented in patients with postpartum mood disorders, and postpartum psychosis is nearly always a marker of bipolar disorder.

Dysthymia

Dysthymia is chronic depression that is milder in severity than major depression. It can be disabling for the person because the depressed mood is present most of the time during at least a 2-year period. Many patients have 1 or 2 associated vegetative signs, such as disturbance of sleep and appetite. Also, patients often feel inadequate, have low self-esteem, and struggle with interpersonal relationships. If onset is in late adolescence, the dysthymia may become intertwined with the person's personality, behavior, and general attitude toward life. Treatment is usually a combination of psychotherapy and pharmacotherapy. Pharmacotherapy may be particularly useful for patients with a family history of mood disorders or for those who have the early-onset form of dysthymia. In patients with dysthymia, superimposed major depressive episodes may develop.

Key Definition

Dysthymia: *chronic depression that is milder in severity than major depression.*

Adjustment Disorder With Depressed Mood

Adjustment disorder with depressed mood is a reaction that develops in response to an identifiable psychosocial stressor (eg, divorce, job loss, family or marital problems). The severity of the adjustment disorder (degree of impairment) does not always parallel the intensity of the precipitating event. The critical factor appears to be the relevance of the event or stressor to the patient and the patient's

ability to cope with the stress. In general, these reactions are relatively transient. Although patients generally can be managed by an empathetic primary care physician, the development of extreme withdrawal, suicidal ideation, or failure to improve as the circumstances improve may prompt psychiatric referral. Treatment includes supportive psychotherapy, psychosocial interventions, and, sometimes, use of antidepressant agents.

Principles of Depression Treatment

There are 3 common major groups of treatment modalities for depression: psychotherapy, pharmacotherapy, and neuromodulation treatments such as ECT. Generally, these therapeutic modalities are used in some combination. Although internists rarely conduct formal psychotherapy, brief cognitive interventions, such as challenging overly perfectionistic beliefs, can be helpful.

The selection of medication is based on the adverse reaction profile of the medication and on the personal or family history of a good response to a particular agent. Initially, the patient should use a low dose, followed by titration to a therapeutic dose based on clinical assessment. Blood level determinations of a drug are meaningful only for tricyclic antidepressants used at higher doses. Treatment duration usually extends for a minimum of 6 to 12 months after the patient noticeably improves. Patients who have a severe depressive episode or who have experienced 2 or more depressive episodes are at high risk of symptom recurrence without prophylactic medication. Use of antidepressants should be tapered rather than stopped abruptly when treatment is discontinued. If the response to the first antidepressant agent is minimal, the clinician should reevaluate the diagnosis, change to a different class of drug, or consider ECT.

Mania and Bipolar Disorder

The essential features of a manic episode are the presence of an abnormally euphoric, expansive, or irritable mood associated with 3 of the criteria in Box 67.2 (4 criteria are required if the mood is only irritable). For a diagnosis of bipolar disorder, the patient must have had at least 1 episode of mania (bipolar I disorder) or hypomania (bipolar II disorder). Most patients with bipolar disorder have had recurrent depressive episodes in addition to manic episodes, although rarely patients have mania exclusively. The prevalence of bipolar disorder is estimated to be about 1%. Bipolar disorder occurs about as frequently in women as in men, and the usual age at onset is from the teens to 30 years. A family history of bipolar or another mood disorder is more common among patients with bipolar disorder than among patients with other mood disorders. Some patients do not experience a fully developed manic

Box 67.2 • Criteria for a Manic Episode[a]

Inflated self-esteem or grandiosity

Less need for sleep (rested after 3 h)

Pressured speech

Flight of ideas

Distractibility

Increase in goal-directed activity or psychomotor agitation

Excessive involvement in pleasurable activities that have a high potential for painful consequences (eg, unrestrained buying sprees, sexual indiscretions, or inappropriate financial investments)

[a] Symptoms must be present for at least 1 week (4 days if hypomanic) unless interrupted by treatment. Mood is persistently elevated, expansive, or irritable. A diagnosis of manic episode requires 3 of the 7 criteria (4 are required if the mood is only irritable).

episode but have fewer symptoms. The term *hypomania* has been introduced to describe this form of bipolar disorder (bipolar II disorder), which generally is challenging to clinicians because its subtle features make it more difficult to recognize and it may be confused with other psychiatric disorders.

Treatment is aimed at mood stabilization with medication and improved social and occupational functioning. Pharmacotherapy of mania includes lithium carbonate, divalproex sodium, other mood stabilizers, and atypical antipsychotics. Lithium has the added benefit of being useful in prevention or treatment of bipolar depression. Lamotrigine is also effective in preventing bipolar depression. Patients with bipolar depression may be treated with lithium carbonate, lamotrigine, or an atypical antipsychotic (lurasidone, quetiapine, and olanzapine/fluoxetine combination have US Food and Drug Administration approval).

Mood Disorders Caused by a General Medical Condition

Mood disorders can be caused by medical illness. Many medical conditions may induce mood changes, so the clinical interview should identify coexisting symptoms such as excessive guilt, social withdrawal, or suicidal ideation, which are more specific for a primary depressive disorder. Medical conditions that may cause mood symptoms include endocrinopathies (Cushing syndrome, Addison disease, hyperthyroidism, hypothyroidism, hyperparathyroidism, and hypoparathyroidism), certain malignancies (lymphomas, pancreatic carcinoma, and astrocytomas), neurologic conditions (Parkinson disease, Huntington disease, and Alzheimer disease), autoimmune conditions

(systemic lupus erythematosus), and infections (chronic hepatitis C, encephalitis, mononucleosis, and human immunodeficiency virus infection).

Substance-Induced Mood Disorders

The essential feature of a substance-induced mood disorder is a mood disturbance, either depressed or manic, due to the direct physiologic effects of a substance. Many substances can induce mood changes, including medications, toxins, and drugs of abuse. The mood symptoms may occur during the use of or exposure to the substance or during withdrawal from the substance. Medications that have been implicated in inducing mood disturbances include corticosteroids, interferon, reserpine, methyldopa, carbonic anhydrase inhibitors, stimulants, sedative-hypnotics, benzodiazepines, and narcotics. Long-term use or abuse of alcohol or hallucinogens has also been implicated in inducing mood disturbances.

KEY FACTS

✓ When assessing psychiatric symptoms, consider whether the symptom interferes with functioning or causes distress

✓ More women (20%) than men (12%) have depression over a lifetime

✓ Seasonal affective disorder—twice as likely in women; characterized by psychomotor retardation, hypersomnia, overeating, and weight gain

✓ If untreated, postpartum depression can keep a mother from bonding with her child

✓ Major treatment modalities for depression—psychotherapy, pharmacotherapy, and neuromodulation treatments such as electroconvulsive therapy

✓ A diagnosis of bipolar disorder requires at least 1 episode of mania (bipolar I disorder) or hypomania (bipolar II disorder)

Anxiety Disorders

Anxiety symptoms may be misinterpreted as those of medical illness because many of the symptoms overlap (eg, tachycardia, diaphoresis, tremor, shortness of breath, nausea, abdominal pain, chest pain). Autonomic arousal and anxious agitation in a medically ill patient can also be attributed quickly to stress or anxiety when the symptoms may represent pulmonary embolus or cardiac arrhythmia. Common sources of anxiety in the medical setting are related to fears of death, abandonment, loss of function, pain, dependency, and loss of control. When to treat or to seek psychiatric consultation depends on the assessment of the degree of anxiety. Is the patient able to function in his or her role without distress or avoidance?

Panic Disorder and Agoraphobia

Panic disorder refers to recurrent, discrete episodes of extreme anxiety accompanied by various somatic symptoms, such as dyspnea, unsteady feelings, palpitations, paresthesias, hyperventilation, trembling, diaphoresis, chest pain or discomfort, or abdominal distress. **Agoraphobia** refers to extreme fear of being in places or situations from which escape may be difficult or embarrassing. This fear may lead to avoidance, ultimately causing severe limitations in daily functioning for the patient. Panic disorder is more common in women (prevalence, 2%–3%) than in men (prevalence, 0.5%–1.5%). The usual age at onset is from the late teens to the early 30s. A history of childhood separation anxiety is reported in 20% to 50% of patients. The incidence is higher in first- and second-degree relatives. Most patients describe their first panic attack as spontaneous. They often go to an emergency department after the first attack, believing that they are having a heart attack or a severe medical problem.

Key Definitions

Panic disorder: *recurrent, discrete episodes of extreme anxiety accompanied by various somatic symptoms.*

Agoraphobia: *extreme fear of being in places or situations from which escape may be difficult or embarrassing.*

Patients with panic attacks may be prone to episodes of major depression. The differential diagnosis of panic disorder includes several medical disorders, such as endocrine disturbances (eg, hyperthyroidism, pheochromocytoma, hypoglycemia), gastrointestinal tract disturbances (eg, colitis, irritable bowel syndrome), cardiopulmonary disturbances (eg, pulmonary embolism, exacerbation of chronic obstructive pulmonary disease, acute allergic reactions), and neurologic conditions (especially conditions such as seizures that are episodic or are associated with paresthesias, faintness, or dizziness).

Several substances of abuse may cause or exacerbate anxiety symptoms. Stimulants (eg, cocaine, amphetamines, caffeine) can fuel anxiety, as can withdrawal from sedating agents (eg, alcohol, benzodiazepines, narcotics). Patients may use alcohol or benzodiazepines to prevent or treat panic symptoms, but regular or high-dose use may result in a cycle of tolerance and withdrawal, paradoxically causing an increase in anxiety symptoms.

Effective treatment for most patients includes the following, alone or in combination: antidepressants (particularly selective serotonin reuptake inhibitor [SSRI] antidepressants and generally not bupropion), cognitive behavioral therapy, or benzodiazepines (short-term). Alcohol and benzodiazepines may reduce the distress of panic attacks, but symptoms may rebound, potentially leading to substance abuse and paradoxically worsening anxiety.

Posttraumatic Stress Disorder

Posttraumatic stress disorder can be a brief reaction that follows an extremely traumatic, overwhelming, or catastrophic experience, or it may be a chronic condition that produces severe disability. The syndrome is characterized by the following:

1. Persistent reexperiencing (intrusive memories, flashbacks, nightmares)
2. Avoidance of reminders of the event and often a restricted range of affect
3. Persistently increased arousal (startle response, hypervigilance)

Posttraumatic stress disorder may occur in adults or children. There is increased comorbidity with substance abuse, depression, and other anxiety disorders. Patients may be more prone to impulsivity, including suicide. As with other anxiety disorders, treatment is usually a combination of psychotherapeutic and, if necessary, pharmacologic interventions. Again, SSRI antidepressants are the mainstay of treatment; prazosin, a centrally acting α-adrenergic antagonist, has been shown to be effective in reducing nightmares.

Generalized Anxiety Disorder

Generalized anxiety disorder is characterized by chronic excessive anxiety and apprehension about life circumstances accompanied by somatic symptoms of anxiety, such as trembling, restlessness, autonomic hyperactivity, and hypervigilance. Treatment is usually a combination of cognitive behavioral psychotherapy and psychopharmacologic modalities.

Obsessive-Compulsive Disorder

Obsessive-compulsive disorder is characterized by 2 features:

1. Obsessions—distressing thoughts, ideas, or impulses experienced as unwanted
2. Compulsions—repetitive, intentional behaviors performed in response to an obsession, usually neutralizing the anxiety caused by the obsession

Prevalence rates are 2% to 3% and are about equal in men and women. The onset of this disorder is usually in adolescence or early adulthood. Obsessive traits are often present before onset of the disorder. The predominant neurobiologic theory for the cause of obsessive-compulsive disorder involves dysfunction of brain serotonin systems.

Pharmacologic treatment of this disorder is with antidepressants that are more selective for effects on the serotonin transmission system. These include clomipramine and SSRIs (fluvoxamine, fluoxetine, citalopram/escitalopram, paroxetine, and sertraline). Behavioral therapies and some forms of psychotherapy can also be helpful as primary or adjunctive therapy.

The Suicidal Patient

Emergency medicine physicians are often the first to deal with patients who have suicidal ideation or who have attempted or completed suicide. The recognition of risk factors for suicide, a thorough assessment of the psychiatric and medical factors, and urgent intervention are critically important. Although the patient who overdoses with a benzodiazepine may be very serious about the intent to die, the person who overdoses with acetaminophen is more at risk for serious medical complications.

Recognition of a suicidal gesture is essential in evaluating a patient in an emergency department. Although drug overdoses are the commonest form, alcohol intoxication, single-vehicle crashes, and falls from heights may merit further investigation. Many suicidal patients see a physician the week before the attempt. Risk factors to be aware of include recent psychiatric hospitalization, an older divorced or widowed man, unemployment, poor physical health, past suicide attempts, family history of suicide (especially a parent), psychosis, alcoholism, drug abuse, chronic pain syndrome, sudden life changes, loneliness, and the anniversary of a significant loss. More than 50% of completed suicide attempts involve guns; access to firearms should be assessed as part of a standard suicide risk assessment.

Psychopharmacology

Medication is rarely the sole treatment of a psychiatric disorder, but rather a component of a comprehensive treatment plan. Because psychoactive medications are used in various circumstances for many different indications, the major groups of these medications are discussed below in general terms. The choice of a medication usually is based on its adverse reaction profile and the clinical profile of the patient. There are many effective drugs in each major group, but they differ in terms of pharmacokinetics, adverse reactions, and available routes of administration.

Antidepressants: General Principles

First-generation antidepressants include tricyclic antidepressants (TCAs) and monoamine oxidase inhibitors (MAOIs). Newer-generation antidepressants are not easily grouped by their chemical structure or function; SSRIs are the most widely used of this group.

Although older-generation antidepressants are effective in treating depression, they are associated with adverse reactions that limit their use. TCAs are associated with orthostatic hypotension, anticholinergic adverse reactions, and altered cardiac conduction. MAOIs are effective antidepressants but require special dietary restrictions and attention to interactions with other medications to avoid a hypertensive crisis caused by unmetabolized tyramine.

Antidepressants can be useful in depression, panic disorder, obsessive-compulsive disorder, generalized anxiety disorder, social anxiety disorder, posttraumatic stress disorder, enuresis, bulimia, and attention-deficit/hyperactivity disorder, among others. TCAs and duloxetine can be beneficial for treating certain pain syndromes.

A complete trial of antidepressant medication consists of 4 to 6 weeks of therapeutic doses before refractoriness is considered. If improvement has occurred with the initial trial of the medication but the patient's condition has not returned to baseline, it may be appropriate to increase the dose of the medication, switch to another medication class, or augment by adding another medication. After clinical improvement has been noted, the medication may need to be used for an extended period.

Concerns about antidepressants potentially causing an increase in suicidal thoughts or behavior have resulted in the development of a black box warning for all antidepressants. This topic is controversial, since several studies have not corroborated this concern. The important clinical point to remember is that patients with depression should be assessed for suicidal thinking whether or not they are taking antidepressant medications.

Benzodiazepines

Benzodiazepines are used most appropriately to treat time-limited anxiety or insomnia related to an identifiable stress or change in sleep cycle. After long-term use (>2–3 months), therapy with benzodiazepines and related substances should be tapered rather than discontinued abruptly to avoid relapse, rebound, and withdrawal.

Relapse is the return of the original anxiety symptoms, often after weeks to months. *Rebound* is the intensification of the original symptoms, which usually last several days and appear within hours to days after abrupt cessation of drug use. *Withdrawal* includes autonomic and central nervous system symptoms that are different from the original presenting symptoms of the disorder.

Several benzodiazepines have metabolites with long half-lives, so smaller doses are needed in the elderly, patients with cognitive dysfunction, and children. These patient groups, especially patients with known brain damage, are prone to paradoxical reactions (anxiety, irritability, aggression, agitation, and insomnia).

Lithium

Lithium is used for bipolar disorder, for recurrent depression, and as an adjunct for depression treatment after ECT. Peak levels occur in 1 to 2 hours, and its half-life is about 24 hours; levels are generally checked 10 to 12 hours after the last dose and 4 to 5 days after a dose change. Common adverse reactions include resting tremor, diarrhea, polyuria, polydipsia, thirst, and nausea (lithium should be taken on a full stomach, or the extended-release form should be considered). Use in the first trimester of pregnancy is associated with a potential increase in the frequency of Ebstein anomaly, although this remains a rare event. Renal effects generally can be reversed with discontinued use of lithium; renal function should be followed. A hematologic effect can be benign leukocytosis. Hypothyroidism is common, and thyroid function should be monitored. Lithium can also affect parathyroid function.

Lithium has a narrow therapeutic index (typically 0.5–1.0 mEq/L), and toxicity (typically >1.5–3.5 mEq/L) can cause renal failure and death. Signs of toxicity include abdominal pain and vomiting, dry mouth, nystagmus and blurred vision, delirium, ataxia, hyperreflexia and fasciculations, and seizures.

Lithium levels are increased by angiotensin-converting enzyme inhibitors, thiazide diuretics, nonsteroidal anti-inflammatory drugs, dehydration, overheating or increased perspiration, and certain antibiotics (tetracycline, spectinomycin, and metronidazole). Levels can be decreased by caffeine and theophylline.

Electroconvulsive Therapy

ECT is the most effective treatment for severely depressed patients, especially those with psychotic features. It is also helpful in treating catatonia and mania and may be used in children and adults. ECT can be administered safely to pregnant women if fetal monitoring is available. A usual course of treatment is 6 to 12 sessions given over 2 to 4 weeks.

ECT no longer has any absolute contraindications, although it has several relative contraindications related to anesthesia risks, intracranial space-occupying lesions, and increased intracranial pressure. Before ECT is administered, the patient should be assessed for cardiovascular function, pulmonary function, electrolyte balance, neurologic status (eg, history of epilepsy), and previous experiences with anesthesia.

KEY FACTS

- ✓ A patient with posttraumatic stress disorder keeps reexperiencing the event, avoids reminders of it, and is easily startled and hypervigilant
- ✓ Obsessive-compulsive disorder is a combination of distressing thoughts, ideas, or impulses (obsessions) and repetitive, intentional behaviors performed in response to an obsession to neutralize anxiety (compulsions)
- ✓ Lithium has a number of common adverse reactions— resting tremor, diarrhea, polyuria, polydipsia, thirst, and nausea
- ✓ For severe depression, especially with psychotic features, the most effective treatment is electroconvulsive therapy

Psychotic and Somatic Symptom and Related Disorders

BRIAN A. PALMER, MD

Psychotic Disorders

Psychosis is a generic term used to describe altered thought and behavior in which the patient is incapable of interpreting his or her situation rationally and accurately. Psychotic symptoms can occur in various medical, neurologic, and psychiatric disorders. Many psychotic reactions seen in medical settings are associated with the use of recreational or prescription drugs. Some of these drug-induced psychotic reactions are nearly indistinguishable from schizophrenia in terms of hallucinations and paranoid delusions (eg, amphetamine and phencyclidine [PCP] psychoses).

Key Definition

Psychosis: *altered thought and behavior in which the patient is incapable of interpreting his or her situation rationally and accurately.*

When evaluating psychotic patients, exploring temporal relationships between illness, medication, and the onset of symptoms is often helpful in determining the cause. As an example, it would be unusual for schizophrenia to initially manifest in a 70-year-old patient; thus, psychotic symptoms that develop at this age likely have a metabolic, medical, or substance-induced cause. Many brain regions may be involved with the production of psychotic symptoms, but abnormalities in the frontal, temporal, and limbic regions are more likely than others to produce psychotic features.

Various disorders throughout a person's life may be associated with schizophrenia-like psychoses. Examples include genetic abnormalities (a microdeletion of chromosome 22, the velocardiofacial syndrome), childhood neurologic disorders (autism and epilepsy), adult neurologic disorders (narcolepsy), medical and metabolic diseases (infections, inflammatory disorders, endocrinopathies, nutritional deficiencies, uremia, and hepatic encephalopathy), drug abuse, and psychologic stressors.

Schizophrenia is a chronic psychotic illness that likely has many interrelated causes. Psychotic symptoms and altered interpersonal skills typically become evident initially in the teens and 20s, although sometimes initial presentations are seen in the late 30s or early 40s, particularly in women. Symptoms can be subdivided into positive (delusions and hallucinations) and negative (apathy and amotivation) symptoms. Diagnostic criteria include the presence of delusions and hallucinations; marked decrement in functional level in areas such as work, school, social relations, and self-care; and continuous signs of the disturbance for at least 6 months. Exclusion criteria include a consistent mood disorder component and evidence of medical cause for the symptoms. Suicide is seen in 5% of patients with schizophrenia, typically early in the illness.

Brief psychotic disorder describes a primary psychotic illness lasting less than 1 month; *schizophreniform disorder* is a primary psychotic illness lasting 1 to 6 months.

Antipsychotic Agents

The most simple and direct mechanism of action of antipsychotic agents involves blockade of postsynaptic dopamine receptors. Older agents are generally more potent dopamine blockers, with the "high-potency" neuroleptics (such as haloperidol) providing the most direct blockade and "low-potency" agents (such as chlorpromazine) more associated with anticholinergic and antiadrenergic effects. The antipsychotic effects of these agents result from their actions on the dopaminergic neurons of the limbic system, midbrain tegmentum, septal nuclei, and mesocortical dopaminergic projections. Blockade of other dopaminergic pathways is responsible for adverse reactions: nigrostriatal (motor activity) blockade leads to extrapyramidal symptoms; tubuloinfundibular (pituitary and hypothalamus) blockade can increase prolactin levels and cause changes in temperature and appetite regulation. Because they have less direct dopamine receptor blockade, atypical antipsychotic agents have a lower rate of extrapyramidal adverse reactions, although they can still occur.

Adverse Reactions

Several types of adverse reactions are common and important. They are described here, and their relationship to specific antipsychotic agents is reviewed in Table 68.1.

Acute dystonic reactions occur within hours or days after treatment is initiated with antipsychotic drugs. Dystonia is an uncontrollable tightening of muscles, such as the sternocleidomastoid muscle (causing a neck twisting, torticollis), the extraocular muscles (oculogyric crisis), or the laryngeal muscles (respiratory difficulties). Treatment is with parenteral administration of an anticholinergic agent (eg, diphenhydramine).

Akathisia is an unpleasant feeling of restlessness and the inability to sit still, which generally occurs within days of initiating or increasing an antipsychotic dose. Akathisia is sometimes mistaken for exacerbation of psychosis. Treatment consists of decreasing the dose of the antipsychotic agent (if possible) or using a β-blocking agent such as propranolol.

Table 68.1 • Review of Antipsychotic Agents

Drug	Toxic/Adverse Effects	Drug Interactions/Comments
Typical agents Chlorpromazine Fluphenazine Haloperidol Loxapine Mesoridazine Molindone Perphenazine Thioridazine Thiothixene Trifluoperazine	EPS—dystonia, pseudoparkinsonism, akathisia; TD, NMS (more with high-potency agents, eg, haloperidol) Anticholinergic effects, sedation, orthostatic hypotension (more with low-potency agents, eg, chlorpromazine) Galactorrhea, amenorrhea, gynecomastia, weight gain, sexual dysfunction Photosensitivity, risk of seizures Pigmentary retinopathy—thioridazine	Exercise caution in patients with QTc >450 ms and coadministration of other drugs that cause QTc prolongation Additive sedative effects with CNS depressants Decreased concentrations in presence of carbamazepine, barbiturates, cigarette smoking Increased concentrations in presence of quinidine, fluoxetine, paroxetine Antihypertensive agents may produce additive hypotensive effects Haloperidol and fluphenazine available as depot, long-acting injectables
Atypical agents[a] Aripiprazole Ziprasidone Asenapine Lurasidone Iloperidone Paliperidone Risperidone Quetiapine Olanzapine Clozapine	Increased risk of DM, weight gain, and elevated triglyceride levels—greatest with clozapine and olanzapine Increased mortality in patients with dementia treated for behavioral disorders Risk of EPS and elevated prolactin levels highest with risperidone and paliperidone (dose related) Anticholinergic effects greatest with clozapine and olanzapine Risk of orthostatic hypotension greatest with clozapine, risperidone, and quetiapine Sedative risks greatest with clozapine, olanzapine, and quetiapine Increased risk of seizures and myocarditis with clozapine (dose related) Mandatory WBC monitoring with clozapine (risk of agranulocytosis)	Less risk of EPS, TD, and prolactin effects than with typical agents All have lower levels when used concurrently with carbamazepine; additive orthostatic hypotension with trazodone Aripiprazole—unique mechanism with both dopamine antagonist and agonist activity Aripiprazole, risperidone—increased levels with paroxetine, fluoxetine, duloxetine Clozapine—increased risk of agranulocytosis with captopril, carbamazepine, sulfonamides Clozapine, olanzapine—increased levels with use of cimetidine, erythromycin, fluoroquinolones, fluoxetine, fluvoxamine; decreased levels with cigarette smoking Paliperidone—cytochrome P-450 interactions unlikely Quetiapine—increased levels with ketoconazole and nefazodone; decreased levels with phenytoin Risperidone, paliperidone, aripiprazole, and olanzapine available as depot, long-acting injectables

Abbreviations: CNS, central nervous system; DM, diabetes mellitus; EPS, extrapyramidal symptoms; NMS, neuroleptic malignant syndrome; QTc, corrected QT interval; TD, tardive dyskinesia; WBC, white blood cell count.

[a] In order of least weight gain to most weight gain.

KEY FACTS

✓ Clues to the cause of psychosis can often be found in the temporal relationships between illness, medication, and symptom onset

✓ Brief psychotic disorder and schizophreniform disorder both are primary psychotic illnesses, but the former lasts less than 1 month and the latter, 1 to 6 months

✓ Antipsychotic agents act most simply and directly by blocking postsynaptic dopamine receptors

✓ Acute dystonic reactions occur within hours or days after the start of antipsychotic drug therapy

✓ Akathisia generally occurs within days of starting or increasing an antipsychotic dose

Neuroleptic malignant syndrome is a potentially life-threatening disorder that may occur after the use of any antipsychotic agent, although it is more common with rapid increases in the dosage of high-potency antipsychotic agents. It is characterized by rigidity, fever, leukocytosis, tachycardia, tachypnea, diaphoresis, blood pressure fluctuations, and marked increase in creatine kinase levels because of muscle breakdown. Treatment consists of discontinuing use of the antipsychotic and providing life-support measures (ventilation and cooling). Pharmacologic interventions include dantrolene, a direct-acting muscle relaxant, or bromocriptine, a centrally acting dopamine agonist. Electroconvulsive therapy is effective.

Parkinsonian symptoms have a more gradual onset and can be treated with oral anticholinergic agents or decreased doses of an antipsychotic agent (or both).

Tardive dyskinesia has an incidence of 3% to 5% annually with first-generation neuroleptics and consists of involuntary movements of the face, trunk, or extremities. The most consistent risk factors for its development are long-term medication use (>6 months) and older age. It is best if treatment with the antipsychotic agent can be discontinued at an early sign of tardive dyskinesia, because the dyskinesia is sometimes reversible. Tardive dyskinesia is rarer with atypical antipsychotics.

Glucose intolerance, weight gain, and *electrophysiologic cardiac changes* have been associated with atypical antipsychotics. Additionally, several studies have shown a lack of efficacy for off-label use in patients with dementia, and safety concerns have arisen related to an increased risk of death among these patients.

Clozapine adverse reactions include seizures, orthostasis, and myocarditis. This atypical antipsychotic also has a 1% to 2% risk of producing agranulocytosis, which is reversible if use of the medication is discontinued immediately. Because of this serious potential reaction, a specific requirement of clozapine use is regular white blood cell counts (weekly for the first 6 months).

Somatic Symptom and Related Disorders

The most meaningful change in the *Diagnostic and Statistical Manual of Mental Disorders* (Fifth Edition) was in the area of somatic symptoms. Diagnoses of somatization disorder, hypochondriasis, pain disorder, and undifferentiated somatoform disorder have been removed, and many patients in whom 1 of those disorders was formerly diagnosed may now be considered to have a somatic symptom disorder. The major conceptual change was a move to descriptive focus that is less concerned with whether a medical cause is or is not known and is more concerned with the impact on functioning.

Somatic Symptom Disorder

Somatic symptom disorder involves somatic symptoms that are either very distressing or markedly disrupt functioning, as well as excessive and disproportionate thoughts, feelings, and behaviors associated with these symptoms. The symptoms may or may not be medically explained. As an example, dizziness may result in a somatic symptom disorder whether or not its cause is known; the focus is on the impact of and reaction to the symptom.

Some patients with heart disease or cancer will experience a normal adjustment to their condition—perhaps some anxiety about medical tests, mild sleep disruption, and worries about their family and future. Others will have a somatic symptom disorder, in which their concerns about their symptoms may make them unusually attuned to subtle somatic experiences, with associated thoughts (ruminative worry), feelings (such as terror), and behaviors (such as avoidance) that are clearly out of proportion to the somatic illness.

Many patients with somatic symptom disorder have multiple somatic symptoms, but some may have only 1 symptom, such as pain. Patients with somatic symptom disorder typically worry excessively and may misinterpret a physician's reassurance as not caring. Good practice, nonetheless, involves providing appropriate—neither excessive nor minimalist—testing for and treatment of medical illnesses. Once 1 medical cause of symptoms has been ruled out, repeating testing is unnecessary and may fuel the patient's problems. Because patients with somatic symptom disorder may seek care from multiple providers, unifying their medical care with a high level of coordination can be helpful.

Illness Anxiety Disorder

Illness anxiety disorder is a preoccupation with and fear of having or acquiring a serious disorder. Patients with illness anxiety may misinterpret body sensations such as borborygmi, heartbeats, or sweating. The disorder is diagnosed when a medical cause has been ruled out and anxiety and functional impairment persist for more than 6 months despite appropriate medical evaluation and reassurance. Patients may either seek frequent care or avoid care in response to their illness anxiety.

Key Definition

Illness anxiety disorder: *a preoccupation with and fear of having or acquiring a serious disorder.*

Conversion Disorder (Functional Neurologic Symptom Disorder)

Conversion disorder is a loss or alteration of neurologic functioning suggestive of a disorder that cannot be explained on the basis of known physiologic mechanisms. It is seen most often in the outpatient setting. One example is loss of vision despite intact visual pathways. Patients often respond to any of several therapeutic modalities that suggest hope of a cure. When conversion disorder becomes chronic, it carries a poorer prognosis and is difficult to treat.

Factitious Disorders

Factitious disorders are characterized by the *deliberate* production of signs or symptoms of disease. The diagnosis of these disorders requires that the physician maintain a high degree of awareness and look for objective data at variance with the patient's history (eg, surgical scars that are inconsistent with past surgical history). The more common form of factitious disorder generally occurs among socially conforming young women of a higher socioeconomic class who are intelligent, educated, and often work in a medically related field. The possibility of a coexisting medical disorder or intercurrent illness needs to be appreciated in the diagnostic and therapeutic management of these difficult cases. Factitious disorders are often found in patients with a history of childhood emotional traumas. The disorder may be imposed on oneself or on another (formerly called "by proxy").

KEY FACTS

✓ Neuroleptic malignant syndrome can occur with any antipsychotic but is more likely to follow rapid increase in dosage of high-potency agents

✓ Long-term antipsychotic use (>6 months) and older age increase the risk of tardive dyskinesia

✓ Somatic symptom disorder includes extremely distressing or disruptive somatic symptoms and associated excessive and disproportionate thoughts, feelings, and behaviors

✓ In factitious disorders, signs and symptoms are intentionally produced

69 Substance Use Disorders, Personality Disorders, and Eating Disorders

BRIAN A. PALMER, MD

Substance Use Disorders

Alcohol and other substance use disorders are a major concern in all age groups and across all ethnic, socioeconomic, and racial groups. Despite high lifetime prevalence (up to 20%), less than 10% of persons with substance use disorders are involved in treatment (either self-help groups or professional care).

Several pharmacologic agents are available to help diminish the craving for alcohol and other drugs or to deter relapse. Although several medications, including disulfiram, acamprosate, and naltrexone, may help prevent relapse, they are adjunctive and not a substitute for comprehensive psychosocial treatment.

A substance use disorder is diagnosed when the patient meets at least 2 of the following criteria (mild, 2 or 3 criteria; moderate, 4 or 5 criteria; severe, 6 or more criteria):

1. Using more of the substance or using over a longer period of time than originally intended
2. Unsuccessful efforts to control use or worries about cutting down or stopping
3. Large amounts of time obtaining, using, or recovering from the substance
4. Failure to meet obligations at home, work, or school
5. Giving up former interests
6. Craving the substance
7. Using despite mental or physical health consequences
8. Using despite relationship consequences
9. Recurrent use of the substance when dangerous (eg, while driving)
10. Developing **tolerance** (needing more of the substance for the same effect)
11. Experiencing withdrawal symptoms after stopping use

Key Definition

Tolerance: *needing more of the substance for the same effect.*

Alcohol Use Disorders

The CAGE questions (related to attempts to *c*ut down on alcohol use, other persons expressing *a*nnoyance, experiencing *g*uilt, and *e*arly-morning drinking) have excellent sensitivity and specificity for alcohol use disorders. *Alcohol withdrawal* can range from mild to quite severe, beginning with tachycardia, hypertension, diaphoresis, and tremors and progressing to withdrawal seizures or delirium tremens (or both).

Psychological functioning issues include impaired cognition and changes in mood and behavior. Interpersonal functioning issues include marital problems, child abuse, and impaired social relationships. Occupational functioning issues include academic, scholastic, or job problems. Legal, financial, and spiritual problems also occur.

Benzodiazepine, Sedative-Hypnotic, and Anxiolytic Use Disorders

Benzodiazepines, sedative-hypnotics, and anxiolytics are widely prescribed in many areas of medicine, so abuse and dependence often have an iatrogenic component. Five characteristics may help distinguish medical use from nonmedical use:

1. Intent: What is the purpose of the use?
2. Effect: What is the effect on the user's life?

3. Control: Is the use controlled by the user only, or does a physician share in the control?
4. Legality: Is the use of the drug legal or illegal? Medical drug use is legal.
5. Pattern: In what settings is the drug used?

Withdrawal of the use of benzodiazepines and barbiturates, in particular, may be serious because of the increased risk of withdrawal seizures; slowly tapered doses are indicated, particularly for long-term use.

Opioid Use Disorder

Opioids are prescribed and abused at historically high rates, despite the limited evidence for their use in most chronic pain conditions. Diversion is a common problem. Opioid withdrawal symptoms include diarrhea, dilated pupils, muscle aches or cramps, nausea, increased pulse rate and blood pressure, and piloerection (gooseflesh).

Personality Disorders

The 10 personality disorders are grouped into 3 clusters (Boxes 69.1 through 69.3).

Patients with borderline personality disorder (BPD) and other Cluster B disorders (antisocial, narcissistic, and histrionic) demand the most from internists. BPD is diagnosed with 9 criteria categorized as interpersonal (chaotic relationships, ideal and devalued; efforts to avoid abandonment), affective (lability, anger problems), self (identity confusion, emptiness), and behavioral (suicide attempts, self-injury, and impulsivity). The disorder is treatable and generally improves, despite common perceptions to the contrary. Internists can be most effective by practicing medicine within appropriate standards of care (holding limits

where necessary), clarifying the patient's experience, and working together in teams.

Eating Disorders

The 2 common eating disorders are *anorexia nervosa* and *bulimia*. Both are markedly more prevalent among women than men. Onset is usually in the teenage or young adult years. Eating disorders are increasingly found across all income, racial, and ethnic groups. Both disorders have a primary symptom of preoccupation with weight and distortion of body image. For example, the patient perceives herself to look less attractive than an observer would. The disorders are not mutually exclusive, and about 50% of

---

Box 69.2 • Personality Disorders, Cluster B (Dramatic, Emotional, or Erratic Character Structure)

Antisocial personality

  Diagnosed in adults who had conduct disorder before age 15 y, pervasive disregard for and violation of the rights of others

Borderline personality

  Instability of interpersonal relationships, self-image, and affects; marked impulsivity

Histrionic personality

  Excessive emotionality and attention-seeking

Narcissistic personality

  Grandiosity (fantasy or behavior), need for admiration, lack of empathy

Adapted from Oldham JM. Personality disorders: current perspectives. JAMA. 1994 Dec 14;272(22):1770–6. Used with permission.

Box 69.1 • Personality Disorders, Cluster A (Odd or Eccentric Character Structure)

Paranoid

  Distrust and suspiciousness, assumes malevolent motives

Schizoid personality

  Social detachment, restricted affect socially, neither needs nor wants social connection

Schizotypal personality

  Interpersonal deficits, difficulties with closeness, cognitive and perceptual disturbances (schizophrenia spectrum), behavioral eccentricities

Adapted from Oldham JM. Personality disorders: current perspectives. JAMA. 1994 Dec 14;272(22):1770–6. Used with permission.

Box 69.3 • Personality Disorders, Cluster C (Anxious or Fearful Character Structure)

Avoidant personality

  Social inhibition, feelings of inadequacy, hypersensitive to negative appraisal

Dependent personality

  Excessive need to be cared for; submissive/clinging behavior, fears separation

Obsessive-compulsive personality

  Orderliness, perfectionism, mental/interpersonal control; inflexible, lacks openness

Adapted from Oldham JM. Personality disorders: current perspectives. JAMA. 1994 Dec 14;272(22):1770–6. Used with permission.

patients with anorexia nervosa also have bulimia. Many patients with bulimia previously had at least a subclinical case of anorexia nervosa. Eating disorders have the highest lethality of all psychiatric illnesses.

Anorexia Nervosa

To meet the diagnostic criteria of anorexia nervosa, weight must be 15% below that expected for age and height. However, weight of 30% to 40% below normal is not uncommon and leads to the medical complications of starvation, such as depletion of fat, muscle wasting, bradycardia, arrhythmias, ventricular tachycardia and sudden death, constipation, abdominal pain, leukopenia, hypercortisolemia, and osteoporosis. Extreme cases are characterized by lanugo (fine hair on the body) and metabolic alterations to conserve energy. Thyroid effects include low levels of triiodothyronine (T_3), cold intolerance, and difficulty maintaining core body temperature. Reproductive effects include a pronounced decrease or cessation of the secretion of luteinizing hormone and follicle-stimulating hormone, often resulting in secondary amenorrhea. Reinitiation of nourishment requires careful monitoring and supplementation of potassium, magnesium, and phosphate levels to avoid refeeding syndrome.

Bulimia

Patients with bulimia often consume large quantities of food followed by purging. Physical complications of the binge-purge cycle may include fluid and electrolyte abnormalities, hypochloremic-hypokalemic metabolic alkalosis, esophageal and gastric irritation and bleeding, colonic abnormalities from laxative abuse, marked erosion of dental enamel with associated decay, parotid and salivary gland hypertrophy, and amylase levels 25% to 40% higher than normal. If bulimia is untreated, it often becomes chronic. Some patients have a gradual spontaneous remission of some symptoms.

KEY FACTS

✓ Available therapies for substance use disorders include pharmacologic agents to help diminish cravings and deter relapse

✓ The CAGE questions are a helpful diagnostic tool for alcohol use disorders, with excellent sensitivity and specificity

✓ Symptoms of alcohol withdrawal can range from mild to quite severe

✓ For diagnosis of anorexia nervosa, patients must weigh at least 15% less than normal

✓ The binge-purge cycle of bulimia may cause a variety of physical complications, from fluid and electrolyte abnormalities to erosion of dental enamel

Questions and Answers

Questions

Multiple Choice (choose the best answer)

XI.1. A 42-year-old woman presents to your office again after 16 years of intermittent, severe left lower quadrant abdominal pain. She reports having no weight loss, fever, or chills. The cause of her symptoms is not apparent from previous workups, which included a complete blood cell count, electrolyte evaluations, urinalysis, computed tomographic scan of the abdomen and pelvis, colonoscopy, and gynecologic examination. She has previously been thoroughly evaluated for episodic dizziness, headaches, flulike syndromes, back pain, and pain with intercourse. The results of all these workups were negative. What is the most likely diagnosis?

a. Conversion disorder
b. Somatization disorder
c. Hypochondriasis
d. Body dysmorphic disorder
e. Factitial disorder

XI.2. A 56-year-old man with a history of schizophrenia has a history of mild congestive heart failure and osteoarthritis. He harbors the paranoid belief that his wife is poisoning him, and he receives special messages from the television. These symptoms have been partially controlled with a second-generation antipsychotic, olanzapine 5 mg orally daily. You recommend increasing the olanzapine dosage to 10 mg daily. Which of the following is *false* about the use of olanzapine in this patient?

a. He is at increased risk for neuroleptic malignant syndrome.
b. He is at increased risk for parkinsonism.
c. He is at increased risk for tardive dyskinesia.
d. He is at increased risk for diabetes mellitus.
e. He is at increased risk for anorexia.

XI.3. A 19-year-old woman is brought to the emergency department by police after she was discovered alone on a rural bike trail dancing nude. "I am the lizard queen!" she joyfully proclaims. You learn that she has been acting quite erratically and sleeping poorly for the past week. Which of the following is the *least* likely diagnosis?

a. Major depression with psychotic features
b. Bipolar disorder
c. Substance dependence
d. Schizophrenia
e. Methamphetamine intoxication

XI.4. You contact the family of the patient in the previous question and learn that she has a strong family history of bipolar disorder. The family asks you questions about management of this patient. Which of the following would *not* be appropriate?

a. Hospitalize in a psychiatric unit.
b. Begin use of amitriptyline 50 mg orally.
c. Begin use of ziprasidone 20 mg orally.
d. Perform a urine drug screen.
e. Begin use of valproate sodium 1,000 mg orally.

Answers

XI.1. Answer b.

Somatization disorder is characterized by physical symptoms without an identifiable organic cause. Patients believe that they have a physical problem and are not consciously generating the symptoms or pretending to have them. Somatization disorder entails a history of multiple somatic complaints over many years, including 4 pain symptoms, 2 gastrointestinal tract symptoms, 1 sexual symptom, and 1 neurologic symptom. Conversion disorder is marked by a neurologic symptom, such as a motor or sensory deficit, and is unconscious in origin (unlike factitial disorder, in which the symptoms are consciously produced). Body dysmorphic disorder is characterized by a perception that a normally appearing body part is misshapen or otherwise has an abnormal appearance. Hypochondriasis is characterized by an irrational fear that one has an illness or serious disease.

XI.2. Answer e.

Second-generation antipsychotics are associated with hyperglycemia and an increased risk of diabetes mellitus. Similar to traditional neuroleptics, second-generation antipsychotics may cause extrapyramidal symptoms, tardive dyskinesia, and neuroleptic malignant syndrome. Olanzapine is not usually associated with anorexia.

XI.3. Answer a.

Although any of the disorders mentioned can cause psychosis and odd behavior, major depression is unlikely. Patients who have major depression with psychotic features would be unlikely to appear animated and joyful; more often, they have ego-dystonic (very unpleasant) delusions, such as a belief that their family hates them or that people are conspiring against them.

XI.4. Answer b.

With this patient's age, behavior, and family history, bipolar disorder is high in the differential diagnosis. Antidepressants, especially tricyclics, would be contraindicated because they can induce or prolong mania. With the severity of her symptoms and her poor judgment, she poses a danger to herself, so hospitalization is necessary. Ziprasidone or valproate sodium is a reasonable initial option to manage her symptom of mood elevation. Substance-induced psychosis or mania is high in the differential diagnosis; thus, a drug screen would be important in the evaluation of this patient.

Pulmonology

Section
XII

70

Critical Care Medicine

CASSIE C. KENNEDY, MD

Respiratory Critical Care

Effective functioning of the respiratory system requires 1) normal central nervous system control, 2) intact neuromuscular transmission and bellows function, 3) patent airways, and 4) normal gas exchange at the alveolar-capillary level. Respiratory failure may be caused by dysfunction at any of these levels, resulting in failure of oxygenation (*hypoxemic respiratory failure*) or ventilation (*hypercapnic respiratory failure*).

Hypoxemic Respiratory Failure

Hypoxemic respiratory failure is typically defined as an arterial oxygen tension of less than 60 mm Hg. The cause of hypoxemic respiratory failure can be further delineated by patient history and by calculation of the alveolar-arterial (A-a) gradient. The A-a gradient reflects the difference between the alveolar and arterial concentrations of oxygen and is calculated as follows:

$$\text{A-a Gradient} = [\text{F}_{\text{IO}_2} \times (\text{P}_{\text{ATM}} - \text{P}_{\text{H}_2\text{O}}) - (\text{Pa}_{\text{CO}_2}/0.8)] - \text{Pa}_{\text{O}_2},$$

where F_{IO_2} is the fraction of inspired oxygen, P_{ATM} is sea level atmospheric pressure (760 mm Hg), and $\text{P}_{\text{H}_2\text{O}}$ is the partial pressure of water vapor (47 mm Hg). Normally, the A-a gradient is less than 10 mm Hg in a young adult; it increases by 10 mm Hg every decade thereafter.

> ### Key Definition
>
> **Hypoxemic respiratory failure:** *arterial oxygen tension <60 mm Hg.*

Hypoxemia may result from processes with either a normal or an abnormal A-a gradient. Hypoxemia with a normal A-a gradient can be caused by a decrease in the inspired P_{O_2} (eg, altitude) or hypoventilation (eg, narcotic use). Hypoxemia with an abnormal A-a gradient can be caused by decreased diffusion (eg, idiopathic pulmonary fibrosis), ventilation-perfusion ratio ($\dot{\text{V}}/\dot{\text{Q}}$) mismatch, or shunt. $\dot{\text{V}}/\dot{\text{Q}}$ mismatch occurs with inadequate ventilation or inadequate perfusion (eg, chronic obstructive pulmonary disease) and responds to supplemental oxygen. Shunting occurs when alveoli are bypassed—called an anatomical shunt (eg, an intracardiac shunt)—or when nonventilated lung is perfused—called a physiologic shunt (eg, as in acute respiratory distress syndrome [ARDS]). A shunt typically does not respond to supplemental oxygen, but a physiologic shunt often responds to recruitment of nonventilated alveoli with positive end-expiratory pressure (PEEP).

Hypercapnic Respiratory Failure

Hypercapnic respiratory failure is caused by inadequate alveolar ventilation that is generally the result of airway obstruction, increased dead space ventilation, or decreased minute ventilation (decreased rate, depth, or drive of breathing) compared to demand (eg, overdose or neuromuscular weakness). **Physiologic dead space** is the portion of a breath that is not involved in gas exchange (ie, in the hypopharynx, trachea, and conducting airways). The amount of dead space increases with several disease states (eg, chronic obstructive pulmonary disease [COPD]).

> ### Key Definition
>
> **Physiologic dead space:** *the portion of a breath that is not involved in gas exchange (ie, in the hypopharynx, trachea, and conducting airways).*

Management of Respiratory Failure

Noninvasive Ventilation

Continuous positive airway pressure (CPAP) machines help alleviate obstruction in obstructive sleep apnea and relieve pulmonary edema and hypoxia in congestive heart failure. Noninvasive ventilation with a bilevel positive airway pressure (BiPAP) machine allows for positive pressure ventilation without endotracheal intubation. The typical indication is treatment of hypercapnic respiratory failure in COPD exacerbation. Contraindications to noninvasive ventilation include high aspiration risk, copious secretions, facial trauma, unstable airway patency, and cardiac or respiratory arrest.

Failure of Airway Patency

Failure of airway patency can occur in cases of obstruction or loss of normal gag and cough reflexes (eg, in a person with a decreased mental status). Patients who have lost airway patency or who could lose it (eg, burn victims with inhalation injury) should undergo endotracheal intubation for airway protection.

Endotracheal Intubation

Endotracheal intubation allows maximal control of the airway, enables delivery of specific inspired oxygen concentrations and positive pressure ventilation, and provides protection from aspiration. Indications for intubation include loss of airway patency or threat of loss, sedation with loss of normal control of ventilation, and respiratory failure requiring mechanical ventilation. Complications of intubation include vomiting and aspiration, hypoxemia or hypotension during the procedure, inadvertent intubation of the esophagus, complications from administered medications (eg, succinylcholine causing hyperkalemia), or an intubation attempt leading to an inability to intubate or ventilate (ie, failed airway management).

Mechanical Ventilation

Patients who require mechanical ventilation usually meet the criteria for ventilator support (Table 70.1). The goals of mechanical ventilation are to 1) correct hypoxia, 2) support or improve ventilation, 3) decrease the work of breathing, and 4) support lung injury healing.

Setting the Ventilator

Oxygen Delivery

Oxygen flow is typically set at the lowest fraction of inspired oxygen (F_{IO_2}) that will keep the oxygen saturation at about 90%. Too much oxygen can lead to damage due to oxygen toxicity.

Rate of Ventilation

The respiratory rate multiplied by the tidal volume (V_T) is the *minute ventilation*. If a patient is hypercapnic, an increase in minute ventilation is necessary to correct the

Table 70.1 • Typical Physiologic Criteria for Mechanical Ventilator Support

Variable	Value
Respiratory rate, breaths/min	>25–30
Minute ventilation, L/min	>10–15
Maximal inspiratory pressure (force), cm H_2O	<20
Vital capacity, mL/kg	<10
Pa_{O_2}, mm Hg	<60 when F_{IO_2} >0.60
Pa_{O_2}/F_{IO_2}	<200
$PA_{O_2} - Pa_{O_2}$, mm Hg	>300 with F_{IO_2} =1.00
V_{DS}/V_T	>0.60
pH	<7.20 (with a predominant respiratory component)

Abbreviations: F_{IO_2}, fraction of inspired oxygen; $PA_{O_2} - Pa_{O_2}$, alveolar-arterial gradient in partial pressure of oxygen; V_{DS}, dead space volume; V_T, tidal volume.

problem. Increases in the set respiratory rate can lead to insufficient time to exhale the full breath before initiation of the next breath (typically when the respiratory rate exceeds 30–35 breaths/min, but it can occur at lower rates in obstructive lung disease). This can lead to increased intrathoracic pressure (called intrinsic PEEP or auto-PEEP) and hemodynamic instability. Conversely, increasing the V_T can lead to volutrauma, especially in lung injury; typically, the ideal V_T is 6 mL/kg ideal body weight in diagnoses such as ARDS. If neither respiratory rate nor V_T can be safely increased, clinicians sometimes tolerate hypercapnia, especially if it is mild (termed *permissive hypercapnia*).

Positive End-Expiratory Pressure

PEEP is intended to increase functional residual capacity, recruit partially collapsed alveoli, improve lung compliance, and improve $\dot{V}/\dot{Q}$ matching. It decreases atelectrauma (recruitment and derecruitment of alveoli). An adverse effect of PEEP is an excessive increase in intrathoracic pressure with decreased cardiac output. Overdistention of lung units may also worsen gas exchange because of ventilator-induced lung injury. At levels of PEEP greater than 10 to 15 cm H_2O, barotrauma is a concern. The optimal PEEP may be defined as the lowest level of PEEP needed to achieve satisfactory oxygen delivery at a nontoxic F_{IO_2} (<0.60).

Mode of Ventilation

The presence or absence of a set ventilator rate, the control (or set upper limit) of either the pressure or the V_T, and the percentage of machine-controlled breaths determine the *mode* of ventilation (Table 70.2). Patients can have all their breaths predetermined (assist-control mode), some of their breaths predetermined (synchronized intermittent

Table 70.2 • Basic Ventilator Modes and Settings

Mode	Description or Mechanism
Volume Control Modes	
A/C, also called CMV	Active inhalation VT is delivered up to a volume threshold and not a pressure threshold Exhalation is passive; after the VT is delivered, the machine releases and exhalation is driven by chest wall and lung elastance (recoil) Patient initiates the respiratory cycle (unless apneic or paralyzed) Machine senses inspiratory effort and then delivers machine-defined VT for every breath Does not allow patient to breathe spontaneously (ie, patient-defined VT) Machine rate (eg, CMV = 8 breaths/min) defines the minimum number of VT breaths per minute that a patient will receive A patient who initiates more breaths per minute than the defined rate will receive those breaths at the machine-defined VT
SIMV	Active inhalation VT is delivered up to a volume threshold and not a pressure threshold Exhalation is passive; after the VT is delivered, the machine releases and exhalation is driven by chest wall and lung elastance (recoil) Patient initiates the respiratory cycle (unless apneic or paralyzed) Machine senses inspiratory effort and then delivers machine-defined VT for only the rate of machine breaths Machine rate (eg, SIMV = 8 breaths/min) defines the actual number of VT breaths per minute that a patient will receive A patient who initiates more breaths per minute than the defined rate will receive those breaths at the patient-defined VT (ie, the VT of the spontaneous breaths can be different from the VT of the machine breaths)
PCV	Can be used with either CMV or SIMV modes Active inhalation VT is delivered up to a pressure threshold and not a volume threshold Exhalation is passive; after the VT is delivered, the machine releases and exhalation is driven by chest wall and lung elastance (recoil) Patient initiates the respiratory cycle (unless apneic or paralyzed)
Additional Support Modes	
CPAP	This is a spontaneous breathing mode (ie, VT and rate are not provided by the mechanical ventilator) Continuous positive pressure is delivered while a patient breathes spontaneously This pressure is continuous, meaning that both inspiratory and expiratory phases of respiration are supplemented with positive pressure CPAP may be delivered invasively (ie, through an endotracheal tube) or noninvasively (ie, with a tightly fitting mask or with high–gas flow nasal prongs)
PSV	PSV augments spontaneous breaths with a machine-defined amount of positive pressure that is delivered only during inspiration The purpose of PSV mode is to improve patient-machine synchrony (comfort) and to decrease the patient work of breathing; in some patients this may facilitate weaning from mechanical ventilation PSV inspiratory positive flow continues while the patient inhales and then stops when the patient's flow decreases to less than a threshold value (usually <25% of the initial inspiratory flow rate) Patients determine their spontaneous VT during PSV breaths by controlling their flow rate. When they have had enough, they simply stop inspiring
Initial Invasive Mechanical Ventilation Settings	
Mode	As indicated: CMV, SIMV, PSV, CPAP
Tidal volume	Standard: approximately 8 mL/kg ideal body weight ARDS: 6 mL/kg ideal body weight
Rate	Titrate to desired VM for P_{CO_2}, PEEP, and TI
F_{IO_2}	Maintain P_{O_2} > target value (usually 60 mm Hg)
TI	Set to meet patient demand Allow adequate time for exhalation
PEEP	As indicated; maintain lower values unless needed for ARDS Do not use as a prevention maneuver for atelectasis

Abbreviations: A/C, assist/control; ARDS, acute respiratory distress syndrome; CMV, controlled mechanical ventilation; CPAP, continuous positive airway pressure; F_{IO_2}, fraction of inspired oxygen; PCV, pressure control ventilation; PEEP, positive end-expiratory pressure; PSV, pressure support ventilation; SIMV, synchronized intermittent mandatory ventilation; TI, inspiratory time; VM, minute ventilation; VT, tidal volume.

mandatory ventilation mode), or none of their breaths pre-determined (spontaneous mode).

In *assist control mode*, physicians control all breaths and choose between either a preset volume (ie, volume-controlled ventilation) or a preset pressure limit (ie, pressure-controlled ventilation). In *pressure support mode* (also called CPAP mode), patients determine the rate of breathing; however, the physician can adjust the amount of pressure support from the ventilator to increase the depth or size of breath or to decrease the work of breathing. This mode is typically used during weaning. In *intermittent mandatory ventilation mode*, patients must take a physician-determined number of preset breaths with preset parameters such as a fixed volume. Between these preset breaths, the patient may breathe spontaneously, typically with a set pressure to decrease the work of breathing.

KEY FACTS

✓ Requirements for effective respiratory system—
- normal central nervous system control
- intact neuromuscular transmission and bellows function
- patent airways
- normal gas exchange at the alveolar-capillary level

✓ Causes of hypercapnic respiratory failure (from inadequate alveolar ventilation)—
- airway obstruction
- increased dead space ventilation
- decreased minute ventilation compared to demand

✓ CPAP machine—
- relieves obstruction in obstructive sleep apnea
- relieves pulmonary edema and hypoxia in congestive heart failure

✓ Indications for intubation—
- loss of airway patency (or threat of loss)
- sedation with loss of normal control of ventilation
- respiratory failure requiring mechanical ventilation

✓ Minute Ventilation = Respiratory Rate × Tidal Volume

✓ PEEP—
- increases functional residual capacity
- recruits partially collapsed alveoli
- improves lung compliance
- improves $\dot{V}/\dot{Q}$ matching

Mechanical Ventilation Concerns

Ventilator-Associated Pneumonia

Ventilator-associated pneumonia (VAP) is a serious, potentially preventable complication of mechanical ventilation. Mortality can be decreased with the use of a VAP bundle

---

Box 70.1 • IHI Ventilator Bundle

Elevation of the head of the bed (to 30°)

Daily cessation of sedation and assessment of readiness for extubation

Peptic ulcer disease prophylaxis

Deep vein thrombosis prophylaxis

Daily oral care with chlorhexidine

Abbreviation: IHI, Institute for Healthcare Improvement.

---

for VAP prevention, as recommended by the Institute for Healthcare Improvement (IHI) (Box 70.1).

Intrinsic PEEP

Intrinsic PEEP (also called auto-PEEP), is an important complication of positive pressure ventilation. Inadequate time during the expiratory phase of the respiratory cycle results in a new machine breath being delivered before the previous breath is completely exhaled. This may worsen hyperinflation, increase intrathoracic pressure, reduce venous return, and worsen associated complications (eg, barotrauma). Intrinsic PEEP may occur in spontaneously breathing patients with obstructive airway disease, but the effect is most important in mechanically ventilated patients. Immediate intervention in a ventilated patient with hemodynamic instability due to intrinsic PEEP includes temporary disconnection of the ventilator circuit to allow the patient to exhale and thus correct the hyperinflation. Subsequent treatment typically involves optimizing bronchodilator therapy and altering the ventilator cycle to allow optimal expiratory time.

Prolonged Intubation and Tracheostomy

Prolonged invasive mechanical ventilation increases the risk of tracheal injury and stenosis, bleeding, tracheoesophageal fistula, and, possibly, increased bronchial or pulmonary infections. For patients who require prolonged mechanical ventilation or airway support, the timing of tracheostomy is controversial. Tracheostomy is commonly considered for patients who have needed or are expected to need intubation and mechanical ventilation for more than 2 to 4 weeks. Tracheostomy has the advantages of decreased laryngeal injury, increased patient comfort, ease of suctioning, and, in certain patients, allowance for oral ingestion and speech.

Endotracheal Tube Problems

Ventilators can measure peak pressures and plateau pressures, and both should be monitored carefully. A high peak pressure alarm in the absence of a high plateau pressure often indicates a problem in the endotracheal tube (eg, mucous plugging, kinking of the tube, or biting of the tube).

The plateau pressure should be maintained at less than 30 cm H_2O to avoid barotrauma. An elevated plateau pressure can reflect abdominal distention (eg, abdominal compartment syndrome) or poor lung compliance (eg, pneumothorax, pneumonia, or pulmonary edema). The underlying cause should be treated (eg, surgery for abdominal compartment syndrome or decompression for pneumothorax). If worsening lung compliance due to underlying lung parenchymal process is the problem, the ventilator settings should be adjusted to decrease the plateau pressure (eg, decrease tidal volume).

Weaning From Mechanical Ventilation

Patients are candidates for weaning (ie, liberation) from mechanical ventilation when they are hemodynamically stable, the underlying pathophysiologic processes (both pulmonary and nonpulmonary) are resolving, and they have adequately recovered from respiratory failure. The most effective and consistent way to wean patients is to use a protocol that involves a nurse or respiratory therapist. Patients receiving mechanical ventilation should have a daily interruption of sedation with a spontaneous breathing trial. This can be done by disconnecting the patient from the ventilator circuit (a T-piece system) or by reducing support to spontaneous mode with a low-pressure support setting (typically, 5 cm H_2O) for 30 minutes to 2 hours. A weaning protocol is presented in Figure 70.1.

Acute Respiratory Distress Syndrome

ARDS is diffuse lung injury that causes acute hypoxic respiratory failure (in <1 week) with bilateral opacities that are not otherwise explained and respiratory failure that is not caused by cardiac failure or volume overload. When PEEP is set at 5 cm H_2O or more, ARDS is described as *mild* (Pao_2:Fio_2 ratio >200 cm H_2O but ≤300 cm H_2O), *moderate* (Pao_2:Fio_2 ratio >100 cm H_2O but ≤200 cm H_2O), or *severe* (Pao_2:Fio_2 ratio ≤100 cm H_2O). Mortality from ARDS has averaged about 43%, with recent studies suggesting a decreasing mortality rate over time. Several conditions are associated with ARDS (Table 70.3).

> **Key Definition**
>
> Acute respiratory distress syndrome: *acute (<1 week), diffuse lung injury that causes hypoxic respiratory failure that is not caused by cardiac failure or volume overload and is accompanied by bilateral opacities that are otherwise unexplained.*

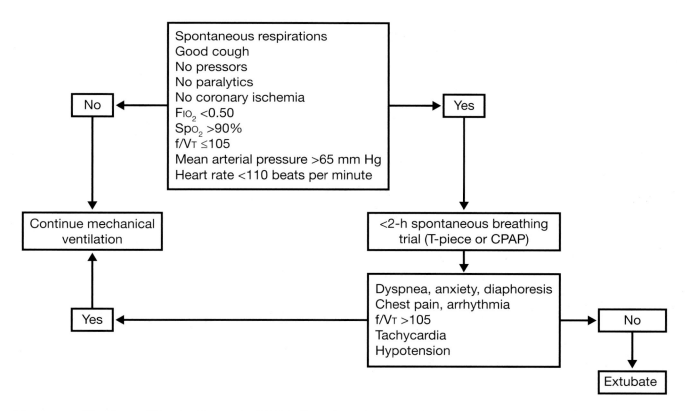

Figure 70.1 *Ventilatory Weaning Protocol. CPAP indicates continuous positive airway pressure; Fio_2, fraction of inspired oxygen; f/V_T, respiratory frequency divided by tidal volume (rapid shallow breathing index); Spo_2, arterial oxygen saturation.*

Table 70.3 • Conditions Associated With Acute Respiratory Distress Syndrome (ARDS)[a]

Disorder or Type of Disorder	Cause
Shock	Any cause
Sepsis	Lung infections, other bacteremic or endotoxic states
Trauma	Head injury, lung contusion, fat embolism
Aspiration	Gastric, near-drowning, tube feedings
Hematologic	*Transfusions,* leukoagglutinin, *disseminated intravascular coagulation,* thrombotic thrombocytopenic purpura
Metabolic	Pancreatitis, uremia
Drug-related	Narcotics, barbiturates, aspirin
Toxic	Inhaled—oxygen, smoke Chemicals—paraquat Irritant gases—nitrogen dioxide, chlorine, sulfur dioxide, ammonia
Miscellaneous	Radiation, air embolism, high altitude

[a] Terms in italics indicate disorders and causes most commonly associated with ARDS.

Treatment involves mechanical ventilation strategies (ie, lung-protective ventilatory strategies) that allow for lung healing. These strategies include maintaining a tidal volume of 6 mL/kg (based on ideal body weight) and maintaining plateau airway pressures at less than 30 cm H_2O. Because ARDS patients have a physiologic shunt, hypoxemia is treated with incremental PEEP levels to increase and maintain alveolar recruitment and prevent alveolar derecruitment. In addition, prone positioning has been used to open flooded dependent alveoli and improve $\dot{V}/\dot{Q}$ matching and oxygenation, with a resultant improvement in mortality. Evidence also supports the use of paralytic medication for 48 hours in patients with severe ARDS, although with concerns of critical illness polyneuropathy, practitioners may be more selective with implementation. A conservative fluid strategy to maintain adequate systemic perfusion is preferred. Throughout the course of critical illness, acute and chronic supplemental nutrition (enteral feeding) is recommended if tolerated. Patient mobilization with ambulation and weaning from the ventilator are also initiated as soon as possible for all patients with ARDS.

The use of corticosteroids in patients with ARDS is controversial. Nitric oxide and other vasodilating agents provide short-term improvement in oxygenation but no mortality benefit for patients with ARDS. High-frequency oscillator ventilators were not effective in reducing mortality in clinical trials. Data are emerging on the use of extracorporeal membrane oxygenation (ECMO) in patients with ARDS; however, consensus has not been reached on its application.

Shock

Shock is defined as the inadequate provision of oxygen and metabolic substrate to the tissues. Oxygen delivery is expressed as the product of cardiac output and arterial oxygen concentration:

$$Do_2 = CO \times [(Hb \times 1.39 \times Sao_2) + (Pao_2 \times 0.003)],$$

where Do_2 is delivery of oxygen, CO is cardiac output, Hb is hemoglobin, Sao_2 is arterial saturation of hemoglobin with oxygen, and Pao_2 is arterial oxygen tension. Early recognition and treatment of hypoperfusion can decrease the ensuing inflammatory response to shock (Figure 70.2). Shock should be recognized as a state of hypoperfusion usually associated with hypotension. Signs of shock include tachycardia, tachypnea, hypotension, oliguria, altered mental status, metabolic acidosis, and abnormal renal or liver function.

> **Key Definition**
>
> Shock: *inadequate provision of oxygen and metabolic substrate to tissues.*

Initial assessment is aimed at determining the cause of shock. The following classification system is widely used: 1) hypovolemic (eg, hemorrhage), 2) distributive (eg, anaphylaxis), 3) cardiogenic (eg, myocardial infarction), and 4) obstructive (eg, cardiac tamponade) (Table 70.4).

Hemodynamic Assessment

The use of pulmonary arterial catheters in critically ill patients has decreased since a landmark study showed that the harm exceeded the benefits.

Central Line Placement

The indications for central venous access are lack of adequate peripheral veins, need for medications or solutions that are hypertonic or phlebitic, need for long-term access,

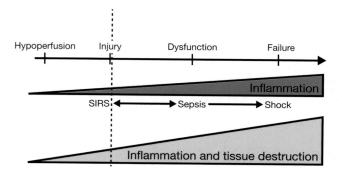

Figure 70.2 *Shock: Time Matters. SIRS indicates systemic inflammatory response syndrome.*

Table 70.4 • Classification of Shock[a]

Shock Type	Preload (Central Venous Pressure)	Wedge Pressure	Systemic Vascular Resistance	Cardiac Output	Examples of Causes
Hypovolemic (hemorrhagic)	↓	↓	↑	↓	Bleeding Vomiting, diarrhea Diuretic use (excess) Burns, exudative skin lesions Diabetes insipidus
Distributive	↔	↔	↓	↑	Sepsis Liver disease Anaphylaxis Thiamine deficiency Spinal cord injury (neurogenic shock)
Cardiogenic	↑↔	↑	↑	↓	Pump failure (right- or left-sided) Acute coronary syndrome Acute mitral regurgitation
Obstructive Tamponade (equalization of pressures)	↔	↔	↔	↔	Cardiac tamponade

[a] Arrows indicate increase (↑), decrease (↓), or no change (↔).

need for measuring central pressures, and access for procedures (hemodialysis and cardiac pacing). The most common locations for central access are the internal jugular, subclavian, and femoral veins.

Relative contraindications include procedural inexperience of the practitioner, significant coagulopathy, inability to identify landmarks, infection or burn at the entry site, and thrombosis of the proposed central venous site. At most institutions, central venous catheters are now inserted with the help of direct ultrasonographic visualization.

Complications of central venous catheterization include bloodstream infections, cardiac arrhythmias, pneumothorax, air embolism, vascular injury, catheter or guidewire embolism, catheter knotting, bleeding, and other potential complications of needle or catheter misplacement.

The IHI has identified prevention of catheter-related bloodstream infections (CR-BSIs) with use of the IHI Central Line Bundle as a key element in improving patient outcomes and preventing morbidity. The key components of the Central Line Bundle are 1) hand hygiene; 2) maximal barrier precautions upon insertion; 3) chlorhexidine skin antisepsis; 4) optimal catheter site selection, with avoidance of the femoral vein for central venous access in adult patients; and 5) daily review of line necessity, with prompt removal of unnecessary lines. CR-BSIs are usually attributed to the migration of bacteria from the skin along the catheter tract. *CR-BSI* is usually defined as more than 15 colony-forming units/mL on semiquantitative culture of the catheter tip. *Catheter-related bacteremia* is defined as bacterial growth and blood cultures that are positive for

KEY FACTS

✓ Criteria for weaning from mechanical ventilation—
- patient is hemodynamically stable
- patient's underlying pathophysiologic processes are resolving
- patient has adequately recovered from respiratory failure

✓ ARDS—use of corticosteroids for treatment is controversial

✓ Indications for central venous access—
- lack of adequate peripheral veins
- need for medications or solutions that are hypertonic or phlebitic
- need for long-term access
- need for measuring central pressures
- access for procedures (hemodialysis and cardiac pacing)

✓ Key components of the IHI Central Line Bundle for preventing CR-BSIs—
- hand hygiene
- maximal barrier precautions upon insertion
- chlorhexidine skin antisepsis
- optimal catheter site selection (with avoidance of femoral vein in adults)
- daily review of line necessity (with prompt removal of unnecessary lines)

the same organism as on the catheter tip. Risk factors include infected catheter site or cutaneous breakdown, multiple manipulations, the number of catheter lumens, and the duration of use of the same site (particularly after 3 or 4 days). Treatment of CR-BSIs should include catheter removal and replacement at another site if necessary.

Sepsis

Sepsis is an exaggerated inflammatory response to a noxious (infectious) stimulus and is characterized by a severe catabolic reaction, widespread endothelial dysfunction, and release of innate inflammatory response components. To achieve a common terminology, *systemic inflammatory response syndrome* (SIRS) was introduced for findings of fever or hypothermia, tachycardia, tachypnea, and leukocytosis or leukopenia regardless of cause. Not all cases of SIRS are caused by infection. *Sepsis* is defined as SIRS with a known or presumed source of infection, and *severe sepsis* is defined as sepsis associated with organ system dysfunction and systemic effects, including hypotension, decreased urine output, or metabolic acidosis. *Septic shock* refers to persistent signs of organ hypoperfusion despite adequate fluid resuscitation.

Severe Sepsis and Septic Shock Treatment

The Surviving Sepsis Campaign 2012 includes treatment guidelines for severe sepsis and septic shock (Box 70.2).

KEY FACTS

✓ Sepsis is an exaggerated inflammatory response to a noxious (infectious) stimulus and is characterized by several features—

- a severe catabolic reaction
- widespread endothelial dysfunction
- release of innate inflammatory response components

✓ SIRS—fever or hypothermia, tachycardia, tachypnea, and leukocytosis or leukopenia regardless of cause

✓ Sepsis—SIRS with a known or presumed source of infection

✓ Severe sepsis—associated with organ system dysfunction and systemic effects (hypotension, decreased urine output, or metabolic acidosis)

✓ Septic shock—persistent signs of organ hypoperfusion despite adequate fluid resuscitation

---

Hemorrhagic Shock

As with sepsis, underresuscitation for shock and hypoperfusion is a common shortfall in the management of intensive care unit (ICU) patients who have clinically significant

---

Box 70.2 • Treatment Guidelines for Severe Sepsis and Septic Shock From the Surviving Sepsis Campaign 2012

1. Start blood cultures before antibiotics
2. Perform studies as indicated for source identification
3. Administer appropriate antibiotics early (within 1 h after recognition of sepsis)
4. De-escalate antibiotic therapy when appropriate
5. Control the source of the infection (insert drains if indicated)
6. Administer an initial fluid challenge of 30 mL/kg of crystalloids
7. Administer norepinephrine as the first-choice vasopressor to maintain mean arterial pressure ≥65 mm Hg (vasopressin or epinephrine is an additional choice)
8. Infuse dobutamine if patient has myocardial dysfunction or signs of hypoperfusion despite adequate volume and mean arterial pressure
9. The goal hemoglobin level should be 7–9 g/dL unless myocardial ischemia, bleeding, or tissue hypoperfusion is present
10. Administer intravenous hydrocortisone in patients who have refractory shock after receiving fluid and vasopressor therapy
11. Manage ARDS as above when ARDS is present
12. Maintain the blood glucose level ≤180 mg/dL
13. Provide appropriate ICU peptic ulcer disease and deep vein thrombosis prophylaxis

Abbreviations: ARDS, acute respiratory distress syndrome; ICU, intensive care unit.

Data from Dellinger RP, Levy MM, Rhodes A, Annane D, Gerlach H, Opal SM, et al; Surviving Sepsis Campaign Guidelines Committee including the Pediatric Subgroup. Surviving sepsis campaign: international guidelines for management of severe sepsis and septic shock: 2012. Crit Care Med. 2013 Feb;41(2):580–637. Used with permission.

---

hemorrhage. When significant blood loss is suspected, the focus should immediately shift to the assessment of perfusion status. Determine whether the patient has shock, either overt or cryptic. Do not exclusively use hemoglobin and hematocrit as quantitative markers of blood loss and determinants of shock. As with other forms of shock, assess factors such as capillary refill time, urine output, presence or absence of altered sensorium, and lactate level and presence of metabolic acidosis. These are nonspecific but valuable indicators that help evaluate how sick the patient is and how aggressive the resuscitation must be.

Blood loss can be classified according to clinical findings (Table 70.5). Identification of the source of hemorrhage is important, but resuscitation has the highest priority. Patients in the ICU are also at risk for acquired bleeding

Table 70.5 • Classification of Blood Loss

Feature	Class			
	I	**II**	**III**	**IV**
Blood loss, mL	<750	750–1,500	1,500–2,000	>2,000
Blood pressure	No change	Systolic: no change Diastolic: increased	Decreased	Hypotension (possibly severe)
Pulse, beats per minute	100	100–120	>120 (thready)	>120–140 (very thready)
Respiratory rate	Normal	Increased	Increased	Increased
Sensorium	Alert, thirsty	Anxious	Anxious or drowsy	Drowsy or obtunded
Urine output	Normal	Decreased	Oliguria	Oliguria or anuria

disorders, especially thrombocytopenia. Patients with thrombocytopenia in the ICU should undergo screening for heparin-induced thrombocytopenia and disseminated intravascular coagulation.

For all patients with clinically significant hemorrhage, several considerations should be addressed on arrival (Box 70.3). These considerations, by various mechanisms, can directly influence the initial diagnosis and management of patients with hemorrhagic shock (Box 70.4).

Upper Gastrointestinal Tract Bleeding

Patients with upper gastrointestinal tract bleeding typically present with hematemesis or melena. Patients should be evaluated as described above with priority given to resuscitation as indicated. Endoscopy should be performed

---

Box 70.3 • Considerations to Address for a Patient With Significant Hemorrhage

Presence of shock

Presence of coagulopathy or thrombocytopenia

Presence of hypothermia

Use of medications that exacerbate bleeding, inhibit clotting, or affect platelets (and consideration for discontinuation or reversal if applicable)

Active alcohol ingestion (for gastrointestinal tract bleeding)

Active comorbidities that worsen the outcome

Prior history of hemorrhage that required admission to an intensive care unit

Presence of severe liver disease (especially with upper gastrointestinal tract bleeding where varices could be a life-threatening concern)

Recent surgery or procedure that can be associated with bleeding

Prior history of relevant conditions, such as peptic ulcer disease, polyps, and diverticular disease (for gastrointestinal tract bleeding)

Box 70.4 • Management Priorities for a Patient With Hemorrhagic Shock

1. Administer necessary fluid and blood resuscitation
2. Correct coagulopathy
3. Reverse or discontinue medications with adverse effects if possible (eg, anticoagulants)
4. Notify the gastroenterology department about the patient and the possible need for emergent endoscopy for gastrointestinal tract bleeding if applicable
5. Consider notifying the surgery department or interventional radiology if applicable

---

within 24 hours. Consideration should be given to administering erythromycin before endoscopy to improve visualization. Typically, proton pump inhibitor therapy is administered as a continuous infusion. The goal of endoscopy is to identify the source of bleeding and, more importantly, to use interventional techniques to stop blood loss (eg, injections, clips, or cauterization). Any inciting risk factors for the gastrointestinal tract bleeding (eg, nonsteroidal anti-inflammatory agents) should be discontinued, and *Helicobacter pylori* infection should be treated if identified.

For variceal bleeding, patients should receive a continuous infusion of intravenous octreotide and antibiotic prophylaxis to prevent spontaneous bacterial peritonitis. Endoscopic therapy is typically performed within 12 hours. Variceal ligation has been shown to be more effective than sclerotherapy. Patients with refractory bleeding may require balloon tamponade (temporizing treatment) or transjugular intrahepatic portosystemic shunt (definitive treatment).

Lower Gastrointestinal Tract Bleeding

The treatment of acute lower gastrointestinal tract hemorrhage is largely supportive: Resuscitate the patient, administer blood, correct the coagulopathy, and involve other providers (eg, in the gastroenterology and surgery departments) with the care plan early in the process. Identifying the source of bleeding can be difficult because active bleeding can be intermittent and elusive. Many patients presenting to an ICU with lower gastrointestinal tract hemorrhage have had a previous episode. The utility of emergent colonoscopy, especially in a patient who has not undergone preparation, is not clearly defined. Various studies have reported widely disparate diagnostic yields with the test when performed under these circumstances. Other diagnostic adjuncts, such as arteriography or nuclear medicine scans, may be needed to more precisely identify the source of bleeding.

Fulminant Hepatic Failure

Patients with fulminant hepatic failure most typically present to the ICU without a known history of liver disease. Common causes include toxins; prescription, over-the-counter (eg, acetaminophen), or herbal medications; shock; acute viral hepatitis; autoimmune disease; and vascular catastrophe (Budd-Chiari syndrome). Patients with acute liver failure typically present with overt hepatic synthetic failure with progressive coagulopathy and then worsening encephalopathy. Patients are at risk for dying of complications of hepatic failure, including infection or sepsis, multiorgan failure, and complications of cerebral edema (with or without central nervous system hemorrhage). In the ICU, management and treatment include providing supportive care (Box 70.5), seeking possible causes that are reversible, and advancing to orthotopic liver transplant quickly when the issues described above develop.

Abdominal Compartment Syndrome

Abdominal compartment syndrome (ACS) (also called intra-abdominal hypertension) is the presence of elevated

---

Box 70.5 • Supportive ICU Care for Patients With Fulminant Hepatic Failure

Close surveillance for infections

Airway protection with endotracheal intubation when encephalopathy or increased intracranial pressure is present

Aggressive management of coagulopathy

Intracranial pressure monitoring and therapies when obtundation and evidence of intracranial pressure elevation are present

Maintenance of the perfusion status of other vital organs (eg, kidneys)

Abbreviation: ICU, intensive care unit.

---

abdominal pressure in the abdominal cavity to the detriment of organ function. Patients at risk include those with severe penetrating and blunt abdominal trauma, ruptured abdominal aortic aneurysm, retroperitoneal hemorrhage, pneumoperitoneum, neoplasm, pancreatitis, massive ascites, liver transplant, abdominal wall burn eschar, abdominal surgery, high-volume fluid resuscitation (>3,500 mL in 24 hours), ileus, and pulmonary, renal, or liver dysfunction.

Patients present with decreased urine output, hypotension, increased respiratory distress with elevated peak pressures, and abdominal distention. Diagnosis can be confirmed with measurement of intra-abdominal pressure (IAP). ACS is defined as a sustained IAP greater than 20 mm Hg (with or without abdominal perfusion pressure <60 mm Hg) that is associated with new organ dysfunction. If elevated IAP is suspected, the bladder pressure can be used to estimate the IAP (keep in mind that flexing or tensing of abdominal musculature can raise the IAP). Treatment of ACS involves surgical decompression of the abdominal cavity.

71 Cystic Fibrosis, Bronchiectasis, and Pleural Effusion

VIVEK N. IYER, MD

Cystic Fibrosis

Cystic fibrosis (CF) is the most common autosomal recessive disease among whites, with a frequency of 1 in 2,000 to 1 in 3,000 live births. The disease is caused by a mutation in the gene that encodes for the CF transmembrane conductance regulator (CFTR) on chromosome 7. This mutation causes production of thick, sticky secretions that clog the airways and the pancreatic and biliary ducts, resulting in chronic cough, frequent sinus and lower respiratory tract infections, progressive bronchiectasis, end-stage lung disease, pancreatic insufficiency, diabetes mellitus, biliary disease, and malabsorption. Infertility is also common in both males and females. Colonization and infections with many organisms are common (eg, *Staphylococcus aureus*, *Pseudomonas aeruginosa*, *Haemophilus influenza*, nontuberculous mycobacteria, and *Aspergillus*). CF is the most common cause of chronic obstructive pulmonary disease (COPD) and pancreatic deficiency in the first 3 decades of life in the United States. Median life expectancy for patients with CF has been increasing (from 31.3 years in 2002 to 41.1 years in 2012).

CF is usually diagnosed before the patient is 2 years old, but for 20% of patients, the diagnosis is not made until adolescence or adulthood. A diagnosis of CF in adults requires the following: 1) clinical symptoms consistent with a diagnosis of CF in at least 1 organ system *and* 2) evidence of CFTR dysfunction as noted by the presence of a sweat chloride level of at least 60 mmol/L on 2 separate occasions, an abnormal nasal potential difference, *or* the identification of 2 disease-causing *CFTR* gene mutations. Sweat chloride testing must be performed with extreme care because inaccurate collection is a common source of misdiagnosis. False-positive results can be from smoking, chronic bronchitis, malnutrition, poor technique, and many other causes. False-negative results can occur in edematous states and in persons receiving corticosteroids. The concentrations of sodium and sweat chloride increase with age.

Treatment of pulmonary manifestations revolves around therapies to promote mucus clearance, including aggressive chest physiotherapy, percussion, postural drainage, and nebulized treatment with hypertonic saline and dornase alfa. Prompt treatment of upper and lower respiratory tract infections, adequate hydration, immunizations, and intensive nutritional, physical, and psychologic support are all essential to improving life span and quality of life. Ivacaftor, a drug that has been recently approved by the US Food and Drug Administration, directly targets a specific mutated CFTR protein; others are in clinical trials. Bilateral lung transplant is an option for patients with end-stage lung disease with progressive bronchiectasis and COPD. Infection with *Burkholderia cepacia* is associated with poor outcomes and is generally considered a contraindication for lung transplant.

Bronchiectasis

Bronchiectasis refers to ectasia, or dilatation, of bronchi and bronchioles that typically occurs from repeated lower respiratory tract infections. Tuberculosis is a common cause of bronchiectasis in the developing world. In the United States, bronchiectasis in adults is often secondary to childhood infections, chronic aspiration, immunodeficiency, hypogammaglobinemia, rheumatoid arthritis, Sjögren syndrome, CF, primary ciliary dyskinesia (eg, Kartagener syndrome), and allergic bronchopulmonary aspergillosis (ABPA). In a substantial percentage of patients (30%–40%), no specific cause can be found. Bronchiectasis most commonly involves the lower lung fields; upper lobe involvement may indicate CF, tuberculosis, or nontuberculous mycobacterial disease. ABPA may result in central bronchiectasis with perihilar involvement (finger-in-glove sign).

Bronchiectasis: *dilatation of bronchi and bronchioles that typically occurs after repeated lower respiratory tract infections.*

Classic symptoms of bronchiectasis include chronic cough and copious expectoration of mucopurulent sputum. Nonpulmonary symptoms include fetor oris, anorexia, weight loss, arthralgia, and clubbing. High-resolution computed tomography (HRCT) of the chest is the preferred test for definitive diagnosis. HRCT may also show bronchial obstruction due to inspissated purulent secretions, loss of lung volume, and air-fluid levels. Lung function studies typically show an obstructive pattern with air trapping. Complications of bronchiectasis include hemoptysis, progressive respiratory failure, cor pulmonale, and secondary infections due to fungi and nontuberculous mycobacteria.

Treatment of bronchiectasis is centered on maintaining excellent pulmonary hygiene with use of adequate hydration, chest percussion therapy, postural drainage, hypertonic saline nebulization along with inhaled bronchodilators, and corticosteroids. Predisposing conditions should be treated aggressively (eg, intravenous immunoglobulin infusions for hypogammaglobinemia, removal of foreign bodies or tumor, and control of aspiration). Cyclic antibiotic treatment is beneficial in select patients who have frequent exacerbations. Surgical resection is reserved for patients with localized disease and complications such as severe hemoptysis.

Pleural Effusion

Patients who have pleural effusions commonly present with dyspnea, nonproductive cough, and pleuritic chest pain. Additional information should be obtained, including a history of weight loss, symptoms of heart failure, malignancy, medication use, and travel and an occupational and exposure history.

The principal causes of pleural effusion are listed in Box 71.1. The diagnosis may be suggested by certain characteristics of the effusion. Pleural fluid testing should be selective and based on clinical suspicion. Despite extensive testing, the cause may remain elusive in up to one-third of patients with pleural effusion.

KEY FACTS

✓ Signs and symptoms of CF—
- chronic cough, frequent sinus and lower respiratory tract infections, progressive bronchiectasis, end-stage lung disease
- pancreatic insufficiency, diabetes mellitus
- biliary disease, malabsorption
- infertility (in males and females)

✓ Sweat chloride testing—perform with extreme care because inaccurate collection is a common source of misdiagnosis

✓ Treatment of CF—
- clear the mucus
- treat upper and lower respiratory tract infections
- provide adequate hydration, immunizations, and intensive nutritional, physical, and psychologic support

✓ Bronchiectasis—
- usually affects lower lung lobes (with upper lobe involvement, consider CF, tuberculosis, or nontuberculous mycobacterial disease)
- classic symptoms: chronic cough and copious expectoration of mucopurulent sputum
- HRCT of the chest for definitive diagnosis

Box 71.1 • Principal Causes of Pleural Effusion

Transudate
  More common
    Congestive heart failure
    Cirrhosis, hepatic hydrothorax
    Atelectasis
    Hypoalbuminemia
    Constrictive pericarditis
    Nephrotic syndrome
  Less common
    Peritoneal dialysis
    Hypothyroidism, myxedema
    Superior vena cava obstruction
    Meigs syndrome
    Urinothorax
Exudate
  Infections
    Parapneumonic (bacterial) effusions
    Bacterial empyema
    Fungal infection
  Tuberculosis
  Neoplasms
    Primary and metastatic lung tumors
    Mesothelioma
  Pulmonary embolism (up to 20% are transudates)
  Esophageal rupture
  Pancreatitis
  Trauma
  Connective tissue diseases
    Rheumatoid arthritis
    Systemic lupus erythematosus
  Drug-induced effusions
  Uremic pleuritis
  Yellow nail syndrome
  Dressler syndrome
  Chylothorax

Distinguishing an Exudate From a Transudate

Traditionally, the Light criteria have been used to identify an exudative effusion, but a meta-analysis found that other findings can also be used to identify fluid as an exudate (Box 71.2). The most common cause of a transudate is congestive heart failure, and the most common cause of an exudate is pneumonia (parapneumonic effusion).

Pleural Fluid Parameters

Glucose and pH

The pleural fluid glucose concentration and pH usually change in the same direction. Glucose levels are low (fluid glucose <60 mg/dL or ratio of fluid glucose to plasma glucose <0.5) in rheumatoid effusion, malignant mesothelioma, systemic lupus erythematosus, esophageal rupture, tuberculous pleurisy, and empyema. Pleural fluid pH is less than 7.30 in empyema, esophageal rupture, rheumatoid effusion, tuberculosis, malignancy, and trauma. A parapneumonic effusion with pH less than 7.20 likely is the result of empyema, and drainage with a chest tube may be required. Empyema caused by *Proteus* species has a pH greater than 7.8 (because of the production of ammonia).

Amylase

The amylase level in pleural fluid is increased in esophageal rupture (because of leakage of salivary amylase), malignancy, pancreatitis, and pancreaticopleural fistula. In any unexplained left-sided effusion, pancreatic disease should be excluded and the pleural fluid amylase level should be estimated.

Chylous Effusion

Chylous effusion is suggested by a turbid or milky white appearance of the fluid. The pleural fluid triglyceride

---

Box 71.3 • Mnemonic for Causes of Chylous Effusion: 5 *T*'s

Thoracic duct
Trauma
Tumor (lymphoma)
Tuberculosis
Tuberous sclerosis (lymphangiomyomatosis)

---

concentration is often greater than 110 mg/dL. A concentration less than 50 mg/dL excludes chylothorax. A helpful mnemonic for causes of chylous effusion is 5 *T*'s (Box 71.3). Lymphoma is the most common nontraumatic cause of chylothorax.

Cell Counts

A **hemorrhagic effusion** (pleural fluid hematocrit >50% of serum hematocrit) occurs in trauma, tumor, asbestos effusion, pancreatitis, pulmonary embolism with infarctions, and other conditions. A bloody effusion in lung cancer usually denotes pleural metastasis, even if the cytologic results are negative. Pleural fluid eosinophilia (>10%) is nonspecific and occurs with air or blood in the pleural space, fungal infections, drug-induced effusions, and malignancy. Pleural fluid lymphocytosis is most commonly associated with tuberculosis but can also occur with chronic effusions, lymphoma, sarcoidosis, chylothorax, and chronic rheumatoid pleurisy.

Key Definition

Hemorrhagic effusion: *bloody pleural fluid with a hematocrit >50% of the serum hematocrit.*

Cytology

Cytologic examination is an important test if patients have a known or suspected malignancy. Diagnostic yields are improved with more than 1 thoracentesis but remain in the 50% to 60% range. A positive fluid cytology finding in primary lung carcinoma implies late-stage, unresectable disease.

Cultures

Pleural fluid should be directly inoculated into aerobic, anaerobic, and fungal blood culture bottles to increase diagnostic yield. For patients with suspected tuberculosis, culture of pleural biopsy specimens is also useful. The diagnosis of pleural tuberculosis often requires the

---

Box 71.2 • Criteria for Identifying an Exudate

Light criteria—fluid is an exudate if any 1 of the following is present:

1. Ratio of pleural fluid protein to serum protein >0.5
2. Ratio of pleural fluid LDH to serum LDH >0.6
3. Pleural fluid LDH >67% of the upper limit of the reference range for serum LDH

Other criteria—fluid is an exudate if any 1 of the following is present:

1. Pleural fluid protein >2.9 g/dL
2. Pleural fluid cholesterol >45 mg/dL
3. Pleural fluid LDH >0.45 times the upper limit of the reference range for serum LDH

Abbreviation: LDH, lactate dehydrogenase.

combination of several techniques, including determining the level of pleural fluid adenosine deaminase.

Pleural Biopsy

Pleural biopsies can be obtained percutaneously or with medical thoracoscopy, which is an outpatient procedure that allows for visualization of the entire pleural lining. Medical thoracoscopy is useful for recurrent effusions of undetermined cause and in certain conditions such as malignancy and tuberculosis.

Complications of Thoracentesis

Complications of thoracentesis have been greatly reduced by the use of sterile technique and ultrasonographic guidance. Complications include pneumothorax, hemothorax, pulmonary edema, intrapulmonary hemorrhage, hemoptysis, vasovagal reaction, air embolism, subcutaneous emphysema empyema, seeding of a needle tract with malignant cells, and puncture of the liver or spleen.

KEY FACTS

✓ Pleural effusion—dyspnea, nonproductive cough, and pleuritic chest pain

✓ Most common cause of transudate—congestive heart failure

✓ Most common cause of exudate—pneumonia (parapneumonic effusion)

✓ Parapneumonic effusion with pH <7.20—likely from empyema that requires drainage with a chest tube

✓ Mnemonic for causes of chylous effusion—5 *T*'s: thoracic duct, trauma, tumor, tuberculosis, tuberous sclerosis

✓ Positive findings on fluid cytology in primary lung carcinoma—late-stage, unresectable disease

✓ Diagnosis of pleural tuberculosis—may need several techniques, including determining the level of pleural fluid adenosine deaminase

72 Interstitial Lung Diseases

FABIEN MALDONADO, MD AND TIMOTHY R. AKSAMIT, MD

Diagnosis

An estimated 1 in 3,000 to 1 in 4,000 persons in the general population have a diagnosis of **interstitial lung disease** (ILD), and ILDs account for about 15% of all consultations for general pulmonologists. These diseases encompass a group of heterogeneous lung conditions characterized by diffuse involvement of the lung parenchyma and pulmonary interstitium. By convention, infections, pulmonary edema, lung malignancies, and emphysema are excluded, but they should be carefully considered as part of the differential diagnosis (Box 72.1).

Key Definition

Interstitial lung disease: *a heterogeneous group of lung conditions that are characterized by diffuse involvement of the lung parenchyma and pulmonary interstitium and that exclude infections, pulmonary edema, lung malignancies, and emphysema.*

Some ILDs are characterized by suggestive or even pathognomonic findings, but the majority are best diagnosed through a dynamic interaction between clinicians, radiologists, and pathologists. Prompt recognition of ILD and initiation of appropriate therapy can greatly improve otherwise potentially life-threatening respiratory conditions. The 4 major categories of ILD are 1) ILDs of known cause (eg, drug-induced lung disease and connective tissue disease–related ILD [CTD-ILD]), 2) idiopathic interstitial pneumonias (Box 72.2), 3) granulomatous ILDs (eg, sarcoidosis and hypersensitivity pneumonitis [HP]), and 4) other ILDs (usually readily recognizable from characteristic findings).

Box 72.1 • Causes of Interstitial Lung Disease

Collagen vascular

Dermatomyositis
Rheumatoid arthritis
Scleroderma
Systemic lupus erythematosus

Drug-induced

Chemotherapy
Drug therapy
Radiotherapy

Genetic

Hermansky-Pudlak syndrome
Metabolic storage disease
Neurofibromatosis
Tuberous sclerosis

Idiopathic

Infectious

Chronic mycobacterial
Chronic mycoses

Malignant

Bronchoalveolar cell carcinoma
Lymphangitic metastases
Lymphoma

Occupational or inhalational

Asbestosis
Coal workers' pneumoconiosis
Hypersensitivity
Silicosis
Toxic gas

Vasculitides

Churg-Strauss syndrome
Giant cell arteritis
Granulomatosis with polyangiitis (formerly known as Wegener granulomatosis)

Box 72.2 • Idiopathic Interstitial Lung Disease

Idiopathic pulmonary fibrosis (IPF) (associated with a histopathologic or radiologic pattern of usual interstitial pneumonia [UIP])

Nonspecific interstitial pneumonia (NSIP)

Sarcoidosis

Cryptogenic organizing pneumonia (COP) (formerly called idiopathic bronchiolitis obliterans with organizing pneumonia [BOOP])

Eosinophilic lung diseases

Lymphocytic interstitial pneumonia (LIP)

Alveolar microlithiasis

Lymphangioleiomyomatosis (LAM)

Langerhans cell histiocytosis (pathologically, eosinophilic granulomatosis)

Pulmonary alveolar proteinosis

Acute respiratory distress syndrome (formerly called acute lung injury)

The strategy for diagnosing ILD should follow a stepwise approach, including 1) comprehensive history and thorough physical examination, 2) pulmonary function tests (PFTs), 3) radiologic studies (usually including high-resolution computed tomography [HRCT]), and, if needed, 4) bronchoscopic or surgical (or both) lung biopsy (Figure 72.1). However, all tests are not necessary for the majority of patients, and the diagnosis may be achieved without histologic confirmation.

History

A detailed history is the most important step in the diagnosis of ILD (Table 72.1). Environmental exposures (eg, pets, organic material, or mineral dust) or occupational exposures should be comprehensively investigated.

Physical Examination

Rales ("dry crackles" or "Velcro crackles") suggest fibrosis but are nonspecific. Clubbing of the digits can be associated with idiopathic pulmonary fibrosis (IPF) and asbestosis but is rare otherwise. Clubbing should raise concerns for alternative diagnoses (eg, lung or pleural malignancies, chronic suppurative lung diseases, or a right-to-left shunt). Careful attention should be paid to extrapulmonary manifestations of systemic diseases, such as musculoskeletal pain, sicca syndrome, and Raynaud phenomenon.

Pulmonary Function Studies

Typically, PFTs show a restrictive pattern, as evidenced by decreased lung volumes and preservation of flows. The diffusing capacity of lung for carbon monoxide (D_{LCO}) is also reduced. When D_{LCO} is reduced out of proportion to the rest of the PFTs, concurrent pulmonary hypertension or emphysema may be present.

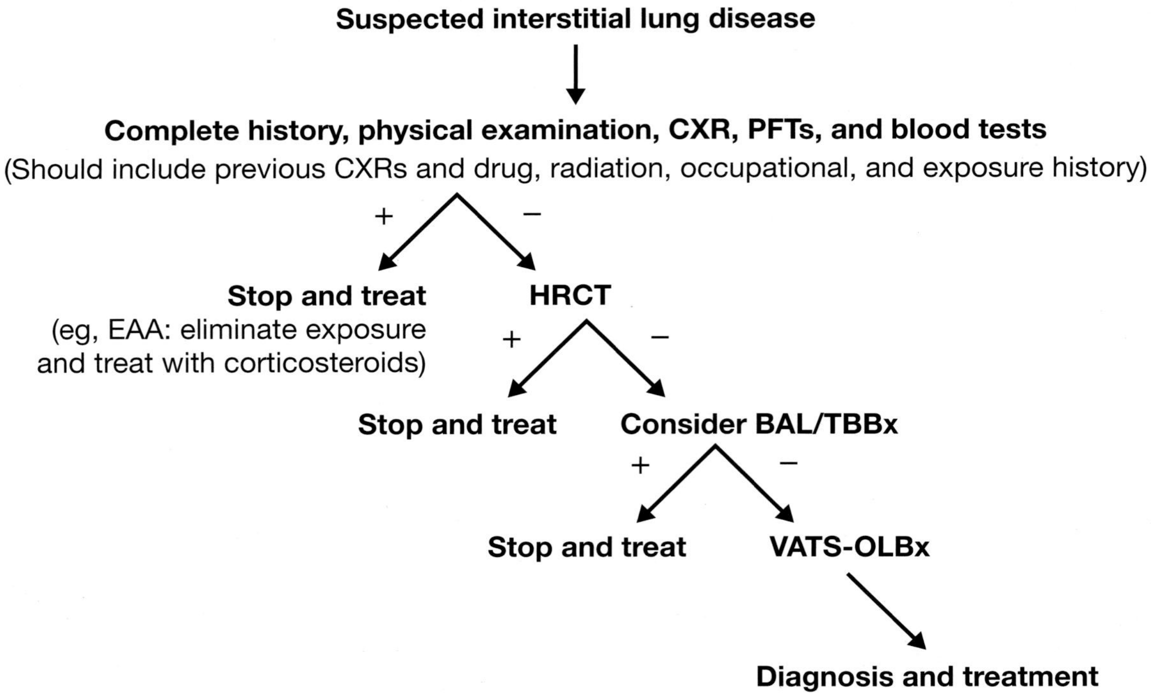

Suspected interstitial lung disease

↓

Complete history, physical examination, CXR, PFTs, and blood tests
(Should include previous CXRs and drug, radiation, occupational, and exposure history)

+ / −

Stop and treat
(eg, EAA: eliminate exposure and treat with corticosteroids)

HRCT

+ / −

Stop and treat

Consider BAL/TBBx

+ / −

Stop and treat

VATS-OLBx

Diagnosis and treatment

Figure 72.1 *Strategy for Diagnosing Interstitial Lung Disease. BAL indicates bronchoalveolar lavage; CXR, chest radiography; EAA, extrinsic allergic alveolitis; HRCT, high-resolution computed tomography; OLBx, open lung biopsy; PFT, pulmonary function test; TBBx, transbronchial biopsy; VATS, video-assisted thoracoscopy; +, positive findings; −, negative findings.*

Table 72.1 • Interstitial Lung Diseases Distinguished by History

Exposure or Feature	Disease
Amiodarone, methotrexate, nitrofurantoin, chemotherapy, radiotherapy	Drug-induced or iatrogenic lung disease
Insulation work, shipbuilding, mining, sandblasting	Pneumoconioses
Birds, indoor hot tubs, moldy humidifiers	Hypersensitivity pneumonitis
Acute onset of disease	Acute eosinophilic pneumonia or organizing pneumonia Virtually rules out IPF and asbestosis (which evolve over months to years)
Current smoker	Desquamative interstitial pneumonia, IPF, pulmonary Langerhans cell histiocytosis
Former smoker or never smoker	Sarcoidosis, hypersensitivity pneumonitis

Abbreviation: IPF, idiopathic pulmonary fibrosis.

Box 72.3 • Characteristic Imaging Findings in Patients With Interstitial Lung Disease

Distribution of infiltrates may provide guidance

Use the mnemonic *CHAPS* to remember predominant upper lung opacities:

C—cystic fibrosis, chronic eosinophilic pneumonia
H—HP, histiocytosis (PLCH)
A—allergic bronchopulmonary aspergillosis, ankylosing spondylitis
P—pneumoconioses
S—sarcoidosis and silicosis

IPF and asbestosis predominate in lower lung areas

Bilateral hilar lymphadenopathy suggests sarcoidosis or silicosis

Alveolar infiltrates in a "bat wing" distribution are typical of PAP (or cardiogenic pulmonary edema)

Peripheral opacities ("photographic negative of pulmonary edema") have been described in chronic eosinophilic pneumonia

Pneumothorax may be the clinical manifestation of PLCH and LAM

Abbreviations: HP, hypersensitivity pneumonitis; IPF, idiopathic pulmonary fibrosis; LAM, lymphangioleiomyomatosis; PAP, pulmonary alveolar proteinosis; PLCH, pulmonary Langerhans cell histiocytosis.

Imaging Studies

Although chest radiography has been largely supplanted by HRCT, several characteristic findings are useful (Box 72.3). HRCT has revolutionized the diagnosis of ILD and often obviates the need for histopathologic examination. Several characteristic features should narrow the differential diagnosis. Alveolar opacities (consolidation or ground-glass infiltrates) suggest reversible disease, while reticular "fibrotic" infiltrates are less likely to resolve. Honeycombing, traction bronchiectases, and basal predominance are typical for usual interstitial pneumonia (UIP), a pattern necessary for the diagnosis of idiopathic pulmonary fibrosis (IPF) (see section on IPF below). Thin-walled cysts suggest pulmonary Langerhans cell histiocytosis (PLCH) (upper lobe predominance) or lymphangioleiomyomatosis (LAM) (diffuse lung involvement). A "crazy-paving" pattern (ground-glass infiltrates with septal thickening) is seen in pulmonary alveolar proteinosis (PAP).

Laboratory Studies

Laboratory studies are rarely helpful in the diagnosis of ILD. Useful tests include a complete blood cell count with a differential blood count and liver and renal function tests. Hepatitis and human immunodeficiency virus serologies may be indicated. Depending on the clinical picture, other laboratory studies can be considered (Box 72.4).

Box 72.4 • Laboratory Studies That May Be Useful in the Diagnosis of ILD

Complete blood cell count with differential blood count

Liver function tests

Renal function tests

Serologies for hepatitis and HIV

Serologies for connective tissue disease in OP and NSIP

Serum protein electrophoresis if amyloidosis is in the differential

Hypersensitivity pneumonitis antibody testing (rarely helpful in practice)

Angiotensin-converting enzyme level (classically used to follow patients with sarcoidosis, but it is neither sensitive nor specific)

Cytoplasmic antineutrophil cytoplasmic autoantibody (c-ANCA)–proteinase 3 antibodies are both sensitive and specific for granulomatosis with polyangiitis (formerly known as Wegener granulomatosis)

Abbreviations: HIV, human immunodeficiency virus; ILD, interstitial lung disease; NSIP, nonspecific interstitial pneumonia; OP, organizing pneumonia.

Histopathologic Diagnosis

Bronchoscopy is often performed, primarily to exclude infection before immunosuppressive therapy is started. Biopsies are typically too small to establish the diagnosis of ILD, but some features on bronchoalveolar lavage may have diagnostic value (Box 72.5). Surgical lung biopsy is still required in a minority of patients (approximately 30%). Although it usually allows for a confident diagnosis, the risks and benefits need to be weighed and discussed with the patient, because acute exacerbations of ILD have occurred postoperatively with dramatic consequences.

KEY FACTS

✓ Diagnosis of ILDs—
- some ILDs have suggestive or pathognomonic findings
- most ILD diagnoses require dynamic interaction between clinicians, radiologists, and pathologists
- collecting a detailed history is the most important step
- thoroughly investigate environmental and occupational exposures
- if clubbing is present, consider another diagnosis (eg, lung or pleural malignancy, chronic suppurative lung disease, or a right-to-left shunt)

✓ PFT findings in ILD—
- restrictive pattern (decreased lung volumes and preservation of flows)
- decreased D$_{LCO}$ (if D$_{LCO}$ is decreased out of proportion to the rest of the PFTs, the patient may have concurrent pulmonary hypertension or emphysema)

✓ Imaging findings in ILD—
- mnemonic *CHAPS* for remembering predominant upper lung opacities
- IPF and asbestosis predominate in lower lung areas
- alveolar infiltrates in a "bat wing" distribution are typical of PAP or cardiogenic pulmonary edema
- pneumothorax may be clinical manifestation of PLCH and LAM

ILDS of Known Cause

Connective Tissue Disease–Related Interstitial Lung Diseases

Virtually all connective tissue diseases may affect the lungs. CTD-ILDs are more common in females, with the exception of rheumatoid arthritis (RA), which is more common in men. The typical histopathologic patterns seen with CTD-ILD are nonspecific interstitial pneumonia (NSIP) and organizing pneumonia (OP).

> ### Box 72.5 • Diagnostic Utility of Bronchoalveolar Lavage Findings in the Diagnosis of ILD
>
> A predominance of lymphocytes is consistent with sarcoidosis (with a classically inverted CD4:CD8 ratio, typically >4) or hypersensitivity pneumonitis (with a normal or decreased CD4:CD8 ratio)
>
> Eosinophilic predominance is seen with acute and chronic eosinophilic pneumonia
>
> Hemosiderin-laden macrophages are seen in diffuse alveolar hemorrhage
>
> Lipid-laden macrophages are seen in aspiration pneumonia and, less commonly, in lipoid pneumonia
>
> A CD1a$^+$ (a marker of Langerhans histiocytes) cell count >5% suggests PLCH as a possibility
>
> Abbreviations: ILD, interstitial lung disease; PLCH, pulmonary Langerhans cell histiocytosis.

Rheumatoid Arthritis

RA-related ILD (RA-ILD) differs from other CTD-ILDs: RA-ILD is more common in males, and a UIP pattern is typically seen in RA-ILD, which is less responsive to treatment and carries a poor prognosis. RA is commonly associated with pleural effusions, pulmonary nodules, and fibrosis (RA-ILD), but it may affect any part of the respiratory system.

Systemic Lupus Erythematosus

Systemic lupus erythematosus typically causes NSIP or OP (or both). A life-threatening, rare, pulmonary complication is acute lupus pneumonitis, characterized by diffuse alveolar damage, which is identified from lung biopsy and is poorly responsive to treatment. Diaphragmatic weakness (myopathy) may result in subsegmental atelectasis (also called platelike atelectasis) or, when severe, the classic shrinking lung syndrome, which is characterized by low lung volumes in the absence of lung infiltrates.

Inflammatory Myopathies

Inflammatory myopathies (dermatomyositis and polymyositis) may cause NSIP and OP, respiratory muscle weakness, and recurrent aspiration. Clinical manifestations include lung fibrosis, arthritis, Raynaud phenomenon, and myositis. The finding of an eczematous condition called mechanic's hands is a clue to lung involvement (Figure 72.2).

Scleroderma

Scleroderma (systemic sclerosis) is associated with fibrosis and pulmonary hypertension (in up to 25% of the patients), particularly in limited scleroderma or **CREST syndrome** (calcinosis cutis, Raynaud phenomenon, esophageal dysfunction, sclerodactyly, and telangiectasia). Scleroderma

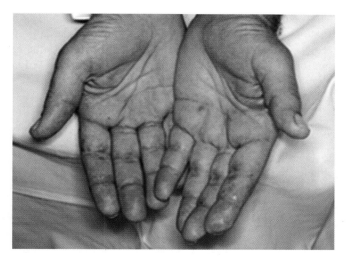

Figure 72.2 *Dermatomyositis. Mechanic's hands are characterized by roughening and fissures of the skin on the lateral and palmar areas of the fingers.*
(Adapted from Khambatta S, Wittich CM. Amyopathic dermatomyositis. Mayo Clin Proc. 2010 Nov;85[11]:e82. Used with permission of Mayo Foundation for Medical Education and Research.)

may also cause recurrent aspiration from esophageal dysmotility. Lymphocytic interstitial pneumonia (thought to be a low-grade lymphoproliferative disorder) is a classic manifestation of Sjögren lung disease.

> ### Key Definition
>
> CREST syndrome: *a limited form of scleroderma that consists of calcinosis cutis, Raynaud phenomenon, esophageal dysfunction, sclerodactyly, and telangiectasia.*

Drug- and Therapy-Induced Lung Diseases

Various pharmacologic agents may cause drug-induced lung disease. Discontinuing use of the drug is mandatory and usually results in prompt clinical improvement. The use of corticosteroids is often recommended, but the evidence for this practice is anecdotal at best. The common offenders discussed below should be presumed to be responsible for lung disease until proved otherwise.

Bleomycin Lung Toxicity

Bleomycin lung toxicity is the prototype of drug-induced lung disease. Bleomycin, an antibiotic chemotherapeutic agent is used in various malignancies, primarily in Hodgkin disease. The toxicity is cumulative, resulting in progressive fibrosis that may be indistinguishable from IPF.

Methotrexate

Methotrexate may cause a sarcoidosis-like reaction, with bilateral hilar lymphadenopathy and diffuse lung infiltrates. Eosinophilia is present in 50% of the patients. Bronchoscopic lung biopsies may show ill-defined granulomas, and the cell count and differential count on bronchoalveolar lavage are similar to those in sarcoidosis with lymphocytic predominance.

Nitrofurantoin

Nitrofurantoin is an antibiotic used to treat and prevent urinary tract infections. It may cause life-threatening, acute forms of lung toxicity (eosinophilic pneumonia) in 1 in 500 to 1 in 5,000 patients. A chronic form, similar in presentation to IPF, occurs in 1 in 50,000 patients. Discontinuing use of the drug is mandatory.

Amiodarone

Amiodarone can cause lung toxicity, which is cumulative in most patients after exposure to amiodarone at a dosage of more than 400 mg daily for 3 to 6 months. One particular radiologic characteristic of amiodarone lung toxicity is the presence of high-attenuation infiltrates on noncontrast HRCT, a result of the high iodine content of amiodarone. Treatment consists of discontinuing use of the drug, but because of its long half-life (2–3 months), clinical improvement may be delayed.

Pneumoconioses

Asbestos-Related Lung Diseases

Asbestos-related lung diseases should be suspected in patients with high-risk occupations (eg, insulation work, shipbuilding, and mining). Most pulmonary manifestations occur after a dormant period of 20 to 40 years, except for benign asbestos-related pleural effusion, which may occur within 10 years of exposure. Calcified pleural (or pericardial) plaques are a marker for asbestos exposure, but they do not generally cause symptoms. Other lung manifestations are listed in Box 72.6.

Silicosis

Silicosis occurs in patients exposed to silica (eg, mining, quarrying, and sandblasting). The disease is distinct from asbestosis, and findings include bilateral hilar lymphadenopathy (occasionally eggshell calcifications) with clustered micronodular infiltrates that typically favor the apices of the lungs. There are 3 characteristic associations: 1) Silicosis is a risk factor for tuberculosis, which should be excluded in patients whose respiratory condition worsens. 2) An association with connective tissue diseases has been described (Caplan syndrome). 3) Silicosis may be an independent risk factor for lung cancer, although to a much lesser extent than asbestos exposure.

KEY FACTS

✓ CTD-ILD—typical histopathologic patterns are NSIP and OP

✓ RA-ILD—typical histopathologic pattern is UIP (less responsive to treatment than other CTD-ILDs and carries a poor prognosis)

✓ Mechanic's hands—a clue to lung involvement in inflammatory myopathies

✓ Drug-induced lung disease—after use of the drug is stopped, clinical improvement is usually prompt

✓ Asbestos exposure—

- calcified pleural (or pericardial) plaques are a marker, but they do not usually cause symptoms

- smoking is not a risk factor for mesothelioma

- smoking acts synergistically with asbestos exposure and exponentially increases the risk of bronchogenic carcinoma

✓ Silicosis—

- a risk factor for tuberculosis (a consideration with a worsening respiratory condition)

- possibly an independent risk factor for lung cancer (but to a much lesser extent than asbestos exposure)

Idiopathic Interstitial Pneumonias

Idiopathic Pulmonary Fibrosis

IPF is the most common idiopathic interstitial pneumonia, and it affects men and women older than 50 years.

Box 72.6 • Lung Manifestations of Asbestos Exposure

Calcified pleural (or pericardial) plaques

Asbestosis

An ILD with similarities to IPF, but asbestosis carries a better prognosis

Treatment is supportive; corticosteroids are not indicated

Rounded atelectasis

A focal subpleural opacity often confused with lung cancer

Malignancy

Mesothelioma—a primary pleural malignancy that carries a poor prognosis; therapeutic options are few

Bronchogenic carcinoma—although smoking is not a risk factor for mesothelioma, it acts synergistically with asbestos exposure and exponentially increases the risk of bronchogenic carcinoma

Abbreviations: ILD, interstitial lung disease; IPF, idiopathic pulmonary fibrosis.

The pathophysiology remains elusive, but the condition is thought to result from poor wound healing of the lung with exuberant fibrosis but without underlying inflammation. No treatment has been approved; corticosteroids should not be used. Lung transplant is an option for select patients.

UIP is a histopathologic diagnosis necessary for the diagnosis of IPF, but it may be seen in other diseases (eg, asbestosis, drug-induced lung disease, HP, and CTD-ILD). Either a radiologic diagnosis (HRCT) or a histopathologic diagnosis of UIP is acceptable (ie, a surgical lung biopsy is not necessary if HRCT shows typical IPF with honeycombing, traction bronchiectases, and basal predominance). Biopsy may precipitate an acute exacerbation, a life-threatening complication of IPF. Other complications include pulmonary hypertension and pneumothorax. The prognosis is poor; median survival is approximately 3 to 5 years. Other conditions associated with UIP should be excluded, since they may be more responsive to treatment.

Nonspecific Interstitial Pneumonia

NSIP is the main differential diagnosis for IPF. Patients with NSIP present at a younger age (<50 years) and females predominate over males (2:1). The frequent presence of autoantibodies suggests that NSIP may be, at least in some patients, an autoimmune process. Radiologically, NSIP shows homogeneous involvement of the lungs, ground-glass opacities, and limited honeycombing and traction bronchiectases. NSIP is also a histopathologic diagnosis that may occur in other diseases (eg, CTD-ILD, HP, and infections). Treatment with corticosteroids is usually effective, and the 5-year survival (about 80%) is much better than with IPF.

Cryptogenic Organizing Pneumonia

Cryptogenic organizing pneumonia (COP) was formerly known as idiopathic bronchiolitis obliterans with organizing pneumonia (BOOP). Typically, COP manifests as a recurrent flulike illness that is resistant to antibiotics and has migratory infiltrates that progress over several months. The radiologic features include consolidation and ground-glass infiltrates (usually peripheral), and the pattern on PFTs is that of restriction rather than obstruction. COP is exquisitely responsive to treatment with corticosteroids, which should be administered for 3 to 6 months. Rebound after discontinuation is common, but COP generally responds to additional treatment with corticosteroids.

Chronic eosinophilic pneumonia manifests much like COP, with recurrent flulike episodes and migratory, peripheral infiltrates (typically described as a "photographic negative of pulmonary edema"). It is also exquisitely responsive to corticosteroids and, like in COP, rebound is frequent after discontinuation of treatment.

Acute Interstitial Pneumonia

Acute interstitial pneumonia (AIP), or Hamman-Rich syndrome, is characterized histologically by diffuse alveolar damage (presence of hyaline membranes), the histologic hallmark of acute respiratory distress syndrome (ARDS). In fact, the term *AIP* is equivalent to *idiopathic ARDS*. As with ARDS, the mortality is high (about 50%), but survivors have the potential for nearly complete respiratory recovery.

Acute Eosinophilic Pneumonia

Another rare type of idiopathic ARDS is acute eosinophilic pneumonia (not to be confused with chronic eosinophilic pneumonia); patients present with acute ARDS and eosinophilic infiltration of the lungs. The presentation is often dramatic and leads to acute respiratory failure and a need for mechanical ventilation. Affected persons are young, and typically, they recently began smoking. The disease has affected military personnel returning from the Middle East. Acute eosinophilic pneumonia responds dramatically to corticosteroids without rebound after discontinued use. Treatment can be short (2 weeks). Pulmonary eosinophilia is common, but peripheral eosinophilia is rare.

KEY FACTS

- ✓ IPF—
  - poor prognosis
  - median survival, 3–5 years
  - exclude other conditions associated with UIP (which may be more responsive to therapy)
- ✓ NSIP—
  - a histopathologic diagnosis that may occur in other diseases (eg, CTD-ILD, HP, and infections)
  - corticosteroid therapy is usually effective
  - 5-year survival, about 80% (much better than with IPF)
- ✓ COP—corticosteroid therapy for 3–6 months

Granulomatous ILDs

Sarcoidosis

Sarcoidosis is a granulomatous disease of unknown cause that typically affects patients younger than 50 years (African American females predominate). Patients may present with acute or gradual-onset lung disease, with possible progression toward end-stage diffuse fibrotic lung disease.

Sarcoidosis is one of the few lung diseases that predominantly affect nonsmokers and former nonsmokers (along with HP). Although the lungs (in >90% of patients) and

---

Box 72.7 • Radiographic Stages of Sarcoidosis

Stage 0—normal chest radiography

Stage I—hilar adenopathy

Stage II—hilar adenopathy with pulmonary infiltrates

Stage III—pulmonary infiltrates without adenopathy

Stage IV—fibrotic lung disease

---

lymph nodes are the most commonly involved organs, the disease can affect virtually any organ, including the heart, liver, spleen, eye, bone, skin, bone marrow, parotid glands, pituitary, and reproductive organs, and the nervous system. Hypercalcemia, anemia, and increased liver enzyme levels may be noted. Familial clusters of sarcoidosis have been reported. The course of the disease is highly variable, from asymptomatic to life-threatening.

Imaging

The radiographic stage of sarcoidosis correlates with the severity of pulmonary disease and prognosis (Box 72.7). Chest radiography may also show characteristic bilateral hilar or mediastinal lymphadenopathy with occasional eggshell calcifications. Computed tomography of the chest may show clustered micronodules.

Diagnosis

In most patients with sarcoidosis, granulomatous inflammation needs to be identified and other causes of granulomatous inflammation excluded (primarily fungal, mycobacterial, and other infections). Thus, sarcoidosis must be considered a diagnosis of exclusion after other causes of granulomatous disease have been ruled out. The serum levels of angiotensin-converting enzyme are not sufficiently sensitive or specific to be of diagnostic value.

Treatment

Corticosteroids are first-line therapy. Other immunosuppressive regimens used as second-line therapy for pulmonary sarcoidosis have included methotrexate, azathioprine, pentoxifylline, and cyclosporine. Treatment is reserved for severe organ disease (including progressive lung disease). In up to 90% of patients with stage I pulmonary sarcoidosis, the disease is expected to remain stable or to resolve spontaneously with no treatment. Stage III pulmonary sarcoidosis is expected to spontaneously remit in only 10% of patients. Pulmonary sarcoidosis is expected to progress within 2 to 5 years after diagnosis, although increased disease activity can occur at any time.

Hypersensitivity Pneumonitis

HP is an uncommon form of ILD. It is considered an allergic reaction to various organic antigens, including molds, grain dusts (farmer's lung), pets and birds (bird fancier's lung), and mycobacterial antigens (hot tub lung). Serum tests for specific antigens have poor sensitivity and specificity. The symptoms and clinical course are related temporally to antigen exposure. With acute disease, patients may have dyspnea, cough, fever, chest pain, headache, malaise, fatigue, and flulike illness. Chronic diffuse fibrotic lung disease may be indistinguishable from IPF.

The histopathologic features of HP show a range of bronchiolar-oriented, ill-defined, noncaseating granulomas. A restrictive pattern is common on PFTs, although an airway component may also be present and result in an obstructive component. Bronchodilators may be needed to treat airflow obstruction. Chest radiography generally shows reticulonodular changes, and HRCT often shows nonspecific nodules and ground-glass opacities predominantly in the upper lobes. Acute symptoms generally improve after the patient is no longer exposed to the antigen. Severe cases require treatment with corticosteroids.

Other Granulomatous Diseases

Other granulomatous diseases include infections, such as fungal or mycobacterial infections. The granulomas are usually necrotizing, as opposed to those in sarcoidosis and HP. Granulomatosis with polyangiitis (formerly known as Wegener granulomatosis) and Churg-Strauss syndrome should also be in the differential diagnosis. Response to intravenous injection of insoluble material, such as intravenous talcosis (as occurs in intravenous drug users), may result in diffuse lung granulomas centered on foreign bodies that are birefringent in polarized light.

Other ILDs

Pulmonary Langerhans Cell Histiocytosis

PLCH is a rare cystic lung disease mostly affecting young white smokers. Spontaneous pneumothoraces are common (in 25% of patients with the systemic variant of the disease, which is more common in children), and there may be bone involvement and pituitary insufficiency (central diabetes insipidus). The combination of exophthalmos, diabetes insipidus, and lytic bone lesions (often in the skull) is known as Hand-Schüller-Christian disease. Absolute cessation of smoking is mandatory.

Lymphangioleiomyomatosis

LAM is a cystic lung disease that affects women of childbearing age and is sometimes associated with tuberous

sclerosis (in up to 20% of patients). It is characterized clinically by a history of recurrent pneumothoraces (in 50%–80% of patients). Hemoptysis is common (in 25%). HRCT typically shows well-defined cysts scattered homogeneously throughout the lungs, without nodules or interstitial fibrosis. The response to hormonal treatment is limited. Currently, lung transplant is the definitive treatment. Sirolimus appears promising in the management of LAM.

Pulmonary Alveolar Proteinosis

PAP is a rare, idiopathic form of diffuse lung disease characterized by the filling of alveoli with proteinaceous material consisting mostly of phospholipoprotein. Most patients are smokers younger than 50 years, with a male predominance (male to female ratio, 3:1). A nonspecific but characteristic alveolar filling pattern seen with HRCT, described as a "crazy-paving" pattern with airspace consolidation and thickened interlobular septa, is suggestive of PAP. The diagnosis is usually indicated by a milky white return of bronchoalveolar lavage fluid or by lung biopsy findings. In addition to smoking cessation, therapy has involved whole-lung lavage and, more recently, trials of granulocyte-macrophage colony-stimulating factor.

KEY FACTS

✓ Sarcoidosis therapy—
- corticosteroids
- reserve for severe organ disease (including progressive lung disease)
- stage I pulmonary sarcoidosis remains stable or resolves spontaneously without treatment in up to 90% of patients

✓ HP—an allergic reaction to organic antigens (molds, grain dusts, pets and birds, and mycobacterial antigens)

✓ PLCH—
- rare cystic lung disease
- mostly in young white smokers
- spontaneous pneumothoraces are common

✓ LAM—
- cystic lung disease
- affects women of childbearing age
- sometimes associated with tuberous sclerosis
- history of recurrent pneumothoraces

73

Obstructive Lung Diseases

VIVEK N. IYER, MD

Obstructive Lung Diseases

Obstructive lung diseases include chronic obstructive pulmonary disease (COPD) (eg, chronic bronchitis and emphysema), asthma, bronchiectasis, cystic fibrosis, obliterative bronchiolitis, and diffuse panbronchiolitis (eg, bullous lung disease, α_1-antitrypsin deficiency, and airway stenosis). The 2 most prevalent obstructive lung diseases are COPD and asthma.

Asthma is a chronic inflammatory disorder of the airways associated with *reversible* airflow obstruction and airway hyperresponsiveness leading to recurrent episodes of wheezing, dyspnea, chest tightness, and cough. **COPD**, in contrast, is characterized by a *persistent* airflow obstruction that is usually progressive and associated with chronic airway inflammation. **Emphysema** is a *pathologic* term that describes alveolar destruction and the presence of giant air spaces (bullae). **Chronic bronchitis** is a *clinical* term that refers to chronic productive cough present for at least 3 months for 2 consecutive years. Chronic bronchitis is an independent risk factor for an accelerated worsening of lung function and an increase in mortality and number of hospitalizations. Some patients have an overlap syndrome with elements of both asthma and COPD. Several characteristics are useful for distinguishing these disorders (Table 73.1). Asthma is discussed in Chapter 2 ("Asthma").

Key Definition

Asthma: *a chronic inflammatory disorder of the airways associated with reversible airflow obstruction and airway hyperresponsiveness leading to recurrent episodes of wheezing, dyspnea, chest tightness, and cough.*

Key Definition

Chronic obstructive pulmonary disease: *a persistent airflow obstruction that is usually progressive and associated with chronic airway inflammation.*

Key Definition

Emphysema: *alveolar destruction and giant air spaces.*

Key Definition

Chronic bronchitis: *presence of a chronic productive cough for ≥3 months for 2 consecutive years.*

A proposed classification of the severity of COPD should guide management at various stages of the disease (Box 73.1). The clinical staging of COPD is based on the severity of airflow obstruction as measured with pulmonary function tests.

Etiology of COPD

Tobacco smoking is the primary cause of COPD in developed countries. Compared to nonsmokers, cigarette smokers have 10 times the risk of dying of COPD, whereas pipe and cigar smokers have between 1.5 and 3 times the risk. Smoking also increases the risk of COPD in persons who have α_1-antitrypsin deficiency. In developing countries, air pollution (both indoor and outdoor) is a major cause

Table 73.1 • Characteristic Features That Are Useful for Distinguishing Emphysema, Chronic Bronchitis, and Asthma

Characteristic	Emphysema	Chronic Bronchitis	Asthma
Age at onset	Typically ≥50 y	Typically ≥50 y	Typically childhood and early adulthood (but can also occur in older adults)
Presence of atopy	No	No	Yes
Smoking history	Yes (typically heavy)	Yes (typically heavy)	No
Classic clinical phenotype	Dyspnea in an older adult with a low body mass index and history of smoking ("pink puffer")	Chronic productive cough with hypoxemia ("blue bloater")	Episodic wheezing, cough, and chest tightness (both daytime and nocturnal)
Need for supplemental oxygen	Yes	Yes	No
Bronchial hyperresponsiveness (positive methacholine challenge test)	No	No	Yes
Exhaled oral nitric oxide	Normal	Normal	Elevated (≥40 parts per billion)
Variable airflow obstruction (eg, morning peak expiratory flow variability)	No	No	Yes
Diffusing capacity	Decreased	Normal or decreased	Normal
Chest radiography	Hyperinflation (teardrop heart, flattened diaphragm, and hyperinflated lungs with decreased markings)	Increased bronchial markings May show features of hyperinflation as seen in emphysema	Usually normal between acute exacerbations Increased bronchial markings may be seen because of bronchial wall thickening

---

Box 73.1 • Practical Aspects of Managing COPD

Steps in management

1. Rule out other diagnoses (asthma, bronchiectasis, bronchiolitis, and α_1-antitrypsin deficiency)
2. Assess extent of lung impairment
3. Assess COPD phenotype (symptom burden, exercise capacity, and exacerbation frequency)
4. Eliminate or address causative or exacerbating factors (with a strong emphasis on smoking cessation, including formal counseling and discussion of nicotine replacement strategies and pharmacologic adjuncts to improve quit rates)
5. Assess need for long-term supplemental oxygen
6. Formulate inhaler and drug treatment plan
7. Enroll patient in a rehabilitation program
8. Educate patient and family

Stepped-care approach

Mild COPD (FEV_1:FVC ratio <70%; FEV_1 ≥80% of predicted value): short-acting bronchodilator as needed
Moderate COPD (FEV_1:FVC ratio <70%; 50% ≤FEV_1 <80% of predicted value): scheduled use of long-acting bronchodilator, short-acting bronchodilator as needed, rehabilitation
Severe COPD (FEV_1:FVC ratio <70%; 30% ≤FEV_1 <50% of predicted value): scheduled use of bronchodilators with or without inhaled corticosteroids if repeated exacerbations or bronchodilator response, short-acting bronchodilator as needed, rehabilitation
Very severe COPD (FEV_1:FVC ratio <70%; FEV_1 <30% of predicted value or presence of respiratory failure or right-sided heart failure): regular use of bronchodilators with or without inhaled corticosteroids, rehabilitation, long-term oxygen if respiratory failure; consider surgical treatments

Abbreviations: COPD, chronic obstructive pulmonary disease; FEV_1, forced expiratory volume in the first second of expiration; FVC, forced vital capacity.

of COPD. Occupational and environmental exposures, heredity (α_1-antitrypsin deficiency), and repeated infections (cystic fibrosis and bronchiectasis) are other factors involved in the development of COPD.

α_1-Antitrypsin is a secretory glycoprotein that maintains a balance between proteolytic and antiproteolytic activity in the lung. α_1-Antitrypsin deficiency is inherited in an autosomal codominant fashion. The most common normal phenotype is MM (2 copies of the M allele). Deficient phenotypes are SZ, MZ, ZZ (severe), and null (severe). Patients often present in the third or fourth decade of life with emphysema and have a family history of COPD. Liver disease occurs in up to 10% to 15% of patients. Smoking-related emphysema is typically upper lobe predominant and centrilobular, whereas α_1-antitrypsin deficiency–related emphysema is predominantly lower lobe and panacinar.

Treatment of COPD

The therapeutic approach to COPD consists of reducing the risk factors (eg, smoking cessation), identifying the severity of COPD, assessing the need for long-term oxygen therapy, quantifying the degree of pulmonary dysfunction and response to bronchodilator therapy, selecting appropriate bronchodilators, anticipating and appropriately treating complications, and educating the patient and family about long-term therapy. Proper inhalation technique is essential

---

KEY FACTS

✓ COPD—
- tobacco smoking is the primary cause in developed countries
- risk of dying of COPD is 10 times higher for cigarette smokers than for nonsmokers
- patients often present in third or fourth decade of life with emphysema and family history of COPD
- 10%–15% of patients have liver disease
- smoking-related emphysema: usually upper lobe predominant and centrilobular
- α_1-antitrypsin deficiency–related emphysema: predominantly lower lobe and panacinar

✓ Treatment of COPD—
- reduce risk factors (eg, smoking cessation)
- identify severity of COPD
- assess need for long-term oxygen therapy
- quantify degree of pulmonary dysfunction and response to bronchodilator therapy
- select appropriate bronchodilators
- anticipate and treat complications
- educate patient and family about long-term therapy

---

in optimal treatment. Practical aspects of managing COPD are outlined in Box 73.1.

Reducing Risk Factors

Because smoking is a major risk factor in the development and progression of COPD, smoking cessation should be discussed and programs offered to those who continue to smoke. Decreased exposure to household air pollution, occupational dusts, gases, and fumes and other pollutants is also important in the management of COPD.

Bronchodilators

Bronchodilator drugs are administered to reverse bronchoconstriction (bronchospasm). Commonly used bronchodilators include 1) β-adrenergic agonists that are short acting (eg, albuterol, isoproterenol, levalbuterol, metaproterenol, and pirbuterol) or long acting (eg, salmeterol, formoterol, indacaterol, olodaterol, and arformoterol) and 2) antimuscarinic agents that are short acting (eg, ipratropium and oxitropium) or long acting (eg, tiotropium, aclidinium and umeclidinium). In addition, several new long-acting β-adrenergic agonists and antimuscarinic agents are in development.

Short-Acting β-Adrenergic (β_2-Selective) Agonists

Short-acting β-adrenergic agonists are the most commonly used bronchodilators. In most patients, single doses of these agents produce clinically important bronchodilation within 5 minutes (peak effect occurs 30–60 minutes after inhalation, with a beneficial effect lasting 3–4 hours). The dosage should be tailored on the basis of clinical features and potential side effects. Adverse effects include tremor, anxiety, restlessness, tachycardia, palpitations, increased blood pressure, and cardiac arrhythmias. Adverse effects are more likely in patients who have cardiovascular, liver, or neurologic disorders and in elderly patients. Rarely, paradoxical bronchospasm results from tachyphylaxis (a rapidly decreasing response to a drug after a few doses) or from exposure to preservatives and propellants. A newer, single-isomer β-agonist, levalbuterol, binds to β-adrenergic receptors with a 100-fold greater affinity than albuterol. Metered dose inhalers are just as effective as nebulized medications, but the total dose of medication is higher in the nebulized formulation.

Long-Acting β-Adrenergic (β_2-Selective) Agonists

Long-acting β-adrenergic agonists are often used in patients who have moderate COPD. Salmeterol is highly lipophilic (albuterol is hydrophilic); hence, it has a depot effect in tissues. Salmeterol has a prolonged duration of action (10–12 hours) and inhibits the release of proinflammatory and spasmogenic mediators from respiratory cells. Salmeterol and formoterol are also effective in preventing exercise-induced asthma, methacholine-induced bronchospasm, and allergen challenge. Adverse effects are similar to those of other β-adrenergic agents.

Anticholinergic Agents

Short-acting anticholinergic agents are useful for achieving immediate bronchodilation. As a single agent, ipratropium is only modestly effective: it prevents bronchoconstriction caused by cholinergic agents, but it does not provide complete protection against bronchoconstriction produced by tobacco smoke, citric acid, sulfur dioxide, or carbon dust. Ipratropium does not cross the blood-brain barrier, and it can aggravate narrow-angle glaucoma, prostatic hypertrophy, and bladder outflow obstruction.

Tiotropium is a long-acting, once-daily, inhaled anticholinergic that provides prolonged bronchodilation in patients with COPD. It decreases the frequency of exacerbations, provides bronchodilation, and improves symptoms, but it does not alter the worsening of lung function in patients with COPD.

Phosphodiesterase Inhibitors

The use of theophylline (a nonspecific phosphodiesterase inhibitor) has greatly diminished with the availability of various inhaled bronchodilators. Theophylline has a narrow therapeutic window and a wide range of toxic effects (eg, cardiac arrhythmias and grand mal seizures), and it interacts with other drugs. Roflumilast is a long-acting, selective phosphodiesterase-4 inhibitor that has shown modest benefit in reducing the exacerbation risk for patients with COPD and the chronic bronchitis phenotype.

Corticosteroids

A short course of systemic corticosteroids serves as a useful adjunct in the treatment of acute COPD exacerbation by reducing the duration and severity of the illness. A short course (5 days) of oral prednisone may have the same efficacy as a longer course (10 days). Inhaled corticosteroids do not slow the worsening of lung function or affect the mortality of patients with COPD, but they may decrease the frequency of exacerbations and modestly improve COPD symptoms. The use of inhaled corticosteroids may also be associated with an increased risk of pneumonia.

Adjuvant Therapy

Long-term azithromycin therapy is beneficial in patients with frequent COPD exacerbations (≥2 per year). Antibiotic therapy is helpful for patients with symptoms suggestive of an acute bacterial infection, especially during COPD exacerbations. Maintenance of good oral hydration, avoidance of tobacco smoking and other respiratory irritants, pneumococcal vaccination, annual influenza vaccination, and prompt treatment of respiratory infections are equally important.

Oxygen

Long-term oxygen therapy (LTOT) is recommended when the Pao_2 is 55 mm Hg or less (corresponding to an oxygen saturation by pulse oximetry [Spo_2] ≤88%). With LTOT, the target Spo_2 should be at least 90%. If there is clinical evidence of cor pulmonale, congestive heart failure, or polycythemia, LTOT can be started at a higher Pao_2 (56–59 mm Hg). Nocturnal oxygen is typically prescribed at a flow rate that is 1 L/min higher than the daytime resting oxygen requirement. When patients have cor pulmonale or suspected sleep apnea, a polysomnogram or nocturnal pulse oximetry may be very useful to exclude sleep apnea and to document adequate nocturnal oxygenation (Spo_2 ≥90%). The need for long-term or indefinite oxygen therapy should be reassessed after 3 months of treatment. Exercise therapy (ie, pulmonary rehabilitation) improves exercise tolerance and maximal oxygen uptake but does not improve spirometry results.

KEY FACTS

✓ Tiotropium for COPD—
  - decreases exacerbation frequency
  - provides bronchodilation
  - improves symptoms
  - does not stop the worsening of lung function

✓ Systemic corticosteroids for COPD—adjunct treatment of acute exacerbation; reduce duration and severity of illness

✓ Inhaled corticosteroids for COPD—
  - do not slow the worsening of lung function
  - do not affect mortality
  - may decrease frequency of exacerbations
  - may modestly improve symptoms
  - may increase risk of pneumonia

✓ Adjuvant therapy for COPD—
  - long-term azithromycin therapy for frequent exacerbations (≥2 per year)
  - good oral hydration
  - avoidance of tobacco smoking and other respiratory irritants
  - pneumococcal vaccination and annual influenza vaccination
  - prompt treatment of respiratory infections

✓ LTOT for COPD—recommended if Pao_2 <55 mm Hg (ie, Spo_2 ≤88%)

✓ Lung volume reduction surgery for COPD—improves exercise capacity, quality of life, and survival of patients with heterogeneous emphysema and poor baseline exercise capacity

Lung Volume Reduction

Surgical and bronchoscopic techniques are available to decrease the volume of poorly functioning emphysematous areas in patients with severe COPD. Lung volume reduction surgery has been shown to improve exercise capacity, quality of life, and survival of patients who have heterogeneous emphysema and poor baseline exercise capacity. Referral to a center with expertise in COPD evaluation is recommended when considering these options.

Causes and Complications of COPD Exacerbations

About half of all COPD exacerbations are caused by viruses. Common bacterial pathogens include *Haemophilus influenzae, Moraxella catarrhalis, Streptococcus pneumoniae,* and other gram-positive and gram-negative species. The result of COPD exacerbations is faster functional decline, poorer quality of life, and accelerated loss of lung function.

74

Pulmonary Evaluation

VIVEK N. IYER, MD

Symptoms and Signs

Cough

Cough is one of the most common reasons for outpatient medical consultation. Cough can be classified according to duration as *acute* (<3 weeks), *subacute* (3–8 weeks), and *chronic* (>8 weeks). Acute cough is usually related to an infectious cause, and symptomatic management usually suffices. Chronic cough, in contrast, is mainly related to postnasal drip, asthma, or gastroeseophageal reflux disease. Angiotensin-converting enzyme inhibitors have been implicated in up to 10% of patients with chronic cough. In about 50% of patients, chronic cough is due to more than 1 cause. For patients with chronic cough, the specific characteristics of the cough (eg, timing, character, and productive or not productive) do not seem to correlate with the underlying cause.

Hemoptysis

Hemoptysis is the expectoration of blood originating from the lower respiratory tract. Bleeding from the upper airways (ie, the nose, mouth, pharynx, and larynx) and the gastrointestinal tract often resembles hemoptysis, but the clinical history can be helpful for differentiation. The pulmonary parenchyma and airways are supplied by pulmonary arteries and bronchial arteries. Causes of hemoptysis can be broadly divided into airway causes (eg, bronchitis, bronchiectasis, neoplasms, foreign body, and trauma); pulmonary parenchymal causes (eg, Goodpasture syndrome, pulmonary vasculitis, and lung infections); and pulmonary

> ### Key Definition
>
> Hemoptysis: *expectoration of blood originating from the lower respiratory tract.*

vascular causes (eg, pulmonary embolism, pulmonary arteriovenous malformations, and mitral stenosis).

History and Examination

An approach to the history and physical examination of patients with pulmonary disease is outlined in Box 74.1. Percussion and auscultation findings associated with various pulmonary conditions are listed in Table 74.1.

> ### Box 74.1 • History and Physical Examination of Patients With Pulmonary Disease
>
> History
>
>   Smoking
>   Occupational exposure
>   Exposure to infected persons or animals
>   Hobbies and pets
>   Family history of diseases of the lung and
>   other organs
>   Past malignancy
>   Systemic (nonpulmonary) diseases
>   Immune status (corticosteroid therapy,
>   chemotherapy, cancer)
>   History of trauma
>   Previous chest radiography
>
> Examination
>
>   Inspection
>   Respiratory rate, hoarseness
>   Respiratory rhythm (abnormal breathing pattern)
>   Accessory muscles in action (FEV_1 <30%)
>   Postural dyspnea (orthopnea, platypnea,
>   trepopnea)
>   Intercostal retraction
>   Paradoxical motions of abdomen or diaphragm
>   Cough (type, sputum, blood)
>   Wheeze (audible with or without stethoscope)
>   Pursed lip breathing or glottic wheeze (patients
>   with COPD)
>   Cyanosis (central vs peripheral)
>   Conjunctival suffusion (CO_2 retention)
>
> (continued on next page)

Clubbing
Thoracic cage (eg, anteroposterior diameter,
  kyphoscoliosis, pectus carinatum)
Trachea, tracheal deviation
Superior vena cava syndrome
Asterixis, central nervous system status
Cardiac impulse, jugular venous pressure, pedal
  edema (signs of cor pulmonale)
Palpation

Clubbing
Lymphadenopathy
Tibial tenderness (hypertrophic pulmonary
  osteoarthropathy)
Motion of thoracic cage (hand or tape measure)
Chest wall tenderness (costochondritis, rib fracture,
  pulmonary embolism)
Tracheal deviation or tenderness, tactile (vocal)
  fremitus
Subcutaneous emphysema
Succussion splash (effusion; air-fluid level in thorax)

Percussion

Thoracic cage (dullness, resonance)
Diaphragmatic motion (normal, 5–7 cm)
Upper abdomen (liver)

Auscultation

Tracheal auscultation
Normal breath sounds
Bronchial breath sounds
Expiratory slowing
Crackles
Wheezes
Pleural rub
Mediastinal noises (mediastinal crunch)
Heart sounds
Miscellaneous (muscle tremor, etc)

Abbreviations: CO_2, carbon dioxide; COPD, chronic
  obstructive pulmonary disease; FEV_1, forced expiratory
  volume in the first second of expiration.

Diagnostic Tests

Plain Chest Radiography

The ability to identify normal radiographic anatomy of the
chest is essential. A step-by-step method should be used to

**Box 74.2 • Systematic Approach for Evaluating
a Chest Radiograph**

1. Check for patient identifier.
2. Evaluate the extrathoracic structures (eg, for
   evidence of destructive arthritis, the absence of a
   breast shadow, or a tracheostomy stoma).
3. Evaluate for infradiaphragmatic abnormalities.
4. Assess skeletal changes (eg, rib fractures, notching,
   osteolytic lesions, or sternal wires).
5. Evaluate intrathoracic but extrapulmonary
   structures and features (eg, mediastinum, thyroid
   calcification, achalasia, aortopulmonary window,
   hila, and calcified adenopathy).
6. Evaluate the pleural surfaces (eg, for blunting or
   calcification).
7. Evaluate the pulmonary parenchyma (eg, for
   infiltrates, air bronchogram, nodules, cysts, abscess,
   or pneumothorax).
8. Evaluate the retrocardiac and retrodiaphragmatic
   spaces on lateral views.

---

interpret chest radiographs so that subtle abnormalities are
not missed (Box 74.2).

Initially, assess the chest radiograph overall without focusing on any specific area or abnormality. Then start with
the extrathoracic structures and move inward. For example,
destructive shoulder arthritis may indicate rheumatoid arthritis and prompt a search for associated pulmonary manifestations; the absence of a breast shadow in a female patient
should prompt evaluation for signs of pulmonary metastases
of breast cancer; visualization of a tracheostomy stoma or
cannula may indicate previous laryngeal cancer (suggesting
the possibility of complications such as aspiration pneumonia and lung metastases); and infradiaphragmatic abnormalities (eg, calcifications in the spleen, displacement of the
gastric bubble and colon, and signs of upper abdominal surgery) may indicate the cause of a pleuropulmonary process.

Then view the skeletal thorax to exclude rib fractures,
osteolytic and other lesions of the ribs, rib notching, missing
ribs, and vertebral abnormalities. Changes due to previous

Table 74.1 • Percussion and Auscultation Findings in Pulmonary Conditions

Condition	Chest Expansion	Fremitus	Resonance	Breath Sounds	Egophony[a]	Bronchophony[a]
Pleural effusion[b]	Decreased	Decreased	Decreased	Decreased	Absent >> present	Absent >> present
Consolidation[c]	Decreased	Increased	Decreased	Bronchial	Present	Present
Atelectasis[d]	Decreased	Decreased	Decreased	Decreased	Absent > present	Absent > present
Pneumothorax	Variable	Decreased	Increased	Decreased	Absent	Absent

[a] Inequality signs indicate *more often than* (>) or *much more often than* (>>).
[b] The trachea is shifted contralaterally in effusion.
[c] Whispered pectoriloquy is present in consolidation.
[d] The trachea is shifted ipsilaterally in atelectasis.

thoracic surgical procedures (eg, coronary artery bypass, thoracotomy, lung resection, or esophageal surgery) may provide clues to the pulmonary disease.

Next assess the intrathoracic but extrapulmonary structures, such as the mediastinum (including the great vessels, esophagus, heart, lymph nodes, and thymus). A calcified mass in the region of the thyroid almost always indicates a goiter. An obliterated aortopulmonary window (a notch below the aortic knob on the left, just above the pulmonary artery) may indicate a tumor or lymphadenopathy. Right paratracheal and paramediastinal lymphadenopathy can be subtle. Hilar regions are difficult to interpret because lymphadenopathy, vascular prominence, or tumor may make the hila appear larger. The retrocardiac region may show hiatal hernia with an air-fluid level; this may be helpful in the diagnosis of reflux or aspiration.

Examine the pleural regions for pleural effusion, pleural thickening (particularly in the apices), blunting of the costophrenic angles, pleural plaques or masses, and pneumothorax. A lateral decubitus radiograph may be necessary to confirm the presence of free fluid in the pleural space. An air bronchogram depicting the major airways may indicate a large tumor (by an abrupt cutoff of the air bronchogram) or consolidation from an infection.

Finally, evaluate the lung parenchyma. Notably, about 15% of the pulmonary parenchyma is located behind the heart and diaphragm; a lateral chest radiograph is helpful in examining this region for retrocardiac or retrodiaphragamatic abnormalities. It is important not to overinterpret increased interstitial lung markings. Generally, bronchovascular markings should be visible throughout the lung parenchyma. The absence of any markings within the lung parenchyma suggests a bulla or an air-containing cyst. Apical areas should be evaluated carefully for the presence of pleural thickening, pneumothorax, small nodules, and subtle infiltrates.

KEY FACTS

✓ Causes of chronic cough—
  * postnasal drip
  * asthma
  * gastroesophageal reflux disease
  * angiotensin-converting enzyme inhibitors (10% of patients)
  * multiple causes (50% of patients)
✓ Interpretation of chest radiographs—use a step-by-step method to avoid missing subtle abnormalities

---

Common radiographic abnormalities of the chest are depicted in Figures 74.1 through 74.26.

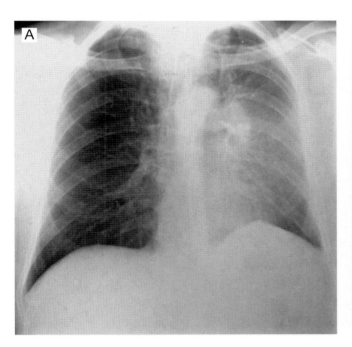

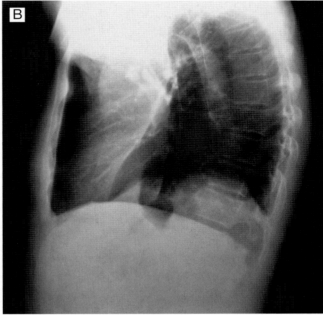

Figure 74.1 *Collapsed Left Upper Lobe. A, Posteroanterior chest radiograph (CXR). B, Lateral CXR. The ground-glass haze over the left hemithorax is typical of a partially collapsed left upper lobe. In more than 50% of patients with collapsed lobes, loss of volume is evidenced by left hemidiaphragmatic elevation; the mediastinum is shifted to the left and the left hilum is pulled cranially. Also, the left main bronchus deviates cranially. Calcification in the left hilar mass is the result of an unrelated, old granulomatous infection. In panel B, the density from the left hilum down toward the anterior portion of the chest is the result of the partially collapsed left upper lobe. The substernal radiolucency is the right lung.*

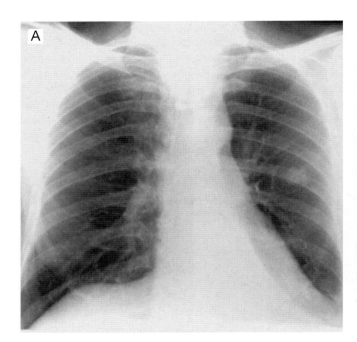
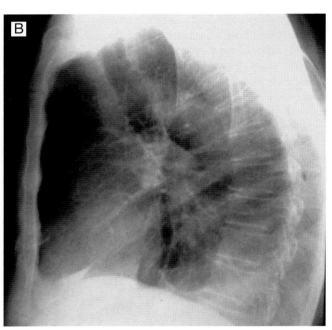

Figure 74.2 *Collapsed Left Lower Lobe. A, Posteroanterior chest radiograph (CXR). B, Lateral CXR. The nodule in the left midlung field and the collapsed left lower lobe (appearing as a density behind the heart) resulted from 2 separate primary lung cancers, which were synchronous bronchogenic carcinomas. Identification of the first evident abnormality, such as the nodule in the midlung field, should not prevent careful evaluation of all other areas. Panel B shows an increased density over the lower thoracic vertebrae without an obvious wedge-shaped infiltrate. Over the anterior portion of the hemidiaphragm, the small wedge-shaped infiltrate is not fluid in the left major fissure because the left major fissure is pulled away posteriorly. Instead, it is an incidental normal variant of fat pushed up into the right major fissure.*

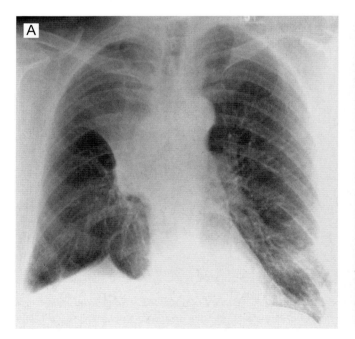
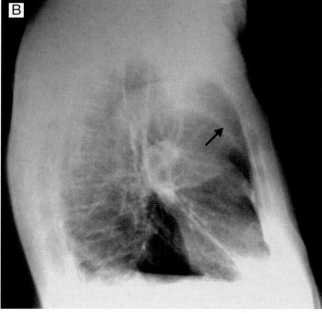

Figure 74.3 *Collapsed Right Upper Lobe. A, Posteroanterior chest radiograph (CXR). B, Lateral CXR. Panel A shows a classic "reversed S" mass in the right hilus with partial collapse of the right upper lobe. Loss of volume is evident with the elevation of the right hemidiaphragm. In panel B, the partially collapsed right upper lobe is faintly seen in the upper anterior portion of the hemithorax (arrow).*

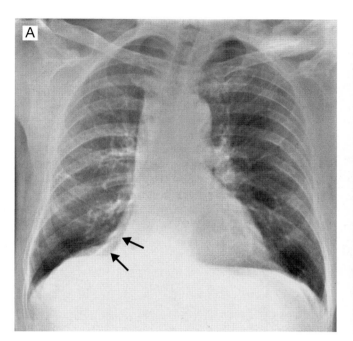
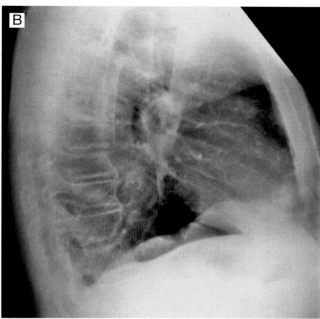

Figure 74.4 *Collapsed Right Lower Lobe. A, Posteroanterior chest radiograph (CXR). B, Lateral CXR. This 75-year-old male smoker had hemoptysis for 1.5 years; his CXR had been read as normal on several occasions. In panel A, the linear density (arrows) projecting downward and laterally along the right border of the heart projects below the diaphragm and is not a normal line. Also, the right hilum is not evident; it has been pulled centrally and downward because of carcinoma obstructing the bronchus of the right lower lobe. The very slight shift in the mediastinum to the right indicates loss of volume. In panel B, the notable collapse of the right lower lobe is indicated by only a subtle, increased density over the lower thoracic vertebrae.*

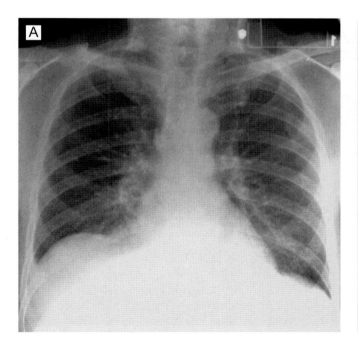
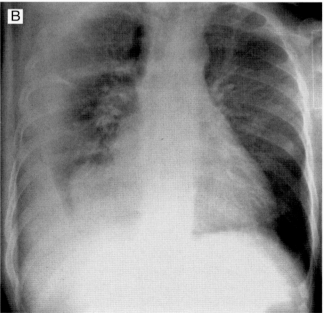

Figure 74.5 *Effusion. A, Posteroanterior chest radiograph (CXR). B, Decubitus CXR. In panel A, an "elevated right hemidiaphragm" is actually an infrapulmonic (or subpulmonic) effusion, as seen in panel B. For unknown reasons, a meniscus is not formed in some people with infrapulmonic pleural effusion. Thus, a seemingly elevated hemidiaphragm should be examined with the suspicion that it could be infrapulmonic effusion. Subpulmonic effusion occurs more frequently in patients with nephrotic syndrome. Decubitus CXR or ultrasonography would disclose the free fluid.*

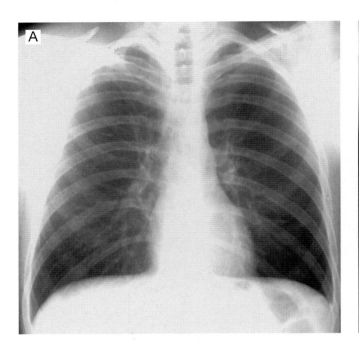

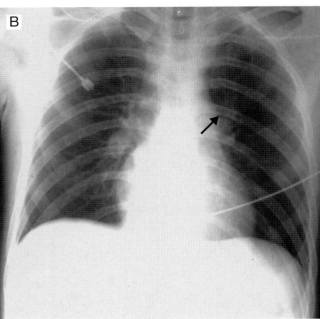

Figure 74.6 *Embolism. A, Prepulmonary embolism on a "normal" posteroanterior chest radiograph (CXR). B, Pulmonary embolism. The CXR is read as normal in up to 30% of patients with angiographically proven pulmonary embolism. In comparison with panel A, panel B shows a subtle elevation of the right hemidiaphragm. In panel A, the right and left hemidiaphragms are equal. In some series, an elevated hemidiaphragm is the most common finding with acute pulmonary embolism. Additional features are the plumpness of the right pulmonary artery, the prominent pulmonary outflow tract on the left (arrow in panel B), and a subtle change in the cardiac diameter. The patient was a 28-year-old man who was in shock from massive pulmonary emboli as a result of major soft tissue trauma from a motorcycle accident 7 days earlier.*

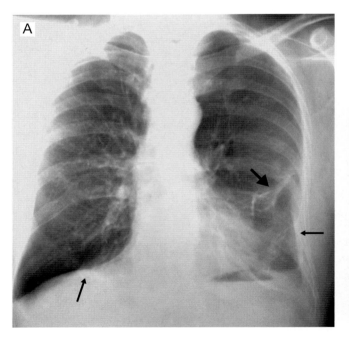

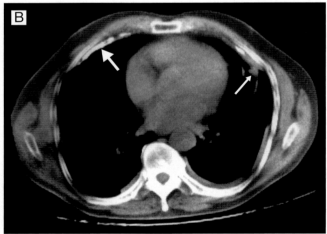

Figure 74.7 *Asbestos Exposure. The patient was a 68-year-old asymptomatic man who smoked. A, Abnormal chest radiograph shows areas of pleural calcification (small arrows), particularly on the right hemidiaphragm. This is a tip-off to previous asbestos exposure. The process in the left midlung was worrisome (large arrow), perhaps indicating a new process such as bronchogenic carcinoma. B, Computed tomography disclosed rounded atelectasis (small arrow). The "comma" extending from this mass is characteristic of rounded atelectasis, which is the result of subacute to chronic pleural effusion resolving and trapping lung as it heals. Pleural calcification is apparent (large arrow).*

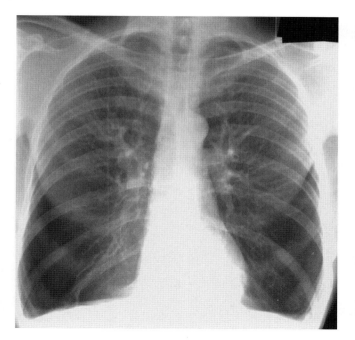

Figure 74.8 *Panlobular Emphysema at the Bases Consistent With the Diagnosis of α₁-Antitrypsin Deficiency. Emphysema should not be read into a chest radiograph because all it usually represents is hyperinflation that can occur with severe asthma as well. However, diminished interstitial markings are at the bases with radiolucency. Also, blood flow is increased to the upper lobes because that is where most of the viable lung tissue is.*

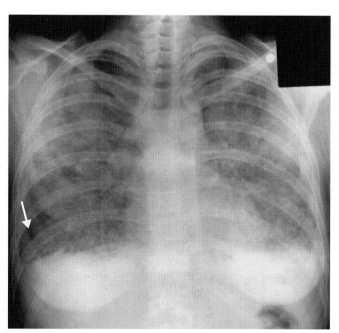

Figure 74.9 *Lymphangitic Carcinoma in a 27-Year-Old Woman. This patient had a 6-week history of progressive dyspnea and weight loss. Because of her young age, neoplasm may not be considered initially. However, the chest radiographic features suggest a neoplasm: bilateral pleural effusions, Kerley B lines as evident in the right base (arrow), and mediastinal and hilar lymphadenopathy in addition to diffuse parenchymal infiltrate.*

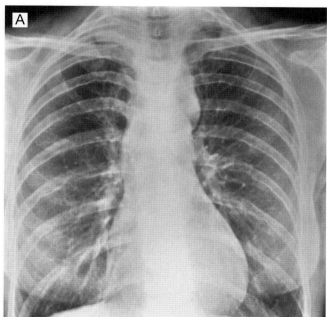

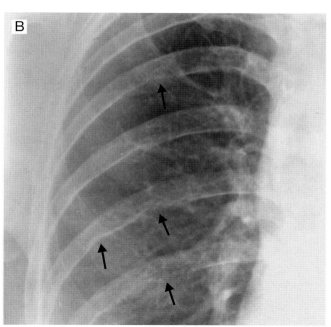

Figure 74.10 *Coarctation. A and B, Posteroanterior chest radiographs show coarctation with a tortuous aorta mimicking a mediastinal mass. This occurs in about one-third of patients with coarctation. The arrows in panel B indicate rib notching.*

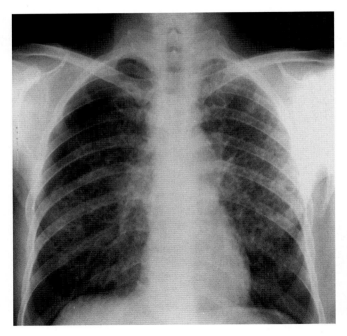

Figure 74.11 *Langerhans Cell Histiocytosis (or Eosinophilic Granuloma). Extensive change is predominantly in the upper two-thirds of the lung fields. Eventually 25% of patients have pneumothorax, as seen on this chest radiograph (right side). The honeycombing, also described as microcysts, is characteristic of advanced Langerhans cell histiocytosis.*

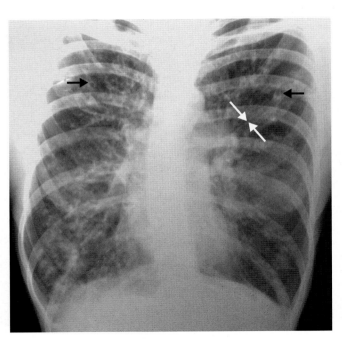

Figure 74.13 *Advanced Cystic Fibrosis. This chest radiograph shows hyperinflation with low-lying hemidiaphragms, bronchiectasis (white arrows pointing to parallel lines), and microabscesses (black arrows), which are small areas of pneumonitis distal to the mucous plug that has been coughed out. Cystic fibrosis almost always begins in the upper lobes.*

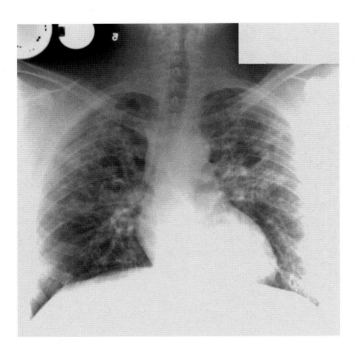

Figure 74.12 *Sarcoidosis in a 35-Year-Old Patient. This chest radiograph shows the predominant parenchymal pattern seen in the upper two-thirds of the lungs in many patients with stage II or III sarcoidosis. The pattern can be interstitial, alveolar (which this one is predominantly), or a combination. Some residual adenopathy is probably in the hila and right paratracheal area.*

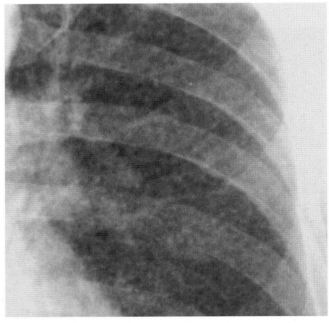

Figure 74.14 *Miliary Tuberculosis. The chest radiograph shows a miliary pattern of relatively discrete micronodules, with little interstitial (linear or reticular) markings. Disseminated fungal disease has a similar appearance, as does bronchoalveolar cell carcinoma; however, the patients do not usually have the systemic manifestations of miliary tuberculosis. Other, less common differential diagnoses include lymphoma, lymphocytic interstitial pneumonitis, and pulmonary edema. Pneumocystis jiroveci pneumonia usually has a more interstitial reaction.*

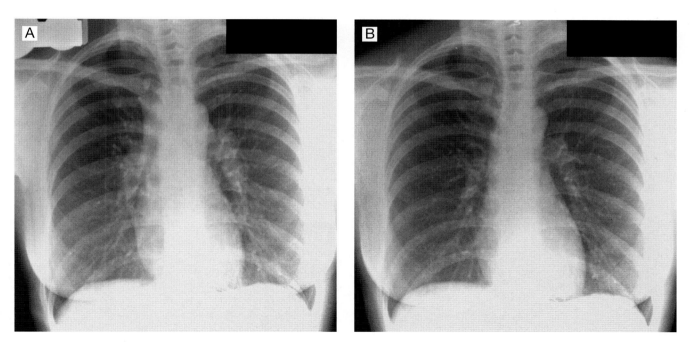

Figure 74.15 *Pulmonary Sarcoidosis. A, Chest radiograph (CXR) of a 30-year-old woman who had stage I pulmonary sarcoidosis with subtle bilateral hilar and mediastinal adenopathy, particularly right paratracheal and left infra-aortic adenopathy. B, CXR 1 year later, after spontaneous regression of sarcoidosis.*

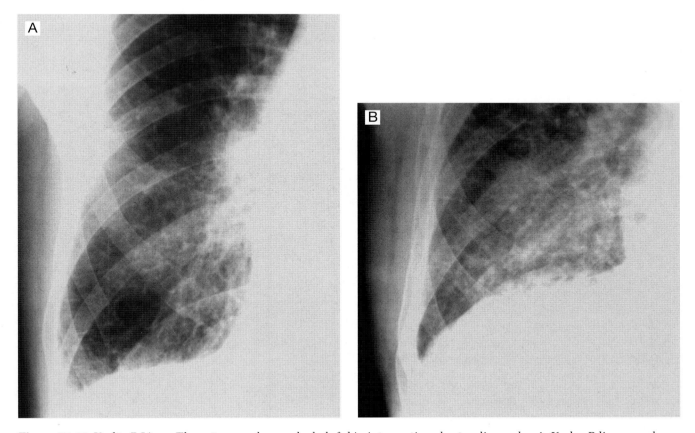

Figure 74.16 *Kerley B Lines. These 2 examples can be helpful in interpreting chest radiographs. A, Kerley B lines are shown in a 75-year-old man with colon cancer. B, The Kerley B lines are from metastatic adenocarcinoma of the colon; they were a tip-off that the parenchymal process in this patient resulted from metastatic carcinoma and not from a primary pulmonary process such as pulmonary fibrosis, which was the working diagnosis.*

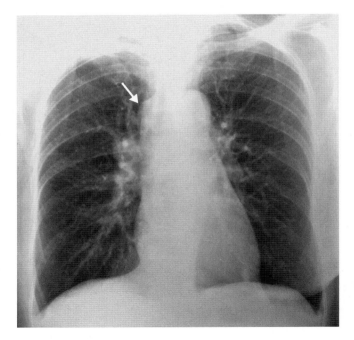

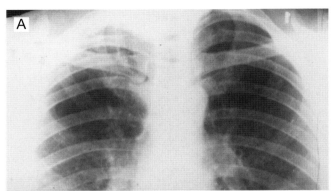

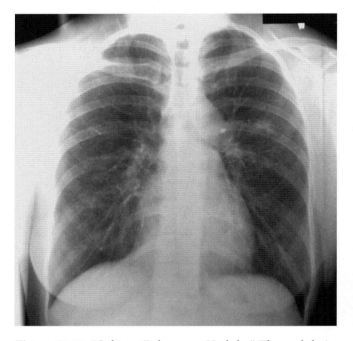

Figure 74.17 *Metastatic Carcinoma of the Breast. This chest radiograph from a 55-year-old woman who had a right mastectomy for breast carcinoma now shows subtle but definite right paratracheal (arrow) and right hilar adenopathy from metastatic carcinoma of the breast.*

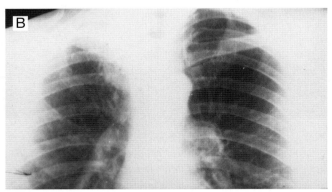

Figure 74.19 *Pancoast Tumor. A, Subtle asymmetry at the apex of the right lung. The patient's symptoms at the initial chest radiography were attributed to a cervical disk. B, The asymmetry was more obvious 3.5 years later when the Pancoast lesion (primary bronchogenic carcinoma) was diagnosed.*

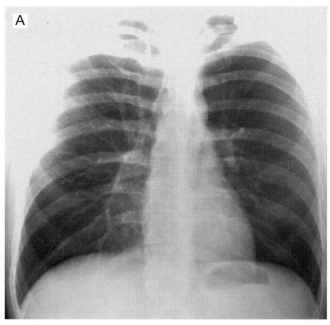

Figure 74.18 *"Solitary Pulmonary Nodule." The nodule in the left midlung field is technically not a solitary pulmonary nodule because of another abnormality in the thorax that might be related: left infra-aortic adenopathy. The differential diagnosis would be bronchogenic carcinoma with hilar nodal metastasis or, as in this patient, acute primary pulmonary histoplasmosis. Had this patient been in an area with coccidioidomycosis, that disease would also be included in the differential diagnosis.*

Figure 74.20 *Bronchial Carcinoid. The adage that "not all that wheezes is asthma" should be remembered every time a patient with asthma is encountered and the condition does not seem to improve. A, In this patient, wheezes were predominant over the left hemithorax. B, The forced expiration film showed air trapping in the left lung. Bronchial carcinoid of the left main bronchus was diagnosed at bronchoscopy.*

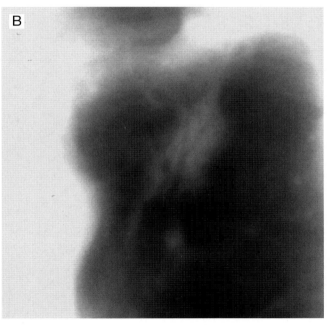

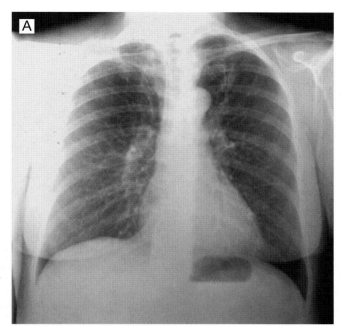

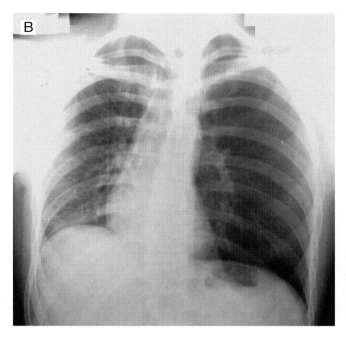

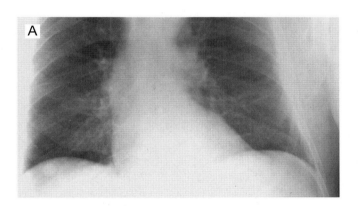

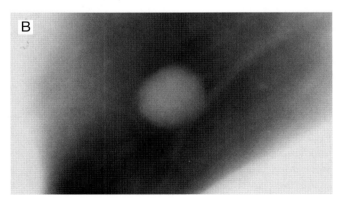

Figure 74.20 *(continued).*

Figure 74.21 *Adenocarcinoma. A, A solitary pulmonary nodule is evident below the right hemidiaphragm, where at least 15% of the lung is obscured. B, Computed tomography shows that the nodule has a discrete border but is noncalcified. The nodule was not present 18 months earlier.*

Figure 74.22 *Infiltrate. A, Solitary infiltrate in the left upper lobe with air bronchogram, as evident on computed tomography or chest radiography. B, Air bronchogram should be considered a sign of bronchoalveolar cell carcinoma or lymphoma until proved otherwise.*

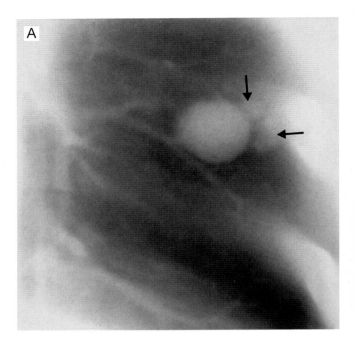

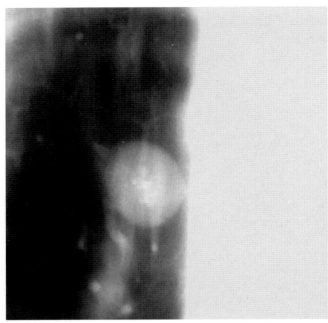

Figure 74.24 *Popcorn Calcification of Hamartoma. This benign process can be seen also with granuloma.*

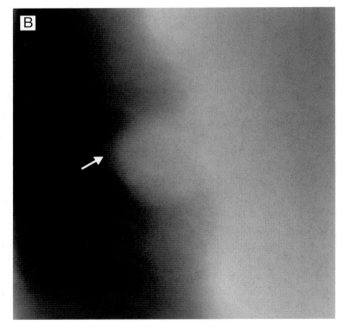

Figure 74.23 *Granuloma. A and B, Computed tomography of solitary pulmonary nodules shows characteristic satellite nodules (arrows).*

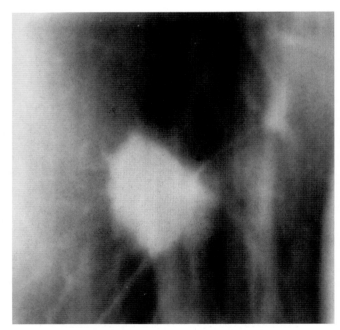

Figure 74.25 *Primary Bronchogenic Carcinoma. Computed tomography of a solitary nodule shows the characteristic spiculation or sunburst effect. Spicules indicate extension of the tumor into the septa. Computed tomography showed a similar appearance.*

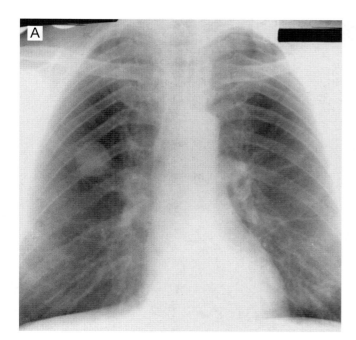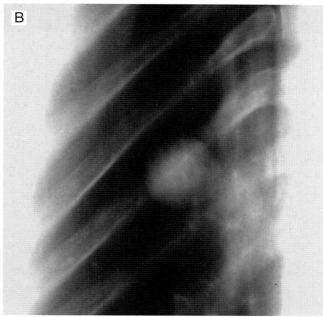

Figure 74.26 *Bull's-Eye Calcification Characteristic of Granuloma in a Solitary Pulmonary Nodule. A and B, These nodules occasionally enlarge but almost never warrant removal.*

Imaging

Computed tomography (CT) is useful in staging lung cancer and in evaluating the presence of solitary pulmonary nodules, multiple (metastatic) lung nodules, diffuse lung disease, and pleural processes. The use of contrast media helps in diagnosing pulmonary embolism and other pulmonary vascular abnormalities. A high-resolution CT scan is helpful in evaluation of interstitial lung diseases and can show characteristic features of pulmonary Langerhans cell granulomatosis, lymphangioleiomyomatosis, idiopathic pulmonary fibrosis, and lymphangitic pulmonary metastasis. Magnetic resonance imaging (MRI) is recommended for the initial evaluation of a superior sulcus tumor (ie, a Pancoast tumor), lesions of the brachial plexus, and paraspinal masses that on chest radiography appear consistent with neurogenic tumors. MRI is superior to CT in evaluating chest wall masses and in searching for small occult mediastinal neoplasms (eg, ectopic parathyroid adenoma).

Pulmonary angiography is useful in detecting pulmonary arteriovenous malformations, fistulas, and pulmonary embolisms. Peripheral or tiny pulmonary emboli, however, may not be detected. Bronchial angiography is used for suspected bronchial arterial bleeding in massive hemoptysis. Radionuclide lung scans (also called ventilation-perfusion scans) are useful in the diagnosis of pulmonary embolism, although CT angiography is used increasingly more often. Quantitative radionuclide scans may be useful in assessing unilateral and regional pulmonary perfusion and function before lung resection in surgical candidates who have preoperative comorbidities.

Fluoroscopy is useful in assessing diaphragmatic motion and in diagnosing diaphragmatic paralysis by the sniff test. Paradoxical motion of the diaphragm suggests diaphragmatic paralysis (but it is present in up to 6% of healthy patients). Bilateral diaphragmatic paralysis diminishes the sensitivity of the test.

Pulmonary Function Tests

Pulmonary function tests (PFTs) are useful in the evaluation of dyspnea (Box 74.3 and Figure 74.27). PFTs can show an obstructive pattern (Figures 74.28–74.31), which suggests diseases such as asthma, chronic obstructive pulmonary disease (COPD), or bronchiectasis. It can also show a restrictive pattern (Figure 74.32) suggestive of interstitial lung disease, chest wall limitation, or neuromuscular weakness. A combination of obstructive and restrictive patterns is also possible (eg, as in patients with combined COPD and pulmonary fibrosis). A **positive bronchodilator response** (ie, an increase of ≥12% *and* a 200-mL increase in either the forced expiratory volume in the first second of expiration [FEV_1] or the forced vital capacity [FVC] after

> ### Key Definition
>
> Positive bronchodilator response: *an increase of ≥12%* and *an increase of ≥200 mL in FEV_1 or FVC after bronchodilator administration.*

Box 74.3 • Interpretation of Pulmonary Function Test Results in the Evaluation of Dyspnea

Airflow obstruction is indicated by an FEV_1:FVC ratio <70%

Severity of airflow obstruction is indicated by the FEV_1, as a percentage of the predicted value
Mild obstruction: FEV_1 ≥80% predicted
Moderate obstruction: 50% ≤ FEV_1 <80% predicted
Severe obstruction: 30% ≤ FEV_1 <50% predicted
Very severe obstruction: FEV_1 <30% predicted

Airflow restriction is indicated by TLC <80% of the predicted value (a restrictive defect is only suggested by a reduced vital capacity; TLC is needed for confirmation)

Severity of restrictive defect is indicated by the TLC as a percentage of the predicted value
Mild restriction: 60% ≤ TLC <80% predicted
Moderate restriction: 50% ≤ TLC <60% predicted
Severe restriction: TLC <50% predicted

A positive bronchodilator response requires both an increase of ≥12% *and* an increase of ≥200 mL in the FEV_1 (or FVC) after bronchodilator therapy

A positive methacholine challenge requires a decrease of ≥20% in the FEV_1 after administration of methacholine

Abbreviations: FEV_1, forced expiratory volume in the first second of expiration; FVC, forced vital capacity; TLC, total lung capacity.

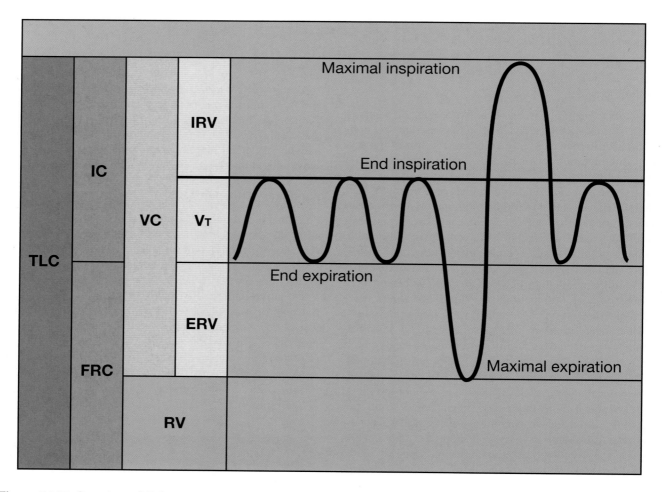

Figure 74.27 *Overview of Pulmonary Function Variables. ERV indicates expiratory reserve volume; FRC, functional residual capacity; IC, inspiratory capacity; IRV, inspiratory reserve volume; RV, residual volume; TLC, total lung capacity; VC, vital capacity; VT, tidal volume.*

Patient 7

The reduction in the FEV_1:FVC ratio suggests the presence of obstructive dysfunction. The decreased TLC suggests additional restrictive lung disease. The MVV is also reduced, and the DLco is severely decreased. This patient has COPD and severe restrictive lung disease. A very low DLco suggests parenchymal disease. Chest radiography showed bilaterally diffuse nodular interstitial changes, especially in the upper two-thirds of the lungs. Biopsy specimens of the bronchial mucosa and lung showed extensive endobronchial sarcoidosis. The clinical diagnosis is severe restrictive lung disease from parenchymal sarcoidosis and obstructive dysfunction caused by endobronchial sarcoidosis.

Patient 8

This patient has normal lung volumes and flow rates. The MVV is slightly decreased but within normal limits. The DLco is very low. The Pao_2 is 56 mm Hg. The clinical diagnosis is primary pulmonary hypertension.

Patient 9

This extremely obese patient has normal lung volumes and flow rates. The DLco is abnormally high. Abnormally high DLco is reported to be a result of increased vital capacity. The clinical diagnosis is obesity-related pulmonary dysfunction.

Exercise Testing

Indications for cardiopulmonary exercise testing include unexplained dyspnea or effort intolerance, disability evaluation, quantification of the severity of pulmonary dysfunction, differentiation between cardiac and pulmonary causes of disability, evaluation of progression of a disease process, estimation of operative risks before cardiopulmonary surgery (eg, lung resection, heart-lung transplant, or lung transplant), rehabilitation, and evaluation of the need for supplemental oxygen during exercise.

Invasive Testing

Bronchoscopy can be used for diagnostic and therapeutic purposes. It can be helpful in the evaluation of persistent cough, hemoptysis, pulmonary nodules, atelectasis, diffuse lung disease, lung infections, suspected cancer, and staging of lung cancer. Therapeutic indications include atelectasis, retained secretions, tracheobronchial foreign bodies, airway stenosis, and obstructive lesions. Bronchoalveolar lavage is helpful in diagnosing lung infections. Lung biopsy can be done with bronchoscopy, thoracoscopy, or thoracotomy.

KEY FACTS

✓ Provocation inhalational challenge with bronchospastic agent (eg, methacholine)—
  - useful when diagnosis of asthma or hyperreactive airway disease is uncertain
  - positive response: decrease of ≥20% in FEV_1 after inhalation of methacholine

✓ FEV_1:FVC ratio—
  - <70% suggests airflow obstruction (FEV_1 is used to classify severity)
  - ≥70% with a decreased FEV_1 should prompt evaluation of TLC (a decreased TLC suggests a restrictive defect)

✓ Causes of disproportionately reduced MVV—poor effort, variable extrathoracic obstruction, or respiratory muscle weakness

✓ Causes of low DLco—
  - anatomical emphysema (smaller area of the alveolar-capillary membrane)
  - anemia (effectively smaller area of the alveolar-capillary membrane); DLco decreases by 7% for each 1-g/dL decrease in hemoglobin
  - restrictive lung diseases (in pulmonary fibrosis or other interstitial lung diseases, alveolar-capillary membrane is smaller in area or thinner)
  - pulmonary hypertension (effectively thinner alveolar-capillary membrane)

✓ Flow curve patterns that help distinguish between intrathoracic and extrathoracic airway obstruction—
  - flattened expiratory flow curve with normal inspiratory flow curve: intrathoracic airway obstruction
  - flattened inspiratory flow curve alone: extrathoracic airway obstruction
  - flattened expiratory and flattened inspiratory flow curves: fixed airway obstruction (undetermined location)

75

Pulmonary Vascular Disease[a]

RODRIGO CARTIN-CEBA, MD, MSc

Pulmonary Hypertension

Pulmonary hypertension (PH) is defined by a mean pulmonary artery pressure (mPAP) of at least 25 mm Hg at rest, as measured during right heart catheterization (RHC). The many causes of PH are classified into 5 groups (Box 75.1).

Key Definition

Pulmonary hypertension: *mPAP ≥25 mm Hg at rest, as measured during RHC.*

Group 1, **pulmonary arterial hypertension** (PAH), is characterized by precapillary PH, normal pulmonary capillary wedge pressure (<15 mm Hg), and increasing vascular resistance, which leads to right-sided heart failure and death. Idiopathic PAH describes a subcategory of PAH. PAH is treated with pulmonary artery–vasodilator therapy. Treatment of other causes of PH (groups 2–5) is predominantly aimed at treating the underlying cause.

Key Definition

Pulmonary arterial hypertension: *precapillary PH, normal pulmonary capillary wedge pressure (<15 mm Hg), and increasing vascular resistance (which leads to right-sided heart failure and death).*

Box 75.1 • Updated Clinical Classification of Pulmonary Hypertension[a]

1. Pulmonary arterial hypertension (PAH)
   1.1. Idiopathic PAH
   1.2. Heritable PAH
      1.2.1. BMPR2
      1.2.2. ALK1, ENG, **SMAD9**, **CAV1**, **KCNK3**
      1.2.3. Unknown
   1.3. Drug and toxin induced
   1.4. Associated with
      1.4.1. Connective tissue disease
      1.4.2. HIV infection
      1.4.3. Portal hypertension
      1.4.4. Congenital heart diseases
      1.4.5. Schistosomiasis
1′. Pulmonary venoocclusive disease or pulmonary capillary hemangiomatosis (or both)
1″. **Persistent pulmonary hypertension of the newborn (PPHN)**
2. Pulmonary hypertension due to left heart disease
   2.1. Left ventricular systolic dysfunction
   2.2. Left ventricular diastolic dysfunction
   2.3. Valvular disease
   2.4. **Congenital or acquired left heart inflow tract or outflow tract obstruction and congenital cardiomyopathies**
3. Pulmonary hypertension due to lung diseases or hypoxia (or both)
   3.1. Chronic obstructive pulmonary disease
   3.2. Interstitial lung disease
   3.3. Other pulmonary diseases with mixed restrictive and obstructive pattern

(Continued on next page)

---

[a] Portions previously published in Cartin-Ceba R, Swanson KL, Krowka MJ. Pulmonary arteriovenous malformations. Chest. 2013 Sep;144(3):1033–44. Used with permission.

3.4. Sleep-disordered breathing

3.5. Alveolar hypoventilation disorders

3.6. Chronic exposure to high altitude

3.7. Developmental lung diseases

4. Chronic thromboembolic pulmonary hypertension (CTEPH)

5. Pulmonary hypertension with unclear multifactorial mechanisms

    5.1. Hematologic disorders: **chronic hemolytic anemia,** myeloproliferative disorders, splenectomy

    5.2. Systemic disorders: sarcoidosis, pulmonary histiocytosis, lymphangioleiomyomatosis

    5.3. Metabolic disorders: glycogen storage disease, Gaucher disease, thyroid disorders

    5.4. Others: tumoral obstruction, fibrosing mediastinitis, chronic renal failure, **segmental PH**

Abbreviations: ALK1, activin receptor-like kinase type 1; BMPR2, bone morphogenic protein receptor type 2; CAV1, caveolin 1; ENG, endoglin; HIV, human immunodeficiency virus; KCNK3, potassium channel, 2-pore domain subfamily K, member 3; SMAD9, SMAD family member 9.

[a] From the 5th World Symposium on Pulmonary Hypertension held in Nice, France, in 2013. The main modifications to the previous Dana Point (2008) classification are in boldface type.

Adapted from Simonneau G, Gatzoulis MA, Adatia I, Celermajer D, Denton C, Ghofrani A, et al. Updated clinical classification of pulmonary hypertension. J Am Coll Cardiol. 2013 Dec 24;62(25 Suppl):D34–41. Erratum in: J Am Coll Cardiol. 2014 Feb 25;63(7):746. Used with permission.

The clinical presentation of patients with PH is non-specific: progressive dyspnea, chest pain, lower extremity edema, and fatigue. Blood testing, which may be helpful for identifying a cause of PH, includes connective tissue serologies, human immunodeficiency virus (HIV) testing, N-terminal pro-brain natriuretic peptide (NT-proBNP), thyroid and liver testing, and a complete blood cell count. Full pulmonary function testing, ventilation-perfusion scanning to assess for chronic thromboembolic disease, and sleep studies are essential in the evaluation.

Typically, a diagnosis of PH is suggested by an increased right ventricular systolic pressure on transthoracic Doppler echocardiography and is confirmed with RHC. Hemodynamic measurements during RHC are important for excluding PH due to left-sided heart failure (with reduced or preserved ejection fraction) and contributions from high cardiac output (eg, liver disease, thyroid disease, or anemia). Acute vasoreactivity testing is mandatory for patients with idiopathic PAH or heritable PAH to identify patients who may respond favorably to treatment with calcium channel blockers.

Table 75.1 • Approved Pulmonary Artery–Targeted Drugs for the Treatment of Pulmonary Arterial Hypertension

Drug Group	Approved Drugs	Administration Route
Prostacyclin analogues	Epoprostenol	Intravenous
	Treprostinil	Intravenous
		Subcutaneous
		Inhaled
		Oral
	Iloprost	Inhaled
Phosphodiesterase type 5 inhibitors	Sildenafil	Oral
	Tadalafil	Oral
Endothelin receptor antagonist	Bosentan	Oral
	Ambrisentan	Oral
	Macitentan	Oral
Guanylate cyclase stimulator	Riociguat	Oral

World Health Organization (WHO) functional class is a powerful predictor of survival. Median survival of patients in WHO functional class I or II is 6 years; for patients in WHO functional class IV, median survival is 6 months. Extremes of age, decreased exercise capacity (6-minute walk distance), syncope, and signs of right ventricular failure carry a poor prognosis.

To date, no cure exists. However, several treatment options that target the pulmonary artery have been shown to improve quality of life and possibly survival. Several pulmonary artery–targeted drugs acting through 4 different mechanisms are currently approved for the treatment of PAH (group 1) (Table 75.1). Combination therapy has become the standard of care in PAH, although the long-term safety and efficacy data are not well defined. A stepwise approach appears beneficial. Drug-drug interactions are common. Oxygen, diuretics, digoxin, and anticoagulation may be useful in the treatment of PAH. Recommendations include participating in supervised exercise training, avoiding pregnancy, and receiving both influenza and pneumococcal vaccinations. Pulmonary artery–targeted therapy in PAH has reduced referral for lung transplant, but transplant is an important option for patients who do not have a response to medical therapy.

Pulmonary Vasculitides and Alveolar Hemorrhage Syndromes

The pulmonary vasculitides are a heterogeneous group of autoimmune disorders characterized by inflammation and necrosis of the small pulmonary vessels. The most common vasculitides affecting the lungs are the antineutrophil cytoplasmic antibody (ANCA)-associated vasculitides, including granulomatosis with polyangiitis (formerly known as Wegener granulomatosis), microscopic polyangiitis, and eosinophilic granulomatosis with polyangiitis (formerly known as Churg-Strauss syndrome). These conditions are reviewed in Chapter 81, "Vasculitis."

Hemorrhage into the alveolar spaces is called diffuse alveolar hemorrhage (DAH) syndrome. DAH is often characterized by the presence of cough, dyspnea, fever, and chest pain with or without hemoptysis. Diagnosis is established with bronchoalveolar lavage (BAL) that shows progressively bloody return or an elevated level of hemosiderin-laden macrophages (>20%) (or both). DAH is often associated with ANCA-associated vasculitides, connective tissue diseases such as systemic lupus erythematosus, and anti–glomerular basement membrane (GBM) disease; these entities can occur as renal-pulmonary syndromes with both DAH and glomerulonephritis. Immunologic-mediated DAH is treated by administering high-dose intravenous methylprednisolone and addressing the underlying cause; plasma exchange may be indicated in certain cases (ie, Goodpasture syndrome).

Anti-GBM Disease (Goodpasture Syndrome)

Anti-GBM disease is a classic example of a cytotoxic (type II) disease in which autoantibodies target the GBM and the alveolar basement membrane. Younger patients with anti-GBM disease typically present with Goodpasture syndrome and recurrent hemoptysis, dyspnea, anemia, hematuria, and renal failure (pulmonary hemorrhage and rapidly progressive glomerulonephritis). The typical patient is a young man in his 20s (male to female ratio, 7:1) with pulmonary symptoms preceding renal manifestations. Among older patients with anti-GBM disease, women are affected more than men, and patients typically present with glomerulonephritis alone.

Kidney biopsy shows diffuse necrotizing crescentic glomerulonephritis, and immunofluorescence staining shows linear deposition of immunoglobulin (Ig)G and complement along basement membranes. Anti-GBM antibody is positive in more than 90% of patients.

Plasmapheresis is the treatment of choice to remove the circulating autoantibodies, and cyclophosphamide and systemic corticosteroids are used to stop production of new autoantibodies. Complete recovery is expected in most patients; relapse occurs in up to 7% of patients.

Pulmonary Arteriovenous Malformation

Pulmonary arteriovenous malformations (PAVMs) are abnormal vascular structures that most often connect a pulmonary artery to a pulmonary vein, resulting in an intrapulmonary right-to-left shunt (Figure 75.1). As a consequence, patients present with hypoxemia and paradoxical embolization complications, including transient ischemic attack (TIA), stroke, and brain abscess. PAVMs lack structural integrity and can rupture, leading to hemorrhagic complications, including hemoptysis and hemothorax. Most PAVMs are hereditary and occur with hereditary hemorrhagic telangiectasia (HHT) or Rendu-Osler-Weber syndrome, an autosomal dominant vascular disorder.

Diagnostic criteria for HHT include telangiectasias (fingers, lips, and tongue), epistaxis (spontaneous and recurrent), visceral arteriovenous malformation (brain, lung, liver, and gastrointestinal tract), and family history. Diagnostic testing involves identifying an intrapulmonary shunt—the most sensitive test is transthoracic contrast echocardiography. Computed tomography of the chest is useful for characterizing PAVM in patients who have positive intrapulmonary shunting. Transcatheter embolotherapy is the treatment of choice for PAVM. Lifelong follow-up is important because recanalization and collateralization may occur after embolization therapy. Surgical resection is rarely necessary, and it is reserved for patients who are not candidates for embolization. Antibiotic prophylaxis for procedures with a risk of bacteremia (eg, dental procedures) is recommended for all patients with PAVM because of the risk of cerebral abscess.

Hepatopulmonary Syndrome

Hepatopulmonary syndrome (HPS) is a complication of portal hypertension. The diagnostic triad includes evidence of portal hypertension, intrapulmonary vascular dilatations, and hypoxemia. Hypoxemia is identified by a low Pao_2 on arterial blood gases (<80 mm Hg on room air) or an increased alveolar-arterial gradient in the partial pressure of oxygen. Classic symptoms of HPS are platypnea-orthodeoxia (dyspnea upon changing to an upright position); clubbing and cyanosis may be seen on examination. The only effective treatment is liver transplant, which resolves hypoxemia and improves survival.

Pulmonary Artery Aneurysm

Pulmonary artery aneurysms are usually asymptomatic and are discovered on routine chest imaging. Many patients do not require treatment other than serial observation. Surgical indications include recurrent hemoptysis, continued growth, or refractory hypoxemia because of right-to-left shunting through the aneurysm.

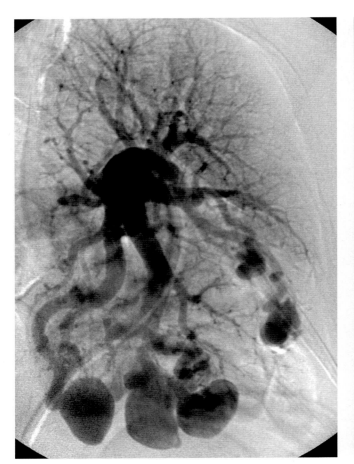 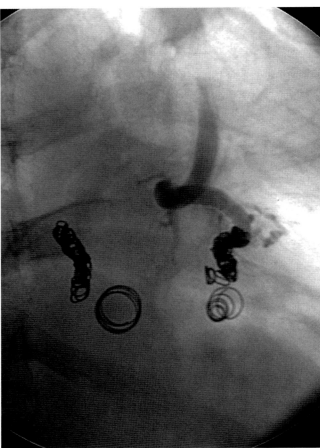

Figure 75.1 *Pulmonary Arteriovenous Malformations. A, Pulmonary angiography documents the presence of multiple, large pulmonary arteriovenous malformations. B, After coil embolization, the pulmonary arteriovenous malformations show a complete lack of flow.*

Pulmonary Capillary Hemangiomatosis

Pulmonary capillary hemangiomatosis is a severe, idiopathic proliferation of pulmonary capillaries that is usually accompanied by PH. Symptoms include dyspnea, hemoptysis, and edema. Computed tomography shows a diffuse reticulonodular pattern with enlarged central pulmonary arteries. The diagnosis requires lung biopsy, which is usually not performed owing to excessive risk. There is no effective treatment. Without transplant, median survival is 3 years.

Pulmonary Vascular Tumors

Pulmonary vascular tumors are rare and are usually metastatic at diagnosis. They may arise from the aorta, inferior vena cava, pulmonary arteries, or veins. Sarcomas and leiomyosarcomas are the most common tumors and may mimic pulmonary embolism. Breast, lung, prostate, pancreas, liver, and stomach cancers may metastasize to the pulmonary vasculature.

KEY FACTS

✓ Tests to identify a cause of PH—

- connective tissue serologies
- HIV testing
- NT-proBNP
- thyroid and liver testing
- complete blood cell count
- pulmonary function testing
- ventilation-perfusion scanning
- sleep studies

✓ Diagnosis of DAH through use of BAL—progressively bloody return and elevated level of hemosiderin-laden macrophages (>20%)

✓ Anti-GBM disease—

- typically younger male patients with Goodpasture syndrome and renal failure (pulmonary hemorrhage and rapidly progressive glomerulonephritis)
- in older patients, glomerulonephritis alone
- kidney biopsy: diffuse necrotizing crescentic glomerulonephritis
- immunofluorescence staining: linear deposition of IgG and complement along basement membranes
- treatment of choice: plasmapheresis (to remove circulating autoantibodies) and cyclophosphamide and systemic corticosteroids (to stop production of new autoantibodies)

✓ PAVMs—hypoxemia and paradoxical embolization complications (eg, TIA, stroke, and brain abscess)

✓ Pulmonary vascular tumors—breast, lung, prostate, pancreas, liver, and stomach cancers may metastasize to the pulmonary vasculature

Pulmonary Lymphatic Disorders

Pulmonary lymphatic disorders include lymphangioma, lymphangiomatosis, lymphangiectasis, and pulmonary lymphatic dysplasia syndromes. Pulmonary lymphatic dysplasia syndromes include idiopathic lymphedema syndromes, idiopathic recurring chylous effusions, and yellow nail syndrome. They are characterized by obstruction of proximal lymphatic channels with a refractory accumulation of chyle. The immunoglobulin loss may result in immunodeficiency, and the protein loss may result in malnutrition. Yellow nail syndrome consists of lymphedema, yellow dystrophic nails, and idiopathic pleural effusions or respiratory tract illness (or both) with bronchiectasis and recurrent pneumonias. The nails usually do not grow, and patients may wonder why the nails do not need to be trimmed.

76 Sleep-Related Breathing Disorders

MITHRI R. JUNNA, MD

Obstructive Sleep Apnea–Hypopnea Syndrome

Obstructive sleep apnea (OSA) is defined as periodic cessation of airflow (duration ≥10 seconds) during sleep with complete obstruction of the upper airway and continued respiratory effort. Typically, the episode is terminated by a temporary arousal from sleep and return of normal upper airway patency. **Hypopnea** is defined as partial obstruction cf the upper airway during sleep (duration ≥10 seconds), usually with a resultant desaturation of at least 4%. Hypopnea is also typically terminated by a temporary arousal. Such periodic episodes of apnea and hypopnea usually result in fragmented sleep and periodic desaturations. OSA should be suspected in patients who are obese, have increased neck circumference, are known to snore, and complain of daytime sleepiness. An overnight in-laboratory polysomnogram or home sleep test is required for making the diagnosis of OSA with documentation of 5 or more episodes of apnea and hypopnea per hour. Although overnight oximetry may suggest the presence of OSA, it is neither sensitive enough to rule out the diagnosis, nor specific enough to confirm it.

OSA has been associated with multisystemic dysfunction (Box 76.1). Several studies suggest that patients with untreated OSA have an increase in postoperative complications and overall mortality.

Key Definition

Obstructive sleep apnea: *periodic cessation of airflow (duration ≥10 seconds) during sleep with complete obstruction of the upper airway and continued respiratory effort.*

Key Definition

Hypopnea: *partial obstruction of the upper airway during sleep (duration ≥10 seconds), usually with a resultant desaturation of at least 4%.*

Box 76.1 • Systemic Disorders That Have Been Associated With Sleep-Related Breathing Disorders

Central nervous system
  Cognitive impairment
  Excessive daytime sleepiness
  Lower seizure threshold
  Recurrent headaches
  Stroke
Cardiovascular system
  Myocardial infarctions
  Hypertension
  Cardiac arrhythmias
  Acceleration of atherosclerosis
  Pulmonary hypertension
Endocrine system
  Insulin insensitivity
  Suppression of growth hormone release
  Alteration of progesterone and testosterone release
  Obesity
Digestive system
  Gastroesophageal reflux disease
Respiratory system
  Hypercapnia
  Dyspnea
  Reduced exercise tolerance
Psychiatric
  Mood disorders
  Insomnia

Central Sleep Apnea Syndromes

Central sleep apnea (CSA) is defined as periodic cessation of airflow (duration ≥10 seconds) during sleep without upper airway obstruction and without respiratory effort (presumably caused by a lack of respiratory muscle stimulation). In contrast to OSA, airflow is gradually resumed and is not always associated with an arousal from sleep. Causes of CSA may be neurologic conditions (eg, stroke, Chiari malformations, or multiple system atrophy), cardiovascular conditions (eg, congestive heart failure or atrial fibrillation), renal failure, opioid use, high altitude, or idiopathic. The respiratory pattern, which cycles between crescendo and decrescendo respirations followed by a pause, is known as *Cheyne-Stokes breathing* or *Cheyne-Stokes respiration,* and typically occurs with congestive heart failure or after a stroke.

Key Definition

Central sleep apnea: *periodic cessation of airflow (duration ≥10 seconds) during sleep without upper airway obstruction and without respiratory effort.*

Sleep-Related Hypoventilation Syndromes

Sleep-related hypoventilation is characterized by decreased minute ventilation with resultant hypercapnia and usually hypoxemia during sleep. Affected persons may also have daytime hypoventilation. Features can include daytime hypercapnia, pulmonary hypertension, and cor pulmonale. Most affected persons are obese (*obesity-hypoventilation syndrome*) or have severe respiratory or neurologic disease.

Treatment

Patients with OSA are treated with noninvasive positive pressure devices, such as continuous positive airway pressure (CPAP) and bilevel positive airway pressure (BPAP) devices. Adequate titration can be achieved during an in-laboratory polysomnogram, but, in certain circumstances, an autotitrating positive airway pressure (PAP) device may be used. Alternatives to PAP therapy can include avoidance of supine sleep (if applicable), use of a mandibular repositioning appliance, oral pressure therapy, surgical treatments, and hypoglossal nerve stimulators. In severe cases, tracheostomy may be required. Treatment of CSA usually requires a specialized BPAP device known as an adaptive servo-ventilator. Weight loss is also helpful in the treatment of OSA and obesity-hypoventilation syndrome.

KEY FACTS

- ✓ Typical features of patients with OSA—obesity, large neck circumference, history of snoring, and complaints of daytime sleepiness
- ✓ Diagnosis of OSA—
  - overnight in-laboratory polysomnogram or home sleep test
  - ≥5 episodes of apnea and hypopnea per hour
- ✓ Causes of CSA—
  - neurologic conditions (eg, stroke, Chiari malformations, or multiple system atrophy)
  - cardiovascular conditions (eg, congestive heart failure or atrial fibrillation)
  - renal failure
  - opioid use
  - high altitude
  - idiopathic
- ✓ Treatment of OSA—if severe, may require tracheostomy
- ✓ Treatment of CSA—usually requires a specialized BPAP device (an adaptive servo-ventilator)

Questions and Answers

Questions

Multiple Choice (choose the best answer)

XII.1. A 25-year-old man is admitted to the intensive care unit (ICU) with deceleration injuries after a motor vehicle collision. The patient required on-scene mechanical extrication from the vehicle. He has bilateral lower extremity fractures that required surgical intervention before he arrived in the ICU. Thus far, he has received 10 L of crystalloid and 2 units of packed red cells. Over the first 4 hours, his blood pressure and urine output decreased and partially responded to an additional 4 L of crystalloid. Currently, his blood pressure is 80/50 mm Hg, his heart rate is 110 beats per minute, his respiratory rate is 18 breaths per minute, and he is normothermic. Other than his lower extremity injuries, no abnormal findings are noted on his examination. His hemoglobin is 9 g/dL, and his coagulation values are normal. His total creatine kinase (CK) is 800 U/L. A computed tomographic scan of the abdomen from the emergency department is normal. What should you do next?
a. Administer a colloid fluid bolus.
b. Obtain an echocardiogram.
c. Administer methylprednisolone.
d. Perform a focused assessment with sonography for trauma (FAST).
e. Begin a bicarbonate infusion.

XII.2. A 25-year-old female nonsmoker presents with a 1-week history of mild cough and dyspnea after a flulike illness with fever, arthralgias, and tender erythematous lesions on the anterior aspects of her legs. She has no history of asthma or significant medical illnesses. No environmental or occupational high-risk exposures are noted. On examination, she has clear lung fields and no other abnormalities. A chest radiograph shows prominent bilateral hilar lymphadenopathy without parenchymal infiltrates. What should you do next?
a. Set up blood cultures.
b. Perform human immunodeficiency virus serology testing.
c. Determine the erythrocyte sedimentation rate.
d. Perform Lyme serology testing.
e. Observe and repeat the chest radiograph in 12 weeks.

XII.3. A 62-year-old man, a former smoker, presents with a 2-year history of progressive dry cough and dyspnea. He has no extrapulmonary symptoms. No occupational or environmental exposures are noted. Findings on examination include bibasilar coarse rales and digital clubbing. A chest radiograph shows prominent interstitial infiltrates in the middle and lower lung fields. The antinuclear antibody titer (1:40) is borderline elevated. Serum protein electrophoresis shows a polyclonal gammopathy. The rheumatoid factor titer (1:40) is also borderline elevated.

A high-resolution computed tomographic (CT) scan of the chest shows subpleural honeycombing with thickened alveolar septa in both lower lobes with bilateral mediastinal 1.5-cm lymph nodes. No ground-glass opacities are present. Which treatment is most likely to result in clinical improvement?
a. Azathioprine
b. Systemic corticosteroids
c. Cyclophosphamide
d. Systemic corticosteroids with azathioprine
e. No treatment

XII.4. A 52-year-old man, a current smoker with a 75–pack-year history, is examined for acute dyspnea and right-sided chest pain. He denies having fever, chills, sweats, cough, sputum production, or hemoptysis. On auscultation of the lungs, diminished breath sounds are heard throughout, with more on the right than the left. The chest radiograph and computed tomographic scan of the chest show scattered interstitial changes with cystic and nodular abnormalities, which are more prominent in the mid and upper lung zones, and a right-sided pneumothorax. What is the most likely diagnosis?
a. Lymphangioleiomyomatosis
b. Pulmonary Langerhans cell histiocytosis (histiocytosis X)
c. Cystic fibrosis
d. Aspiration pneumonia
e. Idiopathic pulmonary fibrosis

XII.5. A 54-year-old woman presents with progressive dyspnea at rest. Chest radiography shows significant left-sided effusion. Results of the thoracentesis and blood tests are shown in Table XII.Q5.

Table XII.Q5

Component	Serum	Thoracentesis Fluid
Protein, g/dL	6.5	2.5
Lactate dehydrogenase, U/L	155	125
pH	...	7.1

Which of the following is *not* a possible cause of the pleural fluid?
a. Pulmonary embolism
b. Empyema
c. Rheumatoid effusion
d. Tuberculosis
e. Malignancy

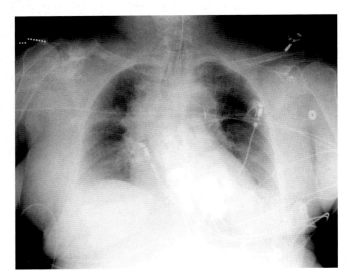

Figure XII.Q6A

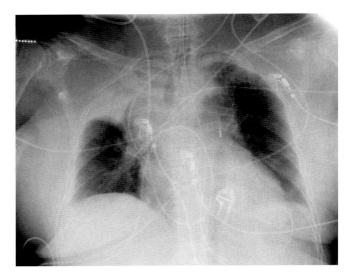

Figure XII.Q6B

XII.6. A 47-year-old man who had been healthy and did not have a significant past medical history is admitted to your intensive care unit with severe shock. Endotracheal intubation was performed before he arrived. The initial chest radiograph is shown in Figure XII.Q6A. Even after receiving several liters of fluid and vasopressors, the patient remains hypotensive. You decide to place a pulmonary artery (PA) catheter. The procedure goes smoothly and the vessel is cannulated at first pass. You request another chest radiography to confirm placement (Figure XII Q6B). Which of the following is the cause of the finding on the second radiograph?

a. Vessel injury resulting in hemothorax
b. Lobar collapse due to mucous plug
c. Pneumothorax
d. Hemopneumothorax
e. Pulmonary infarct due to overwedging of the PA catheter

XII.7. A 19-year-old woman comes to your office with her infant because she is concerned about her recurrent sinusitis. Although she has never been hospitalized, her younger brother was hospitalized for recurrent pancreatitis. She describes a chronic productive cough with dyspnea. Examination reveals wheezing and digital clubbing. What is the recommended initial test to diagnose this disorder?

a. No further testing
b. Sweat chloride testing
c. Testing for a *CFTR* genetic mutation
d. Computed tomographic (CT) scan of the chest with an intravenous contrast agent
e. CT scan of the sinuses followed by magnetic resonance imaging of the brain if abnormalities are detected

XII.8. A 57-year-old man presents for excessive sleepiness and difficulty functioning at his work. His wife has complained of very disruptive snoring and has witnessed frequent apneic episodes. His body mass index is 42. His blood pressure is 155/85 mm Hg. His neck size is 48 cm. Which of the following tests should be performed next to confirm your suspicion?

a. Overnight pulse oximetry
b. Use of a 24-hour ambulatory blood pressure monitor
c. Overnight polysomnography
d. Carotid duplex ultrasonography
e. Adrenal imaging with computed tomography

Answers

XII.1. Answer b.

This patient has myocardial contusion after trauma, with possible left ventricular failure. This is suggested by the mechanism of accident injury and his elevated CK. A bedside echocardiogram can quickly confirm this diagnosis. The other answer choices are less plausible.

XII.2. Answer e.

Sarcoidosis is a granulomatous disease most often affecting the lungs and lymph nodes. It can occur after a flulike illness and may be diagnosed from a specific constellation of symptoms and signs when a patient presents with Löfgren syndrome (erythematous nodosum, bilateral hilar lymphadenopathy, fever, and polyarthritis). In most other instances, a diagnosis of sarcoidosis requires a compatible history, findings of noncaseating granulomas by biopsy, and exclusion of other possible causes of granulomatous inflammation. With systemic involvement, blood tests may show abnormalities, including hypercalcemia, anemia, and elevated liver enzymes. Serum angiotensin-converting enzyme levels are neither specific nor sensitive to use as a diagnostic tool but, when elevated, may be helpful for following disease activity. Bronchoscopy can confirm granulomatous disease in over 90% of patients with hilar adenopathy and parenchymal lung involvement. Rales are uncommon in sarcoidosis even when parenchymal interstitial changes are present. Incidence, clinical course, and prognosis of sarcoidosis are influenced by ethnic and genetic factors. Computed tomographic scan may show nodular opacities with bronchovascular and subpleural distribution, thickened intralobular septa, architectural distortion, or conglomerate masses (late stage). Tobacco use has not been associated with development of sarcoidosis. Extrapulmonary involvement from sarcoidosis may involve the heart, liver, spleen, eyes, bone, skin, bone marrow, parotid glands, pituitary gland, and reproductive organs. This patient's presentation is most consistent with Löfgren syndrome, which carries a very good prognosis; symptoms resolve without treatment. Thus, observation with follow-up chest radiography is appropriate. If symptoms are more bothersome, symptomatic treatment (eg, use of nonsteroidal anti-inflammatory agents) may be considered. For progressive pulmonary and extrapulmonary disease, corticosteroids or immunosuppressive therapy should be considered.

XII.3. Answer e.

The combination of interstitial lung infiltrates predominantly involving the lower lung zones, lack of occupational exposure, duration of symptoms, and peripheral honeycombing make the diagnosis of idiopathic pulmonary fibrosis (IPF) most likely. Favorable prognostic factors in IPF–usual interstitial pneumonia include age younger than 50, female sex, shorter duration of symptoms before presentation, presence of ground-glass opacities on CT scan of the chest, and lymphocytosis on examination of bronchoalveolar lavage fluid. Pulmonary function tests in IPF usually indicate restrictive impairment. Patients with IPF generally do not respond to corticosteroids or other immunosuppressive therapies. No clearly effective treatment options are currently available. Oxygen extends survival among patients with chronic obstructive pulmonary disease, but this benefit has not been shown for IPF patients. Familial clusters of IPF patients suggest a potential genetic predisposition in some cases of IPF.

XII.4. Answer b.

This patient's presentation is most consistent with adult pulmonary Langerhans cell histiocytosis, which, in most cases, is a form of smoking-related interstitial lung disease. Smoking cessation is the primary form of treatment. With smoking cessation alone, stabilization or improvement occurs in up to two-thirds of patients. Other therapies, including systemic corticosteroids and immunosuppressives, have been used with limited success. A role for plasmapheresis has not been described.

XII.5. Answer a.

Pleural fluid analysis and the ratio of pleural fluid lactate dehydrogenase (LDH) to serum LDH (125:155) show that the fluid is an exudate. For fluid to be considered an exudate, the fluid needs to meet only 1 of the Light criteria (ratio of pleural fluid protein to serum protein >0.5; ratio of pleural fluid LDH to serum LDH >0.6; or pleural fluid LDH greater than two-thirds of the upper limit of the reference range for serum LDH). From the results in Table XII.Q5, the protein ratio is less than 0.5, but the LDH ratio is greater than 0.6; thus, the pleural fluid is an exudate. Furthermore, the low pH suggests a certain diagnosis. When thoracentesis fluid pH is less than 7.3, diagnostic possibilities include empyema, esophageal rupture, rheumatoid arthritis, trauma, tuberculosis, and malignancy. Pleural fluid in pulmonary embolism may be either a transudate or an exudate, but the pH of the pleural fluid should not be severely acidic.

XII.6. Answer b.

Although all the answer choices are potential complications of PA catheter placement, careful inspection of the radiograph shows that lobar collapse is the best answer. Note the elevation of the minor fissure and the elevation of the right hemidiaphragm. These are characteristic findings of a lobar collapse. Hemothorax should not be limited to the upper lobes only; rather, fluid would accumulate in the lower portions of the chest, thereby blunting the costophrenic angle. Pneumothorax should result in collapse of the lower lobes as well in this previously healthy patient. Furthermore, pneumothorax should create an air interface and thus appear black, not white, on the radiograph. A hemopneumothorax

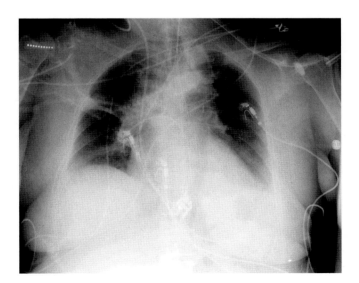

Figure XII.A6

should create an air-liquid interface along the lateral margin of the lung, which is not apparent in this radiograph. The region of involvement would be too large for pulmonary infarct due to overwedging. This patient underwent bronchoscopic clearing of the airways; the chest radiograph 30 minutes later is shown in Figure XII.A6.

XII.7. Answer b.

This patient has recurrent sinusitis, wheezing, digital clubbing, and a family member with recurrent pancreatitis. Cystic fibrosis must be considered as the underlying disorder. Women with cystic fibrosis can be fertile if they have adequate nutritional and pulmonary reserve. In contrast, men often present with azoospermia. The Cystic Fibrosis Foundation recommends sweat chloride testing as the initial diagnostic test. If the sweat chloride concentration is more than 60 mmol/L, the diagnosis of cystic fibrosis is confirmed; if it is 30 to 59 mmol/L, testing for *CFTR* mutations is recommended.

XII.8. Answer c.

This patient has all the risk factors for at least moderately severe obstructive sleep apnea (OSA). Therefore, overnight polysomnography should be performed next to confirm the diagnosis. If OSA is confirmed, treatment should begin with a continuous positive airway pressure device. Overnight oximetry is occasionally used as a screening tool, but the results are not sufficient to establish the diagnosis even though they may be suggestive of OSA. Other tests have no role in establishing the diagnosis of OSA.

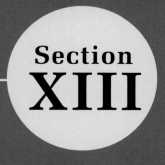

Section

XIII

Rheumatology

Connective Tissue Diseases

FLORANNE C. ERNSTE, MD

Systemic Lupus Erythematosus

Systemic lupus erythematosus (SLE) is a chronic inflammatory disease of unknown cause that affects multiple organ systems. Disease susceptibility is conferred by an interaction between genetics, aberrant immunologic mechanisms, hormonal influences, and environmental factors. SLE has a wide range of heterogeneous clinical manifestations and is characterized by disease flares and remissions. There is a broad spectrum of disease severity, leading to significant morbidity and increased mortality.

> ### Key Definition
>
> Systemic lupus erythematosus: *a chronic, inflammatory autoimmune disease of varying disease severity and organ manifestations characterized by disease flares and remissions.*

Epidemiology

Recent population-based studies in the United States have reported an increased incidence of SLE during the last few decades: incidence is 9 per 100,000 persons, and prevalence is up to 128 per 100,000 persons, although in some nonwhite ethnic groups, the prevalence has been reported to be higher. SLE is more common in females than males, with a female to male ratio ranging from 9:1 to 15:1. SLE is often seen in women of childbearing age; more than half of patients with SLE have disease onset between age 16 years and the mid-40s. In postmenopausal women, the female to male ratio is closer to 2:1. The prevalence of SLE is higher among black, Native American, and Hispanic females. Black females tend to have a younger age of onset and higher incidence of renal complications.

Etiology

The etiology of SLE is unknown, but multiple contributors to the pathogenesis have been identified. These include genetic, hormonal, immunologic, and environmental influences, such as ultraviolet light and viruses.

Genetics

Twin and family studies show a genetic component that contributes to SLE onset. There is a higher concordance rate (>20%) among monozygotic twins than dizygotic twins. Large-scale, genome-wide association studies have identified about 50 gene loci with multiple polymorphisms, including class II HLA genes, complement genes, and immunoglobulin receptor genes. In general, a combination of susceptibility genes, such as HLA-DR2 and HLA-DR3, *STAT4*, and *PTPN22*, and loss of protective genes may predispose individuals to SLE.

Pathogenesis

The pathogenesis of SLE is characterized by a loss of tolerance to self-antigens and autoantibody production. Immune complexes form that bind complement, release inflammatory mediators, and deposit in tissues, leading to injury. Innate immunity is activated by the circulating immune complexes via Toll-like receptors 7 and 9, resulting in type I interferon-α production. This leads to release of downstream proinflammatory cytokines such as tumor necrosis factor α, which is increased in specific SLE manifestations such as lupus nephritis. There are also abnormalities of T and B cells, with a decrease in cytotoxic T cells and suppressor T-cell function and an increase in helper T cells and B-cell hyperactivity, resulting in polyclonal activation and autoantibody production.

Clinical Manifestations

Mucocutaneous

There are 4 common lupus rashes: acute cutaneous rash, subacute cutaneous lupus erythematosus (SCLE) rash, discoid rash, and lupus profundus rash. The acute cutaneous rash is characterized as an erythematous, elevated or flat malar rash (butterfly rash) that spares the nasolabial folds and is exacerbated by sunlight (ie, photosensitive). SCLE is characterized by annular, erythematous rings with serpiginous borders and central hypopigmentation on sun-exposed areas, such as the arms, shoulders, neck, and trunk. SCLE is associated with anti–SS-A (Ro) and anti–SS-B (La) antibodies; it can occur in the absence of SLE manifestations. Discoid lupus is manifested by chronic, erythematous papular or plaquelike lesions involving the face, scalp, and extremities and may occur without SLE manifestations. There is follicular plugging with central atrophy, leading to scarring. Lupus profundus is an inflammatory panniculitis of the subcutaneous fat layer that variably appears on the extremities and/or trunk as painful nodules. Chronic urticaria also may occur in up to 10% of patients.

Alopecia of varying degrees is also a common feature of SLE. Hair loss may be diffuse or patchy and, like the malar rash, is associated with SLE flares. Hair may regrow during disease remissions. Hair loss may also be an adverse effect of cytotoxic drugs, such as methotrexate or cyclophosphamide.

Oral ulcers are another common mucocutaneous feature of active SLE. They usually are painless and occur on the hard palate, buccal mucosa, or tongue. Ulcers also can occur on the nasal septum during active SLE.

Articular

Polyarthralgia and/or inflammatory arthritis are the most common presenting feature of SLE, affecting up to 90% of patients. Unlike rheumatoid arthritis, the arthritis of SLE is classically nondeforming and nonerosive. The arthritis is symmetrical and typically involves the small joints of the hands, wrists, and sometimes knees. A subset of a deforming arthritis called Jaccoud arthropathy is manifested by tendon inflammation and a nonerosive arthritis with joint subluxations and hand/finger contractures.

KEY FACTS

- ✓ SLE has onset during childbearing years and is more prevalent among nonwhite women
- ✓ Alopecia is a common mucocutaneous feature of SLE
- ✓ Ulcers can occur in the mouth and, less often, on the nasal septum in active SLE
- ✓ The most common presenting feature of SLE—polyarthralgia and/or inflammatory arthritis (90% of cases)

Avascular necrosis of the bone may occur. The clinical presentation is acute joint pain and physical disability. The femoral head and tibial plateau are most commonly affected. Plain radiographs of the joint are often insensitive, but radionuclide bone scan or magnetic resonance imaging is useful in detecting avascular necrosis. Conservative therapy with avoidance of excessive weight-bearing activity is usually recommended, but joint replacement may be necessary.

Cardiovascular

Cardiac involvement in SLE is manifested by pericarditis, myocarditis, endocarditis, accelerated coronary atherosclerosis, and rarely coronary vasculitis. The most common cardiac manifestation is pericarditis. It is characterized by chest pain and a pericardial rub, although clinically it may be silent. Nonbacterial vegetations on native valves can range from tiny lesions to large verrucous vegetations and can lead to valvular dysfunction, embolization, or infective endocarditis. Although rare, myocarditis should be suspected in a patient with SLE who has unexplained arrhythmias or cardiomegaly. An association between SLE and premature coronary artery disease has been established and can occur in inactive lupus as a late complication. Women with SLE in their mid-30s to mid-40s have a 50-fold increased risk of premature coronary atherosclerosis and myocardial infarction compared to their age-matched controls. In addition to the traditional cardiovascular risk factors, SLE is an independent cardiovascular risk factor, possibly related to the immune-mediated vascular inflammation.

Pulmonary

Pulmonary involvement may be manifested by any of the following: pleurisy, pleural effusions, acute pneumonitis, pulmonary hypertension, pulmonary embolism, diffuse alveolar hemorrhage, and diaphragmatic dysfunction (ie, shrinking lung syndrome). Pleural manifestations are the most common pulmonary feature of SLE. Patients may give a clinical history of pleuritic chest pain without accompanying chest radiograph abnormalities. When detected, pleural effusions are often small and bilateral but can be massive. The characteristics of lupus effusions are exudative with normal glucose concentration, in contrast to the effusions seen in rheumatoid arthritis, in which the glucose concentration is low. Diffuse alveolar hemorrhage is a serious but uncommon manifestation in SLE and presents with cough and hemoptysis; it is associated with a poor prognosis. Shrinking lung syndrome is rare and poorly understood but thought to be secondary to abnormal respiratory muscles or diaphragmatic dysfunction/weakness.

Renal

Renal involvement in SLE is very common and may occur in approximately 50% to 75% of patients. Nonwhite females with SLE are more often affected. The pathophysiology is primarily that of an immune complex–mediated glomerular disease related to the formation of anti–double-stranded DNA antibodies against nucleosomes that aggregate or directly bind to glomerular basement proteins. Elevated levels of anti–double-stranded DNA antibodies and low levels of complement (C3 and C4) may indicate active renal disease. The highly characteristic immunofluorescence finding on renal biopsy is the so-called full-house pattern: glomerular deposits that stain for immunoglobulin (Ig) G, IgA, IgM, C3, and C1q. The International Society of Nephrology and the Renal Pathology Society have classified lupus nephritis according to renal biopsy findings as follows: minimal mesangial (class I), mesangial proliferative (class II), focal lupus nephritis (class III), diffuse lupus nephritis (class IV), membranous lupus nephritis (class V), and advanced sclerosing lupus nephritis (class VI). In addition, tubulointerstitial disease can coexist with glomerular disease and is seen with an elevated creatinine level, hypertension, and a progressive course. Thrombotic microangiopathy manifested by glomerular and vascular thrombi may occur often, with positive results for anticardiolipin antibodies and lupus anticoagulant. A less common occurrence is renal vein thrombosis with nephrotic syndrome.

Renal involvement may occur in asymptomatic patients; hence, routine monitoring of blood pressure, creatinine, and urinalysis is recommended at frequent intervals. Renal involvement is manifested by proteinuria of greater than 0.5 g/24 h or the presence of casts (eg, red blood cell, heme, granular, tubular, or mixed). Additionally, an elevated creatinine level and the presence of hematuria (>5 red blood cells per high-power field) and/or pyuria (>5 white blood cells per high-power field) in the absence of infection are signs of active renal disease. A strong predictor of lupus nephritis is an elevated level of anti–double-stranded DNA antibodies.

Renal biopsy results have both prognostic and therapeutic implications. Patients with high activity indices on biopsy, such as active inflammation, proliferation, necrosis, and crescent formation, are considered for aggressive therapy. Patients with high chronicity indices, such as tubular atrophy, interstitial fibrosis, scarring, and glomerulosclerosis, are less likely to respond to aggressive therapy. Chronic lesions are associated with decreased renal and patient survival. Patients with mesangial changes alone do not require aggressive immunosuppressive therapy. Active focal or diffuse glomerulonephritis (class III and class IV) and membranous glomerulonephritis with nephrotic-range proteinuria (class V) are treated with induction therapy consisting of pulsed high-dose corticosteroids, then oral corticosteroids with taper, and cyclophosphamide (intravenous route preferred to oral because of fewer complications). Mycophenolate mofetil has shown efficacy equivalent to that of cyclophosphamide with fewer adverse effects and is an option for induction and maintenance therapy in

lupus nephritis. Rituximab, a chimeric monoclonal antibody against CD20 antigen and a B-cell–depleting agent, has gained increased use for induction therapy in refractory proliferative lupus nephritis, but recent trials did not report increased efficacy compared to placebo in achieving primary outcomes. After induction therapy, mycophenolate mofetil or azathioprine is generally used to maintain renal remission; azathioprine is preferred in women with childbearing potential. In approximately 10% to 30% of patients with lupus nephritis, end-stage renal disease will develop within 15 years of diagnosis despite aggressive treatment.

KEY FACTS

✓ Wide range of cardiovascular manifestations in SLE—pericarditis (most common), valvular abnormalities, myocarditis, premature coronary atherosclerosis, myocardial infarction, coronary vasculitis

✓ The most common pulmonary feature of SLE—pleural manifestations

✓ The kidneys are involved in approximately 50% to 75% of patients with SLE

✓ Treatment of class III to V renal involvement in SLE—induction therapy with corticosteroids, cyclophosphamide, or mycophenolate mofetil; maintenance therapy with mycophenolate mofetil, or azathioprine in women of childbearing age

---

In patients with nephrotic-range proteinuria or chronic proteinuria even without evidence of active renal disease, angiotensin-converting enzyme (ACE) inhibitors should be used. They have been shown to reduce proteinuria and have renoprotective effects. Aggressive blood pressure control is paramount to improving renal survival.

Neuropsychiatric

The diagnosis of neuropsychiatric systemic lupus erythematosus (NPSLE) is controversial because of the difficulty in drawing clear associations between heterogeneous neurologic manifestations and active lupus disease. Additionally, numerous metabolic, infectious, or medication-induced mimickers need to be excluded before making an NPSLE diagnosis. SLE has a wide spectrum of manifestations broadly categorized as central nervous system (CNS) or peripheral nervous system abnormalities by the American College of Rheumatology. Among the CNS manifestations are aseptic meningitis, seizure disorder, strokes, demyelinating disease, headache (severe headaches refractory to narcotics), movement disorders such as chorea, myelopathy, acute confusion, anxiety disorder, mood disorder, cognitive dysfunction, and psychosis. Among the peripheral manifestations are polyneuropathy, plexopathy, cranial neuropathy, myasthenia gravis, mononeuropathy, autonomic neuropathy, and Guillain-Barré syndrome. The pathogenesis of CNS lupus is not well understood. On autopsy, common findings are microinfarcts, small-vessel wall thickening, and nerve cell loss; thrombotic occlusion of larger vessels and vasculitis (inflammatory infiltrate with fibrinoid necrosis) are less commonly seen.

The diagnosis of NPSLE is usually clinical. Cerebrospinal fluid analysis is important and may show increased cerebrospinal fluid protein IgG, pleocytosis, increased protein, decreased glucose, antineuronal antibodies, and antiribosomal P antibodies. Results of electroencephalography may be abnormal but nonspecific. Computed tomography (CT) brain studies may show areas of infarctions, hemorrhage, or cortical atrophy. Magnetic resonance imaging studies are superior to CT scans and show areas of increased signal intensity in the periventricular white matter, similar to those found in multiple sclerosis.

Gastrointestinal

Gastrointestinal involvement in SLE ranges from nausea to esophageal reflux, mesenteric vasculitis, liver disease (eg, lupoid hepatitis), and pancreatitis. A gastrointestinal syndrome that occurs during SLE disease exacerbations is manifested by acute abdominal pain, nausea, and anorexia from peritoneal inflammation. Ascites, including massive ascites, may also be present, but infection and/or malignancy must be ruled out with paracentesis. Chronic, painless ascites may occur in a subset of patients without other manifestations of active lupus.

Hematologic

Hematologic abnormalities are frequent manifestations of SLE. Anemia of chronic disease is often seen, but hemolytic anemia (Coombs test positive) is less common. Leukopenia ranges from 2,500 to 4,000 leukocytes/mm³ but usually does not predispose to infections; it may be associated with active SLE secondary to antilymphocyte antibodies. Thrombocytopenia is also common. Idiopathic thrombocytopenic purpura with platelet antibodies can precede a diagnosis of SLE. Patients may have mild petechiae or "easy bruising." Antiphospholipid antibody syndrome should be suspected in patients with chronic, refractory thrombocytopenia. Patients with SLE may have a false-positive VDRL test for syphilis. Patients with SLE also can have false-positive results of the fluorescent treponemal antibody test, but they usually have the beaded pattern of fluorescence. LE cells are present in approximately 70% of patients with SLE caused by an antibody to deoxyribonucleoprotein. The LE cell test is not specific and is no longer performed in many centers.

Diagnosis

The diagnosis of SLE is challenging to make because many features are nonspecific: patients may present with symptoms that mimic other inflammatory disorders, such as infection and malignancy. In general, the diagnosis is based on a variety of clinical manifestations and laboratory findings. Classification criteria developed by expert consensus, such as the 1997 American College of Rheumatology criteria (4 out of 11 criteria must be met) or the 2012 Systemic Lupus International Collaborating Clinics criteria (4 of 17 criteria must be met), aid researchers in categorizing patients, but the criteria may be problematic in confirming a diagnosis because of the heterogeneity of disease manifestations. Classic clinical features in patients with SLE are listed in Box 77.1, adapted from the 1997 American College of Rheumatology criteria.

The significance of autoantibodies in SLE depends on the type and level. Although almost all patients with SLE (>95%) have positive results of antinuclear antibody (ANA) tests, a positive result is not specific for SLE. Asymptomatic individuals without SLE may have low-titer ANA (eg, 1:40) of no clinical significance. Anti–double-stranded DNA levels are specific for SLE; levels fluctuate, and high levels are used as a marker for disease activity, especially in lupus nephritis. Levels of other autoantibodies (eg, ribonucleoprotein [RNP], Smith [Sm], ANA) do not correlate with SLE disease activity. The anti-Sm antibody is highly specific for SLE. ANA patterns are outlined in Table 77.1. Other autoantibodies and disease associations are listed in Table 77.2.

Box 77.1 • Classification Criteria for Diagnosis of Systemic Lupus Erythematosus

Malar rash

Discoid lupus

Photosensitivity

Oral ulcers

Nonerosive arthritis of 2 or more peripheral joints

Serositis: pleuritis or pericarditis

Renal disorder: proteinuria (protein >0.5 g/d) or cellular casts

Neurologic disorder: seizures or psychosis

Hematologic disorder: hemolytic anemia, leukopenia, lymphopenia, or thrombocytopenia

Immunologic disorder: anti–double-stranded DNA, anti-Smith, antiphospholipid antibodies

Positive antinuclear antibody test in the absence of offending drugs

Data from American College of Rheumatology. 1997 Update of the 1982 American College of Rheumatology revised criteria for classification of systemic lupus erythematosus [Internet]. Atlanta (GA): American College of Rheumatology; c1997 [cited 2015 Oct 28]. Available from: http://www.ncbi.nlm.nih.gov/pubmedhealth/PMH0041704/.

Table 77.1 • Antinuclear Antibody Patterns

Fluorescent Pattern	Antigen	Disease Association
Rim, peripheral, shaggy	nDNA	SLE
Homogeneous	DNP	SLE, DIL, others
Speckled	ENA	MCTD, SLE, Sjögren syndrome
Nucleolar	RNA	Scleroderma

Abbreviations: DIL, drug-induced lupus; DNP, deoxyribonucleoprotein; ENA, extractable nuclear antigen; MCTD, mixed connective tissue disease; nDNA, native DNA; SLE, systemic lupus erythematosus.

KEY FACTS

✓ A syndrome of acute abdominal pain, nausea, and anorexia from peritoneal inflammation can occur during SLE exacerbations

✓ Common hematologic manifestations of SLE—anemia of chronic disease, leukopenia, and thrombocytopenia

✓ Anti–double-stranded DNA levels correlate with SLE disease activity; levels of other autoantibodies do not

✓ The anti-Smith antibody is highly specific for SLE

✓ Autoantibodies are prevalent in SLE and other connective tissue diseases but must be interpreted cautiously within the clinical context

Treatment

The SLE disease course is characterized by periods of increased disease activity (flares), chronic persistent symptoms, remission, and cumulative damage of involved organs. Treatment should match disease activity and severity of organ system involvement. Frequent monitoring of disease activity (eg, anti–double-stranded DNA, C3, C4, erythrocyte sedimentation rate, proteinuria) allows for rapid recognition and treatment of SLE flares. Table 77.3 provides guidelines for treatment, and Table 77.4 outlines the complications of treatment. Hydroxychloroquine has been regarded as an essential medication for long-term treatment of SLE because of its low side effect profile, benefits in reducing organ damage and thrombosis, and its association with increased patient survival. Belimumab, a monoclonal antibody that inhibits the B-lymphocyte stimulator, the soluble B-cell–activating factor, has been approved as the only biologic agent available for treating the cutaneous and articular manifestations of SLE nonresponsive to conventional therapy; studies are under way to expand the indications for its use in other SLE manifestations. Rituximab has been gaining use as an off-label alternative for major SLE manifestations, such as in NPSLE and proliferative nephritis, but recent trials have not shown statistically significant benefits.

Table 77.2 • Autoantibodies in Rheumatic Diseases

Antibody	Disease Association
Anti–double-stranded DNA	SLE, 50%–70%
Anti-Sm (Smith)	SLE, 30%
Anti-U1-RNP (ribonucleoprotein)	MCTD, 100% at high titer; SLE, 30%; scleroderma
Anti–SS-A (Ro)	Sjögren syndrome, 70%; SLE, 35%; scleroderma + MCTD; neonatal lupus
Anti–SS-B (La)	Sjögren syndrome, 60%; SLE, 15%; neonatal lupus
Antihistone	Drug-induced SLE, 95%; SLE, 60%; RA, 20%
Anti–Scl-70 (antitopoisomerase I)	Scleroderma, 25%
Anticentromere	CREST, 70%–90%; scleroderma, 10%–15%
Anti-PM1 (polymyositis)	PM, 50%
Anti-Jo1 (antisynthetase)	Antisynthetase syndrome (dermatomyositis, PM, interstitial lung disease, fever, inflammatory arthritis, Raynaud phenomenon), 30%

Abbreviations: CREST, syndrome of *c*alcinosis cutis, *R*aynaud phenomenon, *e*sophageal dysmotility, *s*clerodactyly, *t*elangiectasia; MCTD, mixed connective tissue disease; RA, rheumatoid arthritis; SLE, systemic lupus erythematosus.

Pregnancy and SLE

Women with SLE who become pregnant have a high prevalence of pregnancy-related complications, such as preterm premature rupture of membranes, preeclampsia, thrombosis, and spontaneous abortion. Moreover, patients with SLE typically have increased disease activity during pregnancy, possibly related to fluctuating hormone levels. Predictors of SLE flares during pregnancy are the presence of anti–double-stranded DNA and/or antiphospholipid antibodies, active renal disease, and low complement levels prior to conception. SLE flares should be treated with corticosteroids; however, the risk of hypertension and gestational diabetes is increased with prolonged use. Almost all of the immunosuppressants are contraindicated during pregnancy, with the exception of hydroxychloroquine and azathioprine.

In infants of mothers with SLE, thrombocytopenia and leukopenia can develop from passive transfer of maternal antibodies. Neonatal lupus occurs in approximately 3.5% of SLE pregnancies. Infants may have transient cutaneous lesions after ultraviolet light exposure, complete heart block (about 2% risk), and thrombocytopenia. Mothers usually have anti–SS-A (Ro) and/or anti–SS-B (La) antibodies that cross the placenta and are transiently present in the infant. Mothers are monitored at 16 weeks onward with fetal echocardiography.

Table 77.3 • Commonly Used Treatments for Manifestations of Systemic Lupus Erythematosus

Manifestation	Treatment
Arthritis, fever, mild systemic symptoms	ASA, NSAID, low-dose corticosteroids
Photosensitivity, rash	Avoidance of sun, use of sunscreens with SPF of 50 or higher, topical corticosteroids and/or topical tacrolimus, hydroxychloroquine (Plaquenil), chloroquine
Rash, arthritis	Hydroxychloroquine, methotrexate (Trexall), leflunomide (Arava), azathioprine (Imuran), belimumab (Benlysta)
Significant thrombocytopenia, hemolytic anemia	Corticosteroids, IVIG
Renal disease, CNS disease, pericarditis, other significant organ involvement	Corticosteroids, cyclophosphamide, cyclosporine
Rapidly deteriorating renal function	Cyclophosphamide, mycophenolate mofetil, azathioprine

Abbreviations: ASA, acetylsalicylic acid; CNS, central nervous system; IVIG, intravenous immunoglobulin; NSAID, nonsteroidal anti-inflammatory drug; SPF, sun-protection factor.

Neonatal lupus resolves once the antibodies are cleared from the mother, which may take about 6 months.

Prognosis

The 10-year survival rate is about 90% in newly diagnosed SLE. Yet, despite improved management of SLE and its complications, patients still have a mortality risk 3 times higher than that of the general population and approximately 10% may die within 10 years of diagnosis. Deaths in "early" lupus (about 1 year after diagnosis) are attributed to active disease; deaths in "late" lupus are attributed to premature cardiovascular atherosclerosis and infection. Prognosis is worse in African Americans, Hispanics, and men. Progressive renal disease or CNS disease is associated with decreased survival. SLE also affects work productivity and contributes to increased health care costs, disability, and a poor quality of life. The major causes of death are 1) active SLE disease, 2) infection, and 3) premature cardiovascular disease.

Drug-Induced Lupus

Many drugs have been implicated as causative in drug-induced lupus (DIL). The most common of these are listed

Table 77.4 • Complications of Treatment for Systemic Lupus Erythematosus

Treatment	Complication
Ibuprofen	Aseptic meningitis (headache, fever, stiff neck, CSF pleocytosis)
NSAID	Decreased renal blood flow
ASA	Salicylate hepatitis (common), benign
Corticosteroids	Avascular necrosis, diabetes mellitus, hypertension, osteoporosis, dyslipidemia, obesity
Hydroxychloroquine	Retinal toxicity, skin hyperpigmentation
Methotrexate	Mucositis, hepatitis, nausea, loose stools, hair loss
Leflunomide	Elevated liver enzyme levels, cytopenias, diarrhea
Azathioprine	Nausea, cytopenias, pancreatitis
Immune globulin	Infusion reactions, headaches
Mycophenolate mofetil	Nausea, headaches, hypertension, cytopenias, increased risk of nonopportunistic and opportunistic infections, colitis
Cyclophosphamide	Hemorrhagic cystitis, alopecia, nonopportunistic and opportunistic infections, increased incidence of lymphomas (CNS), sterility (premature ovarian failure)
Cyclosporine	Hypertension, hirsutism, hyperkalemia, hypomagnesemia, renal failure
Belimumab	Nonopportunistic and opportunistic infections, infusion reactions, diarrhea

Abbreviations: ASA, acetylsalicylic acid; CNS, central nervous system; CSF, cerebrospinal fluid; NSAID, nonsteroidal anti-inflammatory drug.

in Box 77.2. Hydralazine, procainamide, and methyldopa have been classically associated with DIL. The pathogenesis is complex, but it is related in part to inhibition of DNA methylation and transformation of the drug to reactive metabolites. A drug-induced lupus syndrome develops in 5% to 10% of patients taking hydralazine and in 15% to 25% of those taking procainamide. DIL may be underreported, since many cases resolve after the offending drug has been removed.

Clinical Manifestations

In contrast to SLE, DIL has an almost equal sex distribution and is predominant in the older population. More cases of DIL in older males are due to hydralazine and procainamide, probably because of increased use among this demographic. The clinical manifestations of DIL include fever, malaise, rash, arthralgias, myalgias, and serositis. Rashes can manifest as purpura or erythematous papular lesions, although subacute cutaneous lupus, discoid lupus,

Box 77.2 • Implicated Agents in Drug-Induced Lupus

Definite

    Procainamide
    Hydralazine
    Isoniazid
    Methyldopa
    Penicillamine
    Diltiazem
    Quinidine
    Minocycline
    Anti-TNF drugs
    Interferon alfa

Probable

    Phenytoin
    Carbamazepine
    Ethosuximide
    Propylthiouracil
    Sulfasalazine
    Captopril
    Lithium carbonate
    Acebutolol
    Terbinafine

Possible

    Penicillin
    Tetracycline
    Valproate
    Statins
    Gemfibrozil
    Hydrochlorothiazide

Abbreviation: TNF, tumor necrosis factor.

and malar rashes may occur. Approximately 30% of patients have serositis, particularly with procainamide use. Pericarditis has been reported in approximately 20% of cases. Asymptomatic pleural effusions may be found on chest radiography. In contrast to SLE, CNS and renal manifestations are rare.

Laboratory Findings

Almost all patients with SLE or DIL have ANA. Anti–double-stranded DNA is found in a small percentage of cases, especially when anti–tumor necrosis factor and interferon alfa agents have been used. In contrast to SLE, serum total hemolytic complement, C3, and C4 values are usually normal. Antibodies such as anti-Sm, anti–SS-A, anti–SS-B, and anti-RNP are also unusual in DIL. The frequency of antihistone antibodies in DIL is high (>95% of cases), but these antibodies also occur in approximately 60% of SLE cases.

Diagnosis

The diagnosis is made by establishing a timeline between onset of symptoms after initiation of drug use, which ranges from 3 weeks to 2 years, and rapid improvement or resolution after discontinuation of the drug, usually within 6 weeks. An ANA test should be obtained. To definitively diagnose DIL, some clinicians may rechallenge patients with the same drug or a similar drug of the same class to determine whether signs/symptoms recur.

Treatment

Patients with DIL should discontinue the offending drug. Symptoms usually subside within several weeks, although the duration for complete resolution varies. Serologic abnormalities (eg, a positive ANA result) can persist for years after resolution of clinical symptoms. Treatment depends on the clinical manifestations and may include nonsteroidal anti-inflammatory drugs or low-dose corticosteroids for arthralgias, fever, and serositis symptoms.

Mixed Connective Tissue Disease

Mixed connective tissue disease (MCTD) is a distinct disease with features that overlap with SLE, systemic sclerosis, polymyositis, and inflammatory arthritis. It is serologically characterized by a positive ANA result and by a high titer of anti-U1-RNP antibody. There is a high female to male predominance (10:1). The clinical manifestations are bilateral hand edema, Raynaud phenomenon, arthritis, and myositis. In some patients with MCTD, phenotype may eventually evolve to be characteristic of systemic sclerosis or SLE. Pulmonary arterial hypertension is associated with MCTD and typically results in a poor prognosis.

KEY FACTS

- ✓ Three drugs classically associated with drug-induced lupus—hydralazine, procainamide, and methyldopa
- ✓ Antihistone antibodies occur in more than 95% of cases of drug-induced lupus, but also in about 60% of SLE cases
- ✓ To diagnose drug-induced lupus, establish that symptoms (eg, fever, rash, arthritis, serositis) began after the drug was started and rapidly improved after it was stopped
- ✓ Characteristic serologic findings in mixed connective tissue disease—antinuclear antibodies and a high titer of anti-U1-ribonucleoprotein antibody

Undifferentiated Connective Tissue Disease

Patients with undifferentiated connective tissue disease have symptoms that do not fulfill the diagnostic criteria for a definite or specific connective tissue disease. Common symptoms include Raynaud phenomenon, arthralgias, sicca, fatigue, and polyarthralgia. The ANA result may be positive, usually of low to medium titer, but other autoantibodies are not present. Surveillance of these patients is required to determine whether progression to a distinct connective tissue disease occurs.

Antiphospholipid Antibody Syndrome

Antiphospholipid antibody syndrome (APS) is a disorder characterized by recurrent venous and arterial thrombosis and/or pregnancy morbidities. The syndrome is diagnosed by clinical and laboratory criteria. Definite APS is diagnosed if at least 1 clinical criterion and 1 laboratory criterion are met. The clinical criteria are as follows: venous, arterial, or small-vessel thrombosis in any organ (superficial venous thrombosis does not satisfy this criterion); or 1 or more fetal losses with normal fetal morphology, unexplained, after 10 weeks' gestation; or 1 or more premature births at or before 34 weeks' gestation due to severe preeclampsia, eclampsia, or placental insufficiency; or 3 or more recurrent fetal losses before 10 weeks' gestation. The laboratory criteria are as follows: 1) medium to high levels of IgG or IgM antiphospholipid antibodies (>40 GPL or MPL units or >99th percentile) on 2 occasions at least 12 weeks apart by enzyme-linked immunosorbent assay; 2) IgG or IgM anti-β_2-glycoprotein-1 antibodies at a titer above the 99th percentile on 2 or more occasions at least 12 weeks apart by enzyme-linked immunosorbent assay; or 3) presence of lupus anticoagulant by dilute Russell viper venom time and activated partial thromboplastin time (aPTT), followed by mixing study and confirmatory testing on 2 occasions 12 weeks apart. These criteria represent a version of the revised Sapporo classification criteria.

Many, but not all, patients with lupus anticoagulant also have increased IgG or IgM antiphospholipid antibody levels. These antibodies may be found in patients with no apparent disease in whom recurrent thrombosis develops; these patients have primary APS. Secondary APS occurs in the setting of an underlying condition, such as SLE, infection, or malignancy. It is also common to see transiently elevated antiphospholipid antibody levels and/or lupus anticoagulant due to infection and/or an inflammatory state; hence the need for confirmatory testing 12 weeks later.

Clinical Features

Multiple organ systems may be affected to varying degrees. Patients with recurrent venous thromboses most often have involvement of the deep and superficial veins of the leg, but other sites have been reported, including cerebral venous sinus, pulmonary, portal, mesenteric, hepatic, pelvic, and inferior vena cava. Patients with recurrent arterial thromboses may have strokes (secondary to valvular emboli) or transient ischemic attacks, as well as retinal, coronary, brachial, or mesenteric thromboses.

Libman-Sacks endocarditis and other valvular abnormalities have been reported, such as thickening, stenosis, and vegetations in up to 50% of patients with APS. A variety of skin abnormalities have been observed, such as livedo reticularis, digital gangrene, nailfold infarcts, and leg ulcers.

The hallmark laboratory features of APS are persistent thrombocytopenia and prolongation of the aPTT. The failure of normal plasma to correct the aPTT distinguishes lupus anticoagulant and antiphospholipid antibody from clotting factor deficiencies. In addition, a Coombs-positive hemolytic anemia is a characteristic finding in APS.

Catastrophic APS refers to development of thrombosis of 3 or more organ systems with positive results for antiphospholipid antibodies and/or lupus anticoagulant in a short time, such as a week. Life-threatening organ ischemia often occurs in the CNS and pulmonary, renal, gastrointestinal, and cardiac systems. Depending on the extent of catastrophic APS and the organs involved, patients may present with acute pulmonary hemorrhage, confusion, acute abdominal pain due to bowel infarction, and renal insufficiency requiring hemodialysis; these patients are best managed in a critical care setting. Prognosis is poor and treatment often involves multiple courses of plasma exchange, high-dose glucocorticoid therapy, and anticoagulation. Data on use of rituximab in refractory APS are limited, but its use has been increasing.

Key Definition

Catastrophic antiphospholipid antibody syndrome: *development of thrombosis of 3 or more organ systems with positive results for antiphospholipid antibodies and/or lupus anticoagulant in a short period of time, such as a week.*

Treatment

The initial approach to treatment involves use of unfractionated heparin or low-molecular-weight heparin (LMWH) in combination with warfarin for 3 to 5 days until the warfarin reaches a therapeutic effect with an increased international normalized ratio (INR) in the range of 2 to 3. For most patients with definite APS and thrombosis, warfarin will need to be taken lifelong. In pregnant women with definite APS, subcutaneous LMWH is used; warfarin is resumed in the postpartum period. In pregnant women with definite APS and a history of prior pregnancy morbidity, low-dose aspirin and LMWH are used in combination. In patients with either antiphospholipid antibodies or lupus anticoagulant, use of estrogen-containing oral contraceptive pills should be avoided, since these patients may be at higher risk for thrombosis. In patients who have recurrent thrombosis despite warfarin treatment with an INR in the 2 to 3 range, additional intensive therapy is suggested, such as increasing the target INR range to 3 to 4 and adding LMWH and low-dose aspirin. Monitoring the INR in patients with APS may be problematic, potentially related to the presence of antiprothrombin antibodies, which may falsely prolong the prothrombin time even without warfarin therapy and/or lupus anticoagulant increasing the INR. Monitoring factor Xa levels may be a solution.

Raynaud Phenomenon

Raynaud phenomenon refers to reversible digital vasospasm characterized by classic, triphasic color changes (pallor, cyanosis, and reactive hyperemia followed by erythema). It is often accompanied by pain and numbness in the fingers, hands, toes, and/or feet. Constriction of the digital vessels leads to pallor, cyanosis results from blood stasis marked by deoxygenation, and reactive hyperemia is due to increased blood flow. Raynaud phenomenon has primary and secondary forms. Primary Raynaud phenomenon is often mild and is characterized by symmetrical involvement in young women. This group of patients may be at risk for a connective tissue disorder if results of an ANA test are positive, even decades after initial occurrence. Cold or emotional stress is a common precipitating agent. Primary Raynaud phenomenon is a clinical diagnosis, although investigation should be made into secondary causes with such tests as a complete blood cell count, ANA, erythrocyte sedimentation rate, C-reactive protein, creatinine, urinalysis, and serum protein electrophoresis.

Key Definition

Raynaud phenomenon: *reversible digital vasospasm characterized by classic, triphasic color changes (pallor, cyanosis, and reactive hyperemia followed by erythema).*

Secondary Raynaud phenomenon is associated with an underlying disorder, such as a connective tissue disease (eg, systemic sclerosis, MCTD). Nailfold capillary microscopy reveals tortuous, enlarged dilated capillary loops in systemic sclerosis, MCTD, and dermatomyositis. These patients may have digital pitting, periungual telangiectasias, scarring, loss of digital pulp, and gangrenous changes. Other causes of secondary Raynaud phenomenon are listed in Box 77.3 and include vasoconstricting effects from drugs, occlusive vascular disorders, and occupational hazards.

Treatment involves conservative management, such as wearing mittens or gloves to keep the core body temperature elevated and avoidance of precipitating factors, such as vasoconstricting drugs. Smoking cessation should be emphasized. Vasodilators, such as calcium channel blockers,

---

Box 77.3 • Causes of Secondary Raynaud Phenomenon

Connective tissue diseases
 Scleroderma
 Mixed connective tissue disease
 Sjögren syndrome
 Systemic lupus erythematosus
 Rheumatoid arthritis
 Polymyositis/dermatomyositis
 Antiphospholipid antibody syndrome
 Cryoglobulinemia
Drugs
 Bleomycin
 Vinblastine
 Bromocriptine
 Cyclosporine
 β-Blockers
 Antimigraine agents, eg, sumatriptan
 Toxins, eg, cocaine
Vascular occlusive disorders
 Increased blood viscosity (paraproteinemia)
 Thoracic outlet obstruction
 Atherosclerosis
 Vasculitis
 Microemboli
 Thromboangiitis obliterans (Buerger disease)
Occupational hazards
 Jackhammer use
 Cold injury
 Polyvinyl chloride exposure
Miscellaneous
 Cold agglutinins
 Hepatitis infection

---

are the mainstays of treatment. Commonly used calcium blockers are nifedipine, amlodipine, and diltiazem. Other, less commonly used agents are 2% nitrate paste, α-blockers, sildenafil, phosphodiesterase-5 inhibitors, and intravenous or oral prostacyclin analogues. Surgical treatment is rarely used but is often necessary in patients with severe Raynaud phenomenon with digital ischemia accompanied by tissue loss and pain; in these patients, a stellate ganglion block, digital nerve block, or surgical digital sympathectomy is done.

Systemic Sclerosis (Scleroderma)

Systemic sclerosis (scleroderma) is divided into several categories: 1) diffuse systemic sclerosis (diffuse scleroderma); 2) limited cutaneous scleroderma, which includes CREST (*c*alcinosis cutis, *R*aynaud phenomenon, *e*sophageal dysmotility, *s*clerodactyly, *t*elangiectasias); 3) localized scleroderma, such as morphea and linear scleroderma manifested by indurated plaques over extremities and torso. Systemic sclerosis sine scleroderma is rare and characterized by internal organ involvement without classic skin manifestations. For the diagnosis of systemic sclerosis (SSc), 1 major criterion or 2 or more minor criteria need to be present. The major criterion is symmetrical induration of the skin of the fingers and the skin proximal to metacarpophalangeal or metatarsophalangeal joints. The minor criteria are sclerodactyly, digital pitting scars in or loss of substance from the finger pad, and bibasilar pulmonary fibrosis. The pathologic hallmarks of scleroderma are an obliterative noninflammatory vasculopathy, proliferation of fibroblasts, and excessive accumulation of collagen in the skin and other organs, leading to fibrosis.

KEY FACTS

✓ For a diagnosis of definite antiphospholipid antibody syndrome, at least 1 clinical criterion and 1 laboratory criterion must be met

✓ Hallmark laboratory features of antiphospholipid antibody syndrome—persistent thrombocytopenia and prolongation of activated partial thromboplastin time

✓ If normal plasma does not correct the activated partial thromboplastin time, the problem is lupus anticoagulant and antiphospholipid antibody, not clotting factor deficiencies

✓ Three categories of systemic sclerosis (scleroderma)—diffuse systemic sclerosis (diffuse scleroderma), limited cutaneous scleroderma (including CREST), and localized scleroderma

---

Clinical Manifestations

Cutaneous

Three skin stages have been described in SSc. In stage 1, there is marked swelling/edema of hands or fingers due to inflammation with a loss of skin folds; decreased sweat and oil production leads to dry, cracked skin refractory to standard moisturizing agents. There may be diffuse pruritus due to elaboration of histamine and bradykinin. Stage 2 is characterized by progressive skin fibrosis resulting in hardened skin at fingertips and progressing proximally; in SSc, the face, chest, abdomen, and upper thighs may be involved in addition to the distal extremities. In stage 3 (late stage), there is skin softening from atrophy with some hair regrowth. Patients with rapidly progressive acral and trunk skin thickening are at risk for early visceral abnormalities, such as scleroderma renal crisis.

Raynaud Phenomenon

Raynaud phenomenon occurs in more than 95% of patients with scleroderma. Onset may be years before cutaneous findings of scleroderma are evident. In some patients, Raynaud phenomenon may occur simultaneously with skin changes. Its lack should trigger an investigation

---

Box 77.4 • Scleroderma Spectrum Disorders

Morphea
Eosinophilic fasciitis
Scleredema
Scleromyxedema
Nephrogenic systemic fibrosis

---

into the other causes of skin induration listed in Box 77.4. Patients with SSc have abnormal nailfold capillaries that can be visualized by an ophthalmoscope; these are manifested by prominent vasculature with dropout. Because of intimal fibrosis and structural abnormalities of the microvasculature, digital pitting, ulcers, and other digital ischemic changes may develop.

Articular

A nondeforming, symmetrical inflammatory polyarthritis similar to rheumatoid arthritis may precede cutaneous manifestations with involvement of the proximal interphalangeal joints, metacarpophalangeal joints, and wrists. Use of immunosuppressants, such as methotrexate or azathioprine, for treatment of the arthritis may be helpful. However, with progressive skin thickening and fibrosis, fixed flexion contractures may occur at multiple proximal interphalangeal joints, leading to structural deformities. Tendon friction rubs may be heard at the wrists, elbows, and/or ankles.

Pulmonary

Pulmonary involvement in the form of interstitial lung disease (ILD) and/or pulmonary arterial hypertension (PAH) is a common cause of morbidity and mortality in SSc. ILD is characterized by a basilar distribution and may occur in approximately 70% to 80% of patients. It is the most common pulmonary abnormality, especially in patients with diffuse SSc. Pulmonary function testing with spirometry should be obtained to screen for ILD. A reduction in diffusing capacity of the lung for carbon monoxide (D_{LCO}) is a sensitive means for detecting early ILD. A reduced D_{LCO} should be investigated with a high-resolution CT scan to determine if active alveolitis is present (ie, ground-glass opacities and reticular densities). The histologic pattern in a majority of patients is nonspecific interstitial pneumonia, which is often fibrotic. Patients who have active alveolitis demonstrated by 1) bronchopulmonary lavage with elevated neutrophil count, 2) high-resolution CT scan showing ground-glass opacities without honeycombing, or 3) lung biopsy may respond to low-dose prednisone and cyclophosphamide therapy. Treatment of ILD is with oral or intravenous (preferred route) cyclophosphamide for 6 to 12 months, which may result in mild to moderate improvement of pulmonary function parameters and stabilize the ILD progression, although treatment effects may not be sustained after 1 to 2 years. Mycophenolate mofetil has been gaining use as an alternative to cyclophosphamide because it has relatively less toxicity, although larger randomized controlled studies are needed to validate that it has similar efficacy compared to cyclophosphamide. Azathioprine is an alternative agent, but less effective than cyclophosphamide.

KEY FACTS

✓ In systemic sclerosis, rapidly progressive acral and trunk skin thickening indicates increased risk of early visceral abnormalities

✓ Common cause of morbidity and mortality in systemic sclerosis—pulmonary involvement (interstitial lung disease and/or pulmonary arterial hypertension)

✓ Interstitial lung disease in systemic sclerosis is treated with oral or intravenous (preferred) cyclophosphamide; may stabilize progression

✓ Pulmonary arterial hypertension in systemic sclerosis is treated with phosphodiesterase-5 inhibitors, prostacyclin analogues, and endothelin receptor antagonists

---

Patients with PAH may have an isolated decrease in D$_{LCO}$ with normal lung volumes. PAH is more common in patients with the CREST, or limited scleroderma, variant. Although echocardiography is helpful for making a diagnosis, right-sided heart catheterization should be performed to confirm the diagnosis and to obtain accurate measurements of pulmonary artery and capillary wedge pressures. PAH is associated with a high mortality rate. Treatment options involve phosphodiesterase-5 inhibitors, such as sildenafil; prostacyclin analogues, such as iloprost, epoprostenol, and treprostinil; and endothelin receptor antagonists, such as bosentan and ambrisentan. These agents have improved patient symptoms and delayed PAH progression.

Cardiac

Cardiac abnormalities occur in up to 70% of patients with SSc. Conduction defects and arrhythmias are the most common abnormalities because of fibrosis of conduction pathways; the most common abnormality is premature ventricular contractions. Other manifestations include pericardial abnormalities such as pericardial effusions and fibrinous pericarditis, diastolic dysfunction, and a dilated cardiomyopathy. Postmortem examination of the myocardium reveals inflammatory infiltrates in muscle cells and fibrosis with contraction band necrosis.

Gastrointestinal

Esophageal dysfunction is the most frequent gastrointestinal abnormality. It occurs in more than 90% of patients with SSc and may be asymptomatic. Lower esophageal sphincter incompetence with decreased sphincter tone results in dyspepsia; chronic injury from acid reflux may produce Barrett esophagus, esophageal strictures, or ulcers. Proton pump inhibitors reduce gastric acid production. Dysphagia can occur from involvement of the smooth muscle of the distal two-thirds of the esophagus. Esophageal dysmotility may respond to therapy with metoclopramide, cisapride, octreotide, or erythromycin. Telangiectasias of the gastric mucosa may result in chronic blood loss leading to iron deficiency anemia; gastric antral vascular ectasias may give the appearance of a "watermelon stomach" on endoscopy. Vascular ectasias may be treated by laser intervention. Small bowel hypomotility may be associated with pseudo-obstruction, bowel dilatation, bacterial overgrowth, and malabsorption. Treatment with rotating antibiotics may be helpful; promotility agents are less effective. Colonic dysmotility also occurs, and wide-mouthed diverticula may be found; intestinal pneumatosis may result from perforation of small or large bowel diverticula. The incidence of primary biliary cirrhosis is increased, especially in limited scleroderma or CREST.

Renal

Scleroderma renal crisis (SRC) is a dreaded organ manifestation of SSc and is typically associated with progressive diffuse skin involvement, use of corticosteroids at dosages greater than 15 mg per day, and other significant immunosuppression several weeks prior to onset. SRC develops in approximately 10% of patients with SSc. It is characterized by intimal proliferation and thrombosis of renal afferent arterioles and a high-renin state. Fulminant hypertension, renal failure leading to hemodialysis, and death may occur if it is not treated aggressively. Patients typically present with newly diagnosed hypertension (although some patients may be normotensive), proteinuria, hematuria, microangiopathic hemolytic anemia, thrombocytopenia, and "onion skinning" manifested by endothelial proliferation, medial hypertrophy, and adventitial fibrosis on renal biopsy. SRC can be easily confused with thrombotic thrombocytopenic purpura; it is imperative to clarify the diagnosis so that appropriate treatment is not delayed, since plasmapheresis is contraindicated with use of ACE inhibitors. Aggressive early antihypertensive therapy with ACE inhibitors can extend life expectancy in SRC. Prognosis was poor and mortality was high before the advent of ACE inhibitors. ACE inhibitors should be continued even if the patient progresses to dialysis because of the potential for recovery of kidney function.

Laboratory Findings

ANA are found in 95% or more of patients with scleroderma. Patients with SSc may have positive results for antitopoisomerase I antibody (anti–Scl-70); the presence of anti–Scl-70 antibody is associated with an increased risk of progressive skin and lung fibrosis. The presence of anti-RNA polymerase III antibody is associated with an increased risk of SRC.

Treatment

Treatment of SSc depends on the organ(s) involved, as discussed in the preceding sections. Aggressive nutritional support, including hyperalimentation, may be required for extensive gastrointestinal disease.

Limited Scleroderma or CREST Syndrome

CREST syndrome is characterized by *c*alcinosis cutis, *R*aynaud phenomenon, *e*sophageal dysmotility, *s*clerodactyly, and *t*elangiectasias. Skin involvement progresses slowly and is limited to the face, neck, and distal extremities. Internal organ involvement occurs but is delayed. Lung involvement occurs in 70% of patients. PAH is more common in CREST than in diffuse scleroderma. Patients with the CREST variant may have a positive result for anticentromere antibodies.

The clinical manifestations of limited and systemic scleroderma are described in Table 77.5.

Sjögren Syndrome

Sjögren syndrome (SS) is an autoimmune disorder characterized by decreased lacrimal and salivary gland function due to lymphocytic infiltration of the glands. The syndrome manifests with dry eyes (keratoconjuctivitis sicca) and dry mouth (xerostomia). It affects less than 1% of the US population and is more common in women than men (9:1 ratio). Onset usually occurs in the 40s to 50s. There are 2 types of SS: primary and secondary. In secondary SS, an underlying connective tissue disease is present, such as rheumatoid arthritis, MCTD, or SLE.

> ### Key Definition
>
> Sjögren syndrome: *an autoimmune disorder characterized by decreased lacrimal and salivary gland function due to lymphocytic infiltration of the glands; manifests with progressive dry eyes (keratoconjuctivitis sicca) and dry mouth (xerostomia).*

Clinical Manifestations

The symptoms and clinical features of SS can be categorized broadly into glandular and extraglandular manifestations. The glandular clinical features are the classic "sicca" symptoms manifested by a sensation of grittiness in the eyes and a dry mouth necessitating frequent sips of fluids during the day; patients often report a history of recurrent dental caries. Parotid gland enlargement may occur in a third of patients. Extraglandular manifestations widely vary in severity and organ system involvement. Some examples of extraglandular involvement include inflammatory arthritis, interstitial pneumonitis, primary biliary cirrhosis, peripheral neuropathy, small vessel vasculitis, and type 1 renal tubular acidosis. Patients who have primary SS are at increased risk for lymphoma: there is a 44-fold increased incidence. Extranodal marginal zone B-cell lymphoma of mucosa-associated tissue is commonly seen. Clinical predictors for lymphoma are a history of cutaneous vasculitis, low C3 and/or C4 levels, cryoglobulinemia, monoclonal gammopathy, and parotid gland enlargement.

Table 77.5 • Clinical Findings in Limited and Diffuse Scleroderma

Clinical Finding	Cutaneous Disease	
	Limited	Diffuse
Raynaud phenomenon	Precedes other symptoms by years	Onset may be simultaneous or associated with other symptoms within 1 y
Nailfold capillaries	Dilated	Dilated with dropout
Skin changes	Distal to elbow	Proximal to elbow with involvement of trunk
Telangiectasia, digital ulcers, calcinosis	Frequent	Rare early, but frequent later in the course
Joint and tendon involvement	Uncommon	Frequent (tendon rubs)
Visceral disease	Pulmonary hypertension	Renal, intestinal, and cardiac disease; pulmonary interstitial fibrosis
Autoantibodies	Anticentromere (70%–90%)	Antitopoisomerase I (anti–Scl-70) (25%)
10-year survival	>70%	<70%

KEY FACTS

✓ Scleroderma renal crisis is typically associated with progressive skin involvement, corticosteroid use >15 mg/day, and other significant immunosuppression

✓ To avoid delay in appropriate treatment, clarify that the diagnosis is scleroderma renal crisis, not thrombotic thrombocytopenic purpura

✓ Angiotensin-converting enzyme inhibitors can extend life expectancy in scleroderma renal crisis; continue therapy even if the patient progresses to dialysis

✓ Antitopoisomerase I antibody (anti–Scl-70) may be present in patients with systemic sclerosis

✓ Primary Sjögren syndrome increases the risk of lymphoma 44-fold

Laboratory Findings

The majority of patients will have a positive result for ANA in a speckled pattern. Approximately 65% to 75% of patients will have a positive result for anti–SS-A antibody, and fewer patients will have a positive result for anti–SS-B antibody, approximately 40% to 50%. It is common to find a polyclonal hypergammaglobulinemia due to increased B-cell activity and an elevated rheumatoid factor level. Cryoglobulins may be detected in approximately 30% of patients.

Diagnosis

Many criteria exist to diagnose SS. Most commonly used in clinical practice are the 2002 American-European Consensus Group classification criteria, which feature the following 6 criteria: dry eye symptoms; dry mouth symptoms; objective evidence of dry eyes (positive result of rose bengal, lissamine green, or Schirmer test); positive lymphocytic histopathologic findings on lip biopsy (focus score of 1 or greater); objective evidence of decreased salivary flow, as seen with salivary scintigraphy; and presence of anti–SS-A and/or anti–SS-B antibodies.

Treatment

Management of glandular manifestations of SS involves symptomatic treatment of dry eyes with use of artificial tears, topical cyclosporine drops, and punctal occlusions. Dry mouth symptoms are treated with lubricating artificial saliva agents, liberal use of sugar-free candies to stimulate salivary flow, and muscarinic agonist medications, such as pilocarpine and cevimeline. Extraglandular manifestations may be treated with immunosuppressive agents according to extent of severity; corticosteroids, antimalarials, disease-modifying antirheumatic drugs, and rituximab have all been used.

Musculoskeletal Disorders

78

ARYA B. MOHABBAT, MD AND CHRISTOPHER M. WITTICH, MD, PharmD

Neck Disorders

Diagnosis

Cervicothoracic complaints can be classified into 3 categories on the basis of etiology: mechanical, neurogenic, and pain secondary to other systemic processes.

Mechanical neck complaints are often secondary to trauma, overuse injury, malposture, and osteoarthritis. The pain is typically described as localized (spinal/paraspinal), dull, aching, and worse with range of motion. Physical examination often reveals point tenderness of the underlying spinous process and paraspinal musculature, as well as a decreased and painful range of motion.

Neurogenic neck complaints are experienced acutely after trauma or gradually as a result of progressive osteoarthritis with subsequent nerve root impingement (Figures 78.1 and 78.2). Classically, patients complain of an underlying dull, deep, and aching sensation with episodes of sharp, stabbing, and burning radicular symptoms. The radicular component is secondary to focal cervical nerve root impingement (Table 78.1), which can be reproduced on physical examination via the Spurling maneuver (Figure 78.3).

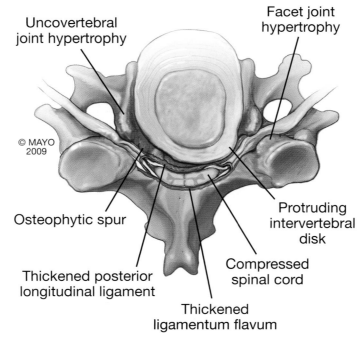

Figure 78.1 *Anatomy of Neck Pain. Classic anatomical changes associated with neck pain.*

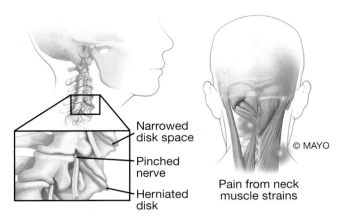

Figure 78.2 Neurogenic and Muscular Neck Pain. Neurogenic and muscular sources of neck pain.

Neck pain *secondary to systemic disease* often is associated with systemic symptoms such as fever, chills, weight loss, rash, polyarthralgia, or polymyalgia. The concomitant symptoms should help to guide the history, examination, and work-up in order to elucidate the underlying illness.

Imaging studies, including plain radiography, computed tomography myelography, and magnetic resonance imaging, are reserved for patients with antecedent trauma, progressive neurologic symptoms (ie, weakness, hyporeflexia/hyperreflexia, spasticity, paresthesia) and those with features concerning for an underlying systemic process.

Treatment

The majority of patients with cervicothoracic complaints recover with conservative therapy. Treatments include medication (acetaminophen, nonsteroidal anti-inflammatories, and muscle relaxants), activity modification, soft cervical collar, and physical therapy. Opioids generally are not recommended, though they can be considered for a short duration in patients with acute moderate-severe pain. Ongoing symptoms despite these modalities would warrant consideration for corticosteroid injection. Intractable pain or progressive neurologic deficits warrant orthopedic consultation.

Lower Back Disorders

Diagnosis

Low back pain (LBP) is one of the most common presenting complaints in the primary care setting. Chronic LBP is the most common compensable work-related injury. Interestingly, LBP is generally a self-limited issue, with the vast majority of patients noting improvement within 6 weeks.

The history and physical examination are essential in making the correct diagnosis. Only 3% of patients presenting with LBP have a cause that is not apparent after the initial history and examination (Tables 78.1 and 78.2). Arthritis (Figure 78.4), spinal stenosis, compression fracture, and malignancy are more commonly seen in older patients, while spondyloarthropathies are primarily seen prior to age 40 years. Physical examination should include assessment for spinal alignment, overlying skin changes, vertebral/paravertebral tenderness, and neurologic function, as well as straight-leg and crossed straight-leg raise tests (pain must radiate below the knee for a positive result; Figures 78.5 and 78.6).

Laboratory and imaging studies should be reserved for patients with concomitant red-flag signs/symptoms (Table 78.2). According to the joint guideline from the American College of Physicians and the American Pain Society, imaging should be obtained in cases of acute LBP only if associated with severe neurologic deficits or features concerning for a serious underlying condition. Common indications for spinal radiography are listed in Box 78.1.

KEY FACTS

✓ Mechanical neck complaints often result from trauma, overuse injury, bad posture, and osteoarthritis

✓ Neurogenic neck complaints may occur acutely after trauma or develop gradually from progressive osteoarthritis with nerve root impingement

✓ When neck pain is secondary to systemic disease, systemic symptoms (eg, fever, chills, weight loss) are often present

✓ Low back pain usually is self-limited and improves within 6 weeks

✓ Reserve laboratory and imaging studies for low back pain for patients with red-flag signs or symptoms

Table 78.1 • Neurologic Examination of the Spine

Nerve Root	C5	C6	C7	C8	T1	L4	L5	S1
Motor function	Deltoid, biceps	Biceps, wrist extensors	Triceps	Finger flexors	Intrinsic hand muscles	Quadriceps	Tibialis anterior	Gastrocnemius
Sensory function	Shoulder, lateral arm	Lateral forearm, thumb	Third digit	Medial forearm, fifth digit	Medial arm	Medial calf and ankle	Dorsal foot	Lateral ankle and foot
Reflex	Biceps	Biceps	Triceps	None	None	Knee	None	Ankle

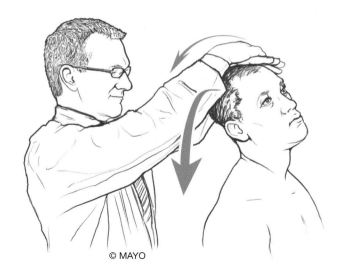

Figure 78.3 Spurling Maneuver. Physical examination maneuver used to elicit cervical nerve root impingement.

Treatment

In the absence of concerning features, treatment of nonspecific LBP involves conservative therapy and reassurance. Conservative therapy includes medication (acetaminophen, nonsteroidal anti-inflammatories, muscle relaxants, and opioids), activity modification, topical medicated agents, local ice and heat therapy, and physical therapy. Bed rest is no longer considered optimal care. Ongoing or radicular symptoms despite therapy warrant consideration for corticosteroid injection. Surgical intervention has documented clear benefit in cases of disk herniation with radiculopathy, cauda equina syndrome (surgical emergency), and severe spinal stenosis.

Shoulder Disorders

Diagnosis

Shoulder pain (Figures 78.7 and 78.8) may arise from intrinsic or extrinsic (referred) sources. An intrinsic (shoulder specific) source is more likely when the patient has pain with range of motion and complaints of shoulder instability, locking, and catching. Common extrinsic sources include referred (radicular) pain from cervical nerve root disorders, gallbladder disease, cardiac ischemia, and apical pulmonary disease. Shoulder pain in younger patients is usually secondary to trauma or overuse. In older patients, shoulder complaints are more likely to be due to degenerative or rotator cuff disorders. Common causes of shoulder disorders are reviewed in Table 78.3.

The examination of the shoulder should be undertaken systematically. Key components include visual inspection, palpation, range of motion, and provocative maneuvers

Table 78.2 • Diagnostic Features of Low Back Pain

Diagnosis	Features
Nerve root disorder	Radiculopathy Sciatica Positive result on straight-leg test Positive result on crossed straight-leg test Provoked via Valsalva maneuver, cough, sneeze
Compression fracture	Elderly History of osteoarthritis History of osteoporosis Trauma Corticosteroid use
Spinal stenosis	Impingement of lumbosacral cord Elderly History of osteoarthritis Buttock and leg pain Pain with standing Relief with forward flexion and sitting Pseudoclaudication
Rheumatologic condition	Young to middle age Family history Morning stiffness Synovitis Polyarthritis
Infection	Fever Drug use Cellulitis Urinary tract infection Other localizable infectious source
Cauda equina syndrome	Rapid neurologic deficits Saddle anesthesia Bowel and bladder dysfunction
Malignancy	Weight loss Nocturnal pain Pain at rest Worsening symptoms

(Table 78.4). Range of motion should be performed both passively and actively. Pain present during both active and passive range of motion is suggestive of an intra-articular source, whereas pain present only with active range of motion is more likely secondary to an extra-articular shoulder source (ie, ligament, tendon, bursa). Furthermore, pain during abduction greater than 120° raises concern for acromioclavicular joint disease, while pain during abduction between 60° and 120° is more commonly associated with rotator cuff and bursal disease, most commonly due to an impingement syndrome.

In rotator cuff disorders, the supraspinatus tendon is most commonly affected. Impingement syndromes involving the rotator cuff are due to compression between the humeral head and acromion process; pain is classically worse with abduction. Weakness or a positive result of the drop-arm test is suggestive of a rotator cuff tear.

Adhesive capsulitis is secondary to progressive thickening of the glenohumeral joint capsule. Classically, this

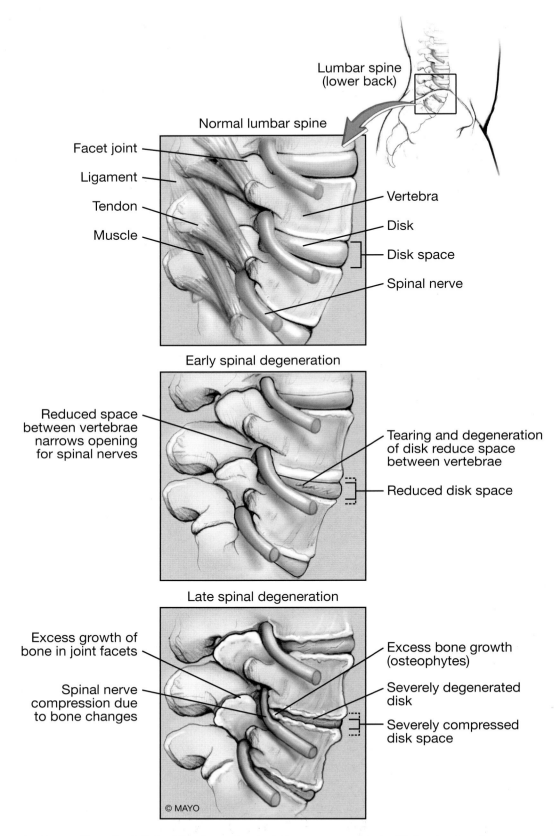

Figure 78.4 *Anatomy of Low Back Pain. Classic anatomical changes associated with low back pain.*

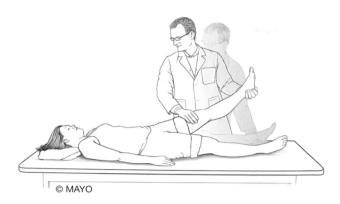

Figure 78.5 Straight-Leg Test, Part 1. Physical examination maneuver used to elicit the presence of lumbar disk herniation.

Box 78.1 • Indications for Radiography in Acute Low Back Pain

Acute back pain after age 50 y
History of back disease
History of back surgery
History of neoplasm
Direct trauma to the back
Fever
Weight loss
Severe pain unrelieved in any position
Neurologic symptoms or signs

is associated with prolonged immobilization (after injury or surgery), diabetes, trauma, hypothyroidism, and stroke. Patients experience loss of both passive and active range of motion and frequently complain of ipsilateral pain when lying on the affected side.

Treatment

Treatment recommendations are reviewed in Table 78.3. Strategies for acromioclavicular disease and bicipital tendinitis require modification of activities and nonsteroidal anti-inflammatories. Physical therapy, corticosteroid injection, and surgical interventions are usually reserved for refractory cases. Treatment of adhesive capsulitis requires prolonged physical therapy. Rotator cuff tendinitis and tear require a combination of rest, activity modification, physical therapy, and nonsteroidal anti-inflammatories; corticosteroid injection and surgery are reserved for refractory cases.

Elbow Disorders

The most common and frequently encountered clinical syndromes of elbow pain are described in Table 78.5 (Figures 78.9 and 78.10).

Hand and Wrist Disorders

Complaints involving the hand and wrist require a thorough history and examination (Table 78.6; Figures 78.11 through 78.13). History should include sites of involvement, symmetrical/asymmetrical nature, duration, presence of systemic symptoms, and history of antecedent trauma. Radiographs should be obtained in all cases of hand/wrist pain that involve antecedent trauma and localized tenderness to palpation in order to exclude fracture. Delay in imaging and treatment of occult fracture can lead to significant morbidity, including avascular necrosis.

Hip Disorders

Diagnosis

Hip pain requires a methodical approach, given the joint's complexity and broad range of differential diagnoses. Numerous extra-articular and nonmusculoskeletal sources can refer pain to the hip. Therefore, a thorough evaluation of the hip should also include evaluation of the abdomen, genitalia, spine, and knee.

Specific Disorders and Treatment

The specific causes of hip pain are best categorized by the actual location of the pain: anterior, lateral, or posterior hip pain. Anterior hip pain, often experienced as groin pain, is most likely secondary to intra-articular osteoarthritis. Symptoms are frequently described as a dull, deep, aching sensation, chronic in nature, and worse with activity.

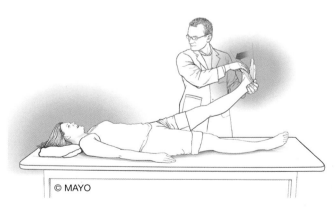

Figure 78.6 Straight-Leg Test, Part 2. Physical examination maneuver used to elicit the presence of lumbar disk herniation.

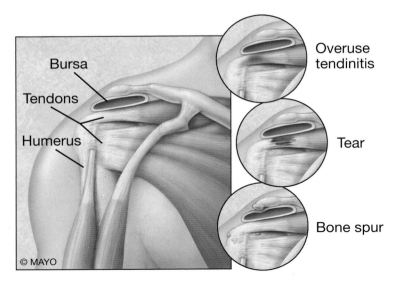

Figure 78.7 Anatomy of Shoulder Pain, Part 1. *Classic anatomical changes associated with shoulder pain.*

Morning stiffness is often present. Other sources of anterior hip pain include fracture, osteonecrosis, and infection (septic arthritis), as well as referred pain from lumbar spinal disease, inguinal hernia, and other abdominal-pelvic sources.

Lateral hip pain is most frequently caused by trochanteric bursitis (Figure 78.14). Causes of trochanteric bursitis include overuse, obesity, trauma, and gait dysfunction. Patients experience a deep, aching lateral hip pain with intermittent radiation of pain to the buttock and lateral knee. Furthermore, patients will complain of point tenderness at the site of the greater trochanter, especially during palpation, as well as when lying on the affected side. Resisted hip abduction also reproduces the discomfort. Treatment options include rest, nonsteroidal anti-inflammatories, physical therapy, corticosteroid injection, and surgery for refractory cases.

Meralgia paresthetica can cause lateral hip pain (Figure 78.15). This condition is due to entrapment of the lateral femoral cutaneous nerve at the level of the inguinal fold. Meralgia paresthetica is frequently associated with obesity, pregnancy, prolonged seated position, and tight-fitting clothing. Symptoms include pain over the anterolateral thigh with concomitant sensory changes (paresthesia and dysesthesia) and tenderness over the inguinal ligament. Treatment includes weight loss, loose-fitting

Key Definition

Meralgia paresthetica: *entrapment neuropathy caused by entrapment of the lateral femoral cutaneous nerve at the level of the inguinal fold.*

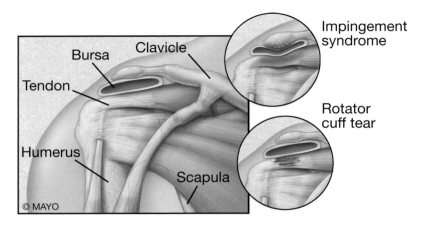

Figure 78.8 Anatomy of Shoulder Pain, Part 2. *Classic anatomical changes associated with shoulder pain.*

Table 78.3 • Shoulder Disorders

	Acromioclavicular Disease	Adhesive Capsulitis	Bicipital Tendinitis	Rotator Cuff Tendinitis/Tear
Cause	Trauma Overuse Osteoarthritis	Immobilization	Overuse Trauma	Overuse Trauma Recurrent tendinitis (tear)
Presentation	Pain at AC joint	Diffuse shoulder pain Decreased range of motion	Anterior shoulder and proximal arm pain	Anterolateral shoulder pain Lateral deltoid pain
Evaluation	Pain at AC joint with palpation Pain at AC joint with abduction >120° Positive result of cross-arm test	Limited and painful range of motion (active and passive)	Bicipital groove tenderness to palpation Positive results of Speed and Yergason tests	Pain with lateral palpation, abduction, internal and external rotation Positive results of impingement tests (Neer, Hawkins, and empty can) Positive drop-arm test (tear)
Treatment	Activity modification NSAIDs Corticosteroid injection Surgery	Physical therapy NSAIDs Corticosteroid injection Surgery	Rest Activity modification NSAIDs Corticosteroid injection Physical therapy	Rest Activity modification NSAIDs Corticosteroid injection Physical therapy Surgery (tear)

Abbreviations: AC, acromioclavicular; NSAID, nonsteroidal anti-inflammatory drug.

Table 78.4 • Shoulder Provocation Tests

Test	Maneuver	Positive Result	Diagnosis
Spurling test	Cervical spine placed in extension with head rotated to affected shoulder while axially loaded	Radiating neck, shoulder, or arm pain	Cervical nerve root disorder
Cross-arm test	Shoulder flexion to 90° and active horizontal adduction	Pain in acromioclavicular joint	Acromioclavicular joint disorder
Yergason test	Elbow flexion to 90°; examiner applies resistance to forearm supination	Pain in bicipital groove	Bicipital tendinitis or instability
Speed test	Shoulder flexion to 90°, forearm supinated; examiner applies resistance to shoulder flexion	Pain in bicipital groove	Bicipital tendinitis or instability
Apley scratch test	Patient reaches overhead and behind to opposite superior and inferior scapular spine	Loss of range of motion	Rotator cuff disorder
Drop-arm test	Examiner passively abducts shoulder to 90°; asks patient to slowly lower arm to waist	Uncontrolled lowering of arm	Rotator cuff tear
Clunk sign	While patient is supine, examiner passively abducts shoulder overhead; with 1 hand, holds distal humerus; places other hand on posterior glenohumeral joint and applies anteriorly directed force on joint while rotating humerus internally and externally	Clunk or grinding sound or sensation	Labral disorder
Neer test	Internal rotation and passive flexion of arm to 180°	Passive painful arc	Subacromial impingement
Hawkins test	Shoulder and elbow flexed to 90°; examiner forces internal rotation of shoulder	Pain	Supraspinatus tendon impingement or tear
Empty can test	Shoulder abducted to 90° and horizontally adducted to 30° (into scapular plane); patient to point thumb downward as if "emptying a can"; examiner applies resisted downward pressure	Pain or weakness	Supraspinatus tendon impingement or tear
Apprehension test	Preferably while patient is supine, examiner passively abducts shoulder and elbow to 90°; applies slight anteriorly directed force to humerus and externally rotates shoulder	Patient has pain or apprehension (muscle guarding). Patient may feel clicking in anterior joint	Anterior glenohumeral joint instability
Relocation test	Performed if positive result on apprehension test. Examiner applies posteriorly directed force on humerus while externally rotating arm	Decrease in or relief of symptoms from previous apprehension test	Anterior glenohumeral joint instability
Sulcus sign	Downward traction applied to humerus	≥1 cm gap between humeral head and acromion	Inferior glenohumeral joint instability

Table 78.5 • Common Elbow Disorders

	Lateral (Tennis) Epicondylitis	Medial (Golfer) Epicondylitis	Ulnar Neuropathy	Radial Neuropathy	Olecranon Bursitis
Cause	Overuse of wrist extensors and forearm supinators Trauma Computer use	Overuse of wrist flexors and forearm pronators Trauma	Trauma Repetitive movements Prolonged elbow resting	Overuse Trauma	Trauma Crystal arthropathy Infection Rheumatoid arthritis
Presentation	Lateral elbow pain with radiation down lateral forearm to dorsal hand	Medial elbow pain with radiation down medial forearm to palmar hand	Cubital tunnel syndrome Elbow pain and paresthesia that radiate down forearm to hand (ulnar distribution)	Proximal forearm pain and paresthesia with radiation to dorsal radial aspect of forearm and hand	Pain and swelling of elbow at bursal site
Evaluation	Lateral epicondyle pain with palpation Pain with forced wrist extension and forearm supination	Medial epicondyle pain with palpation Pain with forced wrist flexion and forearm pronation	Medial elbow pain and paresthesia with elbow flexion Ulnar distribution	Pain with resisted forearm supination Radial distribution	Inflamed olecranon bursa Pain with elbow flexion Fluid aspiration (crystal, Gram stain, culture)
Treatment	Rest Activity modification NSAIDs Corticosteroid injection Physical therapy Bracing Surgery	Same as for lateral epicondylitis	Activity modification NSAIDs Splinting Physical therapy Surgery	Same as for ulnar neuropathy	Treatment of underlying cause Activity modification

Abbreviation: NSAID, nonsteroidal anti-inflammatory drug.

clothes, nonsteroidal anti-inflammatories, physical therapy, and surgical release of the inguinal ligament in refractory cases.

Posterior hip pain is rarely due to an intra-articular source. Rather, posterior hip pain is frequently secondary to lumbosacral spine disease (back pain, paresthesia, and radiculopathy), sacroiliitis (point tenderness and gluteal pain), and piriformis syndrome (gluteal pain with radiculopathy following the sciatic nerve distribution). Imaging in the form of plain radiography and magnetic resonance imaging is very useful in making the diagnosis in cases of sacroiliitis and spinal disease.

Knee Disorders

Diagnosis

Knee pain is a very common complaint in clinical practice. Given the broad range of differential diagnoses (Tables 78.7 and 78.8; Figures 78.16 and 78.17), the history and physical examination are key to establishing the correct diagnosis. The history should include location, chronicity, antecedent trauma, and presence of associated systemic symptoms. The proper knee examination should include bilateral visual inspection, palpation, range of motion, and applicable provocation tests. The anterior drawer and Lachman tests assess for defects of the anterior cruciate ligament. The posterior drawer test assesses for defects of the posterior cruciate ligament. The medial and lateral collateral ligaments can be assessed via an applied valgus and varus stress, respectively. The McMurray and medial-lateral grind tests can detect defects of the menisci. Imaging should

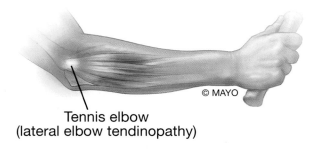

Tennis elbow
(lateral elbow tendinopathy)

Figure 78.9 *Tennis Elbow (Lateral Epicondylitis). Lateral elbow tendinopathy associated with tennis elbow.*

be pursued in cases of trauma, as well as in cases in which examination results are suggestive of ligamentous or meniscal injury.

Treatment

Treatment recommendations are reviewed in Tables 78.7 and 78.8. In general, knee disorders are treated with a combination of rest, activity modifications, physical therapy, and nonsteroidal anti-inflammatories. Corticosteroid injections, referral to orthopedic specialists, and surgical interventions are frequently required for treatment-refractory bursitis and osteoarthritis, as well as in cases of ligamentous and meniscal injury.

Ankle and Foot Disorders

Diagnosis

Successful diagnosis of ankle and foot disorders relies on localization of the focus of pain (Figure 78.18). Providers would be well advised to separate ankle complaints from those of the foot, which in turn should be divided into complaints of the hindfoot, midfoot, and forefoot.

Ankle Disorders

Ankle complaints are generally secondary to trauma (sprain, strain, and fracture) and osteoarthritis. Trauma leading to an ankle sprain is usually due to traumatic inversion and plantar flexion, which most commonly lead to injury of the anterior talofibular ligament. Ankle sprains generally result in pain, swelling, stiffness, and possible instability; the severity of these symptoms helps to grade the degree of sprain. The history should include details of the mechanism of injury, and the examination should include visual inspection, palpation, and assessment for any limitations to range of motion or weight bearing. The need for imaging should be based on antecedent history, examination findings, and the Ottawa ankle rules (Figure 78.19). Treatment of low-grade sprains includes rest, ice, compression, and elevation (RICE) as well as nonsteroidal anti-inflammatories. Higher-grade sprains may require ankle stabilization, physical therapy, limitation of weight bearing, or surgical intervention.

Foot Disorders

Hindfoot pain primarily includes plantar fasciitis (Figure 78.20) and Achilles tendinopathy. Plantar fasciitis (inflammation of the plantar fascia) is caused by overuse and heel spurs, which lead to plantar foot and heel pain that classically is worse with the first few steps and improves with rest. Imaging is generally unnecessary. Treatment includes activity modification, plantar stretching, orthotics/proper footwear, nonsteroidal anti-inflammatories, weight loss,

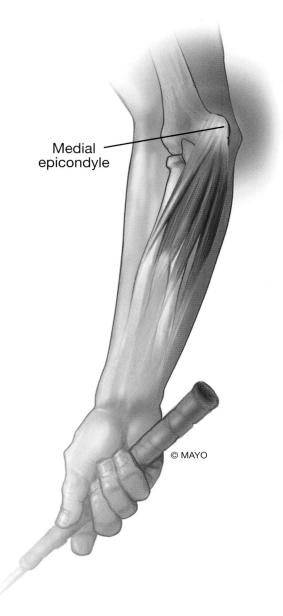

Figure 78.10 Golfer's Elbow (Medial Epicondylitis). Medial elbow tendinopathy associated with golfer's elbow.

KEY FACTS

- ✓ Rotator cuff disorders most commonly affect the supraspinatus tendon
- ✓ Anterior hip pain—most likely due to intra-articular osteoarthritis; often manifested as groin pain
- ✓ Trochanteric bursitis—caused by overuse, obesity, trauma, and gait dysfunction
- ✓ Lateral hip pain may be caused by meralgia paresthetica
- ✓ Components of proper knee examination—bilateral visual inspection, palpation, range of motion, and applicable provocation tests

Table 78.6 • Wrist and Hand Disorders

	Ganglion Cyst	Trigger Finger	Dupuytren Contracture	De Quervain Tenosynovitis	Carpal Tunnel Syndrome	Ulnar Tunnel Syndrome
Cause	Chronic irritation of wrist	Digital flexor tendon inflammation and stenosis	Palmar fascia contracture	Inflammation of abductor pollicis longus and extensor pollicis brevis tendons	Median nerve compression	Ulnar nerve compression
Risk Factors	Age Overuse Trauma	Overuse Diabetes Trauma Rheumatoid arthritis	Familial Diabetes Alcoholism	Overuse Pregnancy	Overuse Obesity Pregnancy Hypothyroidism Diabetes Female sex	Overuse Trauma
Presentation	Swelling overlying wrist joints or tendons	Pain and catching sensation of digital flexor tendon	Flexed digits Difficulty with digital extension	Radial wrist pain when pinching or grasping with thumb	Pain and paresthesia in median nerve distribution Nocturnal symptoms Thenar wasting	Pain and paresthesia in ulnar nerve distribution
Evaluation	Palpable cystic swelling overlying wrist joint or tendons	Digital flexion with pain and palpable catch Palpable nodule along digital flexor tendon	Flexion deformity Palmar fascia thickening	Distal radial styloid process tenderness Finkelstein test	Hand symptom diagram Tinel and Phalen signs Nerve conduction test and EMG	Ulnar Tinel sign Nerve conduction test and EMG
Treatment	No intervention Injection (corticosteroid or hyaluronic acid) Surgery	Hand therapy Corticosteroid injection Surgery	Activity modification Hand therapy Surgery	Splinting Activity modification NSAIDs Corticosteroid injection Surgery	Activity modification Splinting NSAIDs Corticosteroid injection Surgery	Activity modification Splinting NSAIDs Surgery

Abbreviations: EMG, electromyography; NSAID, nonsteroidal anti-inflammatory drug.

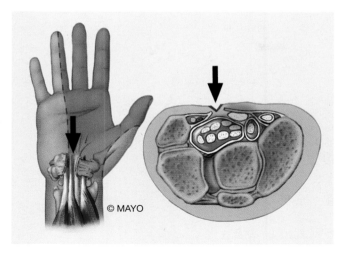

Figure 78.11 *Anatomy of Carpal Tunnel Syndrome. Anatomical changes associated with carpal tunnel syndrome, including nerve pattern distribution.*

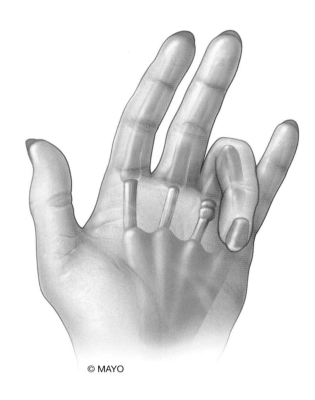

Figure 78.13 *Trigger Finger. Classic presentation of trigger finger.*

corticosteroid injections, and surgical interventions in refractory cases. Achilles tendinopathy is commonly due to overuse, improper footwear, and fluoroquinolone use. Patients complain of tenderness along the tendon and painful foot dorsiflexion. Treatment includes activity modification/rest, heel lift, nonsteroidal anti-inflammatories, and proper stretching. In Achilles tendon rupture, patients often experience a popping or tearing sensation followed by inability to flex the foot, pain, swelling, and an abnormal Thompson test result (failure to plantar flex when the calf is squeezed). Diagnostic ultrasonography can also be used. Orthopedic evaluation is required for cases of tendon rupture.

Midfoot pain most commonly occurs with tarsal tunnel syndrome (entrapment of the posterior tibial nerve behind the medial malleolus). Symptoms include pain and paresthesia along the medial and plantar aspects of the foot, which are worsened by activity. Examination includes assessment for proper distribution of pain and paresthesia and the presence of a posterior medial malleolus Tinel sign. Treatment involves activity modification, orthotics, nonsteroidal anti-inflammatories, and surgical intervention in refractory cases.

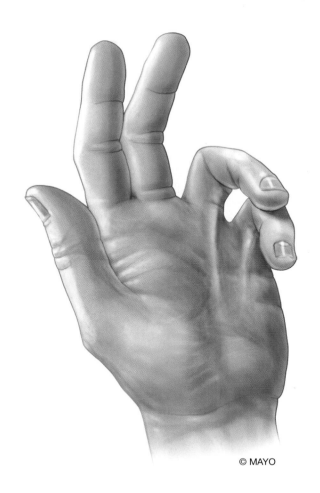

Figure 78.12 *Dupuytren Contracture. Classic presentation of Dupuytren contracture.*

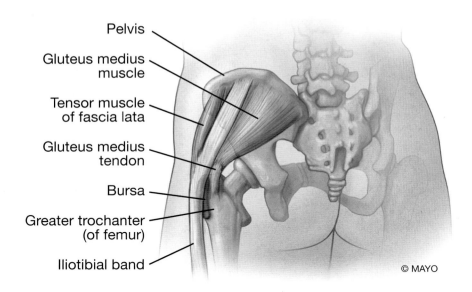

Figure 78.14 Anatomy of the Hip. Normal hip anatomy with applicable adjacent structures.

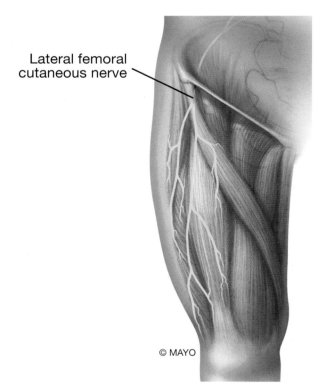

Figure 78.15 Meralgia Paresthetica. Lateral femoral cutaneous nerve impingement leading to meralgia paresthetica.

Forefoot complaints include Morton neuroma and hallux valgus. Morton neuroma (compression of common digital nerves) presents with pain and paresthesia most commonly between the third and fourth toes. This condition is commonly seen in persons who stand for prolonged periods, as well as in women who wear high heels. Examination reveals focal tenderness as well as a palpable neuroma. Avoidance of high heels and prolonged standing, orthotics, corticosteroid injection, and nonsteroidal anti-inflammatories are effective treatment options. Refractory cases may require surgical excision of the neuroma. Hallux valgus (bunion) development leads to pain at the first metatarsophalangeal joint, which worsens with activity, prolonged standing, and wearing high heels. Treatment options include proper footwear, activity modification, nonsteroidal anti-inflammatories, orthotics, bracing, and surgical correction.

Fibromyalgia

Diagnosis

Fibromyalgia is a chronic centralized pain sensitivity syndrome, affecting approximately 2% to 8% of the population. The pathophysiologic basis for fibromyalgia is likely the dysregulation of the thalamus-hypothalamus-amygdala leading to pain and sensory processing abnormalities

Table 78.7 • Knee Disorders: Osteoarthritis, Iliotibial Band Syndrome, Chondromalacia Patellae, and Baker Cyst

	Osteoarthritis	Iliotibial Band Syndrome	Chondromalacia Patellae	Baker (Popliteal) Cyst
Cause	Age Overuse Obesity Corticosteroids	Overuse	Degeneration of patellofemoral cartilage Overuse	Trauma (meniscal injury) Overuse Osteoarthritis Rheumatoid arthritis
Presentation	Pain with use; resolves with rest Morning stiffness	Lateral thigh/knee pain (above joint line); worse with steps	Anterior knee pain; worse with prolonged sitting and stair climbing	Pain and fullness in popliteal fossa
Evaluation	Joint line tenderness Decreased range of motion Effusion Crepitus Radiography	Noble test Tenderness at lateral femoral epicondyle	Patellofemoral compression test	Popliteal swelling, pain, fullness, and palpable effusion Possible ultrasonography to rule out DVT
Treatment	NSAIDs Acetaminophen Topical agents Physical therapy Corticosteroid injection Surgery	Rest NSAIDs Physical therapy Corticosteroid injection	Physical therapy (quadriceps strengthening) NSAIDs Ice Activity modification	Rest NSAIDs Elevation Corticosteroid injection

Abbreviations: DVT, deep vein thrombosis; NSAID, nonsteroidal anti-inflammatory drug.

Table 78.8 • Knee Disorders: Bursitis, Ligament Injury, and Meniscal Injury

	Prepatellar Bursitis	Pes Anserine Bursitis	Anterior Collateral Ligament Injury	Posterior Cruciate Ligament Injury	Collateral Ligament Injury	Meniscal Injury
Cause	Frequent sustained pressure with knee flexed (housemaid's knee) Trauma Infection Gout	Overuse (running, uphill climbing, cycling) Trauma Valgus knee deformity Osteoarthritis	Trauma Knee twisting injury with foot planted	Trauma (dashboard injury) Knee hyper-extension injury	Overuse Trauma	Overuse Trauma
Presentation	Pain, swelling, erythema of anterior knee	Anteromedial knee/leg pain (below medial joint line)	Acute-subacute onset of pain, swelling, and instability	Acute-subacute onset of pain, swelling, and instability	Medial or lateral knee pain	Knee joint line pain Knee lock, buckle, catch, pop
Evaluation	Tenderness, erythema, and pain of prepatellar bursa Aspiration (gout vs infection)	Tenderness at anserine bursa Pain with knee flexion and squatting	Anterior drawer test Lachman test	Posterior drawer test	Varus (lateral collateral) stress test Valgus (medial collateral) stress test	Joint line tenderness Medial-lateral grind test McMurray test
Treatment	Rest Activity modification NSAIDs Treatment of gout or infection	Activity modification Rest NSAIDs Corticosteroid injection	Orthopedic evaluation	Orthopedic evaluation	Rest NSAIDs Physical therapy Orthopedic evaluation	Rest NSAIDs Physical therapy Orthopedic evaluation

Abbreviation: NSAID, nonsteroidal anti-inflammatory drug.

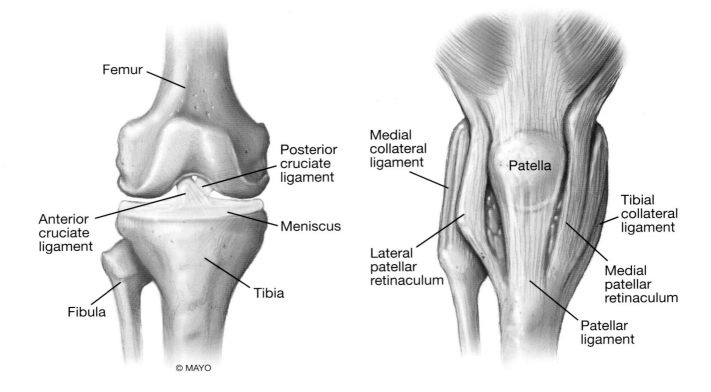

Femur

Posterior
cruciate
ligament

Anterior
cruciate
ligament

Meniscus

Fibula

Tibia

Medial
collateral
ligament

Patella

Tibial
collateral
ligament

Lateral
patellar
retinaculum

Medial
patellar
retinaculum

Patellar
ligament

© MAYO

Figure 78.16 *Anatomy of the Knee, Anterior View. Normal anterior knee anatomy with applicable adjacent structures.*

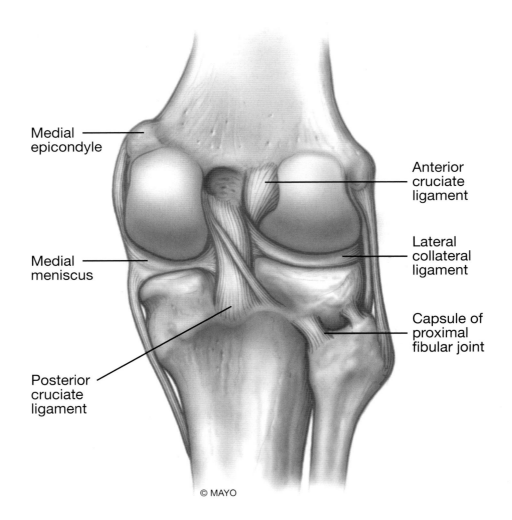

Medial
epicondyle

Anterior
cruciate
ligament

Medial
meniscus

Lateral
collateral
ligament

Capsule of
proximal
fibular joint

Posterior
cruciate
ligament

© MAYO

Figure 78.17 *Anatomy of the Knee, Posterior View. Normal posterior knee anatomy with applicable adjacent structures.*

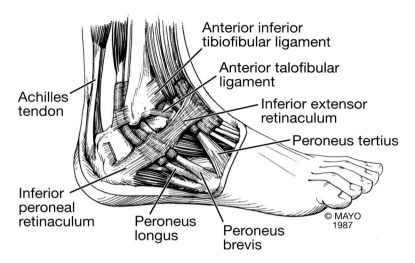

Figure 78.18 *Anatomy of the Foot and Ankle, Lateral View. Normal lateral foot and ankle anatomy with emphasis on tendinous and ligamentous structures.*

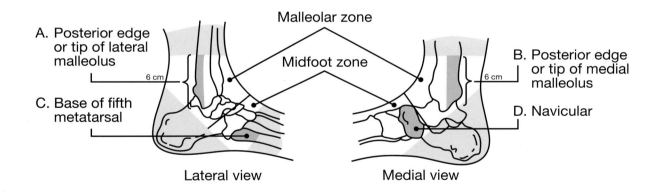

An ankle radiographic series is only required if there is any pain in malleolar zone and any of these findings:

1. Bone tenderness at A or
2. Bone tenderness at B or
3. Inability to bear weight both immediately and in emergency department

A foot radiographic series is only required if there is any pain in midfoot zone and any of these findings:

1. Bone tenderness at C or
2. Bone tenderness at D or
3. Inability to bear weight both immediately and in emergency department

Figure 78.19 *Ottawa Ankle Rules. Risk stratification strategies to determine the need for obtaining imaging in patients with acute ankle injury.*

(Adapted from Stiell IG, McKnight RD, Greenberg GH, McDowell I, Nair RC, Wells GA, et al. Implementation of the Ottawa ankle rules. JAMA. 1994 Mar 16;271[11]:827–32. Used with permission.)

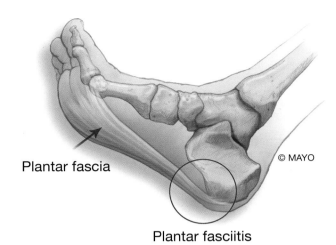

Plantar fascia

© MAYO

Plantar fasciitis

Figure 78.20 *Anatomy of Plantar Fasciitis. Distribution of plantar fascia and associated fasciitis.*

(central sensitization). This results in pain signal generation, pain amplification, hyperalgesia, allodynia, and global sensory hypersensitivity. Recent evidence has also supported a genetic influence, with twin studies having shown a concordance rate up to 50%.

Key Definition
Fibromyalgia: *a chronic centralized pain sensitivity syndrome.*

The hallmark symptom of fibromyalgia is diffuse, multifocal, migratory, waxing and waning pain. The pain is primarily described as widespread arthralgia and myalgia. Concomitantly, patients often complain of fatigue, restless sleep, cognitive deficits ("brain fog"), and other somatic complaints. The majority of patients experience depression or anxiety.

In 1990, the American College of Rheumatology (ACR) put forth the initial diagnostic criteria for fibromyalgia. A thorough tender point examination was required, and the diagnosis was confirmed when 11 or more (out of a total 18) tender points were present (Figure 78.21). In 2010, the ACR revised the diagnostic criteria to implement a global symptomatic approach. Current diagnostic criteria require the following: pain symptoms for ≥3 months; widespread pain index score of ≥7 (the body is divided into 19 areas, with 1 point given for each painful area) and symptom severity score of ≥5 (rated scale of symptoms including fatigue, restless sleep, cognitive complaints, and somatic symptoms); symptoms not due to another underlying cause.

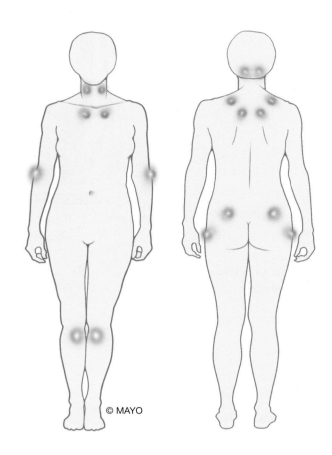

© MAYO

Figure 78.21 *Fibromyalgia. Location of tender points associated with fibromyalgia.*

Treatment

Treatment of fibromyalgia requires a multifaceted approach with the implementation of both medication and nonmedication options. The currently approved agents to treat fibromyalgia include 2 serotonin-norepinephrine reuptake inhibitors (duloxetine and milnacipran) as well as pregabalin. Opioids should be avoided owing to their lack of benefit in fibromyalgia, propensity to lead to opioid-induced hyperalgesia, abuse potential, and side effect profile. When compared to medication options, nonmedication treatments have been shown to be superior in efficacy and to have longer-lasting effects. These options include ongoing patient education, implementation of a graded aerobic exercise program, dietary modifications, physical therapy, occupational therapy, cognitive behavioral therapy, biofeedback therapy, and sleep hygiene.

KEY FACTS

✓ Main causes of hindfoot pain—plantar fasciitis and Achilles tendinopathy

✓ Midfoot pain—most common with tarsal tunnel syndrome

✓ Forefoot complaints—Morton neuroma and hallux valgus

✓ Fibromyalgia's hallmark symptom—diffuse, multifocal, migratory, waxing and waning pain

✓ Fibromyalgia requires multifaceted treatment including both medication and nonmedication options

79

Osteoarthritis, Gout, and Infectious Arthritis

CLEMENT J. MICHET, MD AND FLORANNE C. ERNSTE, MD

Osteoarthritis

Osteoarthritis is the failure of articular cartilage and subsequent degenerative changes in subchondral bone, bony joint margins, synovium, and para-articular fibrous and muscular structures. Osteoarthritis is the most common joint disease; 80% of patients have some limitation of their activities, and 25% are unable to perform major activities of daily living. As a consequence, osteoarthritis is a substantial economic burden to society. The prevalence of osteoarthritis is strongly associated with aging. Joints most commonly affected include the knee, hand, spine, metatarsophalangeal, and hip. Radiologic evidence of the disease greatly exceeds the prevalence of symptomatic cases.

> ### Key Definition
>
> Osteoarthritis: *the failure of articular cartilage and subsequent degenerative changes in subchondral bone, bony joint margins, synovium, and para-articular fibrous and muscular structures.*

Pathogenesis of Osteoarthritis

Two principal changes associated with osteoarthritis are the progressive focal degeneration of articular cartilage and the formation of new bone in the floor of the cartilage lesion at the joint margins (osteophytes). Osteoarthritis represents the interaction of multiple genetic and environmental factors. Not all the mechanisms causing osteoarthritis have been identified. Current theories include 1) mechanical process: cartilage injury, particularly after impact loading, and 2) biochemical process: failure of cartilage repair processes

to adequately compensate for injury. A combination of mechanical and biochemical processes likely contributes in most cases of osteoarthritis. It must be emphasized that osteoarthritis is not just the consequence of "wear and tear" of aging. For example, a person who is genetically prone to generalized osteoarthritis may demonstrate premature disease in the knee related to obesity or trauma.

Clinical Features of Osteoarthritis

The pain of an osteoarthritic joint is usually described as a deep ache. Subchondral bone edema contributes to the pain. The pain occurs with use of the joint and is relieved with rest and cessation of weight bearing. As the disease progresses, the involved joint may be symptomatic with minimal activity or even at rest. The pain originates in the structures around the disintegrating cartilage (there are no nerves in cartilage). There may be stiffness in the joint with initial use, but this initial stiffness is not prolonged as it is in inflammatory arthritis, such as rheumatoid arthritis. Although the symptoms are related predominantly to mechanical failure and motion limits, joint debris and the associated repair process promote mild inflammation, accumulation of synovial fluid, and mild hypertrophy of the synovial membrane. Acute inflammation can transiently occur at Heberden nodes (distal interphalangeal joints with prominent osteophytes as a consequence of osteoarthritis) or at the knee with tearing of a degenerative meniscal cartilage. The pain of osteoarthritis is never generalized, but typically is limited to a few joints at any given time. A new superimposed illness should be considered in an elderly osteoarthritic patient who presents with generalized musculoskeletal pain. Typical scenarios include polymyalgia rheumatica and late-onset rheumatoid arthritis.

Physical examination documents joint margin tenderness, fine crepitus, limits to motion, and enlargement of the joint. The enlargement is usually bony (proliferation of cartilage and bone to form osteophytes), but it can include effusions and mild synovial thickening. Deformity is a late consequence of the osteoarthritis and is associated with atrophy or derangement of the local soft tissues, ligaments, and muscles. Radiographic or physical examination evidence of the severity of osteoarthritis does not reliably predict a patient's symptoms.

Clinical Subsets of Osteoarthritis

Primary Osteoarthritis

Primary osteoarthritis is cartilage failure without a known cause that would predispose to osteoarthritis. It almost never affects the shoulders, elbows, ankles, metacarpophalangeal joints, or ulnar side of the wrist. It is divided into several clinical patterns, as described below.

Generalized osteoarthritis involves the distal interphalangeal joints, proximal interphalangeal joints, first carpometacarpal joints, hips, knees, and spine (Figure 79.1). It occurs most frequently in middle-aged postmenopausal women.

Isolated nodal osteoarthritis is primary osteoarthritis that affects only the distal interphalangeal joints. It occurs predominantly in women and has a familial predisposition. Isolated involvement at the base of the thumb is also common.

Isolated hip osteoarthritis is more common in men than in women. It has no clear association with obesity or activity. Many cases are now thought to be related to mild joint developmental structural abnormalities such as femoral acetabular impingement.

Erosive osteoarthritis affects only the distal and proximal interphalangeal joints. Patients with erosive osteoarthritis

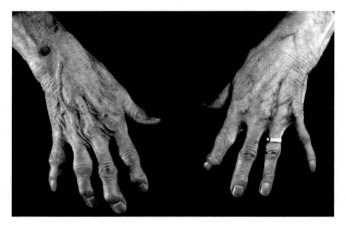

Figure 79.1 *Generalized Osteoarthritis. Note prominent bony hypertrophy at the proximal (Bouchard nodes) and distal (Heberden nodes) interphalangeal joints. The metacarpophalangeal joints are spared. Early hypertrophic changes are seen on profile at the first carpometacarpal joint, giving a slight squaring of the hand deformity, appreciated best in this patient's left hand.*

have episodes of local inflammation. Mucous cyst formation at the distal interphalangeal joint is common. Painful flare-up of the disease recurs for years. Symptoms usually begin about the time of menopause. Bony erosions and collapse of the subchondral plate—features not usually seen in primary osteoarthritis—with osteophytes are markers of erosive osteoarthritis. Angular joint deformity can be severe. Bony ankylosis develops in many cases and is usually associated with relief of pain. This condition may be confused with rheumatoid arthritis, but unlike rheumatoid arthritis, erosive osteoarthritis never affects the metacarpophalangeal or wrist joints.

Diffuse idiopathic skeletal hyperostosis (DISH), also known as Forestier disease, is a diffuse ossification and calcification process involving ligaments and entheses. It occurs chiefly in men older than 50 years. The diagnosis requires the finding of characteristic exuberant, flowing osteophytes that connect 4 or more vertebrae with preservation of the disk space. DISH is radiographically distinguished from typical osteoarthritis of the spine with degenerative disk disease and from ankylosing spondylitis. Extraspinal sites of disease involvement include calcification of the pelvic ligaments, exuberant osteophytosis at the site of peripheral osteoarthritis, well-calcified bony spurs at the calcaneus, and heterotopic bone formation after total joint arthroplasty. Patients with DISH are often obese, and 60% have diabetes mellitus or glucose intolerance. Symptoms include mild back stiffness and, occasionally, back pain. Pathologically and radiologically, DISH is distinct from other forms of primary osteoarthritis.

Key Definition

Diffuse idiopathic skeletal hyperostosis: *a diffuse ossification and calcification process involving ligaments and entheses; also known as Forestier disease.*

Secondary Osteoarthritis

Secondary osteoarthritis is a progressive loss of articular cartilage in unusual distributions (ie, shoulders, wrists, metacarpophalangeal joints, ankles) resulting in degenerative changes and joint failure. Table 79.1 lists some major examples of inherited disorders of connective tissue that predispose to premature or secondary osteoarthritis, including their gene defects and characteristics. For example, Ehlers-Danlos syndrome comprises a rare group of genetic disorders characterized by tissue fragility, skin hyperextensibility, and joint hypermobility; Marfan syndrome is a similar rare genetic syndrome characterized by joint hypermobility and morphologic features of pectus excavatum or pectus carinatum, scoliosis, and disproportionately long extremities. Some metabolic abnormalities that can cause secondary osteoarthritis include ochronosis, hemochromatosis, Wilson disease, and acromegaly. Additionally, Paget disease of bone, involving the femur or pelvis about the hip joint, can predispose to secondary osteoarthritis.

Joint trauma or chronic joint injury also can cause secondary osteoarthritis. The pathogenesis involves stress from repeated impact loading that weakens subchondral bone. Internal joint derangement with ligamentous laxity or meniscal damage alters the normal mechanical alignment of the joint. Chronic rotator cuff tear with subsequent loss of shoulder joint cartilage (ie, rotator cuff arthropathy) and knee osteoarthritis developing years after meniscal cartilage damage are examples of chronic injury leading to secondary osteoarthritis.

Developmental malformations of joints, such as congenital hip dysplasia, femoral acetabular impingement, and epiphyseal dysplasia, lead to premature or secondary osteoarthritis (Table 79.1). Pediatric joint or bone injuries, such as slipped capital femoral epiphysis and Legg-Calvé-Perthes disease (idiopathic avascular necrosis of the femoral head), result in premature or secondary osteoarthritis in young adult patients.

Hemochromatosis Arthropathy

Hereditary hemochromatosis is an autosomal recessive disorder caused by abnormal iron absorption and subsequent iron overload due to point mutations. Most patients are homozygous for C282Y/C282Y, although 5% may be compound heterozygous for the mutations C282Y/H63D of the *HFE* gene on chromosome 6. The compound heterozygous form of the disease is commonly associated with arthropathy.

The classic clinical spectrum of hemochromatosis includes hepatomegaly, bronze skin pigmentation, diabetes mellitus, hypogonadism, cardiomyopathy, and degenerative arthritis. Diabetes, hypogonadism, and cardiomyopathy are considered rare and late manifestations of hemochromatosis. The arthropathy can be an initial manifestation and eventually affects the majority of patients. It symmetrically involves the second and third metacarpophalangeal joints and large joints that are not typically affected by generalized primary osteoarthritis.

Hemochromatosis arthropathy should be considered in patients younger than 50 years who present with pseudogout

Table 79.1 • Inherited Disorders of Connective Tissue

Condition	Gene Defect	Characteristics
Marfan syndrome (autosomal dominant)	Fibrillin gene (*FBN1*)	Hypermobile joints: osteoarthritis, arachnodactyly, kyphoscoliosis Lax skin, striae, ectopic ocular lens Aortic root dilatation (aortic insufficiency), mitral valve prolapse, aneurysms, and aortic dissection
Ehlers-Danlos syndrome (10 subtypes)	Collagen gene defects (*COL5A1, COL5A2*)	Joint hypermobility, friable skin, secondary osteoarthritis; type IV associated with vascular aneurysms
Osteogenesis imperfecta (autosomal dominant and recessive variations; the most common heritable disorder of connective tissue: 1:20,000; 4 subtypes)	Type I collagen gene defects	Brittle bones, blue sclerae, otosclerosis and deafness, joint hypermobility, and tooth malformation
Type II collagenopathies Achondrogenesis type II Hypochondrogenesis Spondyloepiphyseal dysplasia Spondyloepimetaphyseal dysplasia Kniest dysplasia Stickler syndrome Familial precocious osteoarthropathy	Type II collagen gene defects	Spectrum from lethal (achondrogenesis) to premature osteoarthritis (Stickler syndrome); Stickler syndrome is characterized by craniofacial abnormalities (micrognathia, cleft palate), myopia, retinal detachment, hearing loss, joint laxity
Achondroplasia (autosomal dominant)	Fibroblast growth factor III receptor gene defect	Dwarfism, premature osteoarthritis
Pseudoachondroplasia	Cartilage oligomeric matrix protein (COMP) gene defect	Short stature, premature osteoarthritis

or chondrocalcinosis. The iron screening tests look for elevated transferrin saturation and increased serum ferritin levels. Radiographs may reveal chondrocalcinosis and hook-like osteophytes of affected joints such as the metacarpophalangeal joints, as well as uniform joint space narrowing, sclerosis, and subchondral cystic changes. On radiographs, chondrocalcinosis is occasionally seen superimposed on the chronic degenerative changes. The pathogenesis of joint degeneration in hemochromatosis is not well understood and may involve iron inhibition of pyrophosphatase in cartilage; synovial biopsies have revealed ferritin and hemosiderin deposits in synovial cells in addition to calcium pyrophosphate dihydrate crystals. Treatment of hemochromatosis is with phlebotomy, but the arthropathy does not improve with iron removal. Nonsteroidal anti-inflammatory drugs have been used for analgesic treatment of arthropathy.

Neuropathic Arthropathy (Charcot Joint)

Neuropathic arthropathy (Charcot joint) is a progressive joint destruction, usually monarticular, accompanied by sensory loss. It commonly affects patients with diabetic neuropathy. Less common causes are familial peripheral neuropathy, tabes dorsalis, amyloidosis, cervical syringomyelia, and leprosy. The sites of joint involvement depend on the distribution of the underlying disorder but are typically the ankle and midfoot. Patients with diabetic neuropathic arthropathy have had diabetes for an average of 10 years. Frequently, the diabetes is poorly controlled. Diabetic peripheral neuropathy causes blunted pain perception and poor proprioception. The pathogenesis is poorly understood but is believed to be related to repeated microtrauma, overt trauma, small vessel occlusive disease (diabetes), and neuropathic dystrophic effects on bone.

The clinical features of neuropathic arthropathy are distinct. Patients may present with edema, erythema, and warmth of the affected joint, but the pain symptoms often appear mild because of a sensory deficit. Major structural changes occur, involving collapse of the tarsal bones resulting in a convexity of the plantar surface (rocker-bottom foot). Callus formation occurs over the weight-bearing site of bony damage, and the callus may blister and ulcerate. Infection can spread from skin ulcers to the bone. Osteomyelitis frequently complicates diabetic neuropathic arthropathy and should be suspected when an affected patient with diabetes has sudden worsening of glucose control.

Neuropathic arthropathy can be readily diagnosed by plain radiography, although in the early stages the joint may look normal, or there may be swelling of soft tissues or a small joint effusion. In the later stages, radiography shows a disorganized joint architecture with presence of severe joint destruction, bony debris, and simultaneous features of bone resorption and new bone formation. Bone fractures may be seen as free bodies in the joint space; coalescence of bone fragments may then form characteristic sclerotic loose bodies. Progression of a neuropathic joint is rapid and may occur within a few weeks, possibly owing to presence of microfractures leading to considerable bone fragmentation and destruction.

There is no curative treatment for neuropathic arthropathy, but early diagnosis is key to preventing progressive joint destruction. Good local foot care, treatment of secondary infections, and protected weight bearing are important elements of conservative management. Immobilization of the joint with a brace and rest should be done in the early stages to stabilize the joint. Specialist care is necessary.

Osteonecrosis

Osteonecrosis is bone death related to loss of blood supply and may lead to collapse of the articular cartilage surface, ie, secondary osteoarthritis. The most common location for osteonecrosis is the femoral head, but it also occurs in the distal femur, humeral head, bones of the wrist and foot, and ankle. Osteonecrosis occurs more frequently in men than in women (ratio, approximately 8:1). Trauma, such as a femoral neck fracture that interrupts the blood supply to the femoral head, is a common cause of osteonecrosis. There are many nontraumatic causes, and the mechanism of vascular and bone injury remains obscure. Systemic corticosteroid therapy, alcoholism, sickle cell disease, connective tissue diseases such as systemic lupus erythematosus, and antiphospholipid antibodies are common causes (Box 79.1). No underlying cause can be identified in 10% to 25% of patients. Clinical features depend on the location of osteonecrosis but are commonly sudden onset of activity and weight bearing–localized joint pain.

> ### KEY FACTS
>
> ✓ Osteoarthritis causes 2 principal changes—progressive focal degeneration of articular cartilage and formation of osteophytes
>
> ✓ The arthropathy of hemochromatosis affects second and third metacarpophalangeals and large joints not typically involved in primary osteoarthritis
>
> ✓ Neuropathic arthropathy may present with a joint that is swollen, red, and warm, but only mildly painful (sensory deficit)
>
> ✓ Osteonecrosis most commonly occurs in the femoral head, less commonly in the distal femur, humeral head, wrist, foot, and ankle

---

Early diagnosis of osteonecrosis depends on the clinician's index of suspicion, as plain radiographs often show no abnormalities in early stages. Early radiographic changes may involve joint osteopenia with a central area of radiolucency and a sclerotic border; subchondral radiolucency, the so-called crescent sign, may occur, indicating a subchondral fracture. Magnetic resonance imaging is the preferred imaging technique for the diagnosis of preradiographic osteonecrosis.

Treatment is generally conservative and involves reduced weight bearing and analgesics. Progressive bone collapse and pain are treated with joint arthroplasty.

Hemophilic Arthropathy

Hemophilic arthropathy, a form of secondary osteoarthritis, is related to recurrent hemarthroses in patients with hemophilia. The most commonly involved joints include the ankle, knee, and elbow. Bleeding may be provoked by trauma or occur spontaneously. Acute episodes are manifested by a painful monoarthritis with a bloody effusion. They are managed with aspiration, analgesia, joint rest, and factor replacement. Over time, recurrent bleeding leads to synovial hemosiderin deposition, synovitis, and joint destruction. Patients with hemophilia and recurrent acute hemarthroses manifested by severe swelling and pain are at risk for hemophilic arthropathy. Specific radiographic abnormalities found in hemophilic arthropathy include widening of the intercondylar notch of the humeral and femoral areas. Management generally involves treatment of the underlying hemophilia and analgesia.

Radiographic Features of Osteoarthritis

The radiographic features of osteoarthritis do not always predict the extent of symptoms. Weight-bearing images of lower extremity joints should always be obtained to appreciate the degree of joint space loss. Plain radiographs are insensitive for very early disease, and in selected circumstances, magnetic resonance imaging may be needed. However, osteoarthritis is most commonly diagnosed clinically, and extensive imaging is frequently not necessary for management. With aging, radiographic osteoarthritis is far more prevalent than the clinical illness. Radiographic features include osteophyte formation, asymmetric joint-space narrowing, subchondral bony sclerosis, and subchondral cysts. Later bony changes include malalignment and deformity (Figure 79.2). In the spine, the radiographic finding called spondylosis includes anterolateral spinous

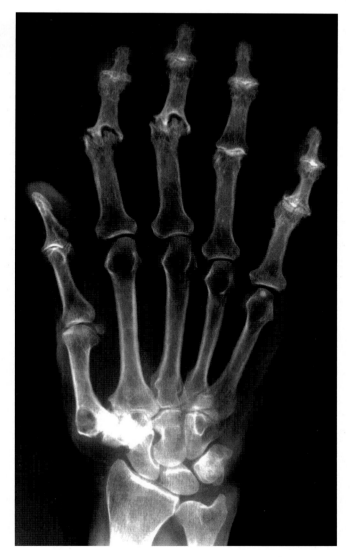

***Figure 79.2** Severe Osteoarthritis. Hypertrophic changes, asymmetric joint-space narrowing, and subchondral sclerosis are prominent at the interphalangeal joints and at the first carpometacarpal joint. Note that the metacarpophalangeal joints are completely spared, distinguishing this arthritis from rheumatoid arthritis. Also, there are joint-space narrowing and sclerosis at the base of the thumb at the first carpometacarpal joint and between the trapezium and the scaphoid. Osteoarthritis does not affect the entire wrist compartment equally. The involvement seen here is the most common. An additional interesting feature seen here is central erosions at the second and third proximal interphalangeal joints. This variant occasionally has been called erosive osteoarthritis.*

osteophytes and degenerative disk disease with disk-space narrowing. There are no laboratory tests useful for diagnosis of osteoarthritis. Evaluation of a painful effusion in an osteoarthritic joint is indicated to exclude an alternative diagnosis, most commonly crystalline arthritis.

Therapy for Osteoarthritis

Therapeutic goals include relieving pain, preserving joint motion and function, and preventing further injury and wear of cartilage. Addressing the patient's ability to cope with the illness may be more helpful than medication therapy alone. Discussion regarding prognosis and reassurance regarding the absence of rheumatoid arthritis are important. Weight loss (especially in knee osteoarthritis), use of canes or crutches, correction of postural abnormalities, and proper shoe support are important measures. Splinting for symptomatic carpometacarpal thumb disease is helpful. Isometric or isotonic range-of-motion exercise, muscle strengthening, and overall aerobic fitness provide para-articular structures with extra support and help reduce symptoms. Relief of muscle spasm with local application of heat or cold to decrease pain can help.

Initial drug therapy should be analgesics, such as acetaminophen. Nonsteroidal anti-inflammatory drugs (NSAIDs) are beneficial for patients with inadequate response to acetaminophen. They are ideally used only as needed and at the lowest dose possible, which should be emphasized to the patient. Proton pump inhibitors should be prescribed for patients at risk of NSAID gastropathy and bleeding. Topical diclofenac or capsaicin may be helpful in patients with hand or knee osteoarthritis and should be considered before systemic NSAID therapy. Selective use of opioid analgesics can be considered for disabling pain, especially in patients who are not surgical candidates. Intra-articular corticosteroids offer temporary relief for joint flares. Hyaluronic acid injections have minimal symptomatic benefit in selected patients with osteoarthritis of the knee. Supplements such as chondroitin and glucosamine sulfate are of no proven benefit.

Joint arthroplasty relieves pain, stabilizes joints, and improves function. Total joint arthroplasty is very successful at the knee, shoulder, or hip. Box 79.2 describes the indications for total joint arthroplasty. In patients with established osteoarthritis of the knee, arthroscopic débridement procedures have no lasting benefit. This surgery is no longer recommended. Herniated disks or spinal stenosis with radicular symptoms may require decompression.

Box 79.2 • Indications for Total Joint Arthroplasty

Radiographically advanced osteoarthritis

Night pain that cannot be modified by changing position

Lockup or giving way of the weight-bearing joint associated with falls or near falls

Joint symptoms that compromise activities of daily living

Crystalline Arthropathies

Hyperuricemia and Gout

Hyperuricemia occurs in 2% to 18% of normal populations. It is associated with hypertension, renal insufficiency, obesity, and arteriosclerotic heart disease. Clinical gouty arthritis ranges in prevalence from 0.1% to 0.4%; it is the most common form of inflammatory arthritis in men. Twenty percent of patients with gouty arthritis have a family history of gout. Because of the rising rates of obesity and metabolic syndrome, gout is becoming even more prevalent. Patients are typically hyperuricemic for years before their first episode of acute gout. Ninety percent of patients with gout have reduced renal clearance of urate. Several abnormalities of renal tubular transport sites have been identified as the cause of urate underexcretion. Estrogen is uricosuric and is the mechanism for the rarity of gout in premenopausal women.

Causes of Secondary Hyperuricemia

Secondary hyperuricemia can be attributed to overproduction or underexcretion of uric acid (Box 79.3). Important causes of overproduction of uric acid include alcohol, cancer, psoriasis, and sickle cell anemia. Excessive dietary purine intake is a common cause of overproduction. Important causes of underexcretion of uric acid include chronic renal insufficiency, lead nephropathy, diabetic ketoacidosis, and drugs, notably thiazide diuretics, nicotinic acid, low-dose aspirin, and calcineurin inhibitors.

Factors Predisposing to Acute Gout

Factors that precipitate gout include ketosis related to fasting, trauma, surgery, dietary indiscretions, and use of alcohol, especially beer.

Clinical Manifestations of Acute Gout

In the majority of patients with gout, the metatarsophalangeal joint of the great toe is involved initially (podagra). Rapid joint swelling is associated with intense pain and extreme tenderness. Symptoms in the foot often awaken the person in the early morning. The attack may last for 2 weeks or more. Immediate treatment shortens the duration of the episode. Urate crystals, which are needle-shaped and strongly negatively birefringent under polarized light, are found in the joint during an acute attack. The diagnosis of gout is established by the demonstration of urate crystals in the joint aspirate.

Gout occurs most commonly in middle-aged men, but, after menopause, the incidence of gout in women increases. Although gout is usually monarticular and usually involves the joints in the lower extremity, attacks may become polyarticular over time. Bursae, such as those at the olecranon, may also be involved. In elderly patients taking diuretics, the first episode of gout may appear in the osteoarthritic hand.

KEY FACTS

✓ Nine of 10 patients with gout have reduced renal clearance of urate

✓ Gout initially involves the metatarsophalangeal joint of the great toe (podagra) in the majority of patients

✓ Finding urate crystals (needle-shaped and strongly negatively birefringent under polarized light) in joint aspirate during an acute attack establishes the diagnosis of gout

✓ Gout may eventually involve multiple joints and also bursae

Treatment of Acute Gouty Arthritis

NSAIDs, such as indomethacin or naproxen, are the drugs of choice for treatment of acute gouty arthritis and should be used for a 7- to 10-day course. These drugs are contraindicated in patients with aspirin hypersensitivity, congestive heart failure, active peptic ulcer disease, or renal insufficiency. Glucocorticoids (oral, intramuscular, intravenous, or intra-articular) are the best choice for a patient who has contraindications to NSAIDs, is taking anticoagulants, or is hospitalized. A typical dose is 30 mg of prednisone daily for up to 5 days. Colchicine should not be given to transplant patients taking cyclosporine or to persons with liver or renal disease.

Treatment During Intercritical Period

Oral colchicine, 0.6 mg twice daily, may be given prophylactically for up to 3 to 6 months when starting uric acid–lowering therapy to prevent exacerbation of acute gout. Long-term use of low-dose colchicine can be associated with a myopathy and neuropathy, especially in patients with renal insufficiency. A myoneuropathy may appear in patients taking medications that affect colchicine metabolism via the cytochrome P-450 system. These include cyclosporine, simvastatin, lovastatin, atorvastatin, diltiazem, cimetidine, verapamil, and amiodarone.

Treatment of Recurrent or Chronic Gout

Uric acid–lowering therapy is indicated in persons with more than 2 gout attacks over the past 12 months, or in patients with soft-tissue tophi, gouty erosions on radiographs, or uric acid nephrolithiasis. The goal of therapy is to consistently maintain a serum uric acid level below 6 mg/dL, thus preventing new joint urate crystallization as well as resorption of the existing deposits.

KEY FACTS

✓ Colchicine, 1.2 mg as a single dose followed in an hour by a 0.6-mg dose, is another therapeutic option for acute gouty arthritis

✓ Indications for uric acid–lowering therapy—more than 2 gout attacks in the past year, or soft-tissue tophi, gouty erosions on radiographs, or uric acid nephrolithiasis

✓ The therapeutic goal for gout—keep the serum uric acid level below 6 mg/dL to prevent new and reduce existing urate deposits

The uricosuric probenecid inhibits tubular reabsorption of filtered and secreted urate. Probenecid should not be used if the patient has a creatinine clearance less than 50 mL/min or a history of kidney stones. This drug requires twice-daily use and has generally been replaced by once-daily xanthine oxidase inhibitors.

Allopurinol is the standard xanthine oxidase inhibitor. Its use should not be started during an acute attack. Allopurinol can cause a rare hypersensitivity syndrome: eosinophilia, fever, hepatitis, renal failure, and erythematous desquamative rash. This syndrome is observed most commonly in patients with renal insufficiency and in Southeast Asians with the genetic marker HLA-B*5801. Allopurinol may be used in patients with renal insufficiency. One suggested guideline for the starting dose is 1.5 times the estimated glomerular filtration rate. The dose of allopurinol is then gradually increased by 50-mg increments until the target serum uric acid level has been reached. Many patients with normal renal function may need more than 300 mg of allopurinol daily to reach an appropriate uric acid level. Febuxostat is a new xanthine oxidase inhibitor that can be used in patients who are allergic to allopurinol. Both of these xanthine oxidase inhibitors will interfere with the metabolism of 6-mercaptopurine and azathioprine, increasing the risk of bone marrow toxicity. Ideally, these drugs should be avoided in persons requiring xanthine oxidase inhibition. In transplant patients, azathioprine is replaced by mycophenolate mofetil in patients requiring allopurinol or febuxostat.

Pegloticase (pegylated uricase), which converts uric acid to allantoin, is approved for chronic gout refractory to conventional therapy. In patients with extensive tophaceous deposits, it promotes more rapid resolution. Pegloticase is a short-term intravenous therapy because inactivating antibodies develop.

Box 79.4 lists important points to remember in management of gout.

Calcium Pyrophosphate Deposition Disease

Classification

Calcium pyrophosphate deposition disease (CPPD) can be divided into 3 main categories: hereditary or familial (eg, Slovakian, Dutch, or Canadian ancestry), secondary, and sporadic. Diseases associated with CPPD include metabolic disorders such as hyperparathyroidism (strong association), hemochromatosis (strong association), hypophosphatasia, hypomagnesemia, and familial hypocalciuric hypercalcemia.

Clinical Features

CPPD has 2 main clinical presentations: acute synovitis and chronic arthropathy. Radiographic evidence of chondrocalcinosis, such as calcifications in hyaline cartilage of the knee and triangular fibrocartilage of the wrist, is often an incidental finding in the elderly. The release of CPPD crystals can induce an acute inflammatory arthritis called **pseudogout**. Pseudogout most commonly affects the knees and wrists, but shoulders, elbows, ankles, and intervertebral disks also can be affected. Pseudogout rarely affects more than 1 joint during an attack, except in hospitalized elderly patients. Acute attacks are self-limiting, generally lasting 1 week. Fever and delirium may occur in the elderly. Chronic CPPD arthropathy is a structural abnormality of cartilage with osteophyte and cyst formation and CPPD crystal deposition within the joint; superimposed pseudogout attacks may occur. The joints most commonly affected are the knees and wrists,

---

Box 79.4 • Important Points in Management of Gout

Treatment of hyperuricemia may slow the decline of the glomerular filtration rate in patients with chronic kidney disease.

Most rheumatologists do not treat asymptomatic hyperuricemia. In the future this recommendation may change in persons with myocardial failure, coronary artery disease, or chronic kidney disease.

Gout and hyperuricemia cannot be treated exclusively with dietary modification. However, patients should be advised to avoid red meat, seafood, beer, and concentrated fructose, as all of these foods may trigger an attack. Dairy proteins, vitamin C, and coffee will help to lower the serum uric acid level. Both losartan and fenofibrate also have mild uricosuric effects and can be helpful in hyperuricemic patients with appropriate indications for their use. Weight loss will also help to reduce the frequency of acute gout.

Up to 33% of patients with acute gout have a normal level of serum uric acid at the time of the acute attack. A serum uric acid determination is not recommended for the evaluation of acute gout. This should be obtained after the attack has remitted.

Half of synovial fluid samples aspirated from first metatarsophalangeal or other previously involved joints of asymptomatic patients with gout have crystals of monosodium urate.

Gout in a premenopausal woman is very unusual.

A septic joint can trigger an attack of gout or pseudogout in a predisposed person. Synovial fluid should always be analyzed for crystals and subjected to Gram stain and culture.

The frequency of gout in patients who have had organ transplant is high (25%). (Both calcineurin inhibitors and diuretics cause hyperuricemia.)

---

followed by the shoulders, hips, metacarpophalangeal joints, and metatarsophalangeal joints. Patients may present with chronic pain and stiffness with limitation of function of the affected joints, which may be misdiagnosed as rheumatoid arthritis.

Key Definition

Pseudogout: *an inflammatory arthritis resulting from the formation of calcium pyrophosphate crystals in articular and hyaline cartilage and fibrocartilage.*

Pathogenesis

The formation of CPPD crystals may be related to effects on the metabolism of inorganic pyrophosphate present in synovial fluid. Local joint factors that may influence CPPD crystal formation include the absence of magnesium, excessive calcium, and the absence of alkaline phosphatase within synovial fluid and tissue. CPPD crystals stimulate inflammation by a mechanism related to elaboration of pro-inflammatory cytokines, similar to that in acute gout; the acute inflammatory reaction is often precipitated by trauma.

Diagnosis of CPPD

For definitive diagnosis, CPPD crystals must be identified in joint fluid obtained by arthrocentesis; CPPD crystals demonstrate weakly positive birefringence under compensated polarized light microscopy. The presence of characteristic calcifications along the hyaline cartilage and fibrocartilage on plain radiographs supports a CPPD diagnosis; however, the acute synovitis of pseudogout may be seen in patients without visible chondrocalcinosis.

Treatment of CPPD

Unlike in gout, there is no treatment that prevents the formation or promotes the elimination of CPPD crystals. If an underlying metabolic disorder associated with CPPD, such as hyperparathyroidism, is present, it should be recognized and treated. For treatment of attacks of pseudogout, NSAIDs, oral prednisone, or an intra-articular injection of a glucocorticoid preparation into the swollen joint can be effective. Low-dose oral colchicine may lead to a decrease in the frequency and severity of attacks, but adverse effects may preclude its prolonged use. Chondrocalcinosis is asymptomatic and therefore is not treated.

KEY FACTS

✓ Diseases associated with CPPD—hyperparathyroidism (strong association), hemochromatosis (strong association), hypophosphatasia, hypomagnesemia, and familial hypocalciuric hypercalcemia

✓ Finding CPPD crystals (weakly positively birefringent under polarized light) in joint aspirate is needed for definitive diagnosis of CPPD disease

✓ Characteristic chondrocalcinosis on plain radiographs supports a CPPD diagnosis but may be absent in pseudogout

✓ Therapies for pseudogout include NSAIDs, oral corticosteroids, and intra-articular corticosteroid injection; adverse effects may limit use of low-dose oral colchicine

---

Basic Calcium Phosphate Deposition Disease

Presentation

The main clinical presentations of basic calcium phosphate disease are 1) acute inflammation, such as calcific tendinitis, bursitis, or periarthritis, and 2) chronic articular inflammation, including Milwaukee shoulder, a noninflammatory pastelike joint fluid containing hydroxyapatite. Subcutaneous deposits of basic calcium phosphate

may be found in the tissues of patients with scleroderma or dermatomyositis, particularly juvenile dermatomyositis (calcinosis cutis).

Diagnosis and Treatment

Diagnosis of basic calcium phosphate disease may be difficult. Individual crystals are not birefringent, so they cannot be seen on routine polarized light microscopy (Table 79.2). Treatment involves NSAIDs and intra-articular corticosteroid injections. Subcutaneous basic calcium phosphate disease is difficult to treat; recently, topical, intra-lesional, and intravenous sodium thiosulfate has been used with mild success, possibly related to the dissolution of calcium salts.

Calcium Oxalate Arthropathy

Calcium oxalate arthropathy occurs in patients with primary oxalosis and in patients with renal failure, usually those undergoing long-term hemodialysis. It can cause acute inflammatory arthritis. Crystals are large, bipyramidal, envelope-shaped, and strongly birefringent. Calcium oxalate can cause calcification of articular structures that is apparent on radiographs.

Other Crystalline Arthropathies

Several other types of crystals have been identified in soft tissues, bursa, and joints. Cholesterol crystals have been found in the synovial fluid and/or olecranon bursa of patients with rheumatoid arthritis and other inflammatory arthritides. The crystals look like broad squares with a notched corner. Corticosteroid crystals have been found after an intra-articular corticosteroid injection; these crystals can induce an inflammatory reaction and synovitis manifested by a painful, swollen joint within 8 hours after

Table 79.2 • Differential Diagnosis of Basic Calcium Phosphate Disease According to Results of Synovial Fluid Analysis

Diagnosis	Leukocyte Count, ×10⁹/L	Differential	Polarization Microscopy
Degenerative joint disease	<1	Mononuclear cells	Negative
Rheumatoid arthritis	5–50	PMNs	Negative
Gout	5–100	PMNs	Monosodium urate
Pseudogout	5–100	PMNs	CPPD
Hydroxyapatite	5–100	PMNs	Negative
Septic arthritis	≥100	PMNs	Negative

Abbreviations: CPPD, calcium pyrophosphate deposition disease; PMNs, polymorphonuclear leukocytes.

injection. Aspiration is often done to exclude infection; the diagnosis of corticosteroid crystalline arthropathy may be supported by the presence of irregular square and rod-shaped crystals. Corticosteroid crystals often have been phagocytosed by neutrophils and macrophages. Charcot-Leyden crystals have been found in hypereosinophilic syndromes; these crystals have a spindle-shaped appearance and are weakly birefringent.

Idiopathic Inflammatory Myopathies

The **idiopathic inflammatory myopathies** are a group of rare systemic inflammatory muscle diseases categorized into 3 main subtypes: dermatomyositis, polymyositis, and inclusion body myositis. They have distinct clinical features and histopathologic abnormalities on muscle biopsies characterized by inflammatory infiltrates composed primarily of T cells, B cells, and macrophages. Patients with idiopathic inflammatory myopathies have progressive muscle weakness, usually symmetric, caused by muscle inflammation and extramuscular organ involvement. Dermatomyositis affects persons in a bimodal distribution, with onset in the juvenile age range of 16 years or younger (called juvenile dermatomyositis) and in the mid-40s to 50s. Inclusion body myositis occurs in persons older than 50 years, and it affects men more often than women (3:1 ratio). Other types of inflammatory myopathies are cancer-associated myositis and connective tissue disease–associated myositis, as seen in patients with scleroderma, mixed connective tissue disease, Sjögren syndrome, and systemic lupus erythematosus. Connective tissue disease–associated myositis generally presents as a mild inflammatory myopathy affecting younger patients (age range, 20s–40s). Cancer-associated myositis is considered a paraneoplastic syndrome triggered by a malignant tumor, typically breast, ovarian, lung, or prostate, in persons older than 50 years.

Key Definition

Idiopathic inflammatory myopathies: *a group of rare systemic inflammatory muscle diseases categorized into 3 main subtypes: dermatomyositis, polymyositis, and inclusion body myositis.*

Clinical Features

Dermatomyositis presents with symmetric proximal muscle weakness and several classic photosensitive rashes, including the following: heliotrope rash of the eyelids with periorbital edema; erythematous papular rash on the metacarpophalangeal and proximal interphalangeal joints (Gottron papules); erythematous, scaly rash over the extensor surfaces of the metacarpophalangeals, proximal interphalangeals, elbows, and knees (Gottron sign); V sign of the chest; shawl sign affecting the upper back and neck; and patchy erythema of the face. Nailfold capillary abnormalities usually occur and can be visualized with an ophthalmoscope as dilated capillary loops with dropout. Although more common in patients with juvenile dermatomyositis, calcinosis may occur over the extensor surfaces, such as elbows and knees. Extramuscular organ involvement may occur in the pulmonary, gastrointestinal, and cardiac systems.

Amyopathic dermatomyositis is a subtype of dermatomyositis with characteristic photosensitive rashes as seen in dermatomyositis, but minimal or no muscle involvement. These patients generally have a less aggressive course than those with dermatomyositis, although a malignancy may be present at diagnosis in approximately 10% of patients. A rare subset of patients with amyopathic dermatomyositis develop progressive pulmonary fibrosis.

Polymyositis also is characterized by symmetric proximal muscle weakness, but without the rashes seen in dermatomyositis. As in dermatomyositis, other organs may be affected by inflammation and/or skeletal muscle weakness. For example, in the lung, interstitial lung disease may occur, typically as nonspecific interstitial pneumonia or progressive respiratory muscle weakness leading to respiratory failure; in the gastrointestinal system, dysphagia from weakness of the cricopharyngeal muscle may be prominent and result in aspiration pneumonia; and in the cardiac system, arrhythmias or myocarditis may occur.

A subset of patients with dermatomyositis or polymyositis have characteristic features that define the antisynthetase syndrome. These patients present with fever; Raynaud phenomenon; arthritis; "mechanic's hands" due to hyperkeratosis of the lateral aspects of the finger pads, primarily in the second and third digits; and interstitial lung disease that may be progressive and refractory to treatment with corticosteroids and other immunosuppressives. Antibodies against the aminoacyl-transfer RNA synthetases may be present in about 35% to 40% of patients: anti-Jo-1 antibodies have been commonly reported with a prevalence of 20% to 40%, but other, rarer (<1%–5% prevalence) autoantibodies exist, such as anti-PL-7, anti-PL-12, anti-EJ, anti-OJ, anti-Ks, anti-Ha, and anti-Zo antibodies.

The characteristic features of inclusion body myositis are insidious onset of weakness with proximal and distal muscle involvement, such as in the finger flexors and wrist muscles. Some patients may have asymmetric muscle involvement. Muscle atrophy of the forearm compartment muscles and/or quadriceps may be seen. Patients often present with frequent falls of unknown cause. Dysphagia is also a prominent symptom and may progress to placement of a feeding tube.

Diagnosis

The work-up for patients suspected of having an idiopathic inflammatory myopathy involves several testing modalities. Serum levels of the following muscle enzymes are measured: creatine kinase, aldolase, aspartate aminotransferase, alanine aminotransferase, and lactate dehydrogenase. Creatine kinase measurement is the most sensitive and accurate laboratory test reflecting muscle inflammation, but its sensitivity diminishes as the muscle disease becomes chronic and muscle inflammation gives way to fibrosis and scarring. In inclusion body myositis, creatine kinase values may be minimally elevated or normal at presentation. Electromyography in patients with dermatomyositis or polymyositis characteristically shows polyphasic motor unit potentials with decreased amplitudes, increased spike frequency, and fibrillation potentials that indicate active disease. Magnetic resonance imaging studies of affected muscle groups have been gaining use as a noninvasive means of detecting muscle inflammation. A muscle biopsy must be obtained on the contralateral side from where electromyography was performed, and preferably the muscle sample should be obtained from an area that demonstrated weakness on examination.

Muscle biopsies are the gold standard for confirming a diagnosis of idiopathic inflammatory myopathy. Muscle biopsies characteristically reveal degeneration, necrosis, and regeneration of myofibrils with a lymphocytic inflammatory infiltrate. The pathogenesis of dermatomyositis and juvenile dermatomyositis involves deposition of C5b-C9 membrane attack complex and complement in the muscle microvasculature, leading to tissue hypoperfusion and fiber atrophy. In dermatomyositis and juvenile dermatomyositis, CD4 T cells, B cells, and plasmacytoid dendritic cells are found in the perivascular and perimysial areas, invading nonnecrotic muscle fibers expressing major histocompatibility complex class I. In polymyositis and inclusion body myositis, CD8 cytotoxic T cells are located within the endomysium; they surround and invade nonnecrotic muscle fibers expressing major histocompatibility complex class I, leading to fiber necrosis and regeneration. In inclusion body myositis, degenerative proteins accumulate in muscle tissue; rimmed vacuoles, congophilic amyloid deposits, and 15- to 18-nm tubulofilament inclusions are characteristic features seen on electron microscopy of the muscle biopsy specimen.

Autoantibodies against nuclear and cytoplasmic antigens are frequently seen in idiopathic inflammatory myopathies. The myositis-specific autoantibodies are useful in defining specific myositis subsets. In addition to the antibodies against the aminoacyl-transfer RNA synthetases that define the antisynthetase syndrome, other myositis-specific antibodies include anti-Mi-2, anti-SRP, and anti-MDA5 antibodies. They are present in approximately 5% to 20% of patients with idiopathic inflammatory myopathies. The anti-Mi-2 antibody is directed against the nuclear helicase protein, Mi2; it is associated with classic dermatomyositis rashes and a milder myositis course. The anti-SRP antibody is directed against the signal recognition particle; it is associated with severe necrotizing myopathy, cardiomyopathy, and a poor prognosis. The anti-MDA5 antibody is an RNA helicase first described in Asians with amyopathic dermatomyositis; it is associated with rapidly progressive interstitial lung disease and a poor prognosis. Myositis-associated autoantibodies, such as the anti-PM-Scl antibody, have been described in forms of myositis that overlap with scleroderma.

There is a well-described association between malignancy and onset of idiopathic inflammatory myopathy. An occult malignancy may be present in up to 25% of patients with dermatomyositis and approximately 10% to 15% of patients with polymyositis within 1 to 3 years of diagnosis. The etiology is not well understood but may involve a paraneoplastic phenomenon manifested by a cross-reaction of cytotoxic T cells against tumor antigens expressed by regenerating muscle fiber cells. The anti-p155/140 antibody has been reported as strongly predictive of cancer-associated myositis. Screening for an occult malignancy is strongly recommended on diagnosis of dermatomyositis or polymyositis, with age- and sex-appropriate testing and computed tomography scans of chest, abdomen, and pelvis or a whole-body positron emission tomography–computed tomography scan. An elevated CA-125 level at diagnosis of dermatomyositis has been strongly predictive of ovarian or primary peritoneal cancer in women.

Treatment

Treatment of idiopathic inflammatory myopathies generally involves high-dose corticosteroids, usually intravenous for 1 to 3 days initially, then oral corticosteroids, such as prednisone 1 mg/kg of body weight, for approximately 4 weeks with tapering every 2 to 4 weeks. The degree and frequency of tapering depend on normalization

---

KEY FACTS

✓ Classic rashes associated with dermatomyositis—heliotrope rash, Gottron papules, Gottron sign, *V* sign of the chest, shawl sign on the upper back and neck, and facial dermatitis

✓ Polymyositis and dermatomyositis both involve symmetric proximal muscle weakness, but only dermatomyositis has characteristic rashes

✓ Characteristic features of inclusion body myositis—insidious onset of weakness with proximal and distal muscle involvement (eg, in finger flexors and wrist muscles)

✓ For confirmation of idiopathic inflammatory myopathy, muscle biopsy remains the gold standard

of the serum muscle enzyme levels and improvement of strength, stamina, and extramuscular organ involvement. A steroid-sparing medication, such as methotrexate, azathioprine, and/or intravenous immunoglobulin, generally is started at diagnosis of idiopathic inflammatory myopathy to allow for quicker tapering. For rashes associated with dermatomyositis, topical corticosteroids, topical tacrolimus, hydroxychloroquine, and photoprotection with sunscreen are all generally effective. Patients with severe, refractory myositis and/or severe extramuscular involvement, such as progressive interstitial lung disease, may be treated with mycophenolate mofetil, cyclophosphamide, rituximab, or oral tacrolimus. There is no effective immunosuppressive treatment to date for inclusion body myositis. Intravenous immunoglobulin is commonly used for supportive treatment of progressive dysphagia in these patients.

KEY FACTS

✓ Malignancy is associated with idiopathic inflammatory myopathy; up to 25% of patients with dermatomyositis and 10% to 15% with polymyositis may have an occult malignancy within 1 to 3 years of diagnosis

✓ Idiopathic inflammatory myopathies generally require high-dose corticosteroid therapy

✓ No effective immunosuppressive treatment is available for inclusion body myositis

---

Drug-Induced Myopathies

Drugs can cause an immune-mediated necrotizing myopathy. The drugs commonly implicated are the lipid-lowering drugs, such as statins, fibrates, and nicotinic acid. Other drugs associated with myopathies include corticosteroids, colchicine, chloroquine, hydroxychloroquine, zidovudine, D-penicillamine, ethanol, cocaine, and heroin. Patients who have a statin-induced myopathy may present with myalgias, increased creatine kinase levels, muscle weakness, and, rarely, rhabdomyolysis. The pathogenesis of statin-induced myopathy is not well understood, but it is related to an antibody-mediated immune mechanism with elaboration of an autoantibody (anti-200/100 kDa protein) directed against hydroxymethylglutaryl-CoA reductase. A muscle biopsy does not reveal an inflammatory infiltrate; rather, T cells and macrophages surrounding necrotic and regenerating muscle fibers have been described.

Infectious Arthritis

Septic arthritis is a medical emergency; rapid recognition and treatment can reduce joint morbidity and patient mortality. A high index of suspicion is required when a patient presents with acute monarticular arthritis and fever. However, it is important to remember that approximately 20% of patients with septic arthritis have multiple-joint involvement, especially those patients who are chronically immunosuppressed.

Bacterial Arthritis

Nongonococcal septic arthritis is commonly caused by spread by a hematogenous route from an infectious source, such as pneumonia, urinary tract infection, infectious endocarditis, disk space infection, and abscesses (including tooth abscesses). Other routes of bacterial spread include dissemination from osteomyelitis, spread from a soft tissue infection such as cellulitis, iatrogenic from diagnostic testing, and trauma. Large joints are more commonly affected, such as the knee (˃50%) and hip; wrists and ankles may also be affected. Predisposing factors for septic arthritis include advanced age, a preexisting inflammatory arthritis such as rheumatoid arthritis, prosthetic joints, diabetes mellitus, alcoholism, intravenous drug use, and cirrhosis.

Rapid onset of a hot, swollen joint that is tender to touch and worsened by movement is the hallmark clinical presentation of septic arthritis. In general, if the affected joint is in the lower extremity, the patient cannot bear weight on it. High fevers with chills and general malaise may be present. In patients with rheumatoid arthritis, the clinical presentation may be abrupt onset of a polyarticular joint flare and/or pain disproportionately greater than indicated by findings on the joint examination.

In addition to blood and urine cultures, the diagnostic work-up for septic arthritis must include joint aspiration. Synovial fluid analysis should include a Gram stain, cultures (typically aerobic, anaerobic, or fungal if clinical

---

KEY FACTS

✓ Nongonococcal septic arthritis commonly arises by hematogenous spread from pneumonia, urinary tract infection, endocarditis, and abscesses

✓ Predisposing factors for septic arthritis—advanced age, preexisting inflammatory arthritis, prosthetic joints, diabetes, alcoholism, intravenous drug use, and cirrhosis

✓ The hallmark clinical presentation of septic arthritis— rapid onset of a hot, swollen joint that is tender to touch and worsened by movement; an affected lower extremity joint generally cannot bear weight

✓ Joint aspiration must be part of the diagnostic work-up for septic arthritis. Synovial fluid analysis should include Gram stain; aerobic, anaerobic, and fungal cultures; and total leukocyte count

✓ The synovial fluid leukocyte count in nongonococcal septic arthritis typically exceeds 50,000/mcL

suspicion is high), and total leukocyte count. Typically, patients with nongonococcal septic arthritis have a leukocyte count of more than 50,000/mcL. The synovial fluid is often purulent. However, synovial Gram stains and cultures may be negative, particularly if antibiotic therapy was initiated prior to aspiration; hence, a high index of suspicion should warrant treatment of septic arthritis even in the absence of positive cultures. Joint radiographs may show associated osteomyelitis or local trauma, but radiographic findings of infection are insensitive and usually lag by weeks behind clinical symptoms. Magnetic resonance imaging with contrast of the affected joint is more sensitive in detecting inflammation, revealing synovial enhancement and joint effusion.

Several organisms commonly cause septic arthritis. *Staphylococcus aureus* is the most common pathogen in adults who have nongonococcal septic arthritis. *Staphylococcus epidermidis* commonly causes prosthetic joint infection. In sickle cell anemia, *Salmonella* is the organism commonly causing septic arthritis. *Pseudomonas* should be considered after cat or dog bites, and an anaerobic infection should be considered in cases of human bites. Intravenous drug users may have bacteremia with unusual organisms, such as *Pseudomonas* or *Serratia*, and the patient may present with septic arthritis in unusual locations, such as the sternoclavicular or sacroiliac joints. Gram-negative bacilli, such as *Escherichia coli* and *Klebsiella*, may cause septic arthritis in patients older than 65 years who have gastrointestinal or genitourinary infections or diabetes or have undergone instrumentation.

Management of septic arthritis involves pharmacologic and surgical therapy. Broad-spectrum antibiotics should be used empirically until culture results are available. The first-line antibiotics for gram-positive cocci are oxacillin/nafcillin or cefazolin; if there is a concern for methicillin-resistant *S aureus*, then vancomycin or linezolid should be used. Antibiotics for gram-negative organisms are ceftriaxone, cefotaxime, ceftazidime, carbapenems, cefepime, piperacillin-tazobactam, or fluoroquinolones. The duration of antibiotic treatment varies and depends on the organism and patient, but is generally 2 to 4 weeks. Surgical management should include daily aspiration and lavage of the affected joint to completely remove the pus; this may be performed by arthroscopy or needle aspiration. If a loculated fluid collection is present or the joint is difficult to aspirate, then open surgical débridement and/or arthroscopic drainage is mandatory.

Gonococcal Arthritis

Disseminated gonococcal infection develops in approximately 0.2% of patients with gonorrhea. Gonococcal arthritis occurs from dissemination of *Neisseria gonorrhoeae* by sexual contact. This is the most common form of septic arthritis in sexually active persons younger than 30 years

who may be asymptomatic carriers of gonococci. Risk factors for disseminated gonococcal infection include female sex, urban residence, prostitution, intravenous drug use, and low socioeconomic status.

There are 2 main clinical presentations. The more common presentation involves the classic triad of dermatitis manifested by a vesiculopustular or pustular rash, tenosynovitis, and migratory polyarthritis. Fever is often present. Skin lesions may be tiny papules with an erythematous base and a hemorrhagic or necrotic center, occurring anywhere on the extremities. The second clinical presentation involves a monarthritis, usually of the knee, wrist, or ankle. These 2 patterns may overlap. Women present with gonococcal arthritis commonly during pregnancy or within 1 week after onset of menses, possibly related to the change in the pH of vaginal secretions. Extra-articular complications of disseminated gonococcal infection include meningitis, myopericarditis, and sepsis.

Testing involves culturing potentially involved mucosa. When a gonococcal infection is suspected, specimens from the pharynx, joints, rectum, blood, and genitourinary tract should be obtained. Specimens should be plated on a Thayer-Martin medium or other specialized media. Synovial fluid cultures are positive in only 30% to 50% of patients with known disseminated gonococcal infection. Specimen samples may be tested by polymerase chain reaction technique to increase sensitivity of detection. Culture of a skin lesion is positive for gonococcus in 40% to 60% of patients with disseminated gonococcal infection. Patients who have recurrent infections may have a congenital terminal complement component deficiency (C5-C9).

First-line antibiotic therapy for gonococcal arthritis is intravenous ceftriaxone for 24 to 48 hours after diagnosis and then transitioning to an oral fluoroquinolone. Treatment typically is given in a 7- to 14-day course. Approximately 30% to 50% of patients infected with *N gonorrhoeae* have a co-infection with *Chlamydia*. *Chlamydia* is not sensitive to ceftriaxone. Empirical azithromycin or doxycycline should be used. It is recommended that the patient's sexual partner(s) be treated empirically for gonorrhea and chlamydial infection as well.

Mycobacterial and Fungal Joint Infections

Although historically uncommon in the United States, mycobacterial joint infections are increasingly being recognized in immunocompromised patients and certain minority groups who have migrated from countries where these infections are endemic. Musculoskeletal involvement occurs in approximately 1% to 2% of patients with tuberculosis; the majority of these patients have pulmonary tuberculosis as well. *Mycobacterium tuberculosis* commonly causes tuberculous arthritis. The clinical presentation is often an indolent, monarticular infection affecting a large joint, such as the knee or hip; the joint infection occurs by direct extension from an adjacent bone infection. *Mycobacterium marinum* lives in saltwater or freshwater. Patients may become infected from direct skin inoculation by handling marine life. Clinical features are skin lesions such as papules or nodules and/or a cellulitis at the area of inoculation accompanied by an inflammatory arthritis and/or tenosynovitis frequently involving the hand and wrist. A high index of suspicion should be present for tuberculous infection; these infections are often diagnosed by synovial fluid aspiration and/or synovial biopsy. Synovial biopsy may reveal caseating granulomas.

Fungal joint infections are often difficult to diagnose unless a high index of suspicion is present. Clinical symptoms are variable and may range from migratory arthralgias, to tenosynovitis of large joints, to monarthritis. Symptoms may be present for several weeks to months before diagnosis. *Candida, Histoplasma, Blastomyces, Coccidioides, Sporothrix, Cryptococcu*s, and *Aspergillus* species have all been reported to cause infections. Sporotrichosis and blastomycosis are the fungal infections most likely to have musculoskeletal manifestations. The classic presentation in sporotrichosis is a gardener or farmer with a rose-thorn penetration that results in a papular, ulcerative rash at the site of inoculation, with lymphatic spread and tenosynovitis and/or monarthritis. Blastomycosis of the bone resembles osteolytic lesions with a periosteal reaction reminiscent of a bone tumor. Synovial fluid aspiration and/or synovial biopsy must be performed for diagnosis; it is important to remember that fungal colonies may grow slowly (days to weeks).

KEY FACTS

✓ *Staphylococcus aureus* is the most common cause of nongonococcal bacterial arthritis in adults

✓ Disseminated gonococcal infection commonly presents as the classic triad of dermatitis (vesiculopustular or pustular rash), tenosynovitis, and migratory polyarthritis

✓ First-line antibiotic therapy for gonococcal arthritis—intravenous ceftriaxone followed by an oral fluoroquinolone

✓ If a gardener has a rose-thorn prick that leads to a papular, ulcerative rash at the site of inoculation, with lymphatic spread and tenosynovitis and/or monarthritis, suspect sporotrichosis

---

Spinal Septic Arthritis

Infectious spondylitis should be suspected in patients with acute or chronic, unrelenting back pain associated with marked local tenderness. Constitutional symptoms, such as fevers, sweats, and weight loss, may be present. The most common organism causing infection is *S aureus*. The thoracolumbar region is commonly affected. An antecedent infection or procedure predisposing to bacteremia may have occurred. Imaging studies usually show an infection crossing the disk space. Vertebral involvement (Pott disease) is the most common manifestation of musculoskeletal tuberculosis due to spread from vascular channels in the lungs and other tissues. In Pott disease, the sites of involvement are commonly T10-L2, and a paraspinal abscess may be coexisting. Vertebral collapse may occur in later stages.

Intravertebral disk infection is often difficult to diagnose because pain patterns may be unusual and localizing signs may be absent. There is usually a concurrent infection, such as a blood or urinary tract infection, or recent spinal surgery. Radiographs of the spine often show no abnormalities, but magnetic resonance imaging often reveals abnormalities of the disk space and soft tissue. The diagnosis may be confirmed by aspiration of the disk space. Surgical drainage and débridement may be necessary, especially if neurologic symptoms are present.

Infected Joint Prostheses

Infection of joint prostheses occurs in 1% to 3% of joint replacements. There may be evidence of loosening of the cement holding the new joint in place, and radiographs may reveal lytic changes around the prosthesis. Aspiration of fluid from the prosthetic joint is necessary to confirm infection. Prosthetic joint infections are usually caused by gram-positive organisms, particularly coagulase-negative staphylococci (eg, *S epidermidis*) and streptococci, in the first 3 to 6 months after the replacement operation and by gram-negative and fungal organisms after 6 months. Bacteria adhere to the prosthetic surface material as a biofilm and become embedded within a layer of glycocalyx that is resistant to the host's immune defenses or antimicrobial agents. If a prosthetic joint infection is suspected, empirical antimicrobial therapy should be initiated; surgical management involves removal of the infected prosthetic material in a 2-stage procedure: insertion of an antibiotic-filled spacer with treatment for weeks to months, then reimplantation of another prosthetic joint. Patients who are not candidates for the staged procedure must have surgical débridement and then lifelong suppressive antibiotic therapy.

Rheumatic Fever and Poststreptococcal Reactive Arthritis

Arthritis affects 75% of patients with rheumatic fever. Joint involvement is more common in children. One-third of patients with acute rheumatic fever have no obvious antecedent pharyngitis. In adults, arthritis may be the only clinical feature of acute rheumatic fever. The arthritis may be migratory, with each joint remaining inflamed for approximately 1 week before another joint becomes inflamed. Monarthritis of the knee or ankle may be present in up to

25% of patients. The arthritis of rheumatic fever is nonerosive and the synovial fluid is sterile. Jaccoud arthropathy is a rare manifestation of arthritis, characterized by ulnar deviation of the metacarpophalangeal joints with hyperextension of the proximal interphalangeal joints as a result of tendon laxity rather than bony damage. This form of arthropathy is also seen in patients with systemic lupus erythematosus. The diagnosis of rheumatic fever is often made by streptococcal antibody tests such as antistreptolysin O and anti-DNase B. Antibody levels peak about 4 weeks after the pharyngeal infection and then decrease over 6 months.

Antimicrobial therapy (eg, penicillin) should be initiated for all patients with streptococcal pharyngeal infection. Patients with joint symptoms without carditis may be treated with high-dose salicylate therapy (3–4 g daily). Monitoring for adverse effects, such as nausea, vomiting, and gastrointestinal bleeding, is advised. Corticosteroids may be required if patients do not respond to salicylates. Joint symptoms may rebound when anti-inflammatory therapy is discontinued.

Viral Arthritis

Viruses associated with arthritis are human immunodeficiency virus (HIV), parvovirus B19, hepatitis B, hepatitis C, rubella, and, less commonly, mumps, herpesvirus, and enterovirus. The common clinical features of viral arthritis are acute onset of a polyarthritis with rash and fever, often self-limited. The pathogenesis involves an immune complex–mediated mechanism or direct viral infection of synovial cells.

KEY FACTS

- ✓ Prosthetic joint infections are usually caused by gram-positive organisms in the first 3 to 6 months after surgery and by gram-negative and fungal organisms after 6 months
- ✓ Two-stage procedure for surgical management of prosthetic joint infection—removal of the infected prosthetic material with insertion of an antibiotic-filled spacer for weeks to months, then reimplantation of another prosthetic joint
- ✓ Rheumatic fever is often diagnosed with streptococcal antibody tests (eg, antistreptolysin O, anti-DNase B)
- ✓ The common clinical features of viral arthritis—acute onset of a polyarthritis with accompanying rash and self-limited fever

---

Parvovirus B19 infection is common. Parvovirus infections are usually mild in children and associated with a "slapped cheek" rash from erythema infectiosum and arthralgias. In adults, arthritis is common, usually without a rash, and may mimic the polyarthritis pattern seen in rheumatoid arthritis. Parvovirus infection also has been associated with cytopenias and aplastic crisis in patients with

hemolytic anemia. The diagnosis of parvovirus infection is made by demonstrating the presence of anti–parvovirus B19 IgM antibodies. IgM antibodies may be present up to 6 weeks after infection and then wane. Parvovirus arthropathy is self-limited and resolves several weeks after an infection, although a subset of patients may develop a chronic arthropathy. Treatment consists of analgesics, such as NSAIDs, or low-dose corticosteroids.

Hepatitis infections are transmitted by parenteral or sexual routes. Hepatitis B arthropathy is associated with a preicteric, prodromal period of general malaise, fever, and nausea. This arthropathy has an immune complex–mediated mechanism that is abrupt in onset, leading to a symmetric polyarthritis of the small joints of the hands, wrists, and knees. Urticaria may be present. Hepatitis C virus infections can mimic autoimmune diseases, including rheumatoid arthritis, Sjögren syndrome, and systemic lupus erythematosus, both clinically and serologically. Numerous autoantibodies may be detected in hepatitis C virus infection, including a positive rheumatoid factor, antinuclear antibody, anti–SS-A and anti–SS-B, and antiphospholipid antibodies. The clinical features of hepatitis C arthropathy are similar to those of hepatitis B infection, with acute onset of polyarthritis of the small joints of hands, wrists, knees, and shoulders. Type 2 cryoglobulinemia or mixed cryoglobulinemia may complicate a hepatitis C infection.

Rubella virus infection may cause fever, cough, lymphadenopathy, and a morbilliform rash in young adults. Joint symptoms occur just before or after the appearance of the characteristic rash. A migratory polyarthralgia may be present.

Rheumatologic Manifestations of HIV Infection

Musculoskeletal complaints can be among the first manifestations of HIV infection (Box 79.5). A wide range of articular symptoms have been described, but the most

---

Box 79.5 • Rheumatologic Manifestations of Human Immunodeficiency Virus (HIV)

Arthralgia

Painful articular syndrome

HIV arthropathy

Reactive arthritis

Psoriatic arthritis

Myositis

Vasculitis

Raynaud phenomenon

Sjögren-like syndrome (diffuse infiltrative lymphocytosis syndrome)

Septic arthritis

Fibromyalgia

common is arthralgias. Articular manifestations can be extremely debilitating. A syndrome described as "painful articular syndrome" is manifested by severe pain in the knees and/or ankles lasting from hours to days. Narcotic analgesia may be needed for control of pain. HIV arthropathy may present as an asymmetric oligoarthritis involving joints in the lower extremities.

Reactive and Psoriatic Arthritis

A reactive arthritis, psoriatic arthritis, or a nonspecific enthesopathy may occur before or simultaneously with the onset of HIV infection. Patients who are HLA-B27 positive often have severe, peripheral psoriatic arthritis, enthesopathy, and dactylitis. Most HIV-infected patients with reactive arthritis have extra-articular manifestations, such as urethritis, keratoderma blennorrhagicum, circinate balanitis, or painless oral ulcers; conjunctivitis is unusual. In approximately one-third of patients, the onset of HIV-associated reactive arthritis has been linked to an antecedent infection caused by *Salmonella, Shigella*, or *Campylobacter* species.

Other Types of Infectious Arthritis

Whipple disease is a rare cause of arthropathy associated with fever, weight loss, neurologic symptoms, malabsorption, lymphadenopathy, and hyperpigmentation. A slow, progressive dementia may develop. The arthritic symptoms may precede the gastrointestinal manifestations. The infectious agent is *Tropheryma whipplei*. Polymerase chain reaction testing of a small-bowel specimen or synovial biopsy or synovial fluid analysis may be necessary to establish the diagnosis. The usual treatment is doxycycline or trimethoprim-sulfamethoxazole for a year.

Rheumatoid Arthritis and Spondyloarthropathies

CLEMENT J. MICHET, MD

Rheumatoid Arthritis

Rheumatoid arthritis is a chronic systemic inflammatory disease characterized by joint destruction. It affects 0.03% to 1.5% of the population worldwide. Women are affected 3 times more frequently than men. Its incidence peaks between the ages of 35 and 45 years; however, the age-related prevalence of the disease increases even after age 65 years. The presentation of an unknown antigen to genetically susceptible persons is believed to trigger rheumatoid arthritis. Recently, cigarette smoking has been identified as a risk factor for seropositive rheumatoid arthritis.

Key Definition

Rheumatoid arthritis: *a chronic systemic inflammatory disease characterized by joint destruction.*

Natural History of Rheumatoid Arthritis

In the majority of patients, the onset of the joint disease is insidious, occurring over weeks to months. However, in a third of patients, the onset is rapid, occurring over days or weeks. Early in the course of the disease, most patients have a predominantly small-joint (hands, wrists, forefeet) oligoarthritis. Their disease becomes polyarticular with time. Spontaneous remissions of rheumatoid arthritis almost never occur after 2 years of disease. Patients who experience a persisting polyarthritis with increased acute-phase reactants and a positive rheumatoid factor or anti–cyclic citrullinated peptide (CCP) antibody are at high risk for early erosive disease within 1 to 2 years of symptom

onset and early disability. The relationship between disease duration and inability to work is nearly linear. After 15 years of rheumatoid arthritis, 15% of patients are completely disabled. Life expectancy in severe seropositive rheumatoid arthritis is shortened, but it may be improving with more aggressive early intervention in the illness. Patients are at increased risk of coronary artery disease, infections, and non-Hodgkin lymphoma.

Pathogenesis of Rheumatoid Arthritis

The inflammation begins in the synovial lining of the joints in a genetically predisposed person. This is an autoimmune process in which rheumatoid arthritis self-antigens are presented to autoreactive T lymphocytes and autoreactive B cells, producing rheumatoid antibodies. This process is cytokine-driven, including tumor necrosis factor alpha, interleukin-6, and interleukin-1, and as a consequence these proinflammatory signaling proteins have provided opportunities for the development of biologic agents inhibiting their roles in disease activation. The joint damage in rheumatoid arthritis is a consequence of synoviocyte, macrophage, and osteoclast activation, leading to synovial "pannus" formation and the destruction of cartilage and bone.

Patients have swelling, pain, and joint stiffness with the onset of clinical disease. Joint warmth, swelling, pain, and limitation of motion worsen as the synovial membrane proliferates and the inflammatory reaction builds. In studies of early arthritis, histologic and radiographic evidence of rheumatoid synovitis is found in clinically unaffected joints, an indication that the disease is present before clinical manifestations appear.

Rheumatoid factor is an immunoglobulin (Ig) directed against the Fc portion of IgG. It is detected in 70% to 80% of patients. It is not specific for rheumatoid arthritis, and the prevalence of rheumatoid factor increases with aging in healthy persons. Rheumatoid factor may be detected in other inflammatory diseases such as primary Sjögren syndrome, systemic lupus erythematosus, mixed cryoglobulinemia, hepatitis C, and systemic vasculitis.

> ### Key Definition
>
> Rheumatoid factor: *an immunoglobulin directed against the Fc portion of IgG. It is detected in 70%–80% of patients.*

Anti-CCP antibodies are detected in the majority of patients with seropositive rheumatoid arthritis. These target antigens are found in peptides containing citrulline, an amino acid resulting from posttranslational enzyme modification of arginine during cell apoptosis. Unlike rheumatoid factor, these antibodies are specific for rheumatoid arthritis. They are present before onset of clinical disease, and in a high titer they are associated with progressive erosive disease.

Clinical Features of Rheumatoid Arthritis

The joints most commonly involved in early rheumatoid arthritis are the metacarpophalangeal, proximal interphalangeal, wrist, and metatarsophalangeal joints (more than 85% of patients) (Figure 80.1). The distal interphalangeal joints are typically spared. The distribution of involvement is symmetric and polyarticular (5 or more joints); predominantly, small joints are involved. Ultimately, multiple other joints may be involved, including the knees, ankles, elbows, shoulders, and the cricoarytenoid and the cervical spine articulations. Joints affected with rheumatoid arthritis are warm and swollen. The joint enlargement feels spongy and occurs with the thickening of the synovium. An associated joint effusion may make the joint feel fluctuant. Patients describe deep aching and soreness in the involved joints, which are aggravated by use and can be present at rest.

Constitutional Features of Rheumatoid Arthritis

Morning stiffness of more than 1 hour, "gelling" throughout the body, and recurrence of the stiffness after resting are some of the many constitutional features that complicate rheumatoid arthritis. Fatigue, weight loss, muscle pain, excessive sweating, or low-grade fever may be reported by patients presenting with rheumatoid arthritis. Adult seropositive rheumatoid arthritis is not a cause of fever of unknown origin because temperatures greater than 38.3°C cannot be attributed to the disease.

Musculoskeletal Complications of Rheumatoid Arthritis

The musculoskeletal complications of rheumatoid arthritis are listed in Box 80.1.

Cervical Spine

Half of all patients with chronic rheumatoid arthritis have radiographic involvement of the atlantoaxial joint. It is diagnosed from cervical flexion and extension radiographs showing subluxation. Alternatively, some patients have

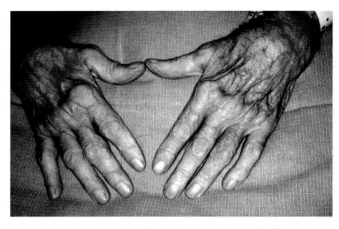

Figure 80.1 *Moderately Active Seropositive Rheumatoid Arthritis. The patient has soft tissue swelling across the entire row of metatarsophalangeal joints and proximal interphalangeal joints bilaterally and soft tissue swelling mounding up over the wrists. Note the nearly complete lack of change at the distal interphalangeal joints.*

> ### Box 80.1 • Musculoskeletal Complications of Rheumatoid Arthritis
>
> Characteristic deformities
>
> Boutonnière deformity of the finger, with hyperextension of the distal interphalangeal joint and flexion of the proximal interphalangeal joint
>
> Swan-neck deformity of the finger, with hyperextension at the proximal interphalangeal joint and flexion of the distal interphalangeal joint
>
> Ulnar deviation of the metacarpophalangeal joints; it can progress to complete volar subluxation of the proximal phalanx from the metacarpophalangeal head
>
> Compression of the carpal bones and radial deviation at the carpus
>
> Subluxation at the wrist
>
> Valgus of the ankle and hindfoot
>
> Pes planus
>
> Forefoot varus and hallux valgus
>
> Cock-up toes from subluxation at the metatarsophalangeal joints

subaxial subluxations, typically at 2 or more levels. The probability of cervical involvement is predicted by the severity and chronicity of peripheral arthritis. The prevalence of this rheumatoid complication is high in patients with rheumatoid arthritis who are referred for orthopedic reconstructive surgery.

The cervical instability is usually asymptomatic; however, patients may have pain and stiffness in the neck and occipital region. Patients may present dramatically with drop attacks or tetraplegia, but more commonly progression can be slow and subtle with symptoms of hand weakness or paresthesias or signs of cervical myelopathy. Interference with blood flow by ischemic compression of the anterior spinal artery or vertebral arteries (vertebrobasilar insufficiency) causes the neurologic symptoms. All patients with destructive rheumatoid arthritis should be managed with intubation precautions and the assumption that cervical instability is present. New neurologic symptoms mandate urgent neurologic evaluation, including magnetic resonance imaging of the cervical spine and consideration of surgical intervention. Indications for surgical treatment include neurologic or vascular compromise and intractable pain. In active patients, prophylactic cervical spine stabilization is recommended when there is evidence of extreme (>8 mm) subluxation of C1 over C2.

Popliteal Cyst

Flexion of the knee markedly increases the intra-articular pressure of a swollen joint. This pressure produces an outpouching of the posterior components of the joint space, termed a *popliteal* or a *Baker cyst*. Ultrasonographic examination of the popliteal space confirms the diagnosis. The cyst can rupture with dissection into the calf resembling acute thrombophlebitis and is called "pseudothrombophlebitis." Premature anticoagulation for possible phlebitis will lead to a hematoma in the calf. Treatment of an acute cyst rupture includes bed rest, elevation of the leg, ice massage or cryocompression, and an intra-articular injection of corticosteroid. Polpliteal cysts require medical management of the knee synovitis. Surgical resection is rarely recommended.

Tenosynovitis

Tenosynovitis of the finger flexor and extensor wrist tendon sheaths is common. Persistent inflammation can produce stenosing tenosynovitis, loss of function, and, ultimately, rupture of tendons. Treatment of acute tenosynovitis includes immobilization, warm soaks, nonsteroidal anti-inflammatory drugs, and local injections of corticosteroid in the tendon sheath.

Carpal Tunnel Syndrome

Rheumatoid arthritis is a common cause of carpal tunnel syndrome. The sudden appearance of bilateral carpal tunnel syndrome should raise the question of an early inflammatory arthritis. This syndrome is associated with paresthesias of the hand in a typical median nerve distribution. Discomfort may radiate up the forearm or into the upper arm. The symptoms worsen with prolonged flexion of the wrist and at night. Late complications include thenar muscle weakness and atrophy and permanent sensory loss. Treatment includes resting splints, control of inflammation, and local injection of glucocorticosteroid. Surgical release is recommended for persistent symptoms.

KEY FACTS

✓ Anti-CCP antibodies—detected in the majority of patients with seropositive rheumatoid arthritis; unlike rheumatoid factor, they are specific for rheumatoid arthritis

✓ Presentation of rheumatoid arthritis—a symmetric, small joint (wrist, metacarpophalangeal, proximal interphalangeal, metatarsophalangeal) polyarthritis lasting for >6 weeks. The presence of a positive CCP antibody increases the likelihood of early rheumatoid arthritis in this setting

✓ Constitutional features complicating rheumatoid arthritis—morning stiffness of >1 hour, "gelling" throughout the body, and recurrence of stiffness after resting

✓ Half of all patients with chronic rheumatoid arthritis have radiographic involvement of the atlantoaxial joint; it is diagnosed from cervical flexion and extension radiographs showing subluxation

---

Extra-articular Complications of Rheumatoid Arthritis

Extra-articular complications of rheumatoid arthritis occur almost exclusively in patients who have high titers of rheumatoid factor. In general, the number and severity of the extra-articular features vary with the duration and severity of disease. Many of the classic extra-articular manifestations of rheumatoid arthritis have become less common with the advent of more aggressive treatment of early disease.

Rheumatoid Nodules

Rheumatoid nodules are the most common extra-articular manifestation of seropositive rheumatoid arthritis. More than 20% of patients have rheumatoid nodules, which occur over extensor surfaces and at pressure points. They are rare in the lungs, heart, sclera, and dura mater. The nodules have characteristic histopathologic features. A collagenous capsule and a perivascular collection of chronic inflammatory cells surround a central area of necrosis encircled by palisading fibroblasts. Breakdown of the skin over rheumatoid nodules, with ulcers and infection, can be a major source of morbidity. The infection can spread to local bursae, infect bone, or spread hematogenously to joints.

Rheumatoid Vasculitis

Rheumatoid vasculitis usually occurs in persons with severe, deforming arthritis and a high titer of rheumatoid factor. It is now rarely encountered with the advent of more aggressive therapies for rheumatoid arthritis. As an immune complex vasculitis, it may present as palpable purpura, mononeuritis multiplex, or a medium-vessel polyarteritis–like syndrome affecting visceral organs.

Neurologic Manifestations

The most common neurologic complication of rheumatoid arthritis is carpal tunnel syndrome. In patients with advanced joint disease, cervical vertebral subluxation can cause myelopathy. The resulting hand paresthesias may be mistaken for carpal tunnel syndrome. Erosive changes may promote basilar invagination of the odontoid process of C2 into the underside of the brain, causing spinal cord compression and death.

Pulmonary Manifestations

Pleural disease has been noted in more than 40% of autopsies in cases of rheumatoid arthritis, but clinically significant pleural disease is less frequent. Characteristically, rheumatoid pleural effusions are asymptomatic until they become large enough to interfere mechanically with respiration. The pleural fluid is an exudate with a concentration of glucose that is low (10–50 mg/dL) because of impaired transport of glucose into the pleural space. Pulmonary nodules may appear singly or in clusters. They typically occur in patients with peripheral rheumatoid nodules. Single nodules have the appearance of a coin lesion. Nodules typically are pleural-based and may cavitate and create a bronchopleural fistula.

Pulmonary interstitial fibrosis is a chronic, slowly progressive process usually occurring later in the course of seropositive rheumatoid arthritis. Interstitial disease is highly associated with smoking. It has physical findings of diffuse dry crackles on lung auscultation and a reticular nodular radiographic pattern affecting both lung fields, initially in the lung bases. A decrease in the diffusing capacity for carbon dioxide and a restrictive pattern on pulmonary function tests are found. Bronchiolitis obliterans with or without cryptogenic organizing pneumonia may occur with rheumatoid arthritis or its treatment. It produces an obstructive picture on pulmonary function testing and typically responds to corticosteroid treatment. High-resolution computed tomography is useful for distinguishing these different interstitial rheumatoid lung syndromes and predicting treatment response. Lung biopsy is rarely necessary. Methotrexate treatment causes a hypersensitivity lung reaction in 1% to 3% of patients. It usually presents in a subacute pattern, which may help to distinguish it from rheumatoid lung disease.

> ### Key Definition
>
> **Pulmonary interstitial fibrosis:** *a chronic, slowly progressive process usually occurring later in the course of seropositive rheumatoid arthritis.*

Cardiac Complications

Patients rarely present with acute pericarditis or tamponade. Recurrent effusive pericarditis without symptoms may evolve to chronic constrictive pericarditis. Signs of unexplained edema, ascites, or right heart failure may be the presenting manifestations in patients with chronic seropositive rheumatoid arthritis. It will not respond to medical therapies. Surgical pericardiectomy is necessary. The most common cardiac complication in patients with rheumatoid arthritis is an increased risk of coronary artery disease.

Liver Abnormalities

Patients with rheumatoid arthritis can have increased levels of liver enzymes, particularly alkaline phosphatase. Increased levels of aspartate aminotransferase, γ-glutamyltransferase, and acute-phase proteins and hypoalbuminemia also occur in active rheumatoid arthritis. Liver biopsy shows nonspecific changes of inflammation. Nodular regenerative hyperplasia is rare and causes portal hypertension and hypersplenism. Many medications used to treat rheumatoid arthritis may cause increased levels of the transaminases.

Ophthalmic Abnormalities

Keratoconjunctivitis sicca, or secondary Sjögren syndrome, is the most common ophthalmic complication in rheumatoid arthritis. Scleritis, although rare, represents an ophthalmologic emergency in patients with seropositive rheumatoid arthritis. It must be distinguished from benign episcleritis. Topical and systemic therapy is necessary in scleritis to avoid potential scleral perforations. Retinopathy is an infrequent complication of long-term hydroxychloroquine therapy.

Laboratory Findings in Rheumatoid Arthritis

Nonspecific alterations in many laboratory values are common. In very active disease, normocytic anemia (hemoglobin value about 10 g/dL), leukocytosis, thrombocytosis, hypoalbuminemia, and hypergammaglobulinemia are common. Rheumatoid factor (IgM) occurs in 90% of patients, but its presence may not be detected for months after the initial joint symptoms occur. A positive rheumatoid factor is not specific for rheumatoid arthritis. Diseases in boldface type in Box 80.2 are most likely to have high titers of rheumatoid factor. Five percent of the general population has a low titer of rheumatoid factor.

Rheumatoid arthritis

Sjögren syndrome

Hepatitis C

Mixed cryoglobulinemia

Idiopathic pulmonary fibrosis

Subacute bacterial endocarditis

Systemic lupus erythematosus

Viral infections

^a Diseases in boldface type are the most likely to have high-titer rheumatoid factor.

Anti-CCP antibodies are more specific for rheumatoid arthritis and may be present when rheumatoid factor is absent. Antinuclear antibodies are common in seropositive rheumatoid disease. C-reactive protein correlates with disease activity, but it is not more helpful than the erythrocyte sedimentation rate. Active rheumatoid arthritis is associated with the chronic disease anemia pattern of low iron-binding capacity, low plasma levels of iron, and an increased ferritin value. A normal ferritin value in this setting suggests a component of iron deficiency anemia.

Synovial fluid is cloudy and light yellow, has poor viscosity, and typically contains 10,000 to 75,000 leukocytes/mL, predominantly neutrophils.

Radiographic Findings in Rheumatoid Arthritis

The radiographic findings in early rheumatoid arthritis are normal or show soft tissue swelling and periarticular osteopenia. Later, the characteristic changes of periarticular osteoporosis, symmetric narrowing of the joint space, and marginal bony erosions become obvious. These signs are most common in radiographs of the hands, wrists, and forefeet. Baseline radiographs of these areas are part of the initial evaluation of newly diagnosed rheumatoid arthritis, both to assess severity of disease at presentation and to monitor progression of disease over time.

Diagnosis of Rheumatoid Arthritis

Adult rheumatoid arthritis should be considered in a person older than 16 years who has inflammatory joint symptoms lasting for more than 6 weeks (Figure 80.2). The time criterion is important because there are viral arthropathies, such as parvovirus B19 infection, that mimic acute rheumatoid arthritis. Hallmark features of early rheumatoid arthritis include morning stiffness lasting for more than 30 minutes, symmetric small joint involvement in the metatarsophalangeal joints (morning first step metatarsalgia), and metacarpophalangeal joints with tenderness and swelling.

The common conditions in the differential diagnosis of seronegative rheumatoid arthritis include the spondyloarthritis disorders. They tend to predominantly involve the lower extremities and spine, are asymmetric, and are associated with single digit involvement (sausage digit or dactylitis). Acute-onset oligoarticular seronegative rheumatoid arthritis needs to be distinguished from reactive arthritis, sarcoid, and Lyme arthritis. A synovial fluid analysis should always be done to exclude crystalline arthritis, gout, and calcium pyrophosphate. The detection of CCP antibody has allowed rheumatologists to identify rheumatoid arthritis very early in the clinical evolution of the disease before patients would meet the classification criteria for established rheumatoid arthritis.

Treatment of Rheumatoid Arthritis

The management of patients with rheumatoid arthritis requires making the correct diagnosis, determining the functional status of the patient, and selecting the goals of management with the patient. Goals of management include relieving inflammation and pain and maintaining function.

The key concept of rheumatoid arthritis therapy is to begin treatment as soon as the diagnosis is made. Using nonsteroidal anti-inflammatory drugs alone for seropositive rheumatoid arthritis is not appropriate. Treatment should be closely managed and advanced with the goal of achieving remission but at a minimum low disease activity based on a targeted disease activity score, so-called "treat to target" strategy.

The choice of first disease-modifying antirheumatic drug is determined by the potential for early joint damage. In seropositive patients, methotrexate is the drug of choice. The dose is gradually increased over 6 to 8 weeks to a target dose of 15 to 25 mg once weekly. Folic acid is given daily as a supplement to reduce toxicities. In persons who do not tolerate methotrexate, leflunomide or sulfasalazine is an alternative. The presence of chronic kidney or liver disease will influence the choice and dose of all 3 agents. Methotrexate and leflunomide are contraindicated in women of childbearing age who are not using reliable contraception.

In patients with seronegative rheumatoid arthritis who do not have erosive disease, hydroxychloroquine is an option as first therapy. Tapered oral corticosteroid therapy is recommended in some protocols for early rheumatoid arthritis while disease-modifying antirheumatic drug therapies are being initiated. In the patient who fails to respond to methotrexate monotherapy over 3 months, add-on intervention is recommended. Options include triple therapy with the addition of hydroxychloroquine and sulfasalazine or, alternatively, a biologic agent such as a tumor necrosis factor inhibitor or others. The decision regarding using biologic therapies should be left up to the consulting rheumatologist.

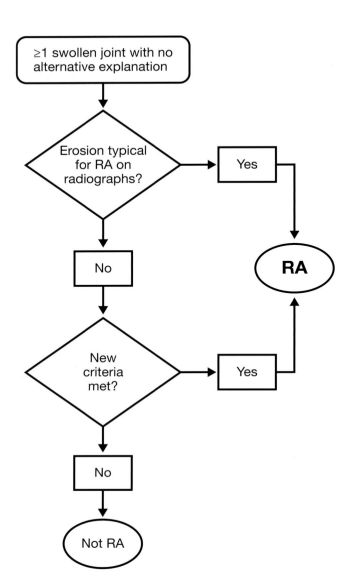

Joint Involvement (0-5)	
1 large joint	0
2-10 large joints	1
1-3 small joints (large joints not counted)	2
4-10 small joints (large joints not counted)	3
>10 joints (at least 1 small joint)	5
Serology (0-3)	
RF negative and ACPA negative	0
RF weakly positive (1-3 x N) or ACPA weakly positive (1-3 x N)	2
RF strongly positive (>3 x N) or ACPA strongly positive (>3 x N)	3
Symptom Duration (0-1)	
<6 weeks	0
≥6 weeks	1
Laboratory Tests for Inflammation (0-1)	
CRP normal **and** ESR normal	0
CRP abnormal **or** ESR abnormal	1

RA if Score ≥6

Figure 80.2 Classification Criteria for Rheumatoid Arthritis (RA), Suggested by the American College of Rheumatology and European League Against Rheumatisim 2010. ACPA indicates anti–citrullinated protein antibodies; CRP, C-reactive protein; ESR, erythrocyte sedimentation rate; N, normal; RF, rheumatoid factor.
(Adapted from Gaujoux-Viala C, Gossec L, Cantagrel A, Dougados M, Fautrel B, Mariette X, et al; French Society for Rheumatology. Recommendations of the French Society for Rheumatology for managing rheumatoid arthritis. Joint Bone Spine. 2014 Jul;81[4]:287–97. Epub 2014 Jun 27 as modified from original: Aletaha D, Neogi T, Silman AJ, Funovits J, Felson DT, Bingham CO 3rd, et al. 2010 rheumatoid arthritis classification criteria: an American College of Rheumatology/European League Against Rheumatism collaborative initiative. Ann Rheum Dis. 2010 Sep;69[9]:1580–8. Erratum in: Ann Rheum Dis. 2010 Oct;69[10]:1892.)

Preventive medical care is essential in the management of rheumatoid arthritis. Assessment for coronary artery risk factors and appropriate interventions are strongly recommended. Patients who have rheumatoid arthritis are at increased risk for osteoporosis. Vaccinations should be current, but patients receiving biologic therapies should not receive live vaccines.

An orthopedic surgical procedure for rheumatoid arthritis still remains an important therapeutic option for preserving or enhancing function. Synovectomy of the extensor wrist and nearby tendon sheaths is beneficial when medication alone fails to control the synovitis. Synovectomy of other joints has become less necessary as medical therapies have advanced. Resection of uncomfortable, draining, or infected nodules and decompression refractory carpal tunnel syndrome are also important surgical treatments for rheumatoid arthritis. Arthroplasty is reserved for patients in whom medical management has failed and in whom intractable pain or compromise in function developed because of a destroyed joint. Joint replacement has had a major impact on reducing patient disability.

Conditions Related to Rheumatoid Arthritis

Seronegative Rheumatoid Arthritis

Rheumatoid factor–negative (seronegative) rheumatoid arthritis is not associated with extra-articular manifestations. However, the arthritis usually can be destructive, deforming, and otherwise indistinguishable from seropositive rheumatoid arthritis. Erosive seronegative rheumatoid arthritis is managed similarly to seropositive disease.

Seronegative Rheumatoid Arthritis of the Elderly

A subgroup of patients older than 60 years with seronegative rheumatoid arthritis may have milder arthritis. In this subgroup, polyarticular inflammation suddenly develops and is controlled best with low doses of prednisone. The presence of anti-CCP antibodies and foot and ankle synovitis may help to distinguish late-onset rheumatoid arthritis from polymyalgia rheumatica. Minimal destructive changes and deformity occur. Some elderly patients with seronegative arthritis, such as men in their 70s, present with acute polyarthritis and pitting edema of the hands and feet, so-called RS3PE (remitting symmetric seronegative synovitis with pitting edema). They have a prompt and gratifying response to low doses of prednisone. RS3PE typically runs a course similar to that of polymyalgia rheumatica. A refractory seronegative inflammatory arthritis in the elderly may also represent a paraneoplastic syndrome.

Adult-Onset Still Disease

Systemic juvenile rheumatoid arthritis is known as Still disease. It has quotidian (fever spike with return to normal all in 1 day) high-spiking fevers, arthralgia, arthritis, seronegativity (negative rheumatoid factor and antinuclear antibody), leukocytosis, macular evanescent rash, serositis, lymphadenopathy, splenomegaly, and hepatomegaly. Fever, rash, and arthritis are the classic triad of Still disease.

Adult-onset Still disease has a slight female predominance. Its onset typically occurs between ages 16 and 35 years. Temperature more than 39°C occurs in a quotidian or double quotidian pattern in 96% of patients. The rash has a typical appearance: a macular salmon-colored eruption on the trunk and extremities. The transient rash is usually noticed at the time of increased temperature. Arthritis occurs in 95% of affected patients. In one-third of patients, the joint disease is progressive and destructive. Adult-onset Still disease has a predilection for the wrists, shoulders, hips, and knees. Sixty percent of patients complain of a sore throat at onset, which can confuse the diagnosis with rheumatic fever; however, the course is much more prolonged than that of acute rheumatic fever. Weight loss is common. Lymphadenopathy occurs in two-thirds of patients and hepatosplenomegaly in about half. Pleurisy, pneumonitis, and abdominal pain occur in less than a third of patients. The serum ferritin level is markedly increased.

Treatment of adult-onset Still disease includes high doses of aspirin or indomethacin. Corticosteroids may be needed to control the systemic symptoms. Half of patients require methotrexate to control the systemic and articular features. Interleukin-1 inhibitor therapy is useful for managing resistant cases.

Felty Syndrome

Felty syndrome has the classic triad of rheumatoid arthritis, leukopenia related to neutropenia, and splenomegaly. Classic Felty syndrome usually occurs after 12 years or more of rheumatoid arthritis. It occurs in less than 1% of patients with seropositive rheumatoid arthritis. Splenomegaly either may not be clinically apparent or may manifest only after the arthritis and leukopenia have been present for some time. Other features of Felty syndrome are listed in Box 80.3. Patients with this syndrome frequently have bacterial infections, particularly of the skin and lungs. Infection related to the cytopenia is the major cause of mortality. High titers of rheumatoid factor are the rule, and two-thirds of patients are positive for antinuclear antibody. Patients often die of sepsis despite vigorous antibacterial treatment. Treatment can include corticosteroids, methotrexate, granulocyte colony-stimulating factor, and splenectomy. Differential diagnosis includes the large granular lymphocyte syndrome. Affected patients frequently have neutropenia with a normal total white cell count related to the lymphocytosis.

KEY FACTS

- ✓ Patients with rheumatoid arthritis are at increased risk of coronary artery disease
- ✓ Serologic testing for acute parvovirus should be done in patients presenting with an acute small joint polyarthritis
- ✓ A diagnosis of seropositive rheumatoid arthritis mandates immediate therapy with a disease-modifying antirheumatic drug, most commonly methotrexate
- ✓ Early therapy of seropositive rheumatoid arthritis has improved survival and reduced the prevalence of many extra-articular complications

---

Box 80.3 • Features of Felty Syndrome

Classic triad
    Seropositive rheumatoid arthritis
    Neutropenia with leukopenia
    Splenomegaly
Other features
    Recurrent fevers with and without infection
    Lower extremity ulcers

Box 80.4 • Rheumatic Diseases Associated With HLA-B27

Ankylosing spondylitis (HLA-B27 in >90%)
Reactive arthritis (>80%)
Enteropathic spondylitis (approximately 75%)
Psoriatic spondylitis (approximately 50%)

Spondyloarthritis

Conditions in the spondyloarthritis spectrum include ankylosing spondylitis, reactive arthritis (Reiter syndrome), arthritis related to inflammatory bowel disease, and psoriatic arthritis. However, most patients are not neatly categorized into any of these classic disorders and are categorized as having undifferentiated spondyloarthritis. These patients may have varied manifestations of spondyloarthritis but do not have one of the classic diseases. An example is refractory Achilles enthesitis and plantar fasciitis, HLA-B27 positive.

Spondyloarthritis is characterized by the following: involvement of the sacroiliac joints (uncommon in rheumatoid arthritis), peripheral arthritis that is usually asymmetric and oligoarticular, absence of rheumatoid factor, acute anterior uveitis, association with HLA-B27, an enthesopathy (disorder of muscle or tendinous attachment to bones), and dactylitis (sausage digit). Family history of similar disorders, psoriasis, or inflammatory bowel disease may be reported.

Spondyloarthritis is associated with the HLA-B27 gene on chromosome 6. The prevalence of HLA-B27 determines the frequency of ankylosing spondylitis in various populations. In randomly selected persons with HLA-B27, the chance of the disease developing is 2%. In B27-positive relatives of B27-positive patients with ankylosing spondylitis, the risk of the disease developing is 20% (Box 80.4).

Ankylosing Spondylitis

Ankylosing spondylitis is a chronic systemic inflammatory disease that affects the sacroiliac joints, the spine, and the peripheral joints. Sacroiliitis and inflammatory low back pain define this disease.

Key Definition

Ankylosing spondylitis: *a chronic systemic inflammatory disease that affects the sacroiliac joints, the spine, and the peripheral joints.*

Features

Characteristic features of inflammatory low back pain in ankylosing spondylitis are the following: age at onset usually between 15 and 40 years, insidious onset, duration of more than 3 months, morning stiffness that improves with exercise but not with rest, and night pain improved by getting out of bed. Response to anti-inflammatory medication is also suggestive of an early spondyloarthritis.

Findings of ankylosing spondylitis on physical examination are listed in Table 80.1. Other physical findings in ankylosing spondylitis are listed in Table 80.2. Radiographic findings in ankylosing spondylitis include sacroiliac sclerosis and possible erosions, spine involvement with squaring of the vertebral bodies, syndesmophytes, and bamboo spine. These findings may take years to appear. In patients with early disease, magnetic resonance imaging can detect inflammation in the sacroiliac joints even when radiographs of the sacroiliac joints are normal.

Laboratory Findings

The erythrocyte sedimentation rate or C-reactive protein value may be increased, there may be an anemia of chronic disease, rheumatoid factor is absent, and 95% of white patients are positive for HLA-B27.

Table 80.1 • Results of Testing in Ankylosing Spondylitis

Test	Method	Results
Schober	Make a mark on the spine at level of L5 and 1 at 10 cm directly above with the patient standing erect. Patient then bends forward maximally and the distance between the 2 marks is measured	An increase of <5 cm indicates early lumbar involvement. Not helpful in older adults with degenerative spondylosis
Chest expansion	Measure maximal chest expansion at nipple line	Chest expansion of <5 cm is clue to early costovertebral involvement

Table 80.2 • Findings in Ankylosing Spondylitis

Characteristic	Finding
Scoliosis	Absent
Decreased range of movement	Symmetric
Tenderness	Diffuse
Hip flexion with straight-leg raising	Normal
Pain with sciatic nerve stretch	Absent
Hip involvement	Frequently present
Neurodeficit	Absent

Extraspinal Involvement

Enthesopathic involvement is characteristic of ankylosing spondylitis and the other spondyloarthropathies and includes plantar fasciitis, Achilles tendinitis, and trochanteric enthesitis. Hip, shoulder, and chest wall involvement are common, but peripheral joints can also be affected, usually with asymmetric involvement of the lower extremities.

Extraskeletal Involvement

Other findings in active disease include 1) fatigue, 2) weight loss, 3) low-grade fever, and 4) uveitis. Uveitis is an important clue to the diagnosis of spondyloarthritis and is not found in adults with rheumatoid arthritis. Osteoporosis is a common complication of ankylosing spondylitis and can occur in early stages of the disease. Late complications can include traumatic spinal fracture leading to cord compression, cauda equina syndrome (symptoms include neurogenic bladder, fecal incontinence, and radicular leg pain), fibrotic changes in upper lung fields, aortic insufficiency, complete heart block, or secondary amyloidosis.

Differential Diagnosis

The differential diagnosis includes diffuse idiopathic skeletal hyperostosis, osteitis condensans ilii, and degenerative spondylosis. The clinical symptoms of diffuse idiopathic skeletal hyperostosis are "stiffness" of spine and relatively good preservation of spine motion. It generally affects middle-aged and elderly men. Patients with diffuse idiopathic skeletal hyperostosis can have dysphagia related to cervical osteophytes. Criteria for the condition are "flowing" ossification along the anterolateral aspect of at least 4 contiguous vertebral bodies, preservation of disk height, absence of apophyseal joint involvement, absence of sacroiliac joint involvement, and extraspinal ossifications, including ligamentous calcifications.

Osteitis condensans ilii affects young to middle-aged females with normal sacroiliac joints. Radiography shows asymptomatic sclerosis on the iliac side of the sacroiliac joint only. The sacroiliac joint also can be involved with 1) tuberculosis, 2) metastatic disease, 3) Paget disease, or 4) other infections (eg, *Brucella, Serratia, Staphylococcus*).

Treatment

Treatment involves physical therapy (upright posture is very important), exercise (low impact), cessation of smoking, genetic counseling, and drug therapy with nonsteroidal anti-inflammatory drugs. Tumor necrosis factor inhibitors can provide benefit for refractory spinal and peripheral joint symptoms. They are also effective for managing refractory uveitis.

Reactive Arthritis

Reactive arthritis is an aseptic arthritis induced by a host response to an infectious agent rather than direct infection. HLA-B27 is associated in 80% of cases. Reactive arthritis develops after infections with *Salmonella, Shigella flexneri, Yersinia enterocolitica, Campylobacter jejuni, Clostridium difficile,* and *Chlamydia trachomatis.* Chlamydia infections may be asymptomatic. Inflammatory eye disease (conjunctivitis or uveitis) and mucocutaneous disease (balanitis, oral ulcerations, or keratoderma) can occur. Keratoderma blennorrhagicum is a characteristic skin disease on the palms and soles that is indistinguishable histologically from psoriasis. Joint predilection is for the toes and asymmetric large joints in the lower extremities. Presentation may be very acute, requiring consideration of gout and septic arthritis in the differential diagnosis. Dactylitis and enthesitis are found and are similar to what occurs in psoriatic arthritis. Reactive arthritis is frequently self-limited, but there is a risk of chronic arthritis.

Treatment is with nonsteroidal anti-inflammatory drugs. Sulfasalazine, methotrexate, and tumor necrosis factor inhibitors are used in patients with persistent disease. Prolonged antibiotic therapy of *Chlamydia*-triggered reactive arthritis remains controversial.

Arthritis Associated With Inflammatory Bowel Disease

Two distinct types of arthritis are associated with chronic inflammatory bowel disease (Box 80.5).

In patients with arthritis, nonsteroidal anti-inflammatory drugs must be used with caution because they may flare the bowel disease. Infliximab or adalimumab are the drugs of choice to treat both spondylitis and Crohn disease. Etanercept is not beneficial for Crohn disease. The peripheral arthritis often remits as the active bowel inflammation is treated.

Psoriatic Arthritis

Psoriatic arthritis develops in approximately 15% of patients with psoriasis. "Sausage" finger or toe (dactylitis) is characteristic of psoriatic arthritis. A patient presenting with dactylitis should be carefully examined for psoriasis, including in the scalp, gluteal cleft, groin, and umbilicus. Patients with HIV infection may present with severe, refractory psoriasis and psoriatic arthritis.

Box 80.5 • Two Distinct Types of Arthritis Associated With Chronic Inflammatory Bowel Disease

Oligoarthritis of the peripheral joints

Tends to correlate with the activity of the bowel disease

At presentation, the bowel disease, especially Crohn disease, may be asymptomatic

Other clues (eg, recurrent erythema nodosa or iron deficiency) may suggest occult inflammatory bowel disease

Enteropathic spondylitis

Does not reflect activity of the bowel disease, and its subsequent progress bears little relationship to the bowel disease

Approximately 75% of patients with enteropathic spondylitis and inflammatory bowel disease are HLA-B27–positive

---

Most patients present with monoarticular or oligoarticular disease but eventually have polyarticular involvement. Involvement of the distal interphalangeal joint with adjacent nail psoriasis is a classic finding, but it is not always present. The extent of psoriasis and joint involvement frequently do not correspond. Axial spinal involvement may be more limited than in ankylosing spondylitis. Unlike rheumatoid arthritis, radiographs often show both new bone formation (periostitis) and erosions. "Pencil-in-cup" deformity of the distal and proximal interphalangeal joints is found on radiography in advanced disease.

Treatment is with nonsteroidal anti-inflammatory drugs, methotrexate, and tumor necrosis factor inhibitors.

Uveitis and Rheumatologic Diseases

Various rheumatologic diseases are associated with uveitis, particularly the spondyloarthritis disorders. Uveitis is uncommon in rheumatoid arthritis and systemic lupus erythematosus. Nongranulomatous uveitis without any other associated symptoms may be associated with HLA-B27 in almost 50% of patients. Other causes of uveitis include sarcoid, Behçet syndrome, polychondritis, and juvenile idiopathic arthritis, especially in young females who are antinuclear antibody–positive.

Behçet Syndrome

The common manifestations of Behçet syndrome include oral and genital ulcers and uveitis. Behçet syndrome is most common in Middle Eastern countries and Japan. HLA-B51 is associated with the syndrome. Uveitis, synovitis, cutaneous vasculitis, and meningoencephalitis may be present. Treatment is with corticosteroids, although more aggressive immunosuppression often is required. In North American white persons, the primary differential diagnosis is Crohn disease.

KEY FACTS

✓ Characteristics of spondyloarthritis—asymmetric, predominantly lower extremity synovitis, involvement of the sacroiliac joints (uncommon in rheumatoid arthritis), peripheral arthritis that is usually oligoarticular, inflammatory spine pain, absence of rheumatoid factor, acute anterior uveitis, association with HLA-B27, an enthesopathy, and dactylitis

✓ Enthesitis, dactylitis, iritis, psoriasis, and inflammatory bowel disease distinguish spondyloarthritis from rheumatoid arthritis

✓ Characteristics of inflammatory low back pain in ankylosing spondylitis: age at onset usually between 15 and 40 years, insidious onset, duration of >3 months, morning stiffness that improves with exercise but not with rest, and night pain improved by getting out of bed

✓ Reactive arthritis—develops after infection with *Salmonella, Shigella flexneri, Yersinia enterocolitica, Campylobacter jejuni, Clostridium difficile,* and *Chlamydia trachomatis*

✓ Involvement of the distal interphalangeal joint with adjacent nail psoriasis—classic finding of psoriatic arthritis, but it is not always present

81

Vasculitis

MATTHEW J. KOSTER, MD AND KENNETH J. WARRINGTON, MD

Vasculitis

Vasculitis refers to a group of autoimmune disorders characterized by inflammation of blood vessels. The inflammatory process results in vascular damage, with stenosis or occlusion of the vessel lumen and consequent end-organ ischemia. Vasculitis may also weaken the arterial wall, resulting in progressive vascular dilatation and aneurysm formation. The distribution of vascular lesions varies considerably among different vasculitic syndromes. Vasculitis can be classified according to the predominant type of vessel involved (referred to as large vessel, medium vessel, or small vessel vasculitis) (Box 81.1). Most forms of vasculitis are chronic systemic disorders that cause multiorgan damage, although vasculitis may be localized to a single organ. The cause of vasculitis is generally unknown, but viral infections, certain medications, and malignancies trigger some forms of vasculitis.

Key Definition

Vasculitis: *autoimmune disorder characterized by inflammation of blood vessels.*

Vasculitis may also occur as a complication of an underlying rheumatologic disorder, such as rheumatoid arthritis or systemic lupus erythematosus. The clinical manifestations of vasculitis are quite variable and depend on the pattern of vascular involvement. Indeed, vasculitis should be considered in the differential diagnosis of any multisystem

Box 81.1 • Names for Vasculitides[a]

Large vessel vasculitis (LVV)
Takayasu arteritis (TAK)
Giant cell arteritis (GCA)

Medium vessel vasculitis (MVV)
Polyarteritis nodosa (PAN)
Kawasaki disease (KD)

Small vessel vasculitis (SVV)
Antineutrophil cytoplasmic antibody (ANCA)-associated vasculitis (AAV)
  Microscopic polyangiitis (MPA)
  Granulomatosis with polyangiitis (GPA) (formerly Wegener granulomatosis)
  Eosinophilic granulomatosis with polyangiitis (EGPA) (Churg-Strauss syndrome)
Immune complex SVV
  Anti–glomerular basement membrane (anti-GBM) disease
  Cryoglobulinemic vasculitis (CV)
  IgA vasculitis (IgAV) (Henoch-Schönlein vasculitis)
  Hypocomplementemic urticarial vasculitis (HUV) (anti-C1q vasculitis)

Variable vessel vasculitis (VVV)
Behçet disease (BD)
Cogan syndrome (CS)

Single-organ vasculitis (SOV)
Cutaneous leukocytoclastic angiitis
Cutaneous arteritis
Primary central nervous system vasculitis
Isolated aortitis
Others

Vasculitis associated with systemic disease
Lupus vasculitis
Rheumatoid vasculitis

(continued on next page)

Portions of "Clinical Features" section for polyarteritis nodosa (PAN) previously published in Friese JL, Warrington KJ, Miller DV, Ytterberg SR, Fleming CJ, Stanson AW. Polyarteritis nodosa (PAN). In: Hendaoui L, Stanson AW, Bouhaouala MH, Joffre F, editors. Systemic vasculitis: imaging features. Berlin (Germany): Springer-Verlag; c2012. p. 189–207. (Medical radiology: diagnostic imaging series). Used with permission.

Sarcoid vasculitis
Others
Vasculitis associated with probable etiology
Hepatitis C virus–associated cryoglobulinemic
vasculitis
Hepatitis B virus–associated vasculitis
Syphilis-associated aortitis
Drug-associated vasculitis
Cancer-associated vasculitis

Abbreviation: Ig, immunoglobulin.

a Adopted by the 2012 International Chapel Hill Consensus
Conference on the Nomenclature of Vasculitides.

Adapted from Jennette JC, Falk RJ, Bacon PA, Basu N, Cid
MC, Ferrario F, et al. 2012 revised International Chapel
Hill Consensus Conference Nomenclature of Vasculitides.
Arthritis Rheum. 2013 Jan;65(1):1–11. Used with permission.

---

illness. Vasculitis mimics are listed in Box 81.2; these conditions should also be considered whenever vasculitis is suspected. The initial evaluation and common test abnormalities for patients with vasculitis are listed in Box 81.3. The ability to recognize characteristic clinical patterns of disease is helpful for making the diagnosis of systemic vasculitis.

Large Vessel Vasculitis

Giant Cell Arteritis

Giant cell arteritis (GCA), previously known as temporal arteritis, predominantly affects persons of northern European ancestry who are older than 50 years. Women

---

Box 81.2 • Conditions That Mimic Vasculitis

Cardiac myxoma with embolization

Fibromuscular dysplasia

Infective endocarditis

Thrombotic thrombocytopenic purpura

Atheroembolism: cholesterol emboli

Ergotism

Hereditary disorders of the connective tissues
(eg, pseudoxanthoma elasticum, vascular type
of Ehlers-Danlos, and Marfan syndrome)

Antiphospholipid syndrome

Livedoid vasculopathy

Arterial coarctation

Bacteremia

Malignancy (eg, intravascular lymphoma)

Rickettsial infection

Chronic infections (eg, hepatitis, HIV, and tuberculosis)

Abbreviation: HIV, human immunodeficiency virus.

Box 81.3 • Initial Evaluation of Patients With Suspected Vasculitis

Complete blood cell count (anemia is common)

ESR (frequently elevated)

CRP (frequently elevated)

Creatinine (elevated with renal involvement)

Urinalysis with microscopic examination (hematuria,
RBC casts, dysmorphic RBCs with renal
involvement)

Liver enzymes (may be elevated)

ANCA screen (positive in some forms of small vessel
vasculitis)

RF, CCP antibody, ANA (may be positive if underlying
rheumatic disease)

Complement (total complement, C3, and C4 may be
low in some forms of vasculitis)

Cryoglobulins (positive in cryoglobulinemic vasculitis)

Hepatitis B and C serologies (if positive, consider
hepatitis-associated vasculitis)

Chest radiograph (evaluate for infiltrates, nodules,
effusion)

Vascular imaging (CTA or MRA) if medium vessel or
large vessel vasculitis is suspected

Nerve conduction studies (if neuropathy is suspected)

Additional imaging or organ-specific evaluation
depending on clinical presentation

Abbreviations: ANA, antinuclear antibody; ANCA,
antineutrophil cytoplasmic antibody; CCP, cyclic
citrullinated peptide; CRP, C-reactive protein; CTA,
computed tomographic angiography; ESR, erythrocyte
sedimentation rate; MRA, magnetic resonance angiography;
RBC, red blood cell; RF, rheumatoid factor.

---

are affected by GCA 2 to 3 times as often as men. GCA is one of the most common forms of vasculitis in adults, with an annual incidence of about 19 cases per 100,000 people who are 50 years or older. The lifetime risk of GCA has been estimated to be around 1% for women and 0.5% for men.

Pathology

The vasculitic process typically involves the extracranial branches of the carotid artery and frequently also affects the aorta and the aortic arch branches. The exact cause of GCA is unknown; however, genetic and environmental factors are likely involved in disease pathogenesis. The histologic findings in GCA consist of mononuclear cell infiltrates that involve all 3 layers of the arterial wall (intima, media, and adventitia). Multinucleated giant cells are seen in 50% of cases, generally in association with a fragmented internal elastic lamina. The inner layer of the artery undergoes concentric fibrointimal proliferation, which results in luminal stenosis.

Clinical Features

Although the clinical features of GCA (Box 81.4) can be variable, patients typically present with new-onset headache and scalp tenderness in the context of a systemic inflammatory syndrome. Polymyalgia rheumatica (PMR) symptoms (aching and stiffness of the neck, shoulders, hips, and proximal extremities) occur in about 40% of patients with GCA. Although present in only about one-third of patients, jaw claudication is highly specific for GCA. Ocular symptoms may occur (eg, decreased vision, diplopia, and amaurosis fugax), and in up to 15% of patients, permanent vision loss results from ischemic optic neuropathy. Neurologic manifestations are uncommon and may include stroke, transient ischemic attack, or neuropathy. Patients with large vessel GCA (involving the aorta and arch branches) often present with constitutional symptoms, claudication of the upper extremities, or asymmetrical blood pressures. Physical examination should include a careful assessment of the temporal arteries and peripheral vessels (for pulses and bruits).

Diagnosis

Markers of inflammation, including the erythrocyte sedimentation rate (ESR) and C-reactive protein (CRP), are often considerably elevated in GCA. Although some patients may have a normal ESR, the CRP level is almost always elevated. Patients may have other nonspecific laboratory abnormalities, such as normocytic anemia, an elevated platelet count, and abnormal liver function test results. The gold standard diagnostic test for GCA is histopathologic examination of a temporal artery biopsy specimen. In a subset of patients with GCA (particularly those with large vessel disease), temporal artery biopsy findings may be negative. In those patients, GCA affecting the aorta and its branches may be diagnosed with magnetic resonance angiography (MRA) or computed tomographic angiography (CTA). In select cases, positron emission tomography (PET) can be used to detect vascular inflammation in large arteries (Figure 81.1). The American College of Rheumatology classification criteria for GCA are listed in Box 81.5.

Treatment

Treatment with corticosteroids should be initiated promptly when the diagnosis of GCA is suspected. Temporal artery biopsy should not delay treatment because histopathologic evidence of arteritis persists for several weeks after corticosteroid therapy has been started. The initial treatment dose of oral prednisone is typically 40 to 60 mg daily. A higher dose of intravenous corticosteroids can be given to patients with impending loss of vision. If patients do not have any contraindications to antiplatelet therapy, low-dose aspirin therapy should be started because it may reduce the risk of vision loss and cerebrovascular events. Measures to prevent or treat steroid-related side effects are also an essential aspect of managing GCA.

Box 81.4 • Clinical Features of Giant Cell Arteritis

Symptoms
  Constitutional
    Fever, fatigue, weight loss, anorexia
  Polymyalgia rheumatica
    Aching and stiffness of the neck, shoulders, hips, and proximal extremities
  Cranial
    Temporal headache
    Scalp tenderness
    Jaw or tongue claudication
    Impaired vision, diplopia, amaurosis fugax, vision loss
  Large vessel disease
    Arm claudication
Signs
  Musculoskeletal
    Pain with range of motion of neck, shoulders, and hips
  Cranial
    Temporal artery tenderness
    Absent temporal artery pulse
  Large vessel disease
    Absent radial artery pulse
    Asymmetrical arm blood pressures
    Bruits (carotid and subclavian arteries)
    Aortic regurgitation murmur (may indicate dilated ascending aorta)

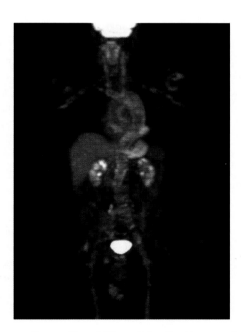

Figure 81.1 *Large Vessel Vasculitis. Positron emission tomographic scan shows fludeoxyglucose F 18 uptake in the aorta and major branches, consistent with large vessel vasculitis.*

Box 81.5 • American College of Rheumatology 1990 Criteria for the Classification of GCA

For the diagnosis of GCA, ≥3 of the following 5 criteria must be present (the presence of ≥3 criteria yields a sensitivity of 93.5% and a specificity of 91.2% for distinguishing GCA from other forms of vasculitis):

1. Age at disease onset ≥50 y—development of symptoms or findings beginning at age 50 y or older

2. New headache—new-onset of or new type of localized pain in the head

3. Temporal artery abnormality—temporal artery tenderness to palpation or decreased pulsation, unrelated to arteriosclerosis of cervical arteries

4. Elevated ESR—ESR ≥50 mm/h by the Westergren method

5. Abnormal artery biopsy findings—biopsy specimen with artery showing vasculitis characterized by a predominance of mononuclear cell infiltration or granulomatous inflammation, usually with multinucleated giant cells

Abbreviations: ESR, erythrocyte sedimentation rate; GCA, giant cell arteritis.

Adapted from Hunder GG, Bloch DA, Michel BA, Stevens MB, Arend WP, Calabrese LH, et al. The American College of Rheumatology 1990 criteria for the classification of giant cell arteritis. Arthritis Rheum. 1990 Aug;33(8):1122–8. Used with permission.

Outcome

GCA is a chronic condition requiring treatment with corticosteroids, often for 1 to 2 years or longer. Disease relapses during corticosteroid tapering are common. An effective steroid-sparing agent has not yet been identified, but methotrexate may decrease the risk of relapse in some patients. Overall, the life expectancy of patients with GCA is similar to that of the general population. However, patients with GCA have an increased risk of aortic aneurysms, particularly of the thoracic aorta. Aneurysms generally develop 3 to 5 years after diagnosis and may lead to aortic dissection, with a high risk of death. Long-term monitoring for aortic aneurysms is therefore recommended.

Takayasu Arteritis

Takayasu arteritis (TAK) is a rare form of large vessel vasculitis that primarily affects the aorta and its major branches. TAK typically occurs in women younger than 40 years. The cause is unknown, but each year, 2 to 3 new cases per million population occur. TAK has a worldwide distribution but is more common in Asians. The histopathologic features are similar to those of GCA. The upper extremity and neck arteries (carotid and vertebral) are most frequently affected. Renal, mesenteric, coronary, pulmonary, and lower extremity arterial involvement may also occur. Vascular inflammation results in arterial thickening

with subsequent narrowing or occlusion of the lumen. Damage to the aorta may lead to dilatation and aneurysm formation.

Key Definition

Takayasu arteritis: *a rare form of large vessel vasculitis that primarily affects the aorta and its major branches.*

Clinical and Laboratory Features

Patients who have TAK often present with nonspecific constitutional symptoms, such as fatigue, malaise, arthralgia, and myalgias. Extremity claudication is a common complaint. Compromise of the cerebral circulation can lead to amaurosis fugax, syncope, transient ischemic attack, or stroke. Patients with coronary artery involvement may present with anginal symptoms. Refractory hypertension may result from renal artery stenosis. Abdominal angina may indicate mesenteric ischemia due to visceral arterial involvement. Other manifestations may include erythema nodosum and inflammatory arthritis. Absence or asymmetry of upper extremity pulses or lower extremity pulses (or both) is often a feature of patients with TAK. Vascular bruits are common, and aortic valvular regurgitation may be present because of dilatation of the ascending aorta.

TAK has no specific biomarker; however, laboratory features of inflammation (eg, elevated ESR and CRP, anemia, and thrombocytosis) are generally detected. About one-third of patients may have normal inflammatory markers. The diagnosis is generally made by MRA or CTA. PET can also be useful to assess for vascular inflammation in the aorta and its main branches. Classification criteria for TAK are listed in Box 81.6.

Treatment and Outcome

Corticosteroids are the initial treatment of choice for TAK. Most patients require the addition of an

Box 81.6 • Classification Criteria for Takayasu Arteritis[a]

Age at disease onset ≤40 y

Claudication of upper extremities

Decreased brachial artery pulse

Blood pressure difference between arms ≥10 mm Hg

Aortic or subclavian bruit

Arteriographic abnormality of aorta, primary branches, or large arteries in the upper or lower extremities

[a] If at least 3 of the 6 criteria are present, the sensitivity for diagnosis is 90% and the specificity is 98%.

immunosuppressive agent (eg, methotrexate, azathio-prine, or mycophenolate mofetil) as the dose of cortico-steroids is tapered. Refractory disease is generally treated with tumor necrosis factor inhibitors, and cyclophospha-mide is used only in life-threatening disease. TAK is gen-erally a chronic disease that requires ongoing treatment and close follow-up. Vascular damage such as arterial stenosis, occlusion, or aneurysm may require open surgi-cal or endovascular repair. Mortality among patients with TAK is increased compared to mortality for the general population. Death is often due to aortic aneurysm or rup-ture or cardiac ischemia.

KEY FACTS

✓ Clinical features of GCA—

- new-onset headache and scalp tenderness in the context of a systemic inflammatory syndrome
- jaw claudication, present in about one-third of patients, is highly specific for GCA
- ocular symptoms may occur (eg, decreased vision, diplopia, and amaurosis fugax)

✓ Treatment of GCA—

- corticosteroids
- begin promptly (do not wait for temporal artery biopsy)
- histopathologic evidence of arteritis persists for weeks after starting therapy

✓ TAK—

- typically in women younger than 40 years
- nonspecific constitutional symptoms (eg, fatigue, malaise, arthralgia, and myalgias)
- extremity claudication is common

Medium Vessel Vasculitis

Polyarteritis Nodosa

Polyarteritis nodosa (PAN) is a systemic necrotizing vascu-litis that predominantly involves medium-sized and small arteries. For most patients, the cause of PAN is unknown, but one-third of cases are related to hepatitis B virus (HBV) infection. Less commonly, PAN may occur as a paraneo-plastic process, or it may be related to drugs (particularly minocycline).

Key Definition

Polyarteritis nodosa: *a systemic necrotizing vasculitis that predominantly involves medium-sized and small arteries.*

Clinical Features

In patients with PAN, the most commonly affected organs are the kidneys, skin, nerves, stomach, and intestines. Patients with PAN generally present with prominent constitutional features, such as fever, fatigue, weight loss, myalgias, and arthralgias. Peripheral neurologic symptoms are frequently present (eg, numbness, paresthesia, and asymmetrical motor deficits). Skin manifestations may include livedo reticu-laris, tender subcutaneous nodules, palpable purpura, digi-tal gangrene, and skin ulcerations. Abdominal pain suggests gastrointestinal tract involvement, such as mesenteric isch-emia, hemorrhage, or bowel perforation. Testicular pain due to ischemia is a characteristic disease manifestation. Renal involvement often leads to arterial hypertension and isch-emic nephropathy with renal insufficiency. Lung involve-ment is typically absent. Some patients have localized PAN involving a single organ such as the skin (cutaneous PAN).

Diagnosis

Abnormal laboratory findings that support a diagnosis of PAN include normocytic anemia, increased ESR and CRP, and thrombocytosis. Testing for antineutrophil cytoplasmic antibodies (ANCAs) is typically negative. Serologic stud-ies for chronic hepatitis should be performed because HBV infection influences treatment. The confirmatory test for PAN is angiography or a biopsy of involved tissue (muscle, nerve, or deep skin) showing vasculitis. Conventional arte-riography is more sensitive than CTA and should include views of the renal and mesenteric arteries. Microaneurysms and stenoses of intraparenchymal arteries are characteristic angiographic findings in patients with PAN (Figure 81.2). The classification criteria for PAN are listed in Table 81.1.

Treatment and Outcome

Prompt initiation of treatment with corticosteroids is es-sential to limit organ damage from vasculitis. Some pa-tients can be treated with prednisone alone. However, in the presence of poor prognostic indicators (eg, renal insuf-ficiency or gastrointestinal tract, cardiac, or neurologic in-volvement), corticosteroids are generally combined with cyclophosphamide. Methotrexate or azathioprine may be used for remission induction in less severe disease or as remission maintenance agents after a course of cyclophos-phamide. For patients with HBV-related PAN, treatment consists of a short course of corticosteroids together with antiviral agents. Although untreated PAN is associated with a poor prognosis, excellent 5-year survival rates (>80%) can be achieved with appropriate immunosuppressive therapy.

Small Vessel Vasculitis

Granulomatosis With Polyangiitis, Microscopic Polyangiitis, and Eosinophilic Granulomatosis With Polyangiitis

Granulomatosis with polyangiitis (GPA) (formerly called Wegener granulomatosis), microscopic polyangiitis (MPA),

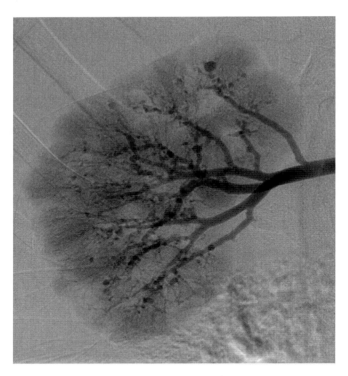

Figure 81.2 Polyarteritis Nodosa. *Renal arteriogram shows characteristic microaneurysms due to polyarteritis nodosa.*

and eosinophilic granulomatosis with polyangiitis (EGPA) (also called Churg-Strauss syndrome) are primary systemic vasculitides that involve mainly small vessels. Patients with these 3 conditions often have circulating ANCAs. ANCAs are specific for antigens in neutrophil granules and monocyte lysosomes. These antibodies can be detected by immunofluorescent techniques, which produce 2 major staining patterns: cytoplasmic ANCA (c-ANCA) and perinuclear ANCA (p-ANCA). About 90% of patients with GPA are c-ANCA positive, and the target antigen is typically proteinase 3 (PR-3). Most patients with MPA and EGPA are p-ANCA positive, owing to reactivity with myeloperoxidase (MPO). Therefore GPA, MPA, and EGPA are also collectively known as the ANCA-associated vasculitides (AAVs).

The incidence of AAV is approximately 10 to 20 per million population per year. GPA is the most common form of AAV (incidence, 8–10 per million population). These conditions occur more frequently in older adults, with a peak onset at age 65 to 70 years, and they affect men and women equally. AAV is more prevalent in whites compared with other populations.

The etiology of AAV is unknown. Genetic and environmental factors, including infections, are thought to be important in disease pathogenesis. Histologically, GPA is characterized by necrotizing granulomatous vasculitis. Necrotizing granulomatous inflammation also occurs in EGPA. However, asthma and eosinophilia are prominent features in EGPA that do not occur in GPA. MPA is characterized by necrotizing small vessel vasculitis without pathologic evidence of granulomatous inflammation, which helps to distinguish this condition from GPA.

Clinical Features

Most patients with AAV present with constitutional symptoms, such as fever and weight loss, in addition to symptoms related to internal organ involvement. The main clinical features of GPA can be summarized by the

Table 81.1 • The American College of Rheumatology 1990 Criteria for the Classification of Polyarteritis Nodosa[a]

Criterion	Definition
1. Weight loss ≥4 kg	Loss of ≥4 kg of body weight since illness began (not from dieting or other factors)
2. Livedo reticularis	Mottled reticular pattern over the skin of portions of the extremities or torso
3. Testicular pain or tenderness	Pain or tenderness of the testicles (not from infection, trauma, or other causes)
4. Myalgias, weakness, or leg tenderness	Diffuse myalgias (excluding shoulder and hip girdle), weakness of muscles, or tenderness of leg muscles
5. Mononeuropathy or polyneuropathy	Development of mononeuropathy, multiple mononeuropathies, or polyneuropathy
6. Diastolic BP >90 mm Hg	Development of hypertension with the diastolic BP >90 mm Hg
7. Elevated SUN or creatinine	Elevation of SUN >40 mg/dL or creatinine >1.5 mg/dL (not from dehydration or obstruction)
8. Hepatitis B virus	Presence of hepatitis B surface antigen or antibody in serum
9. Arteriographic abnormality	Arteriogram showing aneurysms or occlusions of the visceral arteries (not from arteriosclerosis, fibromuscular dysplasia, or other noninflammatory causes)
10. Biopsy of small or medium-sized artery containing PMNs	Histologic changes showing the presence of granulocytes or granulocytes and mononuclear leukocytes in the artery wall

Abbreviations: BP, blood pressure; PMN, polymorphonuclear neutrophil; SUN, serum urea nitrogen.

[a] At least 3 of these 10 criteria are required.

Adapted from Lightfoot RW Jr, Michel BA, Bloch DA, Hunder GG, Zvaifler NJ, McShane DJ, et al. The American College of Rheumatology 1990 criteria for the classification of polyarteritis nodosa. Arthritis Rheum. 1990 Aug;33(8):1088–93. Used with permission.

mnemonic *ELKS*: involvement of the ear, nose, and throat; lung; kidney; and skin. Clinical manifestations may include symptoms of sinusitis or otitis, oral ulcers, and nasal ulcers. The nasal septum may develop necrosis with perforation. Patients with tracheal inflammation can present with stridor and respiratory distress. Pulmonary involvement may include pulmonary nodules or masses, whereas alveolar capillaritis causes pulmonary hemorrhage and lung infiltrates. Massive pulmonary hemorrhage can be a life-threatening manifestation of AAV. In approximately 80% of patients with GPA, glomerulonephritis develops and leads to rapidly progressive renal failure. Other manifestations of the disease may include ocular inflammation, skin vasculitis, peripheral neuropathy, inflammatory arthritis, and gastrointestinal tract vasculitis.

Almost all patients with MPA have renal involvement due to rapidly progressive glomerulonephritis. Alveolar hemorrhage is also a common pulmonary manifestation. Other clinical features of MPA include cutaneous vasculitis, peripheral neuropathy, and vasculitis of the gastrointestinal tract. About 75% of patients with MPA are positive for p-ANCA (MPO).

EGPA typically has 3 main features: allergic rhinitis and asthma; eosinophilic infiltrative disease, such as eosinophilic pneumonia; and systemic small vessel vasculitis. EGPA involves the lungs, peripheral nerves, skin, and, less frequently, the heart and gastrointestinal tract. Compared with GPA and MPA, EGPA typically causes less renal disease, but cardiac involvement is a frequent cause of morbidity and death. All patients with EGPA have eosinophilia (>10% eosinophils in the blood) and about 40% are p-ANCA (MPO) positive.

Diagnosis

The diagnosis of AAV requires an integration of clinical, laboratory, and histopathologic findings. Laboratory assessment should include inflammatory markers (ESR and CRP), liver and renal function, ANCA, and urinalysis. ANCA testing is helpful in reaching a diagnosis of AAV, but some patients with small vessel vasculitis are ANCA negative. In addition, p-ANCA that is negative for MPO antibodies is not specific for vasculitis; it can be present in patients with inflammatory bowel disease, autoimmune liver disease, connective tissue diseases, malignancies, and even drug-induced syndromes. In patients with AAV, serial measurements of ANCA over time do not correlate well with disease activity or risk of relapse.

Patients with suspected AAV should undergo chest imaging for assessment of pulmonary involvement. In patients with neurologic symptoms, nerve conduction studies should be considered to evaluate for peripheral neuropathy. Pathologic examination of involved tissue (eg, skin, muscle, nerve, lung, or kidney) is often necessary to document small vessel vasculitis. A prompt diagnosis of AAV is essential, because damage to internal organs progresses rapidly and can be attenuated with appropriate therapy.

Medical Treatment

Treatment of AAV can be divided into 3 phases: induction of remission, maintenance of remission, and treatment of relapses. Although most therapeutic data come from studies of GPA, the general principles of management also apply to MPA and EGPA.

Remission induction therapy for life-threatening forms of AAV has traditionally consisted of cyclophosphamide and corticosteroids. A typical initial treatment regimen includes oral cyclophosphamide (2 mg/kg daily) in combination with prednisone (1 mg/kg daily). This regimen leads to improvement in more than 90% of patients with GPA and to complete remission in 75%. Rituximab, an anti-CD20 antibody, has now mostly replaced cyclophosphamide as the remission induction agent of choice for AAV. Two randomized clinical trials have shown that rituximab is as effective as cyclophosphamide for the initial treatment of AAV.

Repeated courses of rituximab may also be given for remission maintenance, but the optimal dosing and frequency of administration has not yet been determined. Methotrexate and azathioprine are effective medications for remission maintenance; however, methotrexate is contraindicated in patients with chronic kidney disease. An alternative agent for remission maintenance is mycophenolate mofetil, although it appears to be less effective than azathioprine. Plasma exchange can increase the rate of renal recovery in patients who have acute renal failure secondary to AAV, and ongoing studies are assessing the long-term efficacy of this form of treatment. As with other types of vasculitis, the morbidity associated with therapy is significant, and preventive measures to minimize risk of fractures and infections are essential. In particular, patients should receive prophylaxis against *Pneumocystis jiroveci* pneumonia.

For patients with nonsevere forms of AAV, methotrexate (20–25 mg weekly) in combination with prednisone is effective for inducing disease remission. The treatment of MPA and GPA is essentially the same when major organs are involved. High-dose corticosteroid treatment alone may be adequate for EGPA, although patients with refractory disease often require additional immunosuppressive agents.

Immunoglobulin A Vasculitis

Immunoglobulin (Ig)A vasculitis (Henoch-Schönlein purpura) is characterized by IgA deposition in vessel walls. The clinical features of IgA vasculitis typically include palpable purpura, arthralgia or arthritis, abdominal pain, and hematuria due to renal disease. The vasculitic rash typically involves the lower extremities and buttocks (Figure 81.3). Gastrointestinal tract bleeding occurs in some patients. IgA vasculitis predominantly affects the pediatric population but also occurs in adults. Adult patients with IgA vasculitis have a higher risk of renal disease and should be monitored closely for this complication.

No specific biomarker for IgA vasculitis has been identified, although serum IgA levels may be elevated. The diagnosis is often clinical, and tissue biopsy (usually skin

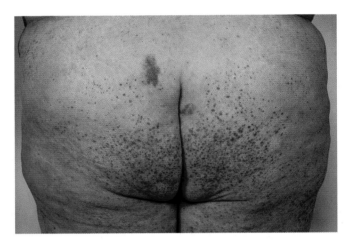

Figure 81.3 *Immunoglobulin (Ig)A Vasculitis. Cutaneous vasculitis (palpable purpura) involving the buttocks in a patient with IgA vasculitis.*

KEY FACTS

✓ PAN—
  • HBV infection is involved in one-third of cases
  • most commonly affected organs: kidneys, skin, nerves, stomach, and intestines
  • characteristic angiographic findings: microaneurysms and stenoses of intraparenchymal arteries

✓ GPA, MPA, and EGPA—
  • primary systemic vasculitides that involve mainly small vessels
  • circulating ANCAs are often present

✓ GPA—90% of patients are c-ANCA positive; target antigen is usually PR-3

✓ MPA and EGPA—most patients are p-ANCA positive, with reactivity to MPO

✓ Mnemonic for GPA clinical features— *ELKS*: involvement of the ear, nose, and throat; lung; kidney; and skin

✓ Clinical features of EGPA—
  • allergic rhinitis and asthma
  • eosinophilic infiltrative disease (eg, eosinophilic pneumonia)
  • systemic small vessel vasculitis

✓ Agent of choice for induction of remission for AAV— rituximab has mostly replaced cyclophosphamide

✓ Clinical features of IgA vasculitis—
  • palpable purpura
  • arthralgia or arthritis
  • abdominal pain
  • hematuria due to renal disease

---

but occasionally kidney) may be required to assess for IgA deposits. In most patients, IgA vasculitis is a self-limiting condition and treatment is mainly supportive. The use of corticosteroids is controversial, but they should be considered for patients with abdominal pain.

Cryoglobulinemia

Cryoglobulins (CGs) are immunoglobulins that precipitate at temperatures less than 37°C. A useful classification scheme for cryoglobulinemia is based on the type of CG present in the patient's serum. Type I CGs are aggregates of a single monoclonal immunoglobulin and generally are associated with hematologic malignancies such as multiple myeloma, Waldenström macroglobulinemia, and lymphomas. Patients with type I CGs are often asymptomatic. However, type I cryoglobulinemia may cause symptoms related to hyperviscosity or thrombosis (or both). Clinical features may include headache, visual disturbances and other neurologic manifestations, Raynaud phenomenon, livedo reticularis, digital ischemia, and skin ulcerations.

Type II and type III CGs consist of more than 1 type of immunoglobulin (associated with mixed cryoglobulinemia). Type II CGs are a mixture of polyclonal immunoglobulin and a monoclonal immunoglobulin. Affected patients often have a positive rheumatoid factor. Type II CGs are mainly due to chronic viral infections (particularly hepatitis C and human immunodeficiency virus) but can also be present with autoimmune disorders and, occasionally, lymphoma. Type III CGs are polyclonal immunoglobulins and are often secondary to connective tissue diseases, such as systemic lupus erythematosus and Sjögren syndrome.

CG-containing immune complexes precipitate on endothelial cells in peripheral blood vessels and fix complement, promoting vasculitic inflammation. The typical clinical presentation includes constitutional symptoms, palpable purpura (due to leukocytoclastic vasculitis), peripheral neuropathy, and arthralgias. Less commonly, mixed cryoglobulinemia is complicated by hepatomegaly, pneumonitis or pulmonary hemorrhage, and glomerulonephritis.

Laboratory Studies

Patients with mixed CGs and small vessel vasculitis usually have an increased ESR, elevated immunoglobulin levels, a positive test for rheumatoid factor, and low levels of complement. Serum protein electrophoresis and immunoelectrophoresis are helpful in determing the type and clonality of the immunoglobulins present. Evidence of chronic hepatitis infection (particularly hepatitis C) is often identified. For cryoglobulin testing, blood must be drawn into a prewarmed syringe or collection tube; failure to prewarm the syringe or collection tube may lead to false-negative results. If cryoglobulins are detected, the laboratory will also report the cryocrit, which is a measure of the volume of the cryoprecipitate as a percentage of the original serum volume. The cryocrit does not correlate well with clinical features.

Treatment

The treatment of cryoglobulinemia depends on the disease severity and the underlying disorder. For example, patients with type I CGs require treatment of the associated hematologic malignancy. Mixed cryoglobulinemia related to chronic hepatitis C is generally treated with antiviral therapy. Patients with mixed cryoglobulinemia related to autoimmune connective tissue diseases are often treated with corticosteroids and rituximab (or cyclophosphamide), particularly if they have severe disease manifestations.

Other Forms of Vasculitis

Vasculitis may occur in association with systemic rheumatologic conditions, such as rheumatoid arthritis, systemic lupus erythematosus, Sjögren syndrome, Behçet disease, and sarcoidosis. The clinical manifestations of these forms of vasculitis are highly variable. Rarely, paraneoplastic vasculitis may accompany solid organ tumors or hematologic malignancies, such as lymphoma, leukemia, and myelodysplastic syndrome. In patients with hematologic malignancies, the most common presentation is a small vessel cutaneous vasculitis. Medications such as antibiotics, allopurinol, propylthiouracil, minocycline, tumor necrosis factor inhibitors, and others have been implicated in triggering vasculitis. Drug-induced vasculitis most often involves the skin, and internal organ manifestations are rare. Patients generally present with petechiae or palpable purpura, and skin biopsy findings include leukocytoclastic vasculitis (small vessel vasculitis with polymorphonuclear fragmentation and necrotic debris). Discontinuation of the inciting medication is often all that is necessary for management, although more severe cases may require immunosuppressive therapy. The differential diagnosis for a patient presenting with palpable purpura is listed in Box 81.7.

Box 81.7 • Differential Diagnosis of Palpable Purpura

Microscopic polyangiitis

Eosinophilic granulomatosis with polyangiitis (Churg-Strauss syndrome)

Granulomatosis with polyangiitis (formerly Wegener granulomatosis)

IgA Vasculitis (Henoch-Schönlein purpura)

Cryoglobulinemic vasculitis

Vasculitis associated with rheumatic diseases (rheumatoid arthritis, Sjögren syndrome, systemic lupus erythematosus)

Drug-associated vasculitis

Cancer-associated vasculitis

Abbreviation: Ig, immunoglobulin.

Polymyalgia Rheumatica

PMR is an inflammatory condition that affects older persons; the mean age at diagnosis is about 73 years. The cause of PMR is unknown, although genetic and environmental factors are likely involved in disease pathogenesis. Patients with PMR typically complain of stiffness and pain that are most prominent in the morning and after inactivity. Symptoms generally localize to the neck, shoulders, hips, and proximal portion of the extremities. Patients often have difficulty finding a comfortable position in bed and have difficulty getting out of bed. Constitutional symptoms, such as low-grade fever, anorexia, and weight loss, are common. On musculoskeletal examination, the patients generally have painful and limited range of motion of the shoulders and hips. Extremity edema or oligoarticular synovitis can occur, particularly at the knees and wrists. Polyarticular small joint arthritis may suggest a diagnosis of elderly-onset rheumatoid arthritis rather than PMR.

No specific biomarker has been identified for the diagnosis of PMR, but classification criteria may be useful to distinguish PMR from other inflammatory disorders (Box 81.8). Patients typically have an increased ESR or CRP (or

---

Box 81.8 • Proposed Provisional Classification Criteria for Polymyalgia Rheumatica (PMR)[a]

Required criteria

Age ≥50 y
Bilateral shoulder pain
Abnormal erythrocyte sedimentation rate or C-reactive protein (or both)

Scoring

Morning stiffness lasting >45 min—2 points
Hip pain or limited range of motion—1 point
Absence of rheumatoid factor or anti-cyclic citrullinated peptide—2 points
Absence of other joint involvement—1 point

Ultrasonography shows subdeltoid bursitis and/or biceps tenosynovitis and/or glenohumeral synovitis in at least 1 shoulder, *and* synovitis and/or trochanteric bursitis in at least 1 hip—1 point

Ultrasonography shows subdeltoid bursitis, biceps tenosynovitis, or glenohumeral synovitis in both shoulders—1 point

[a] With these clinical criteria, a score of ≥4 had a 68% sensitivity and a 78% specificity for discriminating PMR patients from comparison patients. When ultrasonographic criteria were included, a score of ≥5 had a sensitivity of 66% and a specificity of 81% for discriminating PMR patients from comparison patients.

Adapted from Dasgupta B, Cimmino MA, Maradit-Kremers H, Schmidt WA, Schirmer M, Salvarani C, et al. 2012 provisional classification criteria for polymyalgia rheumatica: a European League Against Rheumatism/American College of Rheumatology collaborative initiative. Ann Rheum Dis. 2012 Apr;71(4):484–92. Used with permission.

both), but autoantibodies are usually absent (eg, rheumatoid factor, cyclic citrullinated peptide antibody, and antinuclear antibody). Many patients have a mild normocytic anemia, and some have a normal ESR; the CRP is typically increased in these patients. Imaging is not routinely performed for the diagnosis of PMR. However, in select cases, ultrasononography or magnetic resonance imaging may be helpful for showing articular and periarticular inflammation of the shoulders and hips.

Several conditions should be considered in the differential diagnosis of a patient presenting with polymyalgia symptoms (Box 81.9). Additional laboratory tests and imaging studies may be necessary to distinguish PMR from other conditions. A variant of PMR known as the **RS3PE syndrome** (remitting seronegative symmetrical synovitis with pitting edema) occurs primarily in older men. Patients with this syndrome present with symptoms of PMR but also synovitis and marked edema of the hands or feet.

Key Definition

RS3PE syndrome: *remitting seronegative symmetrical synovitis with pitting edema; a variant of PMR that occurs primarily in older men.*

A well-recognized association exists between PMR and GCA, and it has been suggested that in some patients, PMR is an incomplete form of GCA. PMR may occur before, concurrently with, or after the onset of GCA. Clinically, 40% to 60% of patients with GCA have PMR symptoms, and GCA develops in 15% to 20% of patients who have PMR.

Treatment

Patients with PMR generally have a considerable clinical response within a few days after they begin treatment with prednisone (15–20 mg daily). In some patients, split-dose prednisone (5 mg 3 times daily) is more effective than the comparable single daily dose (15 mg once daily). The initial dose is usually maintained for 2 to 4 weeks, after which the prednisone dose may be decreased by 2.5 mg every 2 to 4 weeks until a dose of 10 mg daily is reached. Subsequently, the prednisone dose is generally tapered by 1 mg each month, although some patients may require an even slower tapering schedule. Patients should be followed clinically, and usually the ESR and CRP are measured monthly to monitor for disease activity. Disease relapses in PMR are common, and most patients require prolonged corticosteroid therapy. The typical duration of treatment is 1 to 2 years (sometimes longer). If polymyalgia symptoms do not improve with corticosteroids or

---

Box 81.9 • Differential Diagnosis of Patients Presenting With Polymyalgia Symptoms

Rheumatologic conditions
  Rheumatoid arthritis
  Spondyloarthropathy
  Vasculitis
  Autoimmune connective tissue diseases
  Inflammatory myopathies
  Crystalline arthritis
Musculoskeletal conditions
  Rotator cuff tendinopathy
  Greater trochanteric pain syndrome
  Degenerative joint disease
  Fibromyalgia
Other
  Thyroid disorders
  Infections (eg, disk space infection, endocarditis)
  Malignancy
  Statin myopathy
  Parkinsonism

---

if markers of inflammation remain persistently elevated, alternative diagnoses should be considered. In particular, careful evaluation for GCA may need to be pursued with temporal artery biopsy or large vessel radiographic imaging (or both). Some patients with PMR are eventually reclassified as having elderly-onset rheumatoid arthritis.

KEY FACTS

✓ Clinical features of cryoglobulinemia—
  • constitutional symptoms
  • palpable purpura (due to leukocytoclastic vasculitis)
  • peripheral neuropathy
  • arthralgias
✓ Laboratory studies for cryoglobulinemia—evidence of chronic hepatitis infection (especially hepatitis C) is often identified
✓ PMR—
  • inflammatory condition
  • affects older persons
  • mean age at diagnosis: 73 years
  • stiffness and pain localized to neck, shoulders, hips, and proximal portion of extremities
✓ Treatment of PMR—
  • prednisone (15–20 mg daily)
  • clinical response is usually evident within a few days after treatment begins

Questions and Answers

Questions

Multiple Choice (choose the best answer)

XIII.1. A 26-year-old woman presents for evaluation of low-grade fevers that have been present about 6 months. She also has lost 3.6 kg and has noted some arthralgias and myalgias. She says that her right arm becomes fatigued if she tries to comb her hair. She is a nonsmoker and reports no respiratory problems. On examination, her temperature is 37.5°C. Her right radial pulse is decreased compared with the left, and the blood pressure in her right arm is decreased compared with the left. Laboratory studies show mild normochromic anemia with a hemoglobin of 11.2 g/dL (reference range >12.0 g/dL), a mildly increased erythrocyte sedimentation rate (ESR) of 36 mm/h (reference range <29 mm/h), a negative antineutrophil cytoplasmic autoantibody (ANCA) test, and normal blood chemistry panel results. Urinalysis and chest radiograph findings are normal. Which of the following is the most likely diagnosis?
   a. Polymyalgia rheumatica (PMR)
   b. Giant cell arteritis (GCA)
   c. Buerger disease
   d. Granulomatosis with polyangiitis (Wegener)
   e. Takayasu arteritis

XIII.2. A 59-year-old man has a 1-week history of low back discomfort. He says that he has been moving furniture over the past several weeks, but he does not recall a specific injury. The pain is worse if he is active; it improves if he is at rest. He reports having no pain radiating to the legs. The patient has been taking ibuprofen 400 mg twice daily with food, and this seems to help. He has no prior history of lower back pain. Neurologic examination findings are normal, with a downgoing Babinski sign, equal and symmetrical knee jerks, and normal strength in the lower extremities. He has somewhat diffuse tenderness over the lumbar spine. Laboratory study results are normal for the complete blood cell count, erythrocyte sedimentation rate, and blood chemistry panel. What would be the most appropriate recommendation at this point?
   a. Bed rest for 2 weeks
   b. Radiograph of the lumbar spine
   c. Electromyographic (EMG) study
   d. Neurologic consultation
   e. HLA-B27 testing

XIII.3. A 26-year-old woman presents to your office because she aches all over. She tells you that this condition has been present for several years but has worsened over the past 6 months. She has problems getting to sleep and does not feel rested when she wakes up. She denies having depression. She is stiff for 5 minutes in the morning and has not noticed any joint swelling. On examination, her body mass index (BMI) is 20. Her muscle strength is normal, and there is no synovitis. There is no rash. She has multiple tender points. Results of the following laboratory studies are normal: complete blood cell count, erythrocyte sedimentation rate, blood chemistry panel, and sensitive thyrotropin. What would be the most appropriate next step?
   a. Obtain an electromyogram (EMG).
   b. Prescribe prednisone 15 mg orally daily.
   c. Prescribe duloxetine 30 mg orally daily.
   d. Obtain overnight oximetry results.
   e. Prescribe oxycodone 5 mg orally every 6 hours, as needed for pain control.

XIII.4. A 50-year-old man has sinus drainage, cough, and hemoptysis. He also says that he has had joint pain for several weeks and swelling in the feet. On examination, he has synovitis of several proximal interphalangeal joints of the hands and bilateral lower extremity edema. Results of laboratory studies show a normochromic anemia (hemoglobin 9.6 mg/dL), an elevated erythrocyte sedimentation rate (67 mm/h), and an elevated creatinine level (1.6 mg/dL). The urinalysis shows proteinuria (2+) and red blood cell casts. Chest radiography shows multiple nodular lesions in both lungs. What would be the most appropriate next test to help establish a diagnosis?
   a. Renal biopsy
   b. Open lung biopsy
   c. Antineutrophil cytoplasmic autoantibody (ANCA) panel for vasculitis
   d. Rheumatoid factor test
   e. Cyclic citrullinated peptide (CCP) antibody test

XIII.5. A 56-year-old woman has bothersome, but not disabling, osteoarthritis of her right knee. She has pain if she walks more than 2 blocks, but she reports no locking, catching, or giving way of the knees. She takes glucosamine chondroitin sulfate (1,200 mg daily) and acetaminophen (up to 1,000 mg 3 times daily as needed for pain). She has hypertension and mild renal insufficiency (serum creatinine 1.6 mg/dL; reference range ≤1.2 mg/dL). She also has a history of coronary artery disease. On examination, she has a small amount of effusion in her right knee, mild genu varus deformity, and mild tenderness along the medial joint line of the right knee. The knees appear stable on examination. Radiographs show medial joint space narrowing of the right knee. Which would be the best next step in her care?
   a. Obtain a magnetic resonance imaging (MRI) scan of the right knee.
   b. Administer an intra-articular corticosteroid injection.
   c. Administer a series of injections with hylan G-F 20.
   d. Prescribe naproxen 500 mg twice daily.
   e. Obtain an orthopedic consultation for possible arthroscopic surgery.

XIII.6. A 57-year-old woman comes to your office for mild knee discomfort. She says that if she walks more than 2 miles, both knees hurt. With daily activity, she is not symptomatic. She currently is not taking any medications for her occasional knee pain. She is most interested in what she can do to prevent progression of her condition. On examination, you note mild varus deformity of both knees and tenderness over the medial joint line. What would be the best advice for her?
a. Take naproxen 500 mg twice daily.
b. Take acetaminophen 1,000 mg 3 times daily.
c. Take glucosamine chondroitin sulfate 1,200 mg daily.
d. Undergo magnetic resonance imaging (MRI) scanning of both knees.
e. Undergo ultrasound-guided aspiration of 1 knee.

XIII.7. A 25-year-old man presents with a 2-week history of pain and swelling of the right Achilles tendon and left ankle. He has a previous history of uveitis on 2 occasions. He describes stiffness in his lower back, which is worse in the morning. Which disease best accounts for his symptoms?
a. Ankylosing spondylitis
b. Rheumatoid arthritis
c. Lupus
d. Gout
e. Pseudogout

XIII.8. A 42-year-old man from Rhode Island has bilateral intermittent painful knee effusions. Synovial fluid analysis is negative with Gram staining and culture, with a leukocyte count of 6.5×10^9/L. No crystals are seen. He has no history of skin rash or low back pain. He has no other joint involvement. After a flulike illness 2 years previously, the patient did have Bell palsy, which resolved. His father has gout. Which of the following diseases is most likely to account for his symptoms?

a. Rheumatoid arthritis
b. Lyme disease
c. Systemic lupus erythematosus (SLE)
d. Gout
e. Spondyloarthropathy

XIII.9. A 32-year-old male intravenous drug user has arthralgias and biopsy-proven cutaneous leukocytoclastic vasculitis. Laboratory study results are shown in Table XIII.Q9.

Table XIII.Q9

Component	Result
Hemoglobin, g/dL	10.2
Leukocyte count, ×10⁹/L	8.2
Erythrocyte sedimentation rate, mm/h	59
Rheumatoid factor	1:640
C4	Low
Aspartate aminotransferase (AST), U/L	3 times upper limit of reference range
Cryoglobulins	Positive

Which of the following tests would be most likely to establish the diagnosis?
a. Anti–cyclic citrullinated peptide
b. Antinuclear antibody
c. Anti-dsDNA antibody
d. Human immunodeficiency virus (HIV)
e. Hepatitis C serology

Answers

XIII.1. Answer e.

Of the choices listed, this patient would most likely have Takayasu arteritis, which is most common in women younger than 40. Weight loss, arthralgias, myalgias, and low-grade fevers are all common features. In addition, patients often present with upper extremity claudication. The decreased radial pulse in the right arm compared with the left and the decreased blood pressure in the right arm suggest upper aortic arch involvement. Typically, mild anemia is present. Some patients have active disease but a normal ESR. Many patients with Takayasu arteritis have a negative ANCA test. Both PMR and GCA occur in older persons. Buerger disease occurs in smokers. Patients with granulomatosis with polyangiitis (Wegener) usually have respiratory symptoms and a positive ANCA test; they often have upper and lower respiratory tract involvement and kidney involvement.

XIII.2. Answer b.

New onset of lower back pain after age 50 would be an indication for radiograph. Bed rest for more than 3 days is not helpful. There is no suggestion of radiculopathy, so EMG and neurologic consultation are not indicated. The patient is not describing inflammatory back pain and is older than 50, so HLA-B27 testing for spondyloarthropathy would not be helpful.

XIII.3. Answer c.

This patient presents with fibromyalgia-like symptoms. She does not have muscle weakness, so an EMG would not be indicated. Her symptoms, physical examination findings, and laboratory test results are not suggestive of inflammation, so prednisone is not indicated. Duloxetine has been shown to be efficacious treatment for fibromyalgia in women. Although the patient's sleep is nonrestorative, she is young and has a low BMI, so sleep apnea is not likely. She has a chronic pain syndrome, and it is usually best to avoid using narcotics to treat fibromyalgia pain.

XIII.4. Answer c.

This patient has features of granulomatosis with polyangiitis (Wegener) with upper and lower respiratory tract involvement and renal involvement. An ANCA panel would likely be positive in a cytoplasmic ANCA pattern with a positive proteinase 3 enzyme-linked immunosorbent assay (PR3 ELISA). A renal biopsy would be expected to show glomerulonephritis, which would not be specific for granulomatosis with polyangiitis (Wegener). An open lung biopsy likely would show histologic features of granulomatosis with polyangiitis (Wegener) (eg, granulomatous vasculitis), but the procedure is invasive and may not be necessary if the ANCA tests are positive. Patients with granulomatosis with polyangiitis (Wegener) can have synovitis. The rheumatoid factor and CCP tests are for rheumatoid arthritis. Patients with rheumatoid arthritis would not typically have hemoptysis, although they could have pulmonary involvement, and they would not usually have glomerulonephritis.

XIII.5. Answer b.

This patient has osteoarthritis. Her examination, history, and radiographs do not suggest another process, so MRI is likely to yield little more information. Because she has renal insufficiency, hypertension, and a history of coronary artery disease, nonsteroidal anti-inflammatory drugs are relatively contraindicated. A corticosteroid injection would be a consideration, especially since she has pain in only 1 joint. If the patient had no response to the corticosteroid injection, viscosupplementation would be a consideration. The patient does not have mechanical symptoms, so there is no clear indication for an arthroscopic procedure.

XIII.6. Answer c.

Nonsteroidal anti-inflammatory drugs and acetaminophen are analgesics, but they do not prevent progression of osteoarthritis. There is some support from evidence-based medicine for the use of glucosamine chondroitin sulfate to retard progression of osteoarthritis of the knee. There is no indication for MRI or ultrasound-guided arthrocentesis of the knee.

XIII.7. Answer a.

Achilles tendinitis (enthesopathy), low back pain with morning stiffness, and uveitis are characteristic of spondyloarthropathies, such as ankylosing spondylitis. The other diseases do not predispose characteristically to back pain, uveitis, or enthesopathy.

XIII.8. Answer b.

Not all patients with Lyme disease recall a tick bite or have erythema chronicum migrans. This patient had flulike symptoms and Bell palsy several years before the onset of his Lyme arthritis, which characteristically involves the knees several years after the initial infection. Bell palsy is a characteristic neurologic manifestation of Lyme disease. Rheumatoid arthritis would be less likely without polyarticular involvement and would not be associated with Bell palsy. No crystals were seen with joint aspiration, which would rule against gout. He has no history of low back pain or uveitis, which would make a spondyloarthropathy unlikely. He has no clinical history to suggest SLE.

XIII.9. Answer e.

Hepatitis C infection can cause cryoglobulinemia, which is responsible for the positive rheumatoid factor and cryoglobulinemic vasculitis. The low C4 is also associated with the cryoglobulinemic vasculitis. The elevated AST is indicative of ongoing hepatitis liver disease. Rheumatoid arthritis, systemic lupus erythematosus, and HIV infection do not characteristically cause cryoglobulinemia.

Index